3rd Edition

HARRISON'S™

NEUROLOGY IN CLINICAL MEDICINE

Derived from Harrison's Principles of Internal Medicine, 18th Edition

Editors

DAN L. LONGO, MD
Professor of Medicine, Harvard Medical School;
Senior Physician, Brigham and Women's Hospital;
Deputy Editor, New England Journal of Medicine,
Boston, Massachusetts

ANTHONY S. FAUCI, MD
Chief, Laboratory of Immunoregulation;
Director, National Institute of Allergy and Infectious Diseases,
National Institutes of Health,
Bethesda, Maryland

DENNIS L. KASPER, MD
William Ellery Channing Professor of Medicine,
Professor of Microbiology and Molecular Genetics,
Harvard Medical School; Director, Channing Laboratory,
Department of Medicine, Brigham and Women's Hospital,
Boston, Massachusetts

STEPHEN L. HAUSER, MD
Robert A. Fishman Distinguished Professor and Chairman,
Department of Neurology,
University of California, San Francisco,
San Francisco, California

J. LARRY JAMESON, MD, PhD
Robert G. Dunlop Professor of Medicine;
Dean, University of Pennsylvania School of Medicine;
Executive Vice-President of the University of Pennsylvania
for the Health System, Philadelphia, Pennsylvania

JOSEPH LOSCALZO, MD, PhD
Hersey Professor of the Theory and Practice of Medicine,
Harvard Medical School; Chairman, Department of Medicine;
Physician-in-Chief, Brigham and Women's Hospital,
Boston, Massachusetts

3rd Edition

HARRISON'S™

NEUROLOGY IN CLINICAL MEDICINE

EDITOR

Stephen L. Hauser, MD
Robert A. Fishman Distinguished
Professor and Chairman, Department of Neurology,
University of California, San Francisco, San Francisco, California

ASSOCIATE EDITOR

S. Andrew Josephson, MD
Associate Professor of Clinical Neurology
C. Castro-Franceschi and G. Mitchell Endowed Neurohospitalist Chair
Vice-Chairman, Parnassus Programs
University of California, San Francisco, San Francisco, California

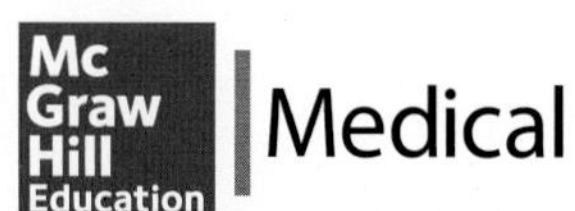

New York Chicago San Francisco Lisbon London Madrid Mexico City
Milan New Delhi San Juan Seoul Singapore Sydney Toronto

Harrison's Neurology in Clinical Medicine, Third Edition

Dr. Fauci's work as an editor and author was performed outside the scope of his employment as a U.S. government employee. This work represents his personal and professional views and not necessarily those of the U.S. government.

2 3 4 5 6 7 8 9 0 CTP/CTP 18 17 16 15 14 13

ISBN 978-0-07-181500-0
MHID 0-07-181500-7

This book was set in Bembo by Cenveo® Publisher Services. The editors were James F. Shanahan and Kim J. Davis. The production supervisor was Catherine H. Saggese. Project management was provided by Tania Andrabi, Cenveo Publisher Services. The cover design was by Thomas DePierro. Cover image, lesion track atrophy, supplied by Dr. Stephen L. Hauser.

China Translation & Printing Services, Ltd. was the printer and binder.

Library of Congress Cataloging-in Publication Data

Harrison's neurology in clinical medicine / editor, Stephen L. Hauser ; associate editor, Scott Andrew Josephson. — 3rd ed.
p. ; cm.
Neurology in clinical medicine
"[B]ased upon the neurology and psychiatry sections from Harrison's principles of internal medicine"—Pref.
Includes bibliographical references and index.
ISBN 978-0-07-181500-0 (pbk. : alk. paper)—
ISBN 0-07-181500-7 (pbk. : alk. paper)
I. Harrison, Tinsley Randolph, 1900-1978. II. Hauser, Stephen L. III. Josephson, Scott Andrew. IV. Harrison's principles of internal medicine. V. Title: Neurology in clinical medicine.
[DNLM: 1. Nervous System Diseases. WL 140]
616—dc23

2012042235

McGraw-Hill Education books are available at special quantity discounts to use as premiums and sales promotions, or for use in corporate training programs. To contact a representative please e-mail us at bulksales@mcgraw-hill.com.

CONTENTS

Contributors ix

Preface xiii

SECTION I
INTRODUCTION TO NEUROLOGY

1 Approach to the Patient with Neurologic Disease 2
Daniel H. Lowenstein, Joseph B. Martin, Stephen L. Hauser

2 The Neurologic Screening Exam 11
Daniel H. Lowenstein

3 Video Atlas of the Detailed Neurologic Examination 12
Martin A. Samuels

4 Neuroimaging in Neurologic Disorders 13
William P. Dillon

5 Electrodiagnostic Studies of Nervous System Disorders: EEG, Evoked Potentials, and EMG 26
Michael J. Aminoff

6 Technique of Lumbar Puncture 35
Elizabeth Robbins, Stephen L. Hauser

SECTION II
CLINICAL MANIFESTATIONS OF NEUROLOGIC DISEASE

7 Pain: Pathophysiology and Management 40
James P. Rathmell, Howard L. Fields

8 Headache 51
Peter J. Goadsby, Neil H. Raskin

9 Back and Neck Pain 71
John W. Engstrom, Richard A. Deyo

10 Syncope 89
Roy Freeman

11 Dizziness and Vertigo 98
Mark F. Walker, Robert B. Daroff

12 Weakness and Paralysis. 103
Michael J. Aminoff

13 Gait and Balance Disorders. 110
Lewis Sudarsky

14 Video Library of Gait Disorders 116
Gail Kang, Nicholas B. Galifianakis, Michael Geschwind

15 Numbness, Tingling, and Sensory Loss 117
Michael J. Aminoff, Arthur K. Asbury

16 Confusion and Delirium 125
S. Andrew Josephson, Bruce L. Miller

17 Coma 132
Allan H. Ropper

18 Aphasia, Memory Loss, and Other Focal Cerebral Disorders. 142
M.-Marsel Mesulam

19 Video Atlas: Primary Progressive Aphasia, Memory Loss, and Other Focal Cerebral Disorders 157
Maria Luisa Gorno-Tempini, Jennifer Ogar, Joel Kramer, Bruce L. Miller, Gil Rabinovici, Maria Carmela Tartaglia

20 Sleep Disorders 158
Charles A. Czeisler, John W. Winkelman, Gary S. Richardson

21 Disorders of Vision 174
Jonathan C. Horton

22 Video Library of Neuro-Ophthalmology 198
Shirley H. Wray

23 Disorders of Smell and Taste 199
Richard L. Doty, Steven M. Bromley

24 Disorders of Hearing 207
Anil K. Lalwani

SECTION III
DISEASES OF THE NERVOUS SYSTEM

25 Mechanisms of Neurologic Diseases 218
Stephen L. Hauser, M. Flint Beal

26 Seizures and Epilepsy. 231
Daniel H. Lowenstein

27 Cerebrovascular Diseases 256
Wade S. Smith, Joey D. English, S. Claiborne Johnston

28 Neurologic Critical Care, Including Hypoxic-Ischemic Encephalopathy, and Subarachnoid Hemorrhage 294
J. Claude Hemphill, III, Wade S. Smith, Daryl R. Gress

29 Alzheimer's Disease and Other Dementias 310
William W. Seeley, Bruce L. Miller

30 Parkinson's Disease and Other Extrapyramidal Movement Disorders 333
C. Warren Olanow, Anthony H. V. Schapira

31 Ataxic Disorders 357
Roger N. Rosenberg

32 Amyotrophic Lateral Sclerosis and Other Motor Neuron Diseases 370
Robert H. Brown, Jr.

33 Disorders of the Autonomic Nervous System 380
Phillip A. Low, John W. Engstrom

34 Trigeminal Neuralgia, Bell's Palsy, and Other Cranial Nerve Disorders 392
M. Flint Beal, Stephen L. Hauser

35 Diseases of the Spinal Cord 400
Stephen L. Hauser, Allan H. Ropper

36 Concussion and Other Head Injuries 415
Allan H. Ropper

37 Primary and Metastatic Tumors of the Nervous System 423
Lisa M. DeAngelis, Patrick Y. Wen

38 Neurologic Disorders of the Pituitary and Hypothalamus 439
Shlomo Melmed, J. Larry Jameson

39 Multiple Sclerosis and Other Demyelinating Diseases. 474
Stephen L. Hauser, Douglas S. Goodin

40 Meningitis, Encephalitis, Brain Abscess, and Empyema 493
Karen L. Roos, Kenneth L. Tyler

41 Chronic and Recurrent Meningitis. 527
Walter J. Koroshetz, Morton N. Swartz

42 HIV Neurology. 536
Anthony S. Fauci, H. Clifford Lane

43 Prion Diseases 549
Stanley B. Prusiner, Bruce L. Miller

44 Paraneoplastic Neurologic Syndromes. 558
Josep Dalmau, Myrna R. Rosenfeld

45 Peripheral Neuropathy. 566
Anthony A. Amato, Richard J. Barohn

46 Guillain-Barré Syndrome and Other Immune-Mediated Neuropathies 599
Stephen L. Hauser, Anthony A. Amato

47 Myasthenia Gravis and Other Diseases of the Neuromuscular Junction 609
Daniel B. Drachman

48 Muscular Dystrophies and Other Muscle Diseases. 618
Anthony A. Amato, Robert H. Brown, Jr.

49 Polymyositis, Dermatomyositis, and Inclusion Body Myositis 648
Marinos C. Dalakas

50 Special Issues in Inpatient Neurologic Consultation 660
S. Andrew Josephson, Martin A. Samuels

51 Atlas of Neuroimaging. 668
Andre Furtado, William P. Dillon

SECTION IV
CHRONIC FATIGUE SYNDROME

52 Chronic Fatigue Syndrome 704
Gijs Bleijenberg, Jos W. M. van der Meer

SECTION V
PSYCHIATRIC DISORDERS

53 Biology of Psychiatric Disorders 710
Robert O. Messing, John H. Rubenstein, Eric J. Nestler

54 Mental Disorders 720
Victor I. Reus

55 Neuropsychiatric Illnesses in War Veterans 742
Charles W. Hoge

SECTION VI
ALCOHOLISM AND DRUG DEPENDENCY

56 Alcohol and Alcoholism. 752
Marc A. Schuckit

57 Opioid Drug Abuse and Dependence 761
Thomas R. Kosten

58 Cocaine and Other Commonly Abused Drugs 767
Nancy K. Mello, Jack H. Mendelson

Appendix
Laboratory Values of Clinical Importance 775
Alexander Kratz, Michael A. Pesce, Robert C. Basner, Andrew J. Einstein

Review and Self-Assessment 801
Charles Wiener, Cynthia D. Brown, Anna R. Hemnes

Index 851

CONTRIBUTORS

Numbers in brackets refer to the chapter(s) written or cowritten by the contributor.

Anthony A. Amato, MD
Professor of Neurology, Harvard Medical School; Department of Neurology, Brigham and Women's Hospital, Boston, Massachusetts [45, 46, 48]

Michael J. Aminoff, MD, DSc
Professor of Neurology, University of California, San Francisco School of Medicine, San Francisco, California [5, 12, 15]

Richard J. Barohn, MD
Chairman, Department of Neurology; Gertrude and Dewey Ziegler Professor of Neurology, University of Kansas Medical Center, Kansas City, Kansas [45]

Robert C. Basner, MD
Professor of Clinical Medicine, Division of Pulmonary, Allergy, and Critical Care Medicine, Columbia University College of Physicians and Surgeons, New York, New York [Appendix]

M. Flint Beal, MD
Chairman of Neurology and Neuroscience; Neurologist-in-Chief, New York Presbyterian Hospital; Weill Cornell Medical College, New York, New York [25, 34]

Gijs Bleijenberg, PhD
Professor; Head, Expert Centre for Chronic Fatigue, Radboud University Nijmegen Medical Centre, Nijmegen, Netherlands [52]

Steven M. Bromley, MD
Clinical Assistant Professor of Neurology, Department of Medicine, New Jersey School of Medicine and Dentistry–Robert Wood Johnson Medical School, Camden, New Jersey [23]

Cynthia D. Brown, MD
Assistant Professor of Medicine, Division of Pulmonary and Critical Care Medicine, University of Virginia, Charlottesville, Virginia [Review and Self-Assessment]

Robert H. Brown, Jr., MD, PhD
Chairman, Department of Neurology, University of Massachusetts Medical School, Worchester, Massachusetts [32, 48]

Charles A. Czeisler, MD, PhD, FRCP
Baldino Professor of Sleep Medicine; Director, Division of Sleep Medicine, Harvard Medical School; Chief, Division of Sleep Medicine, Department of Medicine, Brigham and Women's Hospital, Boston, Massachusetts [20]

Marinos C. Dalakas, MD, FAAN
Professor of Neurology, Department of Pathophysiology, National University of Athens Medical School, Athens, Greece [49]

Josep Dalmau, MD, PhD
ICREA Research Professor, Institute for Biomedical Investigations, August Pi i Sunyer (IDIBAPS)/Hospital Clinic, Department of Neurology, University of Barcelona, Barcelona, Spain; Adjunct Professor of Neurology University of Pennsylvania, Philadelphia, Pennsylvania [44]

Robert B. Daroff, MD
Professor and Chair Emeritus, Department of Neurology, Case Western Reserve University School of Medicine; University Hospitals–Case Medical Center, Cleveland, Ohio [11]

Lisa M. DeAngelis, MD
Professor of Neurology, Weill Cornell Medical College; Chair, Department of Neurology, Memorial Sloan-Kettering Cancer Center, New York, New York [37]

Richard A. Deyo, MD, MPH
Kaiser Permanente Professor of Evidence-Based Family Medicine, Department of Family Medicine, Department of Medicine, Department of Public Health and Preventive Medicine, Center for Research in Occupational and Environmental Toxicology, Oregon Health and Science University; Clinical Investigator, Kaiser Permanente Center for Health Research, Portland, Oregon [9]

William P. Dillon, MD
Elizabeth Guillaumin Professor of Radiology, Neurology and Neurosurgery; Executive Vice-Chair, Department of Radiology and Biomedical Imaging, University of California, San Francisco, San Francisco, California [4, 51]

Richard L. Doty, PhD
Professor, Department of Otorhinolaryngology: Head and Neck Surgery; Director, Smell and Taste Center, University of Pennsylvania School of Medicine, Philadelphia, Pennsylvania [23]

Daniel B. Drachman, MD
Professor of Neurology and Neuroscience, W. W. Smith Charitable Trust Professor of Neuroimmunology, Department of Neurology, Johns Hopkins School of Medicine, Baltimore, Maryland [47]

Andrew J. Einstein, MD, PhD
Assistant Professor of Clinical Medicine, Columbia University College of Physicians and Surgeons; Department of Medicine, Division of Cardiology, Department of Radiology, Columbia University Medical Center and New York-Presbyterian Hospital, New York, New York [Appendix]

Joey D. English, MD
Assistant Clinical Professor, Department of Neurology, Univeristy of California, San Francisco, San Francisco, California [27]

John W. Engstrom, MD
Betty Anker Fife Distinguished Professor of Neurology; Neurology Residency Program Director; Clinical Chief of Service, University of California, San Francisco, San Francisco, California [9, 33]

Anthony S. Fauci, MD, DSc (Hon), DM&S (Hon), DHL (Hon), DPS (Hon), DLM (Hon), DMS (Hon)
Chief, Laboratory of Immunoregulation; Director, National Institute of Allergy and Infectious Diseases, National Institutes of Health, Bethesda, Maryland [42]

Howard L. Fields, MD, PhD
Professor of Neurology, University of California, San Francisco, San Francisco, California [7]

Roy Freeman, MBCHB
Professor of Neurology, Harvard Medical School, Boston, Massachusetts [10]

Andre Furtado, MD
Associate Specialist at the Department of Radiology, Neuroradiology Section, University of California, San Francisco, San Francisco, California [51]

Nicholas B. Galifianakis, MD, MPH
Assistant Clinical Professor, Surgical Movement Disorders Center, Department of Neurology, University of California, San Francisco, San Francisco, California [14]

Michael Geschwind, MD, PhD
Associate Professor of Neurology, Memory and Aging Center, University of California, San Francisco, School of Medicine, San Francisco, California [14]

Peter J. Goadsby, MD, PhD, DSc, FRACP FRCP
Professor of Neurology, University of California, San Francisco, California; Honorary Consultant Neurologist, Hospital for Sick Children, London, United Kingdom [8]

Douglas S. Goodin, MD
Professor of Neurology, University of California, San Francisco School of Medicine, San Francisco, California [39]

Maria Luisa Gorno-Tempini, MD, PhD
Associate Professor of Neurology, Memory and Aging Center, University of California, San Francisco, San Francisco, California [19]

Daryl R. Gress, MD, FAAN, FCCM
Associate Professor of Neurology
University of Virginia, Charlottesville, Virginia [28]

Stephen L. Hauser, MD
Robert A. Fishman Distinguished Professor and Chairman, Department of Neurology, University of California, San Francisco, San Francisco, California [1, 6, 25, 34, 35, 39, 46]

Anna R. Hemnes, MD
Assistant Professor, Division of Allergy, Pulmonary, and Critical Care Medicine, Vanderbilt University Medical Center, Nashville, Tennessee [Review and Self-Assessment]

J. Claude Hemphill, III, MD, MAS
Professor of Clinical Neurology and Neurological Surgery, Department of Neurology, University of California, San Francisco; Director of Neurocritical Care, San Francisco General Hospital, San Francisco, California [28]

Charles W. Hoge, MD
Senior Scientist and Staff Psychiatrist, Center for Psychiatry and Neuroscience, Walter Reed Army Institute of Research and Water Reed Army Medical Center, Silver Spring, Maryland [55]

Jonathan C. Horton, MD, PhD
William F. Hoyt Professor of Neuro-ophthalmology, Professor of Ophthalmology, Neurology and Physiology, University of California, San Francisco School of Medicine, San Francisco, California [21]

J. Larry Jameson, MD, PhD
Robert G. Dunlop Professor of Medicine; Dean, University of Pennsylvania School of Medicine; Executive Vice President of the University of Pennsylvania for the Health System, Philadelphia, Pennsylvania [38]

S. Claiborne Johnston, MD, PhD
Professor of Neurology and Epidemiology, University of California, San Francisco School of Medicine, San Francisco, California [27]

S. Andrew Josephson, MD
Associate Professor, Department of Neurology; Director, Neurohospitalist Program, University of California, San Francisco, San Francisco, California [16, 50]

Gail Kang, MD
Assistant Clinical Professor of Neurology, Memory and Aging Center, University of California, San Francisco, San Francisco, California [14]

Walter J. Koroshetz, MD
National Institute of Neurological Disorders and Stroke, National Institutes of Health, Bethesda, Maryland [41]

Thomas R. Kosten, MD
Baylor College of Medicine; Veteran's Administration Medical Center, Houston, Texas [57]

Joel Kramer, PsyD
Clinical Professor of Neuropsychology in Neurology; Director of Neuropsychology, Memory and Aging Center, University of California, San Francisco, San Francisco, California [19]

Alexander Kratz, MD, PhD, MPH
Associate Professor of Pathology and Cell Biology, Columbia University College of Physicians and Surgeons; Director, Core Laboratory, Columbia University Medical Center, New York, New York [Appendix]

Anil K. Lalwani, MD
Professor, Departments of Otolaryngology, Pediatrics, and Physiology and Neuroscience, New York University School of Medicine, New York, New York [24]

H. Clifford Lane, MD
Clinical Director; Director, Division of Clinical Research; Deputy Director, Clinical Research and Special Projects; Chief, Clinical and Molecular Retrovirology Section, Laboratory of Immunoregulation, National Institute of Allergy and Infectious Diseases, National Institutes of Health, Bethesda, Maryland [42]

Phillip A. Low, MD
Robert D. and Patricia E. Kern Professor of Neurology, Mayo Clinic College of Medicine, Rochester, Minnesota [33]

Daniel H. Lowenstein, MD
Dr. Robert B. and Mrs. Ellinor Aird Professor of Neurology; Director, Epilepsy Center, University of California, San Francisco, San Francisco, California [1, 2, 26]

Joseph B. Martin, MD, PhD
Edward R. and Anne G. Lefler Professor, Department of Neurobiology, Harvard Medical School, Boston, Massachusetts [1]

Nancy K. Mello, PhD
Professor of Psychology (Neuroscience), Harvard Medical School, Boston, Massachusetts; Director, Alcohol and Drug Abuse Research Center, McLean Hospital, Belmont, Massachusetts [58]

Shlomo Melmed, MD
Senior Vice President and Dean of the Medical Faculty, Cedars-Sinai Medical Center, Los Angeles, California [38]

Jack H. Mendelson,[a] MD
Professor of Psychiatry (Neuroscience), Harvard Medical School, Belmont, Massachusetts [58]

Robert O. Messing, MD
Professor, Department of Neurology; Senior Associate Director, Ernest Gallo Clinic and Research Center, University of California, San Francisco, San Francisco, California [53]

M.-Marsel Mesulam, MD
Professor of Neurology, Psychiatry and Psychology, Cognitive Neurology and Alzheimer's Disease Center, Northwestern University Feinberg School of Medicine, Chicago, Illinois [18]

Bruce L. Miller, MD
AW and Mary Margaret Clausen Distinguished Professor of Neurology, University of California, San Francisco School of Medicine, San Francisco, California [16, 19, 29, 43]

---

[a] Deceased

Eric J. Nestler, MD, PhD
Nash Family Professor and Chair, Department of Neuroscience; Director, Friedman Brain Institute, Mount Sinai School of Medicine, New York, New York [53]

Jennifer Ogar, MS
Speech Pathologist, Memory and Aging Center, University of California, San Francisco, San Francisco, California; Acting Chief of Speech Pathology at the Department of Veterans Affairs, Martinez, California [19]

C. Warren Olanow, MD, FRCPC
Department of Neurology and Neuroscience, Mount Sinai School of Medicine, New York, New York [30]

Michael A. Pesce, PhD
Professor Emeritus of Pathology and Cell Biology, Columbia University College of Physicians and Surgeons; Columbia University Medical Center, New York, New York [Appendix]

Stanley B. Prusiner, MD
Director, Institute for Neurodegenerative Diseases; Professor, Department of Neurology, University of California, San Francisco, San Francisco, California [43]

Gil Rabinovici, MD
Attending Neurologist, Memory and Aging Center, University of California, San Francisco, San Francisco, California [19]

Neil H. Raskin, MD
Department of Neurology, University of California, San Francisco, San Francisco, San Francisco, California [8]

James P. Rathmell, MD
Associate Professor of Anesthesia, Harvard Medical School; Chief, Division of Pain Medicine, Massachusetts General Hospital, Boston, Massachusetts [7]

Victor I. Reus, MD, DFAPA, FACP
Department of Psychiatry, University of California, San Francisco School of Medicine; Langley Porter Neuropsychiatric Institute, San Francisco, San Francisco, California [54]

Gary S. Richardson, MD
Senior Research Scientist and Staff Physician, Henry Ford Hospital, Detroit, Michigan [20]

Elizabeth Robbins, MD
Clinical Professor of Pediatrics, University of California, San Francisco, San Francisco, California [6]

Karen L. Roos, MD
John and Nancy Nelson Professor of Neurology and Professor of Neurological Surgery, Indiana University School of Medicine, Indianapolis, Indiana [40]

Allan H. Ropper, MD
Professor of Neurology, Harvard Medical School; Executive Vice Chair of Neurology, Raymond D. Adams Distinguished Clinician, Brigham and Women's Hospital, Boston, Massachusetts [17, 35, 36]

Roger N. Rosenberg, MD
Zale Distinguished Chair and Professor of Neurology, Department of Neurology, University of Texas Southwestern Medical Center, Dallas, Texas [31]

Myrna R. Rosenfeld, MD, PhD
Professor of Neurology and Chief, Division of Neuro-oncology, University of Pennsylvania, Philadelphia, Pennsylvania [44]

John H. Rubenstein, MD, PhD
Nina Ireland Distinguished Professor in Child Psychiatry, Center for Neurobiology and Psychiatry, Department of Psychiatry, University of California, San Francisco, San Francisco, California [53]

Martin A. Samuels, MD, DSc(hon), FAAN, MACP, FRCP
Professor of Neurology, Harvard Medical School; Chairman, Department of Neurology, Brigham and Women's Hospital, Boston, Massachusetts [3, 50]

Anthony H. V. Schapira, DSc, MD, FRCP, FMedSci
University Department of Clinical Neurosciences, University College London; National Hospital for Neurology and Neurosurgery, Queen's Square, London, United Kingdom [30]

Marc A. Schuckit, MD
Distinguished Professor of Psychiatry, University of California, San Diego School of Medicine, La Jolla, California [56]

William W. Seeley, MD
Associate Professor of Neurology, Memory and Aging Center, University of California, San Francisco, San Francisco, California [29]

Wade S. Smith, MD, PhD
Professor of Neurology, Daryl R. Gress Endowed Chair of Neurocritical Care and Stroke; Director, University of California, San Francisco Neurovascular Service, San Francisco, San Francisco, California [27, 28]

Lewis Sudarsky, MD
Associate Professor of Neurology, Harvard Medical School; Director of Movement Disorders, Brigham and Women's Hospital, Boston, Massachusetts [13]

Morton N. Swartz, MD
Professor of Medicine, Harvard Medical School; Chief, Jackson Firm Medical Service and Infectious Disease Unit, Massachusetts General Hospital, Boston, Massachusetts [41]

Maria Carmela Tartaglia, MD, FRCPC
Clinical Instructor of Neurology, Memory and Aging Center, University of California, San Francisco, San Francisco, California [19]

Kenneth L. Tyler, MD
Reuler-Lewin Family Professor and Chair, Department of Neurology; Professor of Medicine and Microbiology, University of Colorado School of Medicine, Denver, Colorado; Chief of Neurology, University of Colorado Hospital, Aurora, Colorado [40]

Jos W. M. van der Meer, MD, PhD
Professor of Medicine; Head, Department of General Internal Medicine, Radboud University, Nijmegen Medical Centre, Nijmegen, Netherlands [52]

Mark F. Walker, MD
Associate Professor, Department of Neurology, Case Western Reserve University School of Medicine; Daroff-Dell' Osso Ocular Motility Laboratory, Louis Stokes Cleveland Department of Veterans Affairs Medical Center, Cleveland, Ohio [11]

Patrick Y. Wen, MD
Professor of Neurology, Harvard Medical School; Dana-Farber Cancer Institute, Boston, Massachusetts [37]

Charles M. Wiener, MD
Dean/CEO Perdana University Graduate School of Medicine, Selangor, Malaysia; Professor of Medicine and Physiology, Johns Hopkins University School of Medicine, Baltimore, Maryland [Review and Self-Assessment]

John W. Winkelman, MD, PhD
Associate Professor of Psychiatry, Harvard Medical School; Medical Director, Sleep Health Centers, Brigham and Women's Hospital, Boston, Massachusetts [20]

Shirley H. Wray, MB, ChB, PhD, FRCP
Professor of Neurology, Harvard Medical School; Department of Neurology, Massachusetts General Hospital, Boston, Massachusetts [22]

PREFACE

The first two editions of *Harrison's Neurology in Clinical Medicine* were unqualified successes. Readers responded enthusiastically to the convenient, attractive, expanded, and updated stand-alone volume, which was based upon the neurology and psychiatry sections from *Harrison's Principles of Internal Medicine*. Our original goal was to provide, in an easy-to-use format, full coverage of the most authoritative information available anywhere of clinically important topics in neurology and psychiatry, while retaining the focus on pathophysiology and therapy that has always been characteristic of *Harrison's*.

This new third edition of *Harrison's Neurology in Clinical Medicine* has been extensively updated to highlight recent advances in the understanding, diagnosis, treatment, and prevention of neurologic and psychiatric diseases. New chapters discuss the pathogenesis and treatment of syncope, dizziness and vertigo, smell and taste disorders, Parkinson's disease, tumors of the nervous system, peripheral neuropathy, and neuropsychiatric problems among war veterans, among other topics. Extensively updated coverage of the dementias highlights new findings from genetics, molecular imaging, cell biology, and clinical research that are transforming our understanding of these common problems. Neuroimmunology is another dynamic and rapidly changing field of neurology, and the new edition of *Harrison's* provides extensive coverage of progress in this area, including a practical guide to navigating the large number of treatment options now available for multiple sclerosis. Another new chapter reviews advances in deciphering the pathogenesis of common psychiatric disorders and discusses challenges to the development of more effective treatments. Many illustrative neuroimaging figures appear throughout the section, and an updated and expanded atlas of neuroimaging findings is also included. We are extremely pleased that readers of the new edition of *Harrison's* will for the first time be able to access a remarkable series of high-definition video presentations including wonderful guides to screening and detailed neurological examinations, as well as video libraries illustrating gait disorders, focal cerebral disorders, and neuro-ophthalmologic disturbances.

For many physicians, neurologic diseases represent particularly challenging problems. Acquisition of the requisite clinical skills is often viewed as time-consuming, difficult to master, and requiring a working knowledge of obscure anatomic facts and laundry lists of diagnostic possibilities. The patients themselves may be difficult, as neurologic disorders often alter an individual's capacity to recount the history of an illness or to even recognize that something is wrong. An additional obstacle is the development of independent neurology services, departments, and training programs at many medical centers, reducing the exposure of trainees in internal medicine to neurologic problems. All of these forces, acting within the fast paced environment of modern medical practice, can lead to an overreliance on unfocused neuroimaging tests, suboptimal patient care, and unfortunate outcomes. Because neurologists represent less than 1% of all physicians, the vast majority of neurologic care must be delivered by nonspecialists who are often generalists and usually internists.

The old adage that neurologists "know everything but do nothing" has been rendered obsolete by advances in molecular medicine, imaging, bioengineering, and clinical research. Examples of new therapies include: thrombolytic therapy for acute ischemic stroke; endovascular recanalization for cerebrovascular disorders; intensive monitoring of brain pressure and cerebral blood flow for brain injury; effective therapies for immune-mediated neurologic disorders; new designer drugs for migraine; the first generation of rational therapies for neurodegenerative diseases; neural stimulators for Parkinson's disease; drugs for narcolepsy and other sleep disorders; and control of epilepsy by surgical resection of small seizure foci precisely localized by functional imaging and electrophysiology. The pipeline continues to grow, stimulated by a quickening tempo of discoveries generating opportunities for rational design of new diagnostics, interventions, and drugs.

The founding editors of *Harrison's Principles of Internal Medicine* acknowledged the importance of neurology but were uncertain as to its proper role in a textbook of internal medicine. An initial plan to exclude neurology from the first edition (1950) was reversed at the eleventh hour, and a neurology section was hastily prepared by Houston Merritt. By the second edition, the section was considerably enlarged by Raymond D. Adams, whose influence on the textbook was profound. The third neurology editor, Joseph B. Martin, brilliantly led the book during the 1980s and 1990s as neurology was transformed from a largely descriptive discipline to one of the most dynamic and rapidly evolving areas of medicine. With these changes, the growth of neurology coverage in *Harrison's* became so pronounced that Harrison suggested the book be retitled, *The Details of Neurology and Some Principles of Internal Medicine*. His humorous comment, now legendary, underscores the depth of coverage of neurologic medicine in *Harrison's* befitting its critical role in the practice of internal medicine.

The Editors are indebted to our authors, a group of internationally recognized authorities who have magnificently distilled a daunting body of information into the essential principles required to understand and manage commonly encountered neurologic problems. Thanks also to Dr. Elizabeth Robbins who has served for more than 15 years as managing editor of the neurology section of *Harrison's*; she has overseen the complex logistics required to produce a multiauthored textbook, and has promoted exceptional standards for clarity, language, and style. Finally, we wish to acknowledge and express our great appreciation to our colleagues at McGraw-Hill. This new volume was championed by James Shanahan and impeccably managed by Kim Davis.

We live in an electronic, wireless age. Information is downloaded rather than pulled from the shelf. Some have questioned the value of traditional books in this new era. We believe that as the volume of information, and the ways to access this information, continues to grow, the need to grasp the essential concepts of medical practice becomes even more challenging. One of our young colleagues recently remarked that he uses the Internet to find facts, but that he reads *Harrison's* to learn medicine. Our aim has always been to provide the reader with an integrated, organic summary of the science and the practice of medicine rather than a mere compendium of chapters, and we are delighted and humbled by the continuing and quite remarkable growth in popularity of *Harrison's* at a time when many "classics" in medicine seem less relevant than in years past. We are of course cognizant of the flexibility in information delivery that today's readers seek, and so we have also made the third edition of *Harrison's Neurology in Clinical Medicine* available in a number of eBook formats for all major devices, including the iPad (available via the iBookstore).

It is our sincere hope that you will enjoy using *Harrison's Neurology in Clinical Medicine,* Third Edition, as an authoritative source for the most up-to-date information in clinical neurology.

Stephen L. Hauser, MD

Review and self-assessment questions and answers were taken from Wiener CM, Brown CD, Hemnes AR (eds). *Harrison's Self-Assessment and Board Review,* 18th ed. New York, McGraw-Hill, 2012, ISBN 978-0-07-177195-5.

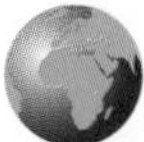
The global icons call greater attention to key epidemiologic and clinical differences in the practice of medicine throughout the world.

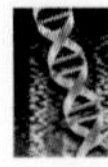
The genetic icons identify a clinical issue with an explicit genetic relationship.

SECTION I

INTRODUCTION TO NEUROLOGY

CHAPTER 1

APPROACH TO THE PATIENT WITH NEUROLOGIC DISEASE

Daniel H. Lowenstein ■ Joseph B. Martin ■ Stephen L. Hauser

Neurologic diseases are common and costly. According to recent estimates by the World Health Organization, neurologic disorders affect over 1 billion people worldwide (Table 1-1), constitute 6.3% of the global burden of disease, and cause 12% of global deaths. Most patients with neurologic symptoms seek care from internists and other generalists rather than from neurologists. Because therapies now exist for many neurologic disorders, a skillful approach to diagnosis is essential. Errors commonly result from an overreliance on costly neuroimaging procedures and laboratory tests, which, while useful, do not substitute for an adequate history and examination. The proper approach to the patient with a neurologic illness begins with the patient and focuses the clinical problem first in anatomic and then in pathophysiologic terms; only then should a specific diagnosis be entertained. This method ensures that technology is judiciously applied, a correct diagnosis is established in an efficient manner, and treatment is promptly initiated.

TABLE 1-1

PREVALENCE OF NEUROLOGIC AND PSYCHIATRIC DISEASES WORLDWIDE

DISORDER	PATIENTS, MILLIONS
Nutritional disorders and neuropathies	352
Migraine	326
Trauma	170
Cerebrovascular diseases	61
Epilepsy	50
Dementia	24
Neurologic infections	18

Source: World Health Organization estimates, 2002–2005.

THE NEUROLOGIC METHOD

LOCATE THE LESION(S)

The first priority is to identify the region of the nervous system that is likely to be responsible for the symptoms. Can the disorder be mapped to one specific location, is it multifocal, or is a diffuse process present? Are the symptoms restricted to the nervous system, or do they arise in the context of a systemic illness? Is the problem in the central nervous system (CNS), the peripheral nervous system (PNS), or both? If in the CNS, is the cerebral cortex, basal ganglia, brainstem, cerebellum, or spinal cord responsible? Are the pain-sensitive meninges involved? If in the PNS, could the disorder be located in peripheral nerves and, if so, are motor or sensory nerves primarily affected, or is a lesion in the neuromuscular junction or muscle more likely?

The first clues to defining the anatomic area of involvement appear in the history, and the examination is then directed to confirm or rule out these impressions and to clarify uncertainties. A more detailed examination of a particular region of the CNS or PNS is often indicated. For example, the examination of a patient who presents with a history of ascending paresthesias and weakness should be directed toward deciding, among other things, if the location of the lesion is in the spinal cord or peripheral nerves. Focal back pain, a spinal cord sensory level, and incontinence suggest a spinal cord origin, whereas a stocking-glove pattern of sensory loss suggests peripheral nerve disease; areflexia usually indicates peripheral neuropathy but may also be present with spinal shock in acute spinal cord disorders.

Deciding "where the lesion is" accomplishes the task of limiting the possible etiologies to a manageable, finite number. In addition, this strategy safeguards against making serious errors. Symptoms of recurrent vertigo, diplopia, and nystagmus should not trigger "multiple sclerosis" as an answer (etiology) but "brainstem" or "pons" (location); then a diagnosis of brainstem arteriovenous malformation will not be missed for lack of consideration. Similarly, the combination of optic neuritis and spastic ataxic paraparesis should initially suggest optic nerve and spinal cord disease; multiple sclerosis (MS), CNS syphilis, and vitamin B_{12} deficiency are treatable disorders that can produce this syndrome. Once the question, "Where is the lesion?" is answered, then the question, "What is the lesion?" can be addressed.

DEFINE THE PATHOPHYSIOLOGY

Clues to the pathophysiology of the disease process may also be present in the history. Primary neuronal (gray matter) disorders may present as early cognitive disturbances, movement disorders, or seizures, whereas white matter involvement produces predominantly "long tract" disorders of motor, sensory, visual, and cerebellar pathways. Progressive and symmetric symptoms often have a metabolic or degenerative origin; in such cases lesions are usually not sharply circumscribed. Thus, a patient with paraparesis and a clear spinal cord sensory level is unlikely to have vitamin B_{12} deficiency as the explanation. A Lhermitte symptom (electric shock–like sensations evoked by neck flexion) is due to ectopic impulse generation in white matter pathways and occurs with demyelination in the cervical spinal cord; among many possible causes, this symptom may indicate MS in a young adult or compressive cervical spondylosis in an older person. Symptoms that worsen after exposure to heat or exercise may indicate conduction block in demyelinated axons, as occurs in MS. A patient with recurrent episodes of diplopia and dysarthria associated with exercise or fatigue may have a disorder of neuromuscular transmission such as myasthenia gravis. Slowly advancing visual scotoma with luminous edges, termed *fortification spectra*, indicates spreading cortical depression, typically with migraine.

THE NEUROLOGIC HISTORY

Attention to the description of the symptoms experienced by the patient and substantiated by family members and others often permits an accurate localization and determination of the probable cause of the complaints, even before the neurologic examination is performed. The history also helps to bring a focus to the neurologic examination that follows. Each complaint should be pursued as far as possible to elucidate the location of the lesion, the likely underlying pathophysiology, and potential etiologies. For example, a patient complains of weakness of the right arm. What are the associated features? Does the patient have difficulty with brushing hair or reaching upward (proximal) or buttoning buttons or opening a twist-top bottle (distal)? Negative associations may also be crucial. A patient with a right hemiparesis without a language deficit likely has a lesion (internal capsule, brainstem, or spinal cord) different from that of a patient with a right hemiparesis and aphasia (left hemisphere). Other pertinent features of the history include the following:

1. *Temporal course of the illness.* It is important to determine the precise time of appearance and rate of progression of the symptoms experienced by the patient. The rapid onset of a neurologic complaint, occurring within seconds or minutes, usually indicates a vascular event, a seizure, or migraine. The onset of sensory symptoms located in one extremity that spread over a few seconds to adjacent portions of that extremity and then to the other regions of the body suggests a seizure. A more gradual onset and less well-localized symptoms point to the possibility of a transient ischemic attack (TIA). A similar but slower temporal march of symptoms accompanied by headache, nausea, or visual disturbance suggests migraine. The presence of "positive" sensory symptoms (e.g., tingling or sensations that are difficult to describe) or involuntary motor movements suggests a seizure; in contrast, transient loss of function (negative symptoms) suggests a TIA. A stuttering onset where symptoms appear, stabilize, and then progress over hours or days also suggests cerebrovascular disease; an additional history of transient remission or regression indicates that the process is more likely due to ischemia rather than hemorrhage. A gradual evolution of symptoms over hours or days suggests a toxic, metabolic, infectious, or inflammatory process. Progressing symptoms associated with the systemic manifestations of fever, stiff neck, and altered level of consciousness imply an infectious process. Relapsing and remitting symptoms involving different levels of the nervous system suggest MS or other inflammatory processes. Slowly progressive symptoms without remissions are characteristic of neurodegenerative disorders, chronic infections, gradual intoxications, and neoplasms.
2. *Patients' descriptions of the complaint.* The same words often mean different things to different patients. "Dizziness" may imply impending syncope, a sense of disequilibrium, or true spinning vertigo. "Numbness" may mean a complete loss of feeling, a positive sensation such as tingling, or even weakness. "Blurred vision" may be used to describe unilateral visual loss, as in transient monocular blindness, or diplopia. The interpretation of the true meaning of the words used by patients to describe symptoms

obviously becomes even more complex when there are differences in primary languages and cultures.

3. *Corroboration of the history by others.* It is almost always helpful to obtain additional information from family, friends, or other observers to corroborate or expand the patient's description. Memory loss, aphasia, loss of insight, intoxication, and other factors may impair the patient's capacity to communicate normally with the examiner or prevent openness about factors that have contributed to the illness. Episodes of loss of consciousness necessitate that details be sought from observers to ascertain precisely what has happened during the event.
4. *Family history.* Many neurologic disorders have an underlying genetic component. The presence of a Mendelian disorder, such as Huntington's disease or Charcot-Marie-Tooth neuropathy, is often obvious if family data are available. More detailed questions about family history are often necessary in polygenic disorders such as MS, migraine, and many types of epilepsy. It is important to elicit family history about all illnesses, in addition to neurologic and psychiatric disorders. A familial propensity to hypertension or heart disease is relevant in a patient who presents with a stroke. There are numerous inherited neurologic diseases that are associated with multisystem manifestations that may provide clues to the correct diagnosis (e.g., neurofibromatosis, Wilson's disease, neuro-ophthalmic syndromes).
5. *Medical illnesses.* Many neurologic diseases occur in the context of systemic disorders. Diabetes mellitus, hypertension, and abnormalities of blood lipids predispose to cerebrovascular disease. A solitary mass lesion in the brain may be an abscess in a patient with valvular heart disease, a primary hemorrhage in a patient with a coagulopathy, a lymphoma or toxoplasmosis in a patient with AIDS, or a metastasis in a patient with underlying cancer. Patients with malignancy may also present with a neurologic paraneoplastic syndrome (Chap. 44) or complications from chemotherapy or radiotherapy. Marfan's syndrome and related collagen disorders predispose to dissection of the cranial arteries and aneurysmal subarachnoid hemorrhage; the latter may also occur with polycystic kidney disease. Various neurologic disorders occur with dysthyroid states or other endocrinopathies. It is especially important to look for the presence of systemic diseases in patients with peripheral neuropathy. Most patients with coma in a hospital setting have a metabolic, toxic, or infectious cause.
6. *Drug use and abuse and toxin exposure.* It is essential to inquire about the history of drug use, both prescribed and illicit. Sedatives, antidepressants, and other psychoactive medications are frequently associated with acute confusional states in the elderly. Aminoglycoside antibiotics may exacerbate symptoms of weakness in patients with disorders of neuromuscular transmission, such as myasthenia gravis, and may cause dizziness secondary to ototoxicity. Vincristine and other antineoplastic drugs can cause peripheral neuropathy, and immunosuppressive agents such as cyclosporine can produce encephalopathy. Excessive vitamin ingestion can lead to disease; for example vitamin A and pseudotumor cerebri, or pyridoxine and peripheral neuropathy. Many patients are unaware that over-the-counter sleeping pills, cold preparations, and diet pills are actually drugs. Alcohol, the most prevalent neurotoxin, is often not recognized as such by patients, and other drugs of abuse such as cocaine and heroin can cause a wide range of neurologic abnormalities. A history of environmental or industrial exposure to neurotoxins may provide an essential clue; consultation with the patient's coworkers or employer may be required.
7. *Formulating an impression of the patient.* Use the opportunity while taking the history to form an impression of the patient. Is the information forthcoming, or does it take a circuitous course? Is there evidence of anxiety, depression, or hypochondriasis? Are there any clues to defects in language, memory, insight, or inappropriate behavior? The neurologic assessment begins as soon as the patient comes into the room and the first introduction is made.

THE NEUROLOGIC EXAMINATION

The neurologic examination is challenging and complex; it has many components and includes a number of skills that can be mastered only through repeated use of the same techniques on a large number of individuals with and without neurologic disease. Mastery of the complete neurologic examination is usually important only for physicians in neurology and associated specialties. However, knowledge of the basics of the examination, especially those components that are effective in screening for neurologic dysfunction, is essential for all clinicians, especially generalists.

There is no single, universally accepted sequence of the examination that must be followed, but most clinicians begin with assessment of mental status followed by the cranial nerves, motor system, sensory system, coordination, and gait. Whether the examination is basic or comprehensive, it is essential that it be performed in an orderly and systematic fashion to avoid errors and serious omissions. Thus, the best way to learn and gain expertise in the examination is to choose one's own approach and practice it frequently and do it in the same exact sequence each time.

The detailed description of the neurologic examination that follows describes the more commonly used parts of the examination, with a particular emphasis on the components that are considered most helpful for the assessment of common neurologic problems. Each section also includes a brief description of the minimal examination necessary for adequate screening for abnormalities in a patient who has no symptoms suggesting neurologic dysfunction. A screening examination done in this way can be completed in 3–5 min.

Several additional points about the examination are worth noting. First, in recording observations, it is important to describe what is found rather than to apply a poorly defined medical term (e.g., "patient groans to sternal rub" rather than "obtunded"). Second, subtle CNS abnormalities are best detected by carefully comparing a patient's performance on tasks that require simultaneous activation of both cerebral hemispheres (e.g., eliciting a pronator drift of an outstretched arm with the eyes closed; extinction on one side of bilaterally applied light touch, also with eyes closed; or decreased arm swing or a slight asymmetry when walking). Third, if the patient's complaint is brought on by some activity, reproduce the activity in the office. If the complaint is of dizziness when the head is turned in one direction, have the patient do this and also look for associated signs on examination (e.g., nystagmus or dysmetria). If pain occurs after walking two blocks, have the patient leave the office and walk this distance and immediately return, and repeat the relevant parts of the examination. Finally, the use of tests that are individually tailored to the patient's problem can be of value in assessing changes over time. Tests of walking a 7.5-m (25-ft) distance (normal, 5–6 s; note assistance, if any), repetitive finger or toe tapping (normal, 20–25 taps in 5 s), or handwriting are examples.

MENTAL STATUS EXAMINATION

- *The bare minimum: During the interview, look for difficulties with communication and determine whether the patient has recall and insight into recent and past events.*

The mental status examination is underway as soon as the physician begins observing and talking with the patient. If the history raises any concern for abnormalities of higher cortical function or if cognitive problems are observed during the interview, then detailed testing of the mental status is indicated. The patient's ability to understand the language used for the examination, cultural background, educational experience, sensory or motor problems, or comorbid conditions need to be factored into the applicability of the tests and interpretation of results.

The Folstein mini-mental status examination (MMSE) (Table 29-5) is a standardized screening examination of cognitive function that is extremely easy to administer and takes <10 min to complete. Using age-adjusted values for defining normal performance, the test is ~85% sensitive and 85% specific for making the diagnosis of dementia that is moderate or severe, especially in educated patients. When there is sufficient time available, the MMSE is one of the best methods for documenting the current mental status of the patient, and this is especially useful as a baseline assessment to which future scores of the MMSE can be compared.

Individual elements of the mental status examination can be subdivided into level of consciousness, orientation, speech and language, memory, fund of information, insight and judgment, abstract thought, and calculations.

Level of consciousness is the patient's relative state of awareness of the self and the environment, and ranges from fully awake to comatose. When the patient is not fully awake, the examiner should describe the responses to the minimum stimulus necessary to elicit a reaction, ranging from verbal commands to a brief, painful stimulus such as a squeeze of the trapezius muscle. Responses that are directed toward the stimulus and signify some degree of intact cerebral function (e.g., opening the eyes and looking at the examiner or reaching to push away a painful stimulus) must be distinguished from reflex responses of a spinal origin (e.g., triple flexion response—flexion at the ankle, knee, and hip in response to a painful stimulus to the foot).

Orientation is tested by asking the person to state his or her name, location, and time (day of the week and date); time is usually the first to be affected in a variety of conditions.

Speech is assessed by observing articulation, rate, rhythm, and prosody (i.e., the changes in pitch and accentuation of syllable and words).

Language is assessed by observing the content of the patient's verbal and written output, response to spoken commands, and ability to read. A typical testing sequence is to ask the patient to name successively more detailed components of clothing, a watch, or a pen; repeat the phrase "No ifs, ands, or buts"; follow a three-step, verbal command; write a sentence; and read and respond to a written command.

Memory should be analyzed according to three main time scales: (1) immediate memory is assessed by saying a list of three items and having the patient repeat the list immediately, (2) short-term memory is tested by asking the patient to recall the same three items 5 and 15 min later, and (3) long-term memory is evaluated by determining how well the patient is able to provide a coherent chronologic history of his or her illness or personal events.

Fund of information is assessed by asking questions about major historic or current events, with special attention to educational level and life experiences.

Abnormalities of *insight and judgment* are usually detected during the patient interview; a more detailed assessment can be elicited by asking the patient to describe how he or she would respond to situations having a variety of potential outcomes (e.g., "What would you do if you found a wallet on the sidewalk?").

Abstract thought can be tested by asking the patient to describe similarities between various objects or concepts (e.g., apple and orange, desk and chair, poetry and sculpture) or to list items having the same attributes (e.g., a list of four-legged animals).

Calculation ability is assessed by having the patient carry out a computation that is appropriate to the patient's age and education (e.g., serial subtraction of 7 from 100 or 3 from 20; or word problems involving simple arithmetic).

CRANIAL NERVE EXAMINATION

- *The bare minimum: Check the fundi, visual fields, pupil size and reactivity, extraocular movements, and facial movements.*

The cranial nerves (CN) are best examined in numerical order, except for grouping together CN III, IV, and VI because of their similar function.

CN I (olfactory)

Testing is usually omitted unless there is suspicion for inferior frontal lobe disease (e.g., meningioma). With eyes closed, ask the patient to sniff a mild stimulus such as toothpaste or coffee and identify the odorant.

CN II (optic)

Check visual acuity (with eyeglasses or contact lens correction) using a Snellen chart or similar tool. Test the visual fields by confrontation, i.e., by comparing the patient's visual fields to your own. As a screening test, it is usually sufficient to examine the visual fields of both eyes simultaneously; individual eye fields should be tested if there is any reason to suspect a problem of vision by the history or other elements of the examination, or if the screening test reveals an abnormality. Face the patient at a distance of approximately 0.6–1.0 m (2–3 ft) and place your hands at the periphery of your visual fields in the plane that is equidistant between you and the patient. Instruct the patient to look directly at the center of your face and to indicate when and where he or she sees one of your fingers moving. Beginning with the two inferior quadrants and then the two superior quadrants, move your index finger of the right hand, left hand, or both hands simultaneously and observe whether the patient detects the movements. A single small-amplitude movement of the finger is sufficient for a normal response. Focal perimetry and tangent screen examinations should be used to map out visual field defects fully or to search for subtle abnormalities. Optic fundi should be examined with an ophthalmoscope, and the color, size, and degree of swelling or elevation of the optic disc noted, as well as the color and texture of the retina. The retinal vessels should be checked for size, regularity, arterial-venous nicking at crossing points, hemorrhage, exudates, etc.

CN III, IV, VI (oculomotor, trochlear, abducens)

Describe the size and shape of pupils and reaction to light and accommodation (i.e., as the eyes converge while following your finger as it moves toward the bridge of the nose). To check extraocular movements, ask the patient to keep his or her head still while tracking the movement of the tip of your finger. Move the target slowly in the horizontal and vertical planes; observe any paresis, nystagmus, or abnormalities of smooth pursuit (saccades, oculomotor ataxia, etc.). If necessary, the relative position of the two eyes, both in primary and multidirectional gaze, can be assessed by comparing the reflections of a bright light off both pupils. However, in practice it is typically more useful to determine whether the patient describes diplopia in any direction of gaze; true diplopia should almost always resolve with one eye closed. Horizontal nystagmus is best assessed at 45° and not at extreme lateral gaze (which is uncomfortable for the patient); the target must often be held at the lateral position for at least a few seconds to detect an abnormality.

CN V (trigeminal)

Examine sensation within the three territories of the branches of the trigeminal nerve (ophthalmic, maxillary, and mandibular) on each side of the face. As with other parts of the sensory examination, testing of two sensory modalities derived from different anatomic pathways (e.g., light touch and temperature) is sufficient for a screening examination. Testing of other modalities, the corneal reflex, and the motor component of CN V (jaw clench—masseter muscle) is indicated when suggested by the history.

CN VII (facial)

Look for facial asymmetry at rest and with spontaneous movements. Test eyebrow elevation, forehead wrinkling, eye closure, smiling, and cheek puff. Look in particular for differences in the lower versus upper facial muscles; weakness of the lower two-thirds of the face with preservation of the upper third suggests an upper motor neuron lesion, whereas weakness of an entire side suggests a lower motor neuron lesion.

CN VIII (vestibulocochlear)

Check the patient's ability to hear a finger rub or whispered voice with each ear. Further testing for air versus mastoid bone conduction (Rinne) and lateralization of a 512-Hz tuning fork placed at the center of the forehead (Weber) should be done if an abnormality is detected by history or examination. Any suspected problem should be followed up with formal audiometry. For further discussion of assessing vestibular nerve function in the setting of dizziness, coma, or hearing loss, see Chaps. 11, 17, and 24, respectively.

CN IX, X (glossopharyngeal, vagus)

Observe the position and symmetry of the palate and uvula at rest and with phonation ("aah"). The pharyngeal ("gag") reflex is evaluated by stimulating the posterior pharyngeal wall on each side with a sterile, blunt object (e.g., tongue blade), but the reflex is often absent in normal individuals.

CN XI (spinal accessory)

Check shoulder shrug (trapezius muscle) and head rotation to each side (sternocleidomastoid) against resistance.

CN XII (hypoglossal)

Inspect the tongue for atrophy or fasciculations, position with protrusion, and strength when extended against the inner surface of the cheeks on each side.

MOTOR EXAMINATION

- *The bare minimum: Look for muscle atrophy and check extremity tone. Assess upper extremity strength by checking for pronator drift and strength of wrist or finger extensors. Tap the biceps, patellar, and Achilles reflexes. Test for lower extremity strength by having the patient walk normally and on heels and toes.*

The motor examination includes observations of muscle appearance, tone, strength, and reflexes. Although gait is in part a test of motor function, it is usually evaluated separately at the end of the examination.

Appearance

Inspect and palpate muscle groups under good light and with the patient in a comfortable and symmetric position. Check for muscle fasciculations, tenderness, and atrophy or hypertrophy. Involuntary movements may be present at rest (e.g., tics, myoclonus, choreoathetosis), during maintained posture (pill-rolling tremor of Parkinson's disease), or with voluntary movements (intention tremor of cerebellar disease or familial tremor).

Tone

Muscle tone is tested by measuring the resistance to passive movement of a relaxed limb. Patients often have difficulty relaxing during this procedure, so it is useful to distract the patient to minimize active movements. In the upper limbs, tone is assessed by rapid pronation and supination of the forearm and flexion and extension at the wrist. In the lower limbs, while the patient is supine the examiner's hands are placed behind the knees and rapidly raised; with normal tone the ankles drag along the table surface for a variable distance before rising, whereas increased tone results in an immediate lift of the heel off the surface. Decreased tone is most commonly due to lower motor neuron or peripheral nerve disorders. Increased tone may be evident as spasticity (resistance determined by the angle and velocity of motion; corticospinal tract disease), rigidity (similar resistance in all angles of motion; extrapyramidal disease), or paratonia (fluctuating changes in resistance; frontal lobe pathways or normal difficulty in relaxing). Cogwheel rigidity, in which passive motion elicits jerky interruptions in resistance, is seen in parkinsonism.

Strength

Testing for pronator drift is an extremely useful method for screening upper limb weakness. The patient is asked to hold both arms fully extended and parallel to the ground with eyes closed. This position should be maintained for ~10 s; any flexion at the elbow or fingers or pronation of the forearm, especially if asymmetric, is a sign of potential weakness. Muscle strength is further assessed by having the patient exert maximal effort for the particular muscle or muscle group being tested. It is important to isolate the muscles as much as possible, i.e., hold the limb so that only the muscles of interest are active. It is also helpful to palpate accessible muscles as they contract. Grading muscle strength and evaluating the patient's effort is an art that takes time and practice. Muscle strength is traditionally graded using the following scale:

0 = no movement
1 = flicker or trace of contraction but no associated movement at a joint
2 = movement with gravity eliminated
3 = movement against gravity but not against resistance
4− = movement against a mild degree of resistance
4 = movement against moderate resistance
4+ = movement against strong resistance
5 = full power

However, in many cases it is more practical to use the following terms:

Paralysis = no movement
Severe weakness = movement with gravity eliminated
Moderate weakness = movement against gravity but not against mild resistance
Mild weakness = movement against moderate resistance
Full strength

Noting the pattern of weakness is as important as assessing the magnitude of weakness. Unilateral or bilateral weakness of the upper limb extensors and lower limb flexors ("pyramidal weakness") suggests a lesion of the pyramidal tract, bilateral proximal weakness suggests myopathy, and bilateral distal weakness suggests peripheral neuropathy.

Reflexes

Muscle stretch reflexes

Those that are typically assessed include the biceps (C5, C6), brachioradialis (C5, C6), and triceps (C7, C8) reflexes in the upper limbs and the patellar or quadriceps (L3, L4) and Achilles (S1, S2) reflexes in the lower limbs. The patient should be relaxed and the muscle positioned midway between full contraction and extension. Reflexes may be enhanced by asking the patient to voluntarily contract other, distant muscle groups (Jendrassik maneuver). For example, upper limb reflexes may be reinforced by voluntary teeth-clenching, and the Achilles reflex by hooking the flexed fingers of the two hands together and attempting to pull them apart. For each reflex tested, the two sides should be tested sequentially, and it is important to determine the smallest stimulus required to elicit a reflex rather than the maximum response. Reflexes are graded according to the following scale:

0 = absent
1 = present but diminished
2 = normoactive
3 = exaggerated
4 = clonus

Cutaneous reflexes

The plantar reflex is elicited by stroking, with a noxious stimulus such as a tongue blade, the lateral surface of the sole of the foot beginning near the heel and moving across the ball of the foot to the great toe. The normal reflex consists of plantar flexion of the toes. With upper motor neuron lesions above the S1 level of the spinal cord, a paradoxical extension of the toe is observed, associated with fanning and extension of the other toes (termed an *extensor plantar response*, or *Babinski sign*). However, despite its popularity, the reliability and validity of the Babinski sign for identifying upper motor neuron weakness is limited—it is far more useful to rely on tests of tone, strength, stretch reflexes, and coordination. Superficial abdominal reflexes are elicited by gently stroking the abdominal surface near the umbilicus in a diagonal fashion with a sharp object (e.g., the wooden end of a cotton-tipped swab) and observing the movement of the umbilicus. Normally, the umbilicus will pull toward the stimulated quadrant. With upper motor neuron lesions, these reflexes are absent. They are most helpful when there is preservation of the upper (spinal cord level T9) but not lower (T12) abdominal reflexes, indicating a spinal lesion between T9 and T12, or when the response is asymmetric. Other useful cutaneous reflexes include the cremasteric (ipsilateral elevation of the testicle following stroking of the medial thigh; mediated by L1 and L2) and anal (contraction of the anal sphincter when the perianal skin is scratched; mediated by S2, S3, S4) reflexes. It is particularly important to test for these reflexes in any patient with suspected injury to the spinal cord or lumbosacral roots.

Primitive reflexes

With disease of the frontal lobe pathways, several primitive reflexes not normally present in the adult may appear. The suck response is elicited by lightly touching the center of the lips, and the root response the corner of the lips, with a tongue blade; the patient will move the lips to suck or root in the direction of the stimulus. The grasp reflex is elicited by touching the palm between the thumb and index finger with the examiner's fingers; a positive response is a forced grasp of the examiner's hand. In many instances stroking the back of the hand will lead to its release. The palmomental response is contraction of the mentalis muscle (chin) ipsilateral to a scratch stimulus diagonally applied to the palm.

Sensory examination

- *The bare minimum: Ask whether the patient can feel light touch and the temperature of a cool object in each distal extremity. Check double simultaneous stimulation using light touch on the hands.*

Evaluating sensation is usually the most unreliable part of the examination, because it is subjective and is difficult to quantify. In the compliant and discerning patient, the sensory examination can be extremely helpful for the precise localization of a lesion. With patients who are uncooperative or lack an understanding of the tests, it may be useless. The examination should be focused on the suspected lesion. For example, in spinal cord, spinal root, or peripheral nerve abnormalities, all major sensory modalities should be tested while looking for a pattern consistent with a spinal level and dermatomal or nerve distribution. In patients with lesions at or above the brainstem, screening the primary sensory modalities in the distal extremities along with tests of "cortical" sensation is usually sufficient.

The five primary sensory modalities—light touch, pain, temperature, vibration, and joint position—are tested in each limb. Light touch is assessed by stimulating the skin with single, very gentle touches of the examiner's finger or a wisp of cotton. Pain is tested using a new pin, and temperature is assessed using a metal object (e.g., tuning fork) that has been immersed in cold and warm water. Vibration is tested using a 128-Hz tuning fork applied to the distal phalanx of the great toe or index finger just below the nail bed. By placing a finger on the opposite side of the joint being tested, the examiner compares the patient's threshold of vibration perception with his or her own. For joint position testing, the examiner grasps the digit or limb laterally and distal to the joint being assessed; small 1- to 2-mm excursions can usually be sensed. The Romberg maneuver is primarily a test of proprioception. The patient is asked to stand with the feet as close together as necessary to maintain balance while the eyes are open, and the eyes are then closed. A loss of balance with the eyes closed is an abnormal response.

"Cortical" sensation is mediated by the parietal lobes and represents an integration of the primary sensory modalities; testing cortical sensation is only meaningful when primary sensation is intact. Double simultaneous stimulation is especially useful as a screening test for cortical function; with the patient's eyes closed, the examiner lightly touches one or both hands and asks the patient to identify the stimuli. With a parietal lobe lesion, the patient may be unable to identify the stimulus on the contralateral side when both hands are touched. Other modalities relying on the parietal cortex include the discrimination of two closely placed stimuli as separate (two-point discrimination), identification of an object by touch and manipulation alone (stereognosis), and the identification of numbers or letters written on the skin surface (graphesthesia).

COORDINATION EXAMINATION

- *The bare minimum: Test rapid alternating movements of the hands and the finger-to-nose and heel-knee-shin maneuvers.*

Coordination refers to the orchestration and fluidity of movements. Even simple acts require cooperation of agonist and antagonist muscles, maintenance of posture, and complex servomechanisms to control the rate and range of movements. Part of this integration relies on normal function of the cerebellar and basal ganglia systems. However, coordination also requires intact muscle strength and kinesthetic and proprioceptive information. Thus, if the examination has disclosed abnormalities of the motor or sensory systems, the patient's coordination should be assessed with these limitations in mind.

Rapid alternating movements in the upper limbs are tested separately on each side by having the patient make a fist, partially extend the index finger, and then tap the index finger on the distal thumb as quickly as possible. In the lower limb, the patient rapidly taps the foot against the floor or the examiner's hand. Finger-to-nose testing is primarily a test of cerebellar function; the patient is asked to touch his or her index finger repetitively to the nose and then to the examiner's outstretched finger, which moves with each repetition. A similar test in the lower extremity is to have the patient raise the leg and touch the examiner's finger with the great toe. Another cerebellar test in the lower limbs is the heel-knee-shin maneuver; in the supine position the patient is asked to slide the heel of each foot from the knee down the shin of the other leg. For all these movements, the accuracy, speed, and rhythm are noted.

GAIT EXAMINATION

- *The bare minimum: Observe the patient while walking normally, on the heels and toes, and along a straight line.*

Watching the patient walk is the most important part of the neurologic examination. Normal gait requires that multiple systems—including strength, sensation, and coordination—function in a highly integrated fashion. Unexpected abnormalities may be detected that prompt the examiner to return in more detail to other aspects of the examination. The patient should be observed while walking and turning normally, walking on the heels, walking on the toes, and walking heel-to-toe along a straight line. The examination may reveal decreased arm swing on one side (corticospinal tract disease), a stooped posture and short-stepped gait (parkinsonism), a broad-based unstable gait (ataxia), scissoring (spasticity), or a high-stepped, slapping gait (posterior column or peripheral nerve disease), or the patient may appear to be stuck in place (apraxia with frontal lobe disease).

NEUROLOGIC DIAGNOSIS

The clinical data obtained from the history and examination are interpreted to arrive at an anatomic localization that best explains the clinical findings (**Table 1-2**), to narrow the list of diagnostic possibilities, and to select the laboratory tests most likely to be informative. The laboratory assessment may include (1) serum electrolytes; complete blood count; and renal, hepatic, endocrine, and immune studies; (2) cerebrospinal fluid examination; (3) focused neuroimaging studies (Chap. 4); or (4) electrophysiologic studies (Chap. 5). The anatomic localization, mode of onset and course of illness, other medical data, and laboratory findings are then integrated to establish an etiologic diagnosis.

TABLE 1-2

FINDINGS HELPFUL FOR LOCALIZATION WITHIN THE NERVOUS SYSTEM

	SIGNS
Cerebrum	Abnormal mental status or cognitive impairment Seizures Unilateral weakness[a] and sensory abnormalities including head and limbs Visual field abnormalities Movement abnormalities (e.g., diffuse incoordination, tremor, chorea)
Brainstem	Isolated cranial nerve abnormalities (single or multiple) "Crossed" weakness[a] and sensory abnormalities of head and limbs, e.g., weakness of right face and left arm and leg
Spinal cord	Back pain or tenderness Weakness[a] and sensory abnormalities sparing the head Mixed upper and lower motor neuron findings Sensory level Sphincter dysfunction
Spinal roots	Radiating limb pain Weakness[b] or sensory abnormalities following root distribution (see Figs. 15-2 and 15-3) Loss of reflexes
Peripheral nerve	Mid or distal limb pain Weakness[b] or sensory abnormalities following nerve distribution (see Figs. 15-2 and 15-3) "Stocking or glove" distribution of sensory loss Loss of reflexes
Neuromuscular junction	Bilateral weakness including face (ptosis, diplopia, dysphagia) and proximal limbs Increasing weakness with exertion Sparing of sensation
Muscle	Bilateral proximal or distal weakness Sparing of sensation

[a]Weakness along with other abnormalities having an "upper motor neuron" pattern, i.e., spasticity, weakness of extensors > flexors in the upper extremity and flexors > extensors in the lower extremity, hyperreflexia.
[b]Weakness along with other abnormalities having a "lower motor neuron" pattern, i.e., flaccidity and hyporeflexia.

The neurologic examination may be normal even in patients with a serious neurologic disease, such as seizures, chronic meningitis, or a TIA. A comatose patient may arrive with no available history, and in such cases the approach is as described in Chap. 17. In other patients, an inadequate history may be overcome by a succession of examinations from which the course of the illness can be inferred. In perplexing cases it is useful to remember that uncommon presentations of common diseases are more likely than rare etiologies. Thus, even in tertiary care settings, multiple strokes are usually due to emboli and not vasculitis, and dementia with myoclonus is usually Alzheimer's disease and not due to a prion disorder or a paraneoplastic cause. Finally, the most important task of a primary care physician faced with a patient who has a new neurologic complaint is to assess the urgency of referral to a specialist. Here, the imperative is to rapidly identify patients likely to have nervous system infections, acute strokes, and spinal cord compression or other treatable mass lesions and arrange for immediate care.

CHAPTER 2

THE NEUROLOGIC SCREENING EXAM

Daniel H. Lowenstein

Knowledge of the basic neurologic examination is an essential clinical skill. A simple neurologic screening examination—assessment of mental status, cranial nerves, motor system, sensory system, coordination, and gait—can be reliably performed in 3–5 min. Although the components of the examination may appear daunting at first, skills usually improve rapidly with repetition and practice. In this video, the technique of performing a simple and efficient screening examination is presented. Videos for this chapter can be accessed at the following link: http://www.mhprofessional.com/mediacenter/.

CHAPTER 3

VIDEO ATLAS OF THE DETAILED NEUROLOGIC EXAMINATION

Martin A. Samuels

The comprehensive neurologic examination is an irreplaceable tool for the efficient diagnosis of neurologic disorders. Mastery of its details requires knowledge of normal nervous system anatomy and physiology combined with personal experience performing orderly and systematic examinations on large numbers of patients and healthy individuals. In the hands of a great clinician, the neurologic examination also becomes a thing of beauty—the pinnacle of the art of medicine. In this video, the most commonly used components of the examination are presented in detail, with a particular emphasis on those elements that are most helpful for assessment of common neurologic problems. Videos for this chapter can be accessed at the following link: http://www.mhprofessional.com/mediacenter/.

CHAPTER 4

NEUROIMAGING IN NEUROLOGIC DISORDERS

William P. Dillon

The clinician caring for patients with neurologic symptoms is faced with myriad imaging options, including computed tomography (CT), CT angiography (CTA), perfusion CT (pCT), magnetic resonance imaging (MRI), MR angiography (MRA), functional MRI (fMRI), MR spectroscopy (MRS), MR neurography (MRN), diffusion and diffusion track imaging (DTI), susceptibility weighted MR imaging (SWI), and perfusion MRI (pMRI). In addition, an increasing number of interventional neuroradiologic techniques are available, including angiography catheter embolization, coiling, and stenting of vascular structures; and spine diagnostic and interventional techniques such as diskography, transforaminal and translaminar epidural and nerve root injections and blood patches. Recent developments such as multidetector CTA (MDCTA) and gadolinium-enhanced MRA, have narrowed the indications for conventional angiography, which is now reserved for patients in whom small-vessel detail is essential for diagnosis or for whom concurrent interventional therapy is planned (Table 4-1).

In general, MRI is more sensitive than CT for the detection of lesions affecting the central nervous system (CNS), particularly those of the spinal cord, cranial nerves, and posterior fossa structures. Diffusion MR, a sequence sensitive to the microscopic motion of water, is the most sensitive technique for detecting acute ischemic stroke of the brain or spinal cord, and it is also useful in the detection of encephalitis, abscesses, and prion diseases. CT, however, is quickly acquired and is widely available, making it a pragmatic choice for the initial evaluation of patients with acute changes in mental status, suspected acute stroke, hemorrhage, and intracranial or spinal trauma. CT is also more sensitive than MRI for visualizing fine osseous detail and is indicated in the initial evaluation of conductive hearing loss as well as lesions affecting the skull base and calvarium. MR may, however, add important diagnostic information regarding bone marrow infiltrative processes that are difficult to detect on CT.

COMPUTED TOMOGRAPHY

TECHNIQUE

The CT image is a cross-sectional representation of anatomy created by a computer-generated analysis of the attenuation of x-ray beams passed through a section of the body. As the x-ray beam, collimated to the desired slice width, rotates around the patient, it passes through selected regions in the body. X-rays that are not attenuated by body structures are detected by sensitive x-ray detectors aligned 180° from the x-ray tube. A computer calculates a "back projection" image from the 360° x-ray attenuation profile. Greater x-ray attenuation (e.g., as caused by bone) results in areas of high "density," while soft tissue structures that have poor attenuation of x-rays such as organs and air-filled cavities are lower in density. The resolution of an image depends on the radiation dose, the detector size, collimation (slice thickness), the field of view, and the matrix size of the display. A modern CT scanner is capable of obtaining sections as thin as 0.5–1 mm with submillimeter resolution at a speed of 0.3–1 s per rotation; complete studies of the brain can be completed in 2–10 s.

Multidetector CT (MDCT) is now standard in most radiology departments. Single or multiple (from 4 to 256) detectors positioned 180° to the x-ray source result in multiple slices per revolution of the beam around the patient. The table moves continuously through the rotating x-ray beam, generating a continuous "helix" of information that can be reformatted into various slice thicknesses and planes. Advantages of MDCT include shorter scan times, reduced patient and organ motion, and the ability to acquire images dynamically during the infusion of intravenous contrast that can be used to

TABLE 4-1

GUIDELINES FOR THE USE OF CT, ULTRASOUND, AND MRI

CONDITION	RECOMMENDED TECHNIQUE
Hemorrhage	
Acute parenchymal	CT, MR
Subacute/chronic	MRI
Subarachnoid hemorrhage	CT, CTA, lumbar puncture → angiography
Aneurysm	Angiography > CTA, MRA
Ischemic infarction	
Hemorrhagic infarction	CT or MRI
Bland infarction	MRI > CT, CTA, angiography
Carotid or vertebral dissection	MRI/MRA
Vertebral basilar insufficiency	CTA, MRI/MRA
Carotid stenosis	CTA > Doppler ultrasound, MRA
Suspected mass lesion	
Neoplasm, primary or metastatic	MRI + contrast
Infection/abscess	MRI + contrast
Immunosuppressed with focal findings	MRI + contrast
Vascular malformation	MRI ± angiography
White matter disorders	MRI
Demyelinating disease	MRI ± contrast
Dementia	MRI > CT
Trauma	
Acute trauma	CT (noncontrast)
Shear injury/chronic hemorrhage	MRI + gradient echo imaging
Headache/migraine	CT (noncontrast)/MRI
Seizure	
First time, no focal neurologic deficits	?CT as screen ± contrast
Partial complex/refractory	MRI with coronal T2W imaging
Cranial neuropathy	MRI with contrast
Meningeal disease	MRI with contrast
Spine	
Low back pain	
No neurologic deficits	MRI or CT after 4 weeks
With focal deficits	MRI > CT
Spinal stenosis	MRI or CT
Cervical spondylosis	MRI or CT myelography
Infection	MRI + contrast, CT
Myelopathy	MRI + contrast
Arteriovenous malformation	MRI, angiography

Abbreviations: CT, computed tomography; CTA, CT angiography; MRA, MR angiography; MRI, magnetic resonance imaging; T2W, T2-weighted.

construct CT angiograms of vascular structures and CT perfusion images (Fig. 4-1*B* and *C*). CTA images are postprocessed for display in three dimensions to yield angiogram-like images (Fig. 4-1*C*, 4-2 *E* and *F*, and *see Fig. 27-4*). CTA has proved useful in assessing the cervical and intracranial arterial and venous anatomy.

Intravenous iodinated contrast is often administered prior to or during a CT study to identify vascular structures and to detect defects in the blood-brain barrier (BBB) that are associated with disorders such as tumors, infarcts, and infections. In the normal CNS, only vessels and structures lacking a BBB (e.g., the pituitary gland, choroid plexus, and dura) enhance after contrast administration. The use of iodinated contrast agents carries a small risk of allergic reaction and adds additional expense. While helpful in characterizing mass lesions as well as essential for the acquisition of CTA studies, the decision to use contrast material should always be considered carefully.

INDICATIONS

CT is the primary study of choice in the evaluation of an acute change in mental status, focal neurologic findings, acute trauma to the brain and spine, suspected subarachnoid hemorrhage, and conductive hearing loss (Table 4-1). CT is complementary to MR in the evaluation of the skull base, orbit, and osseous structures of the spine. In the spine, CT is useful in evaluating patients with osseous spinal stenosis and spondylosis, but MRI is often preferred in those with neurologic deficits. CT can also be obtained following intrathecal contrast injection to evaluate the intracranial cisterns (*CT cisternography*) for cerebrospinal fluid (CSF) fistula, as well as the spinal subarachnoid space (*CT myelography*).

COMPLICATIONS

CT is safe, fast, and reliable. Radiation exposure depends on the dose used but is normally between 2 and 5 mSv (millisievert) for a routine brain CT study. Care must be taken to reduce exposure when imaging children. With the advent of MDCT, CTA, and CT perfusion, care must be taken to appropriately minimize radiation dose whenever possible. Advanced software that permits noise reduction may permit lower radiation doses. The most frequent complications are associated with use of intravenous contrast agents. Two broad categories of contrast media, ionic and nonionic, are in use. Although ionic agents are relatively safe and inexpensive, they are associated with a higher incidence of reactions and side effects. As a result, ionic agents have been largely replaced by safer nonionic compounds.

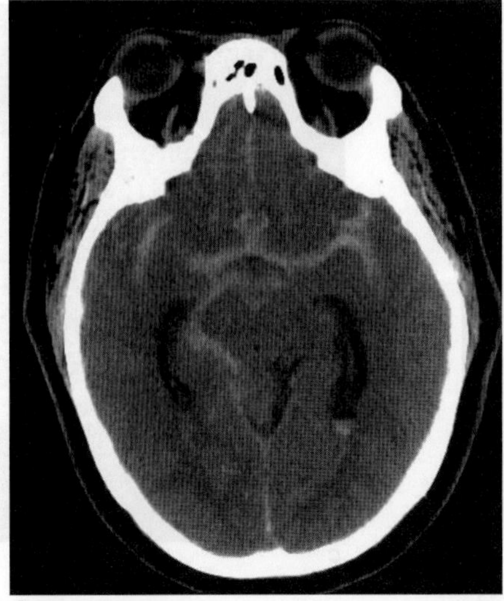
A

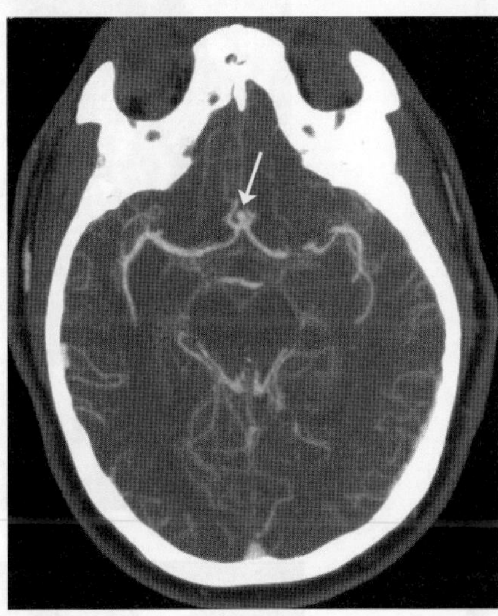
B

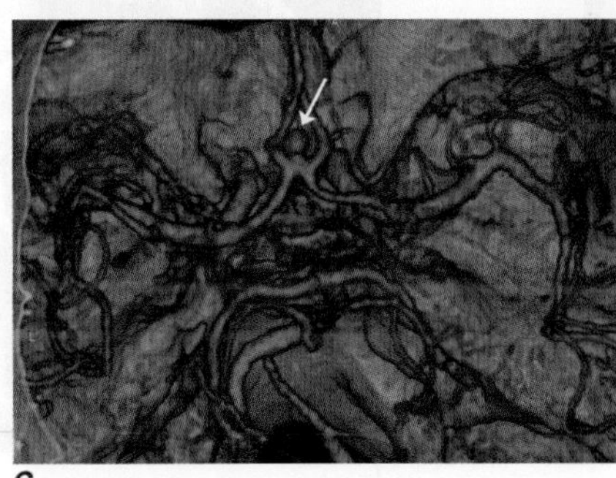
C

FIGURE 4-1
CT angiography (CTA) of ruptured anterior cerebral artery aneurysm in a patient presenting with acute headache. ***A.*** Noncontrast CT demonstrates subarachnoid hemorrhage and mild obstructive hydrocephalus. ***B.*** Axial maximum-intensity projection from CT angiography demonstrates enlargement of the anterior cerebral artery (*arrow*). ***C.*** 3D surface reconstruction using a workstation confirms the anterior cerebral aneurysm and demonstrates its orientation and relationship to nearby vessels (*arrow*). CTA image is produced by 0.5–1-mm helical CT scans performed during a rapid bolus infusion of intravenous contrast medium.

Contrast nephropathy may result from hemodynamic changes, renal tubular obstruction and cell damage, or immunologic reactions to contrast agents. A rise in serum creatinine of at least 85 μmol/L (1 mg/dL) within 48 h of contrast administration is often used as a definition of contrast nephropathy, although other causes of acute renal failure must be excluded. The prognosis is usually favorable, with serum creatinine levels returning to baseline within 1–2 weeks. Risk factors for contrast nephropathy include advanced age (>80 years), preexisting renal disease (serum creatinine exceeding 2 mg/dL), solitary kidney, diabetes mellitus, dehydration, paraproteinemia, concurrent use of nephrotoxic medication or chemotherapeutic agents, and high contrast dose. Patients with diabetes and those with mild renal failure should be well hydrated prior to the administration of contrast agents, although careful consideration should be given to alternative imaging techniques such as MR imaging or noncontrast CT or ultrasound (US) examinations. Nonionic, low-osmolar media produce fewer abnormalities in renal blood flow and less endothelial cell damage but should still be used carefully in patients at risk for allergic reaction. Estimated glomerular filtration rate (eGFR) is a more reliable indicator of renal function compared to creatinine alone as it takes into account age, race, and sex. In one study, 15% of outpatients with a normal serum creatinine had an estimated creatinine clearance of 50 mL/min/1.73 m^2 or less (normal is 90 mL/min/1.73 m^2 or more). The exact eGFR threshold, below which withholding intravenous contrast should be considered, is controversial. The risk of contrast nephropathy increases in patients with an eGFR <60 mL/min/1.73^2; however the majority of these patients will only have a temporary rise in creatinine. The risk of dialysis after receiving contrast significantly increases in patients with eGFR <30 mL/min/1.73^2. Thus, an eGFR threshold between 60 and 30 mL/min/1.73^2 is appropriate; however the exact number is somewhat arbitrary. A creatinine of 1.6 in a 70-year-old, non-African-American male corresponds to an eGFR of approximately 45 mL/min/1.73^2. The American College of Radiology suggests using an eGFR of 45 as a threshold below which iodinated contrast should not be given without serious consideration of the potential for contrast nephropathy. If contrast must be administered to a patient with an eGRF below 45, the patient should be well hydrated, and a reduction in the dose of contrast should be considered. Use of other agents such as bicarbonate and acetylcysteine may reduce the incidence of contrast nephropathy. Other side effects of CT scanning are rare but include a sensation of warmth throughout the body and a metallic taste during intravenous administration of iodinated contrast media. The most serious side effects are anaphylactic reactions, which range from mild hives to bronchospasm, acute anaphylaxis, and death. The pathogenesis of these allergic reactions is not fully

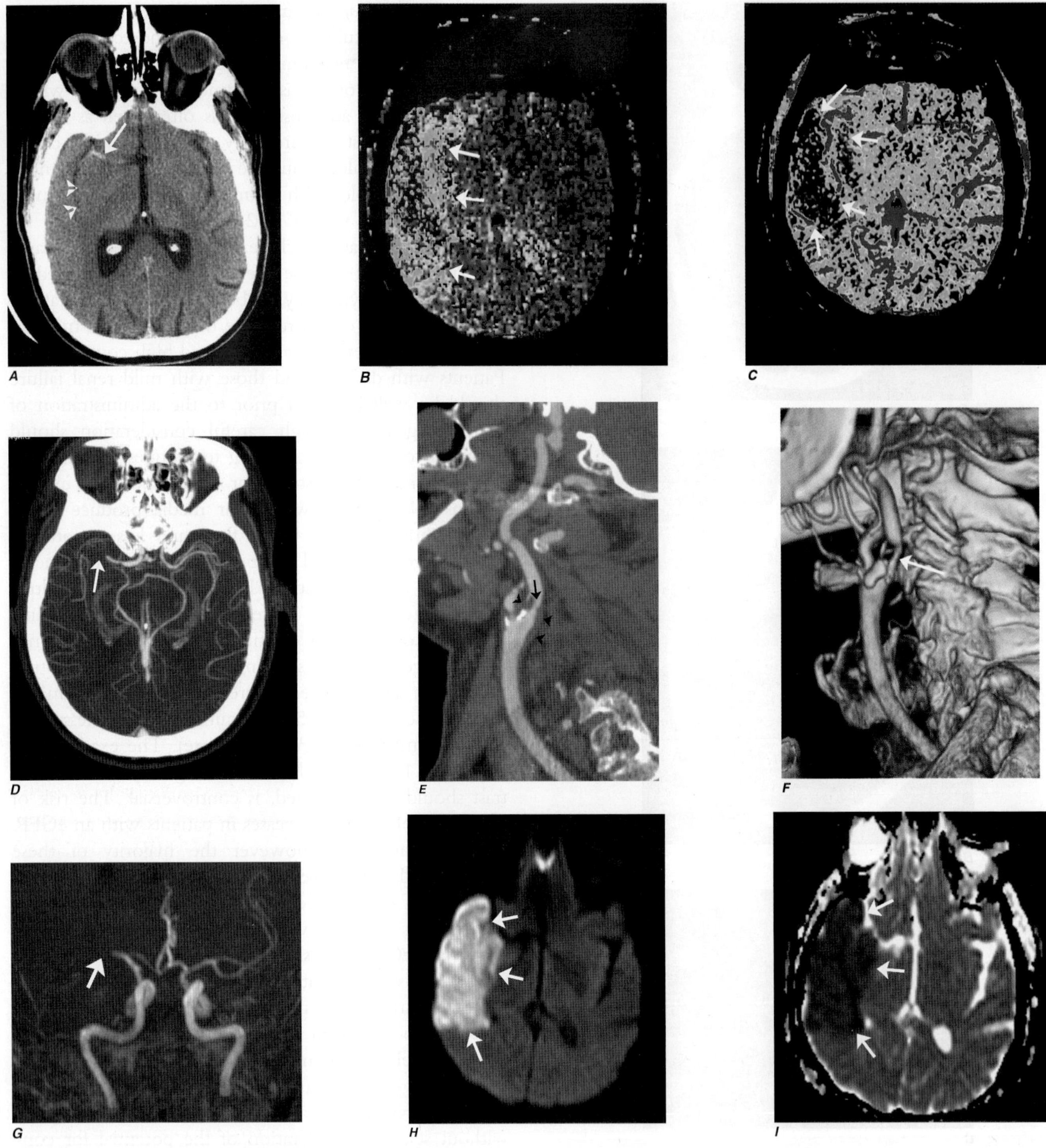

FIGURE 4-2

Acute left hemiparesis due to middle cerebral artery occlusion. *A.* Axial noncontrast CT scan demonstrates high density within the right middle cerebral artery (*arrow*) associated with subtle low density involving the right putamen (*arrowheads*). ***B.*** Mean transit time CT perfusion parametric map indicating prolonged mean transit time involving the right middle cerebral territory (*arrows*). ***C.*** Cerebral blood volume map shows reduced CBV involving an area within the defect shown in ***B***, indicating a high likelihood of infarction (*arrows*). ***D.*** Axial maximum-intensity projection from a CTA study through the circle of Willis demonstrates an abrupt occlusion of the proximal right middle cerebral artery (*arrow*). ***E.*** Sagittal reformation through the right internal carotid artery demonstrates a low-density lipid-laden plaque (*arrowheads*) narrowing the lumen (*black arrow*) ***F.*** 3D surface-rendered CTA image demonstrates calcification and narrowing of the right internal carotid artery (*arrow*), consistent with atherosclerotic disease. ***G.*** Coronal maximum-intensity projection from MRA shows right middle cerebral artery (MCA) occlusion (*arrow*). ***H*** and ***I.*** Axial diffusion-weighted image (***H***) and apparent diffusion coefficient image (***I***) document the presence of a right middle cerebral artery infarction.

TABLE 4-2

GUIDELINES FOR PREMEDICATION OF PATIENTS WITH PRIOR CONTRAST ALLERGY

12 h prior to examination:
Prednisone, 50 mg PO *or* methylprednisolone, 32 mg PO

2 h prior to examination:
Prednisone, 50 mg PO *or* methylprednisolone, 32 mg PO *and* Cimetidine, 300 mg PO *or* ranitidine, 150 mg PO

Immediately prior to examination:
Benadryl, 50 mg IV (alternatively, can be given PO 2 h prior to exam)

understood but is thought to include the release of mediators such as histamine, antibody-antigen reactions, and complement activation. Severe allergic reactions occur in ~0.04% of patients receiving nonionic media, sixfold lower than with ionic media. Risk factors include a history of prior contrast reaction, food allergies to shellfish, and atopy (asthma and hay fever). In such patients, a noncontrast CT or MRI procedure should be considered as an alternative to contrast administration. If iodinated contrast is absolutely required, a nonionic agent should be used in conjunction with pretreatment with glucocorticoids and antihistamines (Table 4-2). Patients with allergic reactions to iodinated contrast material do not usually react to gadolinium-based MR contrast material, although such reactions can occur. It would be wise to pretreat patients with a prior allergic history to MR contrast administration in a similar fashion.

MAGNETIC RESONANCE IMAGING

TECHNIQUE

MRI is a complex interaction between hydrogen protons in biologic tissues, a static magnetic field (the magnet), and energy in the form of radiofrequency (Rf) waves of a specific frequency introduced by coils placed next to the body part of interest. Images are made by computerized processing of resonance information received from protons in the body. Field strength of the magnet is directly related to signal-to-noise ratio. While 1.5-Telsa magnets have become the standard high-field MRI units, 3T–8T magnets are now available and have distinct advantages in the brain and musculoskeletal systems. Spatial localization is achieved by magnetic gradients surrounding the main magnet, which impart slight changes in magnetic field throughout the imaging volume. Rf pulses transiently excite the energy state of the hydrogen protons in the body. Rf is administered at a frequency specific for the field strength of the magnet. The subsequent return to equilibrium energy state (*relaxation*) of the hydrogen protons results in a release of Rf energy (the *echo*), which is detected by the coils that delivered the Rf pulses. The echo is transformed by Fourier analysis into the information used to form an MR image. The MR image thus consists of a map of the distribution of hydrogen protons, with signal intensity imparted by both density of hydrogen protons as well as differences in the relaxation times (see below) of hydrogen protons on different molecules. While clinical MRI currently makes use of the ubiquitous hydrogen proton, research into sodium and carbon imaging appears promising.

T1 and T2 relaxation times

The rate of return to equilibrium of perturbed protons is called the *relaxation rate*. The relaxation rate varies among normal and pathologic tissues. The relaxation rate of a hydrogen proton in a tissue is influenced by local interactions with surrounding molecules and atomic neighbors. Two relaxation rates, T1 and T2, influence the signal intensity of the image. The T1 relaxation time is the time, measured in milliseconds, for 63% of the hydrogen protons to return to their normal equilibrium state, while the T2 relaxation is the time for 63% of the protons to become dephased owing to interactions among nearby protons. The intensity of the signal within various tissues and image contrast can be modulated by altering acquisition parameters such as the interval between Rf pulses (TR) and the time between the Rf pulse and the signal reception (TE). So-called T1-weighted (T1W) images are produced by keeping the TR and TE relatively short. T2-weighted (T2W) images are produced by using longer TR and TE times. Fat and subacute hemorrhage have relatively shorter T1 relaxation rates and thus higher signal intensity than brain on T1W images. Structures containing more water such as CSF and edema, have long T1 and T2 relaxation rates, resulting in relatively lower signal intensity on T1W images and a higher signal intensity on T2W images (Table 4-3). Gray matter contains 10–15%

TABLE 4-3

SOME COMMON INTENSITIES ON T1- AND T2-WEIGHTED MRI SEQUENCES

			SIGNAL INTENSITY			
IMAGE	**TR**	**TE**	**CSF**	**FAT**	**BRAIN**	**EDEMA**
T1W	Short	Short	Low	High	Low	Low
T2W	Long	Long	High	Low	High	High
FLAIR (T2)	Long	Long	Low	Medium	High	High

Abbreviations: CSF, cerebrospinal fluid; TE, interval between Rf pulse and signal reception; TR, interval between radiofrequency (Rf) pulses; T1W and T2W, T1- and T2-weighted.

more water than white matter, which accounts for much of the intrinsic contrast between the two on MRI (Fig. 4-6B). T2W images are more sensitive than T1W images to edema, demyelination, infarction, and chronic hemorrhage, while T1W imaging is more sensitive to subacute hemorrhage and fat-containing structures.

Many different MR pulse sequences exist, and each can be obtained in various planes (Figs. 4-2, 4-3, 4-4). The selection of a proper protocol that will best answer a clinical question depends on an accurate clinical history and indication for the examination. Fluid-attenuated inversion recovery (FLAIR) is a useful pulse sequence that produces T2W images in which the normally high signal intensity of CSF is suppressed (Fig. 4-6*B*). FLAIR images are more than sensitive standard spin echo images for any water-containing lesions or edema. Susceptibility weighted imaging, such as gradient echo imaging, is most sensitive to magnetic susceptibility generated by blood, calcium, and air and is indicated in patients suspected of pathology that might result in microhemorrhages (Fig. 4-5C). MR images can be generated in any plane without changing the patient's position. Each sequence, however, must be obtained separately and takes 1–10 min on average to complete. Three-dimensional volumetric imaging is also possible with MRI, resulting in a 3D volume of data that can be reformatted in any orientation to highlight certain disease processes.

MR contrast material

The heavy-metal element gadolinium forms the basis of all currently approved intravenous MR contrast agents. Gadolinium is a paramagnetic substance, which means that it reduces the T1 and T2 relaxation times of nearby water protons, resulting in a high signal on T1W images and a low signal on T2W images (the latter requires a sufficient local concentration, usually in the form of an intravenous bolus). Unlike iodinated contrast agents, the effect of MR contrast agents depends on the presence of local hydrogen protons on which it must act to achieve the desired effect. Gadolinium is chelated to DTPA (diethylenetriaminepentaacetic acid), which allows safe renal excretion. Approximately 0.2 mL/kg body weight is administered intravenously; the cost is ~$60 per dose. Gadolinium-DTPA does not normally cross the intact BBB immediately but will enhance lesions lacking a BBB (Fig. 4-3*A*) and areas of the brain that normally are devoid of the BBB (pituitary, choroid plexus). However, gadolinium contrast has been noted to slowly cross an intact BBB if given over time and especially in the setting of reduced renal clearance. The agents are generally well tolerated; severe allergic reactions are rare but have been reported. The adverse reaction rate in patients with a prior history of atopy or asthma is 3.7%; however, the reaction rate

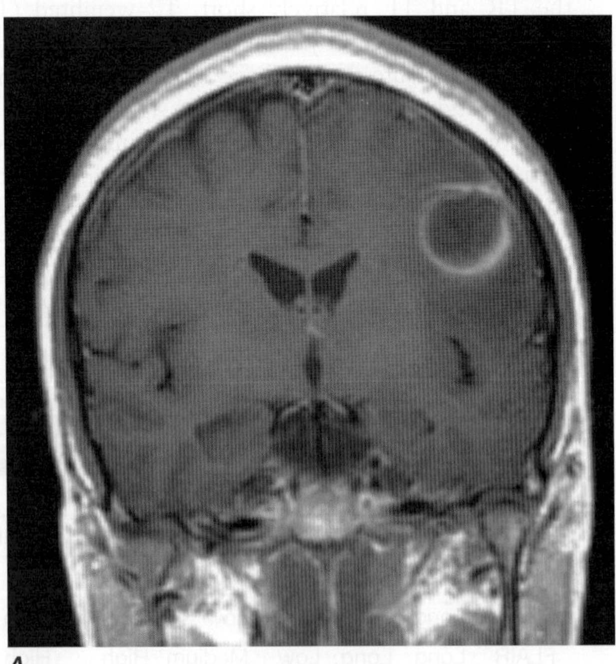

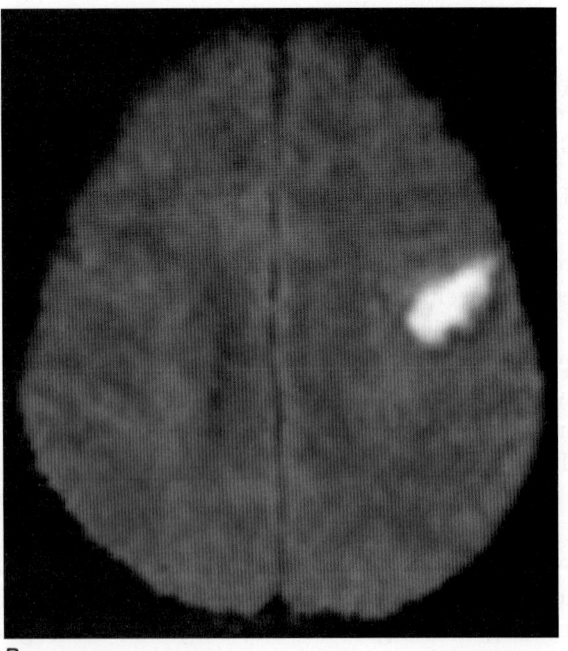

FIGURE 4-3
Cerebral abscess in a patient with fever and a right hemiparesis. *A.* Coronal postcontrast T1-weighted image demonstrates a ring enhancing mass in the left frontal lobe. ***B.*** Axial diffusion-weighted image demonstrates restricted diffusion (high signal intensity) within the lesion, which in this setting is highly suggestive of cerebral abscess.

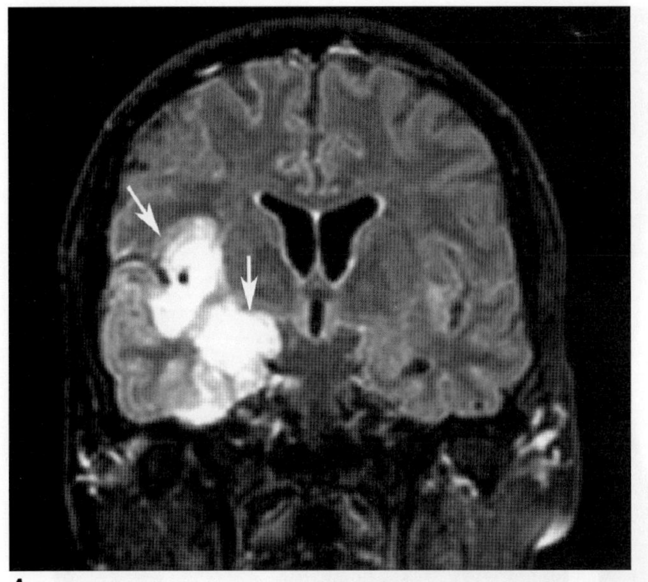

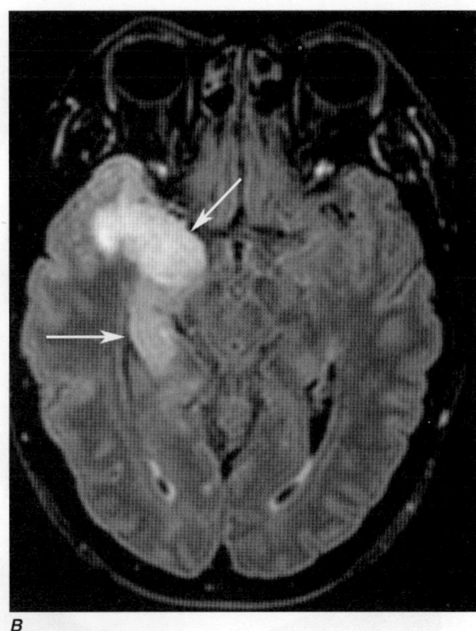

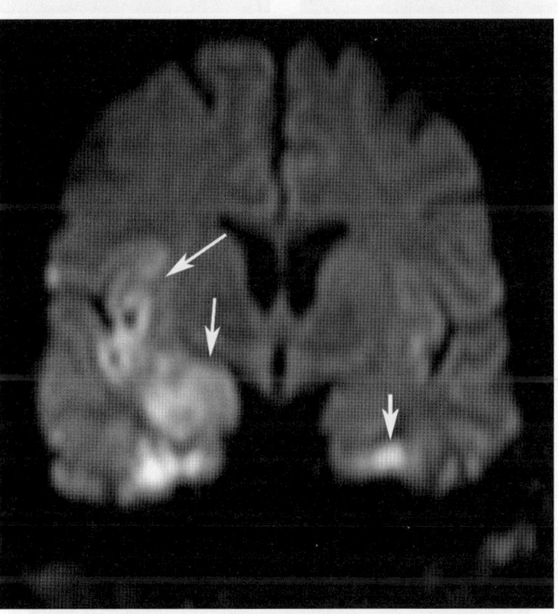

FIGURE 4-4

Herpes simplex encephalitis in a patient presenting with altered mental status and fever. ***A*** **and** ***B*****.** Coronal ***(A)*** and axial ***(B)*** T2-weighted FLAIR images demonstrate expansion and high signal intensity involving the right medial temporal lobe and insular cortex (*arrows*). ***C*****.** Coronal diffusion-weighted image demonstrates high signal intensity indicating restricted diffusion involving the right medial temporal lobe and hippocampus (*arrows*) as well as subtle involvement of the left inferior temporal lobe (*arrowhead*). This is most consistent with neuronal death and can be seen in acute infarction as well as encephalitis and other inflammatory conditions. The suspected diagnosis of herpes simplex encephalitis was confirmed by CSF PCR analysis.

increases to 6.3% in those patients with a prior history of unspecified allergic reaction to iodinated contrast agents. Gadolinium contrast material can be administered safely to children as well as adults, although these agents are generally avoided in those under 6 months of age. Renal failure does not occur.

A rare complication, nephrogenic systemic fibrosis (NSF), has recently been reported in patients with renal insufficiency who have been exposed to gadolinium contrast agents. The onset of NSF has been reported between 5 and 75 days following exposure; histologic features include thickened collagen bundles with surrounding clefts, mucin deposition, and increased numbers of fibrocytes and elastic fibers in skin. In addition to dermatologic symptoms, other manifestations include widespread fibrosis of the skeletal muscle, bone, lungs, pleura, pericardium, myocardium, kidney, muscle, bone, testes, and dura. For this reason, the American

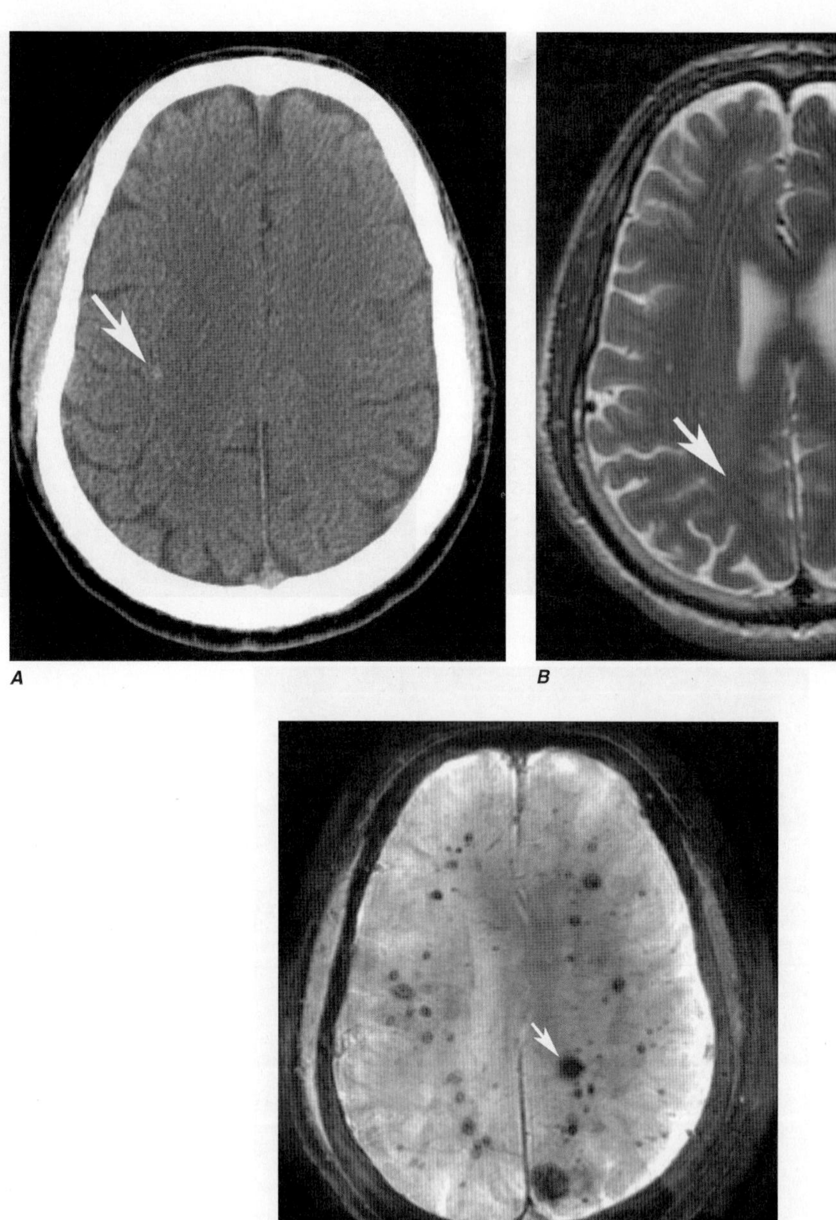

FIGURE 4-5

Susceptibility weighted imaging in a patient with familial cavernous malformations. *A.* Noncontrast CT scan shows one hyperdense lesion in the right hemisphere (*arrow*). ***B.*** T2-weighted fast spin echo image shows subtle low-intensity lesions (*arrows*). ***C.*** Susceptibility weighted image shows numerous low-intensity lesions consistent with hemosiderin-laden cavernous malformations (*arrow*).

College of Radiology recommends that prior to elective gadolinium-based MR contrast agent (GBMCA) administration, a recent (e.g., past 6 weeks) glomerular filtration rate (GFR) assessment be obtained in patients with a history of:

1. Renal disease (including solitary kidney, renal transplant, renal tumor)
2. Age >60 years
3. History of hypertension
4. History of diabetes
5. History of severe hepatic disease/liver transplant/pending liver transplant: for these patients it is recommended that the patient's GFR assessment be nearly contemporaneous with the MR examination.

The incidence of NSF in patients with severe renal dysfunction (GFR <30) varies from 0.19 to 4%. A recent meta-analysis reported an odds ratio of 26.7 (95% CI = 10.3–69.4) for development of NSF after gadolinium administration in patients with impaired renal function (GFR <30 mL/min/1.72 m). Thus, it is not

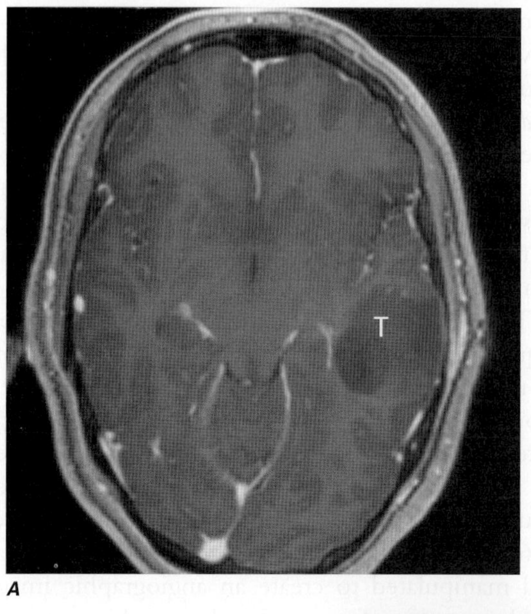

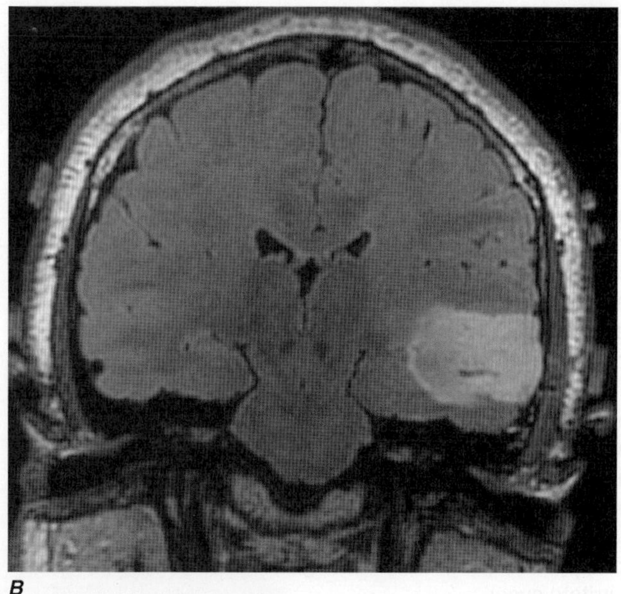

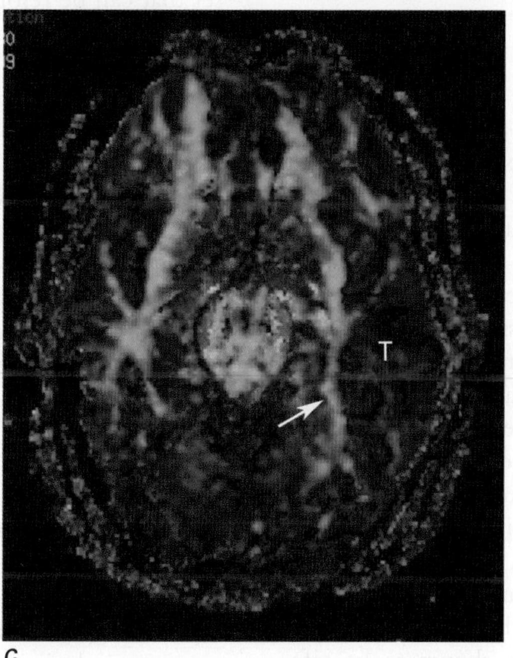

FIGURE 4-6

Diffusion tractography in cerebral glioma. *A.* An axial postcontrast T1-weighted image shows a nonenhancing glioma (T) of the left temporal lobe cortex lateral to the fibers of the internal capsule. ***B.*** Coronal T2 FLAIR image demonstrates high signal glioma in left temporal lobe. ***C.*** Axial diffusion fractional anisotropy image shows the position of the deep white matter fibers (*arrow*) relative to the enhancing tumor (T).

recommended to administer gadolinium to any patient with a GFR below 30. Caution is advised for patients with a GFR below 45.

COMPLICATIONS AND CONTRAINDICATIONS

From the patient's perspective, an MRI examination can be intimidating, and a higher level of cooperation is required than with CT. The patient lies on a table that is moved into a long, narrow gap within the magnet. Approximately 5% of the population experiences severe claustrophobia in the MR environment. This can be reduced by mild sedation but remains a problem for some. Unlike CT, movement of the patient during an MR sequence distorts all the images; therefore, uncooperative patients should either be sedated for the MR study or scanned with CT. Generally, children under the age of 10 years usually require conscious sedation

TABLE 4-4

COMMON CONTRAINDICATIONS TO MR IMAGING
Cardiac pacemaker or permanent pacemaker leads
Internal defibrillatory device
Cochlear prostheses
Bone growth stimulators
Spinal cord stimulators
Electronic infusion devices
Intracranial aneurysm clips (some but not all)
Ocular implants (some) or ocular metallic foreign body
McGee stapedectomy piston prosthesis
Duraphase penile implant
Swan-Ganz catheter
Magnetic stoma plugs
Magnetic dental implants
Magnetic sphincters
Ferromagnetic IVC filters, coils, stents—safe 6 weeks after implantation
Tattooed eyeliner (contains ferromagnetic material and may irritate eyes)

Note: See also *http://www.mrisafety.com.*

in order to complete the MR examination without motion degradation.

MRI is considered safe for patients, even at very high field strengths (>3–4 T). Serious injuries have been caused, however, by attraction of ferromagnetic objects into the magnet, which act as missiles if brought too close to the magnet. Likewise, ferromagnetic implants such as aneurysm clips, may torque within the magnet, causing damage to vessels and even death. Metallic foreign bodies in the eye have moved and caused intraocular hemorrhage; screening for ocular metallic fragments is indicated in those with a history of metal work or ocular metallic foreign bodies. Implanted cardiac pacemakers are generally a contraindication to MRI owing to the risk of induced arrhythmias; however, some newer pacemakers have been shown to be safe. All health care personnel and patients must be screened and educated thoroughly to prevent such disasters as the magnet is always "on." Table 4-4 lists common contraindications for MRI.

MAGNETIC RESONANCE ANGIOGRAPHY

MR angiography is a general term describing several MR techniques that result in vascular-weighted images. These provide a vascular flow map rather than the anatomic map shown by conventional angiography. On routine spin echo MR sequences, moving protons (e.g., flowing blood, CSF) exhibit complex MR signals that range from high- to low-signal intensity relative to background stationary tissue. Fast-flowing blood returns no signal (flow void) on routine T1W or T2W spin echo MR images. Slower-flowing blood, as occurs in veins or distal to arterial stenosis, may appear high in signal. However, using special pulse sequences called *gradient echo sequences*, it is possible to increase the signal intensity of moving protons in contrast to the low signal background intensity of stationary tissue. This creates angiography-like images, which can be manipulated in three dimensions to highlight vascular anatomy and relationships.

Time-of-flight (TOF) imaging, currently the technique used most frequently, relies on the suppression of nonmoving tissue to provide a low-intensity background for the high signal intensity of flowing blood entering the section; arterial or venous structures may be highlighted. A typical TOF angiography sequence results in a series of contiguous, thin MR sections (0.6–0.9 mm thick), which can be viewed as a stack and manipulated to create an angiographic image data set that can be reformatted and viewed in various planes and angles, much like that seen with conventional angiography (Fig. 4-2G).

Phase-contrast MRA has a longer acquisition time than TOF MRA, but in addition to providing anatomic information similar to that of TOF imaging, it can be used to reveal the velocity and direction of blood flow in a given vessel. Through the selection of different imaging parameters, differing blood velocities can be highlighted; selective venous and arterial MRA images can thus be obtained. One advantage of phase-contrast MRA is the excellent suppression of high-signal-intensity background structures.

MRA can also be acquired during infusion of contrast material. Advantages include faster imaging times (1–2 min vs. 10 min), fewer flow-related artifacts, and higher-resolution images. Recently, contrast-enhanced MRA has become the standard for extracranial vascular MRA. This technique entails rapid imaging using coronal three-dimensional TOF sequences during a bolus infusion of 15–20 mL of gadolinium-DTPA. Proper technique and timing of acquisition relative to bolus arrival are critical for success.

MRA has lower spatial resolution compared with conventional film-based angiography, and therefore the detection of small-vessel abnormalities, such as vasculitis and distal vasospasm, is problematic. MRA is also less sensitive to slowly flowing blood and thus may not reliably differentiate complete from near-complete occlusions. Motion, either by the patient or by anatomic structures, may distort the MRA images, creating artifacts. These limitations notwithstanding, MRA has proved useful in evaluation of the extracranial carotid and vertebral circulation as well as of larger-caliber intracranial arteries and dural sinuses. It has also proved useful in the noninvasive detection of intracranial aneurysms and vascular malformations.

ECHO-PLANAR MR IMAGING

Recent improvements in gradients, software, and high-speed computer processors now permit extremely rapid MRI of the brain. With echo-planar MRI (EPI), fast gradients are switched on and off at high speeds to create the information used to form an image. In routine spin echo imaging, images of the brain can be obtained in 5–10 min. With EPI, all of the information required for processing an image is accumulated in 50–150 ms, and the information for the entire brain is obtained in 1–2 min, depending on the degree of resolution required or desired. Fast MRI reduces patient and organ motion, permitting diffusion imaging and tractography (Figs. 4-2*H*, 4-3, 4-4*C*, 4-6; and see Fig. 27-16), perfusion imaging during contrast infusion, fMRI, and kinematic motion studies.

Perfusion and diffusion imaging are EPI techniques that are useful in early detection of ischemic injury of the brain and may be useful together to demonstrate infarcted tissue as well as ischemic but potentially viable tissue at risk of infarction (e.g., the ischemic penumbra). Diffusion-weighted imaging (DWI) assesses microscopic motion of water; restriction of motion appears as relative high-signal intensity on diffusion-weighted images. Infarcted tissue reduces the water motion within cells and in the interstitial tissues, resulting in high signal on DWI. DWI is the most sensitive technique for detection of acute cerebral infarction of <7 days' duration (Fig. 4-2*H*) and is also sensitive to encephalitis and abscess formation, which have reduced diffusion and result in high signal on diffusion-weighted images (Fig. 4-3*B*).

Perfusion MRI involves the acquisition of EPI images during a rapid intravenous bolus of gadolinium contrast material. Relative perfusion abnormalities can be identified on images of the relative cerebral blood volume, mean transit time, and cerebral blood flow. Delay in mean transit time and reduction in cerebral blood volume and cerebral blood flow are typical of infarction. In the setting of reduced blood flow, a prolonged mean transit time of contrast but normal or elevated cerebral blood volume may indicate tissue supplied by collateral flow that is at risk of infarction. Perfusion MRI imaging can also be used in the assessment of brain tumors to differentiate intraaxial primary tumors from extraaxial tumors or metastasis.

Diffusion tensor imaging (DTI) is a diffusion MRI technique that assesses the direction of microscopic motion of water along white matter tracts. This technique has great potential in the assessment of brain maturation as well as disease entities that undermine the integrity of the white matter architecture. It has proven valuable in preoperative assessment of subcortical white matter tract anatomy prior to brain tumor surgery (Fig. 4-6).

Functional MRI of the brain is an EPI technique that localizes regions of activity in the brain following task activation. Neuronal activity elicits a slight increase in the delivery of oxygenated blood flow to a specific region of activated brain. This results in an alteration in the balance of oxyhemoglobin and deoxyhemoglobin, which yields a 2–3% increase in signal intensity within veins and local capillaries. Further studies will determine whether these techniques are cost-effective or clinically useful, but currently preoperative somatosensory and auditory cortex localization is possible. This technique has proved useful to neuroscientists interested in interrogating the localization of certain brain functions.

MAGNETIC RESONANCE NEUROGRAPHY

MRN is a T2-weighted MR technique that shows promise in detecting increased signal in irritated, inflamed, or infiltrated peripheral nerves. Images are obtained with fat-suppressed fast spin echo imaging or short inversion recovery sequences. Irritated or infiltrated nerves will demonstrate high signal on T2W imaging. This is indicated in patients with radiculopathy whose conventional MR studies of the spine are normal, or in those suspected of peripheral nerve entrapment or trauma.

POSITRON EMISSION TOMOGRAPHY (PET)

PET relies on the detection of positrons emitted during the decay of a radionuclide that has been injected into a patient. The most frequently used moiety is 2-[^{18}F] fluoro-2-deoxy-D-glucose (FDG), which is an analogue of glucose and is taken up by cells competitively with 2-deoxyglucose. Multiple images of glucose uptake activity are formed after 45–60 min. Images reveal differences in regional glucose activity among normal and pathologic brain structures. A lower activity of FDG in the parietal lobes has been associated with Alzheimer's disease. FDG PET is used primarily for the detection of extracranial metastatic disease. Combination PET-CT scanners, in which both CT and PET are obtained at one sitting, are replacing PET scans alone for most clinical indications. Functional images superimposed on high-resolution CT scans result in more precise anatomic diagnoses.

MYELOGRAPHY

TECHNIQUE

Myelography involves the intrathecal instillation of specially formulated water-soluble iodinated contrast medium into the lumbar or cervical subarachnoid space.

CT scanning is usually performed after myelography (*CT myelography*) to better demonstrate the spinal cord and roots, which appear as filling defects in the opacified subarachnoid space. *Low-dose CT myelography*, in which CT is performed after the subarachnoid injection of a small amount of relatively dilute contrast material, has replaced conventional myelography for many indications, thereby reducing exposure to radiation and contrast media. Newer multidetector scanners now obtain CT studies quickly so that reformations in sagittal and coronal planes, equivalent to traditional myelography projections, are now routine.

INDICATIONS

Myelography has been largely replaced by CT myelography and MRI for diagnosis of diseases of the spinal canal and cord (Table 4-1). Remaining indications for conventional plain-film myelography include the evaluation of suspected meningeal or arachnoid cysts and the localization of spinal dural arteriovenous or CSF fistulas. Conventional myelography and CT myelography provide the most precise information in patients with prior spinal fusion and spinal fixation hardware.

CONTRAINDICATIONS

Myelography is relatively safe; however, it should be performed with caution in any patient with elevated intracranial pressure, evidence of a spinal block, or a history of allergic reaction to intrathecal contrast media. In patients with a suspected spinal block, MR is the preferred technique. If myelography is necessary, only a small amount of contrast medium should be instilled below the lesion in order to minimize the risk of neurologic deterioration. Lumbar puncture is to be avoided in patients with bleeding disorders, including patients receiving anticoagulant therapy, as well as in those with infections of the overlying soft tissues.

COMPLICATIONS

Headache, nausea, and vomiting are the most frequent complications of myelography and are reported to occur in up to 38% of patients. These symptoms result from either neurotoxic effects of the contrast agent, persistent leakage of CSF at the puncture site, or psychological reactions to the procedure. Vasovagal syncope may occur during lumbar puncture; it is accentuated by the upright position used during lumbar myelography. Adequate hydration before and after myelography will reduce the incidence of this complication. Postural headache (post–lumbar puncture headache) is generally due to leakage of CSF from the puncture site, resulting in CSF hypotension. Management of post–lumbar puncture headache is discussed in Chap. 8.

If significant headache persists for longer than 48 h, placement of an epidural blood patch should be considered. Hearing loss is a rare complication of myelography. It may result from a direct toxic effect of the contrast medium or from an alteration of the pressure equilibrium between CSF and perilymph in the inner ear. Puncture of the spinal cord is a rare but serious complication of cervical (C1–2) or high lumbar puncture. The risk of cord puncture is greatest in patients with spinal stenosis, Chiari malformations, or conditions that reduce CSF volume. In these settings, a low-dose lumbar injection followed by thin-section CT or MRI is a safer alternative to cervical puncture. Intrathecal contrast reactions are rare, but aseptic meningitis and encephalopathy may occur. The latter is usually dose related and associated with contrast entering the intracranial subarachnoid space. Seizures occur following myelography in 0.1–0.3% of patients. Risk factors include a preexisting seizure disorder and the use of a total iodine dose of >4500 mg. Other reported complications include hyperthermia, hallucinations, depression, and anxiety states. These side effects have been reduced by the development of nonionic, water-soluble contrast agents as well as by head elevation and generous hydration following myelography.

SPINE INTERVENTIONS

DISKOGRAPHY

The evaluation of back pain and radiculopathy may require diagnostic procedures that attempt either to reproduce the patient's pain or relieve it, indicating its correct source prior to lumbar fusion. Diskography is performed by fluoroscopic placement of a 22- to 25-gauge needle into the intervertebral disk and subsequent injection of 1–3 mL of contrast media. The intradiskal pressure is recorded, as is an assessment of the patient's response to the injection of contrast material. Typically little or no pain is felt during injection of a normal disk, which does not accept much more than 1 mL of contrast material, even at pressures as high as 415–690 kPa (60–100 lb/in^2). CT and plain films are obtained following the procedure. Concerns have been raised that diskography may contribute to an accelerated rate of disk degeneration.

SELECTIVE NERVE ROOT AND EPIDURAL SPINAL INJECTIONS

Percutaneous selective nerve root and epidural blocks with glucocorticoid and anesthetic mixtures may be both therapeutic as well as diagnostic, especially if a patient's pain is relieved. Typically, 1–2 mL of an equal mixture of a long-acting glucocorticoid such as betamethasone and a long-acting anesthetic such as bupivacaine 0.75% is instilled under CT or fluoroscopic guidance in the intraspinal epidural space or adjacent to an existing nerve root.

ANGIOGRAPHY

Catheter angiography is indicated for evaluating intracranial small-vessel pathology (such as vasculitis), for assessing vascular malformations and aneurysms, and in endovascular therapeutic procedures (Table 4-1). Angiography has been replaced for many indications by CT/CTA or MRI/MRA.

Angiography carries the greatest risk of morbidity of all diagnostic imaging procedures, owing to the necessity of inserting a catheter into a blood vessel, directing the catheter to the required location, injecting contrast material to visualize the vessel, and removing the catheter while maintaining hemostasis. Therapeutic transcatheter procedures (see below) have become important options for the treatment of some cerebrovascular diseases. The decision to undertake a diagnostic or therapeutic angiographic procedure requires careful assessment of the goals of the investigation and its attendant risks.

To improve tolerance to contrast agents, patients undergoing angiography should be well hydrated before and after the procedure. Since the femoral route is used most commonly, the femoral artery must be compressed after the procedure to prevent a hematoma from developing. The puncture site and distal pulses should be evaluated carefully after the procedure; complications can include thigh hematoma or lower extremity emboli.

COMPLICATIONS

A common femoral arterial puncture provides retrograde access via the aorta to the aortic arch and great vessels. The most feared complication of cerebral angiography is stroke. Thrombus can form on or inside the tip of the catheter, and atherosclerotic thrombus or plaque can be dislodged by the catheter or guidewire or by the force of injection and can embolize distally in the cerebral circulation. Risk factors for ischemic complications include limited experience on the part of the angiographer, atherosclerosis, vasospasm, low cardiac output, decreased oxygen-carrying capacity, advanced age, and prior history of migraine. The risk of a neurologic complication varies but is ~4% for transient ischemic attack and stroke, 1% for permanent deficit, and <0.1% for death.

Ionic contrast material injected into the cerebral vasculature can be neurotoxic if the BBB is breached, either by an underlying disease or by the injection of hyperosmolar contrast agent. Ionic contrast media are less well tolerated than nonionic media, probably because they can induce changes in cell membrane electrical potentials. Patients with dolichoectasia of the basilar artery can suffer reversible brainstem dysfunction and acute short-term memory loss during angiography, owing to the slow percolation of the contrast material and the consequent prolonged exposure of the brain. Rarely, an intracranial aneurysm ruptures during an angiographic contrast injection, causing subarachnoid hemorrhage, perhaps as a result of injection under high pressure.

SPINAL ANGIOGRAPHY

Spinal angiography may be indicated to evaluate vascular malformations and tumors and to identify the artery of Adamkiewicz (Chap. 35) prior to aortic aneurysm repair. The procedure is lengthy and requires the use of relatively large volumes of contrast; the incidence of serious complications, including paraparesis, subjective visual blurring, and altered speech, is ~2%. Gadolinium-enhanced MRA has been used successfully in this setting, as has iodinated contrast CTA, which has promise for replacing diagnostic spinal angiography for some indications.

INTERVENTIONAL NEURORADIOLOGY

This rapidly developing field is providing new therapeutic options for patients with challenging neurovascular problems. Available procedures include detachable coil therapy for aneurysms, particulate or liquid adhesive embolization of arteriovenous malformations, balloon angioplasty and stenting of arterial stenosis or vasospasm, transarterial or transvenous embolization of dural arteriovenous fistulas, balloon occlusion of carotid-cavernous and vertebral fistulas, endovascular treatment of vein-of-Galen malformations, preoperative embolization of tumors, and thrombolysis of acute arterial or venous thrombosis. Many of these disorders place the patient at high risk of cerebral hemorrhage, stroke, or death.

The highest complication rates are found with the therapies designed to treat the highest-risk diseases. The advent of electrolytically detachable coils has ushered in a new era in the treatment of cerebral aneurysms. One randomized trial found a 28% reduction of morbidity and mortality at 1 year among those treated for anterior circulation aneurysm with detachable coils compared with neurosurgical clipping. It remains to be determined what the role of coils will be relative to surgical options, but in many centers, coiling has become standard therapy for many aneurysms.

CHAPTER 5

ELECTRODIAGNOSTIC STUDIES OF NERVOUS SYSTEM DISORDERS: EEG, EVOKED POTENTIALS, AND EMG

Michael J. Aminoff

ELECTROENCEPHALOGRAPHY

The electrical activity of the brain (the electroencephalogram [EEG]) is easily recorded from electrodes placed on the scalp. The potential difference between pairs of electrodes on the scalp (bipolar derivation) or between individual scalp electrodes and a relatively inactive common reference point (referential derivation) is amplified and displayed on a computer monitor, oscilloscope, or paper. The characteristics of the normal EEG depend on the patient's age and level of arousal. The rhythmic activity normally recorded represents the postsynaptic potentials of vertically oriented pyramidal cells of the cerebral cortex and is characterized by its frequency. In normal awake adults lying quietly with the eyes closed, an 8- to 13-Hz alpha rhythm is seen posteriorly in the EEG, intermixed with a variable amount of generalized faster (beta) activity (>13 Hz); the alpha rhythm is attenuated when the eyes are opened (Fig. 5-1). During drowsiness, the alpha rhythm is also attenuated; with light sleep, slower activity in the theta (4–7 Hz) and delta (<4 Hz) ranges becomes more conspicuous.

Digital systems are now widely used for recording the EEG. They allow the EEG to be reconstructed and displayed with any desired format and manipulated for more detailed analysis, and also permit computerized techniques to be used to detect certain abnormalities. Activating procedures are generally undertaken while the EEG is recorded in an attempt to provoke abnormalities. Such procedures commonly include hyperventilation (for 3 or 4 min), photic stimulation, sleep, and sleep deprivation on the night prior to the recording.

Electroencephalography is relatively inexpensive and may aid clinical management in several different contexts.

THE EEG AND EPILEPSY

The EEG is most useful in evaluating patients with suspected epilepsy. The presence of electrographic seizure activity—i.e., of abnormal, repetitive, rhythmic activity having an abrupt onset and termination and a characteristic evolution—clearly establishes the diagnosis. The absence of such electrocerebral accompaniment does not exclude a seizure disorder, however, because there may be no change in the scalp-recorded EEG during certain focal seizures. With generalized tonic-clonic seizures, the EEG is always abnormal during the episode. It is often not possible to obtain an EEG during clinical events that may represent seizures, especially when such events occur unpredictably or infrequently. Continuous monitoring for prolonged periods in video-EEG telemetry units has made it easier to capture the electrocerebral accompaniments of such clinical episodes. Monitoring by these means is sometimes helpful in confirming that seizures are occurring, characterizing the nature of clinically equivocal episodes, and determining the frequency of epileptic events.

The EEG findings may also be helpful in the interictal period by showing certain abnormalities that are strongly supportive of a diagnosis of epilepsy. Such *epileptiform activity* consists of bursts of abnormal discharges containing spikes or sharp waves. The presence of epileptiform activity is not specific for epilepsy, but it has a much greater prevalence in epileptic patients than in normal individuals. However, even in an individual who is known to have epilepsy, the initial routine interictal EEG may be normal up to 60% of the time. Thus, the EEG cannot establish the diagnosis of epilepsy in many cases.

The EEG findings have been used in classifying seizure disorders and selecting appropriate anticonvulsant

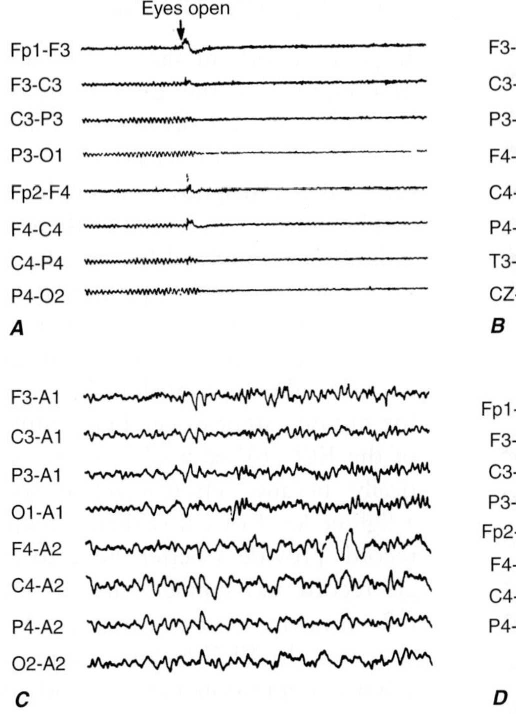

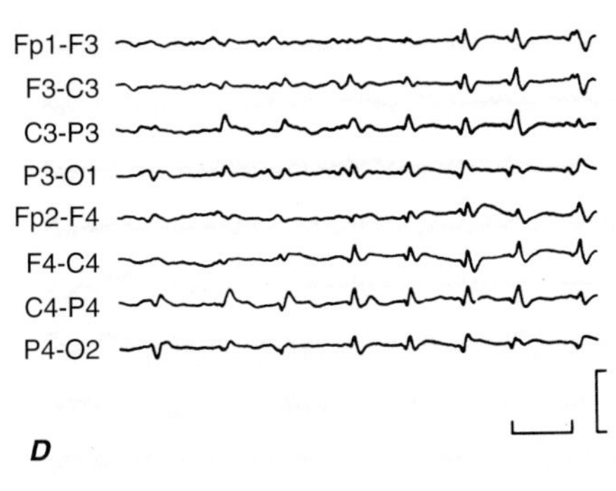

FIGURE 5-1

A. Normal EEG showing a posteriorly situated 9-Hz alpha rhythm that attenuates with eye opening. ***B.*** Abnormal EEG showing irregular diffuse slow activity in an obtunded patient with encephalitis. ***C.*** Irregular slow activity in the right central region, on a diffusely slowed background, in a patient with a right parietal glioma. ***D.*** Periodic complexes occurring once every second in a patient with Creutzfeldt-Jakob disease. Horizontal calibration: 1 s; vertical calibration: 200 μV in A, 300 μV in other panels. (*From MJ Aminoff, ed: Electrodiagnosis in Clinical Neurology, 5th ed. New York, Churchill Livingstone, 2005.*) In this and the following figure, electrode placements are indicated at the left of each panel and accord with the international 10:20 system. A, earlobe; C, central; F, frontal; Fp, frontal polar; P, parietal; T, temporal; O, occipital. Right-sided placements are indicated by even numbers, left-sided placements by odd numbers, and midline placements by Z.

medication for individual patients (Fig. 5-2). The episodic generalized spike-wave activity that occurs during and between seizures in patients with typical absence epilepsy contrasts with focal interictal epileptiform discharges or ictal patterns found in patients with focal seizures. These latter seizures may have no correlates in the scalp-recorded EEG or may be associated with abnormal rhythmic activity of variable frequency, a localized or generalized distribution, and a stereotyped pattern that varies with the patient. Focal or lateralized epileptogenic lesions are important to recognize, especially if surgical treatment is contemplated. Intensive long-term monitoring of clinical behavior and the EEG is required for operative candidates, however, and this generally also involves recording from intracranially placed electrodes (which may be subdural, extradural, or intracerebral in location).

The findings in the routine scalp-recorded EEG may indicate the prognosis of seizure disorders: In general, a normal EEG implies a better prognosis than otherwise, whereas an abnormal background or profuse epileptiform activity suggests a poor outlook. The EEG findings are not helpful in determining which patients with head injuries, stroke, or brain tumors will go on to develop seizures, because in such circumstances epileptiform activity is commonly encountered regardless of whether seizures occur. The EEG findings are sometimes used to determine whether anticonvulsant medication can be discontinued in epileptic patients who have been seizure-free for several years, but the findings provide only a general guide to prognosis. Further seizures may occur after withdrawal of anticonvulsant medication despite a normal EEG or, conversely, may not occur despite a continuing EEG abnormality. The decision to discontinue anticonvulsant medication is made on clinical grounds, and the EEG does not have a useful role in this context except for providing guidance when there is clinical ambiguity or the patient requires reassurance about a particular course of action.

The EEG has no role in the management of tonic-clonic status epilepticus except when there is clinical uncertainty whether seizures are continuing in a comatose patient. In patients treated by pentobarbital-induced coma for refractory status epilepticus, the EEG findings are useful in indicating the level of anesthesia and whether seizures are occurring. During status epilepticus, the EEG shows repeated electrographic seizures or continuous spike-wave discharges. In nonconvulsive status

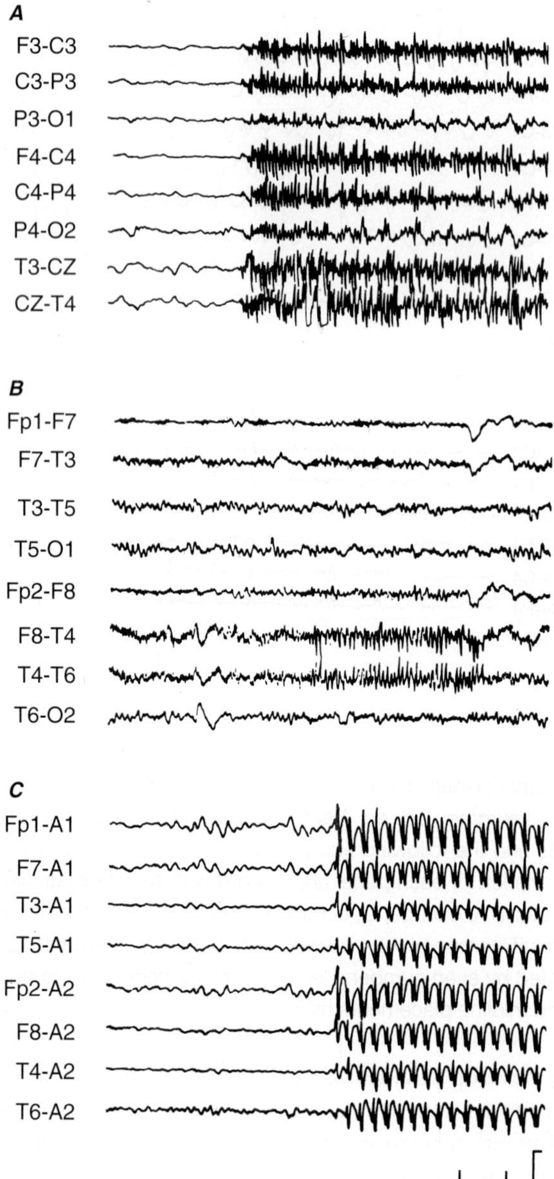

FIGURE 5-2

Electrographic seizures. *A.* Onset of a tonic seizure showing generalized repetitive sharp activity with synchronous onset over both hemispheres. ***B.*** Burst of repetitive spikes occurring with sudden onset in the right temporal region during a clinical spell characterized by transient impairment of external awareness. ***C.*** Generalized 3-Hz spike-wave activity occurring synchronously over both hemispheres during an absence (petit mal) attack. Horizontal calibration: 1 s; vertical calibration: 400 mV in ***A,*** 200 mV in ***B,*** and 750 mV in ***C.*** *(From MJ Aminoff, ed: Electrodiagnosis in Clinical Neurology, 5th ed. New York, Churchill Livingstone, 2005.)*

epilepticus, a disorder that may not be recognized unless an EEG is performed, the EEG may also show continuous spike-wave activity ("spike-wave stupor") or, less commonly, repetitive electrographic seizures (focal status epilepticus).

THE EEG AND COMA

In patients with an altered mental state or some degree of obtundation, the EEG tends to become slower as consciousness is depressed, regardless of the underlying cause (Fig. 5-1). Other findings may also be present and may suggest diagnostic possibilities, as when electrographic seizures are found or there is a focal abnormality indicating a structural lesion. The EEG generally slows in metabolic encephalopathies, and triphasic waves may be present. The findings do not permit differentiation of the underlying metabolic disturbance but help to exclude other encephalopathic processes by indicating the diffuse extent of cerebral dysfunction. The response of the EEG to external stimulation is helpful prognostically because electrocerebral responsiveness implies a lighter level of coma than a nonreactive EEG. Serial records provide a better guide to prognosis than a single record and supplement the clinical examination in following the course of events. As the depth of coma increases, the EEG becomes nonreactive and may show a burst-suppression pattern, with bursts of mixed-frequency activity separated by intervals of relative cerebral inactivity. In other instances there is a reduction in amplitude of the EEG until eventually activity cannot be detected. Such electrocerebral silence does not necessarily reflect irreversible brain damage, because it may occur in hypothermic patients or with drug overdose. The prognosis of electrocerebral silence, when recorded using an adequate technique, depends upon the clinical context in which it is found. In patients with severe cerebral anoxia, for example, electrocerebral silence in a technically satisfactory record implies that useful cognitive recovery will not occur.

In patients with clinically suspected brain death, an EEG, when recorded using appropriate technical standards, may be confirmatory by showing electrocerebral silence. However, complicating disorders that may produce a similar but reversible EEG appearance (e.g., hypothermia or drug intoxication) must be excluded. The presence of residual EEG activity in suspected brain death fails to confirm the diagnosis but does not exclude it. The EEG is usually normal in patients with locked-in syndrome and helps in distinguishing this disorder from the comatose state with which it is sometimes confused clinically.

THE EEG IN OTHER NEUROLOGIC DISORDERS

In the developed countries, CT scanning and MRI have taken the place of EEG as a noninvasive means of screening for focal structural abnormalities of the brain, such as tumors, infarcts, or hematomas (Fig. 5-1). Nonetheless, the EEG is still used for this purpose in many parts of the world, although infratentorial or slowly expanding lesions may fail to cause any abnormalities. Focal slow-wave disturbances, a localized loss of electrocerebral activity, or more generalized electrocerebral disturbances are common findings but provide no reliable indication about the nature of the underlying pathology.

In patients with an acute encephalopathy, focal or lateralized periodic slow-wave complexes, sometimes with a sharpened outline, suggest a diagnosis of herpes simplex encephalitis, and periodic lateralizing epileptiform discharges (PLEDs) are commonly found with acute hemispheric pathology such as a hematoma, abscess, or rapidly expanding tumor. The EEG findings in dementia are usually nonspecific and do not distinguish between the different causes of cognitive decline except in rare instances when, for example, the presence of complexes occurring with a regular repetition rate (so-called periodic complexes) supports a diagnosis of Creutzfeldt-Jakob disease (Fig. 5-1) or subacute sclerosing panencephalitis. In most patients with dementias, the EEG is normal or diffusely slowed, and the EEG findings alone cannot indicate whether a patient is demented or distinguish between dementia and pseudodementia.

CONTINUOUS EEG MONITORING

The brief EEG obtained routinely in the laboratory often fails to reveal abnormalities that are transient and infrequent. Continuous monitoring over 12 or 24 h or longer may detect abnormalities or capture clinical events that would otherwise be missed. The EEG is often recorded continuously in critically ill patients to detect early changes in neurologic status, which is particularly useful when the clinical examination is limited. Continuous EEG recording in this context has been used to detect acute events such as nonconvulsive seizures or developing cerebral ischemia, to monitor cerebral function in patients with metabolic disorders such as liver failure, and to manage the level of anesthesia in pharmacologically induced coma.

MAGNETOENCEPHALOGRAPHY AND MAGNETIC SOURCE IMAGING

Recording the magnetic field of the electrical activity of the brain (magnetoencephalography [MEG]) provides a means of examining cerebral activity that is less subject to distortion by other biologic tissues than the EEG. MEG is used in only a few specialized centers because of the complexity and expense of the necessary equipment. It permits the source of activity to be localized and coregistered with the MRI in a technique that is known as *magnetic source imaging*. In patients with focal epilepsy, MEG is useful in localizing epileptogenic foci for surgery and for guiding the placement of intracranial electrodes for electrophysiologic monitoring. MEG has also been used for mapping brain tumors, identifying the central fissure preoperatively, and localizing functionally eloquent cortical areas such as those concerned with language.

EVOKED POTENTIALS

SENSORY EVOKED POTENTIALS

The noninvasive recording of spinal or cerebral potentials elicited by stimulation of specific afferent pathways is an important means of monitoring the functional integrity of these pathways but does not indicate the pathologic basis of lesions involving them. Such evoked potentials (EPs) are so small compared to the background EEG activity that the responses to a number of stimuli have to be recorded and averaged with a computer in order to permit their recognition and definition. The background EEG activity, which has no fixed temporal relationship to the stimulus, is averaged out by this procedure.

Visual evoked potentials (VEPs) are elicited by monocular stimulation with a reversing checkerboard pattern and are recorded from the occipital region in the midline and on either side of the scalp. The component of major clinical importance is the so-called P100 response, a positive peak having a latency of approximately 100 ms. Its presence, latency, and symmetry over the two sides of the scalp are noted. Amplitude may also be measured, but changes in size are much less helpful for the recognition of pathology. VEPs are most useful in detecting dysfunction of the visual pathways anterior to the optic chiasm. In patients with acute severe optic neuritis, the P100 is frequently lost or grossly attenuated; as clinical recovery occurs and visual acuity improves, the P100 is restored but with an increased latency that generally remains abnormally prolonged indefinitely. The VEP findings are therefore helpful in indicating previous or subclinical optic neuritis. They may also be abnormal with ocular abnormalities and with other causes of optic nerve disease, such as ischemia or compression by a tumor. Normal VEPs may be elicited by flash stimuli in patients with cortical blindness. Routine VEPs record a mass response over a relatively large cortical area and thus may be insensitive to localized waveform abnormalities. A newer technique, *multifocal VEP*, measures responses from 120 individual sectors within each affected eye, and thus is likely to be more sensitive than routine VEP.

Brainstem auditory evoked potentials (BAEPs) are elicited by monaural stimulation with repetitive clicks and are recorded between the vertex of the scalp and the mastoid process or earlobe. A series of potentials, designated by roman numerals, occurs in the first 10 ms after the stimulus and represents in part the sequential activation of different structures in the pathway between the auditory nerve (wave I) and the inferior colliculus (wave V) in the midbrain. The presence, latency, and interpeak latency of the first five positive potentials recorded at the vertex are evaluated. The findings are helpful in screening for acoustic neuromas, detecting brainstem pathology, and evaluating comatose patients. The BAEPs are normal in coma due to metabolic/toxic disorders or bihemispheric disease but abnormal in the presence of brainstem pathology.

Somatosensory evoked potentials (SSEPs) are recorded over the scalp and spine in response to electrical stimulation of a peripheral (mixed or cutaneous) nerve. The configuration, polarity, and latency of the responses depend on the nerve that is stimulated and on the recording arrangements. SSEPs are used to evaluate proximal (otherwise inaccessible) portions of the peripheral nervous system and the integrity of the central somatosensory pathways.

Clinical utility of EPs

EP studies may detect and localize lesions in afferent pathways in the central nervous system (CNS). They have been used particularly to investigate patients with suspected multiple sclerosis (MS), the diagnosis of which requires the recognition of lesions involving several different regions of the central white matter. In patients with clinical evidence of only one lesion, the electrophysiologic recognition of abnormalities in other sites helps to suggest or support the diagnosis but does not establish it unequivocally. Multimodality EP abnormalities are not specific for MS; they may occur in AIDS, Lyme disease, systemic lupus erythematosus, neurosyphilis, spinocerebellar degenerations, familial spastic paraplegia, and deficiency of vitamin E or B_{12}, among other disorders. The diagnostic utility of the electrophysiologic findings therefore depends on the circumstances in which they are found. Abnormalities may aid in the localization of lesions to broad areas of the CNS, but attempts at precise localization on electrophysiologic grounds are misleading because the generators of many components of the EP are unknown.

The EP findings are sometimes of prognostic relevance. Bilateral loss of SSEP components that are generated in the cerebral cortex implies that cognition may not be regained in posttraumatic or postanoxic coma, and EP studies may also be useful in evaluating patients with suspected brain death. In patients who are comatose for uncertain reasons, preserved BAEPs suggest either a metabolic-toxic etiology or bihemispheric disease. In patients with spinal cord injuries, SSEPs have been used to indicate the completeness of the lesion. The presence or early return of a cortically generated response to stimulation of a nerve below the injured segment of the cord indicates an incomplete lesion and thus a better prognosis for functional recovery than otherwise. In surgery, intraoperative EP monitoring of neural structures placed at risk by the procedure may permit the early recognition of dysfunction and thereby permit a neurologic complication to be averted or minimized.

Visual and auditory acuity may be determined using EP techniques in patients whose age or mental state precludes traditional ophthalmologic or audiologic examinations.

COGNITIVE EVOKED POTENTIALS

Certain EP components depend on the mental attention of the subject and the setting in which the stimulus occurs, rather than simply on the physical characteristics of the stimulus. Such "event-related" potentials (ERPs) or "endogenous" potentials are related in some manner to the cognitive aspects of distinguishing an infrequently occurring target stimulus from other stimuli occurring more frequently. For clinical purposes, attention has been directed particularly at the so-called P3 component of the ERP, which is also designated the P300 component because of its positive polarity and latency of approximately 300–400 ms after onset of an auditory target stimulus. The P3 component is prolonged in latency in many patients with dementia, whereas it is generally normal in patients with depression or other psychiatric disorders that might be mistaken for dementia. ERPs are, therefore, sometimes helpful in making this distinction when there is clinical uncertainty, although a response of normal latency does not exclude dementia.

MOTOR EVOKED POTENTIALS

The electrical potentials recorded from muscle or the spinal cord following stimulation of the motor cortex or central motor pathways are referred to as *motor evoked potentials*. For clinical purposes such responses are recorded most often as the compound muscle action potentials elicited by transcutaneous magnetic stimulation of the motor cortex. A strong but brief magnetic field is produced by passing a current through a coil, and this induces stimulating currents in the subjacent neural tissue. The procedure is painless and apparently safe. Abnormalities have been described in several neurologic disorders with clinical or subclinical involvement of central motor pathways, including MS and motor neuron disease. In addition to a possible role in the diagnosis of neurologic disorders or in evaluating the extent of pathologic involvement, the technique provides information of prognostic relevance (e.g., in suggesting the likelihood of recovery of motor function after stroke) and provides a means of monitoring intraoperatively the functional integrity of central motor tracts. Nevertheless, it is not used widely for clinical purposes.

ELECTROPHYSIOLOGIC STUDIES OF MUSCLE AND NERVE

The motor unit is the basic element subserving motor function. It is defined as an anterior horn cell, its axon and neuromuscular junctions, and all the muscle fibers innervated by the axon. The number of motor units in a muscle ranges from approximately 10 in the extraocular muscles to several thousand in the large muscles of the legs. There is considerable variation in the average number of muscle fibers within the motor units of an individual muscle, i.e., in the innervation ratio of different muscles. Thus the innervation ratio is <25 in the human external rectus or platysma muscle and between 1600 and 1700 in the medial head of the gastrocnemius muscle. The muscle fibers of individual motor units are divided into two general types by distinctive contractile properties, histochemical stains, and characteristic responses to fatigue. Within each motor unit, all of the muscle fibers are of the same type.

ELECTROMYOGRAPHY

The pattern of electrical activity in muscle (i.e., the electromyogram [EMG]), both at rest and during activity, may be recorded from a needle electrode inserted into the muscle. The nature and pattern of abnormalities relate to disorders at different levels of the motor unit.

Relaxed muscle normally is electrically silent except in the end plate region, but abnormal spontaneous activity (Fig. 5-3) occurs in various neuromuscular disorders, especially those associated with denervation or inflammatory changes in affected muscle. Fibrillation potentials and positive sharp waves (which reflect muscle fiber irritability) and complex repetitive discharges are most often—but not always—found in denervated muscle and may also occur after muscle injury and in certain myopathic disorders, especially inflammatory disorders such as polymyositis. After an acute neuropathic lesion, they are found earlier in proximal rather than distal muscles and sometimes do not develop distally in the extremities for 4–6 weeks; once present, they may persist indefinitely unless reinnervation occurs or the muscle degenerates so completely that no viable tissue remains. Fasciculation potentials (which reflect

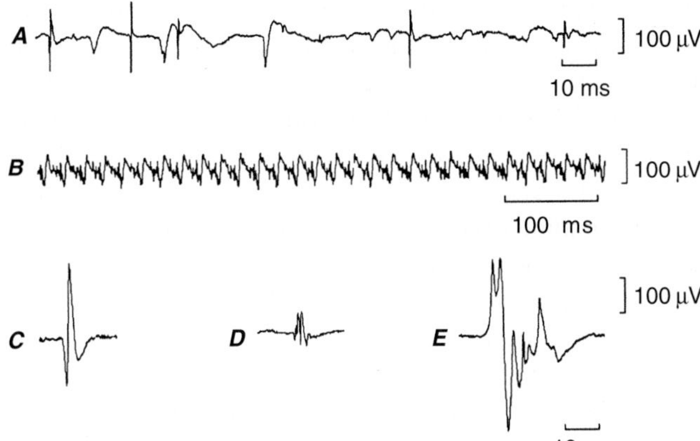

FIGURE 5-3

Activity recorded during EMG. *A.* Spontaneous fibrillation potentials and positive sharp waves. ***B.*** Complex repetitive discharges recorded in partially denervated muscle at rest. ***C.*** Normal triphasic motor unit action potential. ***D.*** Small, short-duration, polyphasic motor unit action potential such as is commonly encountered in myopathic disorders. ***E.*** Long-duration polyphasic motor unit action potential such as may be seen in neuropathic disorders.

the spontaneous activity of individual motor units) are characteristic of slowly progressive neuropathic disorders, especially those with degeneration of anterior horn cells (such as amyotrophic lateral sclerosis). Myotonic discharges—high-frequency discharges of potentials derived from single muscle fibers that wax and wane in amplitude and frequency—are the signature of myotonic disorders such as myotonic dystrophy or myotonia congenita but occur occasionally in polymyositis or other, rarer, disorders.

Slight voluntary contraction of a muscle leads to activation of a small number of motor units. The potentials generated by any muscle fibers of these units that are within the pickup range of the needle electrode will be recorded (Fig. 5-3). The parameters of normal motor unit action potentials depend on the muscle under study and age of the patient, but their duration is normally between 5 and 15 ms, amplitude is between 200 µV and 2 mV, and most are bi- or triphasic. The number of units activated depends on the degree of voluntary activity. An increase in muscle contraction is associated with an increase in the number of motor units that are activated (recruited) and in the frequency with which they discharge. With a full contraction, so many motor units are normally activated that individual motor unit action potentials can no longer be distinguished, and a complete interference pattern is said to have been produced.

The incidence of small, short-duration, polyphasic motor unit action potentials (i.e., having more than four phases) is usually increased in myopathic muscle, and an excessive number of units is activated for a specified degree of voluntary activity. By contrast, the loss of motor units that occurs in neuropathic disorders leads to a reduction in number of units activated during a maximal contraction and an increase in their firing rate, i.e., there is an incomplete or reduced interference pattern. The configuration and dimensions of the potentials may also be abnormal, depending on the duration of the neuropathic process and on whether reinnervation has occurred. The surviving motor units are initially normal in configuration but, as reinnervation occurs, they increase in amplitude and duration and become polyphasic (Fig. 5-3).

Action potentials from the same motor unit sometimes fire with a consistent temporal relationship to each other, so that double, triple, or multiple discharges are recorded, especially in tetany, hemifacial spasm, or myokymia.

Electrical silence characterizes the involuntary, sustained muscle contraction that occurs in phosphorylase deficiency, which is designated a contracture.

EMG enables disorders of the motor units to be detected and characterized as either neurogenic or myopathic. In neurogenic disorders, the pattern of affected muscles may localize the lesion to the anterior horn cells or to a specific site as the axons traverse a nerve root, limb plexus, and peripheral nerve to their terminal arborizations. The findings do not enable a specific etiologic diagnosis to be made, however, except in conjunction with the clinical findings and results of other laboratory studies.

The findings may provide a guide to the severity of an acute disorder of a peripheral or cranial nerve (by indicating whether denervation has occurred and the completeness of the lesion) and whether the pathologic process is active or progressive in chronic or degenerative disorders such as amyotrophic lateral sclerosis. Such information is important for prognostic purposes.

Various quantitative EMG approaches have been developed. The most common is to determine the mean duration and amplitude of 20 motor unit action potentials using a standardized technique. The technique of macro-EMG provides information about the number and size of muscle fibers in a larger volume of the motor unit territory and has also been used to estimate the number of motor units in a muscle. Scanning EMG is a computer-based technique that has been used to study the topography of motor unit action potentials and, in particular, the spatial and temporal distribution of activity in individual units. The technique of single-fiber EMG is discussed separately below.

NERVE CONDUCTION STUDIES

Recording of the electrical response of a muscle to stimulation of its motor nerve at two or more points along its course (Fig. 5-4) permits conduction velocity to be determined in the fastest-conducting motor fibers between the points of stimulation. The latency and amplitude of the electrical response of muscle (i.e., of the compound muscle action potential) to stimulation of its motor nerve at a distal site are also compared with values defined in normal subjects. Sensory nerve conduction studies are performed by determining the conduction velocity and amplitude of action potentials in sensory fibers when these fibers are stimulated at one point and the responses are recorded at another point along the course of the nerve. In adults, conduction velocity in the arms is normally between 50 and 70 m/s, and in the legs is between 40 and 60 m/s.

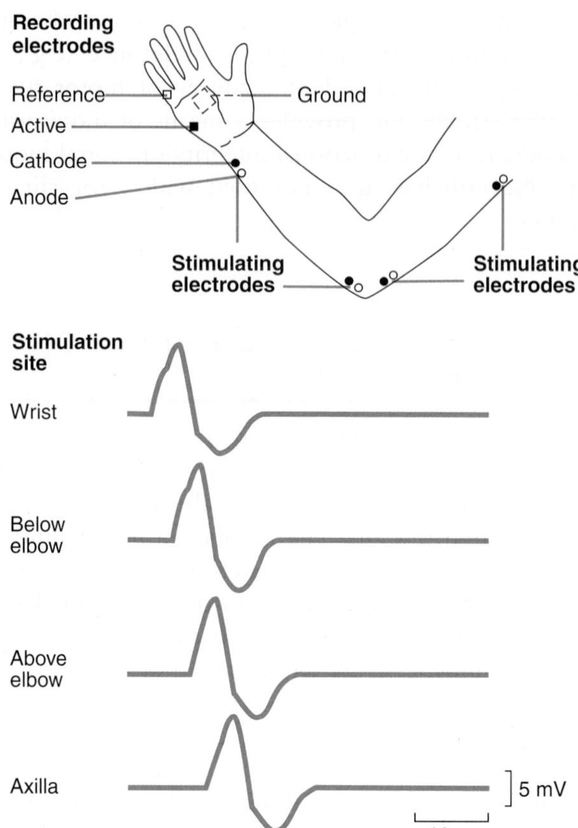

FIGURE 5-4
Arrangement for motor conduction studies of the ulnar nerve. Responses are recorded with a surface electrode from the abductor digiti minimi muscle to supramaximal stimulation of the nerve at different sites, and are shown in the lower panel. (*From Aminoff MJ: Electromyography in Clinical Practice: Electrodiagnostic Aspects of Neuromuscular Disease, 3rd ed. New York, Churchill Livingstone, 1998.*)

Nerve conduction studies complement the EMG examination, enabling the presence and extent of peripheral nerve pathology to be determined. They are particularly helpful in determining whether sensory symptoms are arising from pathology proximal or distal to the dorsal root ganglia (in the former instance, peripheral sensory conduction studies will be normal) and whether neuromuscular dysfunction relates to peripheral nerve disease. In patients with a mononeuropathy, they are invaluable as a means of localizing a focal lesion, determining the extent and severity of the underlying pathology, providing a guide to prognosis, and detecting subclinical involvement of other peripheral nerves. They enable a polyneuropathy to be distinguished from a mononeuropathy multiplex when this is not possible clinically, an important distinction because of the etiologic implications. Nerve conduction studies provide a means of following the progression and therapeutic response of peripheral nerve disorders and are being used increasingly for this purpose in clinical trials. They may suggest the underlying pathologic basis in individual cases. Conduction velocity is often markedly slowed, terminal motor latencies are prolonged, and compound motor and sensory nerve action potentials may be dispersed in the demyelinative neuropathies (such as in Guillain-Barré syndrome, chronic inflammatory polyneuropathy, metachromatic leukodystrophy, or certain hereditary neuropathies); conduction block is frequent in acquired varieties of these neuropathies. By contrast, conduction velocity is normal or slowed only mildly, sensory nerve action potentials are small or absent, and there is EMG evidence of denervation in axonal neuropathies such as occur in association with metabolic or toxic disorders.

The utility and complementary role of EMG and nerve conduction studies are best illustrated by reference to a common clinical problem. Numbness and paresthesias of the little finger and associated wasting of the intrinsic muscles of the hand may result from a spinal cord lesion, C8/T1 radiculopathy, brachial plexopathy (lower trunk or medial cord), or a lesion of the ulnar nerve. If sensory nerve action potentials can be recorded normally at the wrist following stimulation of the digital fibers in the affected finger, the pathology is probably proximal to the dorsal root ganglia (i.e., there is a radiculopathy or more central lesion); absence of the sensory potentials, by contrast, suggests distal pathology. EMG examination will indicate whether the pattern of affected muscles conforms to radicular or ulnar nerve territory, or is more extensive (thereby favoring a plexopathy). Ulnar motor conduction studies will generally also distinguish between a radiculopathy (normal findings) and ulnar neuropathy (abnormal findings) and will often identify the site of an ulnar nerve lesion. The nerve is stimulated at several points along its course to determine whether the compound action potential recorded from a distal muscle that it supplies shows a marked alteration in size or area or a disproportionate change in latency, with stimulation at a particular site. The electrophysiologic findings thus permit a definitive diagnosis to be made and specific treatment instituted in circumstances where there is clinical ambiguity.

F-WAVE STUDIES

Stimulation of a motor nerve causes impulses to travel antidromically (i.e., toward the spinal cord) as well as orthodromically (to the nerve terminals). Such antidromic impulses cause a few of the anterior horn cells to discharge, producing a small motor response that occurs considerably later than the direct response elicited by nerve stimulation. The F wave so elicited is sometimes abnormal (absent or delayed) with proximal pathology of the peripheral nervous system, such as a radiculopathy, and may therefore be helpful in detecting abnormalities when conventional nerve conduction studies are normal. In general, however, the clinical utility of F-wave studies has been disappointing, except perhaps in Guillain-Barré syndrome, where they are often absent or delayed.

H-REFLEX STUDIES

The H reflex is easily recorded only from the soleus muscle (S1) in normal adults. It is elicited by low-intensity stimulation of the tibial nerve and represents a monosynaptic reflex in which spindle (Ia) afferent fibers constitute the afferent arc and alpha motor axons the efferent pathway. The H reflexes are often absent bilaterally in elderly patients or with polyneuropathies and may be lost unilaterally in S1 radiculopathies.

MUSCLE RESPONSE TO REPETITIVE NERVE STIMULATION

The size of the electrical response of a muscle to supramaximal electrical stimulation of its motor nerve relates to the number of muscle fibers that are activated. Neuromuscular transmission can be tested by several different protocols, but the most helpful is to record with surface electrodes the electrical response of a muscle to supramaximal stimulation of its motor nerve by repetitive (2–3 Hz) shocks delivered before and at selected intervals after a maximal voluntary contraction.

There is normally little or no change in size of the compound muscle action potential following repetitive stimulation of a motor nerve at 2–3 Hz with stimuli delivered at intervals after voluntary contraction of the muscle for about 20–30 s, even though preceding activity in the junctional region influences the release of acetylcholine and thus the size of the end-plate potentials elicited by a test stimulus. This is because more acetylcholine is normally released than is required to bring the motor end-plate potentials to the threshold for generating muscle fiber action potentials. In disorders of neuromuscular transmission this safety factor is reduced. Thus in myasthenia gravis, repetitive stimulation, particularly at a rate of between 2 and 5 Hz, may lead to a depression of neuromuscular transmission, with a decrement in size of the response recorded from affected muscles. Similarly, immediately after a period of maximal voluntary activity, single or repetitive stimuli of the motor nerve may elicit larger muscle responses than before, indicating that more muscle fibers are responding. This postactivation facilitation of neuromuscular transmission is followed by a longer-lasting period of depression, maximal between 2 and 4 min after the conditioning period and lasting for as long as 10 min or so, during which responses are reduced in size.

Decrementing responses to repetitive stimulation at 2–5 Hz are common in myasthenia gravis but may also occur in the congenital myasthenic syndromes. In Lambert-Eaton myasthenic syndrome, in which there is defective release of acetylcholine at the neuromuscular junction, the compound muscle action potential elicited by a single stimulus is generally very small. With repetitive stimulation at rates of up to 10 Hz, the first few responses may decline in size, but subsequent responses increase. If faster rates of stimulation are used (20–50 Hz), the increment may be dramatic so that the amplitude of compound muscle action potentials eventually reaches a size that is several times larger than the initial response. In patients with botulism, the response to repetitive stimulation is similar to that in Lambert-Eaton myasthenic syndrome, although the findings are somewhat more variable and not all muscles are affected.

SINGLE-FIBER ELECTROMYOGRAPHY

This technique is particularly helpful in detecting disorders of neuromuscular transmission. A special needle electrode is placed within a muscle and positioned to record action potentials from two muscle fibers belonging to the same motor unit. The time interval between the two potentials will vary in consecutive discharges; this is called the *neuromuscular jitter.* The jitter can be quantified as the mean difference between consecutive interpotential intervals and is normally between 10 and 50 μs. This value is increased when neuromuscular transmission is disturbed for any reason, and in some instances impulses in individual muscle fibers may fail to occur because of impulse blocking at the neuromuscular junction. Single-fiber EMG is more sensitive than repetitive nerve stimulation or determination of acetylcholine receptor antibody levels in diagnosing myasthenia gravis.

Single-fiber EMG can also be used to determine the mean fiber density of motor units (i.e., mean number of muscle fibers per motor unit within the recording area) and to estimate the number of motor units in a muscle, but this is of less immediate clinical relevance.

BLINK REFLEXES

Electrical or mechanical stimulation of the supraorbital nerve on one side leads to two separate reflex responses of the orbicularis oculi—an ipsilateral R1 response having a latency of approximately 10 ms and a bilateral R2 response with a latency in the order of 30 ms. The trigeminal and facial nerves constitute the afferent and efferent arcs of the reflex, respectively. Abnormalities of either nerve or intrinsic lesions of the medulla or pons may lead to uni- or bilateral loss of the response, and the findings may therefore be helpful in identifying or localizing such pathology.

CHAPTER 6

TECHNIQUE OF LUMBAR PUNCTURE

Elizabeth Robbins ■ Stephen L. Hauser

In experienced hands, lumbar puncture (LP) is usually a safe procedure. Major complications are extremely uncommon but can include cerebral herniation, injury to the spinal cord or nerve roots, hemorrhage, or infection. Minor complications occur with greater frequency and can include backache, post-LP headache, and radicular pain or numbness.

IMAGING AND LABORATORY STUDIES PRIOR TO LP

Patients with an altered level of consciousness, a focal neurologic deficit, new-onset seizure, papilledema, or an immunocompromised state are at increased risk for potentially fatal cerebellar or tentorial herniation following LP. Neuroimaging should be obtained in these patients prior to LP to exclude a focal mass lesion or diffuse swelling. Imaging studies should include the spine in patients with symptoms suggesting spinal cord compression, such as back pain, leg weakness, urinary retention, or incontinence. In patients with suspected meningitis who require neuroimaging prior to diagnostic LP, administration of antibiotics, preferably following blood culture, should precede the neuroimaging study.

Patients receiving therapeutic anticoagulation or those with coagulation defects including thrombocytopenia are at increased risk of post-LP spinal subdural or epidural hematomas, either of which can produce permanent nerve injury and/or paralysis. If a bleeding disorder is suspected, the platelet count, international normalized ratio (INR), and partial thromboplastin time should be checked prior to lumbar puncture. There are no data available to assess the safety of LP in patients with low platelet counts; a count of <20,000/μL is considered to be a contraindication to LP. Bleeding complications rarely occur in patients with platelet counts ≥50,000/μL and an INR ≤1.5. Patients receiving low-molecular-weight heparin are at increased risk of post-LP spinal or epidural hematoma, and doses should be held for 24 h before the procedure.

LP should not be performed through infected skin as organisms can be introduced into the subarachnoid space (SAS).

ANALGESIA

Anxiety and pain can be minimized prior to beginning the procedure. Anxiety can be allayed by the use of lorazepam, 1–2 mg given PO 30 min prior to the procedure or IV 5 min prior to the procedure. Topical anesthesia can be achieved by the application of a lidocaine-based cream. Lidocaine 4% is effective when applied 30 min prior to the procedure; lidocaine/prilocaine requires 60–120 min. The cream should be applied in a thick layer so that it completely covers the skin; an occlusive dressing is used to keep the cream in place.

POSITIONING

Proper positioning of the patient is essential. The procedure should be performed on a firm surface; if the procedure is to be performed at the bedside, the patient should be positioned at the edge of the bed and not in the middle. The patient is asked to lie on his or her side, facing away from the examiner, and to "roll up into a ball." The neck is gently ante-flexed and the thighs pulled up toward the abdomen; the shoulders and pelvis should be vertically aligned without forward or backward tilt (Fig. 6-1). The spinal cord terminates at approximately the L1 vertebral level in 94% of individuals. In the remaining 6%, the conus extends to the L2-L3 interspace. LP is therefore performed at or below the L3-L4 interspace. A useful anatomic guide is a line

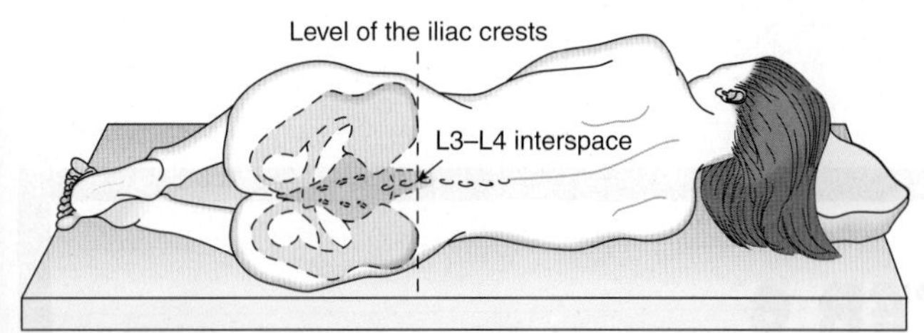

FIGURE 6-1

Proper positioning of a patient in the lateral decubitus position. Note that the shoulders and hips are in a vertical plane; the torso is perpendicular to the bed. (*From RP Simon et al [eds]: Clinical Neurology, 7th ed. New York, McGraw-Hill, 2009.*)

drawn between the posterior superior iliac crests, which corresponds closely to the level of the L3-L4 interspace. The interspace is chosen following gentle palpation to identify the spinous processes at each lumbar level.

An alternative to the lateral recumbent position is the seated position. The patient sits at the side of the bed, with feet supported on a chair. The patient is instructed to curl forward, trying to touch the nose to the umbilicus. It is important that the patient not simply lean forward onto a bedside tabletop, as this is not an optimal position for opening up the spinous processes. LP is sometimes more easily performed in obese patients if they are sitting. A disadvantage of the seated position is that measurement of opening pressure may not be accurate. In situations in which LP is difficult using palpable spinal landmarks, bedside ultrasound to guide needle placement may be employed.

TECHNIQUE

Once the desired target for needle insertion has been identified, the examiner should put on sterile gloves. After cleansing the skin with povidone-iodine or similar disinfectant, the area is draped with a sterile cloth; the needle insertion site is blotted dry using a sterile gauze pad. Proper local disinfection reduces the risk of introducing skin bacteria into the SAS or other sites. Local anesthetic, typically 1% lidocaine, 3–5 mL total, is injected into the subcutaneous tissue; in nonemergency situations a topical anesthetic cream can be applied (see above). When time permits, pain associated with the injection of lidocaine can be minimized by slow, serial injections, each one progressively deeper than the last, over a period of ~5 min. Approximately 0.5–1 mL of lidocaine is injected at a time; the needle is not usually withdrawn between injections. A pause of ~15 s between injections helps to minimize the pain of the subsequent injection. The goal is to inject each mini-bolus of anesthetic into an area of skin that has become numb from the preceding injection. Approximately 5–10 mini-boluses are injected, using a total of ~5 mL of lidocaine.

If possible, the LP should be delayed for 10–15 min following the completion of the injection of anesthetic; this significantly decreases and can even eliminate pain from the procedure. Even a delay of 5 min will help to reduce pain.

The LP needle (typically 20- to 22-gauge) is inserted in the midline, midway between two spinous processes, and slowly advanced. The bevel of the needle should be maintained in a horizontal position, parallel to the direction of the dural fibers and with the flat portion of the bevel pointed upward; this minimizes injury to the fibers as the dura is penetrated. When lumbar puncture is performed in patients who are sitting, the bevel should be maintained in the vertical position. In most adults, the needle is advanced 4–5 cm (1–2 in.) before the SAS is reached; the examiner usually recognizes entry as a sudden release of resistance, a "pop." If no fluid appears despite apparently correct needle placement, then the needle may be rotated 90°–180°. If there is still no fluid, the stylet is reinserted and the needle is advanced slightly. Some examiners halt needle advancement periodically to remove the stylet and check for flow of cerebrospinal fluid (CSF). If the needle cannot be advanced because it hits bone, if the patient experiences sharp radiating pain down one leg, or if no fluid appears ("dry tap"), the needle is partially withdrawn and reinserted at a different angle. If on the second attempt the needle still hits bone (indicating lack of success in introducing it between the spinous processes), then the needle should be completely withdrawn and the patient should be repositioned. The second attempt is sometimes more successful if the patient straightens the spine completely prior to repositioning. The needle can then be reinserted at the same level or at an adjacent one.

Once the SAS is reached, a manometer is attached to the needle and the opening pressure measured. The examiner should look for normal oscillations in CSF pressure associated with pulse and respirations. The upper limit of normal opening pressure with the patient supine is 180 mmH_2O in adults but may be as high as 200–250 mmH_2O in obese adults.

CSF is allowed to drip into collection tubes; it should not be withdrawn with a syringe. Depending on the clinical indication, fluid is then obtained for studies including: (1) cell count with differential; (2) protein and glucose concentrations; (3) culture (bacterial, fungal, mycobacterial, viral); (4) smears (e.g., Gram's and acid-fast stained smears); (5) antigen tests (e.g., latex agglutination); (6) polymerase chain reaction (PCR) amplification of DNA or RNA of microorganisms (e.g., herpes simplex virus, enteroviruses); (7) antibody levels against microorganisms; (8) immunoelectrophoresis for determination of γ-globulin level and oligoclonal banding; and (9) cytology. Although 15 mL of CSF is sufficient to obtain all of the listed studies, the yield of fungal and mycobacterial cultures and cytology increases when larger volumes are sampled. In general 20–30 mL may be safely removed from adults.

A bloody tap due to penetration of a meningeal vessel (a "traumatic tap") may result in confusion with subarachnoid hemorrhage (SAH). In these situations a specimen of CSF should be centrifuged immediately after it is obtained; clear supernatant following CSF centrifugation supports the diagnosis of a bloody tap, whereas xanthochromic supernatant suggests SAH. In general, bloody CSF due to the penetration of a meningeal vessel clears gradually in successive tubes, whereas blood due to SAH does not. In addition to SAH, xanthochromic CSF may also be present in patients with liver disease and when the CSF protein concentration is markedly elevated (>1.5–2 g/L [150–200 mg/dL]).

Prior to removing the LP needle, the stylet is reinserted to avoid the possibility of entrapment of a nerve root in the dura as the needle is being withdrawn; entrapment could result in a dural CSF leak, causing headache. Some practitioners question the safety of this maneuver, with its potential risk of causing a needlestick injury to the examiner. Injury is unlikely, however, given the flexibility of the small-diameter stylet, which tends to bend, rather than penetrate, on contact. Following LP, the patient is customarily positioned in a comfortable, recumbent position for 1 h before rising, although this may be unnecessary as it does not appear to affect the development of headache (see below).

POST-LP HEADACHE

The principal complication of LP is headache, occurring in 10–30% of patients. Younger age and female gender are associated with an increased risk of post-LP headache. Headache usually begins within 48 h but may be delayed for up to 12 days. Head pain is dramatically positional; it begins when the patient sits or stands upright; there is relief upon reclining or with abdominal compression. The longer the patient is upright, the longer the latency before head pain subsides. The pain is usually a dull ache but may be throbbing; its location is occipitofrontal. Nausea and stiff neck often accompany headache, and occasionally, patients report blurred vision, photophobia, tinnitus, and vertigo. In more than three-quarters of patients, symptoms completely resolve within a week, but in a minority they can persist for weeks or even months.

Post-LP headache is caused by a drop in CSF pressure related to persistent leakage of CSF at the site where the needle entered the subarachnoid space. Loss of CSF volume decreases the brain's supportive cushion, so that when a patient is upright there is probably dilation and tension placed on the brain's anchoring structures, the pain-sensitive dural sinuses, resulting in pain. Although intracranial hypotension is the usual explanation for severe LP headache, the syndrome can occur in patients with normal CSF pressure.

Because post-LP headache usually resolves without specific treatment, care is largely supportive with oral analgesics (acetaminophen, nonsteroidal anti-inflammatory drugs, opioids [Chap. 7]) and antiemetics. Patients may obtain relief by lying in a comfortable (especially a recumbent or head-down Trendelenburg) position. For some patients, beverages with caffeine can provide temporary pain relief.

For patients with persistent pain, treatment with IV caffeine (500 mg in 500 mL saline administered over 2 h) may be effective; atrial fibrillation is a rare side effect. Alternatively, an epidural blood patch accomplished by injection of 15 mL of autologous whole blood is usually effective. This procedure is most often performed by a pain specialist or anesthesiologist. The blood patch has an immediate effect, making it unlikely that sealing off a dural hole with blood clot is its sole mechanism of action. The acute benefit may be due to compression of the CSF space by the clot, increasing CSF pressure. Some clinicians reserve epidural blood patch for patients who do not respond to caffeine, while others prefer to use blood patch as initial management for unremitting post-LP symptoms.

Strategies to decrease the incidence of post-LP headache are listed in Table 6-1. Use of a smaller caliber needle is associated with a lower risk: In one study, the risk of headache following use of a 24- to 27-gauge standard (Quincke) needle was 5–12%, compared to 20–40% when a 20- or 22-gauge needle was used. The smallest gauge needles usually require the use of an introducer needle and are associated with a slower CSF flow rate. Use of an "atraumatic" (Sprotte, "pencil point," or "noncutting") needle also reduces the incidence of moderate to severe headache compared

TABLE 6-1

REDUCING THE INCIDENCE OF POST-LP HEADACHE
Effective Strategies
Use of small-diameter needle (22-gauge or smaller)
Use of atraumatic needle (Sprotte and others)
Replacement of stylet prior to removal of needle
Insertion of needle with bevel oriented in a cephalad to caudad direction (when using standard needle)
Ineffective Strategies
Bed rest (up to 4 h) following LP
Supplemental fluids
Minimizing the volume of spinal fluid removed
Immediate mobilization following LP

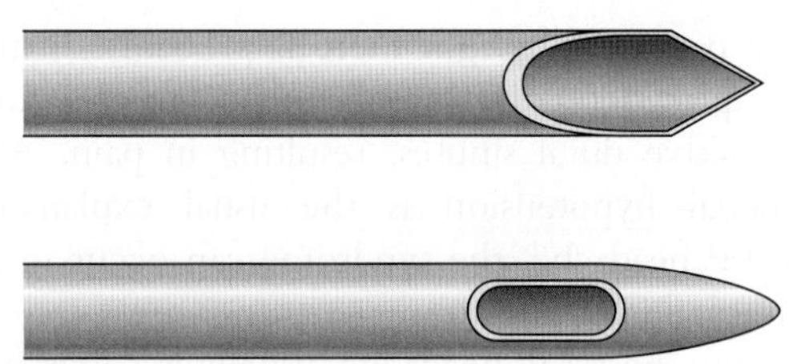

FIGURE 6-2
Comparison of the standard ("traumatic" or Quincke) LP needle with the "atraumatic" (Sprotte). The "atraumatic" needle has its opening on the top surface of the needle, a design intended to reduce the chance of cutting dural fibers that, by protruding through the dura, could be responsible for subsequent CSF fluid leak and post-LP headache. *(From SR Thomas et al: BMJ 321:986, 2000.)*

with standard LP (Quincke, or "traumatic") needles (Fig. 6-2). However, because atraumatic needles are more difficult to use, more attempts may be required to perform the LP, particularly in overweight patients. It may also be necessary to use an introducer with the atraumatic needle, which does not have the customary cutting, beveled tip. There is a low risk of needle damage, e.g., breakage, with the Sprotte atraumatic needle. Another strategy to decrease the incidence of headache is to replace the stylet before removing the LP needle.

Patients are often advised to remain in a recumbent position for up to an hour following lumbar puncture. However, studies comparing mobilization immediately following LP with bed rest for periods up to 4 h show no significant differences in the incidence of headache, suggesting that the customary practice of remaining in a recumbent position post-LP may be unnecessary.

NORMAL VALUES

(See Table 6-2) In uninfected CSF, the normal white blood cell count is fewer than five mononuclear cells (lymphocytes and monocytes) per μL. Polymorphonuclear leukocytes (PMNs) are not found in normal unconcentrated CSF; however, rare PMNs can be found in centrifuged or concentrated CSF specimens such as those utilized for cytologic examination. Red blood cells (RBCs) are not normally present in CSF; if RBCs are present from a traumatic tap, their number decreases as additional CSF is collected. CSF glucose concentrations <2.2 mmol/L (<40 mg/dL) are abnormal.

TABLE 6-2

CEREBROSPINAL FLUID[a]

CONSTITUENT	SI UNITS	CONVENTIONAL UNITS
Glucose	2.22–3.89 mmol/L	40–70 mg/dL
Lactate	1–2 mmol/L	10–20 mg/dL
Total protein		
Lumbar	0.15–0.5 g/L	15–50 mg/dL
Cisternal	0.15–0.25 g/L	15–25 mg/dL
Ventricular	0.06–0.15 g/L	6–15 mg/dL
Albumin	0.066–0.442 g/L	6.6–44.2 mg/dL
IgG	0.009–0.057 g/L	0.9–5.7 mg/dL
IgG index[b]	0.29–0.59	
Oligoclonal bands (OGB)	<2 bands not present in matched serum sample	
Ammonia	15–47 μmol/L	25–80 μg/dL
CSF pressure		50–180 mmH_2O
CSF volume (adult)	~150 mL	
Red blood cells	0	0
Leukocytes		
Total	0–5 mononuclear cells per mm^3	
Differential		
Lymphocytes	60–70%	
Monocytes	30–50%	
Neutrophils	None	

[a]Because cerebrospinal fluid concentrations are equilibrium values, measurements of the same parameters in blood plasma obtained at the same time are recommended. However, there is a time lag in attainment of equilibrium, and cerebrospinal levels of plasma constituents that can fluctuate rapidly (such as plasma glucose) may not achieve stable values until after a significant lag phase.
[b]IgG index = CSF IgG (mg/dL) × serum albumin (g/dL)/serum IgG (g/dL) × CSF albumin (mg/dL).

SECTION II

CLINICAL MANIFESTATIONS OF NEUROLOGIC DISEASE

CHAPTER 7

PAIN: PATHOPHYSIOLOGY AND MANAGEMENT

James P. Rathmell ■ Howard L. Fields

The task of medicine is to preserve and restore health and to relieve suffering. Understanding pain is essential to both of these goals. Because pain is universally understood as a signal of disease, it is the most common symptom that brings a patient to a physician's attention. The function of the pain sensory system is to protect the body and maintain homeostasis. It does this by detecting, localizing, and identifying potential or actual tissue-damaging processes. Because different diseases produce characteristic patterns of tissue damage, the quality, time course, and location of a patient's pain complaint provide important diagnostic clues. It is the physician's responsibility to provide rapid and effective pain relief.

THE PAIN SENSORY SYSTEM

Pain is an unpleasant sensation localized to a part of the body. It is often described in terms of a penetrating or tissue-destructive process (e.g., stabbing, burning, twisting, tearing, squeezing) and/or of a bodily or emotional reaction (e.g., terrifying, nauseating, sickening). Furthermore, any pain of moderate or higher intensity is accompanied by anxiety and the urge to escape or terminate the feeling. These properties illustrate the duality of pain: it is both sensation and emotion. When it is acute, pain is characteristically associated with behavioral arousal and a stress response consisting of increased blood pressure, heart rate, pupil diameter, and plasma cortisol levels. In addition, local muscle contraction (e.g., limb flexion, abdominal wall rigidity) is often present.

PERIPHERAL MECHANISMS

The primary afferent nociceptor

A peripheral nerve consists of the axons of three different types of neurons: primary sensory afferents, motor neurons, and sympathetic postganglionic neurons (Fig. 7-1). The cell bodies of primary sensory afferents are located in the dorsal root ganglia in the vertebral foramina. The primary afferent axon has two branches: one projects centrally into the spinal cord and the other projects peripherally to innervate tissues. Primary afferents are classified by their diameter, degree of myelination, and conduction velocity. The largest-diameter afferent fibers, A-beta (Aβ), respond maximally to light touch and/or moving stimuli; they are present primarily in nerves that innervate the skin. In normal individuals, the activity of these fibers does not produce pain. There are two other classes of primary afferents: the small-diameter myelinated A-delta (Aδ) and the unmyelinated (C fiber) axons (Fig. 7-1). These fibers are present in nerves to the skin and to deep somatic and visceral structures. Some tissues, such as the cornea, are innervated only by Aδ and C fiber afferents. Most Aδ and C fiber afferents respond maximally only to intense (painful) stimuli and produce the subjective experience of pain when they are electrically stimulated; this defines them as *primary afferent nociceptors* (*pain receptors*). The ability to detect painful stimuli is completely abolished when conduction in Aδ and C fiber axons is blocked.

Individual primary afferent nociceptors can respond to several different types of noxious stimuli. For example, most nociceptors respond to heat; intense cold; intense mechanical stimuli, such as a pinch; changes in pH, particularly an acidic environment; and application of chemical irritants including adenosine triphosphate (ATP), serotonin, bradykinin, and histamine.

Sensitization

When intense, repeated, or prolonged stimuli are applied to damaged or inflamed tissues, the threshold for activating primary afferent nociceptors is lowered, and the frequency of firing is higher for all stimulus intensities. Inflammatory mediators such as bradykinin,

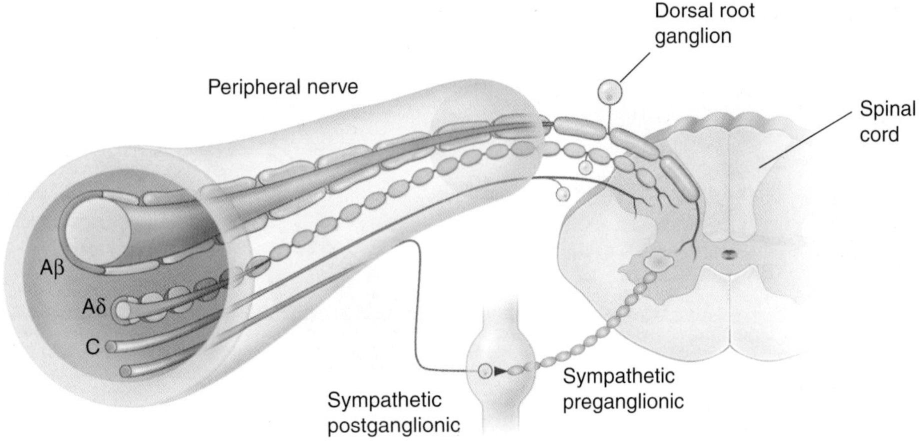

FIGURE 7-1

Components of a typical cutaneous nerve. There are two distinct functional categories of axons: primary afferents with cell bodies in the dorsal root ganglion, and sympathetic postganglionic fibers with cell bodies in the sympathetic ganglion. Primary afferents include those with large-diameter myelinated (Aβ), small-diameter myelinated (Aδ), and unmyelinated (C) axons. All sympathetic postganglionic fibers are unmyelinated.

nerve-growth factor, some prostaglandins, and leukotrienes contribute to this process, which is called *sensitization*. Sensitization occurs at the level of the peripheral nerve terminal *(peripheral sensitization)* as well as at the level of the dorsal horn of the spinal cord *(central sensitization)*. Peripheral sensitization occurs in damaged or inflamed tissues, when inflammatory mediators activate intracellular signal transduction in nociceptors, prompting an increase in the production, transport, and membrane insertion of chemically gated and voltage-gated ion channels. These changes increase the excitability of nociceptor terminals and lower their threshold for activation by mechanical, thermal, and chemical stimuli. Central sensitization occurs when activity, generated by nociceptors during inflammation, enhances the excitability of nerve cells in the dorsal horn of the spinal cord. Following injury and resultant sensitization, normally innocuous stimuli can produce pain. Sensitization is a clinically important process that contributes to tenderness, soreness, and hyperalgesia (increased pain intensity in response to the same noxious stimulus; e.g., moderate pressure causes severe pain). A striking example of sensitization is sunburned skin, in which severe pain can be produced by a gentle slap on the back or a warm shower.

Sensitization is of particular importance for pain and tenderness in deep tissues. Viscera are normally relatively insensitive to noxious mechanical and thermal stimuli, although hollow viscera do generate significant discomfort when distended. In contrast, when affected by a disease process with an inflammatory component, deep structures such as joints or hollow viscera characteristically become exquisitely sensitive to mechanical stimulation.

A large proportion of Aδ and C fiber afferents innervating viscera are completely insensitive in normal noninjured, noninflamed tissue. That is, they cannot be activated by known mechanical or thermal stimuli and are not spontaneously active. However, in the presence of inflammatory mediators, these afferents become sensitive to mechanical stimuli. Such afferents have been termed *silent nociceptors*, and their characteristic properties may explain how, under pathologic conditions, the relatively insensitive deep structures can become the source of severe and debilitating pain and tenderness. Low pH, prostaglandins, leukotrienes, and other inflammatory mediators such as bradykinin play a significant role in sensitization.

Nociceptor-induced inflammation

Primary afferent nociceptors also have a neuroeffector function. Most nociceptors contain polypeptide mediators that are released from their peripheral terminals when they are activated (Fig. 7-2). An example is substance P, an 11-amino-acid peptide. Substance P is released from primary afferent nociceptors and has multiple biologic activities. It is a potent vasodilator, degranulates mast cells, is a chemoattractant for leukocytes, and increases the production and release of inflammatory mediators. Interestingly, depletion of substance P from joints reduces the severity of experimental arthritis. Primary afferent nociceptors are not simply passive messengers of threats to tissue injury but also play an active role in tissue protection through these neuroeffector functions.

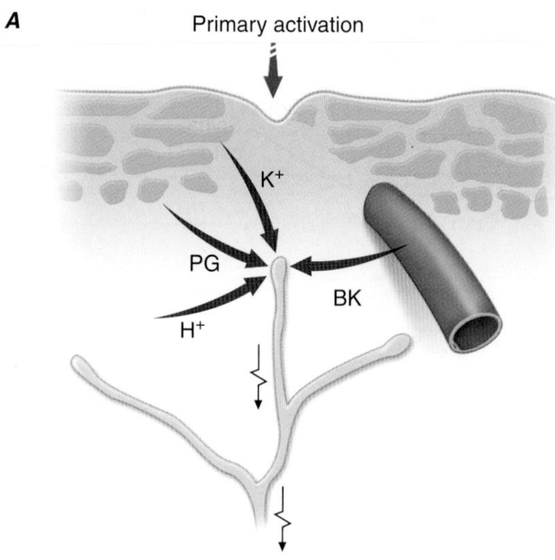

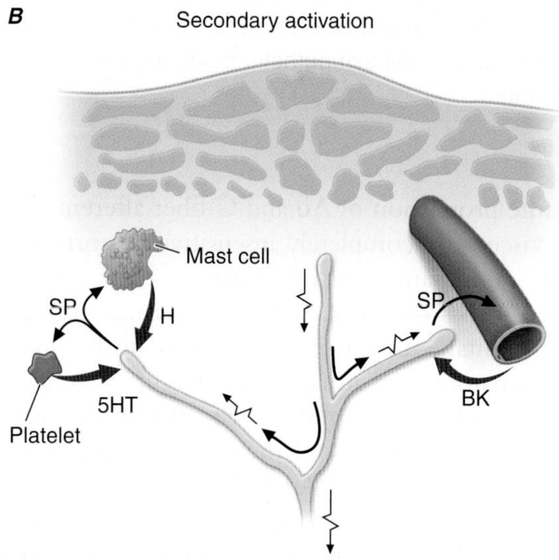

FIGURE 7-2

Events leading to activation, sensitization, and spread of sensitization of primary afferent nociceptor terminals. ***A.*** Direct activation by intense pressure and consequent cell damage. Cell damage induces lower pH (H^+) and leads to release of potassium (K^+) and to synthesis of prostaglandins (PG) and bradykinin (BK). Prostaglandins increase the sensitivity of the terminal to bradykinin and other pain-producing substances. ***B.*** Secondary activation. Impulses generated in the stimulated terminal propagate not only to the spinal cord but also into other terminal branches where they induce the release of peptides, including substance P (SP). Substance P causes vasodilation and neurogenic edema with further accumulation of bradykinin (BK). Substance P also causes the release of histamine (H) from mast cells and serotonin (5HT) from platelets.

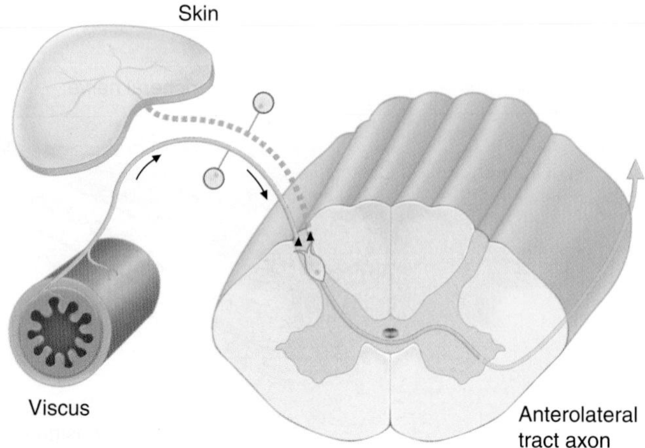

FIGURE 7-3

The convergence-projection hypothesis of referred pain. According to this hypothesis, visceral afferent nociceptors converge on the same pain-projection neurons as the afferents from the somatic structures in which the pain is perceived. The brain has no way of knowing the actual source of input and mistakenly "projects" the sensation to the somatic structure.

CENTRAL MECHANISMS

The spinal cord and referred pain

The axons of primary afferent nociceptors enter the spinal cord via the dorsal root. They terminate in the dorsal horn of the spinal gray matter (Fig. 7-3). The terminals of primary afferent axons contact spinal neurons that transmit the pain signal to brain sites involved in pain perception. When primary afferents are activated by noxious stimuli, they release neurotransmitters from their terminals that excite the spinal cord neurons. The major neurotransmitter released is glutamate, which rapidly excites dorsal horn neurons. Primary afferent nociceptor terminals also release peptides, including substance P and calcitonin gene-related peptide, which produce a slower and longer-lasting excitation of the dorsal horn neurons. The axon of each primary afferent contacts many spinal neurons, and each spinal neuron receives convergent inputs from many primary afferents.

The convergence of sensory inputs to a single spinal pain-transmission neuron is of great importance because it underlies the phenomenon of referred pain. All spinal neurons that receive input from the viscera and deep musculoskeletal structures also receive input from the skin. The convergence patterns are determined by the spinal segment of the dorsal root ganglion that supplies the afferent innervation of a structure. For example, the afferents that supply the central diaphragm are derived from the third and fourth cervical dorsal root ganglia. Primary afferents with cell bodies in these same ganglia supply the skin of the shoulder and lower neck. Thus, sensory inputs from both the shoulder skin and the central diaphragm converge on pain-transmission neurons in the third and fourth cervical spinal segments. *Because of this convergence and the fact that the spinal neurons are most often activated by inputs from the skin, activity evoked in spinal neurons by input from deep structures is mislocalized by the patient to a place that roughly corresponds with the region of skin innervated by the same spinal segment.* Thus, inflammation near the central diaphragm is usually reported as shoulder discomfort. This spatial displacement of pain sensation from the site of the injury that produces it is known as *referred pain.*

Ascending pathways for pain

A majority of spinal neurons contacted by primary afferent nociceptors send their axons to the contralateral thalamus. These axons form the contralateral spinothalamic tract, which lies in the anterolateral white matter of the spinal cord, the lateral edge of the medulla, and the lateral pons and midbrain. The spinothalamic pathway is crucial for pain sensation in humans. Interruption of this pathway produces permanent deficits in pain and temperature discrimination.

Spinothalamic tract axons ascend to several regions of the thalamus. There is tremendous divergence of the pain signal from these thalamic sites to broad areas of the cerebral cortex that subserve different aspects of the pain experience (Fig. 7-4). One of the thalamic projections is to the somatosensory cortex. This projection mediates the purely sensory aspects of pain, i.e., its location, intensity, and quality. Other thalamic neurons project to cortical regions that are linked to emotional responses, such as the cingulate gyrus and other areas of the frontal lobes, including the insular cortex. These pathways to the frontal cortex subserve the affective or unpleasant emotional dimension of pain. This affective dimension of pain produces suffering and exerts potent control of behavior. Because of this dimension, fear is a constant companion of pain. As a consequence, injury or surgical lesions to areas of the frontal cortex activated by painful stimuli diminish the emotional impact of pain while largely preserving the individual's ability to recognize noxious stimuli as painful.

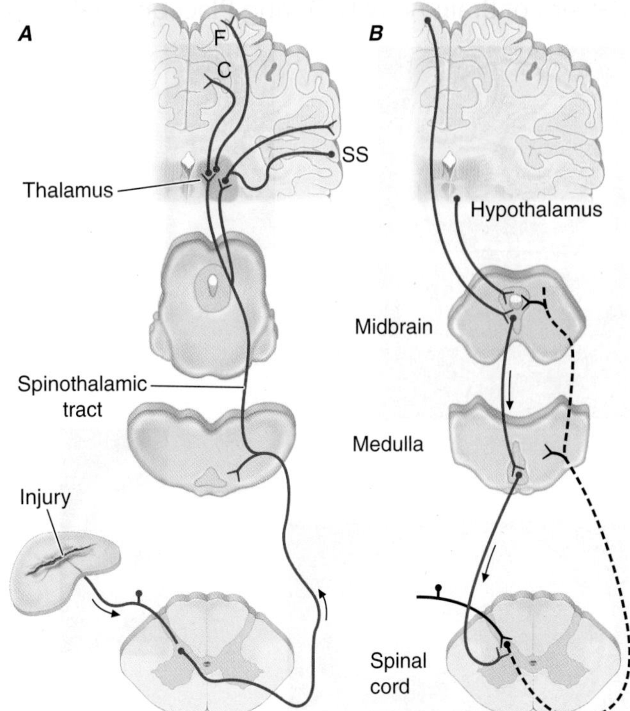

FIGURE 7-4
Pain transmission and modulatory pathways. *A.* Transmission system for nociceptive messages. Noxious stimuli activate the sensitive peripheral ending of the primary afferent nociceptor by the process of transduction. The message is then transmitted over the peripheral nerve to the spinal cord, where it synapses with cells of origin of the major ascending pain pathway, the spinothalamic tract. The message is relayed in the thalamus to the anterior cingulate (C), frontal insular (F), and somatosensory cortex (SS). ***B.*** Pain-modulation network. Inputs from frontal cortex and hypothalamus activate cells in the midbrain that control spinal pain-transmission cells via cells in the medulla.

PAIN MODULATION

The pain produced by injuries of similar magnitude is remarkably variable in different situations and in different individuals. For example, athletes have been known to sustain serious fractures with only minor pain, and Beecher's classic World War II survey revealed that many soldiers in battle were unbothered by injuries that would have produced agonizing pain in civilian patients. Furthermore, even the suggestion that a treatment will relieve pain can have a significant analgesic effect (the placebo effect). On the other hand, many patients find even minor injuries (such as venipuncture) frightening and unbearable, and the expectation of pain can induce pain even without a noxious stimulus. The suggestion that pain will worsen following administration of an inert substance can increase its perceived intensity (the nocebo effect).

The powerful effect of expectation and other psychological variables on the perceived intensity of pain is explained by brain circuits that modulate the activity of the pain-transmission pathways. One of these circuits has links to the hypothalamus, midbrain, and medulla, and it selectively controls spinal pain-transmission neurons through a descending pathway (Fig. 7-4).

Human brain–imaging studies have implicated this pain-modulating circuit in the pain-relieving effect of attention, suggestion, and opioid analgesic medications (Fig. 7-5). Furthermore, each of the component structures of the pathway contains opioid receptors and is sensitive to the direct application of opioid drugs. In animals, lesions of this descending modulatory system reduce the analgesic effect of systemically administered opioids such as morphine. Along with the opioid receptor, the component nuclei of this pain-modulating

Pattern of Brain Activity During Placebo Analgesia

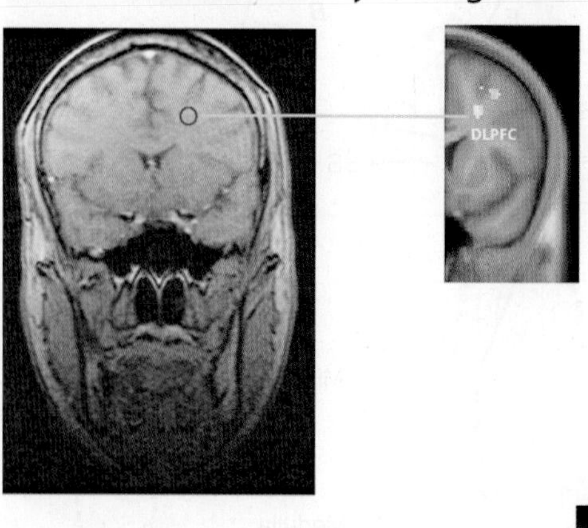

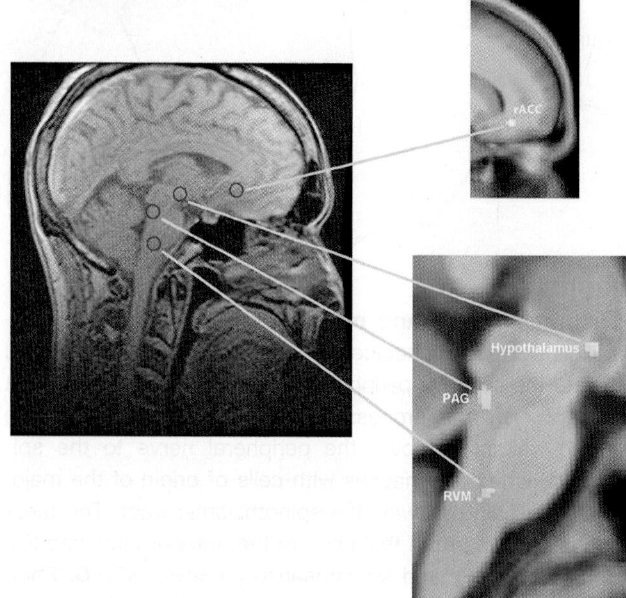

FIGURE 7-5

Functional magnetic resonance imaging (fMRI) demonstrates placebo-enhanced brain activity in anatomic regions correlating with the opioidergic descending pain control system. Top panel, Frontal fMRI image shows placebo-enhanced brain activity in the dorsal lateral prefrontal cortex (DLPFC). Bottom panel, Sagittal fMRI images show placebo-enhanced responses in the rostral anterior cingulate cortex (rACC), the rostral ventral medullae (RVM), the periaqueductal gray (PAG) area, and the hypothalamus. The placebo-enhanced activity in all areas was reduced by naloxone, demonstrating the link between the descending opioidergic system and the placebo analgesic response. (*Adapted with permission from F Eippert et al: Neuron 63:533, 2009.*)

circuit contain endogenous opioid peptides such as the enkephalins and β-endorphin.

The most reliable way to activate this endogenous opioid-mediated modulating system is by suggestion of pain relief or by intense emotion directed away from the pain-causing injury (e.g., during severe threat or an athletic competition). In fact, pain-relieving endogenous opioids are released following surgical procedures and in patients given a placebo for pain relief.

Pain-modulating circuits can enhance as well as suppress pain. Both pain-inhibiting and pain-facilitating neurons in the medulla project to and control spinal pain-transmission neurons. Because pain-transmission neurons can be activated by modulatory neurons, it is theoretically possible to generate a pain signal with no peripheral noxious stimulus. In fact, human functional imaging studies have demonstrated increased activity in this circuit during migraine headaches. A central circuit that facilitates pain could account for the finding that pain can be induced by suggestion or enhanced by expectation and provides a framework for understanding how psychological factors can contribute to chronic pain.

NEUROPATHIC PAIN

Lesions of the peripheral or central nociceptive pathways typically result in a loss or impairment of pain sensation. Paradoxically, damage to or dysfunction of these pathways can also produce pain. For example, damage to peripheral nerves, as occurs in diabetic neuropathy, or to primary afferents, as in herpes zoster, can result in pain that is referred to the body region innervated by the damaged nerves. Pain may also be produced by damage to the central nervous system (CNS), for example, in some patients following trauma or cerebrovascular injury to spinal cord, brainstem, or thalamic areas that contain central nociceptive pathways. Such neuropathic pains are often severe and are typically resistant to standard treatments for pain.

Neuropathic pain typically has an unusual burning, tingling, or electric shock–like quality and may be triggered by very light touch. These features are rare in other types of pain. On examination, a sensory deficit is characteristically present in the area of the patient's pain. Hyperpathia, a greatly exaggerated pain sensation to innocuous or mild nociceptive stimuli, is also characteristic of neuropathic pain; patients often complain that the very lightest moving stimulus evokes exquisite pain (allodynia). In this regard, it is of clinical interest that a topical preparation of 5% lidocaine in patch form is effective for patients with postherpetic neuralgia who have prominent allodynia.

A variety of mechanisms contribute to neuropathic pain. As with sensitized primary afferent nociceptors, damaged primary afferents, including nociceptors, become highly sensitive to mechanical stimulation and may generate impulses in the absence of stimulation. Increased sensitivity and spontaneous activity are due, in part, to an increased concentration of sodium channels. Damaged primary afferents may also develop sensitivity to norepinephrine. Interestingly, spinal cord pain-transmission neurons cut off from their normal input may also become spontaneously active. Thus, both CNS and peripheral nervous system hyperactivity contribute to neuropathic pain.

Sympathetically maintained pain

Patients with peripheral nerve injury occasionally develop spontaneous pain in the region innervated by the nerve. This pain is often described as having a burning quality. The pain typically begins after a delay of hours to days or even weeks and is accompanied by swelling of the extremity, periarticular bone loss, and arthritic changes in the distal joints. The pain may be relieved by a local anesthetic block of the sympathetic innervation to the affected extremity. Damaged primary afferent nociceptors acquire adrenergic sensitivity and can be activated by stimulation of the sympathetic outflow. This constellation of spontaneous pain and signs of sympathetic dysfunction following injury has been termed *complex regional pain syndrome* (CRPS). When this occurs after an identifiable nerve injury, it is termed CRPS type II (also known as posttraumatic neuralgia or, if severe, *causalgia*). When a similar clinical picture appears without obvious nerve injury, it is termed CRPS type I (also known as *reflex sympathetic dystrophy*). CRPS can be produced by a variety of injuries, including fractures of bone, soft tissue trauma, myocardial infarction, and stroke (Chap. 33). CRPS type I typically resolves with symptomatic treatment; however, when it persists, detailed examination often reveals evidence of peripheral nerve injury. Although the pathophysiology of CRPS is poorly understood, the pain and the signs of inflammation, when acute, can be rapidly relieved by blocking the sympathetic nervous system. This implies that sympathetic activity can activate undamaged nociceptors when inflammation is present. Signs of sympathetic hyperactivity should be sought in patients with posttraumatic pain and inflammation and no other obvious explanation.

TREATMENT Acute Pain

The ideal treatment for any pain is to remove the cause; thus, while treatment can be initiated immediately, efforts to establish the underlying etiology should always proceed as treatment begins. Sometimes, treating the underlying condition does not immediately relieve pain. Furthermore, some conditions are so painful that rapid and effective analgesia is essential (e.g., the postoperative state, burns, trauma, cancer, or sickle cell crisis). Analgesic medications are a first line of treatment in these cases, and all practitioners should be familiar with their use.

ASPIRIN, ACETAMINOPHEN, AND NON-STEROIDAL ANTI-INFLAMMATORY AGENTS (NSAIDS) These drugs are considered together because they are used for similar problems and may have a similar mechanism of action (Table 7-1). All these compounds inhibit cyclooxygenase (COX), and, except for acetaminophen, all have anti-inflammatory actions, especially at higher dosages. They are particularly effective for mild to moderate headache and for pain of musculoskeletal origin.

Because they are effective for these common types of pain and are available without prescription, COX inhibitors are by far the most commonly used analgesics. They are absorbed well from the gastrointestinal tract and, with occasional use, have only minimal side effects. With chronic use, gastric irritation is a common side effect of aspirin and NSAIDs and is the problem that most frequently limits the dose that can be given. Gastric irritation is most severe with aspirin, which may cause erosion and ulceration of the gastric mucosa leading to bleeding or perforation. Because aspirin irreversibly acetylates platelet cyclooxygenase and thereby interferes with coagulation of the blood, gastrointestinal bleeding is a particular risk. Older age and history of gastrointestinal disease increase the risks of aspirin and NSAIDs. In addition to the well-known gastrointestinal toxicity of NSAIDs, nephrotoxicity is a significant problem for patients using these drugs on a chronic basis. Patients at risk for renal insufficiency, particularly those with significant contraction of their intravascular volume as occurs with chronic diuretic use or acute hypovolemia, should be monitored closely. NSAIDs can also increase blood pressure in some individuals. Long-term treatment with NSAIDs requires regular blood pressure monitoring and treatment if necessary. Although toxic to the liver when taken in high doses, acetaminophen rarely produces gastric irritation and does not interfere with platelet function.

The introduction of a parenteral form of NSAID, ketorolac, extends the usefulness of this class of compounds in the management of acute severe pain. Ketorolac is sufficiently potent and rapid in onset to supplant opioids for many patients with acute severe headache and musculoskeletal pain.

There are two major classes of COX: COX-1 is constitutively expressed, and COX-2 is induced in the inflammatory state. COX-2–selective drugs have similar analgesic potency and produce less gastric irritation than the nonselective COX inhibitors. The use of COX-2–selective drugs does not appear to lower the risk of nephrotoxicity compared to nonselective NSAIDs. On the other hand, COX-2–selective drugs offer a significant benefit in the management of acute postoperative pain because they do not affect blood coagulation. Nonselective COX inhibitors are usually contraindicated postoperatively because they impair platelet-mediated blood clotting and are thus associated with increased bleeding at the operative site. COX-2 inhibitors, including celecoxib (Celebrex), are associated with increased cardiovascular risk. It is possible that this is a class effect

TABLE 7-1

DRUGS FOR RELIEF OF PAIN

GENERIC NAME	DOSE, mg	INTERVAL	COMMENTS
Nonnarcotic Analgesics: Usual Doses and Intervals			
Acetylsalicylic acid	650 PO	q 4 h	Enteric-coated preparations available
Acetaminophen	650 PO	q 4 h	Side effects uncommon
Ibuprofen	400 PO	q 4–6 h	Available without prescription
Naproxen	250–500 PO	q 12 h	Delayed effects may be due to long half-life
Fenoprofen	200 PO	q 4–6 h	Contraindicated in renal disease
Indomethacin	25–50 PO	q 8 h	Gastrointestinal side effects common
Ketorolac	15–60 IM/IV	q 4–6 h	Available for parenteral use
Celecoxib	100–200 PO	q 12–24 h	Useful for arthritis
Valdecoxib	10–20 PO	q12–24 h	Removed from U.S. market in 2005

GENERIC NAME	PARENTERAL DOSE, mg	PO DOSE, mg	COMMENTS
Narcotic Analgesics: Usual Doses and Intervals			
Codeine	30–60 q 4 h	30–60 q 4 h	Nausea common
Oxycodone	—	5–10 q 4–6 h	Usually available with acetaminophen or aspirin
Morphine	5 q 4 h	30 q 4 h	
Morphine sustained release	—	15–60 bid to tid	Oral slow-release preparation
Hydromorphone	1–2 q 4 h	2–4 q 4 h	Shorter acting than morphine sulfate
Levorphanol	2 q 6–8 h	4 q 6–8 h	Longer acting than morphine sulfate; absorbed well PO
Methadone	5–10 q 6–8 h	5–20 q 6–8 h	Delayed sedation due to long half-life; therapy should not be initiated with greater than 40 mg/day and dose escalation should be made no more frequently than every 3 days
Meperidine	50–100 q 3–4 h	300 q 4 h	Poorly absorbed PO; normeperidine a toxic metabolite; routine use of this agent is not recommended
Butorphanol	—	1–2 q 4 h	Intranasal spray
Fentanyl	25–100 μg/h	—	72-h transdermal patch
Tramadol	—	50–100 q 4–6 h	Mixed opioid/adrenergic action

GENERIC NAME	UPTAKE BLOCKADE 5-HT	UPTAKE BLOCKADE NE	SEDATIVE POTENCY	ANTICHOLINERGIC POTENCY	ORTHOSTATIC HYPOTENSION	CARDIAC ARRHYTHMIA	AVE. DOSE, mg/d	RANGE, mg/d
Antidepressants[a]								
Doxepin	++	+	High	Moderate	Moderate	Less	200	75–400
Amitriptyline	++++	++	High	Highest	Moderate	Yes	150	25–300
Imipramine	++++	++	Moderate	Moderate	High	Yes	200	75–400
Nortriptyline	+++	++	Moderate	Moderate	Low	Yes	100	40–150
Desipramine	+++	++++	Low	Low	Low	Yes	150	50–300
Venlafaxine	+++	++	Low	None	None	No	150	75–400
Duloxetine	+++	+++	Low	None	None	No	40	30–60

GENERIC NAME	PO DOSE, mg	INTERVAL	GENERIC NAME	PO DOSE, mg	INTERVAL
Anticonvulsants and Antiarrhythmics[a]					
Phenytoin	300	daily/qhs	Clonazepam	1	q 6 h
Carbamazepine	200–300	q 6 h	Gabapentin[b]	600–1200	q 8 h
Oxcarbazepine	300	bid	Pregabalin	150–600	bid

[a]Antidepressants, anticonvulsants, and antiarrhythmics have not been approved by the U.S. Food and Drug Administration (FDA) for the treatment of pain.

[b]Gabapentin in doses up to 1800 mg/d is FDA approved for postherpetic neuralgia.

Note: 5-HT, serotonin; NE, norepinephrine.

of NSAIDs, excluding aspirin. These drugs are contraindicated in patients in the immediate period after coronary artery bypass surgery and should be used with caution in patients with a history of or significant risk factors for cardiovascular disease.

OPIOID ANALGESICS Opioids are the most potent pain-relieving drugs currently available. Of all analgesics, they have the broadest range of efficacy and provide the most reliable and effective method for rapid pain relief. Although side effects are common, most are reversible: nausea, vomiting, pruritus, and constipation are the most frequent and bothersome side effects. Respiratory depression is uncommon at standard analgesic doses, but can be life-threatening. Opioid-related side effects can be reversed rapidly with the narcotic antagonist naloxone. The physician should not hesitate to use opioid analgesics in patients with acute severe pain. Table 7-1 lists the most commonly used opioid analgesics.

Opioids produce analgesia by actions in the CNS. They activate pain-inhibitory neurons and directly inhibit pain-transmission neurons. Most of the commercially available opioid analgesics act at the same opioid receptor (μ-receptor), differing mainly in potency, speed of onset, duration of action, and optimal route of administration. Some side effects are due to accumulation of nonopioid metabolites that are unique to individual drugs. One striking example of this is normeperidine, a metabolite of meperidine. Normeperidine produces hyperexcitability and seizures that are not reversible with naloxone. Normeperidine accumulation is increased in patients with renal failure.

The most rapid relief with opioids is obtained by intravenous administration; relief with oral administration is significantly slower. Common side effects include nausea, vomiting, constipation, and sedation. The most serious side effect is respiratory depression. Patients with any form of respiratory compromise must be kept under close observation following opioid administration; an oxygen-saturation monitor may be useful. Opioid-induced respiratory depression is typically accompanied by significant sedation and a reduction in respiratory rate. A fall in oxygen saturation represents a critical level of respiratory depression and the need for immediate intervention to prevent life-threatening hypoxemia. Ventilatory assistance should be maintained until the opioid-induced respiratory depression has resolved. The opioid antagonist naloxone should be readily available whenever opioids are used at high doses or in patients with compromised pulmonary function. Opioid effects are dose-related, and there is great variability among patients in the doses that relieve pain and produce side effects. Because of this, initiation of therapy requires titration to optimal dose and interval. The most important principle is to provide adequate pain relief. This requires determining whether the drug has adequately relieved the pain and frequent reassessment to determine the optimal interval for dosing. *The most common error made by physicians in managing severe pain with opioids is to prescribe an inadequate dose. Because many patients are reluctant to complain, this practice leads to needless suffering.* In the absence of sedation at the expected time of peak effect, a physician should not hesitate to repeat the initial dose to achieve satisfactory pain relief.

An innovative approach to the problem of achieving adequate pain relief is the use of patient-controlled analgesia (PCA). PCA uses a microprocessor-controlled infusion device that can deliver a baseline continuous dose of an opioid drug as well as preprogrammed additional doses whenever the patient pushes a button. The patient can then titrate the dose to the optimal level. This approach is used most extensively for the management of postoperative pain, but there is no reason why it should not be used for any hospitalized patient with persistent severe pain. PCA is also used for short-term home care of patients with intractable pain, such as that caused by metastatic cancer.

It is important to understand that the PCA device delivers small, repeated doses to maintain pain relief; in patients with severe pain, the pain must first be brought under control with a loading dose before transitioning to the PCA device. The bolus dose of the drug (typically 1 mg morphine, 0.2 mg hydromorphone, or 10 μg fentanyl) can then be delivered repeatedly as needed. To prevent overdosing, PCA devices are programmed with a lockout period after each demand dose is delivered (5–10 min) and a limit on the total dose delivered per hour. While some have advocated the use of a simultaneous continuous or basal infusion of the PCA drug, this increases the risk of respiratory depression and has not been shown to increase the overall efficacy of the technique.

Many physicians, nurses, and patients have a certain trepidation about using opioids that is based on an exaggerated fear of addiction. In fact, there is a vanishingly small chance of patients becoming addicted to narcotics as a result of their appropriate medical use.

The availability of new routes of administration has extended the usefulness of opioid analgesics. Most important is the availability of spinal administration. Opioids can be infused through a spinal catheter placed either intrathecally or epidurally. By applying opioids directly to the spinal or epidural space adjacent to the spinal cord, regional analgesia can be obtained using relatively low total doses. Indeed, the dose required to produce effective localized analgesia when using morphine intrathecally (0.1–0.3 mg) is a fraction of that required to produce similar analgesia when administered intravenously (5–10 mg). In this way, side effects such as sedation, nausea, and respiratory depression can be minimized. This approach has been used extensively in obstetric procedures and for postoperative pain relief following surgical procedures on the lower extremities. Continuous intrathecal delivery via implanted spinal drug-delivery systems is now commonly used, particularly for the treatment of cancer-related pain that would require sedating doses for adequate pain control if given systemically. Opioids can also be given intranasally (butorphanol), rectally, and transdermally (fentanyl), thus avoiding the discomfort of frequent injections in patients who cannot be given oral medication. The fentanyl transdermal patch has the advantage of providing fairly steady plasma levels, which maximizes patient comfort.

Recent additions to the armamentarium for treating opioid-induced side effects are the peripherally acting opioid antagonists alvimopan (Entereg) and methylnaltrexone (Rellistor). Alvimopan is available as an orally administered agent that is restricted to the intestinal lumen by limited absorption; methylnaltrexone is available in a subcutaneously administered form that has virtually no penetration into the CNS. Both agents act by binding to peripheral μ-receptors, thereby inhibiting or reversing the effects of opioids at these peripheral sites. The action of both agents is restricted to receptor sites outside of the CNS; thus, these drugs can reverse the adverse effects of opioid analgesics that are mediated through their peripheral receptors without reversing their analgesic effects. Both agents are effective for persistent ileus following abdominal surgery to the extent that opioid analgesics used for postoperative pain control contribute to this serious problem. Likewise, both agents have been tested for their effectiveness in treating opioid-induced bowel dysfunction (constipation) in patients taking opioid analgesics on a chronic basis. Although contradictory, the weight of evidence indicates that alvimopan can reduce the incidence and duration of ileus following major abdominal surgery and methylnaltrexone can produce rapid reversal of constipation in many patients receiving opioids on a chronic basis.

Opioid and COX Inhibitor Combinations

When used in combination, opioids and COX inhibitors have additive effects. Because a lower dose of each can be used to achieve the same degree of pain relief and their side effects are nonadditive, such combinations are used to lower the severity of dose-related side effects. However, fixed-ratio combinations of an opioid with acetaminophen carry a special risk. Dose escalation as a result of increased severity of pain or decreased opioid effect as a result of tolerance may lead to levels of acetaminophen that are toxic to the liver. Although acetaminophen-related hepatotoxicity is uncommon, it remains a leading cause for liver failure. Thus, many practitioners have moved away from the use of opioid-acetaminophen combination analgesics to avoid the risk of excessive acetaminophen exposure as the dose of the analgesic is escalated.

CHRONIC PAIN

Managing patients with chronic pain is intellectually and emotionally challenging. The patient's problem is often difficult or impossible to diagnose with certainty; such patients are demanding of the physician's time and often appear emotionally distraught. The traditional medical approach of seeking an obscure organic pathology is usually unhelpful. On the other hand, psychological evaluation and behaviorally based treatment paradigms are frequently helpful, particularly in the setting of a multidisciplinary pain-management center. Unfortunately, this approach, while effective, remains largely underused in current medical practice.

There are several factors that can cause, perpetuate, or exacerbate chronic pain. First, of course, the patient may simply have a disease that is characteristically painful for which there is presently no cure. Arthritis, cancer, chronic daily headaches, fibromyalgia, and diabetic neuropathy are examples of this. Second, there may be secondary perpetuating factors that are initiated by disease and persist after that disease has resolved. Examples include damaged sensory nerves, sympathetic efferent activity, and painful reflex muscle contraction. Finally, a variety of psychological conditions can exacerbate or even cause pain.

There are certain areas to which special attention should be paid in a patient's medical history. Because depression is the most common emotional disturbance in patients with chronic pain, patients should be questioned about their mood, appetite, sleep patterns, and daily activity. A simple standardized questionnaire, such as the Beck Depression Inventory, can be a useful screening device. It is important to remember that major depression is a common, treatable, and potentially fatal illness.

Other clues that a significant emotional disturbance is contributing to a patient's chronic pain complaint include pain that occurs in multiple, unrelated sites; a pattern of recurrent, but separate, pain problems beginning in childhood or adolescence; pain beginning at a time of emotional trauma, such as the loss of a parent or spouse; a history of physical or sexual abuse; and past or present substance abuse.

On examination, special attention should be paid to whether the patient guards the painful area and whether certain movements or postures are avoided because of pain. Discovering a mechanical component to the pain can be useful both diagnostically and therapeutically. Painful areas should be examined for deep tenderness, noting whether this is localized to muscle, ligamentous structures, or joints. Chronic myofascial pain is very common, and, in these patients, deep palpation may reveal highly localized trigger points that are firm bands or knots in muscle. Relief of the pain following injection of local anesthetic into these trigger points supports the diagnosis. A neuropathic component to the pain is indicated by evidence of nerve damage, such as sensory impairment, exquisitely sensitive skin, weakness, and muscle atrophy, or loss of deep tendon reflexes. Evidence suggesting sympathetic nervous system involvement includes the presence of diffuse swelling, changes in skin color and temperature, and hypersensitive skin and joint tenderness compared with the normal side. Relief of the pain with a sympathetic block is diagnostic.

A guiding principle in evaluating patients with chronic pain is to assess both emotional and organic factors before initiating therapy. Addressing these issues together, rather than waiting to address emotional issues after organic causes of pain have been ruled out, improves compliance in part because it assures patients that a psychological evaluation does not mean that the physician is questioning the validity of their complaint. Even when an organic cause for a patient's pain can be found, it is still wise to look for other factors. For example, a cancer patient with painful bony metastases may have additional pain due to nerve damage and may also be depressed. Optimal therapy requires that each of these factors be looked for and treated.

TREATMENT Chronic Pain

Once the evaluation process has been completed and the likely causative and exacerbating factors identified, an explicit treatment plan should be developed. An important part of this process is to identify specific and realistic functional goals for therapy, such as getting a good night's sleep, being able to go shopping, or returning to work. A multidisciplinary approach that uses medications, counseling, physical therapy, nerve blocks, and even surgery may be required to improve the patient's quality of life. There are also some newer, relatively invasive procedures that can be helpful for some patients with intractable pain. These include image-guided interventions such as epidural injection of glucocorticoids for acute radicular pain, radiofrequency treatment of the facet joints for chronic facet-related pain, percutaneous intradiscal treatments for both axial and radicular pain, and placement of implanted intraspinal electrodes and implantation of intrathecal drug-delivery systems for severe and persistent pain that is unresponsive to more conservative treatments. There are no set criteria for predicting which patients will respond to these procedures. They are generally reserved for patients who have not responded to conventional pharmacologic approaches. Referral to a multidisciplinary pain clinic for a full evaluation should precede any invasive procedures. Such referrals are clearly not necessary for all chronic pain patients. For some, pharmacologic management alone can provide adequate relief.

TABLE 7-2

PAINFUL CONDITIONS THAT RESPOND TO TRICYCLIC ANTIDEPRESSANTS

Postherpetic neuralgia[a]
Diabetic neuropathy[a]
Tension headache[a]
Migraine headache[a]
Rheumatoid arthritis[a,b]
Chronic low back pain[b]
Cancer
Central post-stroke pain

[a]Controlled trials demonstrate analgesia.
[b]Controlled studies indicate benefit but not analgesia.

ANTIDEPRESSANT MEDICATIONS The tricyclic antidepressants (TCAs), particularly nortriptyline and desipramine (Table 7-1), are useful for the management of chronic pain. Although developed for the treatment of depression, the TCAs have a spectrum of dose-related biologic activities that include analgesia in a variety of chronic clinical conditions. Although the mechanism is unknown, the analgesic effect of TCAs has a more rapid onset and occurs at a lower dose than is typically required for the treatment of depression. Furthermore, patients with chronic pain who are not depressed obtain pain relief with antidepressants. There is evidence that TCAs potentiate opioid analgesia, so they may be useful adjuncts for the treatment of severe persistent pain such as occurs with malignant tumors. Table 7-2 lists some of the painful conditions that respond to TCAs. TCAs are of particular value in the management of neuropathic pain such as occurs in diabetic neuropathy and postherpetic neuralgia, for which there are few other therapeutic options.

The TCAs that have been shown to relieve pain have significant side effects (Table 7-1; Chap. 53). Some of these side effects, such as orthostatic hypotension, drowsiness, cardiac-conduction delay, memory impairment, constipation, and urinary retention, are particularly problematic in elderly patients, and several are additive to the side effects of opioid analgesics. The selective serotonin reuptake inhibitors such as fluoxetine (Prozac) have fewer and less serious side effects than TCAs, but they are much less effective for relieving pain. It is of interest that venlafaxine (Effexor) and duloxetine (Cymbalta), which are nontricyclic antidepressants that block both serotonin and norepinephrine reuptake, appear to retain most of the pain-relieving effect of TCAs with a side-effect profile more like that of the selective serotonin reuptake inhibitors. These drugs may be particularly useful in patients who cannot tolerate the side effects of TCAs.

ANTICONVULSANTS AND ANTIARRHYTHMICS These drugs are useful primarily for patients with neuropathic pain. Phenytoin (Dilantin) and carbamazepine (Tegretol) were first shown to relieve the pain of trigeminal neuralgia. This pain has a characteristic brief, shooting, electric shock–like quality. In fact, anticonvulsants seem to be particularly helpful for pains that have such a lancinating quality. Newer anticonvulsants, gabapentin (Neurontin) and pregabalin (Lyrica), are effective for a broad range of neuropathic pains. Furthermore, because of their favorable side-effect profile, these newer anticonvulsants are often used as first-line agents.

CHRONIC OPIOID MEDICATION The long-term use of opioids is accepted for patients with pain due to malignant disease. Although opioid use for chronic pain of nonmalignant origin is controversial, it is clear that for many such patients, opioid analgesics are the best available option. This is understandable because opioids are the most potent and have the broadest range of efficacy of any analgesic medications. Although addiction is rare in patients who first use opioids for pain relief, some degree of tolerance and physical dependence is likely with long-term use. Therefore, before embarking on opioid therapy, other options should be explored, and the limitations and risks of opioids should be explained to the patient. It is also important to point out that some opioid analgesic medications have mixed agonist-antagonist properties (e.g., pentazocine and butorphanol). From a practical standpoint, this means that they may worsen pain by inducing an abstinence syndrome in patients who are physically dependent on other opioid analgesics.

With long-term outpatient use of orally administered opioids, it is desirable to use long-acting compounds such as levorphanol, methadone, or sustained-release morphine (Table 7-1). Transdermal fentanyl is another excellent option. The pharmacokinetic profile of these drug preparations enables prolonged pain relief, minimizes side effects such as sedation that are associated with high peak plasma levels, and reduces the likelihood of rebound pain associated with a rapid fall in plasma opioid concentration. While long-acting opioid preparations may provide superior pain relief in patients with a continuous pattern of ongoing pain, others suffer from intermittent severe episodic pain and experience superior pain control and fewer side effects with the periodic use of short-acting opioid analgesics. Constipation is a virtually universal side effect of opioid use and should be treated expectantly. A recent advance for patients with chronic debilitating conditions is the development of methylnaltrexone, a peripherally acting mu opioid antagonist that blocks the constipation and itching associated with chronic opioid use without interfering with analgesia; the usual dose is 0.15 mg/kg of body weight given subcutaneously no more often than once daily.

TREATMENT OF NEUROPATHIC PAIN It is important to individualize treatment for patients with neuropathic pain. Several general principles should guide therapy: the first is to move quickly to provide relief, and the second is to minimize drug side effects. For example, in patients with postherpetic neuralgia and significant cutaneous hypersensitivity, topical lidocaine (Lidoderm patches) can provide immediate relief without side effects. Anticonvulsants (gabapentin or pregabalin, see above) or antidepressants (nortriptyline, desipramine, duloxetine, or venlafaxine) can be used as first-line drugs for patients with neuropathic pain. Systemically administered antiarrhythmic drugs such as lidocaine and mexiletene are less likely to be effective; although intravenous infusion of lidocaine predictably provides analgesia in those with many forms of neuropathic pain, the relief is usually transient, typically lasting just hours after the cessation of the infusion. The oral lidocaine congener mexiletene is poorly tolerated, producing frequent gastrointestinal adverse effects. There is no consensus on which class of drug should be used as a first-line treatment for any chronically painful condition. However, because relatively high doses of anticonvulsants are required for pain relief, sedation is very common. Sedation is also a problem with TCAs but is much less of a problem with serotonin/norepinephrine reuptake inhibitors (SNRIs, e.g., venlafaxine and duloxetine). Thus, in the elderly or in those patients whose daily activities require high-level mental activity, these drugs should be considered the first line. In contrast, opioid medications should be used as a second- or third-line drug class. While highly effective for many painful conditions, opioids are sedating, and their effect tends to lessen over time, leading to dose escalation and, occasionally, a worsening of pain due to physical dependence. Drugs of different classes can be used in combination to optimize pain control.

It is worth emphasizing that many patients, especially those with chronic pain, seek medical attention primarily because they are suffering and because only physicians can provide the medications required for pain relief. A primary responsibility of all physicians is to minimize the physical and emotional discomfort of their patients. Familiarity with pain mechanisms and analgesic medications is an important step toward accomplishing this aim.

CHAPTER 8

HEADACHE

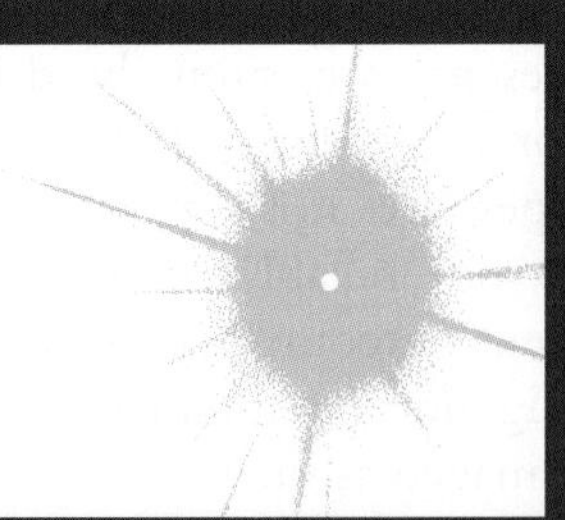

Peter J. Goadsby ■ Neil H. Raskin

Headache is among the most common reasons patients seek medical attention. Diagnosis and management are based on a careful clinical approach augmented by an understanding of the anatomy, physiology, and pharmacology of the nervous system pathways that mediate the various headache syndromes.

GENERAL PRINCIPLES

A classification system developed by the International Headache Society characterizes headache as primary or secondary (Table 8-1). *Primary headaches* are those in which headache and its associated features are the disorder in itself, whereas *secondary headaches* are those caused by exogenous disorders. Primary headache often results in considerable disability and a decrease in the patient's quality of life. Mild secondary headache, such as that seen in association with upper respiratory tract infections, is common but rarely worrisome. Life-threatening headache is relatively uncommon, but vigilance is required in order to recognize and appropriately treat such patients.

TABLE 8-1

COMMON CAUSES OF HEADACHE

PRIMARY HEADACHE		SECONDARY HEADACHE	
TYPE	%	TYPE	%
Tension-type	69	Systemic infection	63
Migraine	16	Head injury	4
Idiopathic stabbing	2	Vascular disorders	1
Exertional	1	Subarachnoid hemorrhage	<1
Cluster	0.1	Brain tumor	0.1

Source: After J Olesen et al: *The Headaches*. Philadelphia, Lippincott, Williams & Wilkins, 2005.

ANATOMY AND PHYSIOLOGY OF HEADACHE

Pain usually occurs when peripheral nociceptors are stimulated in response to tissue injury, visceral distension, or other factors (Chap. 7). In such situations, pain perception is a normal physiologic response mediated by a healthy nervous system. Pain can also result when pain-producing pathways of the peripheral or central nervous system (CNS) are damaged or activated inappropriately. Headache may originate from either or both mechanisms. Relatively few cranial structures are pain-producing; these include the scalp, middle meningeal artery, dural sinuses, falx cerebri, and proximal segments of the large pial arteries. The ventricular ependyma, choroid plexus, pial veins, and much of the brain parenchyma are not pain-producing.

The key structures involved in primary headache appear to be

- the large intracranial vessels and dura mater and the peripheral terminals of the trigeminal nerve that innervate these structures
- the caudal portion of the trigeminal nucleus, which extends into the dorsal horns of the upper cervical spinal cord and receives input from the first and second cervical nerve roots (the trigeminocervical complex)
- rostral pain-processing regions, such as the ventroposteromedial thalamus and the cortex
- the pain-modulatory systems in the brain that modulate input from trigeminal nociceptors at all levels of the pain-processing pathways

The innervation of the large intracranial vessels and dura mater by the trigeminal nerve is known as the *trigeminovascular system*. Cranial autonomic symptoms, such as *lacrimation* and *nasal congestion*, are prominent in the trigeminal autonomic cephalalgias, including cluster headache and paroxysmal hemicrania, and may also be seen in migraine. These autonomic symptoms reflect activation of cranial parasympathetic pathways, and functional imaging studies indicate that vascular changes in migraine and cluster headache, when present, are similarly driven by these cranial autonomic systems. Migraine and other primary headache types are not "vascular headaches"; these disorders do not reliably manifest vascular changes, and treatment outcomes cannot be predicted by vascular effects. Migraine is a brain disorder, and best understood and managed as such.

CLINICAL EVALUATION OF ACUTE, NEW-ONSET HEADACHE

The patient who presents with a new, severe headache has a differential diagnosis that is quite different from the patient with recurrent headaches over many years. In new-onset and severe headache, the probability of finding a potentially serious cause is considerably greater than in recurrent headache. Patients with recent onset of pain require prompt evaluation and appropriate treatment. Serious causes to be considered include meningitis, subarachnoid hemorrhage, epidural or subdural hematoma, glaucoma, tumor, and purulent sinusitis. When worrisome symptoms and signs are present (Table 8-2), rapid diagnosis and management are critical.

A complete neurologic examination is an essential first step in the evaluation. In most cases, patients with an abnormal examination or a history of recent-onset headache should be evaluated by a CT or MRI study. As an initial screening procedure for intracranial pathology in this setting, CT and MRI methods appear to be equally sensitive. In some circumstances, a lumbar puncture (LP) is also required, unless a benign etiology can be otherwise established. A general evaluation of acute headache might include the investigation of cardiovascular and renal status by blood pressure monitoring and urine examination; eyes by funduscopy, intraocular pressure measurement, and refraction; cranial arteries by palpation; and cervical spine by the effect of passive movement of the head and by imaging.

The psychological state of the patient should also be evaluated since a relationship exists between head pain and depression. Many patients in chronic daily pain cycles become depressed, although depression itself is rarely a cause of headache. Drugs with antidepressant actions are also effective in the prophylactic treatment of both tension-type headache and migraine.

Underlying recurrent headache disorders may be activated by pain that follows otologic or endodontic surgical procedures. Thus, pain about the head as the result of diseased tissue or trauma may reawaken an otherwise quiescent migrainous syndrome. Treatment of the headache is largely ineffective until the cause of the primary problem is addressed.

Serious underlying conditions that are associated with headache are described next. Brain tumor is a rare cause of headache and even less commonly a cause of severe pain. The vast majority of patients presenting with severe headache have a benign cause.

TABLE 8-2

HEADACHE SYMPTOMS THAT SUGGEST A SERIOUS UNDERLYING DISORDER
"Worst" headache ever
First severe headache
Subacute worsening over days or weeks
Abnormal neurologic examination
Fever or unexplained systemic signs
Vomiting that precedes headache
Pain induced by bending, lifting, cough
Pain that disturbs sleep or presents immediately upon awakening
Known systemic illness
Onset after age 55
Pain associated with local tenderness, e.g., region of temporal artery

SECONDARY HEADACHE

The management of secondary headache focuses on diagnosis and treatment of the underlying condition.

MENINGITIS

Acute, severe headache with stiff neck and fever suggests meningitis. Lumbar puncture is mandatory. Often there is striking accentuation of pain with eye movement. Meningitis can be easily mistaken for migraine in that the cardinal symptoms of pounding headache, photophobia, nausea, and vomiting are frequently present, perhaps reflecting the underlying biology of some of the patients.

Meningitis is discussed in Chaps. 40 and 41.

INTRACRANIAL HEMORRHAGE

Acute, severe headache with stiff neck but without fever suggests subarachnoid hemorrhage. A ruptured aneurysm, arteriovenous malformation, or intraparenchymal hemorrhage may also present with headache alone. Rarely, if the hemorrhage is small or below the foramen magnum, the head CT scan can be normal.

Therefore, lumbar puncture may be required to diagnose definitively subarachnoid hemorrhage.

Intracranial hemorrhage is discussed in Chap. 28.

BRAIN TUMOR

Approximately 30% of patients with brain tumors consider headache to be their chief complaint. The head pain is usually nondescript—an intermittent deep, dull aching of moderate intensity, which may worsen with exertion or change in position and may be associated with nausea and vomiting. This pattern of symptoms results from migraine far more often than from brain tumor. The headache of brain tumor disturbs sleep in about 10% of patients. Vomiting that precedes the appearance of headache by weeks is highly characteristic of posterior fossa brain tumors. A history of amenorrhea or galactorrhea should lead one to question whether a prolactin-secreting pituitary adenoma (or the polycystic ovary syndrome) is the source of headache. Headache arising de novo in a patient with known malignancy suggests either cerebral metastases or carcinomatous meningitis, or both. Head pain appearing abruptly after bending, lifting, or coughing can be due to a posterior fossa mass, a Chiari malformation, or low CSF volume.

Brain tumors are discussed in Chap. 37.

TEMPORAL ARTERITIS

(See also Chap. 21) Temporal (giant cell) arteritis is an inflammatory disorder of arteries that frequently involves the extracranial carotid circulation. It is a common disorder of the elderly; its annual incidence is 77 per 100,000 individuals age 50 and older. The average age of onset is 70 years, and women account for 65% of cases. About half of patients with untreated temporal arteritis develop blindness due to involvement of the ophthalmic artery and its branches; indeed, the ischemic optic neuropathy induced by giant cell arteritis is the major cause of rapidly developing bilateral blindness in patients >60 years. Because treatment with glucocorticoids is effective in preventing this complication, prompt recognition of the disorder is important.

Typical presenting symptoms include headache, polymyalgia rheumatica, jaw claudication, fever, and weight loss. Headache is the dominant symptom and often appears in association with malaise and muscle aches. Head pain may be unilateral or bilateral and is located temporally in 50% of patients but may involve any and all aspects of the cranium. Pain usually appears gradually over a few hours before peak intensity is reached; occasionally, it is explosive in onset. The quality of pain is only seldom throbbing; it is almost invariably described as dull and boring, with superimposed episodic stabbing pains similar to the sharp pains that appear in migraine. Most patients can recognize that the origin of their head pain is superficial, external to the skull, rather than originating deep within the cranium (the pain site for migraineurs). Scalp tenderness is present, often to a marked degree; brushing the hair or resting the head on a pillow may be impossible because of pain. Headache is usually worse at night and often aggravated by exposure to cold. Additional findings may include reddened, tender nodules or red streaking of the skin overlying the temporal arteries, and tenderness of the temporal or, less commonly, the occipital arteries.

The erythrocyte sedimentation rate (ESR) is often, though not always, elevated; a normal ESR does not exclude giant cell arteritis. A temporal artery biopsy followed by immediate treatment with prednisone 80 mg daily for the first 4–6 weeks should be initiated when clinical suspicion is high. The prevalence of migraine among the elderly is substantial, considerably higher than that of giant cell arteritis. Migraineurs often report amelioration of their headaches with prednisone; thus, caution must be used when interpreting the therapeutic response.

GLAUCOMA

Glaucoma may present with a prostrating headache associated with nausea and vomiting. The headache often starts with severe eye pain. On physical examination, the eye is often red with a fixed, moderately dilated pupil.

Glaucoma is discussed in Chap. 21.

PRIMARY HEADACHE SYNDROMES

Primary headaches are disorders in which headache and associated features occur in the absence of any exogenous cause (Table 8-1). The most common are migraine, tension-type headache, and cluster headache.

MIGRAINE

Migraine, the second most common cause of headache, afflicts approximately 15% of women and 6% of men over a 1-year period. It is usually an episodic headache associated with certain features such as sensitivity to light, sound, or movement; nausea and vomiting often accompany the headache. A useful description of migraine is a benign and recurring syndrome of headache associated with other symptoms of neurologic dysfunction in varying admixtures (Table 8-3). Migraine can often be recognized by its activators, referred to as *triggers*.

The brain of the migraineur is particularly sensitive to environmental and sensory stimuli; migraine-prone patients do not habituate easily to sensory stimuli.

TABLE 8-3

SYMPTOMS ACCOMPANYING SEVERE MIGRAINE ATTACKS IN 500 PATIENTS

SYMPTOM	PATIENTS AFFECTED, %
Nausea	87
Photophobia	82
Lightheadedness	72
Scalp tenderness	65
Vomiting	56
Visual disturbances	36
Paresthesias	33
Vertigo	33
Photopsia	26
Alteration of consciousness	18
Diarrhea	16
Fortification spectra	10
Syncope	10
Seizure	4
Confusional state	4

Source: From NH Raskin, *Headache*, 2nd ed. New York, Churchill Livingston, 1988; with permission.

This sensitivity is amplified in females during the menstrual cycle. Headache can be initiated or amplified by various triggers, including glare, bright lights, sounds, or other afferent stimulation; hunger; excess stress; physical exertion; stormy weather or barometric pressure changes; hormonal fluctuations during menses; lack of or excess sleep; and alcohol or other chemical stimulation. Knowledge of a patient's susceptibility to specific triggers can be useful in management strategies involving lifestyle adjustments.

Pathogenesis

The sensory sensitivity that is characteristic of migraine is probably due to dysfunction of monoaminergic sensory control systems located in the brainstem and thalamus (Fig. 8-1).

Activation of cells in the trigeminal nucleus results in the release of vasoactive neuropeptides, particularly calcitonin gene–related peptide (CGRP), at vascular terminations of the trigeminal nerve and within the trigeminal nucleus. CGRP receptor antagonists have now been shown to be effective in the acute treatment of migraine. Centrally, the second-order trigeminal neurons cross the midline and project to ventrobasal and posterior nuclei of the thalamus for further processing. Additionally, there are projections to the periaqueductal gray and hypothalamus, from which reciprocal descending systems have established antinociceptive effects. Other brainstem regions likely to be involved in descending modulation of trigeminal pain include the nucleus locus coeruleus in the pons and the rostroventromedial medulla.

Pharmacologic and other data point to the involvement of the neurotransmitter 5-hydroxytryptamine (5-HT; also known as serotonin) in migraine. Approximately 60 years ago, methysergide was found to antagonize certain peripheral actions of 5-HT and was introduced as the first drug capable of preventing migraine attacks. The triptans are designed to selectively stimulate subpopulations of 5-HT receptors; at least 14 different 5-HT receptors exist in humans. The triptans are potent agonists of 5-HT_{1B}, 5-HT_{1D}, and 5-HT_{1F} receptors and are less potent at the 5-HT_{1A} receptor. A growing body of data indicates that the antimigraine efficacy of the triptans relates to their ability to stimulate 5-$HT_{1B/1D}$ receptors, which are located on both blood vessels and nerve terminals. Separately, it has now been shown that selective 5-HT_{1F} receptor activation, which has a purely neural effect, can terminate acute migraine.

Data also support a role for dopamine in the pathophysiology of migraine. Most migraine symptoms can be induced by dopaminergic stimulation. Moreover, there is dopamine receptor hypersensitivity in migraineurs, as demonstrated by the induction of yawning, nausea, vomiting, hypotension, and other symptoms of a migraine attack by dopaminergic agonists at doses that do not affect nonmigraineurs. Dopamine receptor antagonists are effective therapeutic agents in migraine, especially when given parenterally or concurrently with other antimigraine agents.

Migraine genes identified by studying families with familial hemiplegic migraine (FHM) reveal involvement of ion channels, suggesting that alterations in membrane excitability can predispose to migraine. Mutations involving the $Ca_v2.1$ (P/Q)–type voltage-gated calcium channel *CACNA1A* gene are now known to cause FHM 1; this mutation is responsible for about 50% of FHM. Mutations in the Na^+-K^+ATPase *ATP1A2* gene, designated FHM 2, are responsible for about 20% of FHM. Mutations in the neuronal voltage-gated sodium channel *SCN1A* cause FHM 3. Functional neuroimaging has suggested that brainstem regions in migraine (Fig. 8-2) and the posterior hypothalamic gray matter region close to the human circadian pacemaker cells of the suprachiasmatic nucleus in cluster headache (Fig. 8-3) are good candidates for specific involvement in primary headache.

Diagnosis and clinical features

Diagnostic criteria for migraine headache are listed in Table 8-4. A high index of suspicion is required to diagnose migraine: the migraine aura, consisting of visual disturbances with flashing lights or zigzag lines

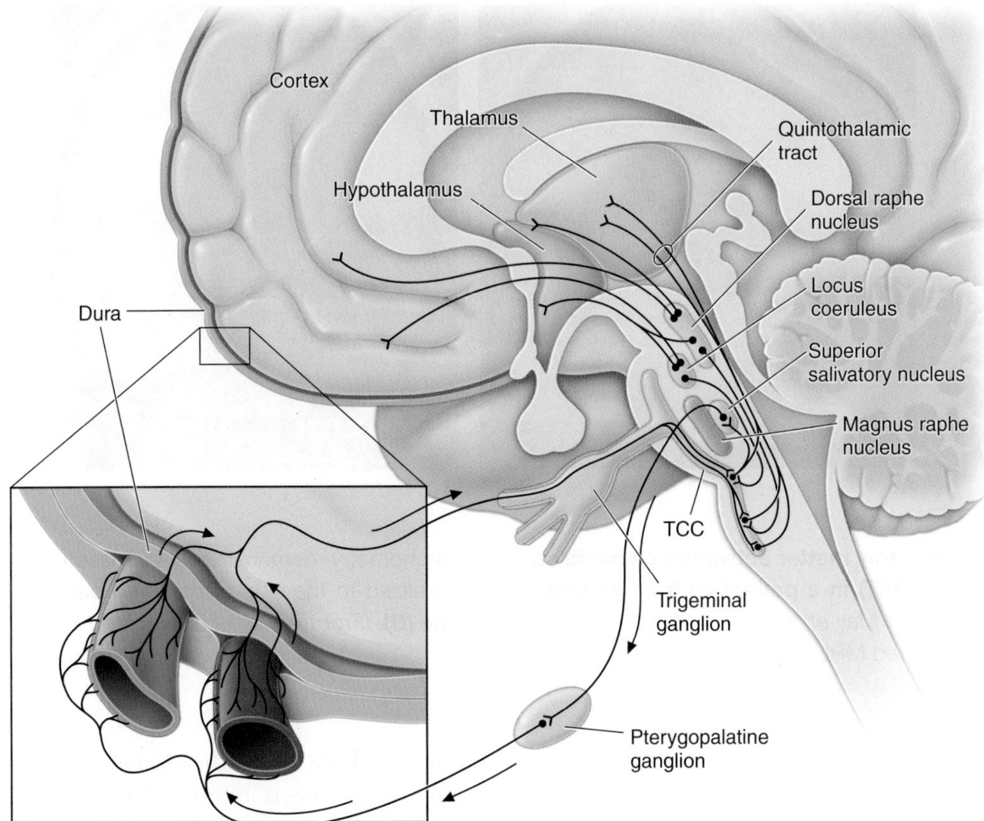

FIGURE 8-1

Brainstem pathways that modulate sensory input. The key pathway for pain in migraine is the trigeminovascular input from the meningeal vessels, which passes through the trigeminal ganglion and synapses on second-order neurons in the trigeminocervical complex (TCC). These neurons in turn project in the quintothalamic tract and, after decussating in the brainstem, synapse on neurons in the thalamus. Important modulation of the trigeminovascular nociceptive input comes from the dorsal raphe nucleus, locus coeruleus, and nucleus raphe magnus.

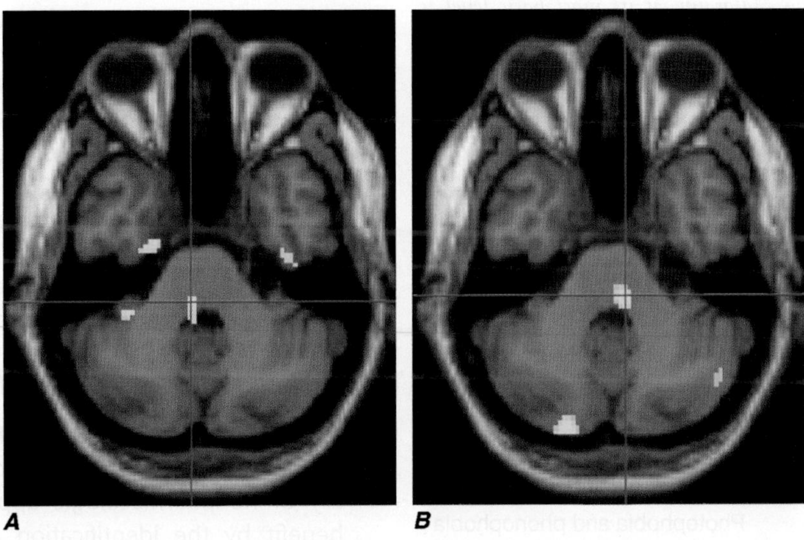

FIGURE 8-2

Positron emission tomography (PET) activation in migraine. In spontaneous attacks of episodic migraine there is activation of the region of the dorsolateral pons; an identical pattern is found in chronic migraine (not shown). This area, which includes the noradrenergic locus coeruleus, is fundamental to the expression of migraine. Moreover, lateralization of changes in this region of the brainstem correlates with lateralization of the head pain in hemicranial migraine; the scans shown in panels ***A*** and ***B*** are of patients with acute migraine headache on the right and left side, respectively. (*From S Afridi et al: Brain 128:932, 2005.*)

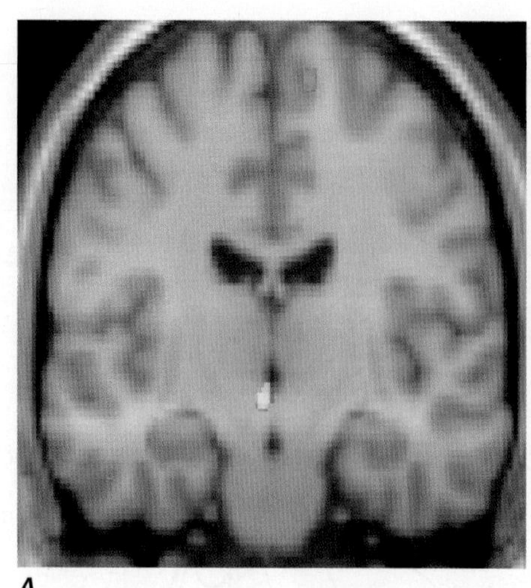

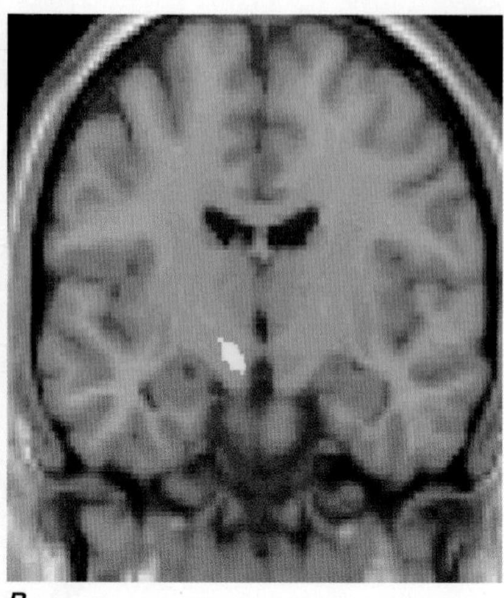

FIGURE 8-3

Posterior hypothalamic gray matter activation on positron emission tomography (PET) in a patient with acute cluster headache *(A)*. (*From A May et al: Lancet 352:275, 1998.*) High-resolution T1-weighted MRI obtained using voxel-based morphometry demonstrates increased gray matter activity, lateralized to the side of pain in a patient with cluster headache ***(B)***. (*From A May et al: Nat Med 5:836, 1999.*)

moving across the visual field or of other neurologic symptoms, is reported in only 20–25% of patients. A headache diary can often be helpful in making the diagnosis; this is also helpful in assessing disability and the frequency of treatment for acute attacks. Patients with episodes of migraine that occur daily or near-daily are considered to have chronic migraine (see "Chronic Daily Headache," later in this chapter). Migraine must be differentiated from tension-type headache (discussed later), the most common primary headache syndrome seen in clinical practice. *Migraine at its most basic level is headache with associated features, and tension-type headache is headache that is featureless. Most patients with disabling headache probably have migraine.*

Patients with acephalgic migraine experience recurrent neurologic symptoms, often with nausea or vomiting, but with little or no headache. Vertigo can be prominent; it has been estimated that one-third of patients referred for vertigo or dizziness have a primary diagnosis of migraine.

TABLE 8-4

SIMPLIFIED DIAGNOSTIC CRITERIA FOR MIGRAINE

Repeated attacks of headache lasting 4–72 h in patients with a normal physical examination, no other reasonable cause for the headache, and:

AT LEAST 2 OF THE FOLLOWING FEATURES:	PLUS AT LEAST 1 OF THE FOLLOWING FEATURES:
Unilateral pain	Nausea/vomiting
Throbbing pain	Photophobia and phonophobia
Aggravation by movement	
Moderate or severe intensity	

Source: Adapted from the International Headache Society Classification (Headache Classification Committee of the International Headache Society, 2004).

TREATMENT Migraine Headaches

Once a diagnosis of migraine has been established, it is important to assess the extent of a patient's disease and disability. The Migraine Disability Assessment Score (MIDAS) is a well-validated, easy-to-use tool (Fig. 8-4).

Patient education is an important aspect of migraine management. Information for patients is available at *www.achenet.org*, the website of the American Council for Headache Education (ACHE). It is helpful for patients to understand that migraine is an inherited tendency to headache; that migraine can be modified and controlled by lifestyle adjustments and medications, but it cannot be eradicated; and that, except in some occasions in women on oral estrogens or contraceptives, migraine is not associated with serious or life-threatening illnesses.

NONPHARMACOLOGIC MANAGEMENT Migraine can often be managed to some degree by a variety of nonpharmacologic approaches. Most patients benefit by the identification and avoidance of specific headache triggers. A regulated lifestyle is helpful, including a healthful diet, regular exercise, regular sleep patterns, avoidance of excess caffeine and alcohol, and avoidance of acute changes in stress levels.

The measures that benefit a given individual should be used routinely since they provide a simple,

***MIDAS Questionnaire**

INSTRUCTIONS: Please answer the following questions about ALL headaches you have had over the last 3 months. Write zero if you did not do the activity in the last 3 months.

1. On how many days in the last 3 months did you miss work or school because of your headaches? .... ____ days
2. How many days in the last 3 months was your productivity at work or school reduced by half or more because of your headaches *(do not include days you counted in question 1 where you missed work or school)*? .... ____ days
3. On how many days in the last 3 months did you **not** do household work because of your headaches? .... ____ days
4. How many days in the last 3 months was your productivity in household work reduced by half or more because of your headaches *(do not include days you counted in question 3 where you did not do household work)*? .... ____ days
5. On how many days in the last 3 months did you miss family, social, or leisure activities because of your headaches? .... ____ days

A. On how many days in the last 3 months did you have a headache? *(If a headache lasted more than one day, count each day.)* .... ____ days

B. On a scale of 0–10, on average how painful were these headaches? *(Where 0 = no pain at all, and 10 = pain as bad as it can be.)* .... ____

*Migraine Disability Assessment Score
(Questions 1–5 are used to calculate the MIDAS score.)
Grade I—Minimal or Infrequent Disability: 0–5
Grade II—Mild or Infrequent Disability: 6–10
Grade III—Moderate Disability: 11–20
Grade IV—Severe Disability: > 20

FIGURE 8-4
MIDAS Questionnaire.

cost-effective approach to migraine management. Patients with migraine do not encounter more stress than headache-free individuals; overresponsiveness to stress appears to be the issue. Since the stresses of everyday living cannot be eliminated, lessening one's response to stress by various techniques is helpful for many patients. These may include yoga, transcendental meditation, hypnosis, and conditioning techniques such as biofeedback. For most patients, this approach is, at best, an adjunct to pharmacotherapy. Nonpharmacologic measures are unlikely to prevent all migraine attacks. If these measures fail to prevent an attack, pharmacologic approaches are then needed to abort an attack.

ACUTE ATTACK THERAPIES FOR MIGRAINE

The mainstay of pharmacologic therapy is the judicious use of one or more of the many drugs that are effective in migraine (Table 8-5). The selection of the optimal regimen for a given patient depends on a number of factors, the most important of which is the severity of the attack. Mild migraine attacks can usually be managed by oral agents; the average efficacy rate is 50–70%. Severe migraine attacks may require parenteral therapy. Most drugs effective in the treatment of migraine are members of one of three major pharmacologic classes: anti-inflammatory agents, 5-$HT_{1B/1D}$ receptor agonists, and dopamine receptor antagonists.

In general, an adequate dose of whichever agent is chosen should be used as soon as possible after the onset of an attack. If additional medication is required within 60 min because symptoms return or have not abated, the initial dose should be increased for subsequent attacks. Migraine therapy must be individualized; a standard approach for all patients is not possible. A therapeutic regimen may need to be constantly refined until one is identified that provides the patient with rapid, complete, and consistent relief with minimal side effects (Table 8-6).

NONSTEROIDAL ANTI-INFLAMMATORY DRUGS (NSAIDs) Both the severity and duration of a migraine attack can be reduced significantly by nonsteroidal anti-inflammatory agents (Table 8-5). Indeed, many undiagnosed migraineurs are self-treated with nonprescription NSAIDs. A general consensus is that NSAIDs are most effective when taken early in the migraine attack. However, the effectiveness of anti-inflammatory agents in migraine is usually less than optimal in moderate or severe migraine attacks. The combination of acetaminophen, aspirin, and caffeine has been approved for use by the U.S. Food and Drug

TABLE 8-5

TREATMENT OF ACUTE MIGRAINE

DRUG	TRADE NAME	DOSAGE
Simple Analgesics		
Acetaminophen, aspirin, caffeine	Excedrin Migraine	Two tablets or caplets q6h (max 8 per day)
NSAIDs		
Naproxen	Aleve, Anaprox, generic	220–550 mg PO bid
Ibuprofen	Advil, Motrin, Nuprin, generic	400 mg PO q3–4h
Tolfenamic acid	Clotam Rapid	200 mg PO. May repeat ×1 after 1–2 h
5-HT$_1$ Agonists		
Oral		
Ergotamine	Ergomar	One 2 mg sublingual tablet at onset and q$^1/_2$h (max 3 per day, 5 per week)
Ergotamine 1 mg, caffeine 100 mg	Ercaf, Wigraine	One or two tablets at onset, then one tablet q$^1/_2$h (max 6 per day, 10 per week)
Naratriptan	Amerge	2.5 mg tablet at onset; may repeat once after 4 h
Rizatriptan	Maxalt Maxalt-MLT	5–10 mg tablet at onset; may repeat after 2 h (max 30 mg/d)
Sumatriptan	Imitrex	50–100 mg tablet at onset; may repeat after 2 h (max 200 mg/d)
Frovatriptan	Frova	2.5 mg tablet at onset, may repeat after 2 h (max 5 mg/d)
Almotriptan	Axert	12.5 mg tablet at onset, may repeat after 2 h (max 25 mg/d)
Eletriptan	Relpax	40 or 80 mg
Zolmitriptan	Zomig Zomig Rapimelt	2.5 mg tablet at onset; may repeat after 2 h (max 10 mg/d)
Nasal		
Dihydroergotamine	Migranal Nasal Spray	Prior to nasal spray, the pump must be primed 4 times; 1 spray (0.5 mg) is administered, followed in 15 min by a second spray
Sumatriptan	Imitrex Nasal Spray	5–20 mg intranasal spray as 4 sprays of 5 mg or a single 20 mg spray (may repeat once after 2 h, not to exceed a dose of 40 mg/d)
Zolmitriptan	Zomig	5 mg intranasal spray as one spray (may repeat once after 2 h, not to exceed a dose of 10 mg/d)
Parenteral		
Dihydroergotamine	DHE-45	1 mg IV, IM, or SC at onset and q1h (max 3 mg/d, 6 mg per week)
Sumatriptan	Imitrex Injection	6 mg SC at onset (may repeat once after 1 h for max of 2 doses in 24 h)
Dopamine Antagonists		
Oral		
Metoclopramide	Reglan,[a] generic[a]	5–10 mg/d
Prochlorperazine	Compazine,[a] generic[a]	1–25 mg/d
Parenteral		
Chlorpromazine	Generic[a]	0.1 mg/kg IV at 2 mg/min; max 35 mg/d
Metoclopramide	Reglan,[a] generic	10 mg IV
Prochlorperazine	Compazine,[a] generic[a]	10 mg IV
Other		
Oral		
Acetaminophen, 325 mg, *plus* dichloralphenazone, 100 mg, *plus* isometheptene, 65 mg	Midrin, Duradrin, generic	Two capsules at onset followed by 1 capsule q1h (max 5 capsules)
Nasal		
Butorphanol	Stadol[a]	1 mg (1 spray in 1 nostril), may repeat if necessary in 1–2 h
Parenteral		
Narcotics	Generic[a]	Multiple preparations and dosages; see Table 7-1

[a]Not all drugs are specifically indicated by the FDA for migraine. Local regulations and guidelines should be consulted.

Note: Antiemetics (e.g., domperidone 10 mg or ondansetron 4 or 8 mg) or prokinetics (e.g., metoclopramide 10 mg) are sometimes useful adjuncts.

Abbreviations: NSAIDs, nonsteroidal anti-inflammatory drugs; 5-HT, 5-hydroxytryptamine.

TABLE 8-6

CLINICAL STRATIFICATION OF ACUTE SPECIFIC MIGRAINE TREATMENTS

CLINICAL SITUATION	TREATMENT OPTIONS
Failed NSAIDs/analgesics	**First tier**
	Sumatriptan 50 mg or 100 mg PO
	Almotriptan 12.5 mg PO
	Rizatriptan 10 mg PO
	Eletriptan 40 mg PO
	Zolmitriptan 2.5 mg PO
	Slower effect/better tolerability
	Naratriptan 2.5 mg PO
	Frovatriptan 2.5 mg PO
	Infrequent headache
	Ergotamine 1–2 mg PO
	Dihydroergotamine nasal spray 2 mg
Early nausea or difficulties taking tablets	Zolmitriptan 5 mg nasal spray
	Sumatriptan 20 mg nasal spray
	Rizatriptan 10 mg MLT wafer
Headache recurrence	Ergotamine 2 mg (most effective PR/usually with caffeine)
	Naratriptan 2.5 mg PO
	Almotriptan 12.5 mg PO
	Eletriptan 40 mg
Tolerating acute treatments poorly	Naratriptan 2.5 mg
	Almotriptan 12.5 mg
Early vomiting	Zolmitriptan 5 mg nasal spray
	Sumatriptan 25 mg PR
	Sumatriptan 6 mg SC
Menses-related headache	**Prevention**
	Ergotamine PO at night
	Estrogen patches
	Treatment
	Triptans
	Dihydroergotamine nasal spray
Very rapidly developing symptoms	Zolmitriptan 5 mg nasal spray
	Sumatriptan 6 mg SC
	Dihydroergotamine 1 mg IM

Administration (FDA) for the treatment of mild to moderate migraine. The combination of aspirin and metoclopramide has been shown to be comparable to a single dose of sumatriptan. Important side effects of NSAIDs include dyspepsia and gastrointestinal irritation.

5-HT$_1$ RECEPTOR AGONISTS

Oral Stimulation of 5-HT$_{1B}$/$_{1D}$ receptors can stop an acute migraine attack. Ergotamine and dihydroergotamine are nonselective receptor agonists, while the triptans are selective 5-HT$_{1B/1D}$ receptor agonists. A variety of triptans, 5-HT$_{1B/1D}$ receptor agonists—naratriptan, rizatriptan, eletriptan, sumatriptan, zolmitriptan, almotriptan, and frovatriptan—are now available for the treatment of migraine.

Each drug in the triptan class has similar pharmacologic properties but varies slightly in terms of clinical efficacy. Rizatriptan and eletriptan are the most efficacious of the triptans currently available in the United States. Sumatriptan and zolmitriptan have similar rates of efficacy as well as time to onset, with an advantage of having multiple formulations, whereas almotriptan, frovatriptan, and naratriptan are somewhat slower in onset and are better tolerated. Clinical efficacy appears to be related more to the t_{max} (time to peak plasma level) than to the potency, half-life, or bioavailability. This observation is consistent with a large body of data indicating that faster-acting analgesics are more effective than slower-acting agents.

Unfortunately, monotherapy with a selective oral 5-HT$_{1B/1D}$ agonist does not result in rapid, consistent, and complete relief of migraine in all patients. Triptans are not effective in migraine with aura unless given after the aura is completed and the headache initiated. Side effects are common though often mild and transient. Moreover, 5-HT$_{1B/1D}$ agonists are contraindicated in individuals with a history of cardiovascular and cerebrovascular disease. Recurrence of headache is another important limitation of triptan use and occurs at least occasionally in most patients. Evidence from randomized controlled trials show that coadministration of a longer-acting NSAID, naproxen 500 mg, with sumatriptan will augment the initial effect of sumatriptan and, importantly, reduce rates of headache recurrence.

Ergotamine preparations offer a nonselective means of stimulating 5-HT$_1$ receptors. A nonnauseating dose of ergotamine should be sought since a dose that provokes nausea is too high and may intensify head pain. Except for a sublingual formulation of ergotamine, oral formulations of ergotamine also contain 100 mg caffeine (theoretically to enhance ergotamine absorption and possibly to add additional analgesic activity). The average oral ergotamine dose for a migraine attack is 2 mg. Since the clinical studies demonstrating the efficacy of ergotamine in migraine predated the clinical trial methodologies used with the triptans, it is difficult to assess the clinical efficacy of ergotamine versus the triptans. In general, ergotamine appears to have a much higher incidence of nausea than triptans, but less headache recurrence.

Nasal The fastest-acting nonparenteral antimigraine therapies that can be self-administered include nasal formulations of dihydroergotamine (Migranal), zolmitriptan (Zomig nasal), or sumatriptan. The nasal sprays result in substantial blood levels within 30–60 min. Although in theory nasal sprays might provide faster and more effective relief of a migraine attack than oral formulations, their reported efficacy is only approximately 50–60%. Studies with an inhalational formulation of dihydroergotamine indicate that its absorption problems can be overcome to produce rapid onset of action with good tolerability.

Parenteral Parenteral administration of drugs such as dihydroergotamine and sumatriptan is approved by the FDA for the rapid relief of a migraine attack. Peak plasma levels of dihydroergotamine are achieved 3 min after IV dosing, 30 min after IM dosing, and 45 min after SC dosing. If an attack has not already peaked, SC or IM administration of 1 mg dihydroergotamine suffices for about 80–90% of patients. Sumatriptan, 6 mg SC, is effective in ~70–80% of patients.

DOPAMINE ANTAGONISTS

Oral Oral dopamine antagonists should be considered as adjunctive therapy in migraine. Drug absorption is impaired during migraine because of reduced gastrointestinal motility. Delayed absorption occurs even in the absence of nausea and is related to the severity of the attack and not its duration. Therefore, when oral NSAIDs and/or triptan agents fail, the addition of a dopamine antagonist such as metoclopramide 10 mg should be considered to enhance gastric absorption. In addition, dopamine antagonists decrease nausea/vomiting and restore normal gastric motility.

Parenteral Parenteral dopamine antagonists (e.g., chlorpromazine, prochlorperazine, metoclopramide) can also provide significant acute relief of migraine; they can be used in combination with parenteral 5-$HT_{1B/1D}$ agonists. A common IV protocol used for the treatment of severe migraine is the administration over 2 min of a mixture of 5 mg of prochlorperazine and 0.5 mg of dihydroergotamine.

OTHER MEDICATIONS FOR ACUTE MIGRAINE

Oral The combination of acetaminophen, dichloralphenazone, and isometheptene, one to two capsules, has been classified by the FDA as "possibly" effective in the treatment of migraine. Since the clinical studies demonstrating the efficacy of this combination analgesic in migraine predated the clinical trial methodologies used with the triptans, it is difficult to compare the efficacy of this sympathomimetic compound to other agents.

Nasal A nasal preparation of butorphanol is available for the treatment of acute pain. As with all narcotics, the use of nasal butorphanol should be limited to a select group of migraineurs, as described next.

Parenteral Narcotics are effective in the acute treatment of migraine. For example, IV meperidine (50–100 mg) is given frequently in the emergency room. This regimen "works" in the sense that the pain of migraine is eliminated. However, this regimen is clearly suboptimal for patients with recurrent headache. Narcotics do not treat the underlying headache mechanism; rather, they act to alter the pain sensation. Moreover, in patients taking oral narcotics such as oxycodone or hydrocodone, narcotic addiction can greatly confuse the treatment of migraine. Narcotic craving and/or withdrawal can aggravate and accentuate migraine. Therefore, it is recommended that narcotic use in migraine be limited to patients with severe, but infrequent, headaches that are unresponsive to other pharmacologic approaches.

MEDICATION-OVERUSE HEADACHE Acute attack medications, particularly codeine or barbiturate-containing compound analgesics, have a propensity to aggravate headache frequency and induce a state of refractory daily or near-daily headache called *medication-overuse headache*. This condition is likely not a separate headache entity but a reaction of the migraine patient to a particular medicine. Migraine patients who have two or more headache days a week should be cautioned about frequent analgesic use (see "Chronic Daily Headache," later in this chapter).

PREVENTIVE TREATMENTS FOR MIGRAINE Patients with an increasing frequency of migraine attacks, or with attacks that are either unresponsive or poorly responsive to abortive treatments, are good candidates for preventive agents. In general, a preventive medication should be considered in the subset of patients with five or more attacks a month. Significant side effects are associated with the use of many of these agents; furthermore, determination of dose can be difficult since the recommended doses have been derived for conditions other than migraine. The mechanism of action of these drugs is unclear; it seems likely that the brain sensitivity that underlies migraine is modified. Patients are usually started on a low dose of a chosen treatment; the dose is then gradually increased, up to a reasonable maximum to achieve clinical benefit.

Drugs that have the capacity to stabilize migraine are listed in Table 8-7. Drugs must be taken daily, and there is usually a lag of at least 2–12 weeks before an effect is seen. The drugs that have been approved by the FDA for the prophylactic treatment of migraine include propranolol, timolol, sodium valproate, topiramate, and methysergide (not available in the United States). In addition, a number of other drugs appear to display prophylactic efficacy. This group includes amitriptyline, nortriptyline, flunarizine, phenelzine, gabapentin, and cyproheptadine. Placebo-controlled trials of onabotulinum toxin type A in episodic migraine were negative, while,

TABLE 8-7

PREVENTIVE TREATMENTS IN MIGRAINE[a]

DRUG	DOSE	SELECTED SIDE EFFECTS
Pizotifen[b]	0.5–2 mg qd	Weight gain Drowsiness
Beta blocker		
Propranolol	40–120 mg bid	Reduced energy Tiredness Postural symptoms Contraindicated in asthma
Tricyclics		
Amitriptyline	10–75 mg at night	Drowsiness
Dothiepin	25–75 mg at night	
Nortriptyline	25–75 mg at night	***Note:*** Some patients may only need a total dose of 10 mg, although generally 1–1.5 mg/kg body weight is required
Anticonvulsants		
Topiramate	25–200 mg/d	Paresthesias Cognitive symptoms Weight loss Glaucoma Caution with nephrolithiasis
Valproate	400–600 mg bid	Drowsiness Weight gain Tremor Hair loss Fetal abnormalities Hematologic or liver abnormalities
Gabapentin	900–3600 mg qd	Dizziness Sedation
Serotonergic drugs		
Methysergide	1–4 mg qd	Drowsiness Leg cramps Hair loss Retroperitoneal fibrosis (1-month drug holiday is required every 6 months)
Flunarizine[b]	5–15 mg qd	Drowsiness Weight gain Depression Parkinsonism
No convincing evidence from controlled trials		
Verapamil		
Controlled trials demonstrate *no effect*		
Nimodipine		
Clonidine		
SSRIs: fluoxetine		

[a]Commonly used preventives are listed with typical doses and common side effects. Not all listed medicines are approved by the FDA; local regulations and guidelines should be consulted.
[b]Not available in the United States.

overall, placebo-controlled trials in chronic migraine were positive. Phenelzine and methysergide are usually reserved for recalcitrant cases because of their serious potential side effects. Phenelzine is a monoamine oxidase inhibitor (MAOI); therefore, tyramine-containing foods, decongestants, and meperidine are contraindicated. Methysergide may cause retroperitoneal or cardiac valvular fibrosis when it is used for >6 months, and thus monitoring is required for patients using this drug; the risk of fibrosis is about 1:1500 and is likely to reverse after the drug is stopped.

The probability of success with any one of the antimigraine drugs is 50–75%. Many patients are managed adequately with low-dose amitriptyline, propranolol, topiramate, gabapentin, or valproate. If these agents fail or lead to unacceptable side effects, second-line agents such as methysergide or phenelzine can be used. Once effective stabilization is achieved, the drug is continued for ~6 months and then slowly tapered to assess the continued need. Many patients are able to discontinue medication and experience fewer and milder attacks for long periods, suggesting that these drugs may alter the natural history of migraine.

TENSION-TYPE HEADACHE

Clinical features

The term *tension-type headache* (TTH) is commonly used to describe a chronic head-pain syndrome characterized by bilateral tight, bandlike discomfort. The pain typically builds slowly, fluctuates in severity, and may persist more or less continuously for many days. The headache may be episodic or chronic (present >15 days per month).

A useful clinical approach is to diagnose TTH in patients whose headaches are completely without accompanying features such as nausea, vomiting, photophobia, phonophobia, osmophobia, throbbing, and aggravation with movement. Such an approach neatly separates migraine, which has one or more of these features and is the main differential diagnosis, from TTH. The International Headache Society's main definition of TTH allows an admixture of nausea, photophobia, or phonophobia in various combinations, although the appendix definition does not; this illustrates the difficulty in distinguishing these two clinical entities. In clinical practice, dichotomizing patients on the basis of the presence of associated features (migraine) and the absence of associated features (TTH) is highly recommended. Indeed patients whose headaches fit the TTH phenotype and who have migraine at other times, along with a family history of migraine, migrainous illnesses of childhood, or typical migraine triggers to their migraine attacks, may be biologically different from those who have TTH headache with none of the features.

Pathophysiology

The pathophysiology of TTH is incompletely understood. It seems likely that TTH is due to a primary disorder of CNS pain modulation alone, unlike migraine, which involves a more generalized disturbance of sensory modulation. Data suggest a genetic contribution to TTH, but this may not be a valid finding: given the current diagnostic criteria, the studies undoubtedly included many migraine patients. The name *tension-type headache* implies that pain is a product of *nervous tension*, but there is no clear evidence for tension as an etiology. Muscle contraction has been considered to be a feature that distinguishes TTH from migraine, but there appear to be no differences in contraction between the two headache types.

TREATMENT Tension-Type Headache

The pain of TTH can generally be managed with simple analgesics such as acetaminophen, aspirin, or NSAIDs. Behavioral approaches including relaxation can also be effective. Clinical studies have demonstrated that triptans in pure TTH are not helpful, although triptans are effective in TTH when the patient also has migraine. For chronic TTH, amitriptyline is the only proven treatment (Table 8-7); other tricyclics, selective serotonin reuptake inhibitors, and the benzodiazepines have not been shown to be effective. There is no evidence for the efficacy of acupuncture. Placebo-controlled trials of onabotulinum toxin type A in chronic TTH have not shown benefit.

TRIGEMINAL AUTONOMIC CEPHALALGIAS, INCLUDING CLUSTER HEADACHE

The trigeminal autonomic cephalalgias (TACs) describe a grouping of primary headaches including cluster headache, paroxysmal hemicrania, and SUNCT (*s*hort-lasting *u*nilateral *n*euralgiform headache attacks with *c*onjunctival injection and *t*earing)/SUNA (*s*hort-lasting *u*nilateral *n*euralgiform headache attacks with cranial *a*utonomic symptoms). TACs are characterized by relatively short-lasting attacks of head pain associated with cranial autonomic symptoms, such as lacrimation, conjunctival injection, or nasal congestion (Table 8-8). Pain is usually severe and may occur more than once a day. Because of the associated nasal congestion or rhinorrhea, patients are often misdiagnosed with "sinus headache" and treated with decongestants, which are ineffective.

TACs must be differentiated from short-lasting headaches that do not have prominent cranial autonomic syndromes, notably trigeminal neuralgia, primary stabbing headache, and hypnic headache. The cycling

TABLE 8-8

CLINICAL FEATURES OF THE TRIGEMINAL AUTONOMIC CEPHALALGIAS

	CLUSTER HEADACHE	PAROXYSMAL HEMICRANIA	SUNCT
Gender	M > F	F = M	F ~ M
Pain			
Type	Stabbing, boring	Throbbing, boring, stabbing	Burning, stabbing, sharp
Severity	Excruciating	Excruciating	Severe to excruciating
Site	Orbit, temple	Orbit, temple	Periorbital
Attack frequency	1/alternate day–8/d	1–40/d (>5/d for more than half the time)	3–200/d
Duration of attack	15–180 min	2–30 min	5–240 s
Autonomic features	Yes	Yes	Yes (prominent conjunctival injection and lacrimation)[a]
Migrainous features[b]	Yes	Yes	Yes
Alcohol trigger	Yes	No	No
Cutaneous triggers	No	No	Yes
Indomethacin effect	—	Yes[c]	—
Abortive treatment	Sumatriptan injection or nasal spray Oxygen	No effective treatment	Lidocaine (IV)
Prophylactic treatment	Verapamil Methysergide Lithium	Indomethacin	Lamotrigine Topiramate Gabapentin

[a]If conjunctival injection and tearing not present, consider SUNA.
[b]Nausea, photophobia, or phonophobia; photophobia and phonophobia are typically unilateral on the side of the pain.
[c]Indicates complete response to indomethacin.
Abbreviation: SUNCT, short-lasting *u*nilateral *n*euralgiform headache attacks with *c*onjunctival injection and *t*earing.

pattern and length, frequency, and timing of attacks are useful in classifying patients. Patients with TACs should undergo pituitary imaging and pituitary function tests as there is an excess of TAC presentations in patients with pituitary tumor–related headache.

Cluster headache

Cluster headache is a rare form of primary headache with a population frequency of approximately 0.1%. The pain is deep, usually retroorbital, often excruciating in intensity, nonfluctuating, and explosive in quality. A core feature of cluster headache is periodicity. At least one of the daily attacks of pain recurs at about the same hour each day for the duration of a cluster bout. The typical cluster headache patient has daily bouts of one to two attacks of relatively short-duration unilateral pain for 8 to 10 weeks a year; this is usually followed by a pain-free interval that averages a little less than 1 year. Cluster headache is characterized as chronic when there is no significant period of sustained remission. Patients are generally perfectly well between episodes. Onset is nocturnal in about 50% of patients, and men are affected three times more often than women. Patients with cluster headache tend to move about during attacks, pacing, rocking, or rubbing their head for relief; some may even become aggressive during attacks. This is in sharp contrast to patients with migraine, who prefer to remain motionless during attacks.

Cluster headache is associated with ipsilateral symptoms of cranial parasympathetic autonomic activation: conjunctival injection or lacrimation, rhinorrhea or nasal congestion, or cranial sympathetic dysfunction such as ptosis. The sympathetic deficit is peripheral and likely to be due to parasympathetic activation with injury to ascending sympathetic fibers surrounding a dilated carotid artery as it passes into the cranial cavity. When present, photophobia and phonophobia are far more likely to be unilateral and on the same side of the pain, rather than bilateral, as is seen in migraine. This phenomenon of unilateral photophobia/phonophobia is characteristic of TACs. Cluster headache is likely to be a disorder involving central pacemaker neurons in the region of the posterior hypothalamus (Fig. 8-3).

TREATMENT Cluster Headache

The most satisfactory treatment is the administration of drugs to prevent cluster attacks until the bout is over. However, treatment of acute attacks is required for all cluster headache patients at some time.

ACUTE ATTACK TREATMENT Cluster headache attacks peak rapidly, and thus a treatment with quick onset is required. Many patients with acute cluster headache respond very well to oxygen inhalation. This should be given as 100% oxygen at 10–12 L/min for 15–20 min. It appears that high flow and high oxygen content are important. Sumatriptan 6 mg SC is rapid in onset and will usually shorten an attack to 10–15 min; there is no evidence of tachyphylaxis. Sumatriptan (20 mg) and zolmitriptan (5 mg) nasal sprays are both effective in acute cluster headache, offering a useful option for patients who may not wish to self-inject daily. Oral sumatriptan is not effective for prevention or for acute treatment of cluster headache.

PREVENTIVE TREATMENTS (Table 8-9) The choice of a preventive treatment in cluster headache depends in part on the length of the bout. Patients with long bouts or those with chronic cluster headache require medicines that are safe when taken for long periods. For patients with relatively short bouts, limited courses of oral glucocorticoids or methysergide (not available in the United States) can be very useful. A 10-day course of prednisone, beginning at 60 mg daily for 7 days and followed by a rapid taper, may interrupt the pain bout for many patients. When ergotamine (1–2 mg) is used, it is most effective when given 1–2 h before an expected attack. Patients who use ergotamine daily must be educated regarding the early symptoms of ergotism, which may include vomiting, numbness, tingling, pain, and cyanosis of the limbs; a weekly limit of 14 mg should be adhered to. Lithium (600–900 mg qd) appears to be particularly useful for the chronic form of the disorder.

Many experts favor verapamil as the first-line preventive treatment for patients with chronic cluster headache or prolonged bouts. While verapamil compares favorably with lithium in practice, some patients require verapamil doses far in excess of those administered for cardiac disorders. The initial dose range is 40–80 mg twice daily; effective doses may be as high as 960 mg/d. Side effects such as constipation and leg swelling can be problematic. Of paramount concern, however, is the cardiovascular safety of verapamil, particularly at high doses. Verapamil can cause heart block by slowing conduction in the atrioventricular node, a condition that can be monitored by following the PR interval on a standard ECG. Approximately 20% of patients treated with verapamil develop ECG abnormalities, which can be observed with doses as low as 240 mg/d; these abnormalities can worsen over time in patients on stable doses. A baseline ECG is recommended for all patients. The ECG is repeated 10 days after a dose change in those patients whose dose is being increased above 240 mg daily. Dose increases are usually made in 80-mg increments. For patients on long-term verapamil, ECG monitoring every 6 months is advised.

NEUROSTIMULATION THERAPY When medical therapies fail in chronic cluster headache, neurostimulation strategies can be employed. Deep-brain stimulation of the region of the posterior hypothalamic gray matter has proven successful in a substantial proportion of patients. Favorable results have also been reported with the less-invasive approach of occipital nerve stimulation.

TABLE 8-9

PREVENTIVE MANAGEMENT OF CLUSTER HEADACHE

SHORT-TERM PREVENTION	LONG-TERM PREVENTION
EPISODIC CLUSTER HEADACHE	EPISODIC CLUSTER HEADACHE & PROLONGED CHRONIC CLUSTER HEADACHE
Prednisone 1 mg/kg up to 60 mg qd, tapering over 21 days	Verapamil 160–960 mg/d
	Lithium 400–800 mg/d
Methysergide 3–12 mg/d	Methysergide 3–12 mg/d
Verapamil 160–960 mg/d	Topiramate[a] 100–400 mg/d
Greater occipital nerve injection	Gabapentin[a] 1200–3600 mg/d
	Melatonin[a] 9–12 mg/d

[a]Unproven but of potential benefit.

PAROXYSMAL HEMICRANIA

Paroxysmal hemicrania (PH) is characterized by frequent unilateral, severe, short-lasting episodes of headache. Like cluster headache, the pain tends to be retroorbital but may be experienced all over the head and is associated with autonomic phenomena such as lacrimation and nasal congestion. Patients with remissions are said to have episodic PH, whereas those with the nonremitting form are said to have chronic PH. The essential features of PH are unilateral, very severe pain; short-lasting attacks (2–45 min); very frequent attacks (usually more than five a day); marked autonomic features ipsilateral to the pain; rapid course (<72 h); and excellent response to indomethacin. In contrast to cluster headache, which predominantly affects males, the male:female ratio in PH is close to 1:1.

Indomethacin (25–75 mg tid), which can completely suppress attacks of PH, is the treatment of choice. Although therapy may be complicated by indomethacin-induced gastrointestinal side effects, currently there are no consistently effective alternatives. Topiramate is helpful in some cases. Piroxicam has been used, although it is not as effective as indomethacin. Verapamil, an effective treatment for cluster headache, does not appear to be useful for PH. In occasional patients, PH can coexist with trigeminal neuralgia (PH-tic syndrome); similar to cluster-tic syndrome, each component may require separate treatment.

Secondary PH has been reported with lesions in the region of the sella turcica, including arteriovenous malformation, cavernous sinus meningioma, and epidermoid tumors. Secondary PH is more likely if the patient requires high doses (>200 mg/d) of indomethacin. In patients with apparent bilateral PH, raised CSF pressure should be suspected. It is important to note that indomethacin reduces CSF pressure. When a diagnosis of PH is considered, MRI is indicated to exclude a pituitary lesion.

SUNCT/SUNA

SUNCT (*s*hort-lasting *u*nilateral *n*euralgiform headache attacks with *c*onjunctival injection and *t*earing) is a rare primary headache syndrome characterized by severe, unilateral orbital or temporal pain that is stabbing or throbbing in quality. Diagnosis requires at least 20 attacks, lasting for 5–240 s; ipsilateral conjunctival injection and lacrimation should be present. In some patients conjunctival injection or lacrimation is missing, and the diagnosis of SUNA (*s*hort-lasting *u*nilateral *n*euralgiform headache attacks with cranial *a*utonomic symptoms) can be made.

Diagnosis

The pain of SUNCT/SUNA is unilateral and may be located anywhere in the head. Three basic patterns can be seen: single stabs, which are usually short-lived; groups of stabs; or a longer attack comprising many stabs between which the pain does not completely resolve, thus giving a "saw-tooth" phenomenon with attacks lasting many minutes. Each pattern may be seen in the context of an underlying continuous head pain. Characteristics that lead to a suspected diagnosis of SUNCT are the cutaneous (or other) triggerability of attacks, a lack of refractory period to triggering between attacks, and the lack of a response to indomethacin. Apart from trigeminal sensory disturbance, the neurologic examination is normal in primary SUNCT.

The diagnosis of SUNCT is often confused with trigeminal neuralgia (TN) particularly in first-division TN (Chap. 34). Minimal or no cranial autonomic symptoms and a clear refractory period to triggering indicate a diagnosis of TN.

Secondary (Symptomatic) SUNCT

SUNCT can be seen with posterior fossa or pituitary lesions. All patients with SUNCT/SUNA should be evaluated with pituitary function tests and a brain MRI with pituitary views.

TREATMENT SUNCT/SUNA

ABORTIVE THERAPY Therapy of acute attacks is not a useful concept in SUNCT/SUNA since the attacks are of such short duration. However, IV lidocaine, which arrests the symptoms, can be used in hospitalized patients.

PREVENTIVE THERAPY Long-term prevention to minimize disability and hospitalization is the goal of treatment. The most effective treatment for prevention is lamotrigine, 200–400 mg/d. Topiramate and gabapentin may also be effective. Carbamazepine, 400–500 mg/d, has been reported by patients to offer modest benefit.

Surgical approaches such as microvascular decompression or destructive trigeminal procedures are seldom useful and often produce long-term complications. Greater occipital nerve injection has produced limited benefit in some patients. Occipital nerve stimulation is probably helpful in an important subgroup of these patients. Complete control with deep-brain stimulation of the posterior hypothalamic region was reported in a single patient. For intractable cases, short-term prevention with IV lidocaine can be effective, as can occipital nerve stimulation.

CHRONIC DAILY HEADACHE

The broad diagnosis of chronic daily headache (CDH) can be applied when a patient experiences headache on 15 days or more per month. CDH is not a single entity; it encompasses a number of different headache syndromes, including chronic TTH as well as headache secondary to trauma, inflammation, infection, medication overuse, and other causes (Table 8-10). Population-based estimates suggest that about 4% of adults have daily or near-daily headache. Daily headache may be primary or secondary, an important consideration in guiding management of this complaint.

APPROACH TO THE PATIENT Chronic Daily Headache

The first step in the management of patients with CDH is to diagnose any underlying condition (Table 8-10). For patients with primary headaches, diagnosis of the headache type will guide therapy. Preventive treatments such as tricyclics, either amitriptyline or nortriptyline at doses up to 1 mg/kg, are very useful in patients

TABLE 8-10

CLASSIFICATION OF CHRONIC DAILY HEADACHE

PRIMARY		
>4 h DAILY	**<4 h DAILY**	**SECONDARY**
Chronic migraine[a]	Chronic cluster headache[b]	Posttraumatic Head injury Iatrogenic Postinfectious
Chronic tension-type headache[a]	Chronic paroxysmal hemicrania	Inflammatory, such as Giant cell arteritis Sarcoidosis Behçet's syndrome
Hemicrania continua[a]	SUNCT/SUNA	Chronic CNS infection
New daily persistent headache[a]	Hypnic headache	Medication-overuse headache[a]

[a]May be complicated by analgesic overuse.
[b]Some patients may have headache >4 h/d.
Abbreviations: SUNA, *s*hort-lasting *u*nilateral *n*euralgiform headache *a*ttacks with cranial autonomic symptoms; SUNCT, *s*hort-lasting *u*nilateral *n*euralgiform headache attacks with *c*onjunctival injection and *t*earing.

with CDH arising from migraine or tension-type headache. Tricyclics are started in low doses (10–25 mg) daily and may be given 12 h before the expected time of awakening in order to avoid excess morning sleepiness. Anticonvulsants, such as topiramate, valproate, and gabapentin, are also useful in migraineurs. Flunarizine can also be very effective for some patients, as can methysergide or phenelzine.

MANAGEMENT OF MEDICALLY INTRACTABLE DISABLING CHRONIC DAILY HEADACHE The management of medically intractable headache is difficult. At this time, the only promising approach is occipital nerve stimulation, which appears to modulate thalamic processing in migraine and has also shown promise in chronic cluster headache, SUNCT/SUNA, and hemicrania continua (see next).

MEDICATION-OVERUSE HEADACHE Overuse of analgesic medication for headache can aggravate headache frequency and induce a state of refractory daily or near-daily headache called *medication-overuse headache*. A proportion of patients who stop taking analgesics will experience substantial improvement in the severity and frequency of their headache. However, even after cessation of analgesic use, many patients continue to have headache, although they may feel clinically improved in some way, especially if they have been using codeine or barbiturates regularly. The residual symptoms probably represent the underlying headache disorder.

Management of Medication Overuse: Outpatients For patients who overuse medications, it is essential that analgesic use be reduced and eliminated. One approach is to reduce the medication dose by 10% every 1–2 weeks. Immediate cessation of analgesic use is possible for some patients, provided there is no contraindication. Both approaches are facilitated by the use of a medication diary maintained during the month or two before cessation; this helps to identify the scope of the problem. A small dose of an NSAID such as naproxen, 500 mg bid, if tolerated, will help relieve residual pain as analgesic use is reduced. NSAID overuse is not usually a problem for patients with daily headache when the dose is taken once or twice daily; however, overuse problems may develop with more frequent dosing schedules. Once the patient has substantially reduced analgesic use, a preventive medication should be introduced. It must be emphasized that *preventives generally do not work in the presence of analgesic overuse*. The most common cause of unresponsiveness to treatment is the use of a preventive when analgesics continue to be used regularly. For some patients, discontinuing analgesics is very difficult; often the best approach is to directly inform the patient that some degree of pain is inevitable during this initial period.

Management of Medication Overuse: Inpatients Some patients will require hospitalization for detoxification. Such patients have typically failed efforts at outpatient withdrawal or have a significant medical condition, such as diabetes mellitus, which would complicate withdrawal as an outpatient. Following admission to the hospital, acute medications are withdrawn completely on the first day, in the absence of a contraindication. Antiemetics and fluids are administered as required; clonidine is used for opiate withdrawal symptoms. For acute intolerable pain during the waking hours aspirin, 1 g IV (not approved in United States), is useful. IM chlorpromazine can be helpful at night; patients must be adequately hydrated. Three to five days into the admission as the effect of the withdrawn substance settles a course of IV dihydroergotamine (DHE) can be employed. DHE, administered every 8 h for 5 consecutive days, can induce a significant remission that allows a preventive treatment to be established. 5-HT_3 antagonists, such as ondansetron or granisetron, are often required with DHE to prevent significant nausea, and domperidone (not approved in the United States) orally or by suppository can be very helpful.

NEW DAILY PERSISTENT HEADACHE New daily persistent headache (NDPH) is a clinically distinct syndrome; its causes are listed in Table 8-11.

CLINICAL PRESENTATION The patient with NDPH presents with headache on most if not all days

TABLE 8-11

DIFFERENTIAL DIAGNOSIS OF NEW DAILY PERSISTENT HEADACHE

PRIMARY	SECONDARY
Migrainous-type	Subarachnoid hemorrhage
Featureless (tension-type)	Low CSF volume headache
	Raised CSF pressure headache
	Posttraumatic headache[a]
	Chronic meningitis

[a]Includes postinfectious forms.

and the patient can clearly, and often vividly, recall the moment of onset. The headache usually begins abruptly, but onset may be more gradual; evolution over 3 days has been proposed as the upper limit for this syndrome. Patients typically recall the exact day and circumstances of the onset of headache; the new, persistent head pain does not remit. The first priority is to distinguish between a primary and a secondary cause of this syndrome. Subarachnoid hemorrhage is the most serious of the secondary causes and must be excluded either by history or appropriate investigation (Chap. 28).

Secondary NDPH

Low CSF Volume Headache In these syndromes, head pain is positional: it begins when the patient sits or stands upright and resolves upon reclining. The pain, which is occipitofrontal, is usually a dull ache but may be throbbing. Patients with chronic low CSF volume headache typically present with a history of headache from one day to the next that is generally not present on waking but worsens during the day. Recumbency usually improves the headache within minutes, but it takes only minutes to an hour for the pain to return when the patient resumes an upright position.

The most common cause of headache due to persistent low CSF volume is CSF leak following lumbar puncture (LP). Post-LP headache usually begins within 48 h but may be delayed for up to 12 days. Its incidence is between 10 and 30%. Beverages with caffeine may provide temporary relief. Besides LP, index events may include epidural injection or a vigorous Valsalva maneuver, such as from lifting, straining, coughing, clearing the eustachian tubes in an airplane, or multiple orgasms. Spontaneous CSF leaks are well recognized, and the diagnosis should be considered whenever the headache history is typical, even when there is no obvious index event. As time passes from the index event, the postural nature may become less apparent; cases in which the index event occurred several years before the eventual diagnosis have been recognized. Symptoms appear to result from low volume rather than low pressure: although low CSF pressures, typically 0–50 mmH_2O, are usually identified, a pressure as high as 140 mmH_2O has been noted with a documented leak.

Postural orthostatic tachycardia syndrome (POTS [Chap. 33]) can present with orthostatic headache similar to low CSF volume headache and is a diagnosis that needs consideration here.

When imaging is indicated to identify the source of a presumed leak, an MRI with gadolinium is the initial study of choice (Fig. 8-5). A striking pattern of diffuse meningeal enhancement is so typical that in the appropriate clinical context the diagnosis is established. Chiari malformations may sometimes be noted on MRI; in such cases, surgery to decompress the posterior fossa usually worsens the headache. Spinal MRI with T2 weighting may reveal a leak and spinal MRI may demonstrate spinal meningeal cysts whose role in these syndromes is yet to be elucidated. The source of CSF leakage may be identified by spinal MRI, by CT, or increasingly with MR myelography, or with ^{111}In-DTPA CSF studies; in the absence of a directly identified site of leakage, early emptying of ^{111}In-DTPA tracer into the bladder or slow progress of tracer across the brain suggests a CSF leak.

Initial treatment for low CSF volume headache is bed rest. For patients with persistent pain, IV caffeine (500 mg in 500 mL saline administered over 2 h) can be very effective. An ECG to screen for arrhythmia should be performed before administration. It is reasonable to administer at least two infusions of caffeine before embarking on additional tests to identify the source of the CSF leak. Since IV caffeine is safe and can be curative,

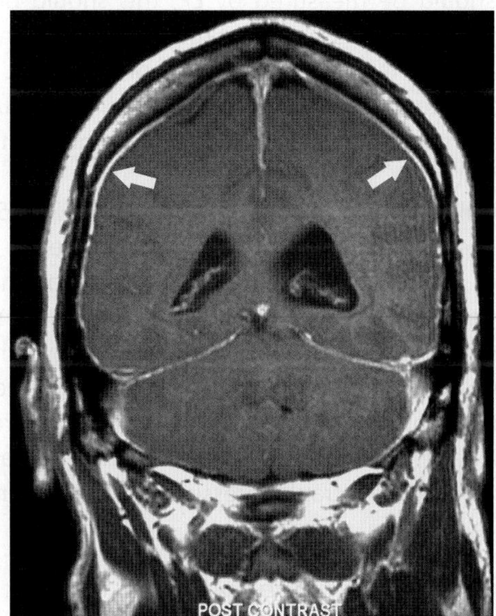

FIGURE 8-5

Magnetic resonance image showing diffuse meningeal enhancement after gadolinium administration in a patient with low CSF volume headache.

it spares many patients the need for further investigations. If unsuccessful, an abdominal binder may be helpful. If a leak can be identified, an autologous blood patch is usually curative. A blood patch is also effective for post-LP headache; in this setting, the location is empirically determined to be the site of the LP. In patients with intractable pain, oral theophylline is a useful alternative; however, its effect is less rapid than caffeine.

Raised CSF Pressure Headache Raised CSF pressure is well recognized as a cause of headache. Brain imaging can often reveal the cause, such as a space-occupying lesion. NDPH due to raised CSF pressure can be the presenting symptom for patients with idiopathic intracranial hypertension (pseudotumor cerebri) without visual problems, particularly when the fundi are normal. Persistently raised intracranial pressure can trigger chronic migraine. These patients typically present with a history of generalized headache that is present on waking and improves as the day goes on. It is generally worse with recumbency. Visual obscurations are frequent. The diagnosis is relatively straightforward when papilledema is present, but the possibility must be considered even in patients without funduscopic changes. Formal visual field testing should be performed even in the absence of overt ophthalmic involvement. Headache on rising in the morning or nocturnal headache is also characteristic of obstructive sleep apnea or poorly controlled hypertension.

Evaluation of patients suspected to have raised CSF pressure requires brain imaging. It is most efficient to obtain an MRI, including an MR venogram, as the initial study. If there are no contraindications, the CSF pressure should be measured by LP; this should be done when the patient is symptomatic so that both the pressure and the response to removal of 20–30 mL of CSF can be determined. An elevated opening pressure and improvement in headache following removal of CSF is diagnostic.

Initial treatment is with acetazolamide (250–500 mg bid); the headache may improve within weeks. If ineffective, topiramate is the next treatment of choice; it has many actions that may be useful in this setting, including carbonic anhydrase inhibition, weight loss, and neuronal membrane stabilization, likely mediated via effects on phosphorylation pathways. Severely disabled patients who do not respond to medical treatment require intracranial pressure monitoring and may require shunting.

Posttraumatic Headache A traumatic event can trigger a headache process that lasts for many months or years after the event. The term *trauma* is used in a very broad sense: headache can develop following an injury to the head, but it can also develop after an infectious episode, typically viral meningitis, a flulike illness, or a parasitic infection. Complaints of dizziness, vertigo, and impaired memory can accompany the headache. Symptoms may remit after several weeks or persist for months and even years after the injury. Typically the neurologic examination is normal and CT or MRI studies are unrevealing. Chronic subdural hematoma may on occasion mimic this disorder. In one series, one-third of patients with NDPH reported headache beginning after a transient flulike illness characterized by fever, neck stiffness, photophobia, and marked malaise. Evaluation reveals no apparent cause for the headache. There is no convincing evidence that persistent Epstein-Barr infection plays a role in this syndrome. A complicating factor is that many patients undergo LP during the acute illness; iatrogenic low CSF volume headache must be considered in these cases. Posttraumatic headache may also be seen after carotid dissection and subarachnoid hemorrhage, and following intracranial surgery. The underlying theme appears to be that a traumatic event involving the pain-producing meninges can trigger a headache process that lasts for many years.

Treatment is largely empirical. Tricyclic antidepressants, notably amitriptyline, and anticonvulsants such as topiramate, valproate, and gabapentin, have been used with reported benefit. The MAOI phenelzine may also be useful in carefully selected patients. The headache usually resolves within 3–5 years, but it can be quite disabling.

Primary NDPH Primary NDPH occurs in both males and females. It can be of the migrainous type, with features of migraine, or it can be featureless, appearing as new-onset TTH (Table 8-11). Migrainous features are common and include unilateral headache and throbbing pain; each feature is present in about one-third of patients. Nausea, photophobia, and/or phonophobia occur in about half of patients. Some patients have a previous history of migraine; however, the proportion of NDPH sufferers with preexisting migraine is no greater than the frequency of migraine in the general population. At 24 months, ~86% of patients are headache-free. Treatment of migrainous-type primary NDPH consists of using the preventive therapies effective in migraine (Table 8-7). Featureless NDPH is one of the primary headache forms most refractory to treatment. Standard preventive therapies can be offered but are often ineffective.

OTHER PRIMARY HEADACHES

Hemicrania continua

The essential features of hemicrania continua are moderate and continuous unilateral pain associated with fluctuations of severe pain; complete resolution of pain with indomethacin; and exacerbations that may be associated with autonomic features, including conjunctival injection, lacrimation, and photophobia on the affected side. The age of onset ranges from 11 to 58 years; women are affected twice as often as men. The cause is unknown.

TREATMENT **Hemicrania Continua**

Treatment consists of indomethacin; other NSAIDs appear to be of little or no benefit. The IM injection of 100 mg indomethacin has been proposed as a diagnostic tool and administration with a placebo injection in a blinded fashion can be very useful diagnostically. Alternatively, a trial of oral indomethacin, starting with 25 mg tid, then 50 mg tid, and then 75 mg tid, can be given. Up to two weeks at the maximal dose may be necessary to assess whether a dose has a useful effect. Topiramate can be helpful in some patients. Occipital nerve stimulation may have a role in patients with hemicrania continua who are unable to tolerate indomethacin.

Primary stabbing headache

The essential features of primary stabbing headache are stabbing pain confined to the head or, rarely, the face, lasting from 1 to many seconds or minutes and occurring as a single stab or a series of stabs; absence of associated cranial autonomic features; absence of cutaneous triggering of attacks; and a pattern of recurrence at irregular intervals (hours to days). The pains have been variously described as "ice-pick pains" or "jabs and jolts." They are more common in patients with other primary headaches, such as migraine, the TACs, and hemicrania continua.

TREATMENT **Primary Stabbing Headache**

The response of primary stabbing headache to indomethacin (25–50 mg two to three times daily) is usually excellent. As a general rule, the symptoms wax and wane, and after a period of control on indomethacin, it is appropriate to withdraw treatment and observe the outcome.

Primary cough headache

Primary cough headache is a generalized headache that begins suddenly, lasts for several minutes, and is precipitated by coughing; it is preventable by avoiding coughing or other precipitating events, which can include sneezing, straining, laughing, or stooping. In all patients with this syndrome, serious etiologies must be excluded before a diagnosis of "benign" primary cough headache can be established. A Chiari malformation or any lesion causing obstruction of CSF pathways or displacing cerebral structures can be the cause of the head pain. Other conditions that can present with cough or exertional headache as the initial symptom include cerebral aneurysm, carotid stenosis, and vertebrobasilar disease. Benign cough headache can resemble benign exertional headache (discussed next), but patients with the former condition are typically older.

TREATMENT **Primary Cough Headache**

Indomethacin 25–50 mg two to three times daily is the treatment of choice. Some patients with cough headache obtain pain relief with LP; this is a simple option when compared to prolonged use of indomethacin, and it is effective in about one-third of patients. The mechanism of this response is unclear.

Primary exertional headache

Primary exertional headache has features resembling both cough headache and migraine. It may be precipitated by any form of exercise; it often has the pulsatile quality of migraine. The pain, which can last from 5 min to 24 h, is bilateral and throbbing at onset; migrainous features may develop in patients susceptible to migraine. Primary exertional headache can be prevented by avoiding excessive exertion, particularly in hot weather or at high altitude.

The mechanism of primary exertional headache is unclear. Acute venous distension likely explains one syndrome, the acute onset of headache with straining and breath holding, as in weightlifter's headache. As exertion can result in headache in a number of serious underlying conditions, these must be considered in patients with exertional headache. Pain from angina may be referred to the head, probably by central connections of vagal afferents, and may present as exertional headache (cardiac cephalgia). The link to exercise is the main clinical clue that headache is of cardiac origin. Pheochromocytoma may occasionally cause exertional headache. Intracranial lesions and stenosis of the carotid arteries are other possible etiologies.

TREATMENT **Primary Exertional Headache**

Exercise regimens should begin modestly and progress gradually to higher levels of intensity. Indomethacin at daily doses from 25 to 150 mg is generally effective in benign exertional headache. Indomethacin (50 mg), ergotamine (1 mg orally), dihydroergotamine (2 mg by nasal spray), or methysergide (1–2 mg orally given 30–45 min before exercise) are useful prophylactic measures.

Primary Sex Headache

Sex headache is precipitated by sexual excitement. The pain usually begins as a dull bilateral headache that suddenly becomes intense at orgasm. The headache can be prevented or eased by ceasing sexual activity before orgasm. Three types of sex headache are reported: a dull ache in the head and neck that intensifies as sexual excitement increases; a sudden, severe, explosive headache occurring at orgasm; and a postural headache developing after coitus that resembles the headache of low CSF pressure. The latter arises from vigorous sexual activity and is a form of low CSF pressure headache. Headaches developing at the time of orgasm are not always benign; 5–12% of cases of subarachnoid hemorrhage are precipitated by sexual intercourse. Sex headache is reported by men more often than women and may occur at any time during the years of sexual activity. It may develop on several occasions in succession and then not trouble the patient again, even without an obvious change in sexual activity. In patients who stop sexual activity when headache is first noticed, the pain may subside within a period of 5 min to 2 h. In about half of patients, sex headache will subside within 6 months. About half of patients with sex headache have a history of exertional headaches, but there is no excess of cough headache. Migraine is probably more common in patients with sex headache.

TREATMENT Primary Sex Headache

Benign sex headaches recur irregularly and infrequently. Management can often be limited to reassurance and advice about ceasing sexual activity if a mild, warning headache develops. Propranolol can be used to prevent headache that recurs regularly or frequently, but the dosage required varies from 40 to 200 mg/d. An alternative is the calcium channel–blocking agent diltiazem, 60 mg tid. Ergotamine (1 mg) or indomethacin (25–50 mg) taken about 30–45 min prior to sexual activity can also be helpful.

Primary thunderclap headache

Sudden onset of severe headache may occur in the absence of any known provocation. The differential diagnosis includes the sentinel bleed of an intracranial aneurysm, cervicocephalic arterial dissection, and cerebral venous thrombosis. Headaches of explosive onset may also be caused by the ingestion of sympathomimetic drugs or of tyramine-containing foods in a patient who is taking MAOIs, or they may be a symptom of pheochromocytoma. Whether thunderclap headache can be the presentation of an unruptured cerebral aneurysm is uncertain. When neuroimaging studies and LP exclude subarachnoid hemorrhage, patients with thunderclap headache usually do very well over the long term. In one study of patients whose CT scans and CSF findings were negative, ~15% had recurrent episodes of thunderclap headache, and nearly half subsequently developed migraine or tension-type headache.

The first presentation of any sudden-onset severe headache should be vigorously investigated with neuroimaging (CT or, when possible, MRI with MR angiography) and CSF examination. Formal cerebral angiography should be reserved for those cases in which no primary diagnosis is forthcoming and for clinical situations that are particularly suggestive of intracranial aneurysm. Reversible segmental cerebral vasoconstriction may be seen in primary thunderclap headache without an intracranial aneurysm. In the presence of posterior leukoencephalopathy, the differential diagnosis includes cerebral angiitis, drug toxicity (cyclosporine, intrathecal methotrexate/cytarabine, pseudoephedrine, or cocaine), posttransfusion effects, and postpartum angiopathy. Treatment with nimodipine may be helpful, although by definition the vasoconstriction of primary thunderclap headache resolves spontaneously.

Hypnic headache

This headache syndrome typically begins a few hours after sleep onset. The headaches last from 15 to 30 min and are typically moderately severe and generalized, although they may be unilateral and can be throbbing. Patients may report falling back to sleep only to be awakened by a further attack a few hours later; up to three repetitions of this pattern occur through the night. Daytime naps can also precipitate head pain. Most patients are female, and the onset is usually after age 60 years. Headaches are bilateral in most, but may be unilateral. Photophobia or phonophobia and nausea are usually absent. The major secondary consideration in this headache type is poorly controlled hypertension; 24-h blood pressure monitoring is recommended to detect this treatable condition.

TREATMENT Hypnic Headache

Patients with hypnic headache generally respond to a bedtime dose of lithium carbonate (200–600 mg). For those intolerant of lithium, verapamil (160 mg) or methysergide (1–4 mg at bedtime) may be alternative strategies. One to two cups of coffee or caffeine, 60 mg orally, at bedtime may be effective in approximately one-third of patients. Case reports suggest that flunarizine, 5 mg nightly, can be effective.

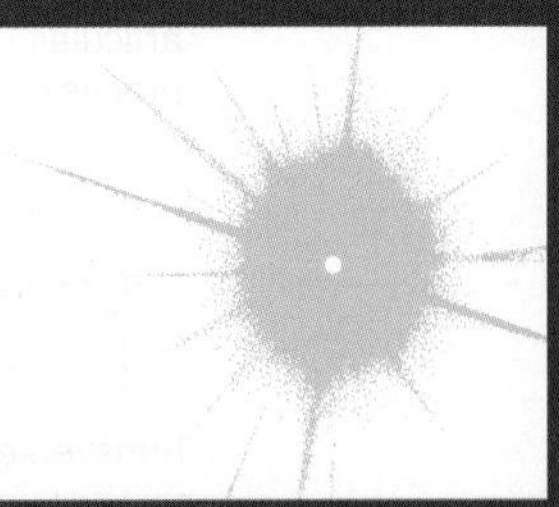

CHAPTER 9
BACK AND NECK PAIN

John W. Engstrom ■ Richard A. Deyo

The importance of back and neck pain in our society is underscored by the following: (1) the cost of back pain in the United States exceeds $100 billion annually; approximately one-third of these costs are direct health care expenses, and two-thirds are indirect costs resulting from loss of wages and productivity; (2) back symptoms are the most common cause of disability in those <45 years; (3) low back pain is the second most common reason for visiting a physician in the United States; and (4) ~1% of the U.S. population is chronically disabled because of back pain.

ANATOMY OF THE SPINE

The anterior portion of the spine consists of cylindrical vertebral bodies separated by intervertebral disks and held together by the anterior and posterior longitudinal ligaments. The intervertebral disks are composed of a central gelatinous nucleus pulposus surrounded by a tough cartilaginous ring, the annulus fibrosis. Disks are responsible for 25% of spinal column length and allow the bony vertebrae to move easily upon each other (Figs. 9-1 and 9-2). Desiccation of the nucleus pulposus and degeneration of the annulus fibrosus increase with age and results in loss of height. The disks are largest in the cervical and lumbar regions where movements of the spine are greatest. The functions of the anterior spine are to absorb the shock of body movements such as walking and running, and to protect the contents of the spinal canal.

The posterior portion of the spine consists of the vertebral arches and processes. Each arch consists of paired cylindrical pedicles anteriorly and paired laminae posteriorly. The vertebral arch also gives rise to two transverse processes laterally, one spinous process posteriorly, plus two superior and two inferior articular facets. The apposition of a superior and inferior facet constitutes a *facet joint*. The functions of the posterior spine are to protect the spinal cord and nerves within the spinal canal and to provide an anchor for the attachment of muscles and ligaments. The contraction of muscles attached to the spinous and transverse processes and laminae works like a system of pulleys and levers that results in flexion, extension, and lateral bending movements of the spine.

Nerve root injury (*radiculopathy*) is a common cause of neck, arm, low back, buttock, and leg pain (Figs. 15-2 and 15-3). The nerve roots exit at a level above their respective vertebral bodies in the cervical region (e.g., the C7 nerve root exits at the C6-C7 level) and below their respective vertebral bodies in the thoracic and lumbar regions (e.g., the T1 nerve root exits at the T1-T2 level). The cervical nerve roots follow a short intraspinal course before exiting. By contrast, because the spinal cord ends at the vertebral L1 or L2 level, the lumbar nerve roots follow a long intraspinal course and can be injured anywhere from the upper lumbar spine to their exit at the intervertebral foramen. For example, disk herniation at the L4-L5 level can produce not only L5 root compression, but also compression of the traversing S1 nerve root (Fig. 9-3).

Pain-sensitive structures of the spine include the periosteum of the vertebrae, dura, facet joints, annulus fibrosus of the intervertebral disk, epidural veins and arteries, and the posterior longitudinal ligament. Disease of these diverse structures may explain many cases of back pain without nerve root compression. The nucleus pulposus of the intervertebral disk is not pain-sensitive under normal circumstances. Pain sensation from within the spinal canal is conveyed partially by the sinuvertebral nerve that arises from the spinal nerve at each spine segment and reenters the spinal canal through the intervertebral foramen at the same level.

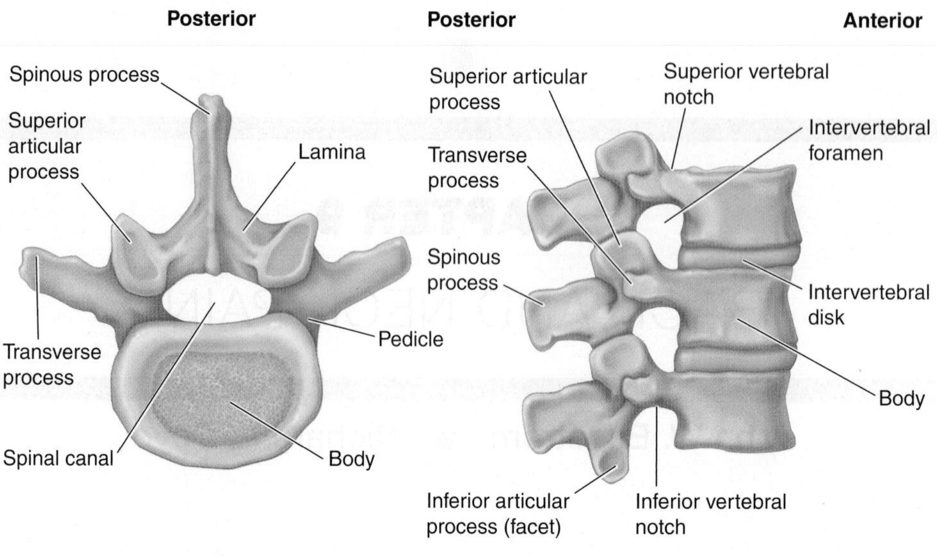

FIGURE 9-1

Vertebral anatomy. (*From A Gauthier Cornuelle, DH Gronefeld: Radiographic Anatomy Positioning. New York, McGraw-Hill, 1998; with permission.*)

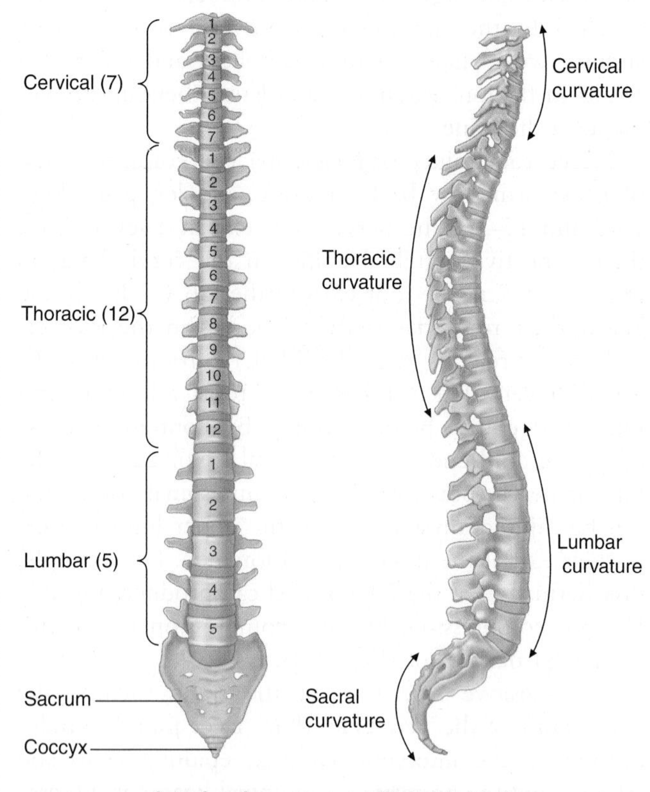

FIGURE 9-2

Spinal column. (*From A Gauthier Cornuelle, DH Gronefeld: Radiographic Anatomy Positioning. New York, McGraw-Hill, 1998; with permission.*)

APPROACH TO THE PATIENT **Back Pain**

TYPES OF BACK PAIN Understanding the types of pain reported by patients is the essential first step. Attention is also focused on identification of risk factors for serious underlying diseases; the majority of these are due to radiculopathy, fracture, tumor, infection, or referred pain from visceral structures (Table 9-1).

Local pain is caused by injury to pain-sensitive structures that compress or irritate sensory nerve endings. The site of the pain is near the affected part of the back.

Pain referred to the back may arise from abdominal or pelvic viscera. The pain is usually described as primarily abdominal or pelvic but is accompanied by back pain and usually unaffected by posture. The patient may occasionally complain of back pain only.

Pain of spine origin may be located in the back or referred to the buttocks or legs. Diseases affecting the upper lumbar spine tend to refer pain to the lumbar region, groin, or anterior thighs. Diseases affecting the lower lumbar spine tend to produce pain referred to the buttocks, posterior thighs, or rarely the calves or feet. Referred or "sclerotomal" pain may explain instances where the pain crosses multiple dermatomes without evidence of nerve root compression.

Radicular back pain is typically sharp and radiates from the low back to a leg within the territory of a nerve root (see "Lumbar Disk Disease," later in this chapter). Coughing, sneezing, or voluntary contraction of abdominal muscles (lifting heavy objects or straining at stool) may elicit the radiating pain. The pain may increase in postures that stretch the nerves and nerve roots. Sitting with the leg outstretched places traction on the sciatic nerve and L5 and S1 roots because the nerve passes posterior to the hip. The femoral nerve (L2, L3, and L4 roots) passes anterior to the hip and is not stretched by sitting. The description of the pain alone often fails to distinguish between sclerotomal pain and radiculopathy.

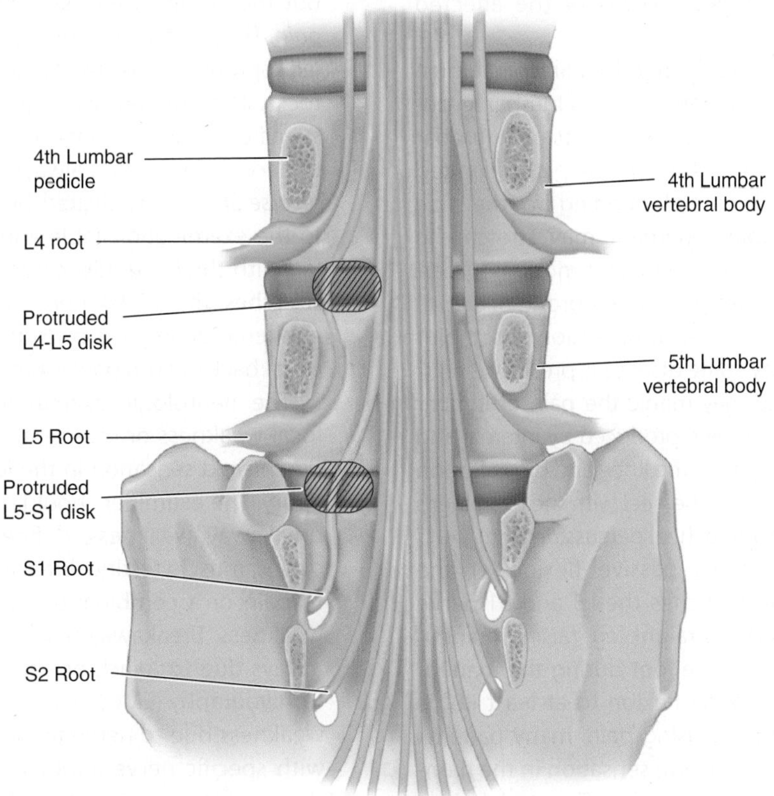

FIGURE 9-3
Compression of L5 and S1 roots by herniated disks. *(From Adams and Victor's Principles of Neurology, 9th ed. New York, McGraw-Hill, 2009; with permission.)*

TABLE 9-1

ACUTE LOW BACK PAIN: RISK FACTORS FOR AN IMPORTANT STRUCTURAL CAUSE
History
Pain worse at rest or at night
Prior history of cancer
History of chronic infection (esp. lung, urinary tract, skin)
History of trauma
Incontinence
Age >70 years
Intravenous drug use
Glucocorticoid use
History of a rapidly progressive neurologic deficit
Examination
Unexplained fever
Unexplained weight loss
Percussion tenderness over the spine
Abdominal, rectal, or pelvic mass
Patrick's sign or heel percussion sign
Straight leg or reverse straight leg–raising signs
Progressive focal neurologic deficit

Pain associated with muscle spasm, although of obscure origin, is commonly associated with many spine disorders. The spasms are accompanied by abnormal posture, tense paraspinal muscles, and dull or achy pain in the paraspinal region.

Knowledge of the circumstances associated with the onset of back pain is important when weighing possible serious underlying causes for the pain. Some patients involved in accidents or work-related injuries may exaggerate their pain for the purpose of compensation or for psychological reasons.

EXAMINATION OF THE BACK A physical examination that includes the abdomen and rectum is advisable. Back pain referred from visceral organs may be reproduced during palpation of the abdomen (pancreatitis, abdominal aortic aneurysm [AAA]) or percussion over the costovertebral angles (pyelonephritis).

The normal spine has a cervical and lumbar lordosis, and a thoracic kyphosis. Exaggeration of these normal alignments may result in hyperkyphosis of the thoracic spine or hyperlordosis of the lumbar spine. Inspection may reveal a lateral curvature of the spine (scoliosis) or an asymmetry in the prominence of the paraspinal muscles, suggesting muscle spasm. Back pain of bony spine origin is often reproduced by palpation or percussion over the spinous process of the affected vertebrae.

Forward bending is often limited by paraspinal muscle spasm; the latter may flatten the usual lumbar lordosis. Flexion at the hips is normal in patients with lumbar spine disease, but flexion of the lumbar spine is limited and sometimes painful. Lateral bending to the side opposite the injured spinal element may stretch the damaged tissues, worsen pain, and limit motion. Hyperextension of the spine (with the patient prone or standing) is limited when nerve root compression, facet joint pathology, or other bony spine disease is present.

Pain from hip disease may mimic the pain of lumbar spine disease. Hip pain can be reproduced by internal and external rotation at the hip with the knee and hip in flexion (Patrick's sign) and by tapping the heel with the examiner's palm while the leg is extended (heel percussion sign).

With the patient supine, passive flexion of the extended leg at the hip stretches the L5 and S1 nerve roots and the sciatic nerve (straight leg–raising maneuver). Passive dorsiflexion of the foot during the maneuver adds to the stretch. While flexion to at least 80° is normally possible without causing pain, many patients normally report a tight, stretching sensation in the hamstring muscles unrelated to back pain. The *straight leg–raising (SLR)* test is positive if the maneuver reproduces the patient's usual back or limb pain. Eliciting the SLR sign in the sitting position can help determine if the finding is reproducible. The patient may describe pain in the low back, buttocks, posterior thigh, or lower leg, but the *key feature is reproduction of the patient's usual pain*. The *crossed SLR sign* is positive when flexion of one leg reproduces the usual pain in the opposite leg or buttocks. The crossed SLR sign is less sensitive but more specific for disk herniation than the SLR sign. The nerve or nerve root lesion is always on the side of the pain. The *reverse SLR sign* is elicited by standing the patient next to the examination table and passively extending each leg with the knee fully extended. This maneuver, which stretches the L2-L4 nerve roots, lumbosacral plexus, and femoral nerve, is considered positive if the patient's usual back or limb pain is reproduced.

The neurologic examination includes a search for focal weakness or muscle atrophy, focal reflex changes, diminished sensation in the legs, or signs of spinal cord injury. The examiner should be alert to the possibility of breakaway weakness, defined as fluctuating strength during muscle testing. Breakaway weakness may be due to pain or a combination of pain and underlying true weakness. Breakaway weakness without pain is almost always due to a lack of effort. In uncertain cases, electromyography (EMG) can determine whether or not true weakness due to nerve tissue injury is present. Findings with specific nerve lumbosacral nerve root lesions are shown in Table 9-2 and are discussed next.

LABORATORY, IMAGING, AND EMG STUDIES Routine laboratory studies are rarely needed for the initial evaluation of nonspecific acute (<3 months duration) low back pain (ALBP). If risk factors for a serious

TABLE 9-2

LUMBOSACRAL RADICULOPATHY—NEUROLOGIC FEATURES

LUMBOSACRAL NERVE ROOTS	EXAMINATION FINDINGS: REFLEX	SENSORY	MOTOR	PAIN DISTRIBUTION
L2[a]	—	Upper anterior thigh	Psoas (hip flexion)	Anterior thigh
L3[a]	—	Lower anterior thigh Anterior knee	Psoas (hip flexion) Quadriceps (knee extension) Thigh adduction	Anterior thigh, knee
L4[a]	Quadriceps (knee)	Medial calf	Quadriceps (knee extension)[b] Thigh adduction Tibialis anterior (foot dorsiflexion)	Knee, medial calf Anterolateral thigh
L5[c]	—	Dorsal surface—foot Lateral calf	Peroneii (foot eversion)[b] Tibialis anterior (foot dorsiflexion) Gluteus medius (hip abduction) Toe dorsiflexors	Lateral calf, dorsal foot, posterolateral thigh, buttocks
S1[c]	Gastrocnemius/soleus (ankle)	Plantar surface—foot Lateral aspect—foot	Gastrocnemius/soleus (foot plantar flexion)[b] Abductor hallucis (toe flexors)[b] Gluteus maximus (hip extension)	Bottom foot, posterior calf, posterior thigh, buttocks

[a]Reverse straight leg–raising sign present—see "Examination of the Back."
[b]These muscles receive the majority of innervation from this root.
[c]Straight leg–raising sign present—see "Examination of the Back."

underlying cause are present (Table 9-1), then laboratory studies (complete blood count [CBC], erythrocyte sedimentation rate [ESR], urinalysis) are indicated.

CT scanning is superior to routine x-rays for the detection of fractures involving posterior spine structures, craniocervical and craniothoracic junctions, C1 and C2 vertebrae, bone fragments within the spinal canal, or misalignment; CT scans are increasingly used as a primary screening modality for moderate to severe trauma. In the absence of risk factors, these imaging studies are rarely helpful in nonspecific ALBP. MRI and CT-myelography are the radiologic tests of choice for evaluation of most serious diseases involving the spine. MRI is superior for the definition of soft tissue structures, whereas CT-myelography provides optimal imaging of the lateral recess of the spinal canal, and is better tolerated by claustrophobic patients. While the added diagnostic value of modern neuroimaging is significant, there is concern that these studies may be overutilized in patients with benign ALBP.

Electrodiagnostic studies can be used to assess the functional integrity of the peripheral nervous system (Chap. 5). Sensory nerve conduction studies are normal when focal sensory loss is due to nerve root damage because the nerve roots are proximal to the nerve cell bodies in the dorsal root ganglia. Injury to nerve tissue distal to the dorsal root ganglion (e.g., plexus or peripheral nerve) results in reduced sensory nerve signals. Needle EMG complements nerve conduction studies by detecting denervation or reinnervation changes in a myotomal (segmental) distribution. Multiple muscles supplied by different nerve roots and nerves are sampled; the pattern of muscle involvement indicates the nerve root(s) responsible for the injury. Needle EMG provides objective information about motor nerve fiber injury when clinical evaluation of weakness is limited by pain or poor effort. EMG and nerve conduction studies will be normal when sensory nerve root injury or irritation is the source of the pain.

CAUSES OF BACK PAIN

(Table 9-3)

CONGENITAL ANOMALIES OF THE LUMBAR SPINE

Spondylolysis is a bony defect in the vertebral pars interarticularis (a segment near the junction of the pedicle with the lamina); the cause is usually a stress microfracture in a congenitally abnormal segment. It occurs in up to 6% of adolescents. The defect (usually bilateral) is best visualized on plain x-rays, CT scan, or bone scan and is frequently asymptomatic. Symptoms may occur

TABLE 9-3

CAUSES OF BACK OR NECK PAIN
Congenital/Developmental
Spondylolysis and spondylolisthesis
Kyphoscoliosis
Spina bifida occulta
Tethered spinal cord
Minor Trauma
Strain or sprain
Whiplash injury
Fractures
Trauma—falls, motor vehicle accidents
Atraumatic fractures—osteoporosis, neoplastic infiltration, exogenous steroids, osteomyelitis
Intervertebral Disk Herniation
Degenerative
Intervertebral foraminal narrowing
Disk-osteophyte complex
Internal disk disruption
LSS with neurogenic claudication
Uncovertebral joint disease
Atlantoaxial joint disease (e.g., rheumatoid arthritis)
Arthritis
Spondylosis
Facet or sacroiliac arthropathy
Neoplasms—metastatic, hematologic, primary bone tumors
Infection/Inflammation
Vertebral osteomyelitis
Spinal epidural abscess
Septic disk (diskitis)
Meningitis
Lumbar arachnoiditis
Autoimmune (e.g., ankylosing spondylitis, reactive arthritis [formerly known as Reiter's syndrome])
Metabolic
Osteoporosis—hyperparathyroidism, immobility
Osteosclerosis (e.g., Paget's disease)
Vascular
Abdominal aortic aneurysm
Vertebral artery dissection
Other
Referred pain from visceral disease
Postural
Psychiatric, malingering, chronic pain syndromes

in the setting of a single injury, repeated minor injuries, or growth. Spondylolysis is the most common cause of persistent low back pain in adolescents and is often associated with sports-related activities.

Spondylolisthesis is the anterior slippage of the vertebral body, pedicles, and superior articular facets, leaving the posterior elements behind. Spondylolisthesis can be associated with spondylolysis, congenital anomalies, degenerative spine disease, or other causes of mechanical weakness of the pars (e.g., infection, osteoporosis, tumor, trauma, prior surgery). The slippage may be asymptomatic or may cause low back pain and hamstring tightness, nerve root injury (the L5 root most frequently), symptomatic spinal stenosis, or cauda equina syndrome (CES) in severe cases. Tenderness may be elicited near the segment that has "slipped" forward (most often L4 on L5 or occasionally L5 on S1). A "step" may be present on deep palpation of the posterior elements of the segment above the spondylolisthetic joint. The trunk may be shortened and the abdomen protuberant as a result. Anterolisthesis or retrolisthesis can also occur at other cervical or lumbar levels in adults and be the source of neck or low back pain. Plain x-rays with the neck or low back in flexion and extension will reveal the movement at the abnormal spinal segment. Surgery is considered for pain symptoms that do not respond to conservative measures (e.g., rest, physical therapy), and in cases with progressive neurologic deficit, postural deformity, slippage >50%, or scoliosis.

Spina bifida occulta is a failure of closure of one or several vertebral arches posteriorly; the meninges and spinal cord are normal. A dimple or small lipoma may overlie the defect. Most cases are asymptomatic and discovered incidentally during an evaluation for back pain.

Tethered cord syndrome usually presents as a progressive cauda equina disorder (see later), although myelopathy may also be the initial manifestation. The patient is often a young adult who complains of perineal or perianal pain, sometimes following minor trauma. MRI studies reveal a low-lying conus (below L1-L2) and a short and thickened filum terminale.

TRAUMA

A patient complaining of back pain and an inability to move the legs may have a spinal fracture or dislocation, and, with fractures above L1, spinal cord compression. Care must be taken to avoid further damage to the spinal cord or nerve roots by immobilizing the back pending the results of radiologic studies.

Sprains and strains

The terms *low back sprain*, *strain*, and *mechanically induced muscle spasm* refer to minor, self-limited injuries associated with lifting a heavy object, a fall, or a sudden deceleration such as in an automobile accident. These terms are used loosely and do not clearly describe a specific anatomic lesion. The pain is usually confined to the lower back, and there is no radiation to the buttocks or legs. Patients with paraspinal muscle spasm often assume unusual postures.

Traumatic vertebral fractures

Most traumatic fractures of the lumbar vertebral bodies result from injuries producing anterior wedging or compression. With severe trauma, the patient may sustain a fracture-dislocation or a "burst" fracture involving the vertebral body and posterior elements. Traumatic vertebral fractures are caused by falls from a height (a pars interarticularis fracture of the L5 vertebra is common), sudden deceleration in an automobile accident, or direct injury. Neurologic impairment is common, and early surgical treatment is indicated. In victims of blunt trauma, CT scans of the chest, abdomen, or pelvis can be reformatted to detect associated vertebral fractures.

LUMBAR DISK DISEASE

This is a common cause of chronic or recurrent low back and leg pain (Figs. 9-3 and 9-4). Disk disease is most likely to occur at the L4-L5 or L5-S1 levels, but upper lumbar levels are involved occasionally. The cause is often unknown; the risk is increased in overweight individuals. Disk herniation is unusual prior to age 20 years and is rare in the fibrotic disks of the elderly. Genetic factors may play a role in predisposing some patients to disk disease. The pain may be located in the low back only or referred to a leg, buttock, or hip. A sneeze, cough, or trivial movement may cause the nucleus pulposus to prolapse, pushing the frayed and weakened annulus posteriorly. With severe disk disease, the nucleus may protrude through the annulus (herniation) or become extruded to lie as a free fragment in the spinal canal.

The mechanism by which intervertebral disk injury causes back pain is controversial. The inner annulus fibrosus and nucleus pulposus are normally devoid of innervation. Inflammation and production of proinflammatory cytokines within the protruding or ruptured disk may trigger or perpetuate back pain. Ingrowth of nociceptive (pain) nerve fibers into inner portions of a diseased disk may be responsible for chronic "diskogenic" pain. Nerve root injury (radiculopathy) from disk herniation may be due to compression, inflammation, or both; pathologically, demyelination and axonal loss are usually present.

A ruptured disk may be asymptomatic or cause back pain, abnormal posture, limitation of spine motion

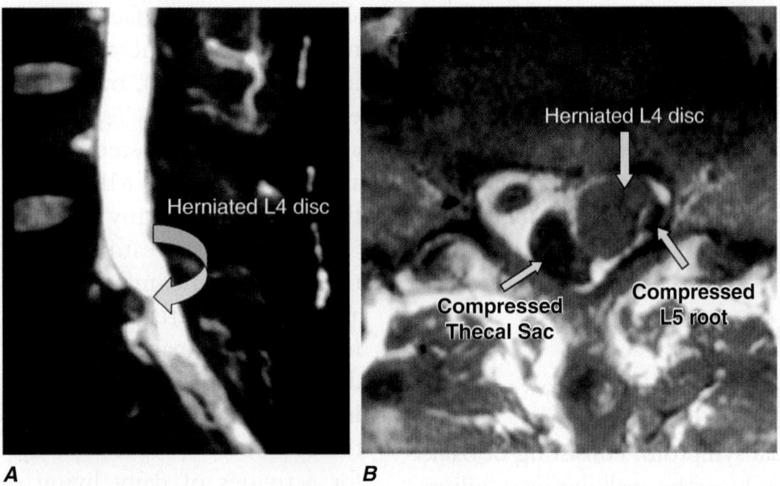

FIGURE 9-4

Left L5 radiculopathy. ***A.*** Sagittal T2-weighted image on the left reveals disk herniation at the L4-L5 level. ***B.*** Axial T1-weighted image shows paracentral disk herniation with displacement of the thecal sac medially and the left L5 nerve root posteriorly in the left lateral recess.

(particularly flexion), a focal neurologic deficit, or radicular pain. A dermatomal pattern of sensory loss or a reduced or absent deep tendon reflex is more suggestive of a specific root lesion than is the pattern of pain. Motor findings (focal weakness, muscle atrophy, or fasciculations) occur less frequently than focal sensory or reflex changes. Symptoms and signs are usually unilateral, but bilateral involvement does occur with large central disk herniations that compress multiple roots or cause inflammation of nerve roots within the spinal canal. Clinical manifestations of specific nerve root lesions are summarized in Table 9-2. There is suggestive evidence that lumbar disk herniation with a nonprogressive nerve root deficit can be managed nonsurgically.

The differential diagnosis covers a variety of serious and treatable conditions, including epidural abscess, hematoma, fracture, or tumor. Fever, constant pain uninfluenced by position, sphincter abnormalities, or signs of spinal cord disease suggest an etiology other than lumbar disk disease. Absence of ankle reflexes can be a normal finding in persons older than age 60 years or a sign of bilateral S1 radiculopathy. An absent deep tendon reflex or focal sensory loss may indicate injury to a nerve root, but other sites of injury along the nerve must also be considered. For example, an absent knee reflex may be due to a femoral neuropathy or an L4 nerve root injury. A loss of sensation over the foot and lateral lower calf may result from a peroneal or lateral sciatic neuropathy or an L5 nerve root injury. Focal muscle atrophy may reflect a nerve root, peripheral nerve, anterior horn cell disease, or disuse.

A lumbar spine MRI scan or CT-myelogram is necessary to establish the location and type of pathology. Spine MRIs yield exquisite views of intraspinal and adjacent soft tissue anatomy. Bony lesions of the lateral recess or intervertebral foramen are optimally visualized by CT-myelography. The correlation of neuroradiologic findings to symptoms, particularly pain, is not simple. Contrast-enhancing tears in the annulus fibrosus or disk protrusions are widely accepted as common sources of back pain; however, studies have found that many asymptomatic adults have similar findings. Asymptomatic disk protrusions are also common and may enhance with contrast. *Furthermore, in patients with known disk herniation treated either medically or surgically, persistence of the herniation 10 years later had no relationship to the clinical outcome.* In summary, MRI findings of disk protrusion, tears in the annulus fibrosus, or contrast enhancement are common incidental findings that, by themselves, should not dictate management decisions for patients with back pain.

The diagnosis of nerve root injury is most secure when the history, examination, results of imaging studies, and the EMG are concordant. The correlation between CT and EMG for localization of nerve root injury is between 65 and 73%. Up to one-third of asymptomatic adults have a lumbar disk protrusion detected by CT or MRI scans.

Management of lumbar disk disease is discussed later in the chapter.

Cauda equina syndrome (CES) signifies an injury of multiple lumbosacral nerve roots within the spinal canal distal to the termination of the spinal cord at L1-2. Low back pain, weakness and areflexia in the legs, saddle anesthesia, or loss of bladder function may occur. The problem must be distinguished from disorders of the lower spinal cord (conus medullaris syndrome), acute transverse myelitis (Chap. 35), and Guillain-Barré syndrome (Chap. 46). Combined involvement of the conus medullaris and cauda equina can occur. CES is commonly due to a ruptured lumbosacral intervertebral disk, lumbosacral spine fracture, hematoma within the spinal canal (e.g., following lumbar puncture in patients with coagulopathy), compressive tumor, or other mass lesion. Treatment options include surgical decompression, sometimes urgently, in an attempt to restore or preserve motor or sphincter function, or radiotherapy for metastatic tumors (Chap. 37).

DEGENERATIVE CONDITIONS

Lumbar spinal stenosis (LSS) describes a narrowed lumbar spinal canal and is frequently asymptomatic. *Neurogenic claudication* is the usual symptom, consisting of back and buttock or leg pain induced by walking or standing and relieved by sitting. Symptoms in the legs are usually bilateral. Lumbar stenosis, by itself, is frequently asymptomatic, and the correlation between the severity of symptoms and degree of stenosis of the spinal canal is poor. Unlike vascular claudication, symptoms are often provoked by standing without walking. Unlike lumbar disk disease, symptoms are usually relieved by sitting. Patients with neurogenic claudication can often walk much farther when leaning over a shopping cart and can pedal a stationary bike while sitting with ease. These flexed positions increase the anteroposterior spinal canal diameter and reduce intraspinal venous hypertension, resulting in pain relief. Focal weakness, sensory loss, or reflex changes may occur when spinal stenosis is associated with neural foraminal narrowing and radiculopathy. Severe neurologic deficits, including paralysis and urinary incontinence, occur only rarely.

LSS can be acquired (75%), congenital, or due to a combination of these factors. Congenital forms (achondroplasia, idiopathic) are characterized by short, thick pedicles that produce both spinal canal and lateral recess stenosis. Acquired factors that contribute to spinal stenosis include degenerative diseases (spondylosis, spondylolisthesis, scoliosis), trauma, spine surgery, metabolic or endocrine disorders (epidural lipomatosis, osteoporosis, acromegaly, renal osteodystrophy, hypoparathyroidism), and Paget's disease. MRI provides the best definition of the abnormal anatomy (Fig. 9-5).

Conservative treatment of symptomatic LSS includes nonsteroidal anti-inflammatory drugs (NSAIDs), acetaminophen, exercise programs, and symptomatic treatment of acute pain episodes. There is insufficient evidence to support the use of epidural glucocorticoid injections. Surgical therapy is considered when medical therapy does not relieve symptoms sufficiently to allow for activities of daily living or when significant focal neurologic signs are present. Most patients with neurogenic claudication treated surgically experience significant relief of back and leg pain within 6 weeks post-operation, and pain relief persists for at least 2 years. Patients treated nonoperatively improve uncommonly. Up to one-quarter develop recurrent stenosis at the same spinal level or an adjacent level 7–10 years after the initial surgery; recurrent symptoms usually respond to a second surgical decompression.

Neural foraminal narrowing with radiculopathy is a common degenerative disorder most often caused by the same processes that cause lumbar spinal stenosis (Figs. 9-1 and 9-6), including osteophytes, lateral disk protrusion, calcified disk-osteophytes, facet joint hypertrophy, uncovertebral joint hypertrophy (cervical spine), congenitally shortened pedicles, or, frequently, a combination of these processes. Neoplasms (primary or metastatic), fractures, infections (epidural abscess), or hematomas are other considerations. These conditions can produce unilateral nerve root symptoms or signs due to bony compression at the intervertebral foramen or lateral recess;

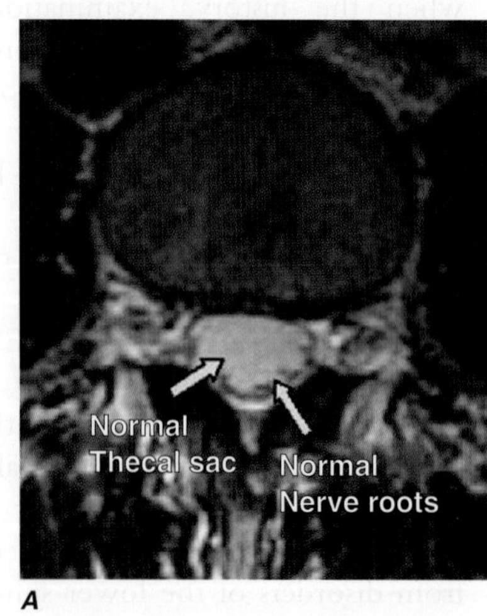

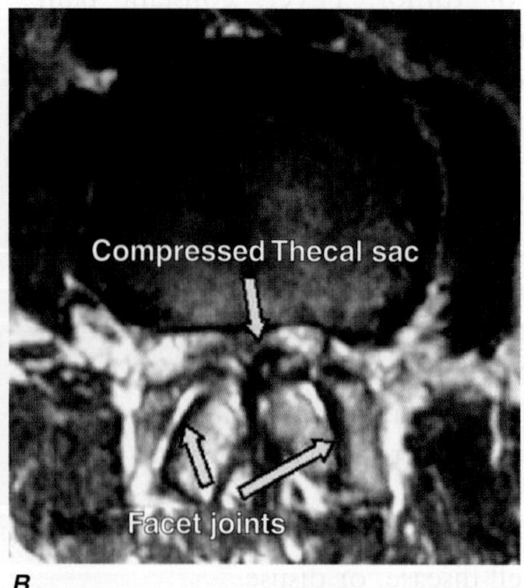

FIGURE 9-5

Axial T2-weighted images of the lumbar spine. *A.* The image shows a normal thecal sac within the lumbar spinal canal. The thecal sac is bright. The lumbar roots are dark punctuate dots in the posterior thecal sac with the patient supine. ***B.*** The thecal sac is not well visualized due to severe lumbar spinal canal stenosis, partially the result of hypertrophic facet joints.

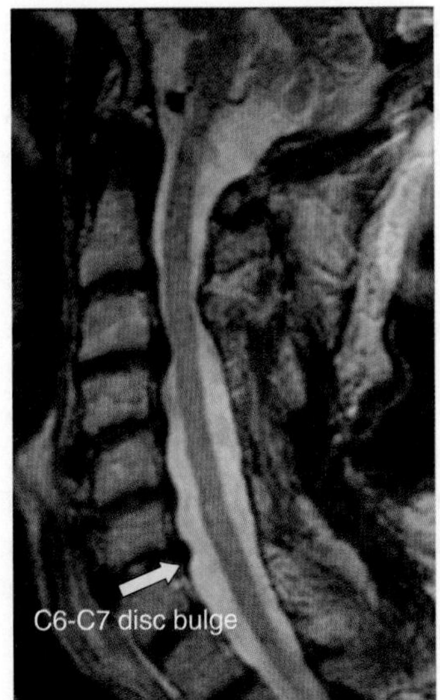

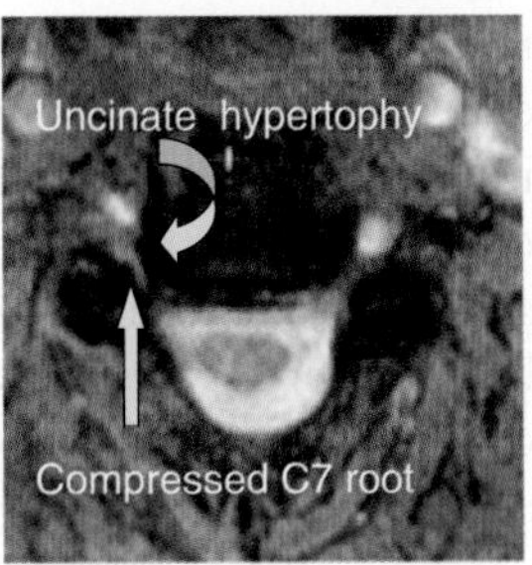

A Sagittal T2 cervical spine B

FIGURE 9-6

Right C7 radiculopathy. *A.* Sagittal T2-weighted image shows mild disk bulging at C6-C7 and a mildly narrowed spinal canal, but no visible nerve root compression. ***B.*** Axial T2-weighted image. The combination of uncinate hypertrophy and facet hypertrophy (ovoid dark space just lateral to the C7 root) narrows the right C6-C7 intervertebral foramen resulting in right C7 nerve root compression.

symptoms are indistinguishable from disk-related radiculopathy, but treatment may differ depending upon the specific etiology. The history and neurologic examination alone cannot distinguish between these possibilities, and a spinal neuroimaging (CT or MRI) procedure is required to identify the underlying cause. Neurologic findings from the examination and EMG can help direct the attention of the radiologist to specific nerve or root structures that are best visualized on axial images. For *facet joint hypertrophy,* surgical foraminotomy produces long-term relief of leg and back pain in 80–90% of patients. The usefulness of therapeutic facet joint blocks for pain has not been rigorously studied.

ARTHRITIS

Spondylosis, or osteoarthritic spine disease, typically occurs in later life and primarily involves the cervical and lumbosacral spine. Patients often complain of back pain that increases with movement and is associated with stiffness. The relationship between clinical symptoms and radiologic findings is usually not straightforward. Pain may be prominent when x-ray, CT, or MRI findings are minimal, and prominent degenerative spine disease can be seen in asymptomatic patients. Osteophytes or combined disk-osteophytes may cause or contribute to central spinal canal stenosis, lateral recess stenosis, or neural foraminal narrowing.

Ankylosing spondylitis

This distinctive arthritic spine disease typically presents with the insidious onset of low back and buttock pain. Patients are often males below age 40. Associated features include morning back stiffness, nocturnal pain, pain unrelieved by rest, an elevated ESR, and the histocompatibility antigen HLA-B27. Onset at a young age and back pain improving with exercise are characteristic. Loss of the normal lumbar lordosis and exaggeration of thoracic kyphosis develop as the disease progresses. Inflammation and erosion of the outer fibers of the annulus fibrosus at the point of contact with the vertebral body are followed by ossification and bony growth that bridges adjacent vertebral bodies and reduces spine mobility in all planes. MRI has been used to assess the presence of inflammation in joints as well as response to treatment and is more sensitive than plain x-rays. In later stages, plain x-rays reveal bridging of vertebral bodies to produce the fused "bamboo spine."

Stress fractures after minimal or no trauma can occur through the spontaneously ankylosed posterior bony elements of the rigid, osteoporotic spine and can produce focal pain, spinal instability, spinal cord compression, or CES. Atlantoaxial subluxation with spinal cord compression can occur in up to 20% of patients over time. Ankylosis of the ribs to the spine and a decrease in the height of the thoracic spine may compromise respiratory function. Therapy with anti–tumor necrosis factor agents is effective in reducing disease activity and improving function. Similar to ankylosing spondylitis, restricted movements may accompany reactive arthritis (formerly known as Reiter's syndrome), psoriatic arthritis, and chronic inflammatory bowel disease.

NEOPLASMS

Back pain is the most common neurologic symptom in patients with systemic cancer and is the presenting symptom in 20%. The cause is usually vertebral body metastasis but can also result from spread of cancer through the intervertebral foramen (especially with lymphoma) or from carcinomatous meningitis. Cancer-related back pain tends to be constant, dull, unrelieved by rest, and worse at night. By contrast, mechanical low back pain usually improves with rest. MRI, CT, and CT-myelography are the studies of choice when spinal metastasis is suspected. Once a metastasis is found, imaging of the entire spine reveals additional tumor deposits in one-third of patients. MRI is preferred for soft tissue definition, but the most rapidly available imaging modality is best because the patient's condition may worsen quickly without intervention. Fewer than 5% of patients who are nonambulatory at the time of diagnosis ever regain the ability to walk; thus, early diagnosis is crucial. The management of spinal metastasis is discussed in detail in Chap. 37.

INFECTIONS/INFLAMMATION

Vertebral osteomyelitis is often caused by staphylococci, but other bacteria or tuberculosis (Pott's disease) may be responsible. The primary source of infection is usually the urinary tract, skin, or lungs. Intravenous drug use is a well-recognized risk factor. Whenever pyogenic osteomyelitis is found, the possibility of bacterial endocarditis should be considered. Back pain unrelieved by rest, spine tenderness over the involved spine segment, and an elevated ESR are the most common findings in vertebral osteomyelitis. Fever or an elevated white blood cell count is found in a minority of patients. MRI and CT are sensitive and specific for early detection of osteomyelitis; CT may be more readily available in emergency settings and better tolerated by some patients with severe back pain. The intervertebral disk can also be affected by infection (diskitis), and very rarely by tumor.

Spinal epidural abscess (Chap. 35) presents with back pain (aggravated by movement or palpation), fever, radiculopathy, or signs of spinal cord compression. The subacute development of two or more of these findings should increase the index of suspicion for spinal epidural abscess. The abscess may track over multiple spinal levels and is best delineated by spine MRI.

Lumbar adhesive arachnoiditis with radiculopathy is due to fibrosis following inflammation within the subarachnoid space. The fibrosis results in nerve root adhesions, and presents as back and leg pain associated with motor, sensory, or reflex changes. Causes of arachnoiditis include multiple lumbar operations, chronic spinal infections (especially tuberculosis in the developing world), spinal cord injury, intrathecal hemorrhage, myelography (rare), intrathecal injections (glucocorticoids, anesthetics, or other agents), and foreign bodies. The MRI shows clumped nerve roots or loculations of cerebrospinal fluid within the thecal sac. Clumped nerve roots may also occur with demyelinating polyneuropathy or neoplastic infiltration. Treatment is usually unsatisfactory. Microsurgical lysis of adhesions, dorsal rhizotomy, dorsal root ganglionectomy, and epidural steroids have been tried, but outcomes have been poor. Dorsal column stimulation for pain relief has produced varying results.

METABOLIC CAUSES

Osteoporosis and osteosclerosis

Immobilization or underlying conditions such as osteomalacia, the postmenopausal state, renal disease, multiple myeloma, hyperparathyroidism, hyperthyroidism, metastatic carcinoma, or glucocorticoid use may accelerate osteoporosis and weaken the vertebral body, leading to compression fractures and pain. Up to two-thirds of compression fractures seen on radiologic imaging are asymptomatic. The most common nontraumatic vertebral body fractures are due to postmenopausal or senile osteoporosis. The risk of an additional vertebral fracture at 1 year following a first vertebral fracture is 20%. The presence of fever, weight loss, fracture at a level above T4, or other conditions described above should increase the suspicion for a cause other than senile osteoporosis. If tumor is suspected, a bone biopsy or diagnostic search for a primary tumor is indicated. The sole manifestation of a compression fracture may be localized back pain or radicular pain exacerbated by movement and often reproduced by palpation over the spinous process of the affected vertebra. The clinical context, neurologic signs, and radiologic appearance of the spine establish the diagnosis.

Relief of acute pain can often be achieved with acetaminophen or a combination of opioids and acetaminophen. The role of NSAIDs is controversial. Both pain and disability are improved with bracing. Antiresorptive drugs, especially bisphosphonates (e.g., alendronate), have been shown to reduce the risk of osteoporotic fractures and are the preferred treatment to prevent additional fractures. Less than one-third of patients with prior compression fractures are adequately treated for osteoporosis despite the increased risk for future fractures; even fewer at-risk patients without a history of fracture are adequately treated. Interventions (percutaneous vertebroplasty [PVP], kyphoplasty) exist for osteoporotic compression fractures associated with debilitating pain. Controlled studies suggest a benefit for pain reduction acutely, but not at 2 months, when compared with conservative care. Relief of pain following PVP has also been reported in patients with vertebral metastases, myeloma, or hemangiomas.

Osteosclerosis, an abnormally increased bone density often due to Paget's disease, is readily identifiable on routine x-ray studies and can sometimes be a source of back pain. It may be associated with an isolated increase in alkaline phosphatase in an otherwise healthy older person. Spinal cord or nerve root compression can result from bony encroachment. It should not be assumed that Paget's disease is the cause of a patient's back pain until other etiologies have been carefully considered.

REFERRED PAIN FROM VISCERAL DISEASE

Diseases of the thorax, abdomen, or pelvis may refer pain to the posterior portion of the spinal segment that innervates the diseased organ. Occasionally, back pain may be the first and only manifestation. Upper abdominal diseases generally refer pain to the lower thoracic or upper lumbar region (eighth thoracic to the first and second lumbar vertebrae), lower abdominal diseases to the midlumbar region (second to fourth lumbar vertebrae), and pelvic diseases to the sacral region. Local signs (pain with spine palpation, paraspinal muscle spasm) are absent, and little or no pain accompanies routine movements of the spine.

Low thoracic or lumbar pain with abdominal disease

Tumors of the posterior wall of the stomach or duodenum typically produce epigastric pain, but midline back or paraspinal pain may occur if retroperitoneal extension is present. Fatty foods occaionally induce back pain associated with biliary disease. Diseases of the pancreas can produce right paraspinal back pain (head of the pancreas involved) or left paraspinal pain (body or tail involved). Pathology in retroperitoneal structures (hemorrhage, tumors, pyelonephritis) can produce paraspinal pain that radiates to the lower abdomen, groin, or anterior thighs. A mass in the iliopsoas region can produce unilateral lumbar pain with radiation toward the groin, labia, or testicle. The sudden appearance of lumbar pain in a patient receiving anticoagulants suggests retroperitoneal hemorrhage.

Isolated low back pain occurs in some patients with a contained rupture of an abdominal aortic aneurysm (AAA). The classic clinical triad of abdominal pain, shock, and back pain occurs in <20% of patients. The typical patient at risk is an elderly male smoker with back pain. Frequently, the diagnosis is initially missed because the symptoms and signs can be nonspecific. Misdiagnoses include nonspecific back pain, diverticulitis, renal colic, sepsis, and myocardial infarction. A careful abdominal examination revealing a pulsatile mass (present in 50–75% of patients) is an important physical finding. Patients with suspected AAA should be evaluated with abdominal ultrasound, CT, or MRI.

Sacral pain with gynecologic and urologic disease

Pelvic organs rarely cause low back pain, except for gynecologic disorders involving the uterosacral ligaments. The pain is referred to the sacral region. Endometriosis or uterine cancers may invade the uterosacral ligaments. Pain associated with endometriosis is typically premenstrual and often continues until it merges with menstrual pain. Uterine malposition may cause uterosacral ligament traction (retroversion, descensus, and prolapse) or produce sacral pain after prolonged standing.

Menstrual pain may be felt in the sacral region. Poorly localized, cramping pain can radiate down the legs. Pain due to neoplastic infiltration of nerves is typically continuous, progressive in severity, and unrelieved by rest at night. Less commonly, radiation therapy of pelvic tumors may produce sacral pain from late radiation necrosis of tissue. Low back pain that radiates into one or both thighs is common in the last weeks of pregnancy.

Urologic sources of lumbosacral back pain include chronic prostatitis, prostate cancer with spinal metastasis, and diseases of the kidney or ureter. Lesions of the bladder and testes do not often produce back pain. Infectious, inflammatory, or neoplastic renal diseases may produce ipsilateral lumbosacral pain, as can renal artery or vein thrombosis. Paraspinal lumbar pain may be a symptom of ureteral obstruction due to nephrolithiasis.

OTHER CAUSES OF BACK PAIN

Postural back pain

There is a group of patients with nonspecific chronic low back pain (CLBP) in whom no specific anatomic lesion can be found despite exhaustive investigation. These individuals complain of vague, diffuse back pain with prolonged sitting or standing that is relieved by rest. Exercises to strengthen the paraspinal and abdominal muscles are sometimes helpful.

Psychiatric disease

CLBP may be encountered in patients who seek financial compensation; in malingerers; or in those with concurrent substance abuse. Many patients with CLBP have a history of psychiatric illness (depression, anxiety states), or childhood trauma (physical or sexual abuse) that antedates the onset of back pain. Preoperative psychological assessment has been used to exclude patients with marked psychological impairments that predict a poor surgical outcome from spine surgery.

IDIOPATHIC

The cause of low back pain occasionally remains unclear. Some patients have had multiple operations for disk disease but have persistent pain and disability. The original indications for surgery may have been questionable, with back pain only, no definite neurologic signs, or a minor disk bulge noted on CT or MRI. Scoring systems based upon neurologic signs, psychological factors, physiologic studies, and imaging studies have been devised to minimize the likelihood of unsuccessful surgery.

TREATMENT Back Pain

ACUTE LOW BACK PAIN (ALBP) WITHOUT RADICULOPATHY ALBP is defined as pain of <3 months' duration. Full recovery can be expected in 85% of adults with ALBP without leg pain. Most have purely "mechanical" symptoms (i.e., pain that is aggravated by motion and relieved by rest).

The initial assessment excludes serious causes of spine pathology that require urgent intervention, including infection, cancer, or trauma. Risk factors for a serious cause of ALBP are shown in Table 9-1. Laboratory and imaging studies are unnecessary if risk factors are absent. CT or plain spine films are rarely indicated in the first month of symptoms unless a spine fracture is suspected.

The prognosis is generally excellent. Many patients do not seek medical care and apparently improve on their own. Even among those seen in primary care, two-thirds report being substantially improved after seven weeks. This spontaneous improvement can mislead clinicians and researchers about the efficacy of treatment interventions. Perhaps as a result, many ineffective treatments have become widespread in the past, such as bed rest, lumbar traction, sacroiliac fusion, and coccygectomy.

Clinicians should reassure patients that improvement is very likely, and instruct them in self-care. Education is an important part of treatment. Satisfaction and the likelihood of follow-up increase when patients are educated about prognosis, treatment methods, activity modifications, and strategies to prevent future exacerbations. In one study, patients who felt they did not receive an adequate explanation for their symptoms wanted further diagnostic tests. In general, bed rest should be avoided, or kept to a day or two at most, for relief of severe symptoms. Several randomized trials suggest that bed rest does not accelerate the pace of recovery. In general, the best activity recommendation is for walking and early resumption of normal physical activity, avoiding only strenuous manual labor. Possible advantages of early ambulation for acute back pain include maintenance of cardiovascular conditioning, improved disk and cartilage nutrition, improved bone and muscle strength, and increased endorphin levels. Specific back exercises or early vigorous exercise have not shown benefits for acute back pain, but may be useful for chronic pain. Application of heat by heating pads or heated blankets is sometimes helpful.

Evidence-based guidelines suggest that over-the-counter medicines such as acetaminophen and NSAIDs are first-line options for the treatment of ALBP. Skeletal muscle relaxants, such as cyclobenzaprine or methocarbamol, may be useful, but sedation is a common side effect. Limiting the use of muscle relaxants to nighttime only may be an option for some patients. Because of the risk of abuse of some drugs in this category, including benzodiazepines and carisoprodol, short courses are generally recommended.

It is unclear whether opioid analgesics and tramadol are more effective than NSAIDs or acetaminophen for treating ALBP; most of the available efficacy data are for treatment of chronic back pain. Their use is best reserved for patients who cannot tolerate acetaminophen or NSAIDs, or for those with severe refractory pain. As with muscle relaxants, these drugs are often sedating, so it may be useful to prescribe them at nighttime only. Side effects of short-term opioid use include nausea, constipation, and pruritis; risks of long-term opioid use include hypersensitivity to pain, hypogonadism, and dependency.

There is no evidence to support use of oral or injected glucocorticoids for acute low back pain without radiculopathy. Antiepileptic drugs, such as gabapentin, are not FDA approved for treating low back pain, and there is insufficient evidence to support their use in this setting.

Nonpharmacologic treatments for acute low back pain include spinal manipulation, physical therapy, massage, acupuncture, transcutaneous electrical nerve stimulation, ultrasound, diathermy, and magnets. Spinal manipulation appears to be roughly equivalent to conventional medical treatments and may be a useful alternative for patients who wish to avoid or who cannot tolerate drug therapy. There is little evidence to support the use of physical therapy, massage, acupuncture, laser therapy, therapeutic ultrasound, magnets, corsets, or lumbar traction. Though important for chronic pain, back exercises for acute back pain are generally not supported by clinical evidence. There is no useful evidence regarding the value of ice or heat applications for ALBP; many patients report temporary symptomatic relief from ice, and heat may produce a short-term reduction in pain after the first week.

CHRONIC LOW BACK PAIN WITHOUT RADICULOPATHY Chronic low back pain is defined as pain lasting >12 weeks; it accounts for 50% of total back pain costs. Risk factors include obesity, female gender, older age, prior history of back pain, restricted spinal mobility, pain radiating into a leg, high levels of psychological distress, poor self-rated health, minimal physical activity, smoking, job dissatisfaction, and widespread pain. In general, the same treatments that are recommended for acute low back pain can be useful for patients with chronic low back pain. In this setting, however, the benefit of opioid therapy or muscle relaxants is less clear.

Evidence supports the use of exercise therapy, and this can be one of the mainstays of treatment for chronic back pain. Effective regimens have generally included a combination of gradually increasing aerobic exercise, strengthening exercises, and stretching exercises. Motivating patients is sometimes challenging, and supervised exercise is best, for example, with a supportive physical therapist. In general, activity tolerance is the primary goal, while pain relief is secondary. Exercise programs can reverse atrophy in paraspinal muscles and strengthen extensors of the trunk. Supervised intensive physical exercise or "work hardening" regimens have been effective in returning some patients to work, improving walking distance, and reducing pain. In addition, some forms of yoga have been evaluated in randomized trials and may be helpful for patients who are interested.

Medications for chronic low back pain may include acetaminophen, NSAIDs, and tricyclic antidepressants. Trials of the latter suggest some benefit even for patients without evidence of depression. Trials do not support the efficacy of selective serotonin reuptake inhibitors for back pain. However, depression is common among patients with chronic pain and should be appropriately treated.

Cognitive-behavioral therapy is based on evidence that psychological and social factors, as well as somatic pathology, are important in the genesis of chronic pain and disability. The patient's attitudes and beliefs, psychological distress, and patterns of illness behavior may all influence responses to chronic pain. Thus, in addition to addressing pathophysiologic mechanisms, psychological treatments are aimed at reducing disability by modifying cognitive processes and environmental contingencies. Cognitive-behavioral therapy includes efforts to identify and modify patients' thinking about their pain and disability by strategies that may involve imagery, attention diversion, or modifying maladaptive thoughts, feelings, and beliefs. This approach includes educating patients about a multidimensional view of pain, identifying pain-eliciting or pain-aggravating thoughts and feelings, using coping strategies and relaxation techniques, and even hypnosis. A systematic review concluded that such treatments are more effective than a waiting list control group for short-term pain relief; however, long-term results remain unclear. Behavioral treatments may have effects similar in magnitude to exercise therapy.

Back pain is the most common reason for seeking complementary and alternative treatments. The most common of these for back pain are spinal manipulation, acupuncture, and massage. The role of complementary and alternative medicine approaches, aside from spinal manipulation, remains unclear. Biofeedback has not been studied rigorously. As with acute back pain, spinal manipulation may on average offer benefits similar to conventional care. Rigorous recent trials of acupuncture suggest that true acupuncture is not superior to sham acupuncture, but that both may offer an advantage over routine care. Whether this is due entirely to placebo effects or to stimulation provided even by sham acupuncture is uncertain. Some trials of massage therapy have been encouraging, but this has been less well studied than manipulation or acupuncture.

Studies of transcutaneous electrical nerve stimulation (TENS) have reached conflicting conclusions, but a recent evidence-based guideline suggested that there was no convincing evidence for its efficacy in treating chronic back pain.

Various injections, including epidural glucocorticoid injections, facet joint injections, and trigger point injections, have been used for treating chronic low back pain. However, in the absence of radiculopathy, there is no evidence that epidural glucocorticoids are effective for treating chronic back pain. Several randomized trials suggest that facet joint injections are not more effective than saline injections, and recent evidence-based guidelines recommend against their use. Similarly, there is little evidence to support the use of trigger point injections. Injection studies are sometimes used diagnostically to help determine the anatomic source of back pain. Reproduction of the patient's typical pain with discography has been used as evidence that a specific disk is the pain generator. Pain relief following a foraminal nerve root block or glucocorticoid injection into a facet has been similarly used as evidence that the facet joint or nerve root is the source. However, the possibility that the injection response was a placebo effect or due to systemic absorption of the glucocorticoids is often not excluded.

Another category of intervention for chronic back pain includes electrothermal and radiofrequency therapies. Intradiskal therapy has been proposed using both types of energy to thermocoagulate and destroy nerves in the intervertebral disk, using specially designed catheters or electrodes. A systematic review has suggested that current evidence does not support the use of these intradiskal therapies.

Radiofrequency denervation is sometimes used to destroy nerves that are thought to mediate pain, and this technique has been used for facet joint pain (with the target nerve being the medial branch of the primary dorsal ramus), for back pain thought to arise from the intervertebral disk (ramus communicans), and radicular back pain (dorsal root ganglia). A few small trials have resulted in conflicting results for facet joint pain. The evidence for presumed diskogenic pain and for radicular pain is similarly meager. A trial for patients with chronic radicular pain found no difference between radiofrequency denervation of the dorsal root ganglia and sham treatment. Recent systematic reviews have thus concluded that there is insufficient evidence to reliably evaluate these interventional therapies.

Surgical intervention for chronic low back pain in the absence of radiculopathy has been evaluated in a small number of randomized trials, all conducted in Europe. Each of these studies included patients with back pain and a degenerative disk, but no sciatica. Three of the four trials concluded that lumbar fusion surgery was no more effective than highly structured, rigorous rehabilitation combined with cognitive-behavioral therapy. The fourth trial found an advantage of fusion surgery over haphazard "usual care," which appeared to be less effective than the structured rehabilitation in other trials. Given conflicting evidence, indications for surgery for chronic back pain alone have remained controversial. Both U.S. and British guidelines suggest considering referral for an opinion on spinal fusion for people who have completed an optimal nonsurgical treatment program (including combined physical and psychological treatment) and who have persistent severe back pain for which they would consider surgery.

The newest surgical treatment for degenerated disks with back pain is disk replacement with prosthetic disks. These are generally designed as metal plates with a polyethylene cushion sandwiched in between. The trials that led to approval of these devices compared them to spine fusion, and concluded that the artificial disks were "not inferior." Serious complications appeared to be somewhat more likely with the artificial disk. This treatment remains controversial for low back pain.

Intensive multidisciplinary rehabilitation programs may involve daily or frequent care involving physical therapy, exercise, cognitive-behavioral therapy, a workplace evaluation, and other interventions. For patients who have not responded to other interventions, such programs appear to offer some benefit. Systematic reviews suggest that the evidence is limited and effects are moderate.

Some observers have raised concern that chronic back pain may often be overtreated. The use of opioids, epidural glucocorticoid injections, facet joint injections, and surgical intervention has increased rapidly in the past decade, without corresponding population-level improvements in pain or functioning among patients with back pain. In each case, randomized trials provide only minimal support for these treatments in the setting of chronic back pain without radiculopathy. For low back pain without radiculopathy, new British guidelines explicitly recommend against use of selective serotonin reuptake inhibitors (SSRIs), any type of injection, TENS, lumbar supports, traction, radiofrequency facet joint denervation, intradiskal electrothermal therapy, or intradiskal radiofrequency thermocoagulation. Similarly, these treatments are not recommended in guidelines from the American College of Physicians and the American Pain Society. On the other hand, exercise therapy and treatment of depression appear to be underused.

LOW BACK PAIN WITH RADICULOPATHY A common cause of back pain with radiculopathy is a herniated disk with nerve root impingement, resulting in back pain with radiation down the leg. The prognosis for acute low back pain with radiculopathy due to disk herniation (sciatica) is generally favorable, with most patients demonstrating substantial improvement over a matter of months. Serial imaging studies suggest spontaneous regression of the herniated portion of the disk in two-thirds of patients over 6 months. Nonetheless, there are several important treatment options for providing symptom relief while this natural healing process unfolds.

Resumption of normal activity as much as possible is usually the best activity recommendation. Randomized trial evidence suggests that bed rest is ineffective for treating sciatica as well as for back pain alone. Acetaminophen and NSAIDs are appropriate for pain relief, although severe pain may require short courses of opioid analgesics.

Epidural glucocorticoid injections have a role in providing temporary symptom relief for sciatica due to a herniated disk. Although randomized trial evidence is conflicting, there appears to be some overall short-term benefit for pain relief of sciatica. However, there does not appear to be a benefit in terms of reducing subsequent surgical interventions. Diagnostic nerve root blocks have been advocated to determine if pain originates from a specific nerve root. However, improvement may result even when the nerve root is not responsible for the pain; this may occur as a placebo effect, from a pain-generating lesion located distally along the peripheral nerve, or from anesthesia of the sinuvertebral nerve. The utility of diagnostic nerve root blocks remains a subject of debate.

Surgical intervention is indicated for patients who have progressive motor weakness, demonstrated on clinical examination or EMG, as a result of nerve root injury. Urgent surgery is recommended for patients who have evidence of the cauda equina syndrome or spinal cord compression, generally suggested by bowel or bladder dysfunction, diminished sensation in a saddle distribution, a sensory level, bilateral leg weakness, or bilateral leg spasticity.

Surgery is also an important option for patients who have disabling radicular pain despite optimal conservative treatment. Sciatica is perhaps the most common reason for recommending spine surgery. Because patients with a herniated disk and sciatica generally experience rapid improvement over a matter of weeks, most experts do not recommend considering surgery unless the patient has failed to respond to 6–8 weeks of appropriate nonsurgical management. For patients who have not improved, randomized trials indicate that, compared to nonsurgical treatment, surgery results in more rapid pain relief. However, after the first year or two of follow-up, patients with sciatica appear to have much the same level of pain relief and functional improvement with or without surgery. Thus, both treatment approaches are reasonable, and patient preferences should play a major role in decision making. Some patients will want the fastest possible relief and find surgical risks acceptable. Others will be more risk-averse and more tolerant of symptoms, and will choose watchful waiting if they understand that improvement is likely in the end.

The usual surgical procedure is a partial hemilaminectomy with excision of the prolapsed disk. Fusion of the involved lumbar segments should be considered only if significant spinal instability is present (i.e., degenerative spondylolisthesis). The costs associated with lumbar interbody fusion have increased dramatically in recent years. There are no large prospective, randomized trials comparing fusion to other types of surgical intervention. In one study, patients with persistent low back pain despite an initial diskectomy fared no better with spine fusion than with a conservative regimen of cognitive intervention and exercise. Artificial disks have been in use in Europe for the past decade; their utility remains controversial in the United States.

PAIN IN THE NECK AND SHOULDER

(Table 9-4) Neck pain, which usually arises from diseases of the cervical spine and soft tissues of the neck, is common. Neck pain arising from the cervical spine is typically precipitated by movement and may be accompanied by focal tenderness and limitation of motion. Pain arising from the brachial plexus, shoulder, or peripheral nerves can be confused with cervical spine disease, but the history and examination usually identify a more distal origin for the pain. Cervical spine trauma, disk disease, or spondylosis with intervertebral foraminal narrowing may be asymptomatic or painful and can produce a myelopathy, radiculopathy, or both. The same risk factors for a serious cause of low back pain are thought to apply to neck pain with the addition that neurologic signs of myelopathy (incontinence, sensory level, spastic legs) may also occur. Lhermitte's sign, an electrical shock down the spine with neck flexion, suggests cervical spinal cord involvement from any cause.

TRAUMA TO THE CERVICAL SPINE

Trauma to the cervical spine (fractures, subluxation) places the spinal cord at risk for compression. Motor vehicle accidents, violent crimes, or falls account for 87% of cervical spinal cord injuries (Chap. 35). Immediate immobilization of the neck is essential to minimize further spinal cord injury from movement of unstable cervical spine segments. The decision to obtain imaging should be based upon the nature of the injury. The NEXUS low-risk criteria established that normally alert patients without palpation tenderness in the midline; intoxication; neurologic deficits; and painful distracting injuries had a very low likelihood of a clinically significant traumatic injury to the cervical spine. The Canadian C-spine rule recommends that imaging should be obtained following neck region trauma if the patient is >65 years old, has limb paresthesias, or a dangerous mechanism for the injury (e.g., bicycle collision with tree or parked car, fall from height >3 feet or 5 stairs, diving accident). A CT scan is the diagnostic procedure of choice for detection of acute fractures. When traumatic injury to the vertebral arteries or cervical spinal cord is suspected, visualization by MRI with MR angiography is preferred.

Whiplash injury is due to rapid flexion and extension of the neck, usually in automobile accidents, and causes cervical musculoligamental injury. This diagnosis should not be applied to patients with fractures, disk herniation, head injury, focal neurologic findings, or altered consciousness. Up to 50% of persons reporting whiplash injury acutely have persistent neck pain 1 year later. Once personal compensation for pain and suffering was removed from the Australian health care system, the prognosis for recovery at 1 year from whiplash injury improved also. Imaging of the cervical spine is not cost-effective acutely but is useful to detect disk herniations when symptoms persist for >6 weeks following the injury. Severe initial symptoms have been associated with a poor long-term outcome.

CERVICAL DISK DISEASE

Herniation of a lower cervical disk is a common cause of neck, shoulder, arm, or hand pain or tingling. Neck pain, stiffness, and a range of motion limited by pain are the usual manifestations. A herniated cervical disk is responsible for ~25% of cervical radiculopathies. Extension and lateral rotation of the neck narrows the ipsilateral intervertebral foramen and may reproduce radicular symptoms (Spurling's sign). In young persons, acute nerve root compression from a ruptured cervical disk is often due to trauma. Cervical disk herniations are usually posterolateral near the lateral recess. The cervical nerve roots most commonly affected are C7 and C6. Typical patterns of reflex, sensory, and motor changes

TABLE 9-4

CERVICAL RADICULOPATHY—NEUROLOGIC FEATURES

CERVICAL NERVE ROOTS	EXAMINATION FINDINGS REFLEX	SENSORY	MOTOR	PAIN DISTRIBUTION
C5	Biceps	Over lateral deltoid	Supraspinatus[a] (initial arm abduction) Infraspinatus[a] (arm external rotation) Deltoid[a] (arm abduction) Biceps (arm flexion)	Lateral arm, medial scapula
C6	Biceps	Thumb, index fingers Radial hand/forearm	Biceps (arm flexion) Pronator teres (internal forearm rotation)	Lateral forearm, thumb, index finger
C7	Triceps	Middle fingers Dorsum forearm	Triceps[a] (arm extension) Wrist extensors[a] Extensor digitorum[a] (finger extension)	Posterior arm, dorsal forearm, lateral hand
C8	Finger flexors	Little finger Medial hand and forearm	Abductor pollicis brevis (abduction D1) First dorsal interosseous (abduction D2) Abductor digiti minimi (abduction D5)	4th and 5th fingers, medial forearm
T1	Finger flexors	Axilla and medial arm	Abductor pollicis brevis (abduction D1) First dorsal interosseous (abduction D2) Abductor digiti minimi (abduction D5)	Medial arm, axilla

[a]These muscles receive the majority of innervation from this root.

that accompany specific cervical nerve root lesions are summarized in Table 9-4. While the classic patterns are clinically helpful, there are numerous exceptions because (1) there is overlap in function between adjacent nerve roots, (2) symptoms and signs may be evident in only part of the injured nerve root territory, and (3) the location of pain is the most variable of the clinical features.

CERVICAL SPONDYLOSIS

Osteoarthritis of the cervical spine may produce neck pain that radiates into the back of the head, shoulders, or arms, or may be the source of headaches in the posterior occipital region (supplied by the C2-C4 nerve roots). Osteophytes, disk protrusions, or hypertrophic facet or uncovertebral joints may alone or in combination compress one or several nerve roots at the intervertebral foramina (Fig. 9-6); this compression accounts for 75% of cervical radiculopathies. The roots most commonly affected are C7 and C6. Narrowing of the spinal canal by osteophytes, ossification of the posterior longitudinal ligament (OPLL), or a large central disk may compress the cervical spinal cord. Combinations of radiculopathy and myelopathy may be present. When little or no neck pain accompanies cord compression, the diagnosis may be confused with amyotrophic lateral sclerosis (Chap. 32), multiple sclerosis (Chap. 39), spinal cord tumors, or syringomyelia (Chap. 35). The possibility of cervical spondylosis should be considered even when the patient presents with symptoms or signs in the legs only. MRI is the study of choice to define the anatomic abnormalities, but plain CT is adequate to assess bony spurs, foraminal narrowing, lateral recess stenosis, or OPLL. EMG and nerve conduction studies can localize and assess the severity of the nerve root injury.

OTHER CAUSES OF NECK PAIN

Rheumatoid arthritis (RA) of the cervical apophyseal joints produces neck pain, stiffness, and limitation of motion. In advanced RA, synovitis of the atlantoaxial joint (C1-C2; Fig. 9-2) may damage the transverse ligament of the atlas, producing forward displacement of the atlas on the axis (atlantoaxial subluxation). Radiologic evidence of atlantoaxial subluxation occurs in 30% of patients with RA. Not surprisingly, the degree of subluxation correlates with the severity of erosive disease. When subluxation is present, careful assessment is important to identify early signs of myelopathy. Occasional patients develop high spinal cord compression leading to quadriparesis, respiratory insufficiency, and death. Surgery should be considered when myelopathy or spinal instability is present. MRI is the imaging modality of choice.

Ankylosing spondylitis can cause neck pain and less commonly atlantoaxial subluxation; surgery may be required to prevent spinal cord compression. Acute *herpes zoster* presents as acute posterior occipital or neck pain prior to the outbreak of vesicles. *Neoplasms* metastatic to the cervical spine, *infections* (osteomyelitis and epidural abscess), and *metabolic bone diseases* may be the cause of neck pain. Neck pain may also be referred from the heart with coronary artery ischemia (cervical angina syndrome).

THORACIC OUTLET

The thoracic outlet contains the first rib, the subclavian artery and vein, the brachial plexus, the clavicle, and the lung apex. Injury to these structures may result in postural or movement-induced pain around the shoulder and supraclavicular region. *True neurogenic thoracic outlet syndrome* (TOS) is an uncommon disorder resulting from compression of the lower trunk of the brachial plexus or ventral rami of the C8 or T1 nerve roots most often by an anomalous band of tissue connecting an elongate transverse process at C7 with the first rib. Pain is mild or absent. Signs include weakness and wasting of intrinsic muscles of the hand and diminished sensation on the palmar aspect of the fifth digit. An anteroposterior cervical spine x-ray will show the elongate C7 transverse process, and EMG and nerve conduction studies confirm the diagnosis. Treatment consists of surgical resection of the anomalous band. The weakness and wasting of intrinsic hand muscles typically does not improve, but surgery halts the insidious progression of weakness. *Arterial TOS* results from compression of the subclavian artery by a cervical rib resulting in poststenotic dilatation of the artery and thrombus formation. Blood pressure is reduced in the affected limb, and signs of emboli may be present in the hand. Neurologic signs are absent. Ultrasound can confirm the diagnosis noninvasively. Treatment is with thrombolysis or anticoagulation (with or without embolectomy) and surgical excision of the cervical rib compressing the subclavian artery. *Venous TOS* is due to subclavian vein thrombosis resulting in swelling of the arm and pain. The vein may be compressed by a cervical rib or anomalous scalene muscle. Venography is the diagnostic test of choice. *Disputed TOS* includes a large number of patients with chronic arm and shoulder pain of unclear cause. The lack of sensitive and specific findings on physical examination or laboratory markers for this condition frequently results in diagnostic uncertainty. The role of surgery in disputed TOS is controversial. Multidisciplinary pain management is a conservative approach, although treatment is often unsuccessful.

BRACHIAL PLEXUS AND NERVES

Pain from injury to the brachial plexus or peripheral nerves of the arm can occasionally mimic pain of cervical spine origin. Neoplastic infiltration of the lower trunk of the brachial plexus may produce shoulder or supraclavicular pain radiating down the arm, numbness of the fourth and fifth fingers or medial forearm, and weakness of intrinsic hand muscles innervated by the ulnar and median nerves. Delayed radiation injury may produce similar findings, although pain is less often present and almost always less severe. A Pancoast tumor of the lung is another cause and should be considered, especially when a Horner's syndrome is present. *Suprascapular neuropathy* may produce severe shoulder pain, weakness, and wasting of the supraspinatus and infraspinatus muscles. *Acute brachial neuritis* is often confused with radiculopathy; the acute onset of severe shoulder or scapular pain is followed typically over days by weakness of the proximal arm and shoulder girdle muscles innervated by the upper brachial plexus. The onset is often preceded by an infection. The long thoracic nerve may be affected; the latter results in a winged scapula. Brachial neuritis may also present as an isolated paralysis of the diaphragm or with involvement of other nerves of the upper limb. Recovery is generally good but may take up to 3 years to be complete.

Occasional cases of carpal tunnel syndrome produce pain and paresthesias extending into the forearm, arm, and shoulder resembling a C5 or C6 root lesion. Lesions of the radial or ulnar nerve can mimic a radiculopathy at C7 or C8, respectively. EMG and nerve conduction studies can accurately localize lesions to the nerve roots, brachial plexus, or peripheral nerves.

For further discussion of peripheral nerve disorders, see Chap. 45.

SHOULDER

Pain arising from the shoulder can on occasion mimic pain from the spine. If symptoms and signs of radiculopathy are absent, then the differential diagnosis includes mechanical shoulder pain (tendonitis, bursitis, rotator cuff tear, dislocation, adhesive capsulitis, and cuff impingement under the acromion) and referred pain (subdiaphragmatic irritation, angina, Pancoast tumor). Mechanical pain is often worse at night, associated with local shoulder tenderness and aggravated by abduction, internal rotation, or extension of the arm. Pain from shoulder disease may radiate into the arm or hand, but sensory, motor, and reflex changes are absent.

TREATMENT Neck Pain without Radiculopathy

The evidence regarding treatment for neck pain is less complete than that for low back pain. As with low back pain, spontaneous improvement is the norm for acute neck pain, and the usual goal of therapy is to provide symptom relief while natural healing processes proceed.

The evidence in support of nonsurgical treatments for whiplash-associated disorders is generally of poor quality and neither supports nor refutes the effectiveness of common treatments used for symptom relief. Gentle mobilization of the cervical spine combined with exercise programs may be more beneficial than usual care. Evidence is insufficient to recommend for or against the use of cervical traction, neck collars, TENS, ultrasound, diathermy, or massage. The role of acupuncture for neck pain also remains ambiguous, with poor-quality studies and conflicting results.

For patients with neck pain unassociated with trauma, supervised exercise, with or without mobilization, appears to be effective. Exercises often include shoulder rolls and neck stretches. Although there is relatively little evidence about the use of muscle relaxants, analgesics, and NSAIDs in neck pain, many clinicians use these medications in much the same way as for low back pain.

Low-level laser therapy directed at areas of tenderness, local acupuncture points, or a grid of predetermined points is a controversial approach to the treatment of neck pain. The putative benefits might be mediated by anti-inflammatory effects, reduction of skeletal muscle fatigue, or inhibition of transmission at neuromuscular junctions. A 2009 meta-analysis suggested that this treatment may provide greater pain relief than sham therapy for both acute and chronic neck pain. Comparison to other conservative treatment measures is needed.

Although some surgical studies have proposed a role for anterior diskectomy and fusion in patients with neck pain, these studies generally have not been rigorously conducted. A systematic review suggested that there was no valid clinical evidence to support either cervical fusion or cervical disk arthroplasty in patients with neck pain without radiculopathy. Similarly, there is no evidence to support radiofrequency neurotomy or cervical facet injections for neck pain without radiculopathy.

TREATMENT Neck Pain with Radiculopathy

The natural history of neck pain even with radiculopathy is favorable, and many patients will improve without specific therapy. Although there are no randomized trials of NSAIDs for neck pain, a course of NSAIDs, with or without muscle relaxants, may be appropriate initial therapy. Other nonsurgical treatments are commonly used, including opioid analgesics, oral glucocorticoids, cervical traction, and immobilization with a hard or soft cervical collar. However, there are no randomized trials to establish the effectiveness of these treatments in comparison to natural history alone. Soft cervical collars can be modestly helpful by limiting spontaneous and reflex neck movements that exacerbate pain.

As for lumbar radiculopathy, epidural glucocorticoids may provide short-term symptom relief in cervical radiculopathy. If cervical radiculopathy is due to bony compression from cervical spondylosis with foraminal narrowing, then surgical decompression is generally indicated to forestall progression of neurologic signs.

Surgical treatment can produce rapid and substantial symptom relief, although it is unclear whether long-term outcomes are improved over nonsurgical therapy. Reasonable indications for cervical disk surgery include a progressive radicular motor deficit, functionally limiting pain that fails to respond to conservative management, or spinal cord compression.

Surgical treatments include anterior cervical diskectomy alone, laminectomy with diskectomy, diskectomy with fusion, and disk arthroplasty (implanting an artificial cervical disk). Fusions can be performed with a variety of techniques. The risk of subsequent radiculopathy or myelopathy at cervical segments adjacent to a fusion is ~3% per year and 26% per decade. Although this risk is sometimes portrayed as a late complication of surgery, it may also reflect the natural history of degenerative cervical disk disease. The durability of disk prostheses is uncertain. Available data do not strongly support one surgical technique over another.

CHAPTER 10

SYNCOPE

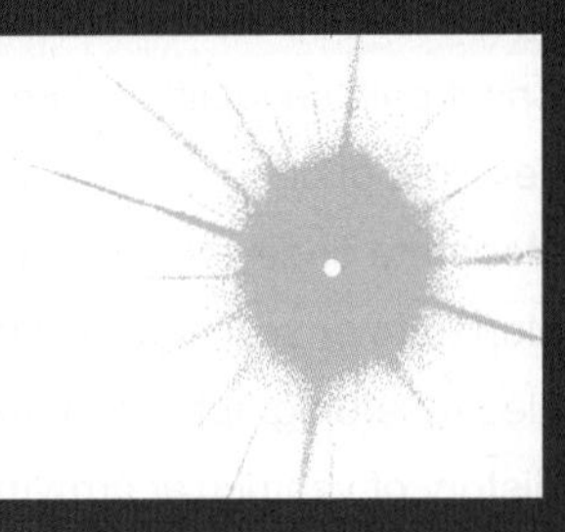

Roy Freeman

Syncope is a transient, self-limited loss of consciousness due to acute global impairment of cerebral blood flow. The onset is rapid, duration brief, and recovery spontaneous and complete. Other causes of transient loss of consciousness need to be distinguished from syncope; these include seizures, vertebrobasilar ischemia, hypoxemia, and hypoglycemia. A syncopal prodrome (*presyncope*) is common, although loss of consciousness may occur without any warning symptoms. Typical presyncopal symptoms include dizziness, lightheadedness or faintness, weakness, fatigue, and visual and auditory disturbances. The causes of syncope can be divided into three general categories: (1) neurally mediated syncope (also called *reflex syncope*), (2) orthostatic hypotension, and (3) cardiac syncope.

Neurally mediated syncope comprises a heterogeneous group of functional disorders that are characterized by a transient change in the reflexes responsible for maintaining cardiovascular homeostasis. Episodic vasodilation and bradycardia occur in varying combinations, resulting in temporary failure of blood pressure control. In contrast, in patients with orthostatic hypotension due to autonomic failure, these cardiovascular homeostatic reflexes are chronically impaired. Cardiac syncope may be due to arrhythmias or structural cardiac diseases that cause a decrease in cardiac output. The clinical features, underlying pathophysiologic mechanisms, therapeutic interventions, and prognoses differ markedly among these three causes.

EPIDEMIOLOGY AND NATURAL HISTORY

Syncope is a common presenting problem, accounting for approximately 3% of all emergency room visits and 1% of all hospital admissions. The annual cost for syncope-related hospitalization in the United States is ~\$2 billion. Syncope has a lifetime cumulative incidence of up to 35% in the general population. The peak incidence in the young occurs between ages 10 and 30 years, with a median peak around 15 years. Neurally mediated syncope is the etiology in the vast majority of these cases. In elderly adults, there is a sharp rise in the incidence of syncope after 70 years.

In population-based studies, neurally mediated syncope is the most common cause of syncope. The incidence is slightly higher in females than males. In young subjects there is often a family history in first-degree relatives. Cardiovascular disease due to structural disease or arrhythmias is the next most common cause in most series, particularly in emergency room settings and in older patients. Orthostatic hypotension also increases in prevalence with age because of the reduced baroreflex responsiveness, decreased cardiac compliance, and attenuation of the vestibulosympathetic reflex associated with aging. In the elderly, orthostatic hypotension is substantially more common in institutionalized (54–68%) than community dwelling (6%) individuals, an observation most likely explained by the greater prevalence of predisposing neurologic disorders, physiologic impairment, and vasoactive medication use among institutionalized patients.

The prognosis after a single syncopal event for all age groups is generally benign. In particular, syncope of noncardiac and unexplained origin in younger individuals has an excellent prognosis; life expectancy is unaffected. By contrast, syncope due to a cardiac cause, either structural heart disease or primary arrhythmic disease, is associated with an increased risk of sudden cardiac death and mortality from other causes. Similarly, mortality rate is increased in individuals with syncope due to orthostatic hypotension related to age and the associated comorbid conditions (Table 10-1).

TABLE 10-1

HIGH-RISK FEATURES INDICATING HOSPITALIZATION OR INTENSIVE EVALUATION OF SYNCOPE
Chest pain suggesting coronary ischemia
Features of congestive heart failure
Moderate or severe valvular disease
Moderate or severe structural cardiac disease
Electrocardiographic features of ischemia
History of ventricular arrhythmias
Prolonged QT interval (>500 ms)
Repetitive sinoatrial block or sinus pauses
Persistent sinus bradycardia
Trifascicular block
Atrial fibrillation
Nonsustained ventricular tachycardia
Family history of sudden death
Preexcitation syndromes
Brugada pattern on ECG

PATHOPHYSIOLOGY

The upright posture imposes a unique physiologic stress upon humans; most, although not all, syncopal episodes occur from a standing position. Standing results in pooling of 500–1000 mL of blood in the lower extremities and splanchnic circulation. There is a decrease in venous return to the heart and reduced ventricular filling that result in diminished cardiac output and blood pressure. These hemodynamic changes provoke a compensatory reflex response, initiated by the baroreceptors in the carotid sinus and aortic arch, resulting in increased sympathetic outflow and decreased vagal nerve activity (Fig. 10-1). The reflex increases peripheral resistance, venous return to the heart, and cardiac output and thus limits the fall in blood pressure. If this response fails, as is the case chronically in orthostatic hypotension and transiently in neurally mediated syncope, cerebral hypoperfusion occurs.

Syncope is a consequence of global cerebral hypoperfusion and thus represents a failure of cerebral blood flow autoregulatory mechanisms. Myogenic factors, local metabolites, and to a lesser extent autonomic neurovascular control are responsible for the autoregulation of cerebral blood flow (Chap. 28). Typically cerebral blood flow ranges from 50 to 60 mL/min per 100 g brain tissue and remains relatively constant over perfusion pressures ranging from 50 to 150 mmHg. Cessation of blood flow for 6–8 s will result in loss of consciousness, while impairment of consciousness ensues when blood flow decreases to 25 mL/min per 100 g brain tissue.

From the clinical standpoint, a fall in systemic systolic blood pressure to ~50 mmHg or lower will result in syncope. A decrease in cardiac output and/or systemic vascular resistance—the determinants of blood pressure—thus underlies the pathophysiology of syncope. Common causes of impaired cardiac output include decreased effective circulating blood volume; increased thoracic pressure; massive pulmonary embolus; cardiac brady- and tachyarrhythmias; valvular heart disease; and myocardial dysfunction. Systemic vascular resistance may be decreased by central and peripheral autonomic nervous system diseases, sympatholytic medications, and transiently during neurally mediated syncope. Increased cerebral vascular resistance, most frequently due to hypocarbia induced by hyperventilation, may also contribute to the pathophysiology of syncope.

The sequence of changes on the electroencephalogram of syncopal subjects during syncope comprises background slowing (often of high amplitude), followed by attenuation or cessation of cortical activity prior to return of slow waves, and then normal activity. Despite the presence of myoclonic movements and other motor activity, electroencephalographic seizure discharges are not present in syncopal subjects.

CLASSIFICATION

NEURALLY MEDIATED SYNCOPE

Neurally mediated syncope is the final pathway of a complex central and peripheral nervous system reflex arc. There is a sudden, transient change in autonomic efferent activity characterized by increased parasympathetic outflow causing bradycardia and sympathoinhibition causing vasodilation. The change in autonomic efferent activity leads to a decrease in blood pressure and a subsequent fall in cerebral blood flow to below the limits of autoregulation (Fig. 10-2). In order to elicit this reflex, a normal or functioning autonomic nervous system is necessary; this is in contrast to the situation in autonomic failure. The triggers of the afferent limb of the reflex arc vary and may be clearly defined, e.g., the carotid sinus, the gastrointestinal tract, or the bladder. In many cases, however, the afferent arc is less easily recognized and, under many circumstances, the cause is multifactorial. Under these circumstances it is likely that multiple afferent pathways converge on the central autonomic network within the medulla that integrates the neural impulses and mediates the vasodepressor-bradycardic response.

Classification of neurally mediated syncope

Neurally mediated syncope may be subdivided based on the afferent pathway and provocative trigger. Vasovagal syncope (the common faint) is provoked by intense emotion, pain, and/or orthostatic stress, whereas the

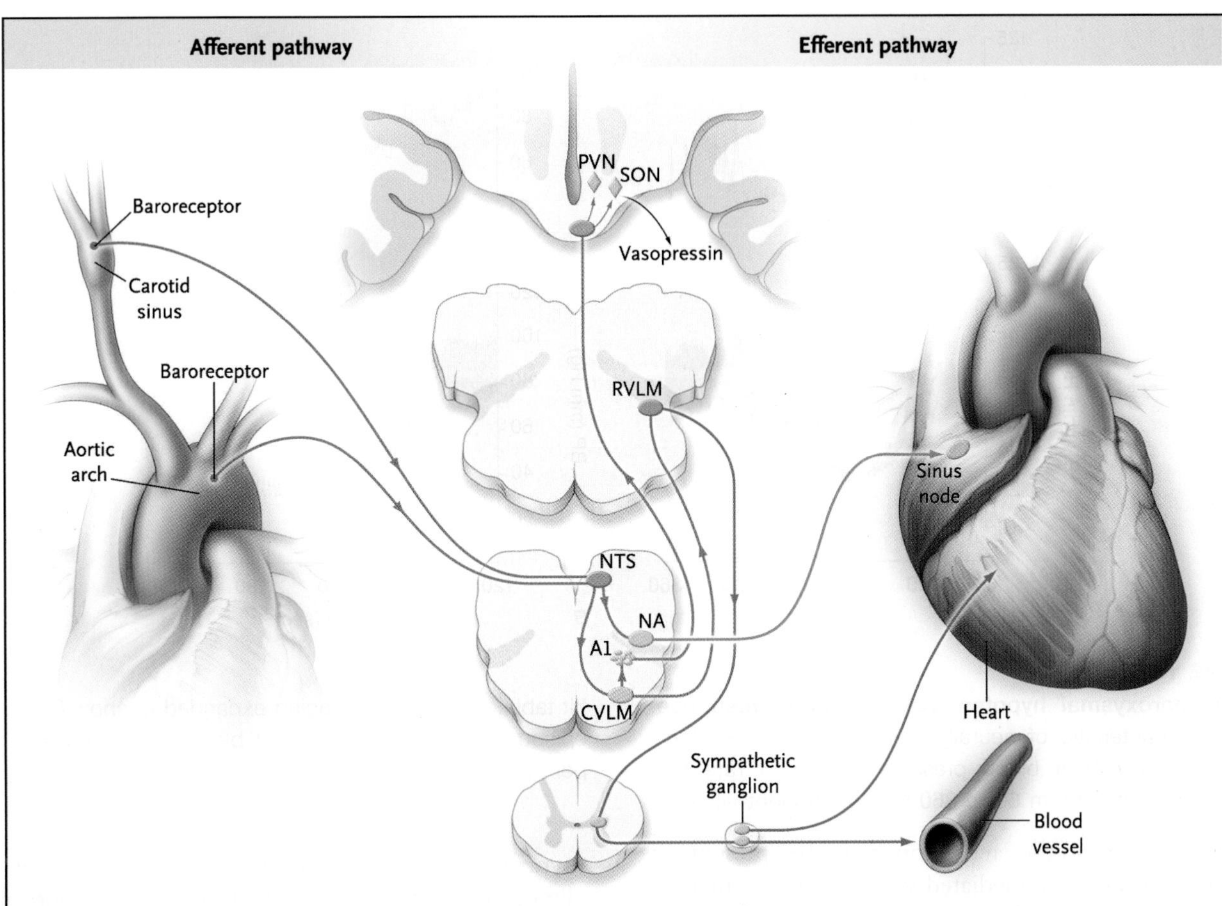

FIGURE 10-1

The Baroreflex. A decrease in arterial pressure unloads the baroreceptors—the terminals of afferent fibers of the glossopharyngeal and vagus nerves—that are situated in the carotid sinus and aortic arch. This leads to a reduction in the afferent impulses that are relayed from these mechanoreceptors through the glossopharyngeal and vagus nerves to the nucleus of the tractus solitarius (NTS) in the dorsomedial medulla. The reduced baroreceptor afferent activity produces a decrease in vagal nerve input to the sinus node that is mediated by the neuroanatomical connections of the NTS to the nucleus ambiguus (NA). There is an increase in sympathetic efferent activity that is mediated by the NTS projections to the caudal ventrolateral medulla (CVLM) (an excitatory pathway) and from there to the rostral ventrolateral medulla (RVLM) (an inhibitory pathway). The activation of RVLM presympathetic neurons in response to hypotension is thus predominantly due to disinhibition. In response to a sustained fall in blood pressure, vasopressin release is mediated by projections from the A1 noradrenergic cell group in the ventrolateral medulla. This projection activates vasopressin-synthesizing neurons in the magnocellular portion of the paraventricular nucleus (PVN) and the supraoptic nucleus (SON) of the hypothalamus. Blue denotes sympathetic neurons and green parasympathetic neurons. (*From R Freeman: N Engl J Med 358:615, 2008.*)

situational reflex syncopes have specific localized stimuli that provoke the reflex vasodilation and bradycardia that leads to syncope. The underlying mechanisms have been identified and pathophysiology delineated for most of these situational reflex syncopes. The afferent trigger may originate in the pulmonary system, gastrointestinal system, urogenital system, heart, and carotid artery (Table 10-2). Hyperventilation leading to hypocarbia and cerebral vasoconstriction, and raised intrathoracic pressure that impairs venous return to the heart, play a central role in many of the situational reflex syncopes. The afferent pathway of the reflex arc differs among these disorders, but the efferent response via the vagus and sympathetic pathways is similar.

Alternately, neurally mediated syncope may be subdivided based on the predominant efferent pathway. Vasodepressor syncope describes syncope predominantly due to efferent, sympathetic, vasoconstrictor failure; cardioinhibitory syncope describes syncope predominantly associated with bradycardia or asystole due to increased vagal outflow; while mixed syncope describes syncope in which there are both vagal and sympathetic reflex changes.

Features of neurally mediated syncope

In addition to symptoms of orthostatic intolerance such as dizziness, lightheadedness, and fatigue, premonitory

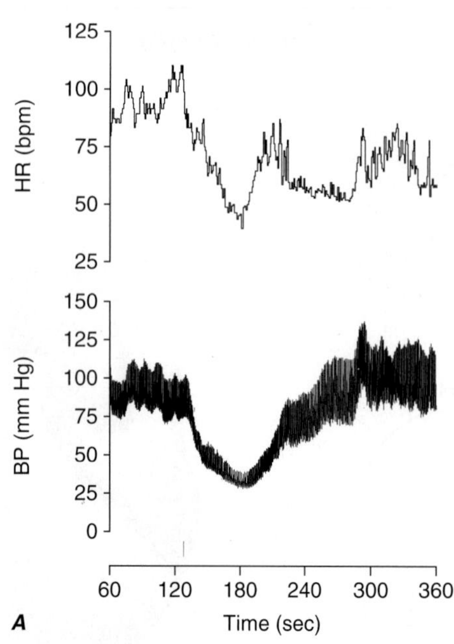

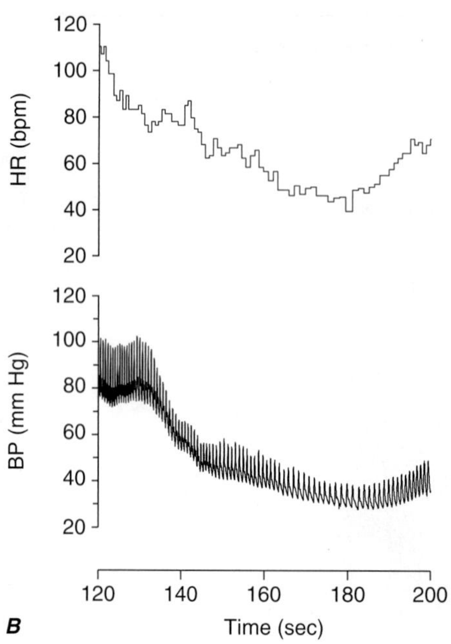

FIGURE 10-2

A.* The paroxysmal hypotensive-bradycardic response** that is characteristic of neurally mediated syncope. Noninvasive beat-to-beat blood pressure and heart rate are shown over 5 min (from 60 to 360 s) of an upright tilt on a tilt table. ***B. The same tracing expanded to show 80 s of the episode (from 80 to 200 s). BP, blood pressure; bpm, beats per minute; HR, heart rate.

features of autonomic activation may be present in patients with neurally mediated syncope. These include diaphoresis, pallor, palpitations, nausea, hyperventilation, and yawning. During the syncopal event, proximal and distal myoclonus (typically arrhythmic and multifocal) may occur, raising the possibility of epilepsy. The eyes typically remain open and usually deviate upward. Urinary but not fecal incontinence may occur. Postictal confusion is rare, although visual and auditory hallucinations are sometimes reported.

While some predisposing factors and provocative stimuli are well established (for example, motionless upright posture, warm ambient temperature, intravascular volume depletion, alcohol ingestion, hypoxemia, anemia, pain, the sight of blood, venipuncture, and intense emotion), the underlying basis for the widely different thresholds for syncope among individuals exposed to the same provocative stimulus is not known. A genetic basis for neurally mediated syncope may exist; several studies have reported an increased incidence of syncope in first-degree relatives of fainters, but no gene or genetic marker has been identified, and environmental, social, and cultural factors have not been excluded by these studies.

TREATMENT Neurally Mediated Syncope

Reassurance, avoidance of provocative stimuli, and plasma volume expansion with fluid and salt are the cornerstones of the management of neurally mediated syncope. Isometric counterpressure maneuvers of the limbs (leg crossing or handgrip and arm tensing) may raise blood pressure and, by maintaining pressure in the autoregulatory zone, avoid or delay the onset of syncope. Randomized controlled trials support this intervention.

Fludrocortisone, vasoconstricting agents, and beta-adrenoreceptor antagonists are widely used by experts to treat refractory patients, although there is no consistent evidence from randomized, controlled trials for any pharmacotherapy to treat neurally mediated syncope. Because vasodilation is the dominant pathophysiologic syncopal mechanism in most patients, use of a cardiac pacemaker is rarely beneficial. Possible exceptions are older patients in whom syncope is associated with asystole or severe bradycardia, and patients with prominent cardioinhibition due to carotid sinus syndrome. In these patients, dual-chamber pacing may be helpful.

ORTHOSTATIC HYPOTENSION

Orthostatic hypotension, defined as a reduction in systolic blood pressure of at least 20 mmHg or diastolic blood pressure of at least 10 mmHg within 3 min of standing or head-up tilt on a tilt table, is a manifestation of sympathetic vasoconstrictor (autonomic) failure (Fig. 10-3). In many (but not all) cases, there is no compensatory increase in heart rate despite hypotension; with partial autonomic failure,

TABLE 10-2

CAUSES OF SYNCOPE

A. Neurally Mediated Syncope

Vasovagal syncope
  Provoked fear, pain, anxiety, intense emotion, sight of blood, unpleasant sights and odors, orthostatic stress
Situational reflex syncope
  Pulmonary
    Cough syncope, wind instrument player's syncope, weightlifter's syncope, "mess trick"[a] and "fainting lark,"[b] sneeze syncope, airway instrumentation
  Urogenital
    Postmicturition syncope, urogenital tract instrumentation, prostatic massage
  Gastrointestinal
    Swallow syncope, glossopharyngeal neuralgia, esophageal stimulation, gastrointestinal tract instrumentation, rectal examination, defecation syncope
  Cardiac
    Swallow syncope, glossopharyngeal neuralgia, esophageal stimulation, gastrointestinal tract instrumentation, rectal examination, defecation syncope
  Carotid sinus
    Carotid sinus sensitivity, carotid sinus massage
  Ocular
    Ocular pressure, ocular examination, ocular surgery

B. Orthostatic Hypotension

Primary autonomic failure due to idiopathic central and peripheral neurodegenerative diseases—the "synucleinopathies"
  Lewy body diseases
    Parkinson's disease
    Lewy body dementia
    Pure autonomic failure
  Multiple system atrophy (the Shy-Drager syndrome)
Secondary autonomic failure due to autonomic peripheral neuropathies
  Diabetes
  Hereditary amyloidosis (familial amyloid polyneuropathy)
  Primary amyloidosis (AL amyloidosis; immunoglobulin light chain associated)
  Hereditary sensory and autonomic neuropathies (HSAN) (especially type III—familial dysautonomia)
  Idiopathic immune-mediated autonomic neuropathy
  Autoimmune autonomic ganglionopathy
  Sjögren's syndrome
  Paraneoplastic autonomic neuropathy
  HIV neuropathy
Postprandial hypotension
Iatrogenic (drug-induced)
Volume depletion

C. Cardiac Syncope

Arrhythmias
  Sinus node dysfunction
  Atrioventricular dysfunction
  Supraventricular tachycardias
  Ventricular tachycardias
  Inherited channelopathies
Cardiac structural disease
  Valvular disease
  Myocardial ischemia
  Obstructive and other cardiomyopathies
  Atrial myxoma
  Pericardial effusions and tamponade

[a]Hyperventilation for 1 min, followed by sudden chest compression.
[b]Hyperventilation (20 breaths) in a squatting position, rapid rise to standing, then Valsalva.

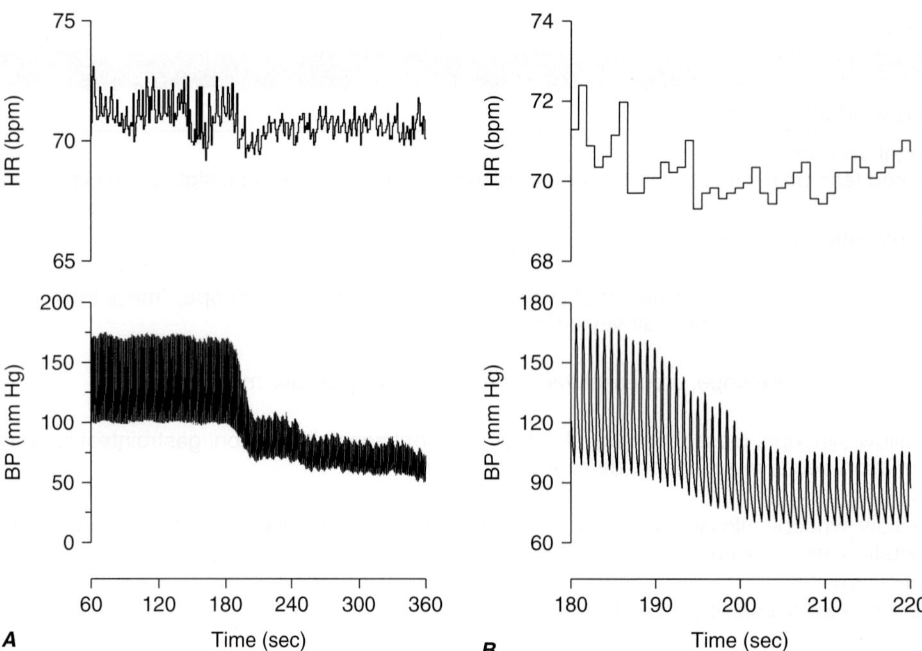

FIGURE 10-3

A.* The gradual fall in blood pressure** without a compensatory heart rate increase that is characteristic of orthostatic hypotension due to autonomic failure. Blood pressure and heart rate are shown over 5 min (from 60 to 360 s) of an upright tilt on a tilt table. ***B. The same tracing expanded to show 40 s of the episode (from 180 to 220 s). BP, blood pressure; bpm, beats per minute; HR, heart rate.

heart rate may increase to some degree but is insufficient to maintain cardiac output. A variant of orthostatic hypotension is "delayed" orthostatic hypotension which occurs beyond 3 min of standing; this may reflect a mild or early form of sympathetic adrenergic dysfunction. In some cases, orthostatic hypotension occurs within 15 s of standing (so-called "initial" orthostatic hypotension), a finding that may represent a transient mismatch between cardiac output and peripheral vascular resistance and does not represent autonomic failure.

Characteristic symptoms of orthostatic hypotension include light-headedness, dizziness, and presyncope (near-faintness) occurring in response to sudden postural change. However, symptoms may be absent or nonspecific, such as generalized weakness, fatigue, cognitive slowing, leg buckling, or headache. Visual blurring may occur, likely due to retinal or occipital lobe ischemia. Neck pain—typically in the suboccipital, posterior cervical, and shoulder region (the "coat-hanger headache")—most likely due to neck muscle ischemia, may be the only symptom. Patients may report orthostatic dyspnea (thought to reflect ventilation-perfusion mismatch due to inadequate perfusion of ventilated lung apices) or angina (attributed to impaired myocardial perfusion even with normal coronary arteries). Symptoms may be exacerbated by exertion, prolonged standing, increased ambient temperature, or meals. Syncope is usually preceded by warning symptoms, but may occur suddenly, suggesting the possibility of a seizure or cardiac cause.

Supine hypertension is common in patients with orthostatic hypotension due to autonomic failure, affecting over 50% of patients in some series. Orthostatic hypotension may present after initiation of therapy for hypertension, and supine hypertension may follow treatment of orthostatic hypotension. However, in other cases, the association of the two conditions is unrelated to therapy; it may in part be explained by baroreflex dysfunction in the presence of residual sympathetic outflow, particularly in patients with central autonomic degeneration.

Causes of neurogenic orthostatic hypotension

Causes of neurogenic orthostatic hypotension include central and peripheral autonomic nervous system dysfunction (Chap. 33). Autonomic dysfunction of other organ systems (including the bladder, bowels, sexual organs, and sudomotor system) of varying severity frequently accompanies orthostatic hypotension in these disorders (Table 10-2).

The primary autonomic degenerative disorders are multiple system atrophy (the Shy-Drager syndrome; Chap. 33), Parkinson's disease (Chap. 30), dementia with Lewy bodies (Chap. 29), and pure autonomic failure (Chap. 33). These are often grouped together as "synucleinopathies" due to the presence of alpha-synuclein, a small protein that precipitates predominantly in the cytoplasm of neurons in the Lewy body disorders (Parkinson's disease, dementia with Lewy bodies, and pure autonomic failure) and in the glia in multiple system atrophy.

Peripheral autonomic dysfunction may also accompany small fiber peripheral neuropathies such as those seen in diabetes, amyloid, immune-mediated neuropathies, hereditary sensory and autonomic neuropathies (HSAN; particularly HSAN type III; familial dysautonomia), and inflammatory neuropathies (Chaps. 46 and 47). Less frequently, orthostatic hypotension is associated with the peripheral neuropathies that accompany vitamin B_{12} deficiency, neurotoxic exposure, HIV and other infections, and porphyria.

Patients with autonomic failure and the elderly are susceptible to falls in blood pressure associated with meals. The magnitude of the blood pressure fall is exacerbated by large meals, meals high in carbohydrate, and alcohol intake. The mechanism of postprandial syncope is not fully elucidated.

Orthostatic hypotension is often iatrogenic. Drugs from several classes may lower peripheral resistance (e.g., alpha-adrenoreceptor antagonists used to treat hypertension and prostatic hypertrophy; antihypertensive agents of several classes; nitrates and other vasodilators; tricyclic agents and phenothiazines). Iatrogenic volume depletion due to diuresis and volume depletion due to medical causes (hemorrhage, vomiting, diarrhea, or decreased fluid intake) may also result in decreased effective circulatory volume, orthostatic hypotension, and syncope.

TREATMENT Orthostatic Hypotension

The first step is to remove reversible causes—usually vasoactive medications (Table 33-6). Next, nonpharmacologic interventions should be introduced. These interventions include patient education regarding staged moves from supine to upright; warnings about the hypotensive effects of meal ingestion; instructions about the isometric counterpressure maneuvers that increase intravascular pressure (see earlier in this chapter); and raising the head of the bed to reduce supine hypertension. Intravascular volume should be expanded by increasing dietary fluid and salt. If these nonpharmacologic measures fail, pharmacologic intervention with fludrocortisone acetate and vasoconstricting agents such as midodrine and pseudoephedrine should be introduced. Some patients with intractable symptoms require additional therapy with supplementary agents that include pyridostigmine, yohimbine, desmopressin acetate (DDAVP), and erythropoietin (Chap. 33).

CARDIAC SYNCOPE

Cardiac (or cardiovascular) syncope is caused by arrhythmias and structural heart disease. These may occur in combination because structural disease renders the heart more vulnerable to abnormal electrical activity.

Arrhythmias

Bradyarrhythmias that cause syncope include those due to severe sinus node dysfunction (e.g., sinus arrest or sinoatrial block) and atrioventricular block (e.g., Mobitz type II, high-grade, and complete AV block). The bradyarrhythmias due to sinus node dysfunction are often associated with an atrial tachyarrhythmia, a disorder known as the tachycardia-bradycardia syndrome. A prolonged pause following the termination of a tachycardic episode is a frequent cause of syncope in patients with the tachycardia-bradycardia syndrome. Medications of several classes may also cause bradyarrhythmias of sufficient severity to cause syncope. Syncope due to bradycardia or asystole is referred to as a Stokes-Adams attack.

Ventricular tachyarrhythmias frequently cause syncope. The likelihood of syncope with ventricular tachycardia is in part dependent on the ventricular rate; rates below 200 beats per min are less likely to cause syncope. The compromised hemodynamic function during ventricular tachycardia is caused by ineffective ventricular contraction, reduced diastolic filling due to abbreviated filling periods, loss of atrioventricular synchrony, and concurrent myocardial ischemia.

Several disorders associated with cardiac electrophysiologic instability and arrhythmogenesis are due to mutations in ion channel subunit genes. These include the long QT syndrome, Brugada syndrome, and catecholaminergic polymorphic ventricular tachycardia. The long QT syndrome is a genetically heterogeneous disorder associated with prolonged cardiac repolarization and a predisposition to ventricular arrhythmias. Syncope and sudden death in patients with long QT syndrome result from a unique polymorphic ventricular tachycardia called torsades des pointes that degenerates into ventricular fibrillation. The long QT syndrome has been linked to genes encoding K^+ channel α-subunits, K^+ channel β-subunits, voltage-gated Na^+ channel, and a scaffolding protein, ankyrin B (ANK2). Brugada syndrome is characterized by idiopathic ventricular fibrillation in association with right ventricular electrocardiogram (ECG) abnormalities without structural heart disease. This disorder is also genetically heterogeneous, although it is most frequently linked to mutations in the Na^+ channel α-subunit, SCN5A. Catecholaminergic polymorphic tachycardia is an inherited, genetically heterogeneous disorder associated with exercise- or stress-induced ventricular arrhythmias, syncope, or sudden death. Acquired QT interval prolongation, most commonly due to drugs, may also result in ventricular arrhythmias and syncope.

Structural disease

Structural heart disease, (e.g., valvular disease, myocardial ischemia, hypertrophic and other cardiomyopathies, cardiac masses such as atrial myxoma, and pericardial effusions) may lead to syncope by compromising cardiac output. Structural disease may also contribute to other pathophysiologic mechanisms of syncope. For example, cardiac structural disease may predispose to arrhythmogenesis; aggressive treatment of cardiac failure with diuretics and/or vasodilators may lead to orthostatic hypotension; and inappropriate reflex vasodilation may occur with structural disorders such as aortic stenosis and hypertrophic cardiomyopathy, possibly provoked by increased ventricular contractility.

TREATMENT Cardiac Syncope

Treatment of cardiac disease depends upon the underlying disorder. Therapies for arrhythmias include cardiac pacing for sinus node disease and AV block, and ablation, anti-arrhythmic drugs, and cardioverter-defibrillators for atrial and ventricular tachyarrhythmias. These disorders are best managed by physicians with specialized skills in this area.

APPROACH TO THE PATIENT Syncope

DIFFERENTIAL DIAGNOSIS Syncope is easily diagnosed when the characteristic features are present; however, several disorders with transient real or apparent loss of consciousness may create diagnostic confusion.

Generalized and partial seizures may be confused with syncope; however, there are a number of differentiating features. Whereas tonic-clonic movements are the hallmark of a generalized seizure, myoclonic and other movements also may occur in up to 90% of syncopal episodes. Myoclonic jerks associated with syncope may be multifocal or generalized. They are typically arrhythmic and of short duration (<30 s). Mild flexor and extensor posturing also may occur. Partial- or partial-complex seizures with secondary generalization are usually preceded by an aura, commonly an unpleasant smell; fear anxiety; abdominal discomfort or other visceral sensations. These phenomena should be differentiated from the premonitory features of syncope.

Autonomic manifestations of seizures (autonomic epilepsy) may provide a more difficult diagnostic challenge. Autonomic seizures have cardiovascular, gastrointestinal, pulmonary, urogenital, pupillary, and cutaneous manifestations that are similar to the premonitory features of syncope. Furthermore, the cardiovascular manifestations of autonomic epilepsy include clinically significant tachycardias and bradycardias that may be of sufficient magnitude to cause loss of consciousness. The presence of accompanying nonautonomic auras may help differentiate these episodes from syncope.

Loss of consciousness associated with a seizure usually lasts longer than 5 min and is associated with prolonged postictal drowsiness and disorientation, whereas reorientation occurs almost immediately after a syncopal event. Muscle aches may occur after both syncope and seizures, although they tend to last longer following a seizure. Seizures, unlike syncope, are rarely provoked by emotions or pain. Incontinence of urine may occur with both seizures and syncope; however, fecal incontinence does not occur with syncope.

Hypoglycemia may cause transient loss of consciousness, typically in individuals with type 1 or type 2 diabetes treated with insulin. The clinical features associated with impending or actual hypoglycemia include tremor, palpitations, anxiety, diaphoresis, hunger, and paresthesias. These symptoms are due to autonomic activation to counter the falling blood glucose. Hunger, in particular, is not a typical premonitory feature of syncope. Hypoglycemia also impairs neuronal function, leading to fatigue, weakness, dizziness, and cognitive and behavioral symptoms. Diagnostic difficulties may occur in individuals in strict glycemic control; repeated hypoglycemia impairs the counterregulatory response and leads to a loss of the characteristic warning symptoms that are the hallmark of hypoglycemia.

Patients with cataplexy experience an abrupt partial or complete loss of muscular tone triggered by strong emotions, typically anger or laughter. Unlike syncope, consciousness is maintained throughout the attacks, which typically last between 30 s and 2 min. There are no premonitory symptoms. Cataplexy occurs in 60–75% of patients with narcolepsy.

The clinical interview and interrogation of eyewitnesses usually allow differentiation of syncope from falls due to vestibular dysfunction, cerebellar disease, extrapyramidal system dysfunction, and other gait disorders. If the fall is accompanied by head trauma, a postconcussive syndrome, amnesia for the precipitating events, and/or the presence of loss of consciousness may contribute to diagnostic difficulty.

Apparent loss of consciousness can be a manifestation of psychiatric disorders such as generalized anxiety, panic disorders, major depression, and somatization disorder. These possibilities should be considered in individuals who faint frequently without prodromal symptoms. Such patients are rarely injured despite numerous falls. There are no clinically significant hemodynamic changes concurrent with these episodes. In contrast, transient loss of consciousness due to vasovagal syncope precipitated by fear, stress, anxiety, and emotional distress is accompanied by hypotension, bradycardia, or both.

INITIAL EVALUATION The goals of the initial evaluation are to determine whether the transient loss of consciousness was due to syncope; to identify the cause; and to assess risk for future episodes and serious harm (Table 10-1). The initial evaluation should include a detailed history, thorough questioning of eyewitnesses, and a complete physical and neurologic examination. Blood pressure and heart rate should be measured in the supine position and after 3 min of standing to determine whether orthostatic hypotension is present. An ECG should be performed if there is suspicion of syncope due to an arrhythmia or underlying cardiac disease. Relevant electrocardiographic abnormalities include bradyarrhythmias or tachyarrhythmias, atrioventricular block, ischemia, old myocardial infarction, long QT syndrome, and bundle branch block. This initial assessment will lead to the identification of a cause of syncope in approximately 50% of patients and also allows stratification of patients at risk for cardiac mortality.

Laboratory Tests Baseline laboratory blood tests are rarely helpful in identifying the cause of syncope. Blood tests should be performed when specific disorders, e.g., myocardial infarction, anemia, and secondary autonomic failure, are suspected (Table 10-2).

Autonomic Nervous System Testing (Chap. 33) Autonomic testing including tilt table testing can be performed in specialized centers. Autonomic testing is helpful to uncover objective evidence of autonomic failure and also to demonstrate a predisposition to neurally mediated syncope. Autonomic testing includes assessments of parasympathetic autonomic nervous system function (e.g., heart rate variability to deep respiration and a Valsalva maneuver), sympathetic cholinergic function (e.g., thermoregulatory sweat response and quantitative sudomotor axon reflex test), and sympathetic adrenergic function (e.g., blood pressure response to a Valsalva maneuver and a tilt table test with beat-to-beat blood pressure measurement). The hemodynamic abnormalities demonstrated on tilt table test (Figs. 10-2 and 10-3) may be useful in distinguishing orthostatic hypotension due to autonomic failure from the hypotensive bradycardic response of neurally mediated syncope. Similarly, the tilt table test may help identify patients with syncope due to delayed or initial orthostatic hypotension.

Carotid sinus massage should be considered in patients with symptoms suggestive of carotid sinus syncope and in patients over age 50 years with recurrent syncope of unknown etiology. This test should only be carried out under continuous ECG and blood pressure monitoring and should be avoided in patients with carotid bruits, plaques, or stenosis.

Cardiac Evaluation ECG monitoring is indicated for patients with a high pretest probability of arrhythmia causing syncope. Patients should be monitored in hospital if the likelihood of a life-threatening arrhythmia is high, e.g., patients with severe structural or coronary artery disease, nonsustained ventricular tachycardia, trifascicular heart block, prolonged QT interval, Brugada's syndrome ECG pattern, and family history of sudden cardiac death. Outpatient Holter monitoring is recommended for patients who experience frequent syncopal episodes (one or more per week), whereas loop recorders, which continually record and erase cardiac rhythm, are indicated for patients with suspected arrhythmias with low risk of sudden cardiac death. Loop recorders may be external (recommended for evaluation of episodes that occur at a frequency of greater than one per month) or implantable (if syncope occurs less frequently).

Echocardiography should be performed in patients with a history of cardiac disease or if abnormalities are found on physical examination or the electrocardiogram. Echocardiographic diagnoses that may be responsible for syncope include aortic stenosis, hypertrophic cardiomyopathy, cardiac tumors, aortic dissection, and pericardial tamponade. Echocardiography also has a role in risk stratification based on the left ventricular ejection fraction.

Treadmill exercise testing with ECG and blood pressure monitoring should be performed in patients who have experienced syncope during or shortly after exercise. Treadmill testing may help identify exercise-induced arrhythmias (e.g., tachycardia-related AV block) and exercise-induced exaggerated vasodilation.

Electrophysiologic studies are indicated in patients with structural heart disease and ECG abnormalities in whom noninvasive investigations have failed to yield a diagnosis. Electrophysiologic studies have low sensitivity and specificity and should only be performed when a high pretest probability exists. Currently, this test is rarely performed to evaluate patients with syncope.

Psychiatric Evaluation Screening for psychiatric disorders may be appropriate in patients with recurrent unexplained syncope episodes. Tilt table testing, with demonstration of symptoms in the absence of hemodynamic change, may be useful in reproducing syncope in patients with suspected psychogenic syncope.

CHAPTER 11

DIZZINESS AND VERTIGO

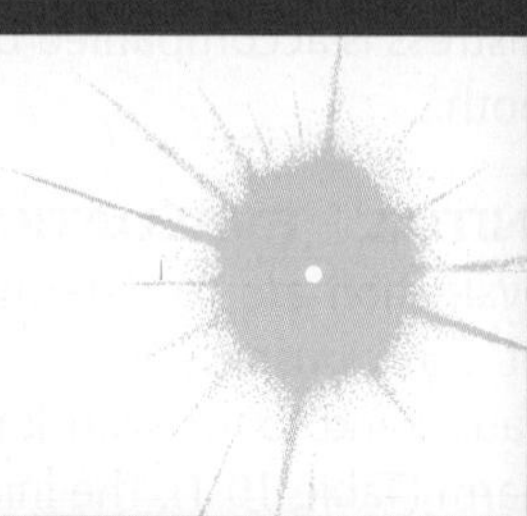

Mark F. Walker ■ Robert B. Daroff

Dizziness is a common, vexing symptom, and epidemiologic data indicate that more than 20% of adults experience dizziness within a given year. The diagnosis is frequently challenging, in part because patients use the term to refer to a variety of different sensations, including feelings of faintness, spinning, and other illusions of motion, imbalance, and anxiety. Other descriptive words, such as *light-headedness*, are equally ambiguous, referring in some cases to a presyncopal sensation due to hypoperfusion of the brain and in others to disequilibrium and imbalance. Patients often have difficulty distinguishing among these various symptoms, and the words they choose do not describe the underlying etiology reliably.

Vascular disorders cause presyncopal dizziness as a result of cardiac dysrhythmia, orthostatic hypotension, medication effects, or another cause. Such presyncopal sensations vary in duration; they may increase in severity until loss of consciousness occurs, or they may resolve before loss of consciousness if the cerebral ischemia is corrected. Faintness and syncope, which are discussed in detail in Chap. 10, should always be considered when one is evaluating patients with brief episodes of dizziness or dizziness that occurs with upright posture.

Vestibular causes of dizziness may be due to peripheral lesions that affect the labyrinths or vestibular nerves or to involvement of the central vestibular pathways. They may be paroxysmal or due to a fixed unilateral or bilateral vestibular deficit. Acute unilateral lesions cause vertigo due to a sudden imbalance in vestibular inputs from the two labyrinths. Bilateral lesions cause imbalance and instability of vision when the head moves (*oscillopsia*). Other causes of dizziness include nonvestibular imbalance and gait disorders (e.g., loss of proprioception from sensory neuropathy, parkinsonism) and anxiety.

In evaluating patients with dizziness, questions to consider include the following: (1) is it dangerous (e.g., arrhythmia, transient ischemic attack/stroke)? (2) is it vestibular? and (3) if vestibular, is it peripheral or central? A careful history and examination often provide enough information to answer these questions and determine whether additional studies or referral to a specialist is necessary.

APPROACH TO THE PATIENT Dizziness

HISTORY When a patient presents with dizziness, the first step is to delineate more precisely the nature of the symptom. In the case of vestibular disorders, the physical symptoms depend on whether the lesion is unilateral or bilateral and whether it is acute or chronic and progressive. Vertigo, an illusion of self or environmental motion, implies asymmetry of vestibular inputs from the two labyrinths or in their central pathways and is usually acute. Symmetric bilateral vestibular hypofunction causes imbalance but no vertigo. Because of the ambiguity in patients' descriptions of their symptoms, diagnosis based simply on symptom character is typically unreliable. The history should focus closely on other features, including whether dizziness is paroxysmal or has occurred only once, the duration of each episode, any provoking factors, and the symptoms that accompany the dizziness.

Causes of dizziness can be divided into episodes that last for seconds, minutes, hours, or days. Common causes of brief dizziness (seconds) include benign paroxysmal positional vertigo (BPPV) and orthostatic hypotension, both of which typically are provoked by changes in position. Attacks of migrainous vertigo and Ménière's disease often last hours. When episodes are of intermediate duration (minutes), transient ischemic attacks of the posterior circulation should be considered, although these episodes also could be due to migraine or a number of other causes.

TABLE 11-1

FEATURES OF PERIPHERAL AND CENTRAL VERTIGO

SIGN OR SYMPTOM	PERIPHERAL (LABYRINTH OR VESTIBULAR NERVE)	CENTRAL (BRAINSTEM OR CEREBELLUM)
Direction of associated nystagmus	Unidirectional; fast phase opposite lesion[a]	Bidirectional (direction-changing) or unidirectional
Purely horizontal nystagmus without torsional component	Uncommon	May be present
Purely vertical or purely torsional nystagmus	Never present[b]	May be present
Visual fixation	Inhibits nystagmus	No inhibition
Tinnitus and/or deafness	Often present	Usually absent
Associated central nervous system abnormalities	None	Extremely common (e.g., diplopia, hiccups, cranial neuropathies, dysarthria)
Common causes	Benign paroxysmal positional vertigo, infection (labyrinthitis), vestibular neuritis, Ménière's disease, labyrinthine ischemia, trauma, toxin	Vascular, demyelinating, neoplasm

[a]In Ménière's disease, the direction of the fast phase is variable.
[b]Combined vertical-torsional nystagmus suggests BPPV.

Symptoms that accompany vertigo may be helpful in distinguishing peripheral vestibular lesions from central causes. Unilateral hearing loss and other aural symptoms (ear pain, pressure, fullness) typically point to a peripheral cause. Because the auditory pathways quickly become bilateral upon entering the brainstem, central lesions are unlikely to cause unilateral hearing loss (unless the lesion lies near the root entry zone of the auditory nerve). Symptoms such as double vision, numbness, and limb ataxia suggest a brainstem or cerebellar lesion.

EXAMINATION Because dizziness and imbalance can be a manifestation of a variety of neurologic disorders, the neurologic examination is important in the evaluation of these patients. Particular focus should be given to assessment of eye movements, vestibular function, and hearing. The range of eye movements and whether they are equal in each eye should be observed. Peripheral eye movement disorders (e.g., cranial neuropathies, eye muscle weakness) are usually *disconjugate* (different in the two eyes). One should check pursuit (the ability to follow a smoothly moving target) and saccades (the ability to look back and forth accurately between two targets). Poor pursuit or inaccurate (*dysmetric*) saccades usually indicates central pathology, often involving the cerebellum. Finally, one should look for spontaneous nystagmus, an involuntary back-and-forth movement of the eyes. Most often nystagmus is of the jerk type, in which a slow drift (*slow phase*) in one direction alternates with a rapid saccadic movement (*quick phase* or *fast phase*) in the opposite direction that resets the position of the eyes in the orbits. Table 11-1 lists features that help distinguish peripheral vestibular nystagmus from central nystagmus. Except in the case of acute vestibulopathy (e.g., vestibular neuritis), if primary position nystagmus is easily seen in the light, it is probably due to a central cause. Two forms of nystagmus that are characteristic of lesions of the cerebellar pathways are vertical nystagmus with downward fast phases (downbeat nystagmus) and horizontal nystagmus that changes direction with gaze (gaze-evoked nystagmus).

Specialists find that the most useful bedside test of peripheral vestibular function is the *head impulse test*, in which the vestibuloocular reflex (VOR) is assessed with small-amplitude (approximately 20 degrees) rapid head rotations; beginning in the primary position, the head is rotated to the left or right while the patient is instructed to fixate on the examiner's face. If the VOR is deficient, a catch-up saccade is seen at the end of the rotation. This test can identify both unilateral (deficient VOR when the head is rotated toward the weak side) and bilateral vestibular hypofunction.

All patients with episodic dizziness, especially if it is provoked by positional change, should be tested with the Dix-Hallpike maneuver. The patient begins in a sitting position with the head turned 45 degrees; holding the back of the head, the examiner then gently lowers the patient into a supine position with the head extended backward by about 20 degrees, and observes for nystagmus; after 30 s the patient is raised to the sitting position and after a 1-min rest the procedure is repeated with the head turned to the other side. Use of Frenzel eyeglasses (self-illuminated goggles with convex lenses that blur the patient's vision but allow the examiner to see the eyes greatly magnified) can improve the sensitivity of the test. If transient upbeating and torsional nystagmus are elicited in the supine position, posterior canal BPPV can be diagnosed confidently and treated with a repositioning maneuver, and additional testing can be avoided.

Dynamic visual acuity is a functional test that can be useful in assessing vestibular function. Visual acuity is measured with the head still and when the head is rotated back and forth by the examiner (about 1–2 Hz). A drop in visual acuity during head motion of more than one line on a near card or Snellen chart is abnormal.

The choice of ancillary tests should be guided by the history and examination findings. Audiometry should be performed whenever a vestibular disorder is suspected. Unilateral sensorineural hearing loss supports a peripheral disorder (e.g., vestibular schwannoma). Predominantly low-frequency hearing loss is characteristic of Ménière's disease. Electro- or videonystagmography includes recordings of spontaneous nystagmus (if present), pursuit, and saccades; caloric testing to assess the responses of the two horizontal semicircular canals; and measurement of positional nystagmus. Patients with unexplained unilateral hearing loss or vestibular hypofunction should undergo magnetic resonance imaging of the internal auditory canals, including administration of gadolinium, to rule out a schwannoma.

TREATMENT Dizziness

Treatment of vestibular symptoms should be driven by the underlying diagnosis. Simply treating dizziness with vestibular suppressant medications is often not helpful and may make the symptoms worse. The diagnostic and specific treatment approaches for the most commonly encountered vestibular disorders are discussed next.

Acute prolonged vertigo

An acute unilateral vestibular lesion causes constant vertigo, nausea, vomiting, oscillopsia (motion of the visual scene), and imbalance. These symptoms are due to a sudden asymmetry of inputs from the two labyrinths or in their central connections, simulating a continuous rotation of the head. Unlike BPPV, the vertigo persists even when the head is not moving.

When a patient presents with an acute vestibular syndrome, the most important question is whether the lesion is central (e.g., a cerebellar or brainstem infarct or hemorrhage), which may be life-threatening, or peripheral, affecting the vestibular nerve or labyrinth. Attention should be given to any symptoms or signs that point to central dysfunction (diplopia, weakness or numbness, dysarthria). The pattern of spontaneous nystagmus, if present, may be helpful (Table 11-1). If the head impulse test is normal, an acute peripheral vestibular lesion is unlikely. However, a central lesion cannot always be excluded with certainly on the basis of symptoms and examination alone; thus, older patients with vascular risk factors who present with an acute vestibular syndrome generally should be evaluated for the possibility of stroke even when there are no specific findings that indicate a central lesion.

Most patients with vestibular neuritis recover spontaneously, but glucocorticoids can improve outcome if administered within 3 days of symptom onset. Antiviral medications are of no proven benefit unless there is evidence to suggest herpes zoster oticus (Ramsay Hunt syndrome). Vestibular suppressant medications may reduce acute symptoms but should be avoided after the first several days as they may impede central compensation and recovery. Patients should be encouraged to resume a normal level of activity as soon as possible, and directed vestibular rehabilitation therapy may accelerate improvement.

Benign paroxysmal positional vertigo

BPPV is a common cause of recurrent vertigo. Episodes are brief (<1 min and typically 15–20 s) and are always provoked by changes in head position relative to gravity, such as lying down, rolling over in bed, rising from a supine position, and extending the head to look upward. The attacks are caused by free-floating otoconia (calcium carbonate crystals) that have been dislodged from the utricular macula and have moved into one of the semicircular canals, usually the posterior canal. When head position changes, gravity causes the otoconia to move within the canal, producing vertigo and nystagmus. With posterior canal BPPV, the nystagmus beats upward and torsionally (the upper poles of the eyes beat toward the affected ear). Less commonly, the otoconia enter the horizontal canal, resulting in a horizontal nystagmus when the patient is lying with either ear down. Superior (also called anterior) canal involvement is rare. BPPV is treated with repositioning maneuvers that utilize gravity to remove the otoconia from the semicircular canal. For posterior canal BPPV, the Epley maneuver is the most commonly used procedure. For more refractory cases of BPPV, patients can be taught a variant of this maneuver that they can perform alone at home.

Vestibular migraine

Vestibular symptoms occur frequently in migraine, sometimes as a headache aura but often independent of headache. The duration of vertigo may be from minutes to hours, and some patients also experience more prolonged periods of disequilibrium (lasting days to weeks). Motion sensitivity and sensitivity to visual motion (e.g., movies) are common in patients with vestibular migraine. Although data from controlled studies are generally lacking, vestibular migraine typically is treated with medications that are used for prophylaxis of migraine headaches. Antiemetics may be helpful to relieve symptoms at the time of an attack.

Ménière's disease

Attacks of Ménière's disease consist of vertigo, hearing loss, and pain, pressure, or fullness in the affected ear. The hearing loss and aural symptoms are key features that distinguish Ménière's disease from other peripheral vestibulopathies. Audiometry at the time of an attack shows a characteristic asymmetric low-frequency hearing loss; hearing commonly improves between attacks, although permanent hearing loss may occur eventually. Ménière's disease is thought to be due to excess fluid (endolymph) in the inner ear, hence the term *endolymphatic hydrops*. Patients suspected of having Ménière's disease should be referred to an otolaryngologist for further evaluation. Diuretics and sodium restriction are the initial treatments. If attacks persist, injections of gentamicin into the middle ear are typically the next line of therapy. Full ablative procedures (vestibular nerve section, labyrinthectomy) seldom are required.

Vestibular schwannoma

Vestibular schwannomas (sometimes less correctly termed *acoustic neuromas*) and other tumors at the cerebellopontine angle cause slowly progressive unilateral sensorineural hearing loss and vestibular hypofunction. These patients typically do not have vertigo, because the gradual vestibular deficit is compensated centrally as it develops. The diagnosis often is not made until there is sufficient hearing loss to be noticed. The examination will show a deficient Halmagyi-Curthoys head impulse response when the head is rotated toward the affected side. Any patient with unexplained asymmetric vestibular function (e.g., no prior history of vestibular neuritis) or asymmetric sensorineural hearing loss (documented on audiometry) should undergo MRI of the internal auditory canals, including gadolinium administration, to rule out a schwannoma.

Bilateral vestibular hypofunction

Patients with bilateral loss of vestibular function also typically do not have vertigo, since vestibular function is lost on both sides simultaneously, thus there is no asymmetry of vestibular input. Symptoms include loss of balance, particularly in the dark, where vestibular input is most critical, and oscillopsia during head movement, such as while walking or riding in a car. Bilateral vestibular hypofunction may be (1) idiopathic and progressive, (2) part of a neurodegenerative disorder, or (3) iatrogenic, due to medication ototoxicity (most commonly gentamicin or other aminoglycoside antibiotics). Other causes include bilateral vestibular schwannomas (neurofibromatosis type 2), autoimmune disease, meningeal-based infection or tumor, and other toxins. It also may occur in patients with peripheral polyneuropathy; in these patients, both vestibular loss and impaired proprioception may contribute to poor balance. Finally, unilateral processes such as vestibular neuritis and Ménière's disease may involve both ears sequentially, resulting in bilateral vestibulopathy.

Examination findings include diminished dynamic visual acuity (see earlier in this chapter) due to loss of stable vision when the head is moving, abnormal head impulse responses in both directions, and a Romberg sign. In the laboratory, responses to caloric testing are reduced. Patients with bilateral vestibular hypofunction should be referred for vestibular rehabilitation therapy. Vestibular suppressant medications should not be used, as they will increase the imbalance. Evaluation by a neurologist is important not only to confirm the diagnosis but also to consider any other associated neurologic abnormalities that may clarify the etiology.

Psychosomatic dizziness

Psychological factors play an important role in chronic dizziness. First, dizziness may be a somatic manifestation of a psychiatric condition such as major depression, anxiety, or panic disorder. Second, patients may develop anxiety and autonomic symptoms as a consequence or comorbidity of an independent vestibular disorder. One particular form of this has been termed variously *phobic postural vertigo*, *psychophysiologic vertigo*, or *chronic subjective dizziness*. These patients have a chronic feeling (months or longer) of dizziness and disequilibrium, an increased sensitivity to self-motion and visual motion (e.g., movies), and a particular intensification of symptoms when moving through complex visual environments such as supermarkets (*visual vertigo*). Although there may be a past history of an acute vestibular disorder (e.g., vestibular neuritis), the neurootologic examination and vestibular testing are normal or indicative of a compensated vestibular deficit, indicating that the ongoing subjective dizziness cannot be explained by a primary vestibular disorder. Anxiety disorders are common in patients with chronic dizziness and contribute substantially to the morbidity. Thus, treatment with antianxiety medications (selective serotonin reuptake inhibitors [SSRIs]) and cognitive/behavioral therapy may be helpful. Vestibular rehabilitation therapy is also sometimes beneficial. Vestibular suppressant medications generally should be avoided. This condition should be suspected when the patient states, "My dizziness is so bad, I'm afraid to leave my house" (agoraphobia). General treatment of vertigo consists of vestibular suppressant medications and vestibular rehabilitation therapy.

TREATMENT Vertigo

Table 11-2 provides a list of commonly used medications for suppression of vertigo. As noted, these medications should be reserved for short-term control of active vertigo, such as during the first few days of acute vestibular neuritis, or for acute attacks of Ménière's disease. They are less helpful for chronic dizziness and, as previously stated, may hinder central compensation. An exception is that benzodiazepines may attenuate psychosomatic dizziness and the associated anxiety, although SSRIs are generally preferable in such patients.

Vestibular rehabilitation therapy promotes central adaptation processes that compensate for vestibular loss and also may help habituate motion sensitivity and other symptoms of psychosomatic dizziness. The general approach is to use a graded series of exercises that progressively challenge gaze stabilization and balance.

TABLE 11-2

TREATMENT OF VERTIGO

AGENT[a]	DOSE[b]
Antihistamines	
Meclizine	25–50 mg 3 times daily
Dimenhydrinate	50 mg 1–2 times daily
Promethazine	25 mg 2–3 times daily (also can be given rectally and IM)
Benzodiazepines	
Diazepam	2.5 mg 1–3 times daily
Clonazepam	0.25 mg 1–3 times daily
Anticholinergic	
Scopolamine transdermal[c]	Patch
Physical therapy	
Repositioning maneuvers[d]	
Vestibular rehabilitation	
Other	
Diuretics and/or low-sodium (1 g/d) diet[e]	
Antimigrainous drugs[f]	
Methylprednisolone[g]	100 mg daily days 1–3; 80 mg daily days 4–6; 60 mg daily days 7–9; 40 mg daily days 10–12; 20 mg daily days 13–15; 10 mg daily days 16–18, 20, 22
Selective serotonin reuptake inhibitors[h]	

[a]All listed drugs are approved by the U.S. Food and Drug Administration, but most are not approved for the treatment of vertigo.
[b]Usual oral (unless otherwise stated) starting dose in adults; a higher maintenance dose can be reached by a gradual increase.
[c]For motion sickness only.
[d]For benign paroxysmal positional vertigo.
[e]For Ménière's disease.
[f]For vestibular migraine.
[g]For acute vestibular neuritis (started within three days of onset).
[h]For psychosomatic vertigo.

CHAPTER 12

WEAKNESS AND PARALYSIS

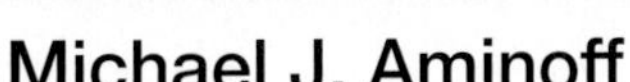
Michael J. Aminoff

Normal motor function involves integrated muscle activity that is modulated by the activity of the cerebral cortex, basal ganglia, cerebellum, and spinal cord. Motor system dysfunction leads to weakness or paralysis, which is discussed in this chapter, or to ataxia (Chap. 31) or abnormal movements (Chap. 30). The mode of onset, distribution, and accompaniments of weakness help suggest its cause.

Weakness is a reduction in the power that can be exerted by one or more muscles. Increased fatigability or limitation in function due to pain or articular stiffness often is confused with weakness by patients. *Increased fatigability* is the inability to sustain the performance of an activity that should be normal for a person of the same age, sex, and size. Increased time is required sometimes for full power to be exerted, and this *bradykinesia* may be misinterpreted as weakness. Severe proprioceptive sensory loss also may lead to complaints of weakness because adequate feedback information about the direction and power of movements is lacking. Finally, *apraxia,* a disorder of planning and initiating a skilled or learned movement unrelated to a significant motor or sensory deficit (Chap. 18), sometimes is mistaken for weakness.

Paralysis indicates weakness that is so severe that a muscle cannot be contracted at all, whereas *paresis* refers to weakness that is mild or moderate. The prefix "hemi-" refers to one-half of the body, "para-" to both legs, and "quadri-" to all four limbs. The suffix "-plegia" signifies severe weakness or paralysis.

The distribution of weakness helps to indicate the site of the underlying lesion. Weakness from involvement of upper motor neurons occurs particularly in the extensors and abductors of the upper limb and the flexors of the lower limb. Lower motor neuron weakness does not have this selectivity but depends on whether involvement is at the level of the anterior horn cells, nerve root, limb plexus, or peripheral nerve—only muscles supplied by the affected structure are weak. Myopathic weakness is generally most marked in proximal muscles, whereas weakness from impaired neuromuscular transmission has no specific pattern of involvement. Weakness often is accompanied by other neurologic abnormalities that help indicate the site of the responsible lesion. These abnormalities include changes in tone, muscle bulk, muscle stretch reflexes, and cutaneous reflexes (**Table 12-1**).

Tone is the resistance of a muscle to passive stretch. Central nervous system (CNS) abnormalities that cause weakness generally produce *spasticity*, an increase in tone associated with disease of upper motor neurons. Spasticity is velocity-dependent, has a sudden release after reaching a maximum (the "clasp-knife" phenomenon), and predominantly affects the antigravity muscles (i.e., upper-limb flexors and lower-limb extensors). Spasticity is distinct from rigidity and paratonia, two other types of hypertonia. *Rigidity* is increased tone that is present throughout the range of motion (a "lead pipe" or "plastic" stiffness) and affects flexors and extensors equally; it sometimes has a cogwheel quality that is enhanced by voluntary movement of the contralateral limb (reinforcement). Rigidity occurs with certain extrapyramidal disorders, such as Parkinson's disease. *Paratonia* (or *gegenhalten*) is increased tone that varies irregularly in a manner that may seem related to the degree of relaxation, is present throughout the range of motion, and affects flexors and extensors equally; it usually results from disease of the frontal lobes. Weakness with *decreased tone* (*flaccidity*) or normal tone occurs with disorders of *motor units*. A motor unit consists of a single lower motor neuron and all the muscle fibers that it innervates.

Muscle bulk generally is not affected in patients with upper motor neuron lesions, although mild disuse atrophy eventually may occur. By contrast, atrophy is often conspicuous when a lower motor neuron lesion is responsible for weakness and also may occur with advanced muscle disease.

TABLE 12-1

SIGNS THAT DISTINGUISH THE ORIGIN OF WEAKNESS

SIGN	UPPER MOTOR NEURON	LOWER MOTOR NEURON	MYOPATHIC
Atrophy	None	Severe	Mild
Fasciculations	None	Common	None
Tone	Spastic	Decreased	Normal/decreased
Distribution of weakness	Pyramidal/regional	Distal/segmental	Proximal
Tendon reflexes	Hyperactive	Hypoactive/absent	Normal/hypoactive
Babinski sign	Present	Absent	Absent

Muscle stretch (tendon) reflexes are usually increased with upper motor neuron lesions, although they may be decreased or absent for a variable period immediately after onset of an acute lesion. This is usually—but not invariably—accompanied by abnormalities of *cutaneous reflexes* (such as superficial abdominals; Chap. 1) and, in particular, by an extensor plantar (Babinski) response. The muscle stretch reflexes are depressed in patients with lower motor neuron lesions when there is direct involvement of specific reflex arcs. The stretch reflexes generally are preserved in patients with myopathic weakness except in advanced stages, when they sometimes are attenuated. In disorders of the neuromuscular junction, the intensity of the reflex responses may be affected by preceding voluntary activity of affected muscles; that activity may lead to enhancement of initially depressed reflexes in Lambert-Eaton myasthenic syndrome and, conversely, to depression of initially normal reflexes in myasthenia gravis (Chap. 47).

The distinction of *neuropathic* (lower motor neuron) from *myopathic* weakness is sometimes difficult clinically, although distal weakness is likely to be neuropathic, and symmetric proximal weakness myopathic. *Fasciculations* (visible or palpable twitch within a muscle due to the spontaneous discharge of a motor unit) and early atrophy indicate that weakness is neuropathic.

PATHOGENESIS

Upper motor neuron weakness

This pattern of weakness results from disorders that affect the upper motor neurons or their axons in the cerebral cortex, subcortical white matter, internal capsule, brainstem, or spinal cord (Fig. 12-1). These lesions produce weakness through decreased activation of the lower motor neurons. In general, distal muscle groups are affected more severely than are proximal ones, and axial movements are spared unless the lesion is severe and bilateral. With corticobulbar involvement, weakness usually is observed only in the lower face and tongue; extraocular, upper facial, pharyngeal, and jaw muscles almost always are spared. With bilateral corticobulbar lesions, *pseudobulbar palsy* often develops: dysarthria, dysphagia, dysphonia, and emotional lability accompany bilateral facial weakness and a brisk jaw jerk. Spasticity accompanies upper motor neuron weakness but may not be present in the acute phase. Upper motor neuron lesions also affect the ability to perform rapid repetitive movements. Such movements are slow and coarse, but normal rhythmicity is maintained. Finger-nose-finger and heel-knee-shin maneuvers are performed slowly but adequately.

Lower motor neuron weakness

This pattern results from disorders of cell bodies of lower motor neurons in the brainstem motor nuclei and the anterior horn of the spinal cord or from dysfunction of the axons of these neurons as they pass to skeletal muscle (Fig. 12-2). Weakness is due to a decrease in the number of muscle fibers that can be activated through a loss of α motor neurons or disruption of their connections to muscle. Loss of γ motor neurons does not cause weakness but decreases tension on the muscle spindles, which decreases muscle tone and attenuates the stretch reflexes elicited on examination. An absent stretch reflex suggests involvement of spindle afferent fibers.

When a motor unit becomes diseased, especially in anterior horn cell diseases, it may discharge spontaneously, producing *fasciculations* that may be seen or felt clinically or recorded by electromyography (EMG). When α motor neurons or their axons degenerate, the denervated muscle fibers also may discharge spontaneously. These single muscle fiber discharges, or *fibrillation potentials,* cannot be seen or felt but can be recorded with EMG. If lower motor neuron weakness is present, recruitment of motor units is delayed or reduced, with fewer than normal activated at a particular discharge frequency. This contrasts with weakness of the upper motor neuron type, in which a normal number of motor units is activated at a given frequency but with a diminished maximal discharge frequency.

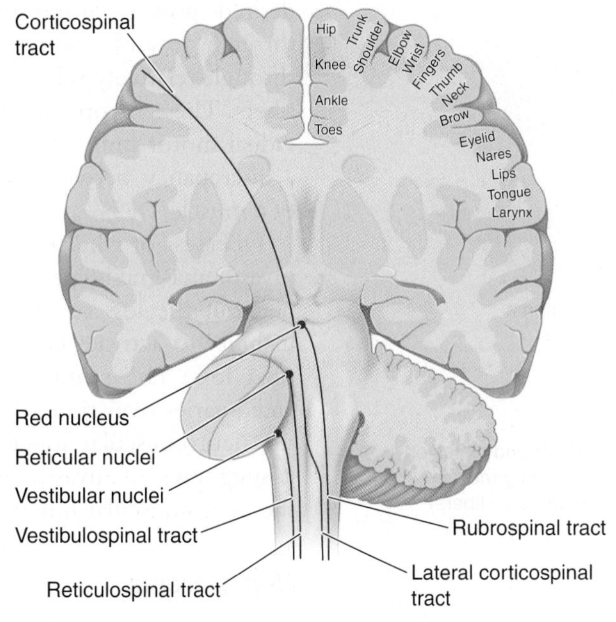

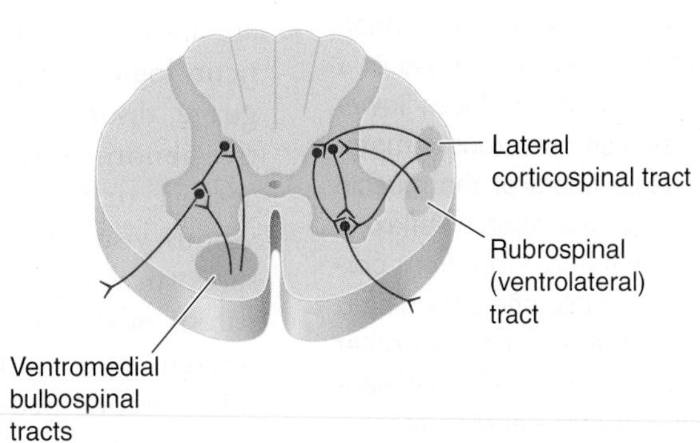

FIGURE 12-1

The corticospinal and bulbospinal upper motor neuron pathways. Upper motor neurons have their cell bodies in layer V of the primary motor cortex (the precentral gyrus, or Brodmann's area 4) and in the premotor and supplemental motor cortex (area 6). The upper motor neurons in the primary motor cortex are somatotopically organized, as illustrated on the right side of the figure.

Axons of the upper motor neurons descend through the subcortical white matter and the posterior limb of the internal capsule. Axons of the *pyramidal* or *corticospinal system* descend through the brainstem in the cerebral peduncle of the midbrain, the basis pontis, and the medullary pyramids. At the cervicomedullary junction, most pyramidal axons decussate into the contralateral corticospinal tract of the lateral spinal cord, but 10–30% remain ipsilateral in the anterior spinal cord. Pyramidal neurons make direct monosynaptic connections with lower motor neurons. They innervate most densely the lower motor neurons of hand muscles and are involved in the execution of learned, fine movements. Corticobulbar neurons are similar to corticospinal neurons but innervate brainstem motor nuclei.

Bulbospinal upper motor neurons influence strength and tone but are not part of the pyramidal system. The descending *ventromedial bulbospinal pathways* originate in the tectum of the midbrain (tectospinal pathway), the vestibular nuclei (vestibulospinal pathway), and the reticular formation (reticulospinal pathway). These pathways influence axial and proximal muscles and are involved in the maintenance of posture and integrated movements of the limbs and trunk. The descending *ventrolateral bulbospinal pathways*, which originate predominantly in the red nucleus (rubrospinal pathway), facilitate distal limb muscles. The bulbospinal system sometimes is referred to as the *extrapyramidal upper motor neuron system*. In all figures, nerve cell bodies and axon terminals are shown, respectively, as closed circles and forks.

Myopathic weakness

Myopathic weakness is produced by disorders of the muscle fibers. Disorders of the neuromuscular junctions also produce weakness, but this is variable in degree and distribution and is influenced by preceding activity of the affected muscle. At a muscle fiber, if the nerve terminal releases a normal number of acetylcholine molecules presynaptically and a sufficient number of postsynaptic

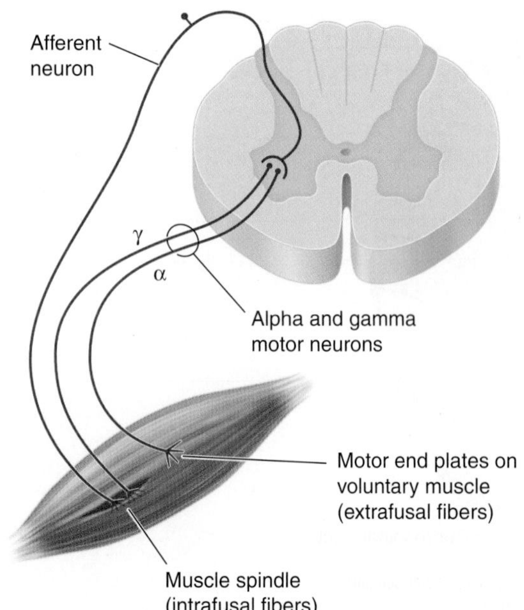

FIGURE 12-2

Lower motor neurons are divided into α and γ types. The larger α motor neurons are more numerous and innervate the extrafusal muscle fibers of the motor unit. Loss of α motor neurons or disruption of their axons produces lower motor neuron weakness. The smaller, less numerous γ motor neurons innervate the intrafusal muscle fibers of the muscle spindle and contribute to normal tone and stretch reflexes. The α motor neuron receives direct excitatory input from corticomotoneurons and primary muscle spindle afferents. The α and γ motor neurons also receive excitatory input from other descending upper motor neuron pathways, segmental sensory inputs, and interneurons. The α motor neurons receive direct inhibition from Renshaw cell interneurons, and other interneurons indirectly inhibit the α and γ motor neurons.

A tendon reflex requires the function of all the illustrated structures. A tap on a tendon stretches muscle spindles (which are tonically activated by γ motor neurons) and activates the primary spindle afferent neurons. These neurons stimulate the α motor neurons in the spinal cord, producing a brief muscle contraction, which is the familiar tendon reflex.

acetylcholine receptors are opened, the end plate reaches threshold and thereby generates an action potential that spreads across the muscle fiber membrane and into the transverse tubular system. This electrical excitation activates intracellular events that produce an energy-dependent contraction of the muscle fiber (excitation-contraction coupling).

Myopathic weakness is produced by a decrease in the number or contractile force of muscle fibers activated within motor units. With muscular dystrophies, inflammatory myopathies, or myopathies with muscle fiber necrosis, the number of muscle fibers is reduced within many motor units. On EMG, the size of each motor unit action potential is decreased, and motor units must be recruited more rapidly than normal to produce the desired power. Some myopathies produce weakness through loss of contractile force of muscle fibers or through relatively selective involvement of type II (fast) fibers. These myopathies may not affect the size of individual motor unit action potentials and are detected by a discrepancy between the electrical activity and force of a muscle.

Diseases of the neuromuscular junction, such as myasthenia gravis, produce weakness in a similar manner, but the loss of muscle fibers is functional (due to inability to activate them) rather than related to muscle fiber loss. The number of muscle fibers that are activated varies over time, depending on the state of rest of the neuromuscular junctions. Thus, fatigable weakness is suggestive of myasthenia gravis or other disorders of the neuromuscular junction.

Hemiparesis

Hemiparesis results from an upper motor neuron lesion above the midcervical spinal cord; most such lesions are above the foramen magnum. The presence of other neurologic deficits helps localize the lesion. Thus, language disorders, cortical sensory disturbances, cognitive abnormalities, disorders of visual-spatial integration, apraxia, or seizures point to a cortical lesion. Homonymous visual field defects reflect either a cortical or a subcortical hemispheric lesion. A "pure motor" hemiparesis of the face, arm, and leg often is due to a small, discrete lesion in the posterior limb of the internal capsule, cerebral peduncle, or upper pons. Some brainstem lesions produce "crossed paralyses," consisting of ipsilateral cranial nerve signs and contralateral hemiparesis (Chap. 27). The absence of cranial nerve signs or facial weakness suggests that a hemiparesis is due to a lesion in the high cervical spinal cord, especially if it is associated with ipsilateral loss of proprioception and contralateral loss of pain and temperature sense (the Brown-Séquard syndrome).

Acute or episodic hemiparesis usually results from ischemic or hemorrhagic stroke but also may relate to hemorrhage occurring into brain tumors or may be a result of trauma; other causes include a focal structural lesion or an inflammatory process as in multiple sclerosis, abscess, or sarcoidosis. Evaluation (Fig. 12-3) begins immediately with a CT scan of the brain and laboratory studies. If the CT is normal and an ischemic stroke is unlikely, MRI of the brain or cervical spine is performed.

Subacute hemiparesis that evolves over days or weeks has an extensive differential diagnosis. A common cause is subdural hematoma, especially in elderly or anticoagulated patients, even when there is no history of trauma. Infectious possibilities include cerebral abscess, fungal granuloma or meningitis, and parasitic infection. Weakness from primary and metastatic neoplasms may evolve

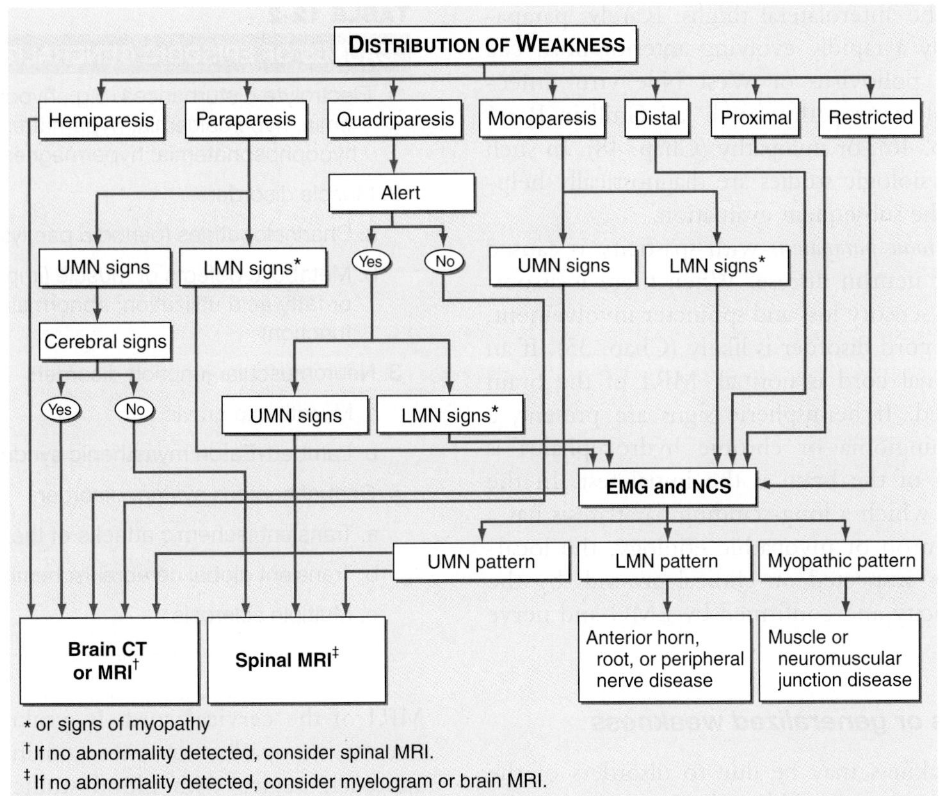

FIGURE 12-3

An algorithm for the initial workup of a patient with weakness. CT, computed tomography; EMG, electromyography; LMN, lower motor neuron; MRI, magnetic resonance imaging; NCS, nerve conduction studies; UMN, upper motor neuron.

over days to weeks. AIDS may present with subacute hemiparesis due to toxoplasmosis or primary CNS lymphoma. Noninfectious inflammatory processes such as multiple sclerosis or, less commonly, sarcoidosis merit consideration. If the brain MRI is normal and there are no cortical and hemispheric signs, MRI of the cervical spine should be undertaken.

Chronic hemiparesis that evolves over months usually is due to a neoplasm or vascular malformation, a chronic subdural hematoma, or a degenerative disease. If an MRI of the brain is normal, the possibility of a foramen magnum or high cervical spinal cord lesion should be considered.

Paraparesis

An intraspinal lesion at or below the upper thoracic spinal cord level is most commonly responsible, but a paraparesis also may result from lesions at other locations that disturb upper motor neurons (especially parasagittal intracranial lesions) and lower motor neurons (anterior horn cell disorders, cauda equina syndromes due to involvement of nerve roots derived from the lower spinal cord [Chap. 35], and peripheral neuropathies).

Acute paraparesis may not be recognized as due to spinal cord disease at an early stage if the legs are flaccid and areflexic. Usually, however, there is sensory loss in the legs with an upper level on the trunk, a dissociated sensory loss suggestive of a central cord syndrome, or exaggerated stretch reflexes in the legs with normal reflexes in the arms. It is important to image the spinal cord (Fig. 12-3). Compressive lesions (particularly epidural tumor, abscess, and hematoma but also a prolapsed intervertebral disk and vertebral involvement by malignancy or infection), spinal cord infarction (proprioception usually is spared), an arteriovenous fistula or other vascular anomaly, and transverse myelitis are among the possible causes (Chap. 35).

Diseases of the cerebral hemispheres that produce acute paraparesis include anterior cerebral artery ischemia (shoulder shrug also is affected), superior sagittal sinus or cortical venous thrombosis, and acute hydrocephalus. If upper motor neuron signs are associated with drowsiness, confusion, seizures, or other hemispheric signs, MRI of the brain should be undertaken.

Paraparesis may result from a cauda equina syndrome, for example, after trauma to the low back, a midline disk herniation, or an intraspinal tumor; although sphincters are affected, hip flexion often is spared, as is sensation over the anterolateral thighs. Rarely, paraparesis is caused by a rapidly evolving anterior horn cell disease (such as poliovirus or West Nile virus infection), peripheral neuropathy (such as Guillain-Barré syndrome; Chap. 46), or myopathy (Chap. 48). In such cases, electrophysiologic studies are diagnostically helpful and refocus the subsequent evaluation.

Subacute or chronic paraparesis with spasticity is caused by upper motor neuron disease. When there is associated lower-limb sensory loss and sphincter involvement, a chronic spinal cord disorder is likely (Chap. 35). If an MRI of the spinal cord is normal, MRI of the brain may be indicated. If hemispheric signs are present, a parasagittal meningioma or chronic hydrocephalus is likely and MRI of the brain is the initial test. In the rare situation in which a long-standing paraparesis has a lower motor neuron or myopathic etiology, the localization usually is suspected on clinical grounds by the absence of spasticity and confirmed by EMG and nerve conduction tests.

Quadriparesis or generalized weakness

Generalized weakness may be due to disorders of the CNS or the motor unit. Although the terms *quadriparesis* and *generalized weakness* often are used interchangeably, quadriparesis is commonly used when an upper motor neuron cause is suspected, and generalized weakness when a disease of the motor unit is likely. Weakness from CNS disorders usually is associated with changes in consciousness or cognition, with spasticity and brisk stretch reflexes, and with alterations of sensation. Most neuromuscular causes of generalized weakness are associated with normal mental function, hypotonia, and hypoactive muscle stretch reflexes. The major causes of intermittent weakness are listed in Table 12-2. A patient with generalized fatigability without objective weakness may have the chronic fatigue syndrome (Chap. 52).

TABLE 12-2

CAUSES OF EPISODIC GENERALIZED WEAKNESS

1. Electrolyte disturbances, e.g., hypokalemia, hyperkalemia, hypercalcemia, hypernatremia, hyponatremia, hypophosphatemia, hypermagnesemia
2. Muscle disorders
   a. Channelopathies (periodic paralyses)
   b. Metabolic defects of muscle (impaired carbohydrate or fatty acid utilization; abnormal mitochondrial function)
3. Neuromuscular junction disorders
   a. Myasthenia gravis
   b. Lambert-Eaton myasthenic syndrome
4. Central nervous system disorders
   a. Transient ischemic attacks of the brainstem
   b. Transient global cerebral ischemia
   c. Multiple sclerosis

Acute quadriparesis

Acute quadriparesis with onset over minutes may result from disorders of upper motor neurons (e.g., anoxia, hypotension, brainstem or cervical cord ischemia, trauma, and systemic metabolic abnormalities) or muscle (electrolyte disturbances, certain inborn errors of muscle energy metabolism, toxins, and periodic paralyses). Onset over hours to weeks may, in addition to these disorders, be due to lower motor neuron disorders. Guillain-Barré syndrome (Chap. 46) is the most common lower motor neuron weakness that progresses over days to 4 weeks; the finding of an elevated protein level in the cerebrospinal fluid is helpful but may be absent early in the course.

In obtunded patients, evaluation begins with a CT scan of the brain. If upper motor neuron signs are present but the patient is alert, the initial test is usually an MRI of the cervical cord. If weakness is lower motor neuron, myopathic, or uncertain in origin, the clinical approach begins with blood studies to determine the level of muscle enzymes and electrolytes and an EMG and nerve conduction study.

Subacute or chronic quadriparesis

When quadriparesis due to upper motor neuron disease develops over weeks, months, or years, the distinction between disorders of the cerebral hemispheres, brainstem, and cervical spinal cord is usually possible clinically. An MRI is obtained of the clinically suspected site of pathology. EMG and nerve conduction studies help distinguish lower motor neuron disease (which usually presents with weakness that is most profound distally) from myopathic weakness, which is typically proximal.

Monoparesis

Monoparesis usually is due to lower motor neuron disease, with or without associated sensory involvement. Upper motor neuron weakness occasionally presents as a monoparesis of distal and nonantigravity muscles. Myopathic weakness rarely is limited to one limb.

Acute monoparesis

If the weakness is predominantly in distal and nonantigravity muscles and is not associated with sensory impairment or pain, focal cortical ischemia is likely (Chap. 27); diagnostic possibilities are similar to those for acute hemiparesis. Sensory loss and pain usually accompany acute lower motor neuron weakness; the weakness commonly is localized to a single nerve root or peripheral nerve within the limb but occasionally reflects plexus involvement. If lower motor neuron weakness is suspected or the pattern of weakness is uncertain, the clinical approach begins with an EMG and a nerve conduction study.

Subacute or chronic monoparesis

Weakness and atrophy that develop over weeks or months are usually of lower motor neuron origin. If they are associated with sensory symptoms, a peripheral cause (nerve, root, or plexus) is likely; in the absence of such symptoms, anterior horn cell disease should be considered. In either case, an electrodiagnostic study is indicated. If weakness is of the upper motor neuron type, a discrete cortical (precentral gyrus) or cord lesion may be responsible, and an imaging study of the appropriate site is performed.

Distal weakness

Involvement of two or more limbs distally suggests lower motor neuron or peripheral nerve disease. Acute distal lower limb weakness results occasionally from an acute toxic polyneuropathy or cauda equina syndrome. Distal symmetric weakness usually develops over weeks, months, or years and, when associated with numbness, is due to diseases of peripheral nerves (Chap. 45). Anterior horn cell disease may begin distally but is typically asymmetric and without accompanying numbness (Chap. 32). Rarely, myopathies present with distal weakness (Chap. 48). Electrodiagnostic studies help localize the disorder (Fig. 12-3).

Proximal weakness

Myopathy often produces symmetric weakness of the pelvic or shoulder girdle muscles (Chap. 48). Diseases of the neuromuscular junction (such as myasthenia gravis [Chap. 47]), may present with symmetric proximal weakness often associated with ptosis, diplopia, or bulbar weakness and fluctuating in severity during the day. The extreme fatigability present in some cases of myasthenia gravis may even suggest episodic weakness, but strength rarely returns fully to normal. In anterior horn cell disease, proximal weakness is usually asymmetric, but it may be symmetric if familial. Numbness does not occur with any of these diseases. The evaluation usually begins with determination of the serum creatine kinase level and electrophysiologic studies.

Weakness in a restricted distribution

Weakness may not fit any of these patterns, being limited, for example, to the extraocular, hemifacial, bulbar, or respiratory muscles. If it is unilateral, restricted weakness usually is due to lower motor neuron or peripheral nerve disease, such as in a facial palsy or an isolated superior oblique muscle paresis. Weakness of part of a limb usually is due to a peripheral nerve lesion such as carpal tunnel syndrome or another entrapment neuropathy. Relatively symmetric weakness of extraocular or bulbar muscles usually is due to a myopathy (Chap. 48) or neuromuscular junction disorder (Chap. 47). Bilateral facial palsy with areflexia suggests Guillain-Barré syndrome (Chap. 46). Worsening of relatively symmetric weakness with fatigue is characteristic of neuromuscular junction disorders. Asymmetric bulbar weakness usually is due to motor neuron disease. Weakness limited to respiratory muscles is uncommon and usually is due to motor neuron disease, myasthenia gravis, or polymyositis/dermatomyositis (Chap. 49).

CHAPTER 13

GAIT AND BALANCE DISORDERS

Lewis Sudarsky

PREVALENCE, MORBIDITY, AND MORTALITY

Gait and balance problems are common in the elderly and contribute to the risk of falls and injury. Gait disorders have been described in 15% of individuals older than age 65 years. By age 80 years, one person in four will use a mechanical aid to assist ambulation. Among those 85 and older, the prevalence of gait abnormality approaches 40%. In epidemiologic studies, gait disorders are consistently identified as a major risk factor for falls and injury.

A substantial number of older persons report insecure balance and experience falls and fear of falling. Prospective studies indicate that 30% of those age >65 years fall each year; the proportion is even higher in frail elderly and nursing home patients. Each year, 8% of individuals age >75 years suffer a serious fall-related injury. Hip fractures often result in hospitalization and nursing home admission. For each person who is physically disabled, there are others whose functional independence is constrained by anxiety and fear of falling. Nearly one in five elderly individuals voluntarily limits activity because of fear of falling. With loss of ambulation, there is a diminished quality of life and increased morbidity and mortality rates.

ANATOMY AND PHYSIOLOGY

Upright bipedal gait depends on the successful integration of postural control and locomotion. These functions are widely distributed in the central nervous system. The biomechanics of bipedal walking are complex, and the performance is easily compromised by neurologic deficit at any level. Command and control centers in the brainstem, cerebellum, and forebrain modify the action of spinal pattern generators to promote stepping. While a form of "fictive locomotion" can be elicited from quadrupedal animals after spinal transection, this capacity is limited in primates. Step generation in primates is dependent on locomotor centers in the pontine tegmentum, midbrain, and subthalamic region. Locomotor synergies are executed through the reticular formation and descending pathways in the ventromedial spinal cord. Cerebral control provides a goal and purpose for walking and is involved in avoidance of obstacles and adaptation of locomotor programs to context and terrain.

Postural control requires the maintenance of the center of mass over the base of support through the gait cycle. Unconscious postural adjustments maintain standing balance: long latency responses are measurable in the leg muscles, beginning 110 ms after a perturbation. Forward motion of the center of mass provides propulsive force for stepping, but failure to maintain the center of mass within stability limits results in falls. The anatomic substrate for dynamic balance has not been well defined, but the vestibular nucleus and midline cerebellum contribute to balance control in animals. Human patients with damage to these structures have impaired balance with standing and walking.

Standing balance depends on good-quality sensory information about the position of the body center with respect to the environment, support surface, and gravitational forces. Sensory information for postural control is primarily generated by the visual system, the vestibular system, and by proprioceptive receptors in the muscle spindles and joints. A healthy redundancy of sensory afferent information is generally available, but loss of two of the three pathways is sufficient to compromise standing balance. Balance disorders in older individuals sometimes result from multiple insults in the peripheral sensory systems (e.g., visual loss, vestibular deficit, peripheral neuropathy), critically degrading the quality of afferent information needed for balance stability.

Older patients with cognitive impairment from neurodegenerative diseases appear to be particularly prone to falls and injury. Frailty, muscle weakness, and deconditioning also contribute to the risk. It has been shown that older people who continue walking while talking are at increased risk for falls. There is a growing literature on the use of attentional resources to manage gait and balance. Walking is generally considered to be unconscious and automatic, but the ability to walk while attending a cognitive task (dual-task walking) may be compromised in frail elderly with a history of falls. Older patients with deficits in executive function may have particular difficulty in managing the attentional resources needed for dynamic balance when distracted.

DISORDERS OF GAIT

The heterogeneity of gait disorders observed in clinical practice reflects the large network of neural systems involved in the task. Walking is vulnerable to neurologic disease at every level. Gait disorders have been classified descriptively, based on the abnormal physiology and biomechanics. One problem with this approach is that many failing gaits look fundamentally similar. This overlap reflects common patterns of adaptation to threatened balance stability and declining performance. *The gait disorder observed clinically must be viewed as the product of a neurologic deficit and a functional adaptation.* Unique features of the failing gait are often overwhelmed by the adaptive response. Some of the common patterns of abnormal gait are summarized next. Gait disorders can also be classified by etiology, as listed in **Table 13-1**.

TABLE 13-1

ETIOLOGY OF GAIT DISORDERS

	CASES	PERCENT
Sensory deficits	22	18.3
Myelopathy	20	16.7
Multiple infarcts	18	15.0
Parkinsonism	14	11.7
Cerebellar degeneration	8	6.7
Hydrocephalus	8	6.7
Toxic/metabolic	3	2.5
Psychogenic	4	3.3
Other	6	5.0
Unknown cause	17	14.2
Total	120	100%

Source: Reproduced with permission from J Masdeu et al: *Gait Disorders of Aging: With Special Reference to Falls*. Boston, Little Brown, 1995.

Cautious gait

The term *cautious gait* is used to describe the patient who walks with an abbreviated stride and lowered center of mass, as if walking on a slippery surface. This disorder is both common and nonspecific. It is, in essence, an adaptation to a perceived postural threat. There may be an associated fear of falling. In one study, this disorder was observed in more than one-third of older patients with a higher level gait disturbance. Physical therapy often improves walking to the degree that follow-up observation may reveal a more specific underlying disorder.

Stiff-legged gait

Spastic gait is characterized by stiffness in the legs, an imbalance of muscle tone, and a tendency to circumduct and scuff the feet. The disorder reflects compromise of corticospinal command and overactivity of spinal reflexes. The patient may walk on his or her toes. In extreme instances, the legs cross due to increased tone in the adductors. Upper motor neuron signs are present on physical examination. Shoes often reflect an uneven pattern of wear across the outside. The disorder may be cerebral or spinal in origin.

Myelopathy from cervical spondylosis is a common cause of spastic or spastic-ataxic gait. Demyelinating disease and trauma are the leading causes of myelopathy in younger patients. In a chronic progressive myelopathy of unknown cause, workup with laboratory and imaging tests may establish a diagnosis. A family history should suggest hereditary spastic paraplegia (HSP; Chap. 32). Genetic testing is now available for some of the common HSP mutations. Tropical spastic paraparesis related to the retrovirus HTLV-I is endemic in parts of the Caribbean and South America. A structural lesion, such as tumor or spinal vascular malformation, should be excluded with appropriate testing. Spinal cord disorders are discussed in detail in Chap. 35.

With cerebral spasticity, asymmetry is common, involvement of the upper extremities is usually observed, and dysarthria is often an associated feature. Common causes include vascular disease (stroke), multiple sclerosis, and perinatal injury to the nervous system (cerebral palsy).

Other stiff-legged gaits include dystonia (Chap. 48) and stiff-person syndrome. Dystonia is a disorder characterized by sustained muscle contractions, resulting in repetitive twisting movements and abnormal posture. It often has a genetic basis. Dystonic spasms produce plantar flexion and inversion of the feet, sometimes with torsion of the trunk. In autoimmune stiff-person syndrome (Chap. 44), there is exaggerated lordosis of the lumbar spine and overactivation of antagonist muscles, which restricts trunk and lower limb movement and results in a wooden or fixed posture.

Parkinsonism and freezing gait

Parkinson's disease (Chap. 30) is common, affecting 1% of the population age >55 years. The stooped posture and shuffling gait are characteristic and distinctive features. Patients sometimes accelerate (festinate) with walking or display retropulsion. There may be difficulty with gait initiation (freezing) and a tendency to turn en bloc. Imbalance and falls may develop as the disease progresses over years. Gait freezing is described in 7% of Parkinson's patients within 2 years of onset and 26% by the end of 5 years. Freezing of gait is even more common in some of the Parkinson's-related neurodegenerative disorders, such as progressive supranuclear palsy, multiple-system atrophy, and corticobasal degeneration. These patients frequently present with axial stiffness, postural instability, and a shuffling gait while lacking the characteristic pill-rolling tremor of Parkinson's disease. Falls within the first year suggest the possibility of progressive supranuclear palsy.

Hyperkinetic movement disorders also produce characteristic and recognizable disturbances in gait. In Huntington's disease (Chap. 29), the unpredictable occurrence of choreic movements gives the gait a dancing quality. Tardive dyskinesia is the cause of many odd, stereotypic gait disorders seen in patients chronically exposed to antipsychotics and other drugs that block the D_2 dopamine receptor.

Frontal gait disorder

Frontal gait disorder, sometimes known as "gait apraxia," is common in the elderly and has a variety of causes. The term is used to describe a shuffling, freezing gait with imbalance and other signs of higher cerebral dysfunction. Typical features include a wide base of support, short stride, shuffling along the floor, and difficulty with starts and turns. Many patients exhibit difficulty with gait initiation, descriptively characterized as the "slipping clutch" syndrome. The term *lower body parkinsonism* is also used to describe such patients. Strength is generally preserved, and patients are able to make stepping movements when not standing and maintaining balance at the same time. This disorder is best considered a higher level motor control disorder, as opposed to an apraxia (Chap. 18).

The most common cause of frontal gait disorder is vascular disease, particularly subcortical small-vessel disease. Lesions are frequently found in the deep frontal white matter and centrum ovale. Gait disorder may be the salient feature in hypertensive patients with ischemic lesions of the deep hemisphere white matter (Binswanger's disease). The clinical syndrome includes mental change (variable in degree), dysarthria, pseudobulbar affect (emotional disinhibition), increased tone, and hyperreflexia in the lower limbs.

Communicating hydrocephalus in adults also presents with a gait disorder of this type. Other features of the diagnostic triad (mental change, incontinence) may be absent in the initial stages. MRI demonstrates ventricular enlargement, an enlarged flow void about the aqueduct, and a variable degree of periventricular white matter change. A lumbar puncture or dynamic test is necessary to confirm the presence of hydrocephalus.

Cerebellar gait ataxia

Disorders of the cerebellum have a dramatic impact on gait and balance. Cerebellar gait ataxia is characterized by a wide base of support, lateral instability of the trunk, erratic foot placement, and decompensation of balance when attempting to walk tandem. Difficulty maintaining balance when turning is often an early feature. Patients are unable to walk tandem heel to toe, and display truncal sway in narrow-based or tandem stance. They show considerable variation in their tendency to fall in daily life.

Causes of cerebellar ataxia in older patients include stroke, trauma, tumor, and neurodegenerative disease, including multiple-system atrophy (Chaps. 30 and 33) and various forms of hereditary cerebellar degeneration (Chap. 31). A short expansion at the site of the fragile X mutation (fragile X pre-mutation) has been associated with gait ataxia in older men. Alcoholic cerebellar degeneration can be screened by history and often confirmed by MRI. In patients with ataxia, MRI demonstrates the extent and topography of cerebellar atrophy.

Sensory ataxia

As reviewed earlier, balance depends on high-quality afferent information from the visual and the vestibular systems and proprioception. When this information is lost or degraded, balance during locomotion is impaired and instability results. The sensory ataxia of tabetic neurosyphilis is a classic example. The contemporary equivalent is the patient with neuropathy affecting large fibers. Vitamin B_{12} deficiency is a treatable cause of large-fiber sensory loss in the spinal cord and peripheral nervous system. Joint position and vibration sense are diminished in the lower limbs. The stance in such patients is destabilized by eye closure; they often look down at their feet when walking and do poorly in the dark. Patients have been described with imbalance from bilateral vestibular loss, caused by disease or by exposure to ototoxic drugs. Table 13-2 compares sensory ataxia with cerebellar ataxia and frontal gait disorder. Some frail older patients exhibit a syndrome of imbalance from the combined effect of multiple sensory deficits. Such patients have disturbances in proprioception, vision, and vestibular sense that impair postural support.

TABLE 13-2

FEATURES OF CEREBELLAR ATAXIA, SENSORY ATAXIA, AND FRONTAL GAIT DISORDERS

	CEREBELLAR ATAXIA	SENSORY ATAXIA	FRONTAL GAIT
Base of support	Wide-based	Narrow base, looks down	Wide-based
Velocity	Variable	Slow	Very slow
Stride	Irregular, lurching	Regular with path deviation	Short, shuffling
Romberg	+/−	Unsteady, falls	+/−
Heel → shin	Abnormal	+/−	Normal
Initiation	Normal	Normal	Hesitant
Turns	Unsteady	+/−	Hesitant, multistep
Postural instability	+	+++	++++
			Poor postural synergies getting up from a chair
Falls	Late event	Frequent	Frequent

Neuromuscular disease

Patients with neuromuscular disease often have an abnormal gait, occasionally as a presenting feature. With distal weakness (peripheral neuropathy) the step height is increased to compensate for footdrop, and the sole of the foot may slap on the floor during weight acceptance. Neuropathy may be associated with a degree of sensory imbalance, as described earlier. Patients with myopathy or muscular dystrophy more typically exhibit proximal weakness. Weakness of the hip girdle may result in a degree of excess pelvic sway during locomotion.

Toxic and metabolic disorders

Alcohol intoxication is the most common cause of acute walking difficulty. Chronic toxicity from medications and metabolic disturbances can impair motor function and gait. Mental status changes may be present, and examination may reveal asterixis or myoclonus. Static equilibrium is disturbed, and such patients are easily thrown off balance. Disequilibrium is particularly evident in patients with chronic renal disease and those with hepatic failure, in whom asterixis may impair postural support. Sedative drugs, especially neuroleptics and long-acting benzodiazepines, affect postural control and increase the risk for falls. These disorders are important to recognize because they are often treatable.

Psychogenic gait disorder

Psychogenic disorders are common in neurologic practice, and the presentation often involves gait. Some patients with extreme anxiety or phobia walk with exaggerated caution with abduction of the arms, as if walking on ice. This inappropriately overcautious gait differs in degree from the gait of the patient who is insecure and making adjustments for imbalance. Depressed patients exhibit primarily slowness, a manifestation of psychomotor retardation, and lack of purpose in their stride. Hysterical gait disorders are among the most spectacular encountered. Odd gyrations of posture with wastage of muscular energy (astasia-abasia), extreme slow motion, and dramatic fluctuations over time may be observed in patients with somatoform disorders and conversion reaction.

APPROACH TO THE PATIENT **Slowly Progressive Disorder of Gait**

When reviewing the history, it is helpful to inquire about the onset and progression of disability. Initial awareness of an unsteady gait often follows a fall. Stepwise evolution or sudden progression suggests vascular disease. Gait disorder may be associated with urinary urgency and incontinence, particularly in patients with cervical spine disease or hydrocephalus. It is always important to review the use of alcohol and medications that affect gait and balance. Information on localization derived from the neurologic examination can be helpful to narrow the list of possible diagnoses.

Gait observation provides an immediate sense of the patient's degree of disability. Characteristic patterns of abnormality are sometimes observed, though failing gaits often look fundamentally similar. Cadence (steps/min), velocity, and stride length can be recorded by timing a patient over a fixed distance. Watching the patient get out of a chair provides a good functional assessment of balance.

Brain imaging studies may be informative in patients with an undiagnosed disorder of gait. MRI is sensitive for cerebral lesions of vascular or demyelinating disease and is a good screening test for occult hydrocephalus. Patients with recurrent falls are at risk for subdural hematoma. Many elderly patients with gait and balance difficulty have white matter abnormalities in the periventricular region and centrum semiovale. While these lesions may be an incidental finding, a substantial burden of white matter disease will ultimately impact cerebral control of locomotion.

DISORDERS OF BALANCE

Balance is the ability to maintain equilibrium: a state in which opposing physical forces cancel. In physiology, this is taken to mean the ability to control the center of mass with respect to gravity and the support surface. In reality, we are not consciously aware of what or where our center of mass is, but everyone, including gymnasts, figure skaters, and platform divers, moves so as to manage it. Imbalance implies a disturbance of equilibrium. Disorders of balance present with difficulty maintaining posture standing and walking and with a subjective sense of disequilibrium, a form of dizziness.

The cerebellum and vestibular system organize antigravity responses needed to maintain the upright posture. As reviewed earlier in this chapter, these responses are physiologically complex, and the anatomic representation is not well understood. Failure, resulting in disequilibrium, can occur at several levels: cerebellar, vestibular, somatosensory, and higher level disequilibrium. Patients with hereditary ataxia or alcoholic cerebellar degeneration do not generally complain of dizziness, but balance is visibly impaired. Neurologic examination will reveal a variety of cerebellar signs. Postural compensation may prevent falls early on, but falls inevitably occur with disease progression. The progression of a neurodegenerative ataxia is often measured by the number of years to loss of stable ambulation. Vestibular disorders (Chap. 11) have symptoms and signs in three categories: (1) vertigo, the subjective appreciation or illusion of movement; (2) nystagmus, a vestibulo-oculomotor sign; and (3) poor standing balance, an impairment of vestibulospinal function. Not every patient has all manifestations. Patients with vestibular deficits related to ototoxic drugs may lack vertigo or obvious nystagmus, but balance is impaired on standing and walking, and the patient cannot navigate in the dark. Laboratory testing is available to explore vestibulo-oculomotor and vestibulospinal deficits.

Somatosensory deficits also produce imbalance and falls. There is often a subjective sense of insecure balance and fear of falling. Postural control is compromised by eye closure (Romberg's sign); these patients also have difficulty navigating in the dark. A dramatic example is the patient with autoimmune subacute sensory neuropathy, sometimes a paraneoplastic disorder (Chap. 44). Compensatory strategies enable such patients to walk in the virtual absence of proprioception, but the task requires active visual monitoring. Patients with higher level disorders of equilibrium have difficulty maintaining balance in daily life and may present with falls. There may be reduced awareness of balance impairment. Classic examples include patients with progressive supranuclear palsy and normal pressure hydrocephalus. Patients on sedating medications are also in this category. In prospective studies, cognitive impairment and the use of sedative medications substantially increase the risk for falls.

FALLS

Falls are common in the elderly; 30% of people older than age 65 years living in the community fall each year. Modest changes in balance function have been described in fit older subjects as a result of normal aging. Subtle deficits in sensory systems, attention, and motor reaction time contribute to the risk, and environmental hazards abound. Epidemiologic studies have identified a number of risk factors for falls, summarized in Table 13-3. A fall is not a neurologic problem, nor reason for referral to a specialist, but there are circumstances in which neurologic evaluation is appropriate. In a classic study, 90% of fall events occurred among 10% of individuals, a group known as *recurrent fallers*. Some of these are frail older persons with chronic diseases. Recurrent falls sometimes indicate the presence of serious balance impairment. Syncope, seizure, or falls related to loss of consciousness require appropriate evaluation and treatment (Chaps. 10 and 26).

The descriptive classification of falls is as difficult as the classification of gait disorders, for many of the same reasons. Postural control systems are widely distributed, and a number of disease-related abnormalities occur. Unlike gait problems that are apparent on observation, falls are rarely observed in the office. The patient and family may have limited information about what triggered the fall. Injuries can complicate the physical examination. While there is no standard nosology of falls, common patterns can be identified.

TABLE 13-3

RISK FACTORS FOR FALLS, A META-ANALYSIS: SUMMARY OF SIXTEEN CONTROLLED STUDIES

RISK FACTOR	MEAN RR (OR)	RANGE
Weakness	4.9	1.9–10.3
Balance deficit	3.2	1.6–5.4
Gait disorder	3.0	1.7–4.8
Visual deficit	2.8	1.1–7.4
Mobility limitation	2.5	1.0–5.3
Cognitive impairment	2.4	2.0–4.7
Impaired functional status	2.0	1.0–3.1
Postural hypotension	1.9	1.0–3.4

Abbreviations: OR, odds ratios from retrospective studies; RR, relative risks from prospective studies.

Source: Reproduced with permission from J Masdeu et al: *Gait Disorders of Aging: With Special Reference to Falls*. Boston, Little Brown, 1995.

Slipping, tripping, and "mechanical falls"

Slipping on icy pavement, tripping on obstacles, and falls related to obvious environmental factors are often termed *mechanical falls*. They occasionally occur in healthy individuals with good balance compensation. Frequent tripping falls raise suspicion about an underlying neurologic deficit. Patients with spasticity, leg weakness, or footdrop experience tripping falls.

Weakness and frailty

Patients who lack strength in antigravity muscles have difficulty rising from a chair, fatigue easily when walking, and have difficulty maintaining their balance after a perturbation. These patients are often unable to get up after a fall and may be on the floor for an hour or more before help arrives. Deconditioning of this sort is often treatable. Resistance strength training can increase muscle mass and leg strength in people in their eighties and nineties.

Drop attacks and collapsing falls

Drop attacks are sudden collapsing falls without loss of consciousness. Patients who collapse from lack of postural tone present a diagnostic challenge. The patient may report that his or her legs just gave out underneath; the family may describe the patient as "collapsing in a heap." Orthostatic hypotension may be a factor in some such falls. Asterixis or epilepsy may impair postural support. A colloid cyst of the third ventricle can present with intermittent obstruction of the foramen of Monroe, resulting in a drop attack. While collapsing falls are more common in older patients with vascular risk factors, they should not be confused with vertebrobasilar ischemic attacks.

Toppling falls

Some patients maintain tone in antigravity muscles but fall over like a tree trunk, as if postural defenses had disengaged. There may be a consistent direction to such falls. The patient with cerebellar pathology may lean and topple over toward the side of the lesion. Patients with lesions of the vestibular system or its central pathways may experience lateral pulsion and toppling falls. Patients with progressive supranuclear palsy often fall over backward. Falls of this nature occur in patients with advanced Parkinson's disease once postural instability has developed.

Gait freezing

Another fall pattern in Parkinson's disease and related disorders is the fall due to freezing of gait. The feet stick to the floor and the center of mass keeps moving, resulting in a disequilibrium from which the patient has difficulty recovering. This sequence of events can result in a forward fall. Gait freezing can also occur as the patient attempts to turn and change direction. Similarly, the patient with Parkinson's disease and festinating gait may find his feet unable to keep up, resulting in a forward fall.

Falls related to sensory deficit

Patients with somatosensory, visual, or vestibular deficits are prone to falls. These patients have particular difficulty dealing with poor illumination or walking on uneven ground. These patients often express subjective imbalance, apprehension, and fear of falling. Deficits in joint position and vibration sense are apparent on physical examination.

TREATMENT **Interventions to Reduce the Risk of Falls and Injury**

Efforts should be made to define the etiology of the gait disorder and mechanism of the falls. Standing blood pressure should be recorded. Specific treatment may be possible, once a diagnosis is established. Therapeutic intervention is often recommended for older patients at substantial risk for falls, even if no neurologic disease is identified. A home visit to look for environmental hazards can be helpful. A variety of modifications may be recommended to improve safety, including improved lighting and the installation of grab bars and nonslip surfaces.

Rehabilitation interventions attempt to improve muscle strength and balance stability and to make the patient more resistant to injury. High-intensity resistance strength training with weights and machines is useful to improve muscle mass, even in frail older patients. Improvements are realized in posture and gait, which should translate to reduced risk of falls and injury. Sensory balance training is another approach to improve balance stability. Measurable gains can be achieved in a few weeks of training, and benefits can be maintained over 6 months by a 10- to 20-min home exercise program. This strategy is particularly successful in patients with vestibular and somatosensory balance disorders. The Yale Health and Aging study used a strategy of targeted, multiple risk factor abatement to reduce falls in the elderly. Prescription medications were adjusted, and home-based exercise programs were tailored to the patients' needs, based on an initial geriatric assessment. The program realized a 44% reduction in falls, compared with a control group of patients who had periodic social visits.

CHAPTER 14

VIDEO LIBRARY OF GAIT DISORDERS

Gail Kang ■ Nicholas B. Galifianakis ■ Michael Geschwind

Problems with gait and balance are major causes of falls, accidents, and resulting disability, especially in later life, and are often harbingers of neurologic disease. Early diagnosis is essential, especially for treatable conditions, as it may permit the institution of prophylactic measures to prevent dangerous falls, and also to reverse or ameliorate the underlying cause. In this video, examples of gait disorders due to Parkinson's disease, other extrapyramidal disorders, and ataxias, as well as other common gait disorders, are presented. Videos for this chapter can be accessed at the following link: http://www.mhprofessional.com/mediacenter/.

CHAPTER 15

NUMBNESS, TINGLING, AND SENSORY LOSS

Michael J. Aminoff ■ Arthur K. Asbury

Normal somatic sensation reflects a continuous monitoring process, little of which reaches consciousness under ordinary conditions. By contrast, disordered sensation, particularly when experienced as painful, is alarming and dominates the patient's attention. Physicians should be able to recognize abnormal sensations by how they are described, know their type and likely site of origin, and understand their implications. Pain is considered separately in Chap. 7.

POSITIVE AND NEGATIVE SYMPTOMS

Abnormal sensory symptoms can be divided into two categories: positive and negative. The prototypical positive symptom is tingling (pins and needles); other positive sensory phenomena include altered sensations that are described as pricking, bandlike, lightning-like shooting feelings (lancinations), aching, knifelike, twisting, drawing, pulling, tightening, burning, searing, electrical, or raw feelings. Such symptoms are often painful.

Positive phenomena usually result from trains of impulses generated at sites of lowered threshold or heightened excitability along a peripheral or central sensory pathway. The nature and severity of the abnormal sensation depend on the number, rate, timing, and distribution of ectopic impulses and the type and function of nervous tissue in which they arise. Because positive phenomena represent excessive activity in sensory pathways, they are not necessarily associated with a sensory deficit (loss) on examination.

Negative phenomena represent loss of sensory function and are characterized by diminished or absent feeling that often is experienced as numbness and by abnormal findings on sensory examination. In disorders affecting peripheral sensation, it is estimated that at least one-half the afferent axons innervating a particular site are lost or functionless before a sensory deficit can be demonstrated by clinical examination. This threshold varies in accordance with how rapidly function is lost in sensory nerve fibers. If the rate of loss is slow, lack of cutaneous feeling may be unnoticed by the patient and difficult to demonstrate on examination, even though few sensory fibers are functioning; if it is rapid, both positive and negative phenomena are usually conspicuous. Subclinical degrees of sensory dysfunction may be revealed by sensory nerve conduction studies or somatosensory evoked potentials (Chap. 5).

Whereas sensory symptoms may be either positive or negative, sensory signs on examination are always a measure of negative phenomena.

TERMINOLOGY

Words used to characterize sensory disturbance are descriptive and based on convention. Paresthesias and dysesthesias are general terms used to denote positive sensory symptoms. The term *paresthesias* typically refers to tingling or pins-and-needles sensations but may include a wide variety of other abnormal sensations, except pain; it sometimes implies that the abnormal sensations are perceived spontaneously. The more general term *dysesthesias* denotes all types of abnormal sensations, including painful ones, regardless of whether a stimulus is evident.

Another set of terms refers to sensory abnormalities found on examination. *Hypesthesia* or *hypoesthesia* refers to a reduction of cutaneous sensation to a specific type of testing such as pressure, light touch, and warm or cold stimuli; *anesthesia,* to a complete absence of skin sensation to the same stimuli plus pinprick; and *hypalgesia* or *analgesia,* to reduced or absent pain perception (nociception), such as perception of the pricking quality elicited by a pin. *Hyperesthesia* means pain or increased sensitivity in response to touch. Similarly, *allodynia* describes the situation in which a nonpainful stimulus, once perceived, is experienced as painful, even excruciating. An example is elicitation of a painful sensation by application of a vibrating tuning fork. *Hyperalgesia* denotes severe pain in response to a mildly noxious stimulus, and *hyperpathia*, a broad term, encompasses all the phenomena described by hyperesthesia, allodynia, and hyperalgesia. With hyperpathia, the threshold for a sensory stimulus is increased and perception is delayed, but once felt, it is unduly painful.

Disorders of deep sensation arising from muscle spindles, tendons, and joints affect proprioception (position sense). Manifestations include imbalance (particularly with eyes closed or in the dark), clumsiness of precision movements, and unsteadiness of gait, which are referred to collectively as *sensory ataxia*. Other findings on examination usually, but not invariably, include reduced or absent joint position and vibratory sensibility and absent deep tendon reflexes in the affected limbs. The Romberg sign is positive, which means that the patient sways markedly or topples when asked to stand with feet close together and eyes closed. In severe states of deafferentation involving deep sensation, the patient cannot walk or stand unaided or even sit unsupported. Continuous involuntary movements (*pseudoathetosis*) of the outstretched hands and fingers occur, particularly with eyes closed.

ANATOMY OF SENSATION

Cutaneous afferent innervation is conveyed by a rich variety of receptors, both naked nerve endings (nociceptors and thermoreceptors) and encapsulated terminals (mechanoreceptors). Each type of receptor has its own set of sensitivities to specific stimuli, size and distinctness of receptive fields, and adaptational qualities. Much of the knowledge about these receptors has come from the development of techniques to study single intact nerve fibers intraneurally in awake, unanesthetized human subjects. It is possible not only to record from but also to stimulate single fibers in isolation. A single impulse, whether elicited by a natural stimulus or evoked by electrical microstimulation in a large myelinated afferent fiber, may be both perceived and localized.

Afferent fibers of all sizes in peripheral nerve trunks traverse the dorsal roots and enter the dorsal horn of the spinal cord (Fig. 15-1). From there the smaller fibers take a route to the parietal cortex different from that of the larger fibers. The polysynaptic projections of the smaller fibers (unmyelinated and small myelinated), which subserve mainly nociception, temperature sensibility, and touch, cross and ascend in the opposite anterior and lateral columns of the spinal cord, through the brainstem, to the ventral posterolateral (VPL) nucleus of the thalamus and ultimately project to the postcentral gyrus of the parietal cortex (Chap. 7). This is the *spinothalamic pathway* or *anterolateral system*. The larger fibers, which subserve tactile and position sense and kinesthesia, project rostrally in the posterior column on the same side of the spinal cord and make their first synapse in the gracile or cuneate nucleus of the lower medulla. Axons of second-order neurons decussate and ascend in the medial lemniscus located medially in the medulla and in the tegmentum of the pons and midbrain and synapse in the VPL nucleus; third-order neurons project to parietal cortex. This large-fiber system is referred to as the *posterior column–medial lemniscal pathway* (lemniscal, for short). Note that although the lemniscal and the anterolateral pathways both project up the spinal cord to the thalamus, it is the (crossed) anterolateral pathway that is referred to as the *spinothalamic tract* by convention.

Although the fiber types and functions that make up the spinothalamic and lemniscal systems are relatively well known, many other fibers, particularly those associated with touch, pressure, and position sense, ascend in a diffusely distributed pattern both ipsilaterally and contralaterally in the anterolateral quadrants of the spinal cord. This explains why a complete lesion of the posterior columns of the spinal cord may be associated with little sensory deficit on examination.

EXAMINATION OF SENSATION

The main components of the sensory examination are tests of primary sensation (pain, touch, vibration, joint position, and thermal sensation [Table 15-1]).

Some general principles pertain. The examiner must depend on patient responses, particularly when testing cutaneous sensation (pin, touch, warm, or cold), and this complicates interpretation. Further, examination may be limited in some patients. In a stuporous patient, for example, sensory examination is reduced to observing the briskness of withdrawal in response to a pinch or another noxious stimulus. Comparison of response on one side of the body to that on the other is essential. In an alert but uncooperative patient, it may not be possible to examine cutaneous sensation, but some idea of proprioceptive function may be gained by noting the patient's best performance of movements requiring balance and precision. Frequently, patients present with sensory symptoms that do not fit an anatomic localization and that are accompanied by either no abnormalities or gross inconsistencies on examination. The examiner should consider whether the sensory symptoms are a disguised request for help with psychological or situational problems. Discretion must be used in pursuing this possibility. Finally, sensory examination of a patient who has no neurologic complaints can be brief and consist of pinprick, touch, and vibration testing in the hands and feet plus evaluation of stance and gait, including the Romberg maneuver. Evaluation of stance and gait also tests the integrity of motor and cerebellar systems.

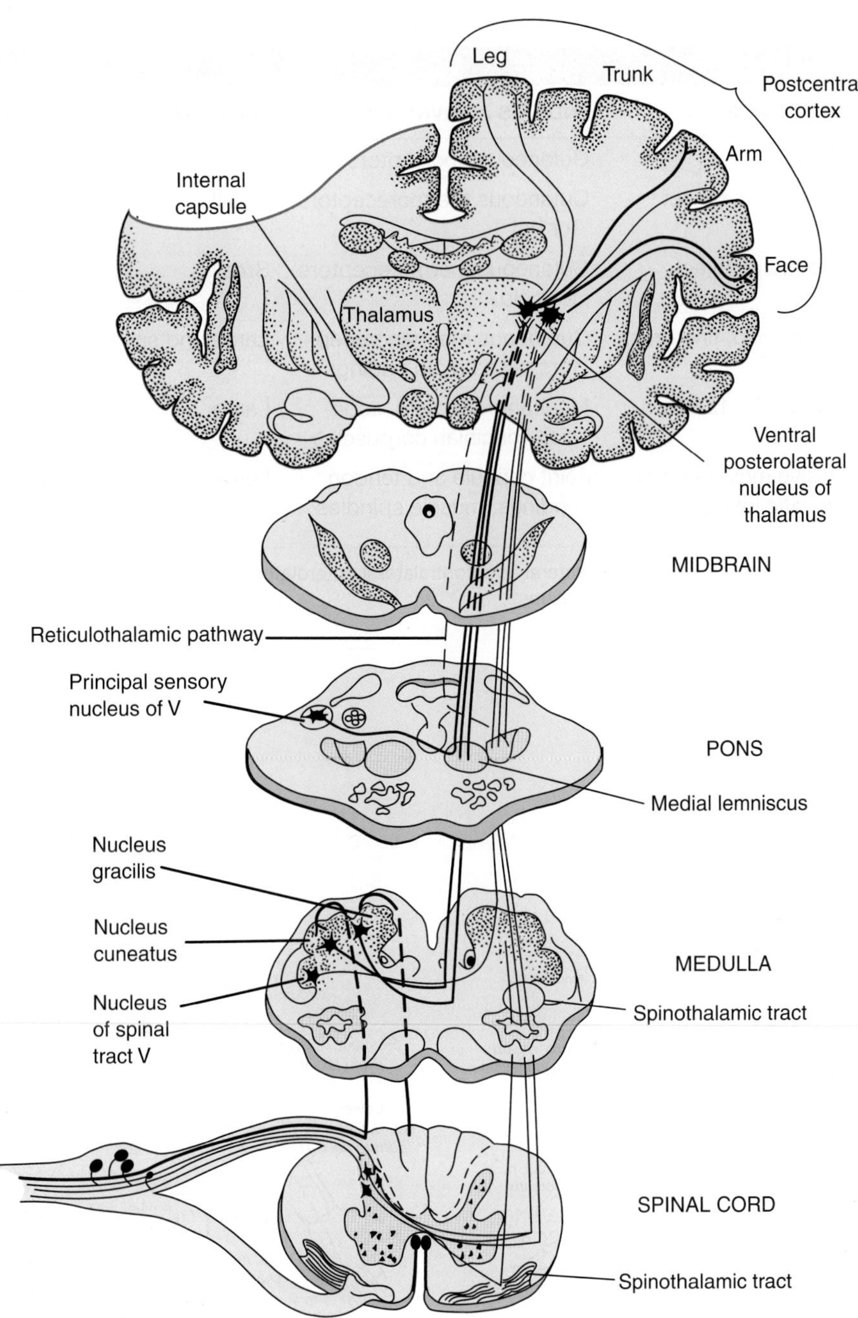

FIGURE 15-1

The main somatosensory pathways. The spinothalamic tract (pain, thermal sense) and the posterior column–lemniscal system (touch, pressure, joint position) are shown. Offshoots from the ascending anterolateral fasciculus (spinothalamic tract) to nuclei in the medulla, pons, and mesencephalon and nuclear terminations of the tract are indicated. (*From AH Ropper, RH Brown, in Adams and Victor's Principles of Neurology, 9th ed. New York, McGraw-Hill, 2009.*)

Primary sensation

(See Table 15-1) The sense of pain usually is tested with a clean pin, with the patient asked to focus on the pricking or unpleasant quality of the stimulus, not just the pressure or touch sensation elicited. Areas of hypalgesia should be mapped by proceeding radially from the most hypalgesic site (Figs. 15-2, 15-3 and 15-4).

Temperature sensation to both hot and cold is best tested with small containers filled with water of the desired temperature. This is impractical in most settings. An alternative way to test cold sensation is to touch a metal object, such as a tuning fork at room temperature, to the skin. For testing warm temperatures, the tuning fork or another metal object may be held under warm water of the desired temperature and then used. The

TABLE 15-1

TESTING PRIMARY SENSATION

SENSE	TEST DEVICE	ENDINGS ACTIVATED	FIBER SIZE MEDIATING	CENTRAL PATHWAY
Pain	Pinprick	Cutaneous nociceptors	Small	SpTh, also D
Temperature, heat	Warm metal object	Cutaneous thermoreceptors for hot	Small	SpTh
Temperature, cold	Cold metal object	Cutaneous thermoreceptors for cold	Small	SpTh
Touch	Cotton wisp, fine brush	Cutaneous mechanoreceptors, also naked endings	Large and small	Lem, also D and SpTh
Vibration	Tuning fork, 128 Hz	Mechanoreceptors, especially pacinian corpuscles	Large	Lem, also D
Joint position	Passive movement of specific joints	Joint capsule and tendon endings, muscle spindles	Large	Lem, also D

Abbreviations: D, diffuse ascending projections in ipsilateral and contralateral anterolateral columns; SpTh, spinothalamic projection, contralateral; Lem, posterior column and lemniscal projection, ipsilateral.

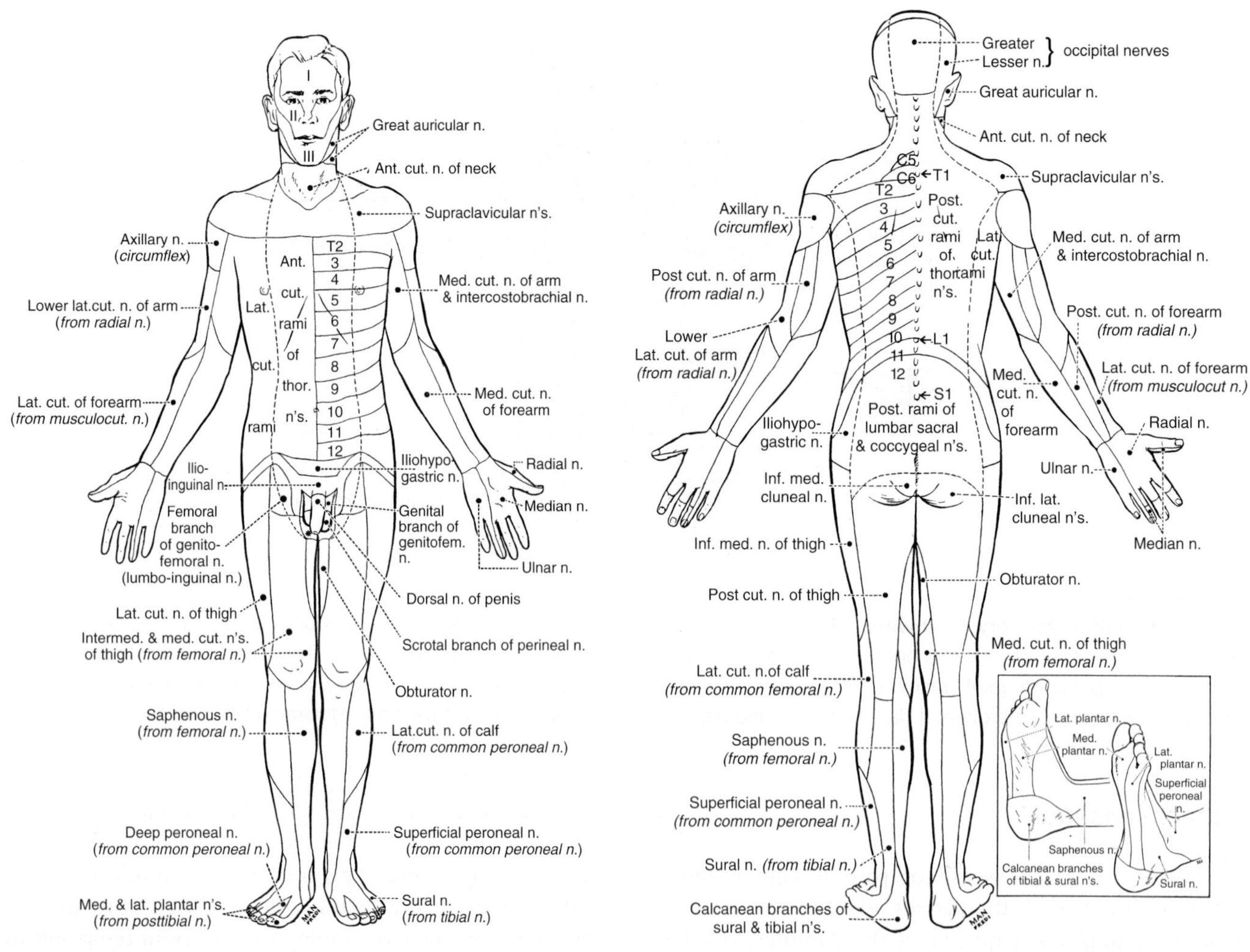

FIGURE 15-2

The cutaneous fields of peripheral nerves. (*Reproduced by permission from W Haymaker, B Woodhall: Peripheral Nerve Injuries, 2nd ed. Philadelphia, Saunders, 1953.*)

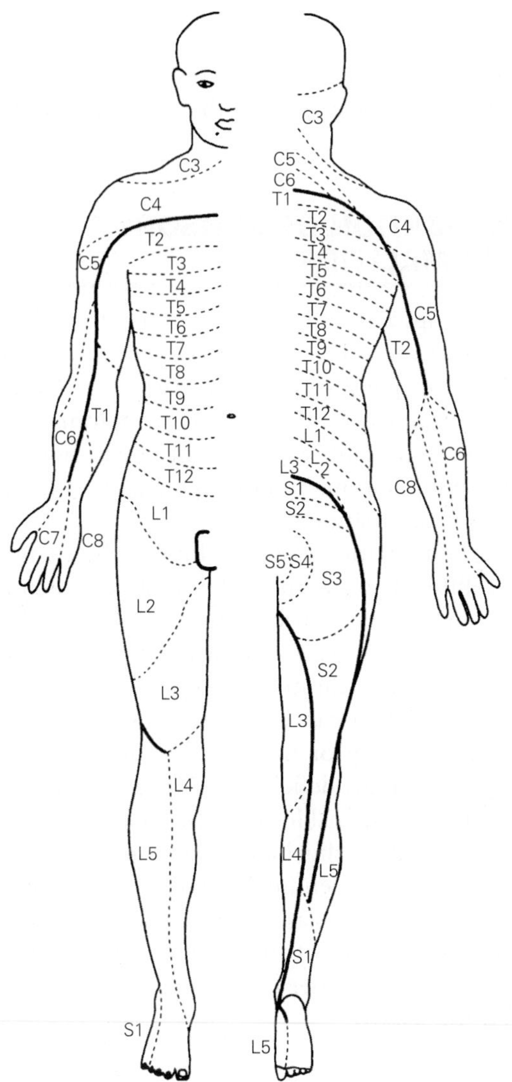

FIGURE 15-3
Distribution of the sensory spinal roots on the surface of the body (dermatomes). *(From D Sinclair: Mechanisms of Cutaneous Sensation. Oxford, UK, Oxford University Press, 1981; with permission from Dr. David Sinclair.)*

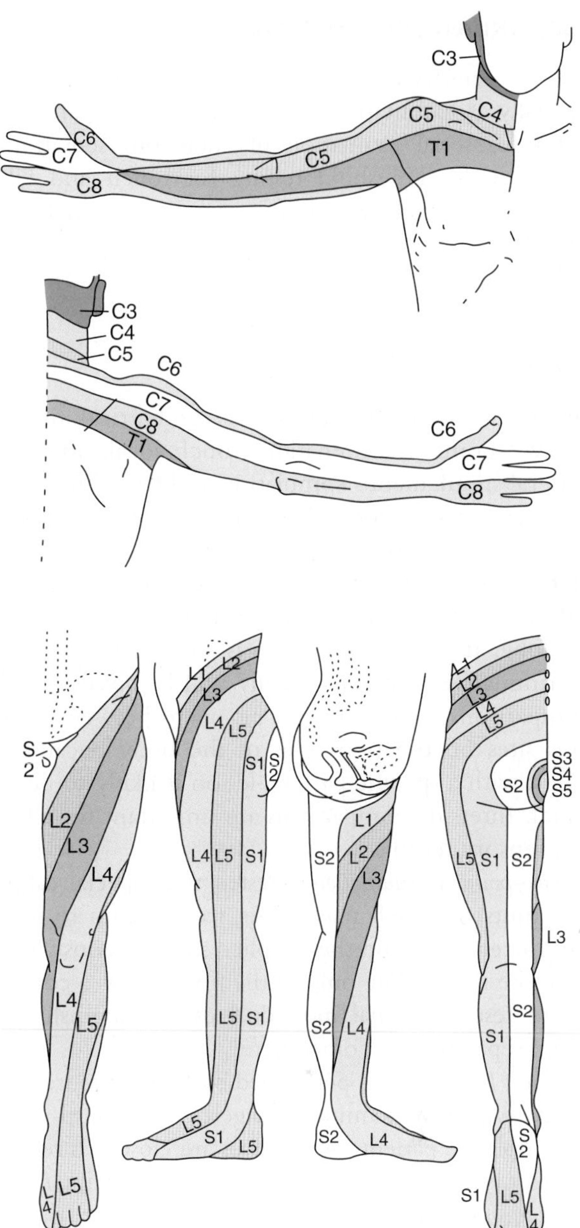

FIGURE 15-4
Dermatomes of the upper and lower extremities, outlined by the pattern of sensory loss following lesions of single nerve roots. *(From JJ Keegan, FD Garrett: Anat Rec 102:409, 1948.)*

appreciation of both cold and warmth should be tested because different receptors respond to each.

Touch usually is tested with a wisp of cotton or a fine camel hair brush. In general, it is better to avoid testing touch on hairy skin because of the profusion of the sensory endings that surround each hair follicle.

Joint position testing is a measure of proprioception, one of the most important functions of the sensory system. With the patient's eyes closed, joint position is tested in the distal interphalangeal joint of the great toe and fingers. If errors are made in recognizing the direction of passive movements, more proximal joints are tested. A test of proximal joint position sense, primarily at the shoulder, is performed by asking the patient to bring the two index fingers together with arms extended and eyes closed. Normal individuals can do this accurately, with errors of 1 cm or less.

The sense of vibration is tested with a tuning fork that vibrates at 128 Hz. Vibration usually is tested over bony points, beginning distally; in the feet it is tested over the dorsal surface of the distal phalanx of the big toes and at the malleoli of the ankles, and in the hands dorsally at the distal phalanx of the fingers. If abnormalities are found, more proximal sites can be examined. Vibratory thresholds at the same site in the patient and the examiner may be compared for control purposes.

Quantitative sensory testing

Effective sensory testing devices are now available commercially. Quantitative sensory testing is particularly useful for serial evaluation of cutaneous sensation in clinical trials. Threshold testing for touch and vibratory and thermal sensation is the most widely used application.

Cortical sensation

The most commonly used tests of cortical function are two-point discrimination, touch localization, and bilateral simultaneous stimulation and tests for graphesthesia and stereognosis. Abnormalities of these sensory tests, in the presence of normal primary sensation in an alert cooperative patient, signify a lesion of the parietal cortex or thalamocortical projections to the parietal lobe. If primary sensation is altered, these cortical discriminative functions usually will be abnormal also. Comparisons should always be made between analogous sites on the two sides of the body because the deficit with a specific parietal lesion is likely to be unilateral. Interside comparisons are important for all cortical sensory testing.

Two-point discrimination is tested with special calipers, the points of which may be set from 2 mm to several centimeters apart and then applied simultaneously to the site to be tested. The pulp of the fingertips is a common site to test; a normal individual can distinguish about 3-mm separation of points there.

Touch localization is performed by light pressure for an instant with the examiner's fingertip or a wisp of cotton wool; the patient, whose eyes are closed, is required to identify the site of touch with the fingertip. *Bilateral simultaneous stimulation* at analogous sites (e.g., the dorsum of both hands) can be carried out to determine whether the perception of touch is extinguished consistently on one side or the other. The phenomenon is referred to as *extinction or neglect*. *Graphesthesia* refers to the capacity to recognize with eyes closed letters or numbers drawn by the examiner's fingertip on the palm of the hand. Once again, interside comparison is of prime importance. Inability to recognize numbers or letters is termed *agraphesthesia*.

Stereognosis refers to the ability to identify common objects by palpation, recognizing their shape, texture, and size. Common standard objects such as keys, paper clips, and coins are best used. Patients with normal stereognosis should be able to distinguish a dime from a penny and a nickel from a quarter without looking. Patients should be allowed to feel the object with only one hand at a time. If they are unable to identify it in one hand, it should be placed in the other for comparison. Individuals who are unable to identify common objects and coins in one hand but can do so in the other are said to have *astereognosis* of the abnormal hand.

LOCALIZATION OF SENSORY ABNORMALITIES

Sensory symptoms and signs can result from lesions at almost any level of the nervous system from the parietal cortex to the peripheral sensory receptor. Noting the distribution and nature of sensory symptoms and signs is the most important way to localize their source. Their extent, configuration, symmetry, quality, and severity are the key observations.

Dysesthesias without sensory findings by examination may be difficult to interpret. To illustrate, tingling dysesthesias in an acral distribution (hands and feet) can be systemic in origin, e.g., secondary to hyperventilation, or induced by a medication such as acetazolamide. Distal dysesthesias also can be an early event in an evolving polyneuropathy or may herald a myelopathy, such as from vitamin B_{12} deficiency. Sometimes distal dysesthesias have no definable basis. In contrast, dysesthesias that correspond in distribution to a particular peripheral nerve territory denote a lesion of that nerve trunk. For instance, dysesthesias restricted to the fifth digit and the adjacent one-half of the fourth finger on one hand reliably point to disorder of the ulnar nerve, most commonly at the elbow.

Nerve and root

In focal nerve trunk lesions severe enough to cause a deficit, sensory abnormalities are readily mapped and generally have discrete boundaries (Figs. 15-2, 15-3 and 15-4). Root ("radicular") lesions frequently are accompanied by deep, aching pain along the course of the related nerve trunk. With compression of a fifth lumbar (L5) or first sacral (S1) root, as from a ruptured intervertebral disk, sciatica (radicular pain relating to the sciatic nerve trunk) is a common manifestation (Chap. 9). With a lesion affecting a single root, sensory deficits may be minimal or absent because adjacent root territories overlap extensively.

Isolated mononeuropathies may cause symptoms beyond the territory supplied by the affected nerve, but abnormalities on examination typically are confined to appropriate anatomic boundaries. In multiple mononeuropathies, symptoms and signs occur in discrete territories supplied by different individual nerves and—as more nerves are affected—may simulate a polyneuropathy if deficits become confluent. With polyneuropathies, sensory deficits are generally graded, distal, and symmetric in distribution (Chap. 45). Dysesthesias, followed by numbness, begin in the toes and ascend symmetrically. When dysesthesias reach the knees, they usually also have appeared in the fingertips. The process appears to be nerve length–dependent, and the deficit is often described as "stocking-glove" in type. Involvement of both hands and feet also occurs with lesions of the upper cervical cord or the brainstem, but an upper level of the sensory disturbance may then be found on the trunk and other evidence of a central lesion may be present, such as sphincter involvement or signs of an upper motor neuron lesion (Chap. 12). Although most polyneuropathies are pansensory and affect all modalities of sensation, selective sensory dysfunction according to nerve fiber size may occur. Small-fiber polyneuropathies are characterized by burning, painful dysesthesias with reduced pinprick and thermal sensation but with sparing of proprioception, motor function, and deep tendon reflexes. Touch is involved variably; when it is spared, the sensory pattern is referred to as exhibiting *sensory dissociation*. Sensory dissociation may occur with spinal cord lesions as well as small-fiber neuropathies. Large-fiber polyneuropathies are characterized by vibration and position sense deficits, imbalance, absent tendon reflexes, and variable motor dysfunction but preservation of most cutaneous sensation. Dysesthesias, if present at all, tend to be tingling or bandlike in quality.

Sensory neuronopathy is characterized by widespread but asymmetric sensory loss occurring in a non-length-dependent manner so that it may occur proximally or distally and in the arms, legs, or both. Pain and numbness progress to sensory ataxia and impairment of all sensory modalities with time. This condition is usually paraneoplastic or idiopathic in origin (Chaps. 44 and 45).

Spinal cord

(See also Chap. 35) If the spinal cord is transected, all sensation is lost below the level of transection. Bladder and bowel function also are lost, as is motor function. Hemisection of the spinal cord produces the Brown-Séquard syndrome, with absent pain and temperature sensation contralaterally and loss of proprioceptive sensation and power ipsilaterally below the lesion (see Figs. 15-1 and 35-1).

Numbness or paresthesias in both feet may arise from a spinal cord lesion; this is especially likely when the upper level of the sensory loss extends to the trunk. When all extremities are affected, the lesion is probably in the cervical region or brainstem unless a peripheral neuropathy is responsible. The presence of upper motor neuron signs (Chap. 12) supports a central lesion; a hyperesthetic band on the trunk may suggest the level of involvement.

A dissociated sensory loss can reflect spinothalamic tract involvement in the spinal cord, especially if the deficit is unilateral and has an upper level on the torso. Bilateral spinothalamic tract involvement occurs with lesions affecting the center of the spinal cord, such as in syringomyelia. There is a dissociated sensory loss with impairment of pinprick and temperature appreciation but relative preservation of light touch, position sense, and vibration appreciation.

Dysfunction of the posterior columns in the spinal cord or of the posterior root entry zone may lead to a bandlike sensation around the trunk or a feeling of tight pressure in one or more limbs. Flexion of the neck sometimes leads to an electric shock–like sensation that radiates down the back and into the legs (Lhermitte's sign) in patients with a cervical lesion affecting the posterior columns, such as from multiple sclerosis, cervical spondylosis, or recent irradiation to the cervical region.

Brainstem

Crossed patterns of sensory disturbance, in which one side of the face and the opposite side of the body are affected, localize to the lateral medulla. Here a small lesion may damage both the ipsilateral descending trigeminal tract and the ascending spinothalamic fibers subserving the opposite arm, leg, and hemitorso (see "Lateral medullary syndrome" in Fig. 27-10). A lesion in the tegmentum of the pons and midbrain, where the lemniscal and spinothalamic tracts merge, causes pansensory loss contralaterally.

Thalamus

Hemisensory disturbance with tingling numbness from head to foot is often thalamic in origin but also can arise from the anterior parietal region. If abrupt in onset, the lesion is likely to be due to a small stroke (lacunar infarction), particularly if localized to the thalamus. Occasionally, with lesions affecting the VPL nucleus or adjacent white matter, a syndrome of thalamic pain, also called *Déjerine-Roussy syndrome*, may ensue. The persistent, unrelenting unilateral pain often is described in dramatic terms.

Cortex

With lesions of the parietal lobe involving either the cortex or the subjacent white matter, the most prominent symptoms are contralateral hemineglect, hemi-inattention, and a tendency not to use the affected hand and arm. On cortical sensory testing (e.g., two-point discrimination, graphesthesia), abnormalities are often found but primary sensation is usually intact. Anterior parietal infarction may present as a pseudothalamic syndrome with contralateral loss of primary sensation from head to toe. Dysesthesias or a sense of numbness may also occur and, rarely, a painful state.

Focal sensory seizures

These seizures generally are due to lesions in the area of the postcentral or precentral gyrus. The principal symptom of focal sensory seizures is tingling, but additional, more complex sensations may occur, such as a rushing feeling, a sense of warmth, or a sense of movement without detectable motion. Symptoms typically are unilateral; commonly begin in the arm or hand, face, or foot; and often spread in a manner that reflects the cortical representation of different bodily parts, as in a Jacksonian march. Duration of seizures is variable; seizures may be transient, lasting only for seconds, or persist for an hour or more. Focal motor features may supervene, often becoming generalized with loss of consciousness and tonic-clonic jerking.

CHAPTER 16

CONFUSION AND DELIRIUM

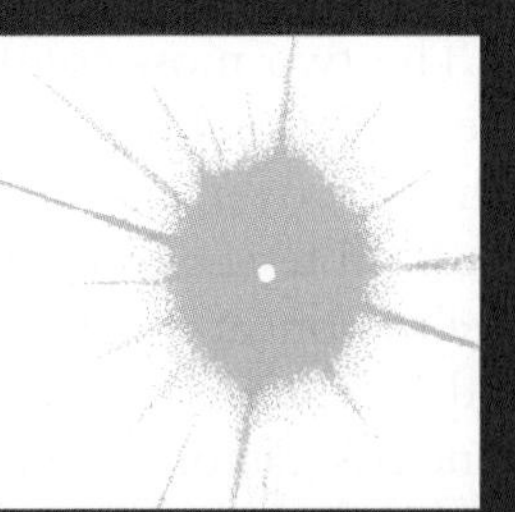

S. Andrew Josephson ■ Bruce L. Miller

Confusion, a mental and behavioral state of reduced comprehension, coherence, and capacity to reason, is one of the most common problems encountered in medicine, accounting for a large number of emergency department visits, hospital admissions, and inpatient consultations. *Delirium*, a term used to describe an acute confusional state, remains a major cause of morbidity and mortality rates, costing billions of dollars yearly in health care costs in the United States alone. Delirium often goes unrecognized despite clear evidence that it is usually the cognitive manifestation of serious underlying medical or neurologic illness.

CLINICAL FEATURES OF DELIRIUM

A multitude of terms are used to describe delirium, including *encephalopathy, acute brain failure, acute confusional state,* and *postoperative or intensive care unit (ICU) psychosis*. Delirium has many clinical manifestations, but essentially it is defined as a relatively acute decline in cognition that fluctuates over hours or days. The hallmark of delirium is a deficit of attention, although all cognitive domains—including memory, executive function, visuospatial tasks, and language—are variably involved. Associated symptoms may include altered sleep-wake cycles, perceptual disturbances such as hallucinations or delusions, affect changes, and autonomic findings that include heart rate and blood pressure instability.

Delirium is a clinical diagnosis that can be made only at the bedside. Two broad clinical categories have been described—the hyperactive and hypoactive subtypes—that are based on differential psychomotor features. The cognitive syndrome associated with severe alcohol withdrawal remains the classic example of the hyperactive subtype, featuring prominent hallucinations, agitation, and hyperarousal, often accompanied by life-threatening autonomic instability. In striking contrast is the hypoactive subtype, exemplified by opiate intoxication, in which patients are withdrawn and quiet, with prominent apathy and psychomotor slowing.

This dichotomy between subtypes of delirium is a useful construct, but patients often fall somewhere along a spectrum between the hyperactive and hypoactive extremes, sometimes fluctuating from one to the other within minutes. Therefore, clinicians must recognize the broad range of presentations of delirium to identify all patients with this potentially reversible cognitive disturbance. Hyperactive patients, such as those with delirium tremens, are easily recognized by their characteristic severe agitation, tremor, hallucinations, and autonomic instability. Patients who are quietly disturbed are overlooked more often on the medical wards and in the ICU, yet multiple studies suggest that this underrecognized hypoactive subtype is associated with worse outcomes.

The reversibility of delirium is emphasized because many etiologies, such as systemic infection and medication effects, can be treated easily. However, the long-term cognitive effects of delirium remain largely unknown and understudied. Some episodes of delirium continue for weeks, months, or even years. The persistence of delirium in some patients and its high recurrence rate may be due to inadequate treatment of the underlying etiology of the syndrome. In some instances, delirium does not disappear because there is underlying permanent neuronal damage. Even after an episode of delirium resolves, there may be lingering effects of the disorder. A patient's recall of events after delirium varies widely, ranging from complete amnesia to repeated reexperiencing of the frightening period of confusion in a disturbing manner, similar to what is seen in patients with posttraumatic stress disorder.

RISK FACTORS

An effective primary prevention strategy for delirium begins with identification of patients at highest risk, including those preparing for elective surgery or being admitted to the hospital. Although no single validated scoring system has been widely accepted as a screen for asymptomatic patients, there are multiple well-established risk factors for delirium.

The two most consistently identified risks are older age and baseline cognitive dysfunction. Individuals who are over age 65 or exhibit low scores on standardized tests of cognition develop delirium upon hospitalization at a rate approaching 50%. Whether age and baseline cognitive dysfunction are truly independent risk factors is uncertain. Other predisposing factors include sensory deprivation, such as preexisting hearing and visual impairment, as well as indices for poor overall health, including baseline immobility, malnutrition, and underlying medical or neurologic illness.

In-hospital risks for delirium include the use of bladder catheterization, physical restraints, sleep and sensory deprivation, and the addition of three or more new medications. Avoiding such risks remains a key component of delirium prevention as well as treatment. Surgical and anesthetic risk factors for the development of postoperative delirium include specific procedures such as those involving cardiopulmonary bypass and inadequate or excessive treatment of pain in the immediate postoperative period.

The relationship between delirium and dementia (Chap. 29) is complicated by significant overlap between the two conditions, and it is not always simple to distinguish between them. Dementia and preexisting cognitive dysfunction serve as major risk factors for delirium, and at least two-thirds of cases of delirium occur in patients with coexisting underlying dementia. A form of dementia with parkinsonism, termed *dementia with Lewy bodies*, is characterized by a fluctuating course, prominent visual hallucinations, parkinsonism, and an attentional deficit that clinically resembles hyperactive delirium. Delirium in the elderly often reflects an insult to the brain that is vulnerable due to an underlying neurodegenerative condition. Therefore, the development of delirium sometimes heralds the onset of a previously unrecognized brain disorder.

EPIDEMIOLOGY

Delirium is a common disease, but its reported incidence has varied widely with the criteria used to define the disorder. Estimates of delirium in hospitalized patients range from 14 to 56%, with higher rates reported for elderly patients and patients undergoing hip surgery. Older patients in the ICU have especially high rates of delirium that range from 70 to 87%. The condition is not recognized in up to one-third of delirious inpatients, and the diagnosis is especially problematic in the ICU environment, where cognitive dysfunction is often difficult to appreciate in the setting of serious systemic illness and sedation. Delirium in the ICU should be viewed as an important manifestation of organ dysfunction not unlike liver, kidney, or heart failure. Outside the acute hospital setting, delirium occurs in nearly two-thirds of patients in nursing homes and in over 80% of those at the end of life. These estimates emphasize the remarkably high frequency of this cognitive syndrome in older patients, a population expected to grow in the upcoming decade with the aging of the "baby boom" generation.

In previous decades an episode of delirium was viewed as a transient condition that carried a benign prognosis. Delirium now has been clearly associated with substantial morbidity rate and increased mortality rate and increasingly is recognized as a sign of serious underlying illness. Recent estimates of in-hospital mortality rates among delirious patients have ranged from 25 to 33%, a rate similar to that of patients with sepsis. Patients with an in-hospital episode of delirium have a higher mortality rate in the months and years after their illness compared with age-matched nondelirious hospitalized patients. Delirious hospitalized patients have a longer length of stay, are more likely to be discharged to a nursing home, and are more likely to experience subsequent episodes of delirium; as a result, this condition has enormous economic implications.

PATHOGENESIS

The pathogenesis and anatomy of delirium are incompletely understood. The attentional deficit that serves as the neuropsychological hallmark of delirium appears to have a diffuse localization with the brainstem, thalamus, prefrontal cortex, and parietal lobes. Rarely, focal lesions such as ischemic strokes have led to delirium in otherwise healthy persons; right parietal and medial dorsal thalamic lesions have been reported most commonly, pointing to the relevance of these areas to delirium pathogenesis. In most cases, delirium results from widespread disturbances in cortical and subcortical regions rather than a focal neuroanatomic cause. Electroencephalogram (EEG) data in persons with delirium usually show symmetric slowing, a nonspecific finding that supports diffuse cerebral dysfunction.

Deficiency of acetylcholine often plays a key role in delirium pathogenesis. Medications with anticholinergic properties can precipitate delirium in susceptible individuals, and therapies designed to boost cholinergic tone such as cholinesterase inhibitors have, in small trials, been shown to relieve symptoms of delirium. Dementia patients are susceptible to episodes of delirium, and those with Alzheimer's pathology are known to have a chronic cholinergic deficiency state due to degeneration of acetylcholine-producing neurons in the basal forebrain. Another common dementia associated with decreased acetylcholine levels, dementia with Lewy bodies, clinically mimics delirium in some patients. Other neurotransmitters are also likely to be involved in this diffuse cerebral disorder. For example, increases in dopamine can also lead to delirium. Patients with Parkinson's disease treated with dopaminergic medications can develop a delirium-like state that features visual hallucinations, fluctuations, and confusion. In contrast, reducing dopaminergic tone with dopamine antagonists such as typical and atypical antipsychotic medications has long been recognized as effective symptomatic treatment in patients with delirium.

Not all individuals exposed to the same insult will develop signs of delirium. A low dose of an anticholinergic medication may have no cognitive effects on a healthy young adult but may produce a florid delirium in an elderly person with known underlying dementia. However, an extremely high dose of the same anticholinergic medication may lead to delirium even in healthy young persons. This concept of delirium developing as the result of an insult in predisposed individuals is currently the most widely accepted pathogenic construct. Therefore, if a previously healthy individual with no known history of cognitive illness develops delirium in the setting of a relatively minor insult such as elective surgery or hospitalization, an unrecognized underlying neurologic illness such as a neurodegenerative disease, multiple previous strokes, or another diffuse cerebral cause should be considered. In this context, delirium can be viewed as the symptom resulting from a "stress test for the brain" induced by the insult. Exposure to known inciting factors such as systemic infection and offending drugs can unmask a decreased cerebral reserve and herald a serious underlying and potentially treatable illness.

APPROACH TO THE PATIENT Delirium

As the diagnosis of delirium is clinical and is made at the bedside, a careful history and physical examination is necessary in evaluating patients with possible confusional states. Screening tools can aid physicians and nurses in identifying patients with delirium, including the Confusion Assessment Method (CAM); the Organic Brain Syndrome Scale; the Delirium Rating Scale; and, in the ICU, the Delirium Detection Score and the ICU version of the CAM. Using the CAM, a diagnosis of delirium is made if there is (1) an acute onset and fluctuating course and (2) inattention accompanied by either (3) disorganized thinking or (4) an altered level of consciousness. These scales are based on criteria from the American Psychiatric Association's *Diagnostic and Statistical Manual of Mental Disorders* (DSM) or the World Health Organization's International Classification of Diseases (ICD). Unfortunately, these scales do not identify the full spectrum of patients with delirium. All patients who are acutely confused should be presumed delirious regardless of their presentation due to the wide variety of possible clinical features. A course that fluctuates over hours or days and may worsen at night (termed *sundowning*) is typical but not essential for the diagnosis. Observation of the patient usually will reveal an altered level of consciousness or a deficit of attention. Other hallmark features that may be present in a delirious patient include alteration of sleep-wake cycles, thought disturbances such as hallucinations or delusions, autonomic instability, and changes in affect.

HISTORY It may be difficult to elicit an accurate history in delirious patients who have altered levels of consciousness or impaired attention. Information from a collateral source such as a spouse or another family member is therefore invaluable. The three most important pieces of history are the patient's baseline cognitive function, the time course of the present illness, and current medications.

Premorbid cognitive function can be assessed through the collateral source or, if needed, via a review of outpatient records. Delirium by definition represents a change that is relatively acute, usually over hours to days, from a cognitive baseline. As a result, an acute confusional state is nearly impossible to diagnose without some knowledge of baseline cognitive function. Without this information, many patients with dementia or depression may be mistaken as delirious during a single initial evaluation. Patients with a more hypoactive, apathetic presentation with psychomotor slowing may be identified as being different from baseline only through conversations with family members. A number of validated instruments have been shown to diagnose cognitive dysfunction accurately by using a collateral source, including the modified Blessed Dementia Rating Scale and the Clinical Dementia Rating (CDR). Baseline cognitive impairment is common in patients with delirium. Even when no such history of cognitive impairment is elicited, there should still be a high suspicion for a previously unrecognized underlying neurologic disorder.

Establishing the time course of cognitive change is important not only to make a diagnosis of delirium but also to correlate the onset of the illness with potentially treatable etiologies such as recent medication changes or symptoms of systemic infection.

Medications remain a common cause of delirium, especially compounds with anticholinergic or sedative properties. It is estimated that nearly one-third of all cases of delirium are secondary to medications, especially in the elderly. Medication histories should include all prescription as well as over-the-counter and herbal substances taken by the patient and any recent changes in dosing or formulation, including substitution of generics for brand-name medications.

Other important elements of the history include screening for symptoms of organ failure or systemic infection, which often contributes to delirium in the elderly. A history of illicit drug use, alcoholism, or toxin exposure is common in younger delirious patients. Finally, asking the patient and collateral source about other symptoms that may accompany delirium, such as depression and hallucinations, may help identify potential therapeutic targets.

PHYSICAL EXAMINATION The general physical examination in a delirious patient should include a careful screening for signs of infection such as fever, tachypnea, pulmonary consolidation, heart murmur, and stiff neck. The patient's fluid status should be assessed; both dehydration and fluid overload with resultant hypoxemia have been associated with delirium, and each is usually easily rectified. The appearance of the skin can be helpful, showing jaundice in hepatic encephalopathy, cyanosis in hypoxemia, or needle tracks in patients using intravenous drugs.

The neurologic examination requires a careful assessment of mental status. Patients with delirium often present with a fluctuating course; therefore, the diagnosis can be missed when one relies on a single time point of evaluation. Some but not all patients exhibit the characteristic pattern of sundowning, a worsening of their condition in the evening. In these cases, assessment only during morning rounds may be falsely reassuring.

An altered level of consciousness ranging from hyperarousal to lethargy to coma is present in most patients with delirium and can be assessed easily at the bedside. In a patient with a relatively normal level of consciousness, a screen for an attentional deficit is in order, as this deficit is the classic neuropsychological hallmark of delirium. Attention can be assessed while taking a history from the patient. Tangential speech, a fragmentary flow of ideas, or inability to follow complex commands often signifies an attentional problem. There are formal neuropsychological tests to assess attention, but a simple bedside test of digit span forward is quick and fairly sensitive. In this task, patients are asked to repeat successively longer random strings of digits beginning with two digits in a row. Average adults can repeat a string of five to seven digits before faltering; a digit span of four or less usually indicates an attentional deficit unless hearing or language barriers are present.

More formal neuropsychological testing can be extraordinarily helpful in assessing a delirious patient, but it is usually too cumbersome and time-consuming in the inpatient setting. A simple Mini Mental Status Examination (MMSE) (see Table 29-5) can provide some information regarding orientation, language, and visuospatial skills; however, performance of some tasks on the MMSE such as spelling "world" backward and serial subtraction of digits will be impaired by delirious patients' attentional deficits alone and are therefore unreliable.

The remainder of the screening neurologic examination should focus on identifying new focal neurologic deficits. Focal strokes or mass lesions in isolation are rarely the cause of delirium, but patients with underlying extensive cerebrovascular disease or neurodegenerative conditions may not be able to cognitively tolerate even relatively small new insults. Patients also should be screened for additional signs of neurodegenerative conditions such as parkinsonism, which is seen not only in idiopathic Parkinson's disease but also in other dementing conditions such as Alzheimer's disease, dementia with Lewy bodies, and progressive supranuclear palsy. The presence of multifocal myoclonus or asterixis on the motor examination is nonspecific but usually indicates a metabolic or toxic etiology of the delirium.

ETIOLOGY Some etiologies can be easily discerned through a careful history and physical examination, whereas others require confirmation with laboratory studies, imaging, or other ancillary tests. A large, diverse group of insults can lead to delirium, and the cause in many patients is often multifactorial. Common etiologies are listed in Table 16-1.

Prescribed, over-the-counter, and herbal medications are common precipitants of delirium. Drugs with anticholinergic properties, narcotics, and benzodiazepines are especially common offenders, but nearly any compound can lead to cognitive dysfunction in a predisposed patient. Whereas an elderly patient with baseline dementia may become delirious upon exposure to a relatively low dose of a medication, less susceptible individuals may become delirious only with very high doses of the same medication. This observation emphasizes the importance of correlating the timing of recent medication changes, including dose and formulation, with the onset of cognitive dysfunction.

In younger patients especially, illicit drugs and toxins are common causes of delirium. In addition to more classic drugs of abuse, the recent rise in availability of so-called club drugs, such as methylenedioxymethamphetamine (MDMA, ecstasy), γ-hydroxybutyrate (GHB), and the phencyclidine (PCP)-like agent ketamine, has led to an increase in delirious young persons presenting to acute care settings. Many common prescription drugs such as oral narcotics and benzodiazepines are often abused and readily available on the street. Alcohol intoxication with high serum levels can cause confusion, but more commonly it is withdrawal from alcohol that leads to a classic hyperactive delirium. Alcohol and

TABLE 16-1

COMMON ETIOLOGIES OF DELIRIUM
Toxins
Prescription medications: especially those with anticholinergic properties, narcotics, and benzodiazepines
Drugs of abuse: alcohol intoxication and alcohol withdrawal, opiates, ecstasy, LSD, GHB, PCP, ketamine, cocaine
Poisons: inhalants, carbon monoxide, ethylene glycol, pesticides
Metabolic conditions
Electrolyte disturbances: hypoglycemia, hyperglycemia, hyponatremia, hypernatremia, hypercalcemia, hypocalcemia, hypomagnesemia
Hypothermia and hyperthermia
Pulmonary failure: hypoxemia and hypercarbia
Liver failure/hepatic encephalopathy
Renal failure/uremia
Cardiac failure
Vitamin deficiencies: B_{12}, thiamine, folate, niacin
Dehydration and malnutrition
Anemia
Infections
Systemic infections: urinary tract infections, pneumonia, skin and soft tissue infections, sepsis
CNS infections: meningitis, encephalitis, brain abscess
Endocrinologic conditions
Hyperthyroidism, hypothyroidism
Hyperparathyroidism
Adrenal insufficiency
Cerebrovascular disorders
Global hypoperfusion states
Hypertensive encephalopathy
Focal ischemic strokes and hemorrhages: especially nondominant parietal and thalamic lesions
Autoimmune disorders
CNS vasculitis
Cerebral lupus
Seizure-related disorders
Nonconvulsive status epilepticus
Intermittent seizures with prolonged postictal states
Neoplastic disorders
Diffuse metastases to the brain
Gliomatosis cerebri
Carcinomatous meningitis
Hospitalization
Terminal end-of-life delirium

Abbreviations: LSD, lysergic acid diethylamide; GHB, γ-hydroxybutyrate; PCP, phencyclidine; CNS, central nervous system.

benzodiazepine withdrawal should be considered in all cases of delirium as even patients who drink only a few servings of alcohol every day can experience relatively severe withdrawal symptoms upon hospitalization.

Metabolic abnormalities such as electrolyte disturbances of sodium, calcium, magnesium, or glucose can cause delirium, and mild derangements can lead to substantial cognitive disturbances in susceptible individuals. Other common metabolic etiologies include liver and renal failure, hypercarbia and hypoxemia, vitamin deficiencies of thiamine and B_{12}, autoimmune disorders including central nervous system (CNS) vasculitis, and endocrinopathies such as thyroid and adrenal disorders.

Systemic infections often cause delirium, especially in the elderly. A common scenario involves the development of an acute cognitive decline in the setting of a urinary tract infection in a patient with baseline dementia. Pneumonia, skin infections such as cellulitis, and frank sepsis also can lead to delirium. This so-called septic encephalopathy, often seen in the ICU, is probably due to the release of proinflammatory cytokines and their diffuse cerebral effects. CNS infections such as meningitis, encephalitis, and abscess are less common etiologies of delirium; however, in light of the high mortality rates associated with these conditions when they are not treated quickly, clinicians must always maintain a high index of suspicion.

In some susceptible individuals, exposure to the unfamiliar environment of a hospital can lead to delirium. This etiology usually occurs as part of a multifactorial delirium and should be considered a diagnosis of exclusion after all other causes have been thoroughly investigated. Many primary prevention and treatment strategies for delirium involve relatively simple methods to address the aspects of the inpatient setting that are most confusing.

Cerebrovascular etiologies are usually due to global hypoperfusion in the setting of systemic hypotension from heart failure, septic shock, dehydration, or anemia. Focal strokes in the right parietal lobe and medial dorsal thalamus rarely can lead to a delirious state. A more common scenario involves a new focal stroke or hemorrhage causing confusion in a patient who has decreased cerebral reserve. In these individuals, it is sometimes difficult to distinguish between cognitive dysfunction resulting from the new neurovascular insult itself and delirium due to the infectious, metabolic, and pharmacologic complications that can accompany hospitalization after stroke.

Because a fluctuating course often is seen in delirium, intermittent seizures may be overlooked when one is considering potential etiologies. Both nonconvulsive status epilepticus and recurrent focal or generalized seizures followed by postictal confusion can cause delirium; EEG remains essential for this diagnosis. Seizure activity spreading from an electrical focus in a mass or infarct can explain global cognitive dysfunction caused by relatively small lesions.

It is very common for patients to experience delirium at the end of life in palliative care settings. This condition, sometimes described as *terminal restlessness*, must be identified and treated aggressively as it is an important cause of patient and family discomfort at the end of life. It should be remembered that these patients also may be suffering from more common etiologies of delirium such as systemic infection.

LABORATORY AND DIAGNOSTIC EVALUATION A cost-effective approach to the diagnostic evaluation of delirium allows the history and physical examination to guide tests. No established algorithm for workup will fit all delirious patients due to the staggering number of potential etiologies, but one stepwise approach is detailed in **Table 16-2**. If a clear precipitant is identified early, such as an offending medication, little further workup is required. If, however, no likely etiology is uncovered with initial evaluation, an aggressive search for an underlying cause should be initiated.

Basic screening labs, including a complete blood count, electrolyte panel, and tests of liver and renal function, should be obtained in all patients with delirium. In elderly patients, screening for systemic infection, including chest radiography, urinalysis and culture, and possibly blood cultures, is important. In younger individuals, serum and urine drug and toxicology screening may be appropriate early in the workup. Additional laboratory tests addressing other autoimmune, endocrinologic, metabolic, and infectious etiologies should be reserved for patients in whom the diagnosis remains unclear after initial testing.

Multiple studies have demonstrated that brain imaging in patients with delirium is often unhelpful. However, if the initial workup is unrevealing, most clinicians quickly move toward imaging of the brain to exclude structural causes. A noncontrast CT scan can identify large masses and hemorrhages but is otherwise relatively insensitive for discovering an etiology of delirium. The ability of MRI to identify most acute ischemic strokes as well as to provide neuroanatomic detail that gives clues to possible infectious, inflammatory, neurodegenerative, and neoplastic conditions makes it the test of choice. Since MRI techniques are limited by availability, speed of imaging, patient cooperation, and contraindications to magnetic exposure, many clinicians begin with CT scanning and proceed to MRI if the etiology of delirium remains elusive.

Lumbar puncture (LP) must be obtained immediately after appropriate neuroimaging in all patients in whom CNS infection is suspected. Spinal fluid examination can also be useful in identifying inflammatory and neoplastic conditions as well as in the diagnosis of hepatic encephalopathy through elevated cerebrospinal fluid (CSF) glutamine levels. As a result, LP should be considered in any delirious patient with a negative workup. EEG does not have a routine role in the workup of delirium, but it remains invaluable if seizure-related etiologies are considered.

TABLE 16-2

STEPWISE EVALUATION OF A PATIENT WITH DELIRIUM

Initial evaluation
- History with special attention to medications (including over-the-counter and herbals)
- General physical examination and neurologic examination
- Complete blood count
- Electrolyte panel including calcium, magnesium, phosphorus
- Liver function tests, including albumin
- Renal function tests

First-tier further evaluation guided by initial evaluation
- Systemic infection screen
  - Urinalysis and culture
  - Chest radiograph
  - Blood cultures
- Electrocardiogram
- Arterial blood gas
- Serum and/or urine toxicology screen (perform earlier in young persons)
- Brain imaging with MRI with diffusion and gadolinium (preferred) or CT
- Suspected CNS infection: lumbar puncture after brain imaging
- Suspected seizure-related etiology: electroencephalogram (EEG) (if high suspicion, should be performed immediately)

Second-tier further evaluation
- Vitamin levels: B_{12}, folate, thiamine
- Endocrinologic laboratories: thyroid-stimulating hormone (TSH) and free T_4; cortisol
- Serum ammonia
- Sedimentation rate
- Autoimmune serologies: antinuclear antibodies (ANA), complement levels; p-ANCA, c-ANCA
- Infectious serologies: rapid plasmin reagin (RPR); fungal and viral serologies if high suspicion; HIV antibody
- Lumbar puncture (if not already performed)
- Brain MRI with and without gadolinium (if not already performed)

Abbreviations: p-ANCA, perinuclear antineutrophil cytoplasmic antibody; c-ANCA, cytoplasmic antineutrophil cytoplasmic antibody.

TREATMENT Delirium

Management of delirium begins with treatment of the underlying inciting factor (e.g., patients with systemic infections should be given appropriate antibiotics, and underlying electrolyte disturbances judiciously corrected). These treatments often lead to prompt resolution of delirium. Blindly targeting the symptoms of delirium pharmacologically only serves to prolong the time patients remain in the confused state and may mask important diagnostic information. Recent trials of medications used to boost cholinergic tone in delirious patients have led to mixed results, and this strategy is not currently recommended.

Relatively simple methods of supportive care can be highly effective in treating patients with delirium. Reorientation by the nursing staff and family combined with visible clocks, calendars, and outside-facing windows can reduce confusion. Sensory isolation should be prevented by providing glasses and hearing aids to patients who need them. Sundowning can be addressed to a large extent through vigilance to appropriate sleep-wake cycles. During the day, a well-lit room should be accompanied by activities or exercises to prevent napping. At night, a quiet, dark environment with limited interruptions by staff can assure proper rest. These sleep-wake cycle interventions are especially important in the ICU setting as the usual constant 24-h activity commonly provokes delirium. Attempting to mimic the home environment as much as possible also has been shown to help treat and even prevent delirium. Visits from friends and family throughout the day minimize the anxiety associated with the constant flow of new faces of staff and physicians. Allowing hospitalized patients to have access to home bedding, clothing, and nightstand objects makes the hospital environment less foreign and therefore less confusing. Simple standard nursing practices such as maintaining proper nutrition and volume status as well as managing incontinence and skin breakdown also help alleviate discomfort and resulting confusion.

In some instances, patients pose a threat to their own safety or to the safety of staff members, and acute management is required. Bed alarms and personal sitters are more effective and much less disorienting than physical restraints. Chemical restraints should be avoided, but when necessary, very low dose typical or atypical antipsychotic medications administered on an as-needed basis are effective. The recent association of antipsychotic use in the elderly with increased mortality rates underscores the importance of using these medications judiciously and only as a last resort. Benzodiazepines are not as effective as antipsychotics and often worsen confusion through their sedative properties. Although many clinicians still use benzodiazepines to treat acute confusion, their use should be limited to cases in which delirium is caused by alcohol or benzodiazepine withdrawal.

PREVENTION

In light of the high morbidity associated with delirium and the tremendously increased health care costs that accompany it, development of an effective strategy to prevent delirium in hospitalized patients is extremely important. Successful identification of high-risk patients is the first step, followed by initiation of appropriate interventions. One trial randomized more than 850 elderly inpatients to simple standardized protocols used to manage risk factors for delirium, including cognitive impairment, immobility, visual impairment, hearing impairment, sleep deprivation, and dehydration. Significant reductions in the number and duration of episodes of delirium were observed in the treatment group, but unfortunately, delirium recurrence rates were unchanged. Recent trials in the ICU have focused on identifying sedatives, such as dexmedetomidine, that are less likely to lead to delirium in critically ill patients. All hospitals and health care systems should work toward developing standardized protocols to address common risk factors with the goal of decreasing the incidence of delirium.

ACKNOWLEDGMENT

In the 16th edition of Harrison's Principles of Internal Medicine, Allan H. Ropper contributed to a section on acute confusional states that was incorporated into this current chapter.

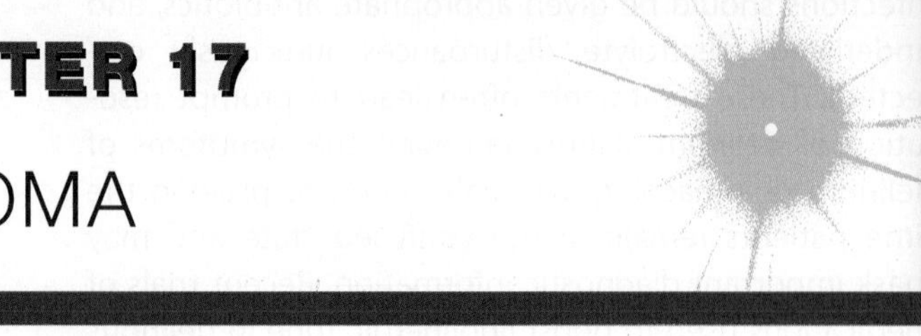

CHAPTER 17
COMA

Allan H. Ropper

Coma is among the most common and striking problems in general medicine. It accounts for a substantial portion of admissions to emergency wards and occurs on all hospital services. Coma demands immediate attention and requires an organized approach.

There is a continuum of states of reduced alertness, the most severe form being *coma*, defined as a deep sleeplike state from which the patient cannot be aroused. *Stupor* refers to a higher degree of arousability in which the patient can be transiently awakened only by vigorous stimuli, accompanied by motor behavior that leads to avoidance of uncomfortable or aggravating stimuli. *Drowsiness*, which is familiar to all persons, simulates light sleep and is characterized by easy arousal and the persistence of alertness for brief periods. Drowsiness and stupor are usually accompanied by some degree of confusion (Chap. 16). A precise narrative description of the level of arousal and of the type of responses evoked by various stimuli as observed at the bedside is preferable to ambiguous terms such as *lethargy*, *semicoma*, or *obtundation*.

Several other conditions that render patients unresponsive and thereby simulate coma are considered separately because of their special significance. The *vegetative state* signifies an awake but nonresponsive state in a patient who has emerged from coma. In the vegetative state, the eyelids may open, giving the appearance of wakefulness. Respiratory and autonomic functions are retained. Yawning, coughing, swallowing, as well as limb and head movements persist and the patient may follow visually presented objects, but there are few, if any, meaningful responses to the external and internal environment—in essence, an "awake coma." The term *vegetative* is unfortunate as it is subject to misinterpretation. There are always accompanying signs that indicate extensive damage in both cerebral hemispheres, e.g., decerebrate or decorticate limb posturing and absent responses to visual stimuli (see later). In the closely related but less severe *minimally conscious state*, the patient has rudimentary vocal or motor behaviors, often spontaneous, but some in response to touch, visual stimuli, or command. Cardiac arrest with cerebral hypoperfusion and head injuries are the most common causes of the vegetative and minimally conscious states (Chap. 28). The prognosis for regaining mental faculties once the vegetative state has supervened for several months is very poor, and after a year, almost nil, hence the term *persistent vegetative state*. Most reports of dramatic recovery, when investigated carefully, are found to yield to the usual rules for prognosis but there have been rare instances in which recovery has occurred to a severely disabled condition and, in rare childhood cases, to an even better state. The possibility of incorrectly attributing meaningful behavior to patients in the vegetative and minimally conscious states has created inordinate problems and anguish for families. On the other hand, the question of whether these patients lack any capability for cognition has been reopened by functional imaging studies demonstrating, in a small proportion of posttraumatic cases, cerebral activation in response to external stimuli.

Apart from the above conditions, several syndromes that affect alertness are prone to be misinterpreted as stupor or coma. *Akinetic mutism* refers to a partially or fully awake state in which the patient is able to form impressions and think, as demonstrated by later recounting of events, but remains virtually immobile and mute. The condition results from damage in the regions of the medial thalamic nuclei or the frontal lobes (particularly lesions situated deeply or on the orbitofrontal surfaces) or from extreme hydrocephalus. The term *abulia* describes a milder form of akinetic mutism characterized by mental and physical slowness and diminished ability to initiate activity. It is also usually the result of damage to the frontal lobes and its connections (Chap. 18). *Catatonia* is a curious hypomobile and mute syndrome that occurs as part of a major psychosis, usually schizophrenia or major depression. Catatonic patients make few voluntary or responsive movements, although they blink, swallow, and may not appear distressed. There are nonetheless signs that the patient is responsive, although it may take ingenuity on the part of the examiner to demonstrate them. For example, eyelid elevation is actively resisted, blinking occurs in response to a visual threat, and the eyes move concomitantly with head rotation, all of which are inconsistent with the presence of a brain lesion causing unresponsiveness. It is characteristic but not invariable in catatonia for the limbs to retain the postures in which they have been placed by the examiner ("waxy flexibility," or catalepsy). With recovery, patients often have some memory of events that occurred during their catatonic stupor. Catatonia is superficially similar to akinetic mutism, but clinical evidence of cerebral damage such as Babinski signs and hypertonicity of the limbs is lacking. The special problem of coma in brain death is discussed later in this chapter.

The *locked-in state* describes yet another type of pseudocoma in which an awake patient has no means of producing speech or volitional movement but retains voluntary vertical eye movements and lid elevation, thus allowing the patient to signal with a clear mind. The pupils are normally reactive. Such individuals have written entire treatises using Morse code. The usual cause is an infarction or hemorrhage of the ventral pons that transects all descending motor (corticospinal and corticobulbar) pathways. A similar awake but deefferented state occurs as a result of total paralysis of the musculature in severe cases of Guillain-Barré syndrome (Chap. 46), critical illness neuropathy (Chap. 28), and pharmacologic neuromuscular blockade.

THE ANATOMY AND PHYSIOLOGY OF COMA

Almost all instances of diminished alertness can be traced to widespread abnormalities of the cerebral hemispheres or to reduced activity of a special thalamocortical alerting system termed the *reticular activating system* (RAS). The proper functioning of this system, its ascending projections to the cortex, and the cortex itself are required to maintain alertness and coherence of thought. It follows that the principal causes of coma are (1) lesions that damage the RAS in the upper midbrain or its projections; (2) destruction of large portions of both cerebral hemispheres; and (3) suppression of reticulocerebral function by drugs, toxins, or metabolic derangements such as hypoglycemia, anoxia, uremia, and hepatic failure.

The proximity of the RAS to midbrain structures that control pupillary function and eye movements permits clinical localization of the cause of coma in many cases. Pupillary enlargement with loss of light reaction and loss of vertical and adduction movements of the eyes suggests that the lesion is in the upper brainstem. Conversely, preservation of pupillary light reactivity and of eye movements absolves the upper brainstem and indicates that widespread structural lesions or metabolic suppression of the cerebral hemispheres is responsible for coma.

Coma due to cerebral mass lesions and herniations

The cranial cavity is separated into compartments by infoldings of the dura. The two cerebral hemispheres are separated by the falx, and the anterior and posterior fossae by the tentorium. Herniation refers to displacement of brain tissue into a compartment that it normally does not occupy. Coma and many of its associated signs can be attributed to these tissue shifts, and certain clinical features are characteristic of specific herniations (Fig. 17-1). They are in essence "false localizing" signs since they derive from compression of brain structures at a distance from the mass.

The most common herniations are those in which a part of the brain is displaced from the supratentorial to the infratentorial compartment through the tentorial opening; this is referred to as *transtentorial* herniation. *Uncal transtentorial* herniation refers to impaction of the anterior medial temporal gyrus (the uncus) into the tentorial opening just anterior to and adjacent to the midbrain (Fig. 17-1A). The uncus compresses the third nerve as it traverses the subarachnoid space, causing enlargement of the ipsilateral pupil (putatively because

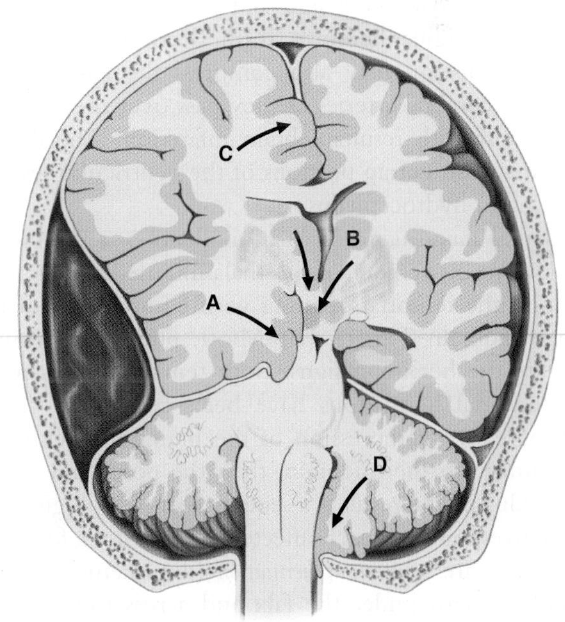

FIGURE 17-1
Types of cerebral herniation. (***A***) Uncal; (***B***) central; (***C***) transfalcial; (***D***) foraminal.

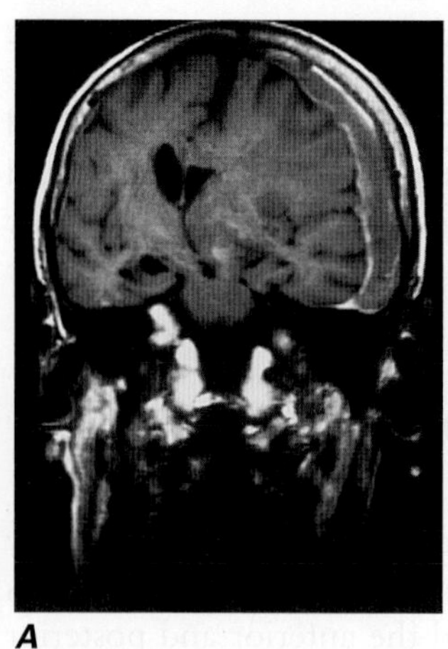
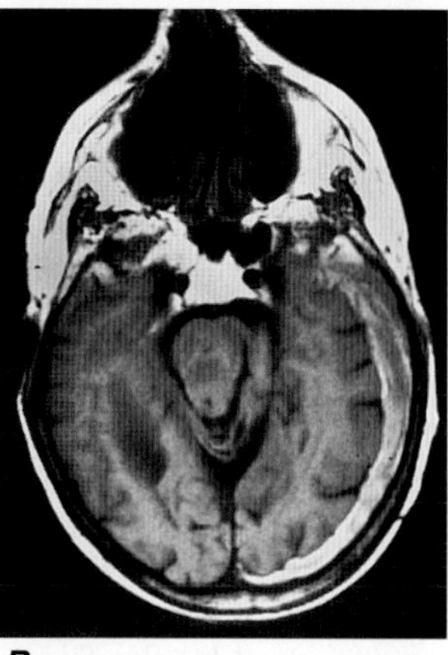

A *B*

FIGURE 17-2

Coronal (*A*) and axial (*B*) magnetic resonance images from a stuporous patient with a left third nerve palsy as a result of a large left-sided subdural hematoma (seen as a gray-white rim). The upper midbrain and lower thalamic regions are compressed and displaced horizontally away from the mass, and there is transtentorial herniation of the medial temporal lobe structures, including the uncus anteriorly. The lateral ventricle opposite to the hematoma has become enlarged as a result of compression of the third ventricle.

the fibers subserving parasympathetic pupillary function are located peripherally in the nerve). The coma that follows is due to compression of the midbrain against the opposite tentorial edge by the displaced parahippocampal gyrus (Fig. 17-2). Lateral displacement of the midbrain may compress the opposite cerebral peduncle, producing a Babinski's sign and hemiparesis contralateral to the original hemiparesis (the Kernohan-Woltman sign). Herniation may also compress the anterior and posterior cerebral arteries as they pass over the tentorial reflections, with resultant brain infarction. The distortions may also entrap portions of the ventricular system, resulting in hydrocephalus.

Central transtentorial herniation denotes a symmetric downward movement of the thalamic medial structures through the tentorial opening with compression of the upper midbrain (Fig. 17-1B). Miotic pupils and drowsiness are the heralding signs. Both temporal and central transtentorial herniations have been considered causes of progressive compression of the brainstem, with initial damage to the midbrain, then the pons, and finally the medulla. The result is a sequence of neurologic signs that corresponds to each affected level. Other forms of herniation are *transfalcial herniation* (displacement of the cingulate gyrus under the falx and across the midline, Fig. 17-1C), and *foraminal herniation* (downward forcing of the cerebellar tonsils into the foramen magnum, Fig. 17-1D), which causes compression of the medulla, respiratory arrest, and death.

A direct relationship between the various configurations of transtentorial herniation and coma is not always found. Drowsiness and stupor can occur with moderate horizontal displacement of the diencephalon (thalamus), before transtentorial herniation is evident. This lateral shift may be quantified on axial images of CT and MRI scans (Fig. 17-2). In cases of *acutely appearing masses*, horizontal displacement of the pineal calcification of 3–5 mm is generally associated with drowsiness, 6–8 mm with stupor, and >9 mm with coma. Intrusion of the medial temporal lobe into the tentorial opening is also apparent on MRI and CT scans as obliteration of the cisterna that surround the upper brainstem.

Coma due to metabolic disorders

Many systemic metabolic abnormalities cause coma by interrupting the delivery of energy substrates (e.g., hypoxia, ischemia, hypoglycemia) or by altering neuronal excitability (drug and alcohol intoxication, anesthesia, and epilepsy). The same metabolic abnormalities that produce coma may, in milder forms, induce an acute confusional state. Thus, in metabolic encephalopathies, clouded consciousness and coma are in a continuum.

Cerebral neurons are fully dependent on cerebral blood flow (CBF) and the delivery of oxygen and glucose. CBF is ~75 mL per 100 g/min in gray matter and 30 mL per 100 g/min in white matter (mean ~55 mL per 100 g/min); oxygen consumption is 3.5 mL per 100 g/min, and glucose utilization is 5 mg per 100 g/min. Brain stores of glucose provide energy for ~2 min after blood flow is interrupted, and oxygen stores last 8–10 s after the cessation of blood flow. Simultaneous hypoxia and ischemia exhaust glucose more rapidly. The electroencephalogram (EEG) rhythm in these circumstances becomes diffusely slowed, typical of metabolic encephalopathies, and as conditions of substrate delivery worsen, eventually brain electrical activity ceases.

Unlike hypoxia-ischemia, which causes neuronal destruction, most metabolic disorders such as hypoglycemia, hyponatremia, hyperosmolarity, hypercapnia, hypercalcemia, and hepatic and renal failure cause only minor neuropathologic changes. The causes of the reversible effects of these conditions on the brain are not understood but may result from impaired energy supplies, changes in ion fluxes across neuronal membranes, and neurotransmitter abnormalities. For example, the high ammonia concentration of hepatic coma interferes with cerebral energy metabolism and with the Na^+, K^+-ATPase pump, increases the number and size of astrocytes, and causes increased concentrations of potentially toxic products of ammonia metabolism; it may also affect neurotransmitters, including the production of putative "false" neurotransmitters that are active at receptor sites. Apart from hyperammonemia, which of these mechanisms is of critical importance is not clear. The mechanism of the encephalopathy of renal failure is also not known. Unlike ammonia, urea does not produce central nervous system (CNS) toxicity and a multifactorial causation has been proposed for the encephalopathy, including increased permeability of the blood-brain barrier to toxic substances such as organic acids and an increase in brain calcium and cerebrospinal fluid (CSF) phosphate content.

Coma and seizures are common accompaniments of large shifts in sodium and water balance in the brain. These changes in osmolarity arise from systemic medical disorders, including diabetic ketoacidosis, the nonketotic hyperosmolar state, and hyponatremia from any cause (e.g., water intoxication, excessive secretion of antidiuretic hormone, or atrial natriuretic peptides). Sodium levels <125 mmol/L induce confusion, and levels <115 mmol/L are associated with coma and convulsions. In hyperosmolar coma, the serum osmolarity is generally >350 mosmol/L. Hypercapnia depresses the level of consciousness in proportion to the rise in carbon dioxide (CO_2) tension in the blood. *In all of these metabolic encephalopathies, the degree of neurologic change depends to a large extent on the rapidity with which the serum changes occur.* The pathophysiology of other metabolic encephalopathies such as hypercalcemia, hypothyroidism, vitamin B_{12} deficiency, and hypothermia are incompletely understood but must also reflect derangements of CNS biochemistry, membrane function, and neurotransmitters.

Epileptic coma

Generalized electrical discharges of the cortex (*seizures*) are associated with coma, even in the absence of epileptic motor activity (*convulsions*). The self-limited coma that follows a seizure, the *postictal state*, may be due to exhaustion of energy reserves or effects of locally toxic molecules that are the by-product of seizures. The postictal state produces a pattern of continuous, generalized slowing of the background EEG activity similar to that of other metabolic encephalopathies.

Toxic (including drug-induced) coma

This common class of encephalopathy is in large measure reversible and leaves no residual damage provided there has not been cardiorespiratory failure. Many drugs and toxins are capable of depressing nervous system function. Some produce coma by affecting both the brainstem nuclei, including the RAS, and the cerebral cortex. The combination of cortical and brainstem signs, which occurs in certain drug overdoses, may lead to an incorrect diagnosis of structural brainstem disease. Overdose of medications that have atropinic actions produces signs such as dilated pupils, tachycardia, and dry skin; opiate overdose produces pinpoint pupils <1 mm in diameter.

Coma due to widespread damage to the cerebral hemispheres

This category, comprising a number of unrelated disorders, results from widespread structural cerebral damage, thereby simulating a metabolic disorder of the cortex. Hypoxia-ischemia is perhaps the best known and one in which it is not possible initially to distinguish the acute reversible effects of hypoperfusion and oxygen deprivation of the brain from the subsequent effects of neuronal damage. Similar bihemispheral damage is produced by disorders that occlude small blood vessels throughout the brain; examples include cerebral malaria, thrombotic thrombocytopenic purpura, and hyperviscosity. Diffuse white matter damage from cranial trauma or inflammatory demyelinating diseases causes a similar syndrome of coma.

APPROACH TO THE PATIENT Coma

Acute respiratory and cardiovascular problems should be attended to prior to neurologic assessment. In most instances, a complete medical evaluation, except for vital signs, funduscopy, and examination for nuchal rigidity, may be deferred until the neurologic evaluation has established the severity and nature of coma. The approach to the patient with coma from cranial trauma is discussed in Chap. 36.

HISTORY In many cases, the cause of coma is immediately evident (e.g., trauma, cardiac arrest, or reported drug ingestion). In the remainder, certain points are especially useful: (1) the circumstances and rapidity with which neurologic symptoms developed; (2) the antecedent symptoms (confusion, weakness, headache, fever, seizures, dizziness, double vision, or vomiting); (3) the use of medications, illicit drugs, or alcohol; and (4) chronic liver, kidney, lung, heart, or other medical disease. Direct interrogation of family, observers, and ambulance technicians on the scene, in person or by telephone, is an important part of the evaluation.

GENERAL PHYSICAL EXAMINATION Fever suggests a systemic infection, bacterial meningitis, encephalitis, heat stroke, neuroleptic malignant syndrome, malignant hyperthermia due to anesthetics or anticholinergic drug intoxication; only rarely is it attributable to a lesion that has disturbed hypothalamic temperature-regulating centers (*"central fever"*). A slight elevation in temperature may follow vigorous convulsions. Hypothermia is observed with exposure; alcoholic, barbiturate, sedative, or phenothiazine intoxication; hypoglycemia; peripheral circulatory failure; or extreme hypothyroidism. Hypothermia itself causes coma only when the temperature is <31°C (87.8°F). Tachypnea may indicate systemic acidosis or pneumonia or rarely infiltration of the brain with lymphoma. Aberrant respiratory patterns that reflect brainstem disorders are discussed later. Marked hypertension suggests hypertensive encephalopathy, but it may also be secondary to a rapid rise in intracranial pressure (ICP) (the Cushing response) most often after cerebral hemorrhage or head injury. Hypotension is characteristic of coma from alcohol or barbiturate intoxication, internal hemorrhage, myocardial infarction, sepsis, profound hypothyroidism, or Addisonian crisis.

The funduscopic examination can detect subarachnoid hemorrhage (subhyaloid hemorrhages), hypertensive encephalopathy (exudates, hemorrhages, vessel-crossing changes, papilledema), and increased ICP (papilledema). Cutaneous petechiae suggest thrombotic thrombocytopenic purpura, meningococcemia, or a bleeding diathesis associated with an intracerebral hemorrhage. Cyanosis, reddish or anemic skin coloration are other indications of an underlying systemic disease responsible for the coma.

NEUROLOGIC EXAMINATION The patient should first be observed without intervention by the examiner. Tossing about in the bed, reaching up toward the face, crossing legs, yawning, swallowing, coughing, or moaning reflect a drowsy state that is close to normal awakeness. Lack of restless movements on one side or an outturned leg suggests a hemiplegia. Intermittent twitching movements of a foot, finger, or facial muscle may be the only sign of seizures. Multifocal myoclonus almost always indicates a metabolic disorder, particularly uremia, anoxia, drug intoxication (especially with lithium or haloperidol), or a prion disease (Chap. 43). In a drowsy and confused patient, bilateral *asterixis* is a certain sign of metabolic encephalopathy or drug intoxication.

Decorticate rigidity and *decerebrate rigidity*, or "posturing," describe stereotyped arm and leg movements occurring spontaneously or elicited by sensory stimulation. Flexion of the elbows and wrists and supination of the arm (decortication) suggests bilateral damage rostral to the midbrain, whereas extension of the elbows and wrists with pronation (decerebration) indicates damage to motor tracts in the midbrain or caudal diencephalon. The less frequent combination of arm extension with leg flexion or flaccid legs is associated with lesions in the pons. These concepts have been adapted from animal work and cannot be applied with precision to coma in humans. In fact, acute and widespread disorders of any type, regardless of location, frequently cause limb extension, and almost all extensor posturing becomes predominantly flexor as time passes.

LEVEL OF AROUSAL A sequence of increasingly intense stimuli is used to determine the threshold for arousal and the motor response of each side of the body. The results of testing may vary from minute to minute, and serial examinations are most useful. Tickling the nostrils with a cotton wisp is a moderate stimulus to arousal—all but deeply stuporous and comatose patients will move the head away and arouse to some degree. An even greater degree of responsiveness is present if the patient uses his hand to remove an offending stimulus. Pressure on the knuckles or bony prominences and pinprick stimulation are humane forms of noxious stimuli; pinching the skin causes unsightly ecchymoses and is generally not necessary but may be useful in eliciting abduction withdrawal movements of the limbs. Posturing in response to noxious stimuli indicates severe damage to the corticospinal system, whereas abduction-avoidance movement of a limb is usually purposeful and denotes an intact corticospinal system. Posturing may also be unilateral and coexists with purposeful limb movements, reflecting incomplete damage to the motor system.

BRAINSTEM REFLEXES Assessment of brainstem function is essential to localization of the lesion in coma (Fig. 17-3). The brainstem reflexes that are conveniently examined are pupillary size and reaction to light, spontaneous and elicited eye movements, corneal responses, and the respiratory pattern. As a rule, coma is due to bilateral hemispheral disease when these brainstem activities are preserved, particularly the pupillary reactions and eye movements. However, the presence of abnormal brainstem signs does not always indicate that the primary lesion is in the brainstem because hemispheral masses can cause secondary brainstem pathology by transtentorial herniation.

Pupillary Signs Pupillary reactions are examined with a bright, diffuse light (not an ophthalmoscope). Reactive and round pupils of midsize (2.5–5 mm) essentially exclude midbrain damage, either primary or secondary to compression. A response to light may be difficult to appreciate in pupils <2 mm in diameter, and bright room lighting mutes pupillary reactivity. One enlarged and poorly reactive pupil (>6 mm) signifies compression or stretching of the third nerve from the effects of a cerebral mass above. Enlargement of the pupil contralateral to a hemispheral mass may occur but is infrequent. An oval and slightly eccentric pupil is a transitional sign that accompanies early midbrain–third nerve compression. The most extreme pupillary sign, bilaterally dilated and unreactive pupils, indicates

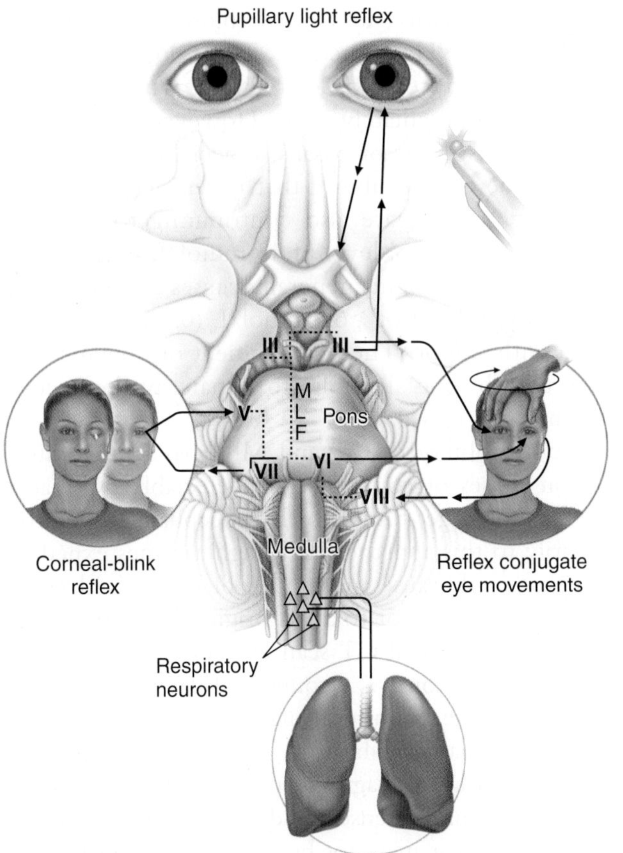

FIGURE 17-3

Examination of brainstem reflexes in coma. Midbrain and third nerve function are tested by pupillary reaction to light, pontine function by spontaneous and reflex eye movements and corneal responses, and medullary function by respiratory and pharyngeal responses. Reflex conjugate, horizontal eye movements are dependent on the medial longitudinal fasciculus (MLF) interconnecting the sixth and contralateral third nerve nuclei. Head rotation (oculocephalic reflex) or caloric stimulation of the labyrinths (oculovestibular reflex) elicits contraversive eye movements (for details, see text).

severe midbrain damage, usually from compression by a supratentorial mass. Ingestion of drugs with anticholinergic activity, the use of mydriatic eye drops, and direct ocular trauma are among the causes of misleading pupillary enlargement.

Unilateral miosis in coma has been attributed to dysfunction of sympathetic efferents originating in the posterior hypothalamus and descending in the tegmentum of the brainstem to the cervical cord. It is therefore of limited localizing value but is an occasional finding in patients with a large cerebral hemorrhage that affects the thalamus. Reactive and bilaterally small (1–2.5 mm) but not pinpoint pupils are seen in metabolic encephalopathies or in deep bilateral hemispheral lesions such as hydrocephalus or thalamic hemorrhage. Even smaller reactive pupils (<1 mm) characterize narcotic or barbiturate overdoses but also occur with extensive pontine hemorrhage. The response to naloxone and the presence of reflex eye movements (see next) assist in distinguishing these.

Ocular Movements The eyes are first observed by elevating the lids and noting the resting position and spontaneous movements of the globes. Lid tone, tested by lifting the eyelids and noting their resistance to opening and the speed of closure, is progressively reduced as unresponsiveness progresses. Horizontal divergence of the eyes at rest is normal in drowsiness. As coma deepens, the ocular axes may become parallel again.

Spontaneous eye movements in coma often take the form of conjugate horizontal roving. This finding alone exonerates damage in the midbrain and pons and has the same significance as normal reflex eye movements (see next). Conjugate horizontal ocular deviation to one side indicates damage to the pons on the opposite side or alternatively, to the frontal lobe on the same side. This phenomenon is summarized by the following maxim: *The eyes look toward a hemispheral lesion and away from a brainstem lesion.* Seizures also drive the eyes to one side but usually with superimposed clonic movements of the globes. The eyes may occasionally turn paradoxically away from the side of a deep hemispheral lesion ("wrong-way eyes"). The eyes turn down and inward with thalamic and upper midbrain lesions, typically thalamic hemorrhage. "Ocular bobbing" describes brisk downward and slow upward movements of the eyes associated with loss of horizontal eye movements and is diagnostic of bilateral pontine damage, usually from thrombosis of the basilar artery. "Ocular dipping" is a slower, arrhythmic downward movement followed by a faster upward movement in patients with normal reflex horizontal gaze; it indicates diffuse cortical anoxic damage.

The oculocephalic reflexes, elicited by moving the head from side to side or vertically and observing eye movements in the direction opposite to the head movement, depend on the integrity of the ocular motor nuclei and their interconnecting tracts that extend from the midbrain to the pons and medulla (Fig. 17-3). The movements, called somewhat inappropriately "doll's eyes" (which refers more accurately to the reflex elevation of the eyelids with flexion of the neck), are normally suppressed in the awake patient. The ability to elicit them therefore indicates both reduced cortical influence on the brainstem and intact brainstem pathways, indicating that coma is caused by a lesion or dysfunction in the cerebral hemispheres. The opposite, an absence of reflex eye movements, usually signifies damage within the brainstem but can result infrequently from overdoses of certain drugs. Normal pupillary size and light reaction distinguishes most drug-induced comas from structural brainstem damage.

Thermal, or "caloric," stimulation of the vestibular apparatus (oculovestibular response) provides a more intense stimulus for the oculocephalic reflex but provides essentially the same information. The test is performed by irrigating the external auditory canal with cool water in order to induce convection currents in the labyrinths. After a brief latency, the result is tonic deviation of both eyes to the side of cool-water irrigation and nystagmus in the opposite direction. (The acronym "COWS" has been used to remind generations of medical students of the direction of nystagmus—"cold water opposite, *w*arm water *s*ame.") The loss of induced conjugate ocular movements indicates brainstem damage. The presence of corrective nystagmus indicates that the frontal lobes are functioning and connected to the brainstem; thus functional or hysterical coma is likely.

By touching the cornea with a wisp of cotton, a response consisting of brief bilateral lid closure is normally observed. The corneal reflex depends on the integrity of pontine pathways between the fifth (afferent) and both seventh (efferent) cranial nerves; in conjunction with reflex eye movements, it is a useful test of pontine function. CNS-depressant drugs diminish or eliminate the corneal responses soon after reflex eye movements are paralyzed but before the pupils become unreactive to light. The corneal (and pharyngeal) response may be lost for a time on the side of an acute hemiplegia.

Respiratory Patterns These are of less localizing value in comparison to other brainstem signs. Shallow, slow, but regular breathing suggests metabolic or drug depression. Cheyne-Stokes respiration in its classic cyclic form, ending with a brief apneic period, signifies bihemispheral damage or metabolic suppression and commonly accompanies light coma. Rapid, deep (Kussmaul) breathing usually implies metabolic acidosis but may also occur with pontomesencephalic lesions. Tachypnea occurs with lymphoma of the CNS. Agonal gasps are the result of lower brainstem (medullary) damage and are recognized as the terminal respiratory pattern of severe brain damage. A number of other cyclic breathing variations have been described but are of lesser significance.

LABORATORY STUDIES AND IMAGING

The studies that are most useful in the diagnosis of coma are: chemical-toxicologic analysis of blood and urine, cranial CT or MRI, EEG, and CSF examination. Arterial blood gas analysis is helpful in patients with lung disease and acid-base disorders. The metabolic aberrations commonly encountered in clinical practice require measurement of electrolytes, glucose, calcium, osmolarity, and renal (blood urea nitrogen) and hepatic (NH_3) function. Toxicologic analysis is necessary in any case of acute coma where the diagnosis is not immediately clear. However, the presence of exogenous drugs or toxins, especially alcohol, does not exclude the possibility that other factors, particularly head trauma, are also contributing to the clinical state. An ethanol level of 43 mmol/L (0.2 g/dL) in nonhabituated patients generally causes impaired mental activity; a level of >65 mmol/L (0.3 g/dL) is associated with stupor. The development of tolerance may allow the chronic alcoholic to remain awake at levels >87 mmol/L (0.4 g/dL).

The availability of CT and MRI has focused attention on causes of coma that are detectable by imaging (e.g., hemorrhage, tumor, or hydrocephalus). Resorting primarily to this approach, although at times expedient, is imprudent because most cases of coma (and confusion) are metabolic or toxic in origin. Furthermore, the notion that a normal CT scan excludes anatomic lesion as the cause of coma is erroneous. Bilateral hemisphere infarction, acute brainstem infarction, encephalitis, meningitis, mechanical shearing of axons as a result of closed head trauma, sagittal sinus thrombosis, and subdural hematoma isodense to adjacent brain are some of the disorders that may not be detected. Nevertheless, if the source of coma remains unknown, a scan should be obtained.

The EEG (Chap. 5) is useful in metabolic or drug-induced states but is rarely diagnostic, except when coma is due to clinically unrecognized seizure, to herpesvirus encephalitis, or to prion (Creutzfeldt-Jakob) disease. The amount of background slowing of the EEG is a reflection of the severity of an encephalopathy. Predominant high-voltage slowing (δ or triphasic waves) in the frontal regions is typical of metabolic coma, as from hepatic failure, and widespread fast (β) activity implicates sedative drugs (e.g., diazepines, barbiturates). A special pattern of "alpha coma," defined by widespread, variable 8- to 12-Hz activity, superficially resembles the normal α rhythm of waking but, unlike normal α activity, is not altered by environmental stimuli. Alpha coma results from pontine or diffuse cortical damage and is associated with a poor prognosis. Normal α activity on the EEG, which is suppressed by stimulating the patient, also alerts the clinician to the locked-in syndrome or to hysteria or catatonia. The most important use of EEG recordings in coma is to reveal clinically inapparent epileptic discharges.

Lumbar puncture is performed less frequently than in the past for coma diagnosis because neuroimaging effectively excludes intracerebral and extensive subarachnoid hemorrhage. However, examination of the CSF remains indispensable in the diagnosis of meningitis and encephalitis. For patients with an altered level of consciousness, it is generally recommended that an imaging study be performed prior to lumbar puncture to exclude a large intracranial mass lesion. Blood culture and antibiotic administration usually precede the imaging study if meningitis is suspected (Chap. 6).

DIFFERENTIAL DIAGNOSIS OF COMA

(Table 17-1) The causes of coma can be divided into three broad categories: those without focal neurologic signs (e.g., metabolic and toxic encephalopathies); meningitis syndromes, characterized by fever or stiff neck and an excess of cells in the spinal fluid (e.g., bacterial meningitis, subarachnoid hemorrhage); and conditions associated with prominent focal signs (e.g., stroke, cerebral hemorrhage). In most instances, coma is part of an obvious medical problem, such as drug ingestion, hypoxia, stroke, trauma, or liver or kidney failure. Conditions that cause sudden coma include drug ingestion, cerebral hemorrhage, trauma, cardiac arrest, epilepsy, or basilar artery embolism. Coma that appears subacutely is usually related to a preexisting medical or neurologic problem or, less often, to secondary brain swelling of a mass such as tumor or cerebral infarction.

When cerebrovascular disease is the cause of coma, diagnosis can be difficult (Chap. 27). The most common diseases are (1) basal ganglia and thalamic hemorrhage (acute but not instantaneous onset, vomiting, headache, hemiplegia, and characteristic eye signs); (2) pontine hemorrhage (sudden onset, pinpoint pupils, loss of reflex eye movements and corneal responses, ocular bobbing, posturing, hyperventilation, and excessive sweating); (3) cerebellar hemorrhage (occipital headache, vomiting, gaze paresis, and inability to stand); (4) basilar artery thrombosis (neurologic prodrome or warning spells, diplopia, dysarthria, vomiting, eye movement and corneal response abnormalities, and asymmetric limb paresis); and (5) subarachnoid hemorrhage (precipitous coma after headache and vomiting). The most common stroke, infarction in the territory of the middle cerebral artery, does not generally cause coma, but edema surrounding large infarctions may expand during the first few days and act as a mass.

The syndrome of acute hydrocephalus accompanies many intracranial diseases, particularly subarachnoid hemorrhage. It is characterized by headache and sometimes vomiting that may progress quickly to coma with extensor posturing of the limbs, bilateral Babinski signs, small unreactive pupils, and impaired oculocephalic movements in the vertical direction.

If the history and examination do not indicate the cause of coma, then information obtained from CT or MRI is needed. The majority of medical causes of coma can be established without a neuroimaging study.

TABLE 17-1

DIFFERENTIAL DIAGNOSIS OF COMA

1. Diseases that cause no focal or lateralizing neurologic signs, usually with normal brainstem functions; CT scan and cellular content of the CSF are normal
   a. Intoxications: alcohol, sedative drugs, opiates, etc.
   b. Metabolic disturbances: anoxia, hyponatremia, hypernatremia, hypercalcemia, diabetic acidosis, nonketotic hyperosmolar hyperglycemia, hypoglycemia, uremia, hepatic coma, hypercarbia, addisonian crisis, hypo- and hyperthyroid states, profound nutritional deficiency
   c. Severe systemic infections: pneumonia, septicemia, typhoid fever, malaria, Waterhouse-Friderichsen syndrome
   d. Shock from any cause
   e. Postseizure states, status epilepticus, subclinical epilepsy
   f. Hypertensive encephalopathy, eclampsia
   g. Severe hyperthermia, hypothermia
   h. Concussion
   i. Acute hydrocephalus
2. Diseases that cause meningeal irritation with or without fever, and with an excess of WBCs or RBCs in the CSF, usually without focal or lateralizing cerebral or brainstem signs; CT or MRI shows no mass lesion
   a. Subarachnoid hemorrhage from ruptured aneurysm, arteriovenous malformation, trauma
   b. Acute bacterial meningitis
   c. Viral encephalitis
   d. Miscellaneous: fat embolism, cholesterol embolism, carcinomatous and lymphomatous meningitis, etc.
3. Diseases that cause focal brainstem or lateralizing cerebral signs, with or without changes in the CSF; CT and MRI are abnormal
   a. Hemispheral hemorrhage (basal ganglionic, thalamic) or infarction (large middle cerebral artery territory) with secondary brainstem compression
   b. Brainstem infarction due to basilar artery thrombosis or embolism
   c. Brain abscess, subdural empyema
   d. Epidural and subdural hemorrhage, brain contusion
   e. Brain tumor with surrounding edema
   f. Cerebellar and pontine hemorrhage and infarction
   g. Widespread traumatic brain injury
   h. Metabolic coma (see earlier) with preexisting focal damage
   i. Miscellaneous: cortical vein thrombosis, herpes simplex encephalitis, multiple cerebral emboli due to bacterial endocarditis, acute hemorrhagic leukoencephalitis, acute disseminated (postinfectious) encephalomyelitis, thrombotic thrombocytopenic purpura, cerebral vasculitis, gliomatosis cerebri, pituitary apoplexy, intravascular lymphoma, etc.

Abbreviations: CSF, cerebrospinal fluid; RBCs, red blood cells; WBCs, white blood cells.

Sometimes imaging results can be misleading such as when small subdural hematomas or old strokes are found, but the patient's coma is due to intoxication.

BRAIN DEATH

This is a state of cessation of cerebral function with preservation of cardiac activity and maintenance of somatic function by artificial means. It is the only type of brain damage recognized as equivalent to death. Several sets of criteria have been advanced for the diagnosis of brain death and it is essential to adhere to those standards endorsed by the local medical community. Ideal criteria are simple, can be assessed at the bedside, and allow no chance of diagnostic error. They contain three essential elements: (1) widespread cortical destruction that is reflected by deep coma and unresponsiveness to all forms of stimulation; (2) global brainstem damage demonstrated by absent pupillary light reaction and by the loss of oculovestibular and corneal reflexes; and (3) destruction of the medulla, manifested by complete apnea. The heart rate is invariant and unresponsive to atropine. Diabetes insipidus is often present but may only develop hours or days after the other clinical signs of brain death. The pupils are usually midsized but may be enlarged; they should not, however, be small. Loss of deep tendon reflexes is not required because the spinal cord remains functional. Babinski signs are generally absent and the toe response is often flexor.

Demonstration that apnea is due to irreversible medullary damage requires that the P_{CO_2} be high enough to stimulate respiration during a test of spontaneous breathing. *Apnea testing* can be done safely by the use of diffusion oxygenation prior to removing the ventilator. This is accomplished by preoxygenation with 100% oxygen, which is then sustained during the test by oxygen administered through a tracheal cannula. CO_2 tension increases ~0.3–0.4 kPa/min (2–3 mmHg/min) during apnea. At the end of a period of observation, typically several minutes, arterial P_{CO_2} should be at least >6.6–8.0 kPa (50–60 mmHg) for the test to be valid. Apnea is confirmed if no respiratory effort has been observed in the presence of a sufficiently elevated P_{CO_2}. Other techniques, including the administration of CO_2 to accelerate the test, are used in special circumstances. The test is usually stopped if there is serious cardiovascular instability.

An isoelectric EEG may be used as a confirmatory test for total cerebral damage. Radionuclide brain scanning, cerebral angiography, or transcranial Doppler measurements may also be included to demonstrate the absence of CBF but they have not been extensively correlated with pathologic changes.

The possibility of profound drug-induced or hypothermic depression of the nervous system should be excluded, and some period of observation, usually 6–24 h, is desirable, during which the clinical signs of brain death are sustained. It is advisable to delay clinical testing for at least 24 h if a cardiac arrest has caused brain death or if the inciting disease is not known.

Although it is largely accepted in Western society that the respirator can be disconnected from a brain-dead patient, problems frequently arise because of poor communication and inadequate preparation of the family by the physician. Reasonable medical practice, ideally with the agreement of the family, allows the removal of support or transfer out of an intensive care unit of patients who are not brain dead but whose neurologic conditions are nonetheless hopeless.

TREATMENT Coma

The immediate goal in a comatose patient is prevention of further nervous system damage. Hypotension, hypoglycemia, hypercalcemia, hypoxia, hypercapnia, and hyperthermia should be corrected rapidly. An oropharyngeal airway is adequate to keep the pharynx open in a drowsy patient who is breathing normally. Tracheal intubation is indicated if there is apnea, upper airway obstruction, hypoventilation, or emesis, or if the patient is liable to aspirate because of coma. Mechanical ventilation is required if there is hypoventilation or a need to induce hypocapnia in order to lower ICP. IV access is established, and naloxone and dextrose are administered if narcotic overdose or hypoglycemia are possibilities; thiamine is given along with glucose to avoid provoking Wernicke's disease in malnourished patients. In cases of suspected basilar thrombosis with brainstem ischemia, IV heparin or a thrombolytic agent is often utilized, after cerebral hemorrhage has been excluded by a neuroimaging study. Physostigmine may awaken patients with anticholinergic-type drug overdose but should be used only with careful monitoring; many physicians believe that it should only be used to treat anticholinergic overdose–associated cardiac arrhythmias. The use of benzodiazepine antagonists offers some prospect of improvement after overdose of soporific drugs and has transient benefit in hepatic encephalopathy.

Administration of hypotonic solutions should be monitored carefully in any serious acute brain illness because of the potential for exacerbating brain swelling. Cervical spine injuries must not be overlooked, particularly before attempting intubation or evaluation of oculocephalic responses. Fever and meningismus indicate an urgent need for examination of the CSF to diagnose meningitis. If the lumbar puncture in a case of suspected meningitis is delayed, an antibiotic such as a third-generation cephalosporin may be administered, preferably after obtaining blood cultures. The management of raised ICP is discussed in Chap. 28.

PROGNOSIS

One hopes to avoid the anguishing outcome of a patient who is left severely disabled or vegetative. The uniformly poor outcome of the persistent vegetative state has already been mentioned. Children and young adults may have ominous early clinical findings such as abnormal brainstem reflexes and yet recover; temporization in offering a prognosis in this group of patients is wise. Metabolic comas have a far better prognosis than traumatic ones. All systems for estimating prognosis in adults should be taken as approximations, and medical judgments must be tempered by factors such as age, underlying systemic disease, and general medical condition. In an attempt to collect prognostic information from large numbers of patients with head injury, the Glasgow Coma Scale was devised; empirically, it has predictive value in cases of brain trauma (Table 36-2). For anoxic and metabolic coma, clinical signs such as the pupillary and motor responses after 1 day, 3 days, and 1 week have been shown to have predictive value (Fig. 28-4). Other studies suggest that the absence of corneal responses may have the most discriminative value. The absence of the cortical waves of the somatosensory evoked potentials has also proved a strong indicator of poor outcome in coma from any cause.

There have been recent advances using functional imaging that demonstrate some preserved cognitive abilities of vegetative and minimally conscious patients. In one series, about 10% of such patients could be trained to activate the frontal or temporal lobes in response to requests by an examiner to imagine certain visuospatial tasks. In one case, a rudimentary form of one-way communication could be established. There are also reports in a limited number of patients of improvement in cognitive function with the implantation of thalamic-stimulating electrodes. It is prudent to avoid generalizations from these experiments.

CHAPTER 18

APHASIA, MEMORY LOSS, AND OTHER FOCAL CEREBRAL DISORDERS

M.-Marsel Mesulam

The cerebral cortex of the human brain contains approximately 20 billion neurons spread over an area of 2.5 m^2. The *primary sensory* areas provide an obligatory portal for the entry of sensory information into cortical circuitry, and the *primary motor* areas provide a final common pathway for coordinating complex motor acts. The primary sensory and motor areas constitute 10% of the cerebral cortex. The rest is subsumed by modality-selective, heteromodal, paralimbic, and limbic areas collectively known as the *association cortex* (Fig. 18-1). The association cortex mediates the integrative processes that subserve cognition, emotion, and behavior. A systematic testing of these mental functions is necessary for the effective clinical assessment of the association cortex and its diseases.

According to current thinking, there are no centers for "hearing words," "perceiving space," or "storing memories." Cognitive and behavioral functions (domains) are coordinated by intersecting *large-scale neural networks* that contain interconnected cortical and subcortical components. The network approach to higher cerebral function has at least four implications of clinical relevance: (1) A single domain such as language or memory can be disrupted by damage to any one of several areas as long as those areas belong to the same network, (2) damage confined to a single area can give rise to multiple deficits involving the functions of all the networks that intersect in that region, (3) damage to a network component may give rise to minimal or transient deficits if other parts of the network undergo compensatory reorganization, and (4) individual anatomic sites within a network display a relative (but not absolute) specialization for different behavioral aspects of the relevant function. Five anatomically defined large-scale networks are most relevant to clinical practice: (1) a perisylvian network for language, (2) a parietofrontal network for spatial cognition, (3) an occipitotemporal network for face and object recognition, (4) a limbic network for retentive memory, and (5) a prefrontal network for cognitive and behavioral control.

THE LEFT PERISYLVIAN NETWORK FOR LANGUAGE: APHASIAS AND RELATED CONDITIONS

Language allows the communication and elaboration of thoughts and experiences by linking them to arbitrary symbols known as words. The neural substrate of language is composed of a distributed network centered in the perisylvian region of the *left* hemisphere. The posterior pole of this network is located at the temporoparietal junction and includes a region known as *Wernicke's area*. An essential function of Wernicke's area is to transform sensory inputs into their neural word representations so that they can establish the distributed associations that give a word its meaning. The anterior pole of the language network is located in the inferior frontal gyrus and includes a region known as *Broca's area*. An essential function of this area is to transform neural word representations into their articulatory sequences so that the words can be uttered in the form of spoken language. The sequencing function of Broca's area also appears to involve the ordering of words into sentences that contain a meaning-appropriate *syntax* (grammar). Wernicke's and Broca's areas are interconnected with each other and with additional perisylvian, temporal, prefrontal, and posterior parietal regions, making up a neural network that subserves the various aspects of language function. Damage to any one of these components or to their interconnections can give rise to language disturbances (*aphasia*). Aphasia should be diagnosed only when there are deficits in the formal aspects

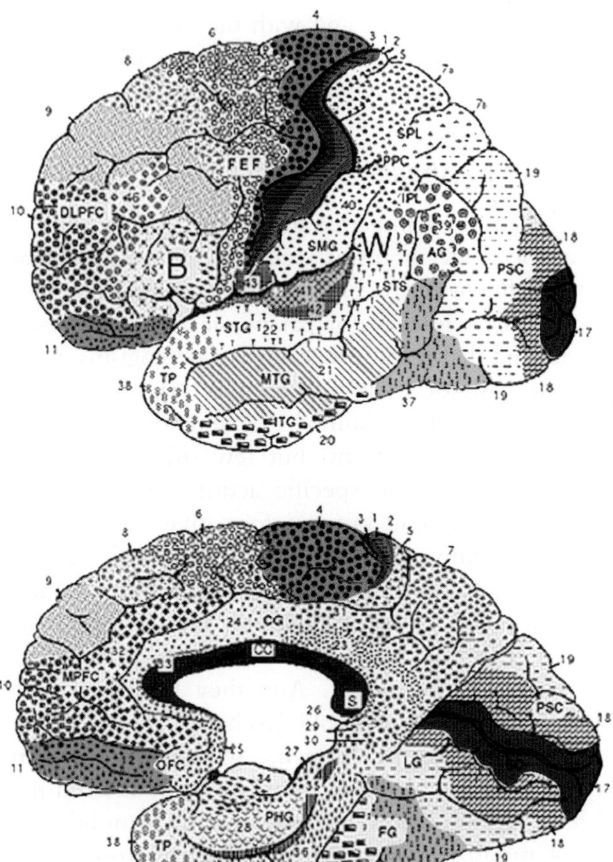

FIGURE 18-1

Lateral *(top)* and medial (*bottom*) views of the cerebral hemispheres. The numbers refer to the Brodmann cytoarchitectonic designations. Area 17 corresponds to the primary visual cortex, 41–42 to the primary auditory cortex, 1–3 to the primary somatosensory cortex, and 4 to the primary motor cortex. The rest of the cerebral cortex contains association areas. AG, angular gyrus; B, Broca's area; CC, corpus callosum; CG, cingulate gyrus; DLPFC, dorsolateral prefrontal cortex; FEF, frontal eye fields (premotor cortex); FG, fusiform gyrus; IPL, inferior parietal lobule; ITG, inferior temporal gyrus; LG, lingual gyrus; MPFC, medial prefrontal cortex; MTG, middle temporal gyrus; OFC, orbitofrontal cortex; PHG, parahippocampal gyrus; PPC, posterior parietal cortex; PSC, peristriate cortex; SC, striate cortex; SMG, supramarginal gyrus; SPL, superior parietal lobule; STG, superior temporal gyrus; STS, superior temporal sulcus; TP, temporopolar cortex; W, Wernicke's area.

of language, such as naming, word choice, comprehension, spelling, and syntax. Dysarthria and mutism do not by themselves lead to a diagnosis of aphasia. The language network shows a left hemisphere dominance pattern in the vast majority of the population. In approximately 90% of right-handers and 60% of left-handers, aphasia occurs only after lesions of the left hemisphere. In some individuals no hemispheric dominance for language can be discerned, and in some others (including a small minority of right handers) there is a right hemisphere dominance for language. A language disturbance that occurs after a right hemisphere lesion in a right hander is called *crossed aphasia*.

CLINICAL EXAMINATION

The clinical examination of language should include the assessment of naming, spontaneous speech, comprehension, repetition, reading, and writing. A deficit of naming (*anomia*) is the single most common finding in aphasic patients. When asked to name a common object (pencil or wristwatch), the patient may fail to come up with the appropriate word, may provide a circumlocutious description of the object ("the thing for writing"), or may come up with the wrong word (*paraphasia*). If the patient offers an incorrect but related word ("pen" for "pencil"), the naming error is known as a *semantic paraphasia*; if the word approximates the correct answer but is phonetically inaccurate ("plentil" for "pencil"), it is known as a *phonemic paraphasia*. Asking the patient to name body parts, geometric shapes, and component parts of objects (lapel of coat, cap of pen) can elicit mild forms of anomia in patients who otherwise can name common objects. In most anomias, the patient cannot retrieve the appropriate name when shown an object but can point to the appropriate object when the name is provided by the examiner. This is known as a one-way (or retrieval-based) naming deficit. A two-way naming deficit exists if the patient can neither provide nor recognize the correct name, indicating the likely presence of a comprehension impairment for the word. *Spontaneous speech* is described as "fluent" if it maintains appropriate output volume, phrase length, and melody or as "nonfluent" if it is sparse and halting and average utterance length is below four words. The examiner also should note if the speech is paraphasic or circumlocutious; if it shows a relative paucity of substantive nouns and action verbs versus function words (prepositions, conjunctions); and if word order, tenses, suffixes, prefixes, plurals, and possessives are appropriate. *Comprehension* can be tested by assessing the patient's ability to follow conversation, asking yes-no questions ("Can a dog fly?", "Does it snow in summer?") or asking the patient to point to appropriate objects ("Where is the source of illumination in this room?"). Statements with embedded clauses or a passive voice construction ("If a tiger is eaten by a lion, which animal stays alive?") help assess the ability to comprehend complex syntactic structure. Commands to close or open the eyes, stand up, sit down, or roll over should not be used to assess overall comprehension since appropriate responses aimed at such axial movements can be preserved in patients who otherwise have profound comprehension deficits.

Repetition is assessed by asking the patient to repeat single words, short sentences, or strings of words such as "No ifs, ands, or buts." The testing of repetition with tongue twisters such as "hippopotamus" and "Irish constabulary" provides a better assessment of dysarthria and pallilalia than of aphasia. Aphasic patients who have little difficulty with tongue twisters may have a particularly hard time repeating a string of function words. It is important to make sure that the number of words does not exceed the patient's attention span. Otherwise, the failure of repetition becomes a reflection of the narrowed attention span rather than an indication of an aphasic deficit. *Reading* should be assessed for deficits in reading aloud as well as comprehension. *Writing* is assessed for spelling errors, word order, and grammar. *Alexia* describes an inability to either read aloud or comprehend single words and simple sentences; *agraphia* (or dysgraphia) is used to describe an acquired deficit in the spelling or grammar of written language.

The correspondence between individual deficits of language function and lesion location does not display a rigid one-to-one relationship and should be conceptualized within the context of the distributed network model. Nonetheless, the classification of aphasias into specific clinical syndromes helps determine the most likely anatomic distribution of the underlying neurologic disease and has implications for etiology and prognosis (Table 18-1). The syndromes listed in Table 18-1 are most applicable to aphasias caused by cerebrovascular accidents (CVAs). They can be divided into "central" syndromes, which result from damage to the two epicenters of the language network (Broca's and Wernicke's areas), and "disconnection" syndromes, which arise from lesions that interrupt the functional connectivity of those centers with each other and with the other components of the language network. The syndromes outlined next are idealizations; pure syndromes occur rarely.

Wernicke's aphasia

Comprehension is impaired for spoken and written language, for single words as well as sentences. Language output is fluent but is highly paraphasic and circumlocutious. The tendency for paraphasic errors may be so pronounced that it leads to strings of neologisms, which form the basis of what is known as "jargon aphasia." Speech contains large numbers of function words (e.g., prepositions, conjunctions) but few substantive nouns or verbs that refer to specific actions. The output is therefore voluminous but uninformative. For example, a patient attempts to describe how his wife accidentally threw away something important, perhaps his dentures: "We don't need it anymore, she says. And with it when that was downstairs was my teeth-tick...a... den...dentith...my dentist. And they happened to be in that bag...see? How could this have happened? How could a thing like this happen...So she says we won't need it anymore...I didn't think we'd use it. And now if I have any problems anybody coming a month from now, 4 months from now, or 6 months from now, I have a new dentist. Where my two...two little pieces of dentist that I use...that I...all gone. If she throws the whole thing away...visit some friends of hers and she can't throw them away."

Gestures and pantomime do not improve communication. The patient does not seem to realize that his or her language is incomprehensible and may appear angry and impatient when the examiner fails to decipher the

TABLE 18-1

CLINICAL FEATURES OF APHASIAS AND RELATED CONDITIONS

	COMPREHENSION	REPETITION OF SPOKEN LANGUAGE	NAMING	FLUENCY
Wernicke's	Impaired	Impaired	Impaired	Preserved or increased
Broca's	Preserved (except grammar)	Impaired	Impaired	Decreased
Global	Impaired	Impaired	Impaired	Decreased
Conduction	Preserved	Impaired	Impaired	Preserved
Nonfluent (motor) transcortical	Preserved	Preserved	Impaired	Impaired
Fluent (sensory) transcortical	Impaired	Preserved	Impaired	Preserved
Isolation	Impaired	Echolalia	Impaired	No purposeful speech
Anomic	Preserved	Preserved	Impaired	Preserved except for word-finding pauses
Pure word deafness	Impaired only for spoken language	Impaired	Preserved	Preserved
Pure alexia	Impaired only for reading	Preserved	Preserved	Preserved

meaning of a severely paraphasic statement. In some patients this type of aphasia can be associated with severe agitation and paranoid behaviors. One area of comprehension that may be preserved is the ability to follow commands aimed at axial musculature. The dissociation between the failure to understand simple questions ("What is your name?") in a patient who rapidly closes his or her eyes, sits up, or rolls over when asked to do so is characteristic of Wernicke's aphasia and helps differentiate it from deafness, psychiatric disease, or malingering. Patients with Wernicke's aphasia cannot express their thoughts in meaning-appropriate words and cannot decode the meaning of words in any modality of input. This aphasia therefore has expressive as well as receptive components. Repetition, naming, reading, and writing also are impaired.

The lesion site most commonly associated with Wernicke's aphasia is the posterior portion of the language network and tends to involve at least parts of Wernicke's area. An embolus to the inferior division of the middle cerebral artery, to the posterior temporal or angular branches in particular, is the most common etiology. Intracerebral hemorrhage, severe head trauma, and neoplasm are other causes. A coexisting right hemianopia or superior quadrantanopia is common and mild right nasolabial flattening may be found, but otherwise the examination is often unrevealing. The paraphasic, neologistic speech in an agitated patient with an otherwise unremarkable neurologic examination may lead to the suspicion of a primary psychiatric disorder such as schizophrenia or mania, but the other components characteristic of acquired aphasia and the absence of prior psychiatric disease usually settle the issue. Some patients with Wernicke's aphasia due to intracerebral hemorrhage or head trauma may improve as the hemorrhage or the injury heals. In most other patients, prognosis for recovery of language function is guarded.

Broca's aphasia

Speech is nonfluent, labored, interrupted by many word-finding pauses, and usually dysarthric. It is impoverished in function words but enriched in meaning-appropriate nouns and verbs. Abnormal word order and the inappropriate deployment of *bound morphemes* (word endings used to denote tenses, possessives, or plurals) lead to a characteristic agrammatism. Speech is telegraphic and pithy but quite informative. In the following passage, a patient with Broca's aphasia describes his medical history: "I see...the dotor, dotor sent me... Bosson. Go to hospital. Dotor...kept me beside. Two, tee days, doctor send me home."

Output may be reduced to a grunt or single word ("yes" or "no"), which is emitted with different intonations in an attempt to express approval or disapproval. In addition to fluency, naming and repetition are impaired. Comprehension of spoken language is intact except for syntactically difficult sentences with a passive voice structure or embedded clauses. Reading comprehension also is preserved with the occasional exception of a specific inability to read small grammatical words such as conjunctions and pronouns. The last two features indicate that Broca's aphasia is not just an "expressive" or "motor" disorder and that it also may involve a comprehension deficit for function words and syntax. Patients with Broca's aphasia can be tearful, easily frustrated, and profoundly depressed. Insight into their condition is preserved, in contrast to Wernicke's aphasia. Even when spontaneous speech is severely dysarthric, the patient may be able to display a relatively normal articulation of words when singing. This dissociation has been used to develop specific therapeutic approaches (melodic intonation therapy) for Broca's aphasia. Additional neurologic deficits usually include right facial weakness, hemiparesis or hemiplegia, and a buccofacial apraxia characterized by an inability to carry out motor commands involving oropharyngeal and facial musculature (e.g., patients are unable to demonstrate how to blow out a match or suck through a straw). Visual fields are intact. The cause is most often infarction of Broca's area (the inferior frontal convolution; "B" in Fig. 18-1) and surrounding anterior perisylvian and insular cortex due to occlusion of the superior division of the middle cerebral artery. Mass lesions, including tumor, intracerebral hemorrhage, and abscess, also may be responsible. Small lesions confined to the posterior part of Broca's area may lead to a nonaphasic and often reversible deficit of speech articulation that usually is accompanied by mild right facial weakness. When the cause of Broca's aphasia is stroke, recovery of language function generally peaks within 2 to 6 months, after which time further progress is limited.

Global aphasia

Speech output is nonfluent, and comprehension of spoken language is severely impaired. Naming, repetition, reading, and writing also are impaired. This syndrome represents the combined dysfunction of Broca's and Wernicke's areas and usually results from strokes that involve the entire middle cerebral artery distribution in the left hemisphere. Most patients are initially mute or say a few words, such as "hi" or "yes." Related signs include right hemiplegia, hemisensory loss, and homonymous hemianopia. Occasionally, a patient with a lesion in Wernicke's area will present with a global aphasia that soon resolves into Wernicke's aphasia.

Conduction aphasia

Speech output is fluent but paraphasic, comprehension of spoken language is intact, and repetition is severely impaired. Naming and writing also are impaired. Reading aloud is impaired, but reading comprehension is preserved. The lesion sites spare Broca's and Wernicke's areas but may induce a functional disconnection between the two so that neural word representations formed in Wernicke's area and adjacent regions cannot be conveyed to Broca's area for assembly into corresponding articulatory patterns. Occasionally, a Wernicke's area lesion gives rise to a transient Wernicke's aphasia that rapidly resolves into a conduction aphasia. The paraphasic output in conduction aphasia interferes with the ability to express meaning, but this deficit is not nearly as severe as the one displayed by patients with Wernicke's aphasia. Associated neurologic signs in conduction aphasia vary according to the primary lesion site.

Nonfluent transcortical aphasia (transcortical motor aphasia)

The features are similar to those of Broca's aphasia, but repetition is intact and agrammatism may be less pronounced. The neurologic examination may be otherwise intact, but a right hemiparesis also can exist. The lesion site disconnects the intact language network from prefrontal areas of the brain and usually involves the anterior watershed zone between anterior and middle cerebral artery territories or the supplementary motor cortex in the territory of the anterior cerebral artery.

Fluent transcortical aphasia (transcortical sensory aphasia)

Clinical features are similar to those of Wernicke's aphasia, but repetition is intact. The lesion site disconnects the intact core of the language network from other temporoparietal association areas. Associated neurologic findings may include hemianopia. Cerebrovascular lesions (e.g., infarctions in the posterior watershed zone) and neoplasms that involve the temporoparietal cortex posterior to Wernicke's area are the most common causes.

Isolation aphasia

This rare syndrome represents a combination of the two transcortical aphasias. Comprehension is severely impaired, and there is no purposeful speech output. The patient may parrot fragments of heard conversations (*echolalia*), indicating that the neural mechanisms for repetition are at least partially intact. This condition represents the pathologic function of the language network when it is isolated from other regions of the brain. Broca's and Wernicke's areas tend to be spared, but there is damage to the surrounding frontal, parietal, and temporal cortex. Lesions are patchy and can be associated with anoxia, carbon monoxide poisoning, or complete watershed zone infarctions.

Anomic aphasia

This form of aphasia may be considered the "minimal dysfunction" syndrome of the language network. Articulation, comprehension, and repetition are intact, but confrontation naming, word finding, and spelling are impaired. Speech is enriched in function words but impoverished in substantive nouns and verbs denoting specific actions. Language output is fluent but paraphasic, circumlocutious, and uninformative. Fluency may be interrupted by word-finding hesitations. The lesion sites can be anywhere within the left hemisphere language network, including the middle and inferior temporal gyri. *Anomic aphasia is the single most common language disturbance seen in head trauma, metabolic encephalopathy, and Alzheimer's disease.*

Pure word deafness

The most common causes are either bilateral or left-sided middle cerebral artery (MCA) strokes affecting the superior temporal gyrus. The net effect of the underlying lesion is to interrupt the flow of information from the auditory association cortex to Wernicke's area. Patients have no difficulty understanding written language and can express themselves well in spoken or written language. They have no difficulty interpreting and reacting to environmental sounds since primary auditory cortex and subcortical auditory relays are intact. Since auditory information cannot be conveyed to the language network, however, it cannot be decoded into neural word representations, and the patient reacts to speech as if it were in an alien tongue that cannot be deciphered. Patients cannot repeat spoken language but have no difficulty naming objects. In time, patients with pure word deafness teach themselves lipreading and may appear to have improved. There may be no additional neurologic findings, but agitated paranoid reactions are common in the acute stages. Cerebrovascular lesions are the most common cause.

Pure alexia without agraphia

This is the visual equivalent of pure word deafness. The lesions (usually a combination of damage to the left occipital cortex and to a posterior sector of the corpus callosum—the splenium) interrupt the flow of visual input into the language network. There is usually a right hemianopia, but the core language network remains unaffected. The patient can understand and produce spoken language, name objects in the left visual hemifield, repeat, and write. However, the patient acts as if illiterate when asked to read even the simplest sentence because the visual information from the written words (presented to the intact left visual hemifield) cannot reach the language network. Objects in the left hemifield may be named accurately because they activate nonvisual associations in the right hemisphere, which in turn can access the language network through transcallosal pathways anterior to the splenium. Patients with this syndrome also may lose the ability to name colors, although they can match colors. This is known as a *color anomia*. The most common etiology of pure alexia is a vascular lesion in the territory of the posterior cerebral artery or an infiltrating neoplasm in the left occipital cortex that involves the optic radiations as well as the crossing fibers of the splenium. Since the posterior cerebral artery also supplies medial temporal components of the limbic system, a patient with pure alexia also may experience an amnesia, but this is usually transient because the limbic lesion is unilateral.

Aphemia

There is an acute onset of severely impaired fluency (often mutism), which cannot be accounted for by corticobulbar, cerebellar, or extrapyramidal dysfunction. Recovery is the rule and involves an intermediate stage of hoarse whispering. Writing, reading, and comprehension are intact, and so this is not a true aphasic syndrome. Partial lesions of Broca's area or subcortical lesions that undercut its connections with other parts of the brain may be present. Occasionally, the lesion site is on the medial aspects of the frontal lobes and may involve the supplementary motor cortex of the left hemisphere.

Apraxia

This generic term designates a complex motor deficit that cannot be attributed to pyramidal, extrapyramidal, cerebellar, or sensory dysfunction and that does not arise from the patient's failure to understand the nature of the task. The form that is encountered most frequently in clinical practice is known as *ideomotor apraxia*. Commands to perform a specific motor act ("cough," "blow out a match") or pantomime the use of a common tool (a comb, hammer, straw, or toothbrush) in the absence of the real object cannot be followed. The patient's ability to comprehend the command is ascertained by demonstrating multiple movements and establishing that the correct one can be recognized. Some patients with this type of apraxia can imitate the appropriate movement (when it is demonstrated by the examiner) and show no impairment when handed the real object, indicating that the sensorimotor mechanisms necessary for the movement are intact. Some forms of ideomotor apraxia represent a disconnection of the language network from pyramidal motor systems: commands to execute complex movements are understood but cannot be conveyed to the appropriate motor areas even though the relevant motor mechanisms are intact. *Buccofacial apraxia* involves apraxic deficits in movements of the face and mouth. *Limb apraxia* encompasses apraxic deficits in movements of the arms and legs. Ideomotor apraxia almost always is caused by lesions in the left hemisphere and is commonly associated with aphasic syndromes, especially Broca's aphasia and conduction aphasia. Its presence cannot be ascertained in patients with language comprehension deficits. The ability to follow commands aimed at axial musculature ("close the eyes," "stand up") is subserved by different pathways and may be intact in otherwise severely aphasic and apraxic patients. Since the handling of real objects is not impaired, ideomotor apraxia by itself causes no major limitation of daily living activities. Patients with lesions of the anterior corpus callosum can display ideomotor apraxia confined to the left side of the body, a sign known as *sympathetic dyspraxia*. A severe form of sympathetic dyspraxia known as the *alien hand* syndrome is characterized by additional features of motor disinhibition on the left hand.

Ideational apraxia refers to a deficit in the execution of a goal-directed sequence of movements in patients who have no difficulty executing the individual components of the sequence. For example, when the patient is asked to pick up a pen and write, the sequence of uncapping the pen, placing the cap at the opposite end, turning the point toward the writing surface, and writing may be disrupted, and the patient may be seen trying to write with the wrong end of the pen or even with the removed cap. These motor sequencing problems usually are seen in the context of confusional states and dementias rather than focal lesions associated with aphasic conditions. *Limb-kinetic apraxia* involves a clumsiness in the actual use of tools that cannot be attributed to sensory, pyramidal, extrapyramidal, or cerebellar dysfunction. This condition can emerge in the context of focal premotor cortex lesions or *corticobasal degeneration*.

Gerstmann's syndrome

The combination of *acalculia* (impairment of simple arithmetic), *dysgraphia* (impaired writing), *finger anomia* (an inability to name individual fingers such as the index and thumb), and *right-left confusion* (an inability to tell whether a hand, foot, or arm of the patient or examiner is on the right or left side of the body) is known as Gerstmann's syndrome. In making this diagnosis it is important to establish that the finger and left-right naming deficits are not part of a more generalized anomia and that the patient is not otherwise aphasic. When Gerstmann's syndrome is seen in isolation, it is commonly associated with damage to the inferior parietal lobule (especially the angular gyrus) in the left hemisphere.

Aprosodia

Variations of melodic stress and intonation influence the meaning and impact of spoken language. For example, the two statements "He *is* clever." and "He is *clever*?" contain an identical word choice and syntax but convey vastly different messages because of differences in the intonation and stress with which the statements are uttered. This aspect of language is known as *prosody*. Damage to perisylvian areas in the right hemisphere can interfere with speech prosody and can lead to syndromes of aprosodia. Damage to right hemisphere regions corresponding to Wernicke's area can selectively impair decoding of speech prosody, whereas damage to right hemisphere regions corresponding to Broca's area yields a greater impairment in the ability to introduce meaning-appropriate prosody into spoken language. The latter deficit is the most common type of aprosodia identified in clinical practice; the patient produces grammatically correct language with accurate word choice, but the statements are uttered in a monotone that interferes with the ability to convey the intended stress and affect. Patients with this type of aprosodia give the mistaken impression of being depressed or indifferent.

Subcortical aphasia

Damage to subcortical components of the language network (e.g., the striatum and thalamus of the left hemisphere) also can lead to aphasia. The resulting syndromes contain combinations of deficits in the various aspects of language but rarely fit the specific patterns described in Table 18-1. In a patient with a CVA, an anomic aphasia accompanied by dysarthria or a fluent aphasia with hemiparesis should raise the suspicion of a subcortical lesion site.

Progressive aphasias

Aphasias caused by cerebrovascular accidents start suddenly and display maximal deficits at the onset. The underlying lesion is relatively circumscribed and is associated with a total loss of neural function in at least part of the lesion site. These are the "classic" aphasias described earlier in this chapter. Aphasias caused by neurodegenerative diseases have an insidious onset and a relentless progression so that the symptomatology changes over time. Since the neuronal loss within the areas encompassed by the neurodegeneration is partial and since it tends to include multiple components of the language network, the clinico-anatomic patterns are different from those described in Table 18-1.

Clinical presentation and diagnosis of primary progressive aphasia (PPA)

When a neurodegenerative disease selectively undermines language function, a clinical diagnosis of PPA is made. A patient with PPA comes to medical attention because of word-finding difficulties, abnormal speech patterns, word-comprehension impairments, or spelling errors of recent onset. PPA is diagnosed when other mental faculties, such as memory for daily events, visuospatial skills (assessed by tests of drawing and face recognition), and comportment (assessed by history obtained from a third party), remain relatively intact; when language is the major area of dysfunction for the first few years of the disease; and when structural brain imaging does not reveal a specific lesion, other than atrophy, that accounts for the language deficit. Impairments in other cognitive functions may emerge eventually, but the language dysfunction remains the most salient feature and deteriorates most rapidly throughout the illness.

Language in PPA

The language impairment in PPA varies from patient to patient. Some patients cannot find the right words to express thoughts; others cannot understand the meaning of heard or seen words; still others cannot name objects in the environment. The language impairment can be fluent (that is, with normal articulation, flow, and number of words per utterance) or nonfluent. The single most common sign of primary progressive aphasia is an inability to come up with the right word during conversation and/or an inability to name objects shown by the examiner (anomia). Distinct forms of agrammatism and/or word comprehension deficits also can arise. The agrammatism consists of inappropriate word order and misuse of small grammatical words. Comprehension deficits, if present, start with an occasional inability to understand single low-frequency words and gradually progress to encompass the comprehension of conversational speech.

The impairments of syntax, comprehension, naming, or writing in PPA form slightly different patterns from those seen in CVA-caused aphasias. Three subtypes of PPA can be recognized: an agrammatic variant characterized by poor fluency and impaired grammar, a semantic variant characterized by preserved fluency and syntax but poor single word comprehension, and a logopenic variant characterized by preserved syntax and comprehension but frequent word-finding pauses during spontaneous speech. The agrammatic variant also is known as *progressive nonfluent aphasia* and displays similarities to Broca's aphasia. However, dysarthria is usually absent. The semantic variant of PPA displays similarities to Wernicke's aphasia, but the comprehension difficulty tends to be most profound for single words denoting concrete objects.

Pathophysiology

The three variants of PPA display overlapping distributions of neuronal loss, but the agrammatic variant is most closely associated with atrophy in the anterior parts of the language network (where Broca's area is located), the semantic variant with atrophy in the anterior temporal components of the language network, and the logopenic variant with atrophy in the temporoparietal component of the language network. The abnormalities may remain confined to the left hemisphere perisylvian and anterior temporal cortices initially, but gradual deterioration in PPA leads to a loss of syndromic specificity as the disease progresses.

Neuropathology

In the majority of PPA cases, the neuropathology falls within the family of frontotemporal lobar degenerations (FTLDs) and displays various combinations of focal neuronal loss, gliosis, tau-positive inclusions including Pick bodies, and tau-negative TDP-43 inclusions. Familial forms of PPA with TDP-43 inclusions recently were linked to mutations of the progranulin gene on chromosome 17. The agrammatic variant most frequently is associated with tauopathy, whereas the semantic variant is most closely associated with TDP-43 inclusions. Alzheimer's pathology is seen most frequently in the logopenic variant. The clinical subtyping of PPA thus may help predict the nature of the underlying neuropathology. The intriguing possibility has been raised that a personal or family history of dyslexia may be a risk factor for primary progressive aphasia, at least in some patients, suggesting that this disease may arise on a background of genetic or developmental vulnerability that affects language-related areas of the brain.

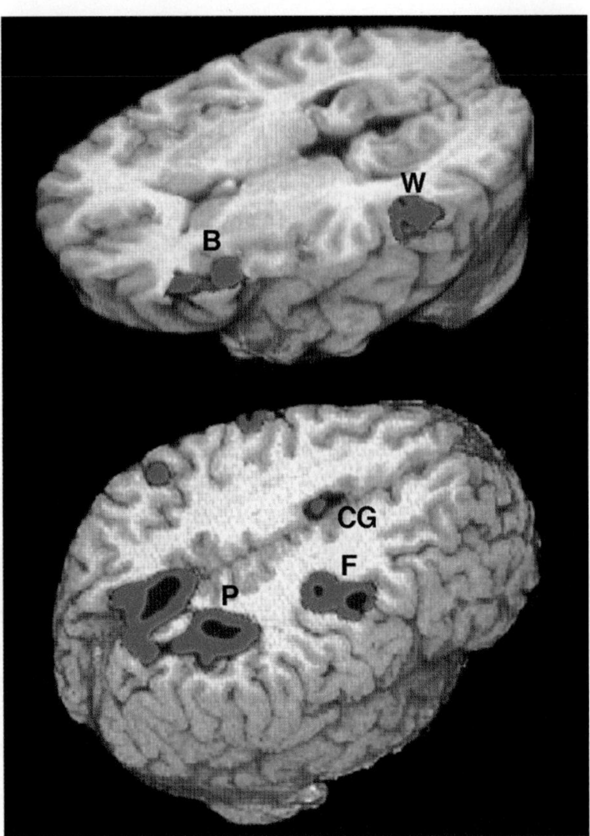

FIGURE 18-2
Functional magnetic resonance imaging of language and spatial attention in neurologically intact subjects. The red and black areas show regions of task-related significant activation. (*Top*) The subjects were asked to determine if two words were synonymous. This language task led to the simultaneous activation of the two epicenters of the language network, Broca's area (B) and Wernicke's area (W). The activations are exclusively in the left hemisphere. (*Bottom*) The subjects were asked to shift spatial attention to a peripheral target. This task led to the simultaneous activation of the three epicenters of the attentional network: the posterior parietal cortex (P), the frontal eye fields (F), and the cingulate gyrus (CG). The activations are predominantly in the right hemisphere. (*Courtesy of Darren Gitelman, MD; with permission*.)

THE PARIETOFRONTAL NETWORK FOR SPATIAL ORIENTATION: NEGLECT AND RELATED CONDITIONS

HEMISPATIAL NEGLECT

Adaptive orientation to significant events within the extrapersonal space is subserved by a large-scale network containing three major cortical components. The *cingulate cortex* provides access to a motivational mapping of the extrapersonal space, the *posterior parietal cortex* to a sensorimotor representation of salient extrapersonal events, and the *frontal eye fields* to motor strategies for attentional behaviors (Fig. 18-2). Subcortical components of this network include the striatum and the thalamus. Contralesional hemispatial neglect represents one outcome of damage to any of the cortical or subcortical components of this network. *The traditional view that hemispatial neglect always denotes a parietal lobe lesion is inaccurate.* In keeping with this anatomic organization, the clinical manifestations of neglect display three behavioral components: sensory events (or their mental representations) within the neglected hemispace have a lesser impact on overall awareness, there is a paucity of exploratory and orienting acts directed toward the neglected hemispace, and the patient behaves as if the neglected hemispace were motivationally devalued.

According to one model of spatial cognition, the right hemisphere directs attention within the *entire* extrapersonal space, whereas the left hemisphere directs attention mostly within the contralateral right hemispace. Consequently, unilateral left hemisphere lesions do not give rise to much contralesional neglect since the global attentional mechanisms of the right hemisphere can compensate for the loss of the *contralaterally* directed attentional functions of the left hemisphere. Unilateral right hemisphere lesions, however, give rise to severe contralesional left hemispatial neglect because the unaffected left hemisphere does not contain ipsilateral attentional mechanisms. This model is consistent with clinical experience, which shows that contralesional neglect is more common, severe, and lasting after damage to the right hemisphere than after damage to the left hemisphere. Severe neglect for the right hemispace is rare, even in left-handers with left hemisphere lesions.

Clinical examination

Patients with severe neglect may fail to dress, shave, or groom the left side of the body; fail to eat food placed on the left side of the tray; and fail to read the left half of sentences. When the examiner draws a large circle (12 to 15 cm [5 to 6 in.] in diameter) and asks the patient to place the numbers 1 to 12 as if the circle represented the face of a clock, there is a tendency to crowd the numbers on the right side and leave the left side empty. When asked to copy a simple line drawing, the patient fails to copy detail on the left, and when the patient is asked to write, there is a tendency to leave an unusually wide margin on the left.

Two bedside tests that are useful in assessing neglect are *simultaneous bilateral stimulation* and *visual target cancellation*. In the former, the examiner provides either unilateral or simultaneous bilateral stimulation in the visual, auditory, and tactile modalities. After right hemisphere injury, patients who have no difficulty detecting unilateral stimuli on either side experience the bilaterally presented stimulus as coming only from the right. This phenomenon is known as *extinction* and is a manifestation of the sensory-representational aspect of hemispatial neglect. In the target detection task, targets (e.g., A's) are interspersed with foils (e.g., other letters of the alphabet) on a 21.5- to 28.0-cm (8.5 to 11 in.) sheet of paper, and the patient is asked to circle all the targets. A failure to detect targets on the left is a manifestation of the exploratory deficit in hemispatial neglect (Fig. 18-3*A*). Hemianopia is not by itself sufficient to cause the target detection failure since the patient is free to turn the head and eyes to the left. Target detection failures therefore reflect a distortion of spatial attention, not just of sensory input. The normal tendency in target detection tasks is to start from the left upper quadrant and move systematically in horizontal or vertical sweeps. Some patients show a tendency to start the process from the right and proceed in a haphazard fashion. This represents a subtle manifestation of left neglect even if the patient eventually manages to detect all the appropriate targets. Some patients with neglect also may deny the existence of hemiparesis and may even deny ownership of the paralyzed limb, a condition known as *anosognosia*.

BÁLINT'S SYNDROME, SIMULTANAGNOSIA, DRESSING APRAXIA, AND CONSTRUCTION APRAXIA

Bilateral involvement of the network for spatial attention, especially its parietal components, leads to a state of severe spatial disorientation known as *Bálint's syndrome*. Bálint's syndrome involves deficits in the orderly visuomotor scanning of the environment (*oculomotor apraxia*) and in accurate manual reaching toward visual targets (*optic ataxia*). The third and most dramatic component of Bálint's syndrome is known as *simultanagnosia* and reflects an inability to integrate visual information in the center of gaze with more peripheral information. The patient gets stuck on the detail that falls in the center of gaze without attempting to scan the visual environment for additional information. A patient with simultanagnosia "misses the forest for the trees." Complex visual scenes cannot be grasped in their entirety, leading to severe limitations in the visual identification of objects and scenes. For example, a patient who is shown a table lamp and asked to name the object may look at its circular base and call it an ashtray. Some patients with simultanagnosia report that objects they look at may vanish suddenly, probably indicating an inability to look back at the original point of gaze after brief saccadic displacements. Movement and distracting stimuli greatly exacerbate the difficulties of visual perception. Simultanagnosia sometimes can occur without the other two components of Bálint's syndrome.

A modification of the letter cancellation task described earlier can be used for the bedside diagnosis of simultanagnosia. In this modification, some of the targets (e.g., A's) are made to be much larger than the others (7.5 to 10 cm vs. 2.5 cm [3 to 4 in. vs. 1 in.] in height), and all targets are embedded among foils. Patients with simultanagnosia display a counterintuitive but characteristic tendency to miss the larger targets (Fig. 18-3*B*). This occurs because the information needed for the identification of the larger targets cannot be confined to the immediate line of gaze and requires the integration of visual information across a more extensive field of view. The greater difficulty in the detection of the larger targets also indicates that poor acuity is not responsible for the impairment of visual function and that the problem is central rather than peripheral.

Another manifestation of bilateral (or right-sided) dorsal parietal lobe lesions is *dressing apraxia*. A patient with this condition is unable to align the body axis with the axis of the garment and can be seen struggling as he or she holds a coat from its bottom or extends his or her arm into a fold of the garment rather than into its sleeve. Lesions that involve the posterior parietal cortex also lead to severe difficulties in copying simple line drawings. This is known as a *construction apraxia* and

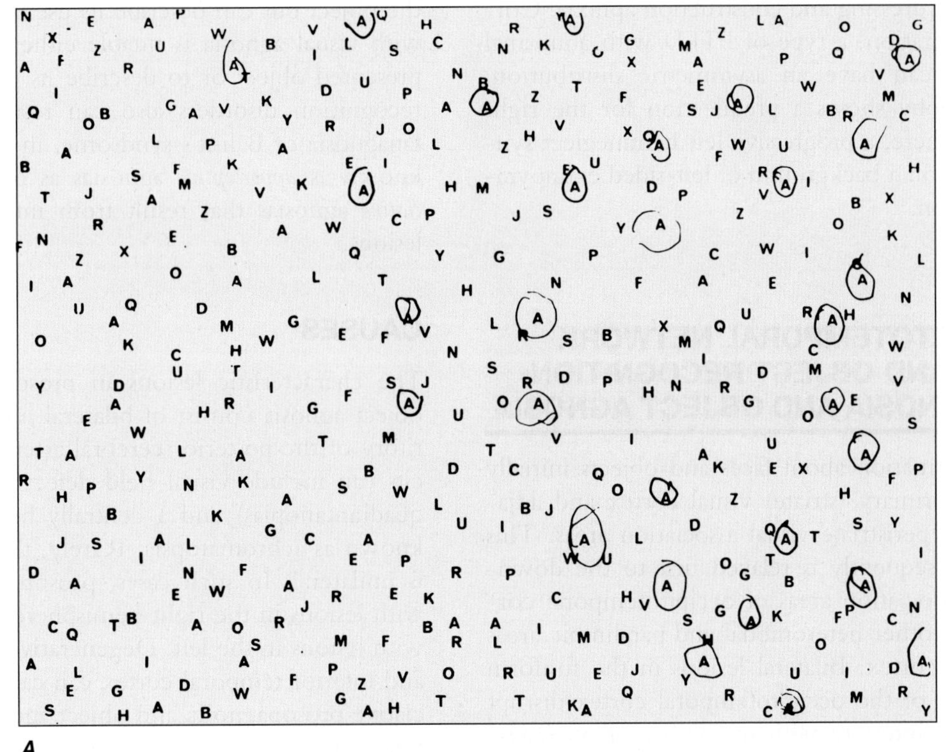

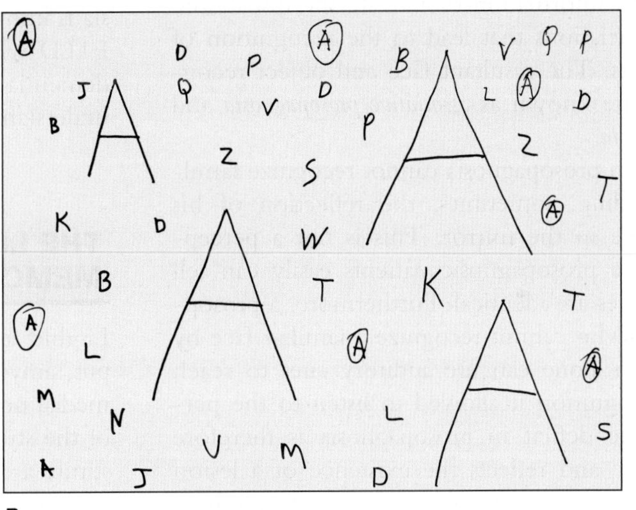

FIGURE 18-3
A. A 47-year-old man with a large frontoparietal lesion in the right hemisphere was asked to circle all the A's. Only targets on the right are circled. This is a manifestation of left hemispatial neglect. ***B.*** A 70-year-old woman with a 2-year history of degenerative dementia was able to circle most of the small targets but ignored the larger ones. This is a manifestation of simultanagnosia.

is much more severe if the lesion is in the right hemisphere. In some patients with right hemisphere lesions, the drawing difficulties are confined to the left side of the figure and represent a manifestation of hemispatial neglect; in others, there is a more universal deficit in reproducing contours and three-dimensional perspective. Dressing apraxia and construction apraxia represent special instances of a more general disturbance in spatial orientation.

Causes of spatial disorientation

Cerebrovascular lesions and neoplasms in the right hemisphere are the most common causes of hemispatial neglect. Depending on the site of the lesion, a patient with neglect also may have hemiparesis, hemihypesthesia, and hemianopia on the left, but these are not invariant findings. The majority of these patients display considerable improvement of hemispatial neglect, usually within the first several weeks. Bálint's syndrome results from bilateral dorsal parietal lesions; common settings include watershed infarction between the middle and posterior cerebral artery territories, hypoglycemia, and sagittal sinus thrombosis.

A progressive form of spatial disorientation known as the *posterior cortical atrophy* syndrome most commonly represents a variant of Alzheimer's disease with unusual concentrations of neurofibrillary degeneration in the parieto-occipital cortex and the superior colliculus. The patient displays a progressive Bálint's syndrome, usually accompanied by dressing and construction apraxia. Corticobasal degeneration, a type of FTLD with abnormal tau inclusions, can have an asymmetric distribution. When the atrophy shows a predilection for the right cerebral hemisphere, a progressive left hemineglect syndrome emerges on a background of left-sided extrapyramidal dysfunction.

THE OCCIPITOTEMPORAL NETWORK FOR FACE AND OBJECT RECOGNITION: PROSOPAGNOSIA AND OBJECT AGNOSIA

Perceptual information about faces and objects initially is encoded in primary (striate) visual cortex and adjacent (upstream) peristriate visual association areas. This information subsequently is relayed first to the downstream visual association areas of occipitotemporal cortex and then to other heteromodal and paralimbic areas of the cerebral cortex. Bilateral lesions in the fusiform and lingual gyri of the occipitotemporal cortex disrupt this process and interfere with the ability of otherwise intact perceptual information to activate the distributed multimodal associations that lead to the recognition of faces and objects. The resultant face and object recognition deficits are known as *associative prosopagnosia* and *visual object agnosia*.

A patient with prosopagnosia cannot recognize familiar faces, including, sometimes, the reflection of his or her own face in the mirror. This is not a perceptual deficit since prosopagnosic patients easily can tell whether two faces are identical. Furthermore, a prosopagnosic patient who cannot recognize a familiar face by visual inspection alone can use auditory cues to reach appropriate recognition if allowed to listen to the person's voice. The deficit in prosopagnosia is therefore modality-specific and reflects the existence of a lesion that prevents the activation of otherwise intact multimodal templates by relevant visual input. The deficit in prosopagnosia is not limited to the recognition of faces but also can extend to the recognition of individual members of larger generic object groups. For example, prosopagnosic patients characteristically have no difficulty with the generic identification of a face as a face or a car as a car, but they cannot recognize the identity of an individual face or the make of an individual car. This reflects a visual recognition deficit for proprietary features that characterize individual members of an object class. When recognition problems become more generalized and extend to the generic identification of common objects, the condition is known as *visual object agnosia*. In contrast to prosopagnosic patients, those with object agnosia cannot recognize a face as a face or a car as a car. It is important to distinguish visual object agnosia from anomia. A patient with anomia cannot name the object but can describe its use. In contrast, a patient with visual agnosia is unable either to name a visually presented object or to describe its use. Face and object recognition disorders also can result from the simultanagnosia of Bálint's syndrome, in which case they are known as *apperceptive* agnosias as opposed to the *associative* agnosias that result from inferior temporal lobe lesions.

CAUSES

The characteristic lesions in prosopagnosia and visual object agnosia consist of bilateral infarctions in the territory of the posterior cerebral arteries. Associated deficits can include visual field defects (especially superior quadrantanopias) and a centrally based color blindness known as achromatopsia. Rarely, the responsible lesion is unilateral. In such cases, prosopagnosia is associated with lesions in the right hemisphere, and object agnosia with lesions in the left. Degenerative diseases of anterior and inferior temporal cortex can cause progressive associative prosopagnosia and object agnosia. The combination of progressive associative agnosia and a fluent aphasia is known as *semantic dementia* and usually is caused by FTLD with TDP-43 inclusions. Patients with semantic dementia fail to recognize faces and objects and cannot understand the meaning of words denoting objects.

THE LIMBIC NETWORK FOR EPISODIC MEMORY: AMNESIAS

Limbic and paralimbic areas (such as the hippocampus, amygdala, and entorhinal cortex), the anterior and medial nuclei of the thalamus, the medial and basal parts of the striatum, and the hypothalamus collectively constitute a distributed network known as the *limbic system*. The behavioral affiliations of this network include the coordination of emotion, motivation, autonomic tone, and endocrine function. An additional area of specialization for the limbic network and the one that is of most relevance to clinical practice is that of declarative (conscious) memory for recent episodes and experiences. A disturbance in this function is known as an *amnestic state*. In the absence of deficits in motivation, attention, language, or visuospatial function, the clinical diagnosis of a persistent global amnestic state is always associated with bilateral damage to the limbic network, usually within the hippocampo-entorhinal complex or the thalamus.

Although the limbic network is the site of damage for amnestic states, it is almost certainly not the storage site for memories. Memories are stored in widely distributed form throughout the cerebral cortex. The role attributed to the limbic network is to bind these distributed fragments into coherent events and experiences that can sustain conscious recall. Damage to the limbic network does not necessarily destroy memories but interferes with their conscious (declarative) recall in coherent form. The individual fragments of information remain preserved despite the limbic lesions and can sustain what is known as *implicit memory*. For example, patients with amnestic states can acquire new motor or perceptual skills even though they may have no conscious knowledge of the experiences that led to the acquisition of these skills.

The memory disturbance in the amnestic state is multimodal and includes retrograde and anterograde components. The *retrograde amnesia* involves an inability to recall experiences that occurred before the onset of the amnestic state. Relatively recent events are more vulnerable to retrograde amnesia than are more remote and more extensively consolidated events. A patient who comes to the emergency room complaining that he cannot remember his or her identity but can remember the events of the previous day almost certainly does not have a neurologic cause of memory disturbance. The second and most important component of the amnestic state is the *anterograde amnesia*, which indicates an inability to store, retain, and recall new knowledge. Patients with amnestic states cannot remember what they ate a few minutes ago or the details of an important event they may have experienced a few hours ago. In the acute stages, there also may be a tendency to fill in memory gaps with inaccurate, fabricated, and often implausible information. This is known as *confabulation*. Patients with the amnestic syndrome forget that they forget and tend to deny the existence of a memory problem when questioned.

CLINICAL EXAMINATION

A patient with an amnestic state is almost always disoriented, especially to time. Accurate temporal orientation and accurate knowledge of current news rule out a major amnestic state. The anterograde component of an amnestic state can be tested with a list of four to five words read aloud by the examiner up to five times or until the patient can immediately repeat the entire list without an intervening delay. In the next phase of testing, the patient is allowed to concentrate on the words and rehearse them internally for 1 min before being asked to recall them. Accurate performance in this phase indicates that the patient is motivated and sufficiently attentive to hold the words online for at least 1 min. The final phase of the testing involves a retention period of 5 to 10 min during which the patient is engaged in other tasks. Adequate recall at the end of this interval requires offline storage, retention, and retrieval. Amnestic patients fail this phase of the task and may even forget that they were given a list of words to remember. Accurate recognition of the words by multiple choice in a patient who cannot recall them indicates a less severe memory disturbance that affects mostly the retrieval stage of memory. The retrograde component of an amnesia can be assessed with questions related to autobiographical or historic events. The anterograde component of amnestic states is usually much more prominent than the retrograde component. In rare instances, usually associated with temporal lobe epilepsy or benzodiazepine intake, the retrograde component may dominate.

The assessment of memory can be quite challenging. Bedside evaluations may detect only the most severe impairments. Less severe memory impairments, as in the case of patients with temporal lobe epilepsy, mild head injury, or early dementia, require quantitative evaluations by neuropsychologists. Confusional states caused by toxic-metabolic encephalopathies and some types of frontal lobe damage interfere with attentional capacity and lead to secondary memory impairments, even in the absence of any limbic lesions. This sort of memory impairment can be differentiated from the amnestic state by the presence of additional impairments in the attention-related tasks described in the section on the frontal lobes.

CAUSES, INCLUDING ALZHEIMER'S DISEASE

Many neurologic diseases can give rise to an amnestic state. They include tumors (of the sphenoid wing, posterior corpus callosum, thalamus, or medial temporal lobe), infarctions (in the territories of the anterior or posterior cerebral arteries), head trauma, herpes simplex encephalitis, Wernicke-Korsakoff encephalopathy, paraneoplastic limbic encephalitis, and degenerative dementias such as Alzheimer's disease and Pick's disease. The one common denominator of all these diseases is the presence of bilateral lesions within one or more components in the limbic network. Occasionally, unilateral left-sided hippocampal lesions can give rise to an amnestic state, but the memory disorder tends to be transient. Depending on the nature and distribution of the underlying neurologic disease, the patient also may have visual field deficits, eye movement limitations, or cerebellar findings.

Alzheimer's disease (AD) and its prodromal state of mild cognitive impairment (MCI) are the most common causes of progressive memory impairments. Temporal disorientation and poor recall of recent conversations are early manifestations. The predilection of the entorhinal cortex and hippocampus for early neurofibrillary degeneration in the MCI-AD spectrum is responsible for the initially selective impairment of episodic memory. In time, a full amnestic state emerges, but usually with additional impairments in language, attention, and visuospatial skills as the neurofibrillary degeneration spreads to additional neocortical areas.

Transient global amnesia is a distinctive syndrome usually seen in late middle age. Patients become acutely disoriented and repeatedly ask who they are, where they are, and what they are doing. The spell is characterized by anterograde amnesia (inability to retain new information) and a retrograde amnesia for relatively recent events that occurred before the onset. The syndrome usually resolves within 24 to 48 h and is followed by the filling in of the period affected by the retrograde amnesia, although there is persistent loss of memory for the events that occurred during the ictus. Recurrences are noted in approximately 20% of patients. Migraine, temporal lobe seizures, and perfusion abnormalities in the posterior cerebral territory have been postulated as causes of transient global amnesia. The absence of associated neurologic findings occasionally may lead to the incorrect diagnosis of a psychiatric disorder.

THE PREFRONTAL NETWORK FOR ATTENTION AND BEHAVIOR

Approximately one-third of all the cerebral cortex in the human brain is situated in the frontal lobes. The frontal lobes can be subdivided into motor-premotor, dorsolateral prefrontal, medial prefrontal, and orbitofrontal components. The terms *frontal lobe syndrome* and *prefrontal cortex* refer only to the last three of these four components. These are the parts of the cerebral cortex that show the greatest phylogenetic expansion in primates, especially in humans. The dorsolateral prefrontal, medial prefrontal, and orbitofrontal areas, along with the subcortical structures with which they are interconnected (i.e., the head of the caudate and the dorsomedial nucleus of the thalamus), collectively make up a large-scale network that coordinates exceedingly complex aspects of human cognition and behavior.

The prefrontal network plays an important role in behaviors that require multitasking and the integration of thought with emotion. Its integrity appears important for the simultaneous awareness of context, options, consequences, relevance, and emotional impact that allows the formulation of adaptive inferences, decisions, and actions. Damage to this part of the brain impairs mental flexibility, reasoning, hypothesis formation, abstract thinking, foresight, judgment, the online (attentive) holding of information, and the ability to inhibit inappropriate responses. Cognitive operations impaired by prefrontal cortex lesions often are referred to as "executive functions."

Even very large bilateral prefrontal lesions may leave all sensory, motor, and basic cognitive functions intact while leading to isolated but dramatic alterations of personality and behavior. The most common clinical manifestations of damage to the prefrontal network take the form of two relatively distinct syndromes. In the *frontal abulic syndrome*, the patient shows a loss of initiative, creativity, and curiosity and displays a pervasive emotional blandness and apathy. In the *frontal disinhibition syndrome*, the patient becomes socially disinhibited and shows severe impairments of judgment, insight, and foresight. The dissociation between intact intellectual function and a total lack of even rudimentary common sense is striking. Despite the preservation of all essential memory functions, the patient cannot learn from experience and continues to display inappropriate behaviors without appearing to feel emotional pain, guilt, or regret when those behaviors repeatedly lead to disastrous consequences. The impairments may emerge only in real-life situations when behavior is under minimal external control and may not be apparent within the structured environment of the medical office. Testing judgment by asking patients what they would do if they detected a fire in a theater or found a stamped and addressed envelope on the road is not very informative since patients who answer these questions wisely in the office may still act very foolishly in the more complex real-life setting. The physician must therefore be prepared to make a diagnosis of frontal lobe disease on the basis of historic information alone even when the mental state is quite intact in the office examination.

CLINICAL EXAMINATION

The emergence of developmentally primitive reflexes, also known as frontal release signs, such as grasping (elicited by stroking the palm) and sucking (elicited by stroking the lips) are seen primarily in patients with large structural lesions that extend into the premotor components of the frontal lobes or in the context of metabolic encephalopathies. The vast majority of patients with prefrontal lesions and frontal lobe behavioral syndromes do not display these reflexes.

Damage to the frontal lobe disrupts a variety of attention-related functions, including working memory (the transient online holding of information), concentration span, the scanning and retrieval of stored information, the inhibition of immediate but inappropriate responses, and mental flexibility. The capacity for focusing on a trend of thought and the ability to shift the focus of attention voluntarily from one thought or stimulus to another can become impaired. Digit span (which should be seven forward and five reverse) is decreased; the recitation of the months of the year in reverse order (which should take less than 15 s) is slowed; and the fluency in producing words starting with the letter a, f, or s that can be generated in 1 min (normally ≥ 12 per letter) is diminished even in nonaphasic patients. Characteristically, there is a progressive slowing of performance as the task proceeds; e.g., a patient asked to count backward by threes may say "100, 97, 94,...91,...88," etc., and may not complete the task. In "go–no go" tasks (where the instruction is to raise the finger upon hearing one tap but keep it still upon hearing two taps), the patient shows a characteristic inability to keep still in response to the "no go" stimulus. Mental flexibility (tested by the ability to shift from one criterion to another in sorting or matching tasks) is impoverished; distractibility by irrelevant stimuli is increased; and there is a pronounced tendency for impersistence and perseveration.

These attentional deficits disrupt the orderly registration and retrieval of new information and lead to *secondary* memory deficits. Those memory deficits can be differentiated from the *primary* memory impairments of the amnestic state by showing that they improve when the attentional load of the task is decreased. Working memory (also known as immediate memory) is an attentional function based on the temporary online holding of information. It is closely associated with the integrity of the prefrontal network and the ascending reticular activating system. Retentive memory, in contrast, depends on the stable (offline) storage of information and is associated with the integrity of the limbic network. The distinction of the underlying neural mechanisms is illustrated by the observation that severely amnestic patients who cannot remember events that occurred a few minutes ago may have intact if not superior working memory capacity as shown in tests of digit span.

CAUSES: TRAUMA, NEOPLASM, AND FRONTOTEMPORAL DEMENTIA

The abulic syndrome tends to be associated with damage in dorsal prefrontal cortex, and the disinhibition syndrome with damage in ventral prefrontal cortex. These syndromes tend to arise almost exclusively after bilateral lesions. Unilateral lesions confined to the prefrontal cortex may remain silent until the pathology spreads to the other side; this explains why thromboembolic CVA is an unusual cause of the frontal lobe syndrome. Common settings for frontal lobe syndromes include head trauma, ruptured aneurysms, hydrocephalus, tumors (including metastases, glioblastoma, and falx or olfactory groove meningiomas), and focal degenerative diseases. A major clinical form of FTLD known as the behavioral variant of frontotemporal dementia (bvFTD) causes a progressive frontal lobe syndrome that can start as early as the fifth decade of life. In these patients, the anterior temporal lobe and caudate nucleus are also atrophic. The behavioral changes can include shoplifting, compulsive gambling, sexual indiscretions, and obsessive-compulsive preoccupations, arising on a background of indifference. In many patients with Alzheimer's disease, neurofibrillary degeneration eventually spreads to prefrontal cortex and gives rise to components of the frontal lobe syndrome, but almost always on a background of severe memory impairment.

Lesions in the caudate nucleus or in the dorsomedial nucleus of the thalamus (subcortical components of the prefrontal network) also can produce a frontal lobe syndrome. This is one reason why the changes in mental state associated with degenerative basal ganglia diseases such as Parkinson's disease and Huntington's disease may take the form of a frontal lobe syndrome. Because of its widespread connections with other regions of association cortex, one essential computational role of the prefrontal network is to function as an integrator, or "orchestrator," for other networks. Bilateral multifocal lesions of the cerebral hemispheres, none of which are individually large enough to cause specific cognitive deficits such as aphasia and neglect, can collectively interfere with the connectivity and integrating function of the prefrontal cortex. A frontal lobe syndrome is the single most common behavioral profile associated with a variety of bilateral multifocal brain diseases, including metabolic encephalopathy, multiple sclerosis, and vitamin B_{12} deficiency, among others. Many patients with the clinical diagnosis of a frontal lobe syndrome tend to have lesions that do not involve prefrontal cortex but involve either the subcortical components of the prefrontal network or its connections with other parts of the brain. To avoid making a diagnosis of "frontal lobe syndrome" in a patient with no evidence of frontal cortex disease, it is advisable to use the diagnostic term *frontal network syndrome*, with the understanding that the responsible lesions can lie anywhere within this distributed network.

A patient with frontal lobe disease raises potential dilemmas in differential diagnosis: the abulia and blandness may be misinterpreted as depression, and the disinhibition as idiopathic mania or acting out. Appropriate intervention may be delayed while a treatable tumor keeps expanding. An informed approach to frontal lobe disease and its behavioral manifestations may help prevent such errors.

CARING FOR PATIENTS WITH DEFICITS OF HIGHER CEREBRAL FUNCTION

Some of the deficits described in this chapter are so complex that they may bewilder not only the patient and family but also the physician. It is imperative to carry out a systematic clinical evaluation to characterize the nature of the deficits and explain them in lay terms to the patient and family. Such an explanation can allay at least some of the anxieties, address the mistaken impression that the deficit (e.g., social disinhibition or inability to recognize family members) is psychologically motivated, and lead to practical suggestions for daily living activities. The consultation of a skilled neuropsychologist may aid in the formulation of diagnosis and management. Patients with simultanagnosia, for example, may benefit from the counterintuitive instruction to stand back when they cannot find an item so that a greater search area falls within the immediate field of gaze. Some patients with frontal lobe disease can be extremely irritable and abusive to spouses yet display all the appropriate social graces during a visit to the medical office. In such cases, the history may be more important than the bedside examination in charting a course of treatment.

Reactive depression is common in patients with higher cerebral dysfunction and should be treated. These patients may be overly sensitive to the usual doses of antidepressants or anxiolytics and require a careful titration of dosage. Brain damage may cause a dissociation between feeling states and their expression so that a patient who may superficially appear jocular could still be suffering from an underlying depression that needs to be treated. In many cases, agitation may be controlled with reassurance. In other cases, treatment with benzodiazepines, antiepilectics, or sedating antidepressants may become necessary. If neuroleptics become absolutely necessary for the control of agitation, atypical neuroleptics are preferable because of their lower extrapyramidal side effects. Treatment with neuroleptics in elderly patients with dementia requires weighing the potential benefits against the potentially serious side effects.

Spontaneous improvement of cognitive deficits due to acute neurologic lesions is common. It is most rapid in the first few weeks but may continue for up to 2 years, especially in young individuals with single brain lesions. The mechanisms for this recovery are incompletely understood. Some of the initial deficits appear to arise from remote dysfunction (diaschisis) in parts of the brain that are interconnected with the site of initial injury. Improvement in these patients may reflect, at least in part, a normalization of the remote dysfunction. Other mechanisms may involve functional reorganization in surviving neurons adjacent to the injury or the compensatory use of homologous structures, e.g., the right superior temporal gyrus with recovery from Wernicke's aphasia. In some patients with large lesions involving Broca's and Wernicke's areas, only Wernicke's area may show contralateral compensatory reorganization (or bilateral functionality), giving rise to a situation in which a lesion that should have caused a global aphasia becomes associated with a residual Broca's aphasia. Prognosis for recovery from aphasia is best when Wernicke's area is spared. Cognitive rehabilitation procedures have been used in the treatment of higher cortical deficits. There are few controlled studies, but some show a benefit of rehabilitation in the recovery from hemispatial neglect and aphasia. Some types of deficits may be more prone to recovery than others. For example, patients with CVA and nonfluent aphasias are more likely to benefit from speech therapy than are patients with fluent aphasias and comprehension deficits. In general, lesions that lead to a denial of illness (e.g., anosognosia) are associated with cognitive deficits that are more resistant to rehabilitation. Periodic neuropsychological assessment is necessary for quantifying the pace of the improvement (or of the progression in the case of dementias) and for generating specific recommendations for cognitive rehabilitation, modifications in the home environment, the timetable for returning to work in patients recovering from acute lesions, and the scheduling of retirement or disability status in patients with degenerative diseases. Determining driving competence is challenging, especially in the early stages of dementing diseases. The diagnosis of a neurodegenerative disease is not by itself sufficient for asking the patient to stop driving. An on-the-road driving test and reports from family members may help time decisions related to this very important activity.

There is a mistaken belief that dementias are anatomically diffuse and that they cause global cognitive impairments. This is true only at the terminal stages. During most of the clinical course, dementias are exquisitely selective with respect to anatomy and cognitive pattern. Alzheimer's disease, for example, causes the greatest destruction in medial temporal areas belonging to the memory network and is clinically characterized by a correspondingly severe amnesia. There are other dementias in which memory is intact. Selective degeneration of the frontal lobes in FTLD leads to a gradual dissolution of behavior and executive functions. Primary progressive aphasia is characterized by a gradual atrophy of the left perisylvian language network and a selective dissolution of language that can remain isolated for up to 10 years. An enlightened approach to the differential diagnosis and to the individualized care of patients with acute and progressive damage to the cerebral cortex requires an understanding of the principles that link neural networks to higher cerebral functions.

CHAPTER 19

VIDEO ATLAS: PRIMARY PROGRESSIVE APHASIA, MEMORY LOSS, AND OTHER FOCAL CEREBRAL DISORDERS

Maria Luisa Gorno-Tempini ■ Jennifer Ogar ■ Joel Kramer ■ Bruce L. Miller ■ Gil Rabinovici ■ Maria Carmela Tartaglia

Language and memory are essential human functions. For the experienced clinician, the recognition of different types of language and memory disturbances often provides essential clues to the anatomic localization and diagnosis of neurologic disorders. This video illustrates classic disorders of language and speech (including the aphasias), memory (the amnesias), and other disorders of cognition that are commonly encountered in clinical practice. Videos for this chapter can be accessed at the following link: http://www.mhprofessional.com/mediacenter/.

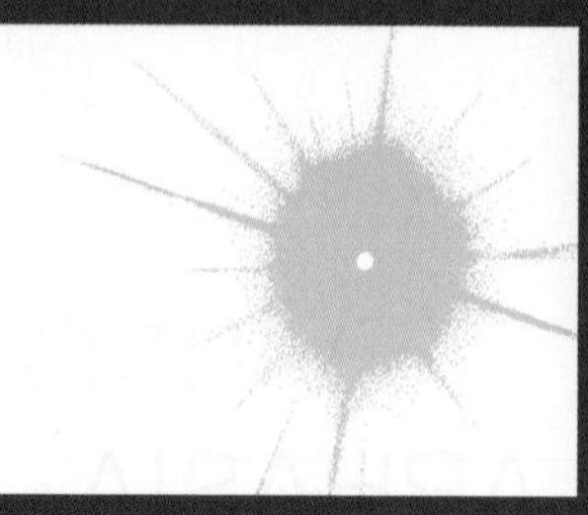

CHAPTER 20
SLEEP DISORDERS

Charles A. Czeisler ■ John W. Winkelman ■ Gary S. Richardson

Disturbed sleep is among the most frequent health complaints physicians encounter. More than one-half of adults in the United States experience at least intermittent sleep disturbance. For most, it is an occasional night of poor sleep or daytime sleepiness. However, the Institute of Medicine has estimated that 50–70 million Americans suffer from a chronic disorder of sleep and wakefulness, which can lead to serious impairment of daytime functioning. In addition, such problems may contribute to or exacerbate medical or psychiatric conditions. Thirty years ago, many such complaints were treated with hypnotic medications without further diagnostic evaluation. Since then, a distinct class of sleep and arousal disorders has been identified.

PHYSIOLOGY OF SLEEP AND WAKEFULNESS

Given the opportunity, most adults will sleep 7–8 h per night, although the timing, duration, and internal structure of sleep vary among healthy individuals and as a function of age. At the extremes, infants and the elderly have frequent interruptions of sleep. In the United States, adults tend to have one consolidated sleep episode per day, although in some cultures sleep may be divided into a mid-afternoon nap and a shortened night sleep. Two principal neural systems govern the expression of the sleep and wakefulness states within the daily cycle. The first potentiates sleep in proportion to the duration of wakefulness (the "sleep homeostat"), while the second rhythmically modulates sleep and wakefulness tendencies at appropriate phases of the 24-h day (the circadian clock). Intrinsic abnormalities in the function of either of these systems, or extrinsic disturbances (environmental, drug- or illness-related) that supersede their normal expression, can lead to clinically recognizable sleep disorders.

STATES AND STAGES OF SLEEP

States and stages of human sleep are defined on the basis of characteristic patterns in the electroencephalogram (EEG), the electrooculogram (EOG—a measure of eye-movement activity), and the surface electromyogram (EMG) measured on the chin and neck. The continuous recording of this array of electrophysiologic parameters to define sleep and wakefulness is termed *polysomnography*.

Polysomnographic profiles define two states of sleep: (1) rapid-eye-movement (REM) sleep and (2) non-rapid-eye-movement (NREM) sleep. NREM sleep is further subdivided into three stages, characterized by increasing arousal threshold and slowing of the cortical EEG. REM sleep is characterized by a low-amplitude, mixed-frequency EEG similar to that of NREM stage N1 sleep. The EOG shows bursts of REM similar to those seen during eyes-open wakefulness. Chin EMG activity is absent, reflecting the brainstem-mediated muscle atonia that is characteristic of that state.

ORGANIZATION OF HUMAN SLEEP

Normal nocturnal sleep in adults displays a consistent organization from night to night (Fig. 20-1). After sleep onset, sleep usually progresses through NREM stages N1–N3 sleep within 45–60 min. Slow-wave sleep (NREM stage N3 sleep) predominates in the first third of the night and comprises 15–25% of total nocturnal sleep time in young adults. The percentage of slow-wave sleep is influenced by several factors, most notably age (see later). Prior sleep deprivation increases the rapidity of sleep onset and both the intensity and amount of slow-wave sleep.

The first REM sleep episode usually occurs in the second hour of sleep. More rapid onset of REM sleep in an adult (particularly if <30 min) may suggest pathology such as endogenous depression, narcolepsy,

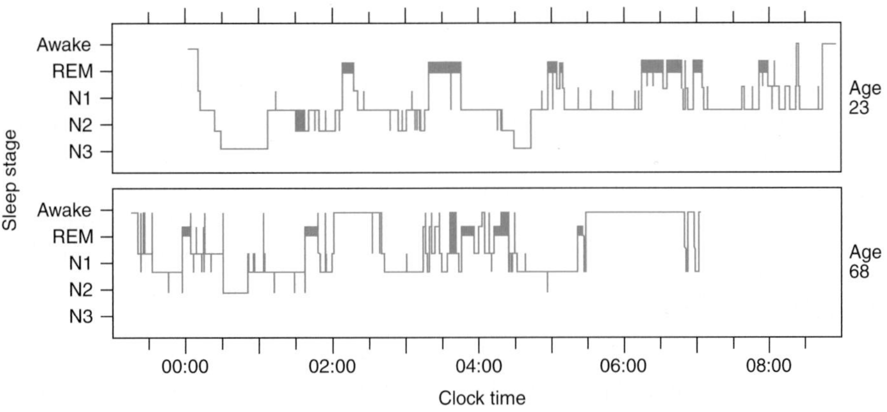

FIGURE 20-1
Stages of REM sleep (solid bars), the three stages of NREM sleep, and wakefulness over the course of the entire night for representative young and older adult men. Characteristic features of sleep in older people include reduction of slow-wave sleep, frequent spontaneous awakenings, early sleep onset, and early morning awakening. *(From the Division of Sleep Medicine, Brigham and Women's Hospital.)*

circadian rhythm disorders, or drug withdrawal. NREM and REM alternate through the night with an average period of 90–110 min (the "ultradian" sleep cycle). Overall, REM sleep constitutes 20–25% of total sleep, and NREM stages N1 and N2 are 50–60%.

Age has a profound impact on sleep state organization (Fig. 20-1). Slow-wave sleep is most intense and prominent during childhood, decreasing sharply coincident with puberty and across the second and third decades of life. After age 30, there is a continued decline in the amount of slow-wave sleep, and the amplitude of delta EEG activity comprising slow-wave sleep is profoundly reduced. The depth of slow-wave sleep, as measured by the arousal threshold to auditory stimulation, also decreases with age. In the otherwise healthy older person, slow-wave sleep may be completely absent, particularly in males. Paradoxically, older people are better able to tolerate acute sleep deprivation than young adults, maintaining reaction time and sustaining vigilance with fewer lapses of attention.

A different age profile exists for REM sleep than for slow-wave sleep. In infancy, REM sleep may comprise 50% of total sleep time, and the percentage is inversely proportional to developmental age. The amount of REM sleep falls off sharply over the first postnatal year as a mature REM-NREM cycle develops; thereafter, REM sleep occupies a relatively constant percentage of total sleep time.

NEUROANATOMY OF SLEEP

Experimental studies in animals have variously implicated the medullary reticular formation, the thalamus, and the basal forebrain in the generation of sleep, while the brainstem reticular formation, the midbrain, the subthalamus, the thalamus, and the basal forebrain have all been suggested to play a role in the generation of wakefulness or EEG arousal.

Current models suggest that the capacity for sleep and wakefulness generation is distributed along an axial "core" of neurons extending from the brainstem rostrally to the basal forebrain. A cluster of γ-aminobutyric acid (GABA) and galaninergic neurons in the ventrolateral preoptic (VLPO) hypothalamus is selectively activated coincident with sleep onset. These neurons project to and inhibit the multiple neural wakefulness centers that comprise the ascending arousal system, and selective cell-specific lesions of VLPO substantially reduce sleep time, indicating that the hypothalamic VLPO neurons play an executive role in sleep regulation. More recent data have identified another sleep center, the median preoptic nucleus (MnPOn) of the hypothalamus with similar activation patterns and projections, suggesting that, like that of wakefulness, executive control of sleep may also be multicentric.

Specific regions in the pons are associated with the neurophysiologic correlates of REM sleep. Small lesions in the dorsal pons result in the loss of the descending muscle inhibition normally associated with REM sleep; microinjections of the cholinergic agonist carbachol into the pontine reticular formation produce a state with all of the features of REM sleep. These experimental manipulations are mimicked by pathologic conditions in humans and animals. A prominent feature of narcolepsy, for example, is abrupt, complete, or partial paralysis (cataplexy) in response to a variety of stimuli, a pathologic activation of neural systems mediating the atonia of normal REM sleep. In narcoleptic dogs, physostigmine, a central cholinesterase inhibitor, increases the frequency of cataplexy episodes, while atropine decreases their frequency. Conversely, in REM sleep behavior disorder (see later), patients suffer from a failure of normal motor inhibition during REM sleep, resulting in involuntary, occasionally violent, movement arising out of dream episodes.

NEUROCHEMISTRY OF SLEEP

Early experimental studies that focused on the raphe nuclei of the brainstem appeared to implicate serotonin as the primary sleep-promoting neurotransmitter, while catecholamines were considered to be responsible for wakefulness. Simple neurochemical models have given way to more complex formulations involving multiple parallel waking systems. Pharmacologic studies suggest that histamine, acetylcholine, dopamine, serotonin, and noradrenaline are all involved in wake promotion. A novel neuropeptide, orexin (also known as hypocretin), localized to a cluster of neurons in the lateral hypothalamus and originally identified based on its pathogenic role in narcolepsy (see later), also appears to be involved in the control of wakefulness.

In the basal forebrain (BF), adenosine receptors on cholinergic neurons are thought to play a role in assessing homeostatic sleep need by providing an index of cellular energy status. Projections from these BF neurons to executive sleep centers such as VLPO thus allow incorporation of homeostatic sleep need into the control of sleep state expression. At a practical level, this model suggests that the alerting effects of caffeine, an adenosine receptor antagonist, reflect the attenuation of the homeostatic signal from the basal forebrain.

The prominent hypnotic effects of benzodiazepine receptor agonists suggest that endogenous ligands of this receptor may be involved in normal sleep physiology. While neurosteroids with activity at this receptor have been identified, their role in normal sleep-wake control remains unclear. In addition, a broad array of endogenous sleep- and wake-promoting substances have been identified, the role of which in normal sleep-wake control remains unclear. These include corticotropin-releasing hormone (CRH), prostaglandin D_2, delta sleep–inducing peptide, muramyl dipeptide, interleukin 1, fatty acid primary amides, and melatonin.

PHYSIOLOGY OF CIRCADIAN RHYTHMICITY

The sleep-wake cycle is the most evident of the many 24-h rhythms in humans. Prominent daily variations also occur in endocrine, thermoregulatory, cardiac, pulmonary, renal, gastrointestinal, and neurobehavioral functions. At the molecular level, endogenous circadian rhythmicity is driven by self-sustaining transcriptional/translational feedback loops (Fig. 20-2). In evaluating a daily variation in humans, it is important to distinguish between those rhythmic components passively evoked by periodic environmental or behavioral changes (e.g., the increase in blood pressure and heart rate that occurs upon assumption of the upright posture) and those actively driven by an endogenous oscillatory process (e.g., the circadian variation in plasma cortisol that persists under a variety of environmental and behavioral conditions).

While it is now recognized that many peripheral tissues in mammals have circadian clocks that regulate diverse physiologic processes, these independent tissue-specific oscillations are coordinated by a central neural pacemaker located in the suprachiasmatic nuclei (SCN)

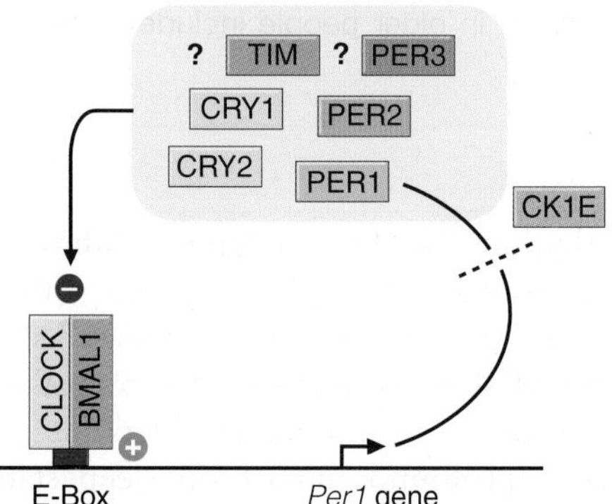

FIGURE 20-2

Model of the molecular feedback loop at the core of the mammalian circadian clock. The positive element of the feedback loop (+) is the transcriptional activation of the Per1 gene (and probably other clock genes) by a heterodimer of the transcription factors CLOCK and BMAL1 (also called MOP3) bound to an E-box DNA regulatory element. The Per1 transcript and its product, the clock component PER1 protein, accumulate in the cell cytoplasm. As it accumulates, the PER1 protein is recruited into a multiprotein complex thought to contain other circadian clock component proteins such as cryptochromes (CRYs), Period proteins (PERs), and others. This complex is then transported into the cell nucleus (across the dotted line), where it functions as the negative element in the feedback loop (–) by inhibiting the activity of the CLOCK-BMAL1 transcription factor heterodimer. As a consequence of this action, the concentration of PER1 and other clock proteins in the inhibitory complex falls, allowing CLOCK-BMAL1 to activate transcription of Per1 and other genes and begin another cycle. The dynamics of the 24-h molecular cycle are controlled at several levels, including regulation of the rate of PER protein degradation by casein kinase-1 epsilon (CK1E). Additional limbs of this genetic regulatory network, omitted for the sake of clarity, are thought to contribute stability. Question marks denote putative clock proteins, such as Timeless (TIM), as yet lacking genetic proof of a role in the mammalian clock mechanism. *(Copyright Charles J. Weitz, PhD, Department of Neurobiology, Harvard Medical School.)*

of the hypothalamus. Bilateral destruction of these nuclei results in a loss of the endogenous circadian rhythm of locomotor activity, which can be restored only by transplantation of the same structure from a donor animal. The genetically determined period of this endogenous neural oscillator, which averages ~24.2 h in humans, is normally synchronized to the 24-h period of the environmental light-dark cycle. Small differences in circadian period underlie variations in diurnal preference, with the circadian period shorter in individuals who typically rise early compared to those who typically go to bed late. Entrainment of mammalian circadian rhythms by the light-dark cycle is mediated via the retinohypothalamic tract, a monosynaptic pathway that links specialized, photoreceptive retinal ganglion cells directly to the SCN. Humans are exquisitely sensitive to the resetting effects of light, particularly the shorter wavelengths (~460–500 nm) of the visible spectrum.

The timing and internal architecture of sleep are directly coupled to the output of the endogenous circadian pacemaker. Paradoxically, the endogenous circadian rhythms of sleep tendency, sleepiness, and REM sleep propensity all peak near the habitual wake time, just after the nadir of the endogenous circadian temperature cycle, whereas the circadian wake propensity rhythm peaks 1–3 h before the habitual bedtime. These rhythms are thus timed to oppose the homeostatic decline of sleep tendency during the habitual sleep episode and the rise of sleep tendency throughout the usual waking day, respectively. Misalignment of the output of the endogenous circadian pacemaker with the desired sleep-wake cycle can, therefore, induce insomnia, decreased alertness, and impaired performance evident in night-shift workers and airline travelers.

BEHAVIORAL CORRELATES OF SLEEP STATES AND STAGES

Polysomnographic staging of sleep correlates with behavioral changes during specific states and stages. During the transitional state between wakefulness and sleep (stage N1 sleep), subjects may respond to faint auditory or visual signals without "awakening." Short-term memory incorporation is inhibited at the onset of NREM stage N1 sleep, which may explain why individuals aroused from that transitional sleep stage frequently deny having been asleep. Such transitions may intrude upon behavioral wakefulness after sleep deprivation, notwithstanding attempts to remain continuously awake (see "Shift-Work Disorder," later in this chapter).

Awakenings from REM sleep are associated with recall of vivid dream imagery >80% of the time. The reliability of dream recall increases with REM sleep episodes occurring later in the night. Imagery may also be reported after NREM sleep interruptions, though these typically lack the detail and vividness of REM sleep dreams. The incidence of NREM sleep dream recall can be increased by selective REM sleep deprivation, suggesting that REM sleep and dreaming per se are not inexorably linked.

PHYSIOLOGIC CORRELATES OF SLEEP STATES AND STAGES

All major physiologic systems are influenced by sleep. Changes in cardiovascular function include a decrease in blood pressure and heart rate during NREM and particularly during slow-wave sleep. During REM sleep, phasic activity (bursts of eye movements) is associated with variability in both blood pressure and heart rate mediated principally by the vagus nerve. Cardiac dysrhythmias may occur selectively during REM sleep. Respiratory function also changes. In comparison to relaxed wakefulness, respiratory rate becomes more regular during NREM sleep (especially slow-wave sleep) and tonic REM sleep and becomes very irregular during phasic REM sleep. Minute ventilation decreases in NREM sleep out of proportion to the decrease in metabolic rate at sleep onset, resulting in a higher PCO_2.

Endocrine function also varies with sleep. Slow-wave sleep is associated with secretion of growth hormone in men, while sleep in general is associated with augmented secretion of prolactin in both men and women. Sleep has a complex effect on the secretion of luteinizing hormone (LH): during puberty, sleep is associated with increased LH secretion, whereas sleep in the postpubertal female inhibits LH secretion in the early follicular phase of the menstrual cycle. Sleep onset (and probably slow-wave sleep) is associated with inhibition of thyroid-stimulating hormone and of the adrenocorticotropic hormone–cortisol axis, an effect that is superimposed on the prominent circadian rhythms in the two systems.

The pineal hormone melatonin is secreted predominantly at night in both day- and night-active species, reflecting the direct modulation of pineal activity by the circadian pacemaker through a circuitous neural pathway from the SCN to the pineal gland. Melatonin secretion is not dependent upon the occurrence of sleep, persisting in individuals kept awake at night. Secretion is inhibited by ambient light, an effect mediated by a neural connection from the retina via the SCN. The role of endogenous melatonin in normal sleep-wake regulation is unclear, but administration of exogenous melatonin can potentiate sleepiness and facilitate sleep onset when administered in the afternoon or evening, at a time when endogenous melatonin levels are low. The efficacy of melatonin as a sleep-promoting therapy for patients with insomnia is currently not known.

Sleep is also accompanied by alterations of thermoregulatory function. NREM sleep is associated with an attenuation of thermoregulatory responses to either heat or cold stress, and animal studies of thermosensitive neurons in the hypothalamus document an NREM-sleep-dependent reduction of the thermoregulatory set-point. REM sleep is associated with complete absence of thermoregulatory responsiveness, resulting in functional poikilothermy. However, the potential adverse impact of this failure of thermoregulation is blunted by inhibition of REM sleep by extreme ambient temperatures.

DISORDERS OF SLEEP AND WAKEFULNESS

APPROACH TO THE PATIENT Sleep Disorders

Patients may seek help from a physician because of one of several symptoms: (1) an acute or chronic inability to initiate or maintain sleep adequately at night (insomnia); (2) chronic fatigue, sleepiness, or tiredness during the day; or (3) a behavioral manifestation associated with sleep itself. The specific approach to an insomnia complaint will depend on the nature of comorbid medical or psychiatric disease, if present. In general, however, the insomnia complaint should be specifically addressed as soon as it is recognized. This more aggressive approach reflects growing evidence that chronic insomnia may contribute to comorbid disease processes. For example, specific management of symptomatic insomnia at the time of diagnosis of major depressive disorder (MDD) has been shown to positively impact the response to antidepressants. Evidence that insomnia and sleep loss affect the perception of pain suggests that a similar approach is warranted in acute and chronic pain management. In general, at least for chronic insomnia, there is little evidence justifying an expectant approach in which specific insomnia therapy is deferred while comorbid disease is first addressed.

Table 20-1 outlines the diagnostic and therapeutic approach to the patient with a complaint of excessive daytime sleepiness.

A careful history is essential. In particular, the duration, severity, and consistency of the symptoms are important, along with the patient's estimate of the consequences of the sleep disorder on waking function. Information from a friend or family member can be invaluable; some patients may be unaware of, or will underreport, such potentially embarrassing symptoms as heavy snoring or falling asleep while driving.

Patients with excessive sleepiness should be advised to avoid all driving until effective therapy has been achieved.

Completion by the patient of a day-by-day sleep-work-drug log for at least 2 weeks can help the physician better understand the nature of the complaint. Work times and sleep times (including daytime naps and nocturnal awakenings) as well as drug and alcohol use, including caffeine and hypnotics, should be noted each day.

Polysomnography is necessary for the diagnosis of specific disorders such as narcolepsy and sleep apnea and may be of utility in other settings as well.

EVALUATION OF INSOMNIA

Insomnia is the complaint of inadequate sleep; it can be classified according to the nature of sleep disruption and the duration of the complaint. Insomnia is subdivided into difficulty falling asleep (*sleep onset insomnia*), frequent or sustained awakenings (*sleep maintenance insomnia*), or early morning awakenings (*sleep offset insomnia*), though most insomnia patients present with two or more of these symptoms. Other insomnia patients present with persistent sleepiness/fatigue despite sleep of adequate duration (*nonrestorative sleep*). Similarly, the duration of the symptom influences diagnostic and therapeutic considerations. An insomnia complaint lasting one to several nights (within a single episode) is termed *transient insomnia* and is typically the result of situational stress or a change in sleep schedule or environment (e.g., jet lag disorder). *Short-term insomnia* lasts from a few days to 3 weeks. Disruption of this duration is usually associated with more protracted stress, such as recovery from surgery or short-term illness. *Long-term insomnia*, or *chronic insomnia*, lasts for months or years and, in contrast with short-term insomnia, requires a thorough evaluation of underlying causes (see later in this chapter). Chronic insomnia is often a waxing and waning disorder, with spontaneous or stressor-induced exacerbations.

An occasional night of poor sleep, typically in the setting of stress or excitement about external events, is both common and without lasting consequences. However, persistent insomnia can lead to impaired daytime function, injury due to accidents, and the development of major depression. In addition, there is emerging evidence that individuals with chronic insomnia have increased utilization of health care resources, even after controlling for comorbid medical and psychiatric disorders.

All insomnias can be exacerbated and perpetuated by behaviors that are not conducive to initiating or maintaining sleep. *Inadequate sleep hygiene* is characterized by a behavior pattern prior to sleep or a bedroom

TABLE 20-1

EVALUATION OF THE PATIENT WITH THE COMPLAINT OF EXCESSIVE DAYTIME SOMNOLENCE

FINDINGS ON HISTORY AND PHYSICAL EXAMINATION	DIAGNOSTIC EVALUATION	DIAGNOSIS	THERAPY
Obesity, snoring, hypertension	Polysomnography with respiratory monitoring	Obstructive sleep apnea	Continuous positive airway pressure; ENT surgery (e.g., uvulopalatopharyngoplasty); dental appliance; pharmacologic therapy (e.g., protriptyline); weight loss
Cataplexy, hypnogogic hallucinations, sleep paralysis, family history	Polysomnography with multiple sleep latency testing	Narcolepsy-cataplexy syndrome	Stimulants (e.g., modafinil, methylphenidate); REM-suppressant antidepressants (e.g., protriptyline); genetic counseling
Restless legs, disturbed sleep, predisposing medical condition (e.g., iron deficiency or renal failure)	Assessment for predisposing medical conditions	Restless legs syndrome	Treatment of predisposing condition, if possible; dopamine agonists (e.g., pramipexole, ropinirole)
Disturbed sleep, predisposing medical conditions (e.g., asthma), and/or predisposing medical therapies (e.g., theophylline)	Sleep-wake diary recording	Insomnias (see text)	Treatment of predisposing condition and/or change in therapy, if possible; behavioral therapy; short-acting benzodiazepine receptor agonist (e.g., zolpidem)

Abbreviations: EMG, electromyogram; ENT, ears, nose, throat; REM, rapid eye movement.

environment that is not conducive to sleep, or irregularity in the timing or duration of the nightly sleep episode. Noise, light, or technology (e.g., television, radio, cell phone, mobile email device or computer) in the bedroom can interfere with sleep, as can a bed partner with periodic limb movements during sleep or one who snores loudly. Clocks can heighten the anxiety about the time it has taken to fall asleep. Drugs that act on the central nervous system, large meals, vigorous exercise, or hot showers just before sleep may all interfere with sleep onset. Many individuals participate in stressful work-related activities in the evening, producing a state incompatible with sleep onset. In preference to hypnotic medications, patients should be counseled to avoid stressful activities before bed, develop a soporific bedtime ritual, and prepare and reserve the bedroom environment for sleeping. Consistent, regular bedtimes and rising times should be maintained daily, including weekends.

PRIMARY INSOMNIA

Many patients with chronic insomnia have no clear, single identifiable underlying cause for their difficulties with sleep. Rather, such patients often have multiple etiologies for their insomnia, which may evolve over the years. In addition, the chief sleep complaint may change over time, with initial insomnia predominating at one point, and multiple awakenings or nonrestorative sleep occurring at other times. Subsyndromal psychiatric disorders (e.g., anxiety and mood complaints), negative conditioning to the sleep environment (psychophysiologic insomnia, see next), amplification of the time spent awake (paradoxical insomnia), physiologic hyperarousal, and poor sleep hygiene (see earlier) may all be present. As these processes may be both causes and consequences of chronic insomnia, many individuals will have a progressive course to their symptoms in which the severity is proportional to the chronicity, and much of the complaint may persist even after effective treatment of the initial inciting etiology. Treatment of insomnia is often directed to each of the putative contributing factors: behavior therapies for anxiety and negative conditioning (see later), pharmacotherapy and/or psychotherapy for mood/anxiety disorders, and an emphasis on maintenance of good sleep hygiene.

If insomnia persists after treatment of these contributing factors, empirical pharmacotherapy is often used on a nightly or intermittent basis. A variety of sedative compounds are used for this purpose. Alcohol and antihistamines are the most commonly used nonprescription sleep aids. The former may help with sleep onset but is associated with sleep disruption during the night and can escalate into abuse, dependence, and withdrawal in the predisposed individual. Antihistamines, which are the primary active ingredient in most over-the-counter sleep aids, may be of benefit when used intermittently but often produce rapid tolerance and may have multiple side effects (especially anticholinergic), which limit their use, particularly in the elderly. Benzodiazepine-receptor agonists are the most effective and well-tolerated class of medications for insomnia. The broad range of half-lives allows flexibility in the duration of sedative action. The most commonly prescribed agents in this family are zaleplon (5–20 mg), with a half-life of 1–2 h; zolpidem (5–10 mg) and triazolam (0.125–0.25 mg), with half-lives of 2–3 h; eszopiclone (1–3 mg), with a half-life of 5.5–8 h; and temazepam (15–30 mg) and lorazepam (0.5–2 mg), with half-lives of 6–12 h. Generally, side effects are minimal when the dose is kept low and the serum concentration is minimized during the waking hours (by using the shortest-acting effective agent). At least one benzodiazepine receptor agonist (eszopiclone) continues to be effective for 6 months of nightly use. However, longer durations of use have not been evaluated, and it is unclear whether this is true of other agents in this class. Moreover, with even brief continuous use of benzodiazepine receptor agonists, rebound insomnia can occur upon discontinuation. The likelihood of rebound insomnia and tolerance can be minimized by short durations of treatment, intermittent use, or gradual tapering of the dose. For acute insomnia, nightly use of a benzodiazepine receptor agonist for a maximum of 2–4 weeks is advisable. For chronic insomnia, intermittent use is recommended, unless the consequences of untreated insomnia outweigh concerns regarding chronic use. Benzodiazepine receptor agonists should be avoided, or used very judiciously, in patients with a history of substance or alcohol abuse. The heterocyclic antidepressants (trazodone, amitriptyline, and doxepin) are the most commonly prescribed alternatives to benzodiazepine receptor agonists due to their lack of abuse potential and lower cost. Trazodone (25–100 mg) is used more commonly than the tricyclic antidepressants as it has a much shorter half-life (5–9 h), has much less anticholinergic activity (sparing patients, particularly the elderly, constipation, urinary retention, and tachycardia), is associated with less weight gain, and is much safer in overdose. The risk of priapism is small (~1 in 10,000).

Psychophysiologic insomnia

Persistent *psychophysiologic insomnia* is a behavioral disorder in which patients are preoccupied with a perceived inability to sleep adequately at night. This sleep disorder begins like any other acute insomnia; however, the poor sleep habits and sleep-related anxiety ("insomnia phobia") persist long after the initial incident. Such patients become hyperaroused by their own efforts to sleep or by the sleep environment, and the insomnia becomes a conditioned or learned response. Patients may be able to fall asleep more easily at unscheduled times (when not trying) or outside the home environment. Polysomnographic recording in patients with psychophysiologic insomnia reveals an objective sleep disturbance, often with an abnormally long sleep latency; frequent nocturnal awakenings; and an increased amount of stage N1 transitional sleep. Rigorous attention should be paid to improving sleep hygiene, correction of counterproductive, arousing behaviors before bedtime, and minimizing exaggerated beliefs regarding the negative consequences of insomnia. Behavioral therapies are the treatment modality of choice, with intermittent use of medications. When patients are awake for >20 min, they should read or perform other relaxing activities to distract themselves from insomnia-related anxiety. In addition, bedtime and wake time should be scheduled to restrict time in bed to be equal to their perceived total sleep time. This will generally produce sleep deprivation, greater sleep drive, and, eventually, better sleep. Time in bed can then be gradually expanded. In addition, methods directed toward producing relaxation in the sleep setting (e.g., meditation, muscle relaxation) are encouraged.

Adjustment insomnia (acute insomnia)

This typically develops after a change in the sleeping environment (e.g., in an unfamiliar hotel or hospital bed) or before or after a significant life event, such as a change of occupation, loss of a loved one, illness, or anxiety over a deadline or examination. Increased sleep latency, frequent awakenings from sleep, and early morning awakening can all occur. Recovery is generally rapid, usually within a few weeks. Treatment is symptomatic, with intermittent use of hypnotics and resolution of the underlying stress. *Altitude insomnia* describes a sleep disturbance that is a common consequence of exposure to high altitude. Periodic breathing of the Cheyne-Stokes type occurs during NREM sleep about half the time at high altitude, with restoration of a regular breathing pattern during REM sleep. Both hypoxia and hypocapnia are thought to be involved in the development of periodic breathing. Frequent awakenings and poor quality sleep characterize altitude insomnia, which is generally worse on the first few nights at high altitude but may persist. Treatment with acetazolamide can decrease time spent in periodic breathing and substantially reduce hypoxia during sleep.

COMORBID INSOMNIA

Insomnia associated with mental disorders

Approximately 80% of patients with psychiatric disorders describe sleep complaints. There is considerable heterogeneity, however, in the nature of the sleep disturbance both between conditions and among patients with the same condition. *Depression* can be associated with sleep onset insomnia, sleep maintenance insomnia, or early morning wakefulness. However, hypersomnia occurs in some depressed patients, especially adolescents and those with either bipolar or seasonal (fall/winter) depression (Chap. 54). Indeed, sleep disturbance is an important vegetative sign of depression and may commence before any mood changes are perceived by the patient. Consistent polysomnographic findings in depression include decreased REM sleep latency, lengthened first REM sleep episode, and shortened first NREM sleep episode; however, these findings are not specific for depression, and the extent of these changes varies with age and symptomatology. Depressed patients also show decreased slow-wave sleep and reduced sleep continuity.

In *mania* and *hypomania*, sleep latency is increased and total sleep time can be reduced. Patients with *anxiety disorders* tend not to show the changes in REM sleep and slow-wave sleep seen in endogenously depressed patients. *Chronic alcoholics* lack slow-wave sleep, have decreased amounts of REM sleep (as an acute response to alcohol), and have frequent arousals throughout the night. This is associated with impaired daytime alertness. The sleep of chronic alcoholics may remain disturbed for years after discontinuance of alcohol usage. Sleep architecture and physiology are disturbed in *schizophrenia*, with a decreased amount of slow-wave sleep (NREM stage N3 sleep) and a lack of augmentation of REM sleep following REM sleep deprivation; chronic schizophrenics often show day-night reversal, sleep fragmentation, and insomnia.

Insomnia associated with neurologic disorders

A variety of neurologic diseases result in sleep disruption through both indirect, nonspecific mechanisms (e.g., pain in cervical spondylosis or low back pain) or by impairment of central neural structures involved in the generation and control of sleep itself. For example, *dementia* from any cause has long been associated with disturbances in the timing of the sleep-wake cycle, often characterized by nocturnal wandering and an exacerbation of symptomatology at night (so-called sundowning).

Epilepsy may rarely present as a sleep complaint (Chap. 26). Often the history is of abnormal behavior, at times with convulsive movements during sleep. The differential diagnosis includes REM sleep behavior disorder, sleep apnea syndrome, and periodic movements of sleep (see earlier in this chapter). Diagnosis requires nocturnal polysomnography with a full EEG montage. Other neurologic diseases associated with abnormal movements, such as *Parkinson's disease*, *hemiballismus*, *Huntington's chorea*, and *Tourette's syndrome* (Chap. 30), are also associated with disrupted sleep, presumably through secondary mechanisms. However, the abnormal movements themselves are greatly reduced during sleep. Headache syndromes (*migraine* or *cluster headache*) may show sleep-associated exacerbations (Chap. 8) by unknown mechanisms.

Fatal familial insomnia is a rare hereditary disorder caused by degeneration of anterior and dorsomedial nuclei of the thalamus. Insomnia is a prominent early symptom. Patients develop progressive autonomic dysfunction, followed by dysarthria, myoclonus, coma, and death. The pathogenesis is a mutation in the prion gene (Chap. 43).

Insomnia associated with other medical disorders

A number of medical conditions are associated with disruptions of sleep. The association is frequently nonspecific, e.g., sleep disruption due to chronic pain from rheumatologic disorders. Attention to this association is important in that sleep-associated symptoms are often the presenting or most bothersome complaint. Treatment of the underlying medical problem is the most useful approach. Sleep disruption can also result from the use of medications such as glucocorticoids (see later).

One prominent association is between sleep disruption and *asthma*. In many asthmatics there is a prominent daily variation in airway resistance that results in marked increases in asthmatic symptoms at night, especially during sleep. In addition, treatment of asthma with theophylline-based compounds, adrenergic agonists, or glucocorticoids can independently disrupt sleep. When sleep disruption is a side effect of asthma treatment, inhaled glucocorticoids (e.g., beclomethasone) that do not disrupt sleep may provide a useful alternative.

Cardiac ischemia may also be associated with sleep disruption. The ischemia itself may result from increases in sympathetic tone as a result of sleep apnea. Patients may present with complaints of nightmares or vivid, disturbing dreams, with or without awareness of the more classic symptoms of angina or of the sleep-disordered breathing. Treatment of the sleep apnea may substantially improve the angina and the nocturnal sleep quality. *Paroxysmal nocturnal dyspnea* can also occur as a consequence of sleep-associated cardiac ischemia that causes pulmonary congestion exacerbated by the recumbent posture.

Chronic obstructive pulmonary disease is also associated with sleep disruption, as are *cystic fibrosis*, *menopause*, *hyperthyroidism*, *gastroesophageal reflux*, *chronic renal failure*, and *liver failure*.

MEDICATION-, DRUG-, OR ALCOHOL-DEPENDENT INSOMNIA

Disturbed sleep can result from ingestion of a wide variety of agents. Caffeine is perhaps the most common pharmacologic cause of insomnia. It produces increased latency to sleep onset, more frequent arousals during sleep, and a reduction in total sleep time for up to 8–14 h after ingestion. Even small amounts of coffee can significantly disturb sleep in some patients; therefore, a 1- to 2-month trial without caffeine should be attempted in patients with these symptoms. Similarly, alcohol and nicotine can interfere with sleep, despite the fact that many patients use them to relax and promote sleep. Although alcohol can increase drowsiness and shorten sleep latency, even moderate amounts of alcohol increase awakenings in the second half of the night. In addition, alcohol ingestion prior to sleep is contraindicated in patients with sleep apnea because of the inhibitory effects of alcohol on upper airway muscle tone. Acutely, amphetamines and cocaine suppress both REM sleep and total sleep time, which return to normal with chronic use. Withdrawal leads to an REM sleep rebound. A number of prescribed medications can produce insomnia. Antidepressants, sympathomimetics, and glucocorticoids are common causes. In addition, severe rebound insomnia can result from the acute withdrawal of hypnotics, especially following the use of high doses of benzodiazepines with a short half-life. For this reason, hypnotic doses should be low to moderate, and prolonged drug tapering is encouraged.

RESTLESS LEGS SYNDROME (RLS)

Patients with this sensorimotor disorder report an irresistible urge to move the legs, or sometimes the upper extremities, that is often associated with creepy-crawling or aching dysesthesias deep within the affected limbs. For most patients with RLS, the dysesthesias and restlessness are much worse in the evening or night compared to the daytime and frequently interfere with the ability to fall asleep. The symptoms appear with inactivity and are temporarily relieved by movement. In contrast, paresthesias secondary to peripheral neuropathy persist with activity. The severity of this chronic disorder may wax and wane over time and can be exacerbated by sleep deprivation, caffeine, alcohol, serotonergic antidepressants, and pregnancy. The prevalence is 1–5% of young to middle-age adults and 10–20% of those aged >60 years. There appear to be important differences in RLS prevalence among racial groups, with higher prevalence in those of Northern European ancestry. Roughly one-third of patients (particularly those with an early age of onset) will have multiple affected family members. At least three separate chromosomal loci have been identified in familial RLS, though no gene has been identified to date. Iron deficiency and renal failure may cause RLS, which is then considered secondary RLS. The symptoms of RLS are exquisitely sensitive to dopaminergic drugs (e.g., pramipexole 0.25–0.5 mg q8PM or ropinirole 0.5–4 mg q8PM), which are the treatments of choice. Opioids, benzodiazepines, and gabapentin may also be of therapeutic value. Most patients with restless legs also experience periodic limb movements of sleep, although the reverse is not the case.

PERIODIC LIMB MOVEMENT DISORDER (PLMD)

Periodic limb movements of sleep (PLMS), previously known as *nocturnal myoclonus*, consists of stereotyped, 0.5- to 5.0-s extensions of the great toe and dorsiflexion of the foot, which recur every 20–40 s during NREM sleep, in episodes lasting from minutes to hours, as documented by bilateral surface EMG recordings of the anterior tibialis on polysomnography. PLMS is the principal objective polysomnographic finding in 17% of patients with insomnia and 11% of those with excessive daytime somnolence (Fig. 20-3). It is often unclear whether it is an incidental finding or the cause of disturbed sleep. When deemed to be the latter, PLMS is called PLMD. PLMS occurs in a wide variety of sleep disorders (including narcolepsy, sleep apnea, REM sleep behavior disorder, and various forms of insomnia) and may be associated with frequent arousals and an increased number of sleep-stage transitions. The pathophysiology is not well understood, though individuals with high spinal transections can exhibit periodic leg movements during sleep, suggesting the existence of a spinal generator. Treatment options include dopaminergic medications or benzodiazepines.

EVALUATION OF DAYTIME SLEEPINESS

Daytime impairment due to sleep loss may be difficult to quantify for several reasons. First, patients may be unaware of the extent of sleep deprivation. In obstructive sleep apnea, for example, the brief arousals from sleep associated with respiratory recovery after each apneic episode results in daytime sleepiness, despite the fact that the patient may be unaware of the sleep fragmentation. Second, subjective descriptions of waking impairment vary from patient to patient. Patients may describe themselves as "sleepy," "fatigued," or "tired" and may have a clear sense of the meaning of those terms, while others may use the same terms to describe a completely different condition. Third, sleepiness, particularly when profound, may affect judgment in a manner analogous to ethanol, such that subjective awareness of the condition and the consequent cognitive and motor impairment is reduced. Finally, patients may be reluctant to admit that sleepiness is a problem, both because they are generally unaware of what constitutes normal alertness and because sleepiness is generally

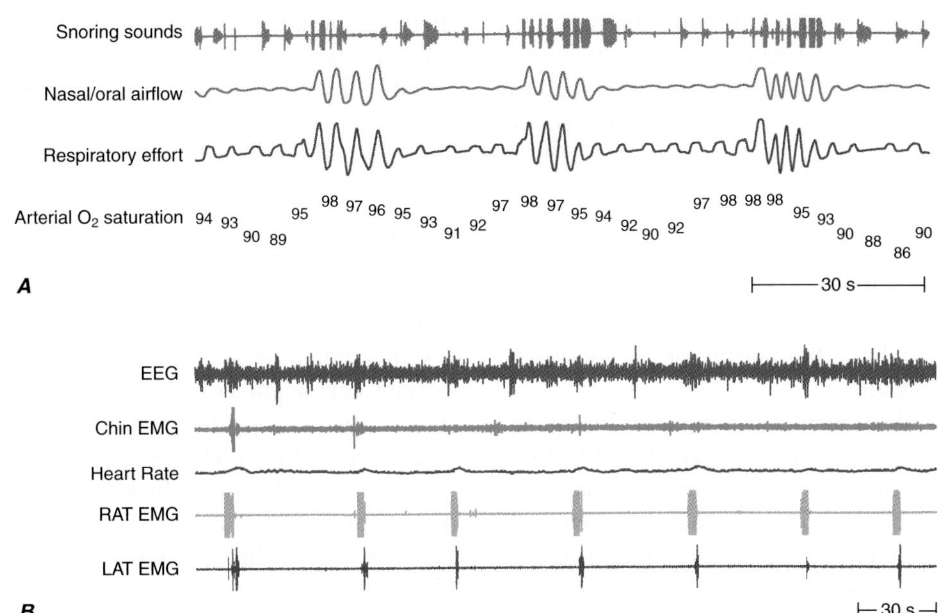

FIGURE 20-3

Polysomnographic recordings of (*A*) obstructive sleep apnea and (*B*) periodic limb movement of sleep. Note the snoring and reduction in air flow in the presence of continued respiratory effort, associated with the subsequent oxygen desaturation (upper panel). Periodic limb movements occur with a relatively constant intermovement interval and are associated with changes in the EEG and heart rate acceleration (lower panel). RAT, right anterior tibialis; LAT, left anterior tibialis. (*From the Division of Sleep Medicine, Brigham and Women's Hospital.*)

viewed pejoratively, ascribed more often to a deficit in motivation than to an inadequately addressed physiologic sleep need.

Specific questioning about the occurrence of sleep episodes during normal waking hours, both intentional and unintentional, is necessary to determine the extent of the adverse effects of sleepiness on a patient's daytime function. Specific areas to be addressed include the occurrence of inadvertent sleep episodes while driving or in other safety-related settings, sleepiness while at work or school (and the relationship of sleepiness to work and school performance), and the effect of sleepiness on social and family life. Standardized questionnaires, e.g., the Epworth Sleepiness Scale, are now commonly used in clinical and research settings to quantify daytime sleep tendency and screen for excessive sleepiness.

Driving is particularly hazardous for patients with increased sleepiness. Reaction time is equally impaired by 24 h of sleep loss as by a blood alcohol level of 0.10 g/dL. More than half of Americans admit to having fallen asleep while driving. An estimated 250,000 motor vehicle crashes per year are due to drowsy drivers, causing about 20% of all serious crash injuries and deaths. Drowsy driving legislation, aimed at improving education of all drivers about the hazards of driving drowsy and establishing sanctions comparable to those for drunk driving, has been enacted in New Jersey and is pending in several other states. Screening for sleep disorders, provision of an adequate number of safe highway rest areas, maintenance of unobstructed shoulder rumble strips, and strict enforcement and compliance monitoring of hours-of-service policies are needed to reduce the risk of sleep-related transportation crashes. Evidence for significant daytime impairment in association either with the diagnosis of a primary sleep disorder, such as narcolepsy or sleep apnea, or with imposed or self-selected sleep-wake schedules (see "Shift-Work Disorder") raises the issue of the physician's responsibility to notify motor vehicle licensing authorities of the increased risk of sleepiness-related motor vehicle crashes. As with epilepsy, legal requirements vary from state to state, and existing legal precedents do not provide a consistent interpretation of the balance between the physician's responsibility and the patient's right to privacy. At a minimum, physicians should inform patients who report a history of nodding off or falling asleep at the wheel or who have excessive daytime sleepiness about the increased risk of operating a motor vehicle, advise such patients not to drive a motor vehicle until the cause of the excessive sleepiness has been diagnosed and successful treatment has been implemented, and reevaluate the patient to determine when it is safe for the patient to resume driving. Each of those steps should be documented in the patient's medical record.

The distinction between fatigue and sleepiness can be useful in the differentiation of patients with complaints of fatigue or tiredness in the setting of disorders such as fibromyalgia, chronic fatigue syndrome (Chap. 52), or endocrine deficiencies such as hypothyroidism or Addison's disease. While patients with these disorders can typically distinguish their daytime symptoms from the sleepiness that occurs with sleep deprivation, substantial overlap can occur. This is particularly true when the primary disorder also results in chronic sleep disruption (e.g., sleep apnea in hypothyroidism) or in abnormal sleep (e.g., fibromyalgia).

While clinical evaluation of the complaint of excessive sleepiness is usually adequate, objective quantification is sometimes necessary. Assessment of daytime functioning as an index of the adequacy of sleep can be made with the multiple sleep latency test (MSLT), which utilizes repeated measurement of sleep latency (time to onset of sleep) under standardized conditions during a day following quantified nocturnal sleep. The average latency across four to six tests (administered every 2 h across the waking day) provides an objective measure of daytime sleep tendency. Disorders of sleep that result in pathologic daytime somnolence can be reliably distinguished with the MSLT. In addition, the multiple measurements of sleep onset may identify direct transitions from wakefulness to REM sleep that are suggestive of specific pathologic conditions (e.g., narcolepsy).

NARCOLEPSY

Narcolepsy is both a disorder of the ability to sustain wakefulness voluntarily and a disorder of REM sleep regulation (Table 20-2). The classic "narcolepsy tetrad" consists of excessive daytime somnolence plus three specific symptoms related to an intrusion of REM sleep characteristics (e.g., muscle atonia, vivid dream imagery) into the transition between wakefulness and sleep: (1) sudden weakness or loss of muscle tone without loss of consciousness, often elicited by emotion (cataplexy); (2) hallucinations at sleep onset (hypnagogic hallucinations) or upon awakening (hypnopompic hallucinations); and (3) muscle paralysis upon awakening (sleep paralysis). The severity of cataplexy varies, as patients may have two to three attacks per day or per decade. Some patients with objectively confirmed narcolepsy (see later) may show no evidence of cataplexy. In those with cataplexy, the extent and duration of an attack may also vary, from a transient sagging of the jaw lasting a few seconds to rare cases of flaccid paralysis of the entire voluntary musculature for up to 20–30 min. Symptoms of narcolepsy typically begin in the second decade, although the onset ranges from ages 5–50 years. Once established, the disease is chronic without remissions. Secondary forms of narcolepsy have been described (e.g., after head trauma).

TABLE 20-2

PREVALENCE OF SYMPTOMS IN NARCOLEPSY

SYMPTOM	PREVALENCE, %
Excessive daytime somnolence	100
Disturbed sleep	87
Cataplexy	76
Hypnagogic hallucinations	68
Sleep paralysis	64
Memory problems	50

Source: Modified from TA Roth, L Merlotti, in SA Burton et al (eds): *Narcolepsy 3rd International Symposium: Selected Symposium Proceedings.* Chicago, Matrix Communications, 1989.

Narcolepsy affects about 1 in 4000 people in the United States and appears to have a genetic basis. Recently, several convergent lines of evidence suggest that the hypothalamic neuropeptide hypocretin (orexin) is involved in the pathogenesis of narcolepsy: (1) a mutation in the hypocretin receptor 2 gene has been associated with canine narcolepsy; (2) hypocretin "knockout" mice that are genetically unable to produce this neuropeptide exhibit behavioral and electrophysiologic features resembling human narcolepsy; and (3) cerebrospinal fluid levels of hypocretin are reduced in most patients who have narcolepsy with cataplexy. The inheritance pattern of narcolepsy in humans is more complex than in the canine model. However, almost all narcoleptics with cataplexy are positive for HLA DQB1*0602, suggesting that an autoimmune process may be responsible.

Diagnosis

The diagnostic criteria continue to be a matter of debate. Certainly, objective verification of excessive daytime somnolence, typically with MSLT mean sleep latencies <8 min, is an essential if nonspecific diagnostic feature. Other conditions that cause excessive sleepiness, such as sleep apnea or chronic sleep deprivation, must be rigorously excluded. The other objective diagnostic feature of narcolepsy is the presence of REM sleep in at least two of the naps during the MSLT. Abnormal regulation of REM sleep is also manifested by the appearance of REM sleep immediately or within minutes after sleep onset in 50% of narcoleptic patients, a rarity in unaffected individuals maintaining a conventional sleep-wake schedule. The REM-related symptoms of the classic narcolepsy tetrad are variably present. There is increasing evidence that narcoleptics with cataplexy (one-half to two-thirds of patients) may represent a more homogeneous group than those without this symptom. However, a history of cataplexy can be difficult to establish reliably. Hypnagogic and hypnopompic hallucinations and sleep paralysis are often found in nonnarcoleptic individuals and may be present in only one-half of narcoleptics. Nocturnal sleep disruption is commonly observed in narcolepsy but is also a nonspecific symptom. Similarly, a history of "automatic behavior" during wakefulness (a trancelike state during which simple motor behaviors persist) is not specific for narcolepsy and serves principally to corroborate the presence of daytime somnolence.

TREATMENT Narcolepsy

The treatment of narcolepsy is symptomatic. Somnolence is treated with wake-promoting therapeutics. Modafinil is now the drug of choice, principally because it is associated with fewer side effects than older stimulants and has a long half-life; 200–400 mg is given as a single daily dose. Older drugs such as methylphenidate (10 mg bid to 20 mg qid) or dextroamphetamine (10 mg bid) are still used as alternatives, particularly in refractory patients.

These latter medications are now available in slow-release formulations, extending their duration of action and allowing once-daily dosing.

Treatment of the REM-related phenomena of cataplexy, hypnagogic hallucinations, and sleep paralysis requires the potent REM sleep suppression produced by antidepressant medications. The tricyclic antidepressants (e.g., protriptyline [10–40 mg/d] and clomipramine [25–50 mg/d]) and the selective serotonin reuptake inhibitors (SSRIs) (e.g., fluoxetine [10–20 mg/d]) are commonly used for this purpose. Efficacy of the antidepressants is limited largely by anticholinergic side effects (tricyclics) and by sleep disturbance and sexual dysfunction (SSRIs). Alternately, gamma hydroxybutyrate (GHB), given at bedtime, and 4 h later, is effective in reducing daytime cataplectic episodes. Adequate nocturnal sleep time and planned daytime naps (when possible) are important preventive measures.

SLEEP APNEA SYNDROMES

Respiratory dysfunction during sleep is a common, serious cause of excessive daytime somnolence as well as of disturbed nocturnal sleep. An estimated 2–5 million individuals in the United States have a reduction or cessation of breathing for 10–150 s from 30 to several hundred times every night during sleep. These episodes may be due to either an occlusion of the airway (*obstructive sleep apnea*), absence of respiratory effort (*central sleep apnea*), or a combination of these factors (*mixed sleep apnea*) (Fig. 20-3). Failure to recognize and treat these conditions appropriately may lead to impairment of daytime alertness, increased risk of sleep-related motor vehicle accidents, hypertension and other serious cardiovascular complications, and increased mortality. Sleep apnea is particularly prevalent in overweight men and in the elderly, yet it is estimated to remain undiagnosed in 80–90% of affected individuals. This is unfortunate since effective treatments are available.

PARASOMNIAS

The term *parasomnia* refers to abnormal behaviors or experiences that arise from or occur during sleep. A continuum of parasomnias arise from NREM sleep, from brief confusional arousals to sleepwalking and night terrors. The presenting complaint is usually related to the behavior itself, but the parasomnias can disturb sleep continuity or lead to mild impairments in daytime alertness. Two main parasomnias occur in REM sleep: REM sleep behavior disorder (RBD), which will be described later in this chapter, and nightmare disorder.

Sleepwalking (somnambulism)

Patients affected by this disorder carry out automatic motor activities that range from simple to complex. Individuals may walk, urinate inappropriately, eat, or exit from the house while remaining only partially aware. Full arousal may be difficult, and individuals may rarely respond to attempted awakening with agitation or even violence. Sleepwalking arises from slow-wave sleep (NREM stage N3 sleep), usually in the first 2 h of the night, and is most common in children and adolescents, when these sleep stages are most robust. Episodes are usually isolated but may be recurrent in 1–6% of patients. The cause is unknown, though it has a familial basis in roughly one-third of cases.

Sleep terrors

This disorder, also called *pavor nocturnus*, occurs primarily in young children during the first several hours after sleep onset, in slow-wave sleep (NREM stage N3 sleep). The child suddenly screams, exhibiting autonomic arousal with sweating, tachycardia, and hyperventilation. The individual may be difficult to arouse and rarely recalls the episode on awakening in the morning. Parents are usually reassured to learn that the condition is self-limited and benign and that no specific therapy is indicated. Both sleep terrors and sleepwalking represent abnormalities of arousal. In contrast, *nightmares* occur during REM sleep and cause full arousal, with intact memory for the unpleasant episode.

Sleep bruxism

Bruxism is an involuntary, forceful grinding of teeth during sleep that affects 10–20% of the population. The patient is usually unaware of the problem. The typical age of onset is 17–20 years, and spontaneous remission usually occurs by age 40. Sex distribution appears to be equal. In many cases, the diagnosis is made during dental examination, damage is minor, and no treatment is indicated. In more severe cases, treatment with a rubber tooth guard is necessary to prevent disfiguring tooth injury. Stress management or, in some cases, biofeedback can be useful when bruxism is a manifestation of psychological stress. There are anecdotal reports of benefit using benzodiazepines.

Sleep enuresis

Bedwetting, like sleepwalking and night terrors, is another parasomnia that occurs during sleep in the young. Before age 5 or 6 years, nocturnal enuresis should probably be considered a normal feature of development. The condition usually improves spontaneously by puberty, has a prevalence in late adolescence of 1–3%, and is rare in adulthood. In older patients with enuresis, a distinction must be made between primary and secondary enuresis, the latter being defined as bedwetting in patients who have previously been fully continent for 6–12 months. Treatment of primary enuresis is reserved for patients of appropriate age (>5 or 6 years) and consists of bladder training exercises and behavioral therapy. Urologic abnormalities are more common in primary enuresis and must be assessed by urologic examination. Important causes of secondary enuresis include emotional disturbances, urinary tract infections or malformations, cauda equina lesions, epilepsy, sleep apnea, and certain medications. Symptomatic pharmacotherapy is usually accomplished with desmopressin (0.2 mg qhs), oxybutynin chloride (5–10 mg qhs), or imipramine (10–50 mg qhs).

Miscellaneous parasomnias

Other clinical entities may be characterized as a parasomnia or a sleep-related movement disorder in that they occur selectively during sleep and are associated with some degree of sleep disruption. Examples include *jactatio capitis nocturna* (nocturnal headbanging, rhythmic movement disorder), confusional arousals, sleep-related eating disorder, and nocturnal leg cramps.

REM sleep behavior disorder (RBD)

RBD is a rare condition that is distinct from other parasomnias in that it occurs during REM sleep. It primarily afflicts men of middle age or older, many of whom have an existing, or developing, neurologic disease. Approximately one-half of patients with RBD will develop Parkinson's disease (Chap. 30) within 10–20 years. Presenting symptoms consist of agitated or violent behavior during sleep, as reported by a bed partner. In contrast to typical somnambulism, injury to the patient or bed partner is not uncommon, and, upon awakening, the patient reports vivid, often unpleasant, dream imagery. The principal differential diagnosis is nocturnal seizures, which can be excluded with polysomnography. In RBD, seizure activity is absent on the EEG, and disinhibition of the usual motor atonia is observed in the EMG during REM sleep, at times associated with complex motor behaviors. The pathogenesis is unclear, but damage to brainstem areas mediating descending motor inhibition during REM sleep may be responsible. In support of this hypothesis are the remarkable similarities between RBD and the sleep of animals with bilateral lesions of the pontine tegmentum in areas controlling REM sleep motor inhibition. Treatment with clonazepam (0.5–1.0 mg qhs) provides sustained improvement in almost all reported cases.

CIRCADIAN RHYTHM SLEEP DISORDERS

A subset of patients presenting with either insomnia or hypersomnia may have a disorder of sleep *timing* rather than sleep *generation*. Disorders of sleep timing can be either organic (i.e., due to an abnormality of circadian pacemaker[s] or its input from entraining stimuli) or environmental (i.e., due to a disruption of exposure to entraining stimuli from the environment). Regardless of etiology, the symptoms reflect the influence of the underlying circadian pacemaker on sleep-wake function. Thus, effective therapeutic approaches should aim to entrain the oscillator at an appropriate phase.

Jet lag disorder

More than 60 million persons experience transmeridian air travel annually, which is often associated with excessive daytime sleepiness, sleep onset insomnia, and frequent arousals from sleep, particularly in the latter half of the night. Gastrointestinal discomfort is common. The syndrome is transient, typically lasting 2–14 d depending on the number of time zones crossed, the direction of travel, and the traveler's age and phase-shifting capacity. Travelers who spend more time outdoors reportedly adapt more quickly than those who remain in hotel rooms, presumably due to brighter (outdoor) light exposure. Avoidance of antecedent sleep loss and obtaining nap sleep on the afternoon prior to overnight travel greatly reduce the difficulty of extended wakefulness. Laboratory studies suggest that sub milligram doses of the pineal hormone melatonin can enhance sleep efficiency, but only if taken when endogenous melatonin concentrations are low (i.e., during biologic daytime), and that melatonin may induce phase shifts in human rhythms. A large-scale clinical trial evaluating the safety and efficacy of melatonin as a treatment for jet lag disorder and other circadian sleep disorders is needed.

In addition to jet lag associated with travel across time zones, many patients report a behavioral pattern that has been termed *social jet lag*, in which their bedtimes and wake times on weekends or days off occur 4–8 h later than they do during the week. This recurrent displacement of the timing of the sleep-wake cycle is common in adolescents and young adults and is associated with sleep onset insomnia, poorer academic performance, increased risk of depressive symptoms, and excessive daytime sleepiness.

Shift-work disorder

More than 7 million workers in the United States regularly work at night, either on a permanent or rotating schedule. Many more begin work between 4 A.M. and 7 A.M., requiring them to commute and then work during the time of day that they would otherwise be asleep. In addition, each week millions more elect to remain awake at night to meet deadlines, drive long distances, or participate in recreational activities. This results in both sleep loss and misalignment of the circadian rhythm with respect to the sleep-wake cycle.

Studies of regular night-shift workers indicate that the circadian timing system usually fails to adapt successfully to such inverted schedules. This leads to a misalignment between the desired work-rest schedule and the output of the pacemaker and in disturbed daytime sleep in most individuals. Sleep deprivation, increased length of time awake prior to work, and misalignment of circadian phase produce decreased alertness and performance, increased reaction time, and increased risk of performance lapses, thereby resulting in greater safety hazards among night workers and other sleep-deprived individuals. Sleep disturbance nearly doubles the risk of a fatal work accident. Additional problems include higher rates of breast, colorectal, and prostate cancer and of cardiac, gastrointestinal, and reproductive disorders in long-term night-shift workers. Recently, the World Health Organization has added night-shift work to its list of probable carcinogens.

Sleep onset is associated with marked attenuation in perception of both auditory and visual stimuli and lapses of consciousness. The sleepy individual may thus attempt to perform routine and familiar motor tasks during the transition state between wakefulness and sleep (stage N1 sleep) in the absence of adequate processing of sensory input from the environment. Motor vehicle operators are especially vulnerable to sleep-related accidents since the sleep-deprived driver or operator often fails to heed the warning signs of fatigue. Such attempts to override the powerful biologic drive for sleep by the sheer force of will can yield a catastrophic outcome when sleep processes intrude involuntarily upon the waking brain. Such sleep-related attentional failures typically last only seconds but are known on occasion to persist for longer durations. These frequent brief intrusions of stage N1 sleep into behavioral wakefulness are a major component of the impaired psychomotor performance seen with sleepiness. There is a significant increase in the risk of sleep-related, fatal-to-the-driver highway crashes in the early morning and late afternoon hours, coincident with bimodal peaks in the daily rhythm of sleep tendency.

Resident physicians constitute another group of workers at risk for accidents and other adverse consequences of lack of sleep and misalignment of the circadian rhythm. Recurrent scheduling of resident physicians to work shifts of 24 h or more consecutive hours impairs psychomotor performance to a degree that is comparable to alcohol intoxication, doubles the risk of attentional failures among intensive care unit interns working at night, and significantly increases the risk of serious medical errors in intensive care units, including a fivefold increase in the risk of serious diagnostic mistakes. Some 20% of hospital interns report making a fatigue-related mistake that injured a patient, and 5% admit making a fatigue-related mistake that results in the death of a patient. Moreover, working for >24 h consecutively increases the risk of percutaneous injuries and more than doubles the risk of motor vehicle crashes on the commute home. For these reasons, in 2008 the Institute of Medicine concluded that the practice of scheduling resident physicians to work for more than 16 consecutive hours without sleep is hazardous for both resident physicians and their patients.

From 5 to 10% of individuals scheduled to work at night or in the early morning hours have much greater than average difficulties remaining awake during night work and sleeping during the day; these individuals are diagnosed with chronic and severe shift-work disorder (SWD). Patients with this disorder have a level of excessive sleepiness during night work and insomnia during day sleep that the physician judges to be clinically significant; the condition is associated with an increased risk of sleep-related accidents and with some of the illnesses associated with night-shift work. Patients with chronic and severe SWD are profoundly sleepy at night. In fact, their sleep latencies during night work average just 2 min, comparable to mean sleep latency durations of patients with narcolepsy or severe daytime sleep apnea.

TREATMENT Shift-Work Disorder

Caffeine is frequently used to promote wakefulness. However, it cannot forestall sleep indefinitely, and it does not shield users from sleep-related performance lapses. Postural changes, exercise, and strategic placement of nap opportunities can sometimes temporarily reduce the risk of fatigue-related performance lapses. Properly timed exposure to bright light can facilitate rapid adaptation to night-shift work.

While many techniques (e.g., light treatment) used to facilitate adaptation to night-shift work may help patients with this disorder, modafinil is the only therapeutic intervention that has ever been evaluated as a treatment for this specific patient population. Modafinil (200 mg, taken 30–60 min before the start of each night shift) is approved by the U.S. Food and Drug Administration as a treatment for the excessive sleepiness during night work in patients with SWD. Although treatment with modafinil significantly increases sleep latency and reduces the risk of lapses of attention during night work, SWD patients remain excessively sleepy at night, even while being treated with modafinil.

Safety programs should promote education about sleep and increase awareness of the hazards associated with night work. The goal should be to minimize both sleep deprivation and circadian disruption. Work schedules should be designed to minimize (1) exposure to night work, (2) the frequency of shift rotation so that shifts do not rotate more than once every 2–3 weeks, (3) the number of consecutive night shifts, and (4) the duration of night shifts. Shift durations of >16 h should be universally recognized as increasing the risk of sleep-related errors and performance lapses to a level that is unacceptable in nonemergency circumstances. At least 11 h off duty should be provided between work shifts, with at least 1 day off every week and 2 consecutive days off every month. Additional off duty time should be allocated after night work, since sleep efficiency is much lower during daytime hours.

Delayed sleep phase disorder

Delayed sleep phase disorder is characterized by (1) reported sleep onset and wake times intractably later than desired, (2) actual sleep times at nearly the same clock hours daily, and (3) essentially normal all-night polysomnography except for delayed sleep onset. Patients exhibit an abnormally delayed endogenous circadian phase, with the temperature minimum during the constant routine occurring later than normal. This delayed phase could be due to (1) an abnormally long, genetically determined intrinsic period of the endogenous circadian pacemaker; (2) an abnormally reduced phase-advancing capacity of the pacemaker; (3) a slower rate of buildup of homeostatic sleep drive during wakefulness; or (4) an irregular prior sleep-wake schedule, characterized by frequent nights when the patient chooses to remain awake well past midnight (for social, school, or work reasons). In most cases, it is difficult to distinguish among these factors, since patients with an abnormally long intrinsic period are more likely to "choose" such late-night activities because they are unable to sleep at that time. Patients tend to be young adults. This self-perpetuating condition can persist for years and does not usually respond to attempts to reestablish normal bedtime hours. Treatment methods involving bright-light phototherapy during the morning hours or melatonin administration in the evening hours show promise in these patients, although the relapse rate is high.

Advanced sleep phase disorder

Advanced sleep phase disorder (ASPD) is the converse of the delayed sleep phase syndrome. Most commonly, this syndrome occurs in older people, 15% of whom report that they cannot sleep past 5 A.M., with twice that number complaining that they wake up too early at least several times per week. Patients with ASPD experience excessive daytime sleepiness during the evening hours, when they have great difficulty remaining awake, even in social settings. Typically, patients awaken from 3 to 5 A.M. each day, often several hours before their desired wake times. In addition to age-related ASPD, an early-onset familial variant of this condition has also been reported. In one such family, autosomal dominant ASPD was due to a missense mutation in a circadian clock component (PER2, as shown in Fig. 20-2) that altered the circadian period. Patients with ASPD may benefit from bright-light phototherapy during the evening hours, designed to reset the circadian pacemaker to a later hour.

Non-24-h sleep-wake disorder

This condition can occur when the synchronizing input (i.e., the light-dark cycle) from the environment to the circadian pacemaker is compromised (as in many blind people with no light perception) or when the maximal phase-advancing capacity of the circadian pacemaker is not adequate to accommodate the difference between the 24-h geophysical day and the intrinsic period of the pacemaker in the patient. Alternatively, patients' self-selected exposure to artificial light may drive the circadian pacemaker to a >24-h schedule. Affected patients are not able to maintain a stable phase relationship between the output of the pacemaker and the 24-h day. Such patients typically present with an incremental pattern of successive delays in sleep propensity, progressing in and out of phase with local time. When the patient's endogenous circadian rhythms are out of phase with the local environment, insomnia coexists with excessive daytime sleepiness. Conversely, when the endogenous circadian rhythms are in phase with the local environment, symptoms remit. The intervals between symptomatic periods may last several weeks to several months. Blind individuals unable to perceive light are particularly susceptible to this disorder, although it can occur in sighted patients. Nightly low-dose (0.5 mg) melatonin administration has been reported to improve sleep and, in some cases, to induce synchronization of the circadian pacemaker.

MEDICAL IMPLICATIONS OF CIRCADIAN RHYTHMICITY

Prominent circadian variations have been reported in the incidence of acute myocardial infarction, sudden cardiac death, and stroke, the leading causes of death in the United States. Platelet aggregability is increased in the early morning hours, coincident with the peak incidence of these cardiovascular events. Misalignment of circadian phase, such as occurs during night-shift work, induces insulin resistance and higher glucose levels in response to a standard meal. Blood pressure of night workers with sleep apnea is higher than that of day workers. A better understanding of the possible role of circadian rhythmicity in the acute destabilization of a chronic condition such as atherosclerotic disease could improve the understanding of its pathophysiology.

Diagnostic and therapeutic procedures may also be affected by the time of day at which data are collected. Examples include blood pressure, body temperature, the dexamethasone suppression test, and plasma cortisol levels. The timing of chemotherapy administration has been reported to have an effect on the outcome of treatment. In addition, both the toxicity and effectiveness of drugs can vary during the day. For example, more than a fivefold difference has been observed in mortality rates following administration of toxic agents to experimental animals at different times of day. Anesthetic agents are particularly sensitive to time-of-day effects. Finally, the physician must be increasingly aware of the public health risks associated with the ever-increasing demands made by the duty-rest-recreation schedules in our round-the-clock society.

CHAPTER 21
DISORDERS OF VISION

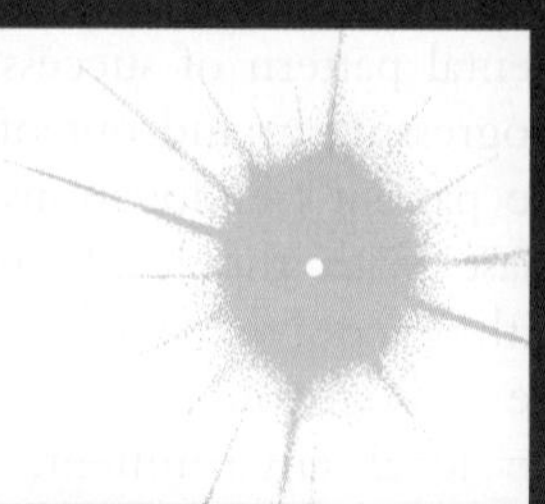

Jonathan C. Horton

THE HUMAN VISUAL SYSTEM

The visual system provides a supremely efficient means for the rapid assimilation of information from the environment to aid in the guidance of behavior. The act of seeing begins with the capture of images focused by the cornea and lens on a light-sensitive membrane in the back of the eye called the *retina*. The retina is actually part of the brain, banished to the periphery to serve as a transducer for the conversion of patterns of light energy into neuronal signals. Light is absorbed by photopigment in two types of receptors: rods and cones. In the human retina there are 100 million rods and 5 million cones. The rods operate in dim (scotopic) illumination. The cones function under daylight (photopic) conditions. The cone system is specialized for color perception and high spatial resolution. The majority of cones are within the macula, the portion of the retina that serves the central 10° of vision. In the middle of the macula a small pit termed the *fovea*, packed exclusively with cones, provides the best visual acuity.

Photoreceptors hyperpolarize in response to light, activating bipolar, amacrine, and horizontal cells in the inner nuclear layer. After processing of photoreceptor responses by this complex retinal circuit, the flow of sensory information ultimately converges on a final common pathway: the ganglion cells. These cells translate the visual image impinging on the retina into a continuously varying barrage of action potentials that propagates along the primary optic pathway to visual centers within the brain. There are a million ganglion cells in each retina and hence a million fibers in each optic nerve.

Ganglion cell axons sweep along the inner surface of the retina in the nerve fiber layer, exit the eye at the optic disc, and travel through the optic nerve, optic chiasm, and optic tract to reach targets in the brain. The majority of fibers synapse on cells in the lateral geniculate body, a thalamic relay station. Cells in the lateral geniculate body project in turn to the primary visual cortex. This massive afferent retinogeniculocortical sensory pathway provides the neural substrate for visual perception. Although the lateral geniculate body is the main target of the retina, separate classes of ganglion cells project to other subcortical visual nuclei involved in different functions. Ganglion cells that mediate pupillary constriction and circadian rhythms are light sensitive owing to a novel visual pigment, melanopsin. Pupil responses are mediated by input to the pretectal olivary nuclei in the midbrain. The pretectal nuclei send their output to the Edinger-Westphal nuclei, which in turn provide parasympathetic innervation to the iris sphincter via an interneuron in the ciliary ganglion. Circadian rhythms are timed by a retinal projection to the suprachiasmatic nucleus. Visual orientation and eye movements are served by retinal input to the superior colliculus. Gaze stabilization and optokinetic reflexes are governed by a group of small retinal targets known collectively as the *brainstem accessory optic system*.

The eyes must be rotated constantly within their orbits to place and maintain targets of visual interest on the fovea. This activity, called *foveation*, or looking, is governed by an elaborate efferent motor system. Each eye is moved by six extraocular muscles that are supplied by cranial nerves from the oculomotor (III), trochlear (IV), and abducens (VI) nuclei. Activity in these ocular motor nuclei is coordinated by pontine and midbrain mechanisms for smooth pursuit, saccades, and gaze stabilization during head and body movements. Large regions of the frontal and parietooccipital cortex control these brainstem eye movement centers by providing descending supranuclear input.

CLINICAL ASSESSMENT OF VISUAL FUNCTION

REFRACTIVE STATE

In approaching a patient with reduced vision, the first step is to decide whether refractive error is responsible. In *emmetropia*, parallel rays from infinity are focused perfectly on the retina. Sadly, this condition is enjoyed by only a minority of the population. In *myopia*, the globe is too long, and light rays come to a focal point in front of the retina. Near objects can be seen clearly, but distant objects require a diverging lens in front of the eye. In *hyperopia*, the globe is too short, and hence a converging lens is used to supplement the refractive power of the eye. In *astigmatism*, the corneal surface is not perfectly spherical, necessitating a cylindrical corrective lens. In recent years it has become possible to correct refractive error with the excimer laser by performing LASIK (laser in situ keratomileusis) to alter the curvature of the cornea.

With the onset of middle age, *presbyopia* develops as the lens within the eye becomes unable to increase its refractive power to accommodate on near objects. To compensate for presbyopia, an emmetropic patient must use reading glasses. A patient already wearing glasses for distance correction usually switches to bifocals. The only exception is a myopic patient, who may achieve clear vision at near simply by removing glasses containing the distance prescription.

Refractive errors usually develop slowly and remain stable after adolescence, except in unusual circumstances. For example, the acute onset of diabetes mellitus can produce sudden myopia because of lens edema induced by hyperglycemia. Testing vision through a pinhole aperture is a useful way to screen quickly for refractive error. If visual acuity is better through a pinhole than it is with the unaided eye, the patient needs refraction to obtain best corrected visual acuity.

ROSENBAUM POCKET VISION SCREENER

	Point	Jaeger	distance equivalent
95			20/800
874			20/400
2843	26	16	20/200
638 E Ш Ǝ X O O	14	10	20/100
8 7 4 5 Ǝ m Ш O X O	10	7	20/70
6 3 9 2 5 m E Ǝ X O X	8	5	20/50
4 2 8 3 6 5 Ш E m O X O	6	3	20/40
3 7 4 2 5 8 Ǝ Ш Ǝ X X O	5	2	20/30
9 3 7 8 2 6 Ш m E X O O	4	1	20/25
4 2 8 7 3 9 E Ш m O O X	3	1+	20/20

Card is held in good light 14 inches from eye. Record vision for each eye separately with and without glasses. Presbyopic patients should read thru bifocal segment. Check myopes with glasses only.

DESIGN COURTESY J. G. ROSENBAUM, M.D.

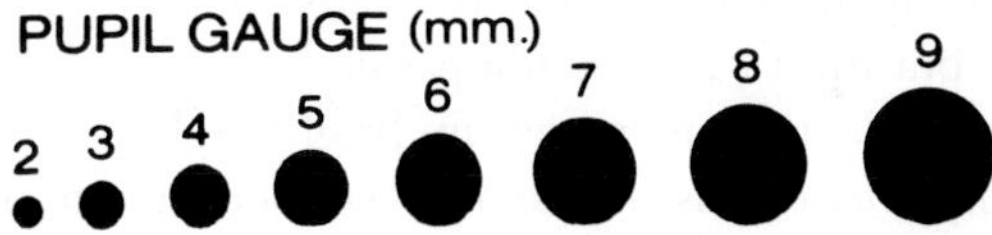

FIGURE 21-1

The Rosenbaum card is a miniature, scale version of the Snellen chart for testing visual acuity at near. When the visual acuity is recorded, the Snellen distance equivalent should bear a notation indicating that vision was tested at near, not at 6 m (20 ft), or else the Jaeger number system should be used to report the acuity.

VISUAL ACUITY

The Snellen chart is used to test acuity at a distance of 6 m (20 ft). For convenience, a scale version of the Snellen chart called the Rosenbaum card is held at 36 cm (14 in.) from the patient (Fig. 21-1). All subjects should be able to read the 6/6 m (20/20 ft) line with each eye using their refractive correction, if any. Patients who need reading glasses because of presbyopia must wear them for accurate testing with the Rosenbaum card. If 6/6 (20/20) acuity is not present in each eye, the deficiency in vision must be explained. If it is worse than 6/240 (20/800), acuity should be recorded in terms of counting fingers, hand motions, light perception, or no light perception. Legal blindness is defined by the Internal Revenue Service as a best corrected acuity of 6/60 (20/200) or less in the better eye or a binocular visual field subtending 20° or less. For driving the laws vary by state, but most states require a corrected acuity of 6/12 (20/40) in at least one eye for unrestricted privileges. Patients with a homonymous hemianopia should not drive.

PUPILS

The pupils should be tested individually in dim light with the patient fixating on a distant target. If the pupils respond briskly to light, there is no need to check the near response, because isolated loss of constriction (miosis) to accommodation does not occur. For this reason, the ubiquitous abbreviation PERRLA (pupils equal, round, and reactive to light and accommodation) implies a wasted effort with the last step. However, it is important to test the near response if the light response is poor or absent. Light-near dissociation occurs with neurosyphilis (Argyll Robertson pupil), with lesions of the dorsal midbrain (obstructive hydrocephalus, pineal region tumors), and after aberrant regeneration (oculomotor nerve palsy, Adie's tonic pupil).

An eye with no light perception has no pupillary response to direct light stimulation. If the retina or optic nerve is only partially injured, the direct pupillary response will be weaker than the consensual pupillary response evoked by shining a light into the other eye. This *relative afferent pupillary defect* (Marcus Gunn pupil) can be elicited with the swinging flashlight test (Fig. 21-2). It is an extremely useful sign in retrobulbar optic neuritis and other optic nerve diseases, in which it may be the sole objective evidence for disease.

Subtle inequality in pupil size, up to 0.5 mm, is a fairly common finding in normal persons. The diagnosis of essential or physiologic anisocoria is secure as long as the relative pupil asymmetry remains constant as ambient lighting varies. Anisocoria that increases in dim light indicates a sympathetic paresis of the iris dilator muscle. The triad of miosis with ipsilateral ptosis and anhidrosis constitutes *Horner's syndrome*, although anhidrosis is an inconstant feature. Brainstem stroke, carotid dissection, and neoplasm impinging on the sympathetic chain occasionally are identified as the cause of Horner's syndrome, but most cases are idiopathic.

Anisocoria that increases in bright light suggests a parasympathetic palsy. The first concern is an oculomotor nerve paresis. This possibility is excluded if the eye movements are full and the patient has no ptosis or diplopia. Acute pupillary dilation (mydriasis) can result from damage to the ciliary ganglion in the orbit. Common mechanisms are infection (herpes zoster, influenza), trauma (blunt, penetrating, surgical), and ischemia (diabetes, temporal arteritis). After denervation of the iris sphincter the pupil does not respond well to light, but the response to near is often relatively intact. When the near stimulus is removed, the pupil redilates very slowly compared with the normal pupil, hence the term *tonic pupil*. In *Adie's syndrome*, a tonic pupil occurs in conjunction with weak or absent tendon reflexes in the lower extremities. This benign disorder, which occurs predominantly in healthy young women, is assumed to represent a mild dysautonomia. Tonic pupils are also associated with Shy-Drager syndrome, segmental hypohidrosis, diabetes, and amyloidosis. Occasionally, a tonic pupil is discovered incidentally in an otherwise completely normal, asymptomatic individual. The diagnosis is confirmed by placing a drop of dilute (0.125%) pilocarpine into each eye. Denervation hypersensitivity produces pupillary constriction in a tonic pupil, whereas the normal pupil shows no response. Pharmacologic dilatation from accidental or deliberate instillation of anticholinergic agents (atropine, scopolamine drops) into the eye also can produce pupillary mydriasis. In this situation, normal strength (1%) pilocarpine causes no constriction.

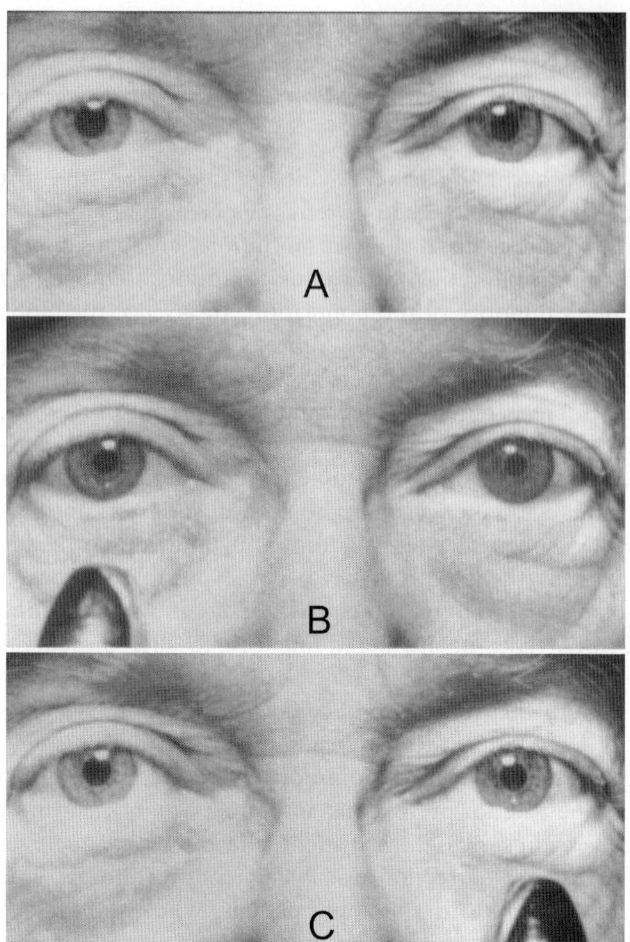

FIGURE 21-2

Demonstration of a relative afferent pupil defect (Marcus Gunn pupil) in the left eye, done with the patient fixating on a distant target. ***A.*** With dim background lighting, the pupils are equal and relatively large. ***B.*** Shining a flashlight into the right eye evokes equal, strong constriction of both pupils. ***C.*** Swinging the flashlight over to the damaged left eye causes dilation of both pupils, although they remain smaller than in ***A.*** Swinging the flashlight back over to the healthy right eye would result in symmetric constriction back to the appearance shown in ***B.*** Note that the pupils always remain equal; the damage to the left retina/optic nerve is revealed by weaker bilateral pupil constriction to a flashlight in the left eye compared with the right eye. (*From P Levatin: Arch Ophthalmol 62:768, 1959. Copyright © 1959 American Medical Association. All rights reserved.*)

Both pupils are affected equally by systemic medications. They are small with narcotic use (morphine, heroin) and large with anticholinergics (scopolamine). Parasympathetic agents (pilocarpine, demecarium bromide) used to treat glaucoma produce miosis. In any patient with an unexplained pupillary abnormality, a slit-lamp examination is helpful to exclude surgical trauma to the iris, an occult foreign body, perforating injury, intraocular inflammation, adhesions (synechia), angle-closure glaucoma, and iris sphincter rupture from blunt trauma.

EYE MOVEMENTS AND ALIGNMENT

Eye movements are tested by asking the patient, with both eyes open, to pursue a small target such as a penlight into the cardinal fields of gaze. Normal ocular versions are smooth, symmetric, full, and maintained in all directions without nystagmus. Saccades, or quick refixation eye movements, are assessed by having the patient look back and forth between two stationary targets. The eyes should move rapidly and accurately in a single jump to their target. Ocular alignment can be judged by holding a penlight directly in front of the patient at about 1 m. If the eyes are straight, the corneal light reflex will be centered in the middle of each pupil. To test eye alignment more precisely, the cover test is useful. The patient is instructed to gaze upon a small fixation target in the distance. One eye is covered suddenly while the second eye is observed. If the second eye shifts to fixate on the target, it was misaligned. If it does not move, the first eye is uncovered and the test is repeated on the second eye. If neither eye moves, the eyes are aligned orthotropically. If the eyes are orthotropic in primary gaze but the patient complains of diplopia, the cover test should be performed with the head tilted or turned in whatever direction elicits diplopia. With practice the examiner can detect an ocular deviation (heterotropia) as small as 1–2° with the cover test. Deviations can be measured by placing prisms in front of the misaligned eye to determine the power required to neutralize the fixation shift evoked by covering the other eye.

STEREOPSIS

Stereoacuity is determined by presenting targets with retinal disparity separately to each eye by using polarized images. The most popular office tests measure a range of thresholds from 800–40 s of arc. Normal stereoacuity is 40 s of arc. If a patient achieves this level of stereoacuity, one is assured that the eyes are aligned orthotropically and that vision is intact in each eye. Random dot stereograms have no monocular depth cues and provide an excellent screening test for strabismus and amblyopia in children.

COLOR VISION

The retina contains three classes of cones, with visual pigments of differing peak spectral sensitivity: red (560 nm), green (530 nm), and blue (430 nm). The red and green cone pigments are encoded on the X chromosome, and the blue cone pigment on chromosome 7. Mutations of the blue cone pigment are exceedingly rare. Mutations of the red and green pigments cause congenital X-linked color blindness in 8% of males. Affected individuals are not truly color blind; rather, they differ from normal subjects in the way they perceive color and the way they combine primary monochromatic lights to match a particular color. Anomalous trichromats have three cone types, but a mutation in one cone pigment (usually red or green) causes a shift in peak spectral sensitivity, altering the proportion of primary colors required to achieve a color match. Dichromats have only two cone types and therefore will accept a color match based on only two primary colors. Anomalous trichromats and dichromats have 6/6 (20/20) visual acuity, but their hue discrimination is impaired. Ishihara color plates can be used to detect red-green color blindness. The test plates contain a hidden number that is visible only to subjects with color confusion from red-green color blindness. Because color blindness is almost exclusively X-linked, it is worth screening only male children.

The Ishihara plates often are used to detect acquired defects in color vision, although they are intended as a screening test for congenital color blindness. Acquired defects in color vision frequently result from disease of the macula or optic nerve. For example, patients with a history of optic neuritis often complain of color desaturation long after their visual acuity has returned to normal. Color blindness also can result from bilateral strokes involving the ventral portion of the occipital lobe (cerebral achromatopsia). Such patients can perceive only shades of gray and also may have difficulty recognizing faces (prosopagnosia). Infarcts of the dominant occipital lobe sometimes give rise to color anomia. Affected patients can discriminate colors but cannot name them.

VISUAL FIELDS

Vision can be impaired by damage to the visual system anywhere from the eyes to the occipital lobes. One can localize the site of the lesion with considerable accuracy by mapping the visual field deficit by finger confrontation and then correlating it with the topographic anatomy of the visual pathway (**Fig. 21-3**). Quantitative visual field mapping is performed by computer-driven perimeters (Humphrey, Octopus) that present a target of variable intensity at fixed positions in the visual field (Fig. 21-3*A*). By generating an automated printout of

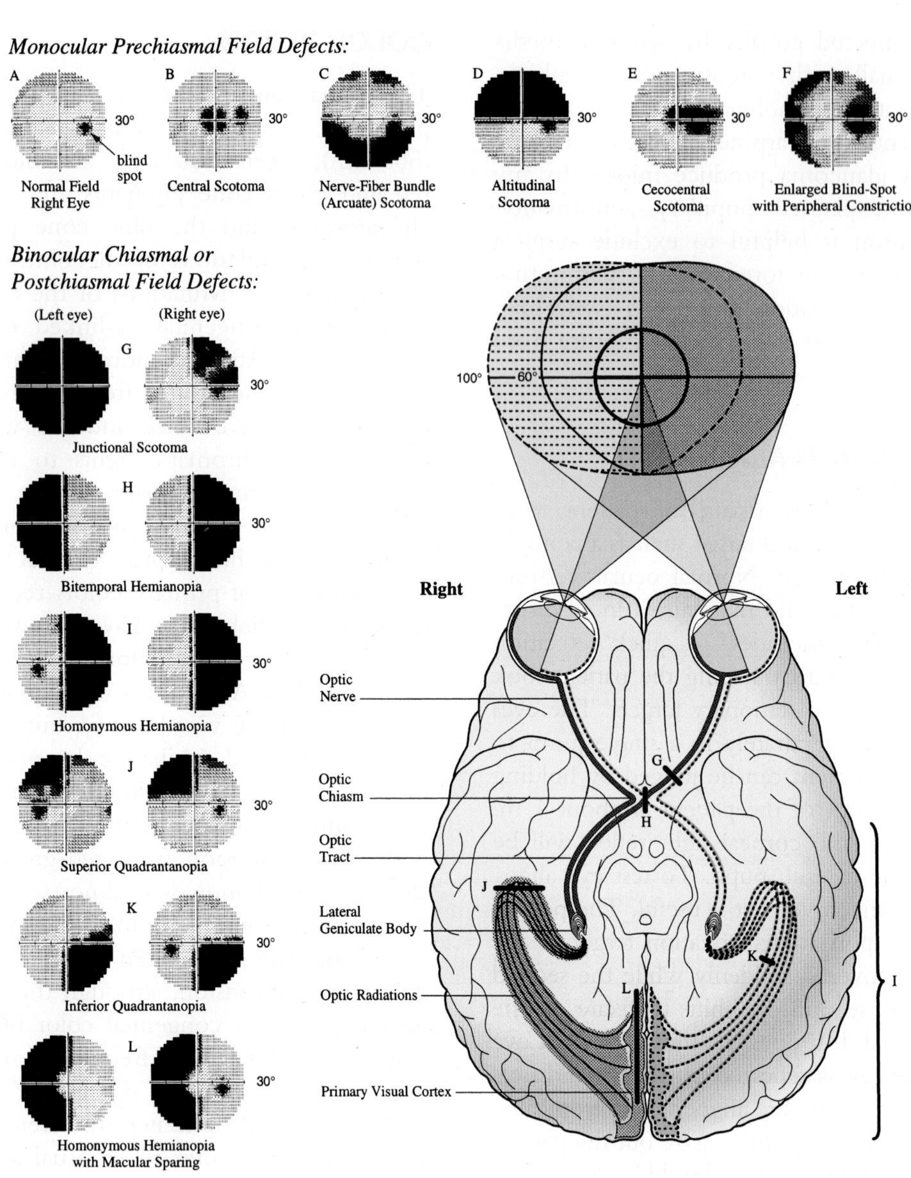

FIGURE 21-3

Ventral view of the brain, correlating patterns of visual field loss with the sites of lesions in the visual pathway. The visual fields overlap partially, creating 120° of central binocular field flanked by a 40° monocular crescent on either side. The visual field maps in this figure were done with a computer-driven perimeter (Humphrey Instruments, Carl Zeiss, Inc.). It plots the retinal sensitivity to light in the central 30° by using a gray scale format. Areas of visual field loss are shown in black. The examples of common monocular, prechiasmal field defects are all shown for the right eye. By convention, the visual fields are always recorded with the left eye's field on the left and the right eye's field on the right, just as the patient sees the world.

light thresholds, these static perimeters provide a sensitive means of detecting scotomas in the visual field. They are exceedingly useful for serial assessment of visual function in chronic diseases such as glaucoma and pseudotumor cerebri.

The crux of visual field analysis is to decide whether a lesion is before, at, or behind the optic chiasm. If a scotoma is confined to one eye, it must be due to a lesion anterior to the chiasm, involving either the optic nerve or the retina. Retinal lesions produce scotomas that correspond optically to their location in the fundus. For example, a superior-nasal retinal detachment results in an inferior-temporal field cut. Damage to the macula causes a central scotoma (Fig. 21-3*B*).

Optic nerve disease produces characteristic patterns of visual field loss. Glaucoma selectively destroys axons that enter the superotemporal or inferotemporal poles of the optic disc, resulting in arcuate scotomas shaped like a Turkish scimitar, which emanate from the blind spot and curve around fixation to end flat against the horizontal meridian (Fig. 21-3*C*). This type of field defect mirrors the arrangement of the nerve fiber layer in the temporal retina. Arcuate or nerve fiber layer scotomas also result from optic neuritis, ischemic optic neuropathy, optic disc drusen, and branch retinal artery or vein occlusion.

Damage to the entire upper or lower pole of the optic disc causes an altitudinal field cut that follows the horizontal meridian (Fig. 21-3*D*). This pattern of visual field loss is typical of ischemic optic neuropathy but also results from retinal vascular occlusion, advanced glaucoma, and optic neuritis.

About half the fibers in the optic nerve originate from ganglion cells serving the macula. Damage to papillomacular fibers causes a cecocentral scotoma that encompasses the blind spot and macula (Fig. 21-3*E*). If the damage is irreversible, pallor eventually appears in the temporal portion of the optic disc. Temporal pallor from a cecocentral scotoma may develop in optic neuritis, nutritional optic neuropathy, toxic optic neuropathy, Leber's hereditary optic neuropathy, and compressive optic neuropathy. It is worth mentioning that the temporal side of the optic disc is slightly more pale than the nasal side in most normal individuals. Therefore, it sometimes can be difficult to decide whether the temporal pallor visible on fundus examination represents a pathologic change. Pallor of the nasal rim of the optic disc is a less equivocal sign of optic atrophy.

At the optic chiasm, fibers from nasal ganglion cells decussate into the contralateral optic tract. Crossed fibers are damaged more by compression than are uncrossed fibers. As a result, mass lesions of the sellar region cause a temporal hemianopia in each eye. Tumors anterior to the optic chiasm, such as meningiomas of the tuberculum sella, produce a junctional scotoma characterized by an optic neuropathy in one eye and a superior-temporal field cut in the other eye (Fig. 21-3*G*). More symmetric compression of the optic chiasm by a pituitary adenoma (Fig. 38-4), meningioma, craniopharyngioma, glioma, or aneurysm results in a bitemporal hemianopia (Fig. 21-3*H*). The insidious development of a bitemporal hemianopia often goes unnoticed by the patient and will escape detection by the physician unless each eye is tested separately.

It is difficult to localize a postchiasmal lesion accurately, because injury anywhere in the optic tract, lateral geniculate body, optic radiations, or visual cortex can produce a homonymous hemianopia (i.e., a temporal hemifield defect in the contralateral eye and a matching nasal hemifield defect in the ipsilateral eye) (Fig. 21-3*I*). A unilateral postchiasmal lesion leaves the visual acuity in each eye unaffected, although the patient may read the letters on only the left or right half of the eye chart. Lesions of the optic radiations tend to cause poorly matched or incongruous field defects in each eye. Damage to the optic radiations in the temporal lobe (Meyer's loop) produces a superior quadrantic homonymous hemianopia (Fig. 21-3*J*), whereas injury to the optic radiations in the parietal lobe results in an inferior quadrantic homonymous hemianopia (Fig. 21-3*K*). Lesions of the primary visual cortex give rise to dense, congruous hemianopic field defects. Occlusion of the posterior cerebral artery supplying the occipital lobe is a common cause of total homonymous hemianopia. Some patients with hemianopia after occipital stroke have macular sparing, because the macular representation at the tip of the occipital lobe is supplied by collaterals from the middle cerebral artery (Fig. 21-3*L*). Destruction of both occipital lobes produces cortical blindness. This condition can be distinguished from bilateral prechiasmal visual loss by noting that the pupil responses and optic fundi remain normal.

DISORDERS

RED OR PAINFUL EYE

Corneal abrasions

Corneal abrasions are seen best by placing a drop of fluorescein in the eye and looking with the slit lamp, using a cobalt-blue light. A penlight with a blue filter will suffice if a slit lamp is not available. Damage to the corneal epithelium is revealed by yellow fluorescence of the exposed basement membrane underlying the epithelium. It is important to check for foreign bodies. To search the conjunctival fornices, the lower lid should be pulled down and the upper lid everted. A foreign body can be removed with a moistened cotton-tipped applicator after a drop of a topical anesthetic such as proparacaine has been placed in the eye. Alternatively, it may be possible to flush the foreign body from the eye by irrigating copiously with saline or artificial tears. If the corneal epithelium has been abraded, antibiotic ointment and a patch should be applied to the eye. A drop of an intermediate-acting cycloplegic such as cyclopentolate hydrochloride 1% helps reduce pain by relaxing the ciliary body. The eye should be reexamined the next day. Minor abrasions may not require patching and cycloplegia.

Subconjunctival hemorrhage

This results from rupture of small vessels bridging the potential space between the episclera and the conjunctiva. Blood dissecting into this space can produce a spectacular red eye, but vision is not affected and the hemorrhage resolves without treatment. Subconjunctival hemorrhage is usually spontaneous but can result from blunt trauma, eye rubbing, or vigorous coughing. Occasionally it is a clue to an underlying bleeding disorder.

Pinguecula

Pinguecula is a small, raised conjunctival nodule at the temporal or nasal limbus. In adults such lesions are extremely common and have little significance unless they become inflamed (pingueculitis). A *pterygium* resembles a pinguecula but has crossed the limbus to encroach on the corneal surface. Removal is justified when symptoms of irritation or blurring develop, but recurrence is a common problem.

Blepharitis

This refers to inflammation of the eyelids. The most common form occurs in association with acne rosacea or seborrheic dermatitis. The eyelid margins usually are colonized heavily by staphylococci. Upon close inspection, they appear greasy, ulcerated, and crusted with scaling debris that clings to the lashes. Treatment consists of warm compresses, strict eyelid hygiene, and topical antibiotics such as bacitracin/polymyxin B ophthalmic ointment. An external *hordeolum* (sty) is caused by staphylococcal infection of the superficial accessory glands of Zeis or Moll located in the eyelid margins. An internal hordeolum occurs after suppurative infection of the oil-secreting meibomian glands within the tarsal plate of the eyelid. Systemic antibiotics, usually tetracyclines or azithromycin, sometimes are necessary for treatment of meibomian gland inflammation (meibomitis) or chronic, severe blepharitis. A *chalazion* is a painless, granulomatous inflammation of a meibomian gland that produces a pealike nodule within the eyelid. It can be incised and drained or injected with glucocorticoids. Basal cell, squamous cell, or meibomian gland carcinoma should be suspected with any nonhealing ulcerative lesion of the eyelids.

Dacryocystitis

An inflammation of the lacrimal drainage system, dacryocystitis can produce epiphora (tearing) and ocular injection. Gentle pressure over the lacrimal sac evokes pain and reflux of mucus or pus from the tear puncta. Dacryocystitis usually occurs after obstruction of the lacrimal system. It is treated with topical and systemic antibiotics, followed by probing or surgery to reestablish patency. *Entropion* (inversion of the eyelid) or *ectropion* (sagging or eversion of the eyelid) can also lead to epiphora and ocular irritation.

Conjunctivitis

Conjunctivitis is the most common cause of a red, irritated eye. Pain is minimal, and visual acuity is reduced only slightly. The most common viral etiology is adenovirus infection. It causes a watery discharge, a mild foreign-body sensation, and photophobia. Bacterial infection tends to produce a more mucopurulent exudate. Mild cases of infectious conjunctivitis usually are treated empirically with broad-spectrum topical ocular antibiotics such as sulfacetamide 10%, polymyxin-bacitracin, or a trimethoprim-polymyxin combination. Smears and cultures usually are reserved for severe, resistant, or recurrent cases of conjunctivitis. To prevent contagion, patients should be admonished to wash their hands frequently, not to touch their eyes, and to avoid direct contact with others.

Allergic conjunctivitis

This condition is extremely common and often is mistaken for infectious conjunctivitis. Itching, redness, and epiphora are typical. The palpebral conjunctiva may become hypertropic with giant excrescences called cobblestone papillae. Irritation from contact lenses or any chronic foreign body also can induce formation of cobblestone papillae. *Atopic conjunctivitis* occurs in subjects with atopic dermatitis or asthma. Symptoms caused by allergic conjunctivitis can be alleviated with cold compresses, topical vasoconstrictors, antihistamines, and mast cell stabilizers such as cromolyn sodium. Topical glucocorticoid solutions provide dramatic relief of immune-mediated forms of conjunctivitis, but their long-term use is ill advised because of the complications of glaucoma, cataract, and secondary infection. Topical nonsteroidal anti-inflammatory drugs (NSAIDs) (e.g., ketorolac tromethamine) are better alternatives.

Keratoconjunctivitis sicca

Also known as dry eye, this produces a burning foreign-body sensation, injection, and photophobia. In mild cases the eye appears surprisingly normal, but tear production measured by wetting of a filter paper (Schirmer strip) is deficient. A variety of systemic drugs, including antihistaminic, anticholinergic, and psychotropic medications, result in dry eye by reducing lacrimal secretion. Disorders that involve the lacrimal gland directly, such as sarcoidosis and Sjögren's syndrome, also cause dry eye. Patients may develop dry eye after radiation therapy if the treatment field includes the orbits. Problems with ocular drying are also common after lesions affecting cranial nerve V or VII. Corneal anesthesia is particularly dangerous, because the absence of a normal blink reflex exposes the cornea to injury without pain to warn the patient. Dry eye is managed by frequent and liberal application of artificial tears and ocular lubricants. In severe cases the tear puncta can be plugged or cauterized to reduce lacrimal outflow.

Keratitis

Keratitis is a threat to vision because of the risk of corneal clouding, scarring, and perforation. Worldwide, the two leading causes of blindness from keratitis are trachoma from chlamydial infection and vitamin A deficiency related to malnutrition. In the United States, contact lenses play a major role in corneal infection and ulceration. They should not be worn by anyone with an active eye infection. In evaluating the cornea, it is important to differentiate between a superficial infection (*keratoconjunctivitis*) and a deeper, more serious ulcerative process. The latter is accompanied by greater visual loss, pain, photophobia, redness, and discharge. Slit-lamp examination shows disruption of the corneal epithelium, a cloudy infiltrate or abscess in the stroma, and an inflammatory cellular reaction in the anterior chamber. In severe cases, pus settles at the bottom of the anterior chamber, giving rise to a hypopyon. Immediate empirical antibiotic therapy should be initiated after corneal scrapings are obtained for Gram's stain, Giemsa stain, and cultures. Fortified topical antibiotics are most effective, supplemented with subconjunctival antibiotics as required. A fungal etiology should always be considered in a patient with keratitis. Fungal infection is common in warm humid climates, especially after penetration of the cornea by plant or vegetable material.

Herpes simplex

The *herpesviruses* are a major cause of blindness from keratitis. Most adults in the United States have serum antibodies to herpes simplex, indicating prior viral infection. Primary ocular infection generally is caused by herpes simplex type 1 rather than type 2. It manifests as a unilateral follicular blepharoconjunctivitis that is easily confused with adenoviral conjunctivitis unless telltale vesicles appear on the periocular skin or conjunctiva. A dendritic pattern of corneal epithelial ulceration revealed by fluorescein staining is pathognomonic for herpes infection but is seen in only a minority of primary infections. Recurrent ocular infection arises from reactivation of the latent herpesvirus. Viral eruption in the corneal epithelium may result in the characteristic herpes dendrite. Involvement of the corneal stroma produces edema, vascularization, and iridocyclitis. Herpes keratitis is treated with topical antiviral agents, cycloplegics, and oral acyclovir. Topical glucocorticoids are effective in mitigating corneal scarring but must be used with extreme caution because of the danger of corneal melting and perforation. Topical glucocorticoids also carry the risk of prolonging infection and inducing glaucoma.

Herpes zoster

Herpes zoster from reactivation of latent varicella (chickenpox) virus causes a dermatomal pattern of painful vesicular dermatitis. Ocular symptoms can occur after zoster eruption in any branch of the trigeminal nerve but are particularly common when vesicles form on the nose, reflecting nasociliary (V1) nerve involvement (Hutchinson's sign). Herpes zoster ophthalmicus produces corneal dendrites, which can be difficult to distinguish from those seen in herpes simplex. Stromal keratitis, anterior uveitis, raised intraocular pressure, ocular motor nerve palsies, acute retinal necrosis, and postherpetic scarring and neuralgia are other common sequelae. Herpes zoster ophthalmicus is treated with antiviral agents and cycloplegics. In severe cases, glucocorticoids may be added to prevent permanent visual loss from corneal scarring.

Episcleritis

This is an inflammation of the episclera, a thin layer of connective tissue between the conjunctiva and the sclera. Episcleritis resembles conjunctivitis, but it is a more localized process and discharge is absent. Most cases of episcleritis are idiopathic, but some occur in the setting of an autoimmune disease. *Scleritis* refers to a deeper, more severe inflammatory process that frequently is associated with a connective tissue disease such as rheumatoid arthritis, lupus erythematosus, polyarteritis nodosa, granulomatosis with polyangiitis (Wegener's) or relapsing polychondritis. The inflammation and thickening of the sclera can be diffuse or nodular. In anterior forms of scleritis, the globe assumes a violet hue and the patient complains of severe ocular tenderness and pain. With posterior scleritis the pain and redness may be less marked, but there is often proptosis, choroidal effusion, reduced motility, and visual loss. Episcleritis and scleritis should be treated with NSAIDs. If these agents fail, topical or even systemic glucocorticoid therapy may be necessary, especially if an underlying autoimmune process is active.

Uveitis

Involving the anterior structures of the eye, uveitis also is called *iritis* or *iridocyclitis*. The diagnosis requires slit-lamp examination to identify inflammatory cells floating in the aqueous humor or deposited on the corneal endothelium (keratic precipitates). Anterior uveitis develops in sarcoidosis, ankylosing spondylitis, juvenile rheumatoid arthritis, inflammatory bowel disease, psoriasis, reactive arthritis (formerly known as Reiter's syndrome), and Behçet's disease. It also is associated with herpes infections, syphilis, Lyme disease, onchocerciasis, tuberculosis, and leprosy. Although anterior uveitis can occur in conjunction with many diseases, no cause is found to explain the majority of cases. For this reason, laboratory evaluation usually is reserved for patients with recurrent or severe anterior uveitis. Treatment is aimed at reducing inflammation and scarring by judicious use of topical glucocorticoids. Dilatation of the pupil reduces pain and prevents the formation of synechiae.

Posterior uveitis

This is diagnosed by observing inflammation of the vitreous, retina, or choroid on fundus examination. It is more likely than anterior uveitis to be associated with an identifiable systemic disease. Some patients have panuveitis, or inflammation of both the anterior and posterior segments of the eye. Posterior uveitis is a manifestation of autoimmune diseases such as sarcoidosis, Behçet's disease, Vogt-Koyanagi-Harada syndrome, and inflammatory bowel disease (Fig. 21-4). It also accompanies diseases such as toxoplasmosis, onchocerciasis, cysticercosis, coccidioidomycosis, toxocariasis, and histoplasmosis; infections caused by organisms such as *Candida*, *Pneumocystis carinii*, *Cryptococcus*, *Aspergillus*, herpes, and cytomegalovirus; and other diseases, such as syphilis, Lyme disease, tuberculosis, cat-scratch disease, Whipple's disease, and brucellosis. In multiple sclerosis, chronic inflammatory changes can develop in the extreme periphery of the retina (pars planitis or intermediate uveitis).

Acute angle-closure glaucoma

This is a rare and frequently misdiagnosed cause of a red, painful eye. Susceptible eyes have a shallow anterior chamber because the eye has either a short axial length (hyperopia) or a lens enlarged by the gradual development of cataract. When the pupil becomes mid-dilated, the peripheral iris blocks aqueous outflow via the anterior chamber angle and the intraocular pressure rises abruptly, producing pain, injection, corneal edema, obscurations, and blurred vision. In some patients, ocular symptoms are overshadowed by nausea, vomiting, or headache, prompting a fruitless workup for abdominal or neurologic disease. The diagnosis is made by measuring the intraocular pressure during an acute attack or by observing a narrow chamber angle by means of a specially mirrored contact lens. Acute angle closure is treated with acetazolamide (PO or IV), topical beta blockers, prostaglandin analogues, α_2-adrenergic agonists, and pilocarpine to induce miosis. If these measures fail, a laser can be used to create a hole in the peripheral iris to relieve pupillary block. Many physicians are reluctant to dilate patients routinely for fundus examination because they fear precipitating an angle-closure glaucoma. The risk is actually remote and more than outweighed by the potential benefit to patients of discovering a hidden fundus lesion visible only through a fully dilated pupil. Moreover, a single attack of angle closure after pharmacologic dilatation rarely causes any permanent damage to the eye and serves as an inadvertent provocative test to identify patients with narrow angles who would benefit from prophylactic laser iridectomy.

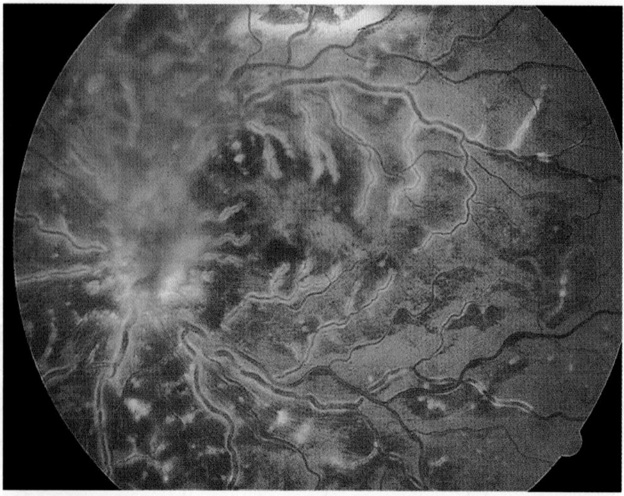

FIGURE 21-4
Retinal vasculitis, uveitis, and hemorrhage in a 32-year-old woman with Crohn's disease. Note that the veins are frosted with a white exudate. Visual acuity improved from 20/400 to 20/20 after treatment with intravenous methylprednisolone.

Endophthalmitis

This results from bacterial, viral, fungal, or parasitic infection of the internal structures of the eye. It usually is acquired by hematogenous seeding from a remote site. Chronically ill, diabetic, or immunosuppressed patients, especially those with a history of indwelling IV catheters or positive blood cultures, are at greatest risk for endogenous endophthalmitis. Although most patients have ocular pain and injection, visual loss is sometimes the only symptom. Septic emboli from a diseased heart valve or a dental abscess that lodge in the retinal circulation can give rise to endophthalmitis. White-centered retinal hemorrhages (Roth's spots) are considered pathognomonic for subacute bacterial endocarditis, but they also appear in leukemia, diabetes, and many other conditions. Endophthalmitis also occurs as a complication of ocular surgery, occasionally months or even years after the operation. An occult penetrating foreign body or unrecognized trauma to the globe should be considered in any patient with unexplained intraocular infection or inflammation.

TRANSIENT OR SUDDEN VISUAL LOSS

Amaurosis fugax

This term refers to a transient ischemic attack of the retina (Chap. 27). Because neural tissue has a high rate of metabolism, interruption of blood flow to the retina for more than a few seconds results in *transient monocular blindness*, a term used interchangeably with amaurosis fugax. Patients describe a rapid fading of vision like a curtain descending, sometimes affecting only a portion of the visual field. Amaurosis fugax usually results from

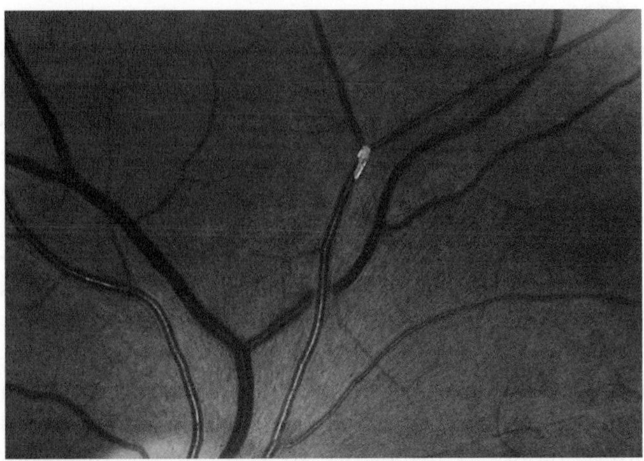

FIGURE 21-5
Hollenhorst plaque lodged at the bifurcation of a retinal arteriole proves that a patient is shedding emboli from the carotid artery, great vessels, or heart.

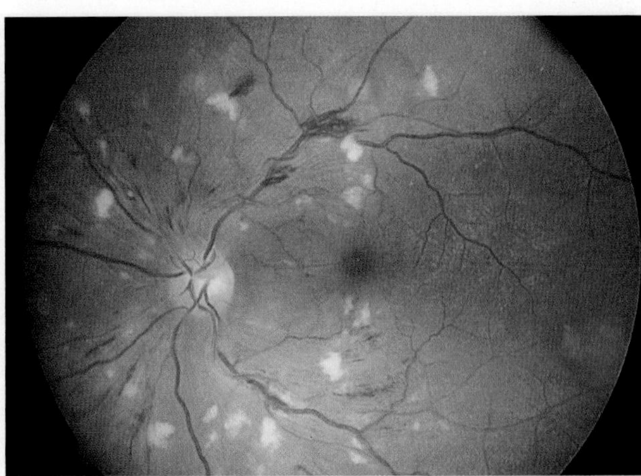

FIGURE 21-7
Hypertensive retinopathy with scattered flame (splinter) hemorrhages and cotton-wool spots (nerve fiber layer infarcts) in a patient with headache and a blood pressure of 234/120.

an embolus that becomes stuck within a retinal arteriole (Fig. 21-5). If the embolus breaks up or passes, flow is restored and vision returns quickly to normal without permanent damage. With prolonged interruption of blood flow, the inner retina suffers infarction. Ophthalmoscopy reveals zones of whitened, edematous retina following the distribution of branch retinal arterioles. Complete occlusion of the central retinal artery produces arrest of blood flow and a milky retina with a cherry-red fovea (Fig. 21-6). Emboli are composed of cholesterol (Hollenhorst plaque), calcium, or platelet-fibrin debris. The most common source is an atherosclerotic plaque in the carotid artery or aorta, although emboli also can arise from the heart, especially in patients with diseased valves, atrial fibrillation, or wall motion abnormalities.

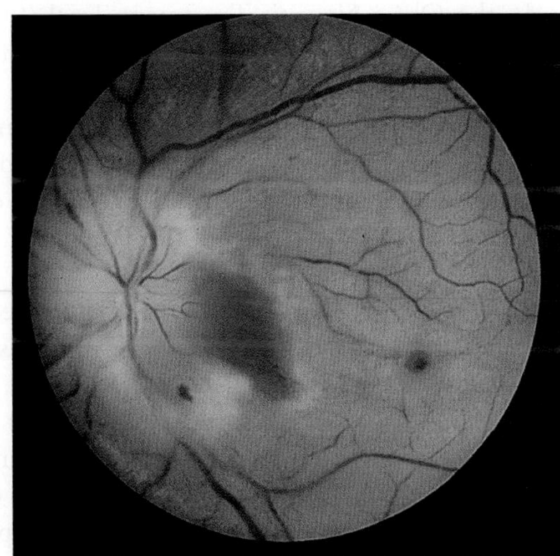

FIGURE 21-6
Central retinal artery occlusion combined with ischemic optic neuropathy in a 19-year-old woman with an elevated titer of anticardiolipin antibodies. Note the orange dot (rather than cherry red) corresponding to the fovea and the spared patch of retina just temporal to the optic disc.

In rare instances, amaurosis fugax results from low central retinal artery perfusion pressure in a patient with a critical stenosis of the ipsilateral carotid artery and poor collateral flow via the circle of Willis. In this situation, amaurosis fugax develops when there is a dip in systemic blood pressure or a slight worsening of the carotid stenosis. Sometimes there is contralateral motor or sensory loss, indicating concomitant hemispheric cerebral ischemia.

Retinal arterial occlusion also occurs rarely in association with retinal migraine, lupus erythematosus, anticardiolipin antibodies (Fig. 21-6), anticoagulant deficiency states (protein S, protein C, and antithrombin deficiency), pregnancy, IV drug abuse, blood dyscrasias, dysproteinemias, and temporal arteritis.

Marked *systemic hypertension* causes sclerosis of retinal arterioles, splinter hemorrhages, focal infarcts of the nerve fiber layer (cotton-wool spots), and leakage of lipid and fluid (hard exudate) into the macula (Fig. 21-7). In hypertensive crisis, sudden visual loss can result from vasospasm of retinal arterioles and retinal ischemia. In addition, acute hypertension may produce visual loss from ischemic swelling of the optic disc. Patients with acute hypertensive retinopathy should be treated by lowering the blood pressure. However, the blood pressure should not be reduced precipitously, because there is a danger of optic disc infarction from sudden hypoperfusion.

Impending *branch* or *central retinal vein occlusion* can produce prolonged visual obscurations that resemble those described by patients with amaurosis fugax. The veins appear engorged and phlebitic, with numerous retinal hemorrhages (Fig. 21-8). In some patients venous blood flow recovers spontaneously, whereas

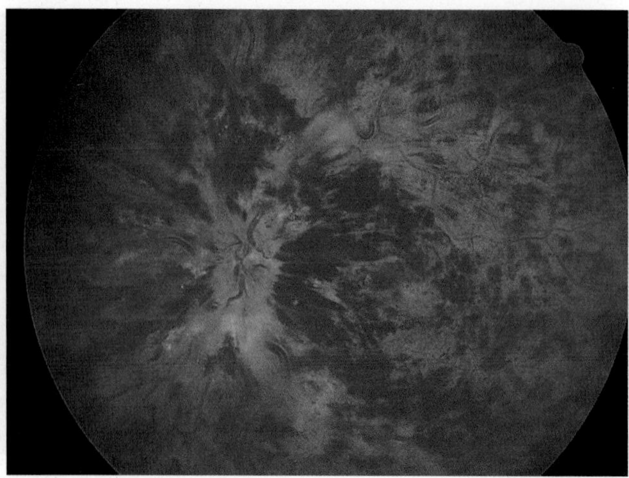

FIGURE 21-8
Central retinal vein occlusion can produce massive retinal hemorrhage ("blood and thunder"), ischemia, and vision loss.

others evolve a frank obstruction with extensive retinal bleeding ("blood and thunder" appearance), infarction, and visual loss. Venous occlusion of the retina is often idiopathic, but hypertension, diabetes, and glaucoma are prominent risk factors. Polycythemia, thrombocythemia, or other factors leading to an underlying hypercoagulable state should be corrected; aspirin treatment may be beneficial.

Anterior ischemic optic neuropathy (AION)

This is caused by insufficient blood flow through the posterior ciliary arteries that supply the optic disc. It produces painless, monocular visual loss that is usually sudden, although some patients have progressive worsening. The optic disc appears swollen and surrounded by nerve fiber layer splinter hemorrhages (Fig. 21-9).

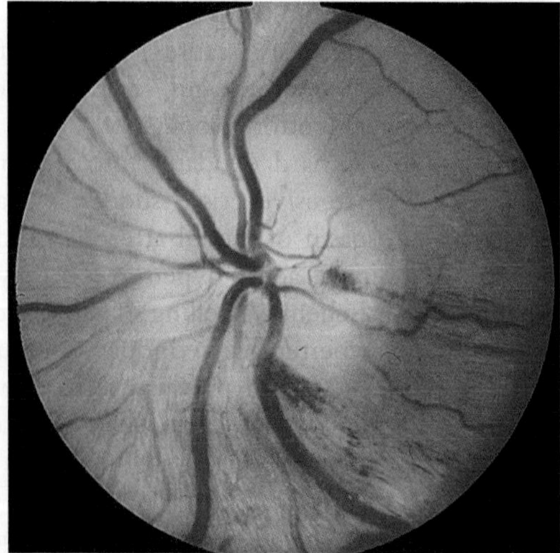

FIGURE 21-9
Anterior ischemic optic neuropathy from temporal arteritis in a 78-year-old woman with pallid disc swelling, hemorrhage, visual loss, myalgia, and an erythrocyte sedimentation rate of 86 mm/h.

AION is divided into two forms: arteritic and nonarteritic. The nonarteritic form is most common. No specific cause can be identified, although diabetes and hypertension are common risk factors. No treatment is available. About 5% of patients, especially those >age 60, develop the arteritic form of AION in conjunction with giant cell (temporal) arteritis. It is urgent to recognize arteritic AION so that high doses of glucocorticoids can be instituted immediately to prevent blindness in the second eye. Symptoms of polymyalgia rheumatica may be present; the sedimentation rate and C-reactive protein level are usually elevated. In a patient with visual loss from suspected arteritic AION, temporal artery biopsy is mandatory to confirm the diagnosis. Glucocorticoids should be started immediately, without waiting for the biopsy to be completed. The diagnosis of arteritic AION is difficult to sustain in the face of a negative temporal artery biopsy, but such cases do occur rarely.

Posterior ischemic optic neuropathy

This is an uncommon cause of acute visual loss, induced by the combination of severe anemia and hypotension. Cases have been reported after major blood loss during surgery, exsanguinating trauma, gastrointestinal bleeding, and renal dialysis. The fundus usually appears normal, although optic disc swelling develops if the process extends far enough anteriorly. Vision can be salvaged in some patients by prompt blood transfusion and reversal of hypotension.

Optic neuritis

This is a common inflammatory disease of the optic nerve. In the Optic Neuritis Treatment Trial (ONTT), the mean age of patients was 32 years, 77% were female, 92% had ocular pain (especially with eye movements), and 35% had optic disc swelling. In most patients, the demyelinating event was retrobulbar and the ocular fundus appeared normal on initial examination (Fig. 21-10), although optic disc pallor slowly developed over subsequent months.

Virtually all patients experience a gradual recovery of vision after a single episode of optic neuritis, even without treatment. This rule is so reliable that failure of vision to improve after a first attack of optic neuritis casts doubt on the original diagnosis. Treatment with high-dose IV methylprednisolone (250 mg every 6 h for 3 days) followed by oral prednisone (1 mg/kg per day for 11 days) makes no difference in final acuity (measured 6 months after the attack), but the recovery of visual function occurs more rapidly.

For some patients, optic neuritis remains an isolated event. However, the ONTT showed that the 15-year cumulative probability of developing clinically definite

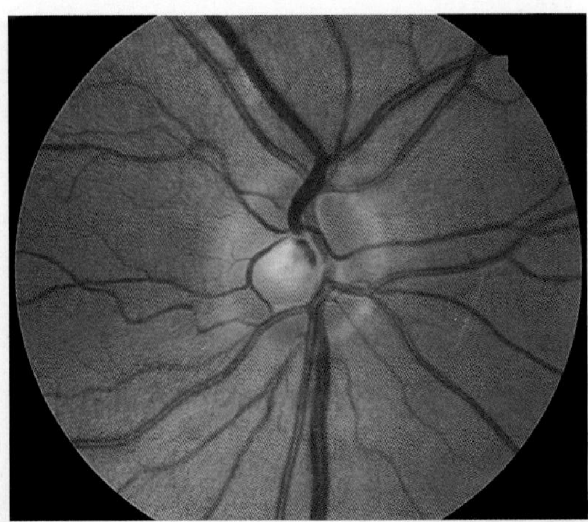

FIGURE 21-10
Retrobulbar optic neuritis is characterized by a normal fundus examination initially, hence the rubric "the doctor sees nothing, and the patient sees nothing." Optic atrophy develops after severe or repeated attacks.

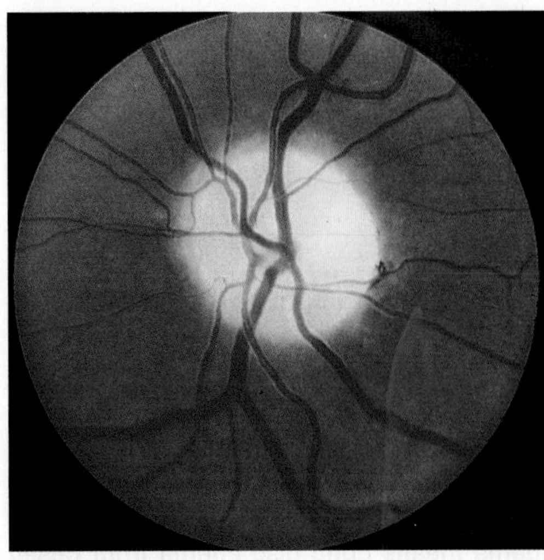

FIGURE 21-11
Optic atrophy is not a specific diagnosis but refers to the combination of optic disc pallor, arteriolar narrowing, and nerve fiber layer destruction produced by a host of eye diseases, especially optic neuropathies.

multiple sclerosis after optic neuritis is 50%. In patients with two or more demyelinating plaques on brain magnetic resonance (MR) imaging, treatment with interferon β-1a can retard the development of more lesions. In summary, an MR scan is recommended in every patient with a first attack of optic neuritis. When visual loss is severe (worse than 20/100), treatment with IV followed by oral glucocorticoids hastens recovery. If multiple lesions are present on the MR scan, treatment with interferon β-1a should be considered.

Leber's hereditary optic neuropathy

This disease usually affects young men, causing gradual, painless, severe central visual loss in one eye, followed weeks or months later by the same process in the other eye. Acutely, the optic disc appears mildly plethoric with surface capillary telangiectases but no vascular leakage on fluorescein angiography. Eventually optic atrophy ensues. Leber's optic neuropathy is caused by a point mutation at codon 11778 in the mitochondrial gene encoding nicotinamide adenine dinucleotide dehydrogenase (NADH) subunit 4. Additional mutations responsible for the disease have been identified, most in mitochondrial genes that encode proteins involved in electron transport. Mitochondrial mutations that cause Leber's neuropathy are inherited from the mother by all her children, but usually only sons develop symptoms.

Toxic optic neuropathy

This can result in acute visual loss with bilateral optic disc swelling and central or cecocentral scotomas. Such cases have been reported to result from exposure to ethambutol, methyl alcohol (moonshine), ethylene glycol (antifreeze), or carbon monoxide. In toxic optic neuropathy, visual loss also can develop gradually and produce optic atrophy (Fig. 21-11) without a phase of acute optic disc edema. Many agents have been implicated as a cause of toxic optic neuropathy, but the evidence supporting the association for many is weak. The following is a partial list of potential offending drugs or toxins: disulfiram, ethchlorvynol, chloramphenicol, amiodarone, monoclonal anti-CD3 antibody, ciprofloxacin, digitalis, streptomycin, lead, arsenic, thallium, d-penicillamine, isoniazid, emetine, and sulfonamides. Deficiency states induced by starvation, malabsorption, or alcoholism can lead to insidious visual loss. Thiamine, vitamin B_{12}, and folate levels should be checked in any patient with unexplained bilateral central scotomas and optic pallor.

Papilledema

This connotes bilateral optic disc swelling from raised intracranial pressure (Fig. 21-12). Headache is a common but not invariable accompaniment. All other forms of optic disc swelling (e.g., from optic neuritis or ischemic optic neuropathy) should be called "optic disc edema." This convention is arbitrary but serves to avoid confusion. Often it is difficult to differentiate papilledema from other forms of optic disc edema by fundus examination alone. Transient visual obscurations are a classic symptom of papilledema. They can occur in only one eye or simultaneously in both eyes. They usually last seconds but can persist longer. Obscurations follow abrupt shifts in posture or happen spontaneously. When obscurations are prolonged or spontaneous, the papilledema is more threatening. Visual acuity is not affected by papilledema unless the papilledema is severe, long-standing, or accompanied by macular edema and

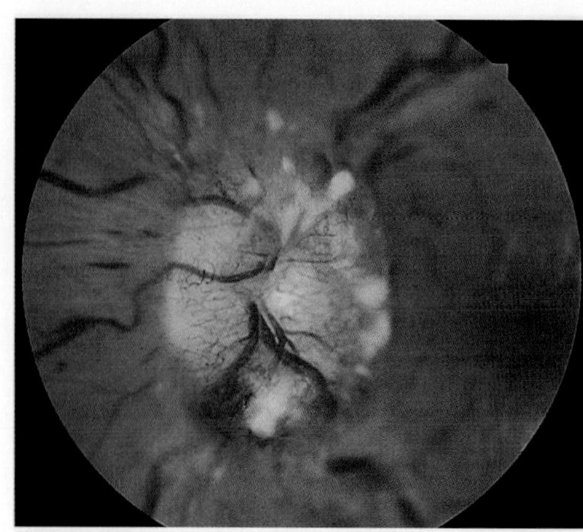

FIGURE 21-12
Papilledema means optic disc edema from raised intracranial pressure. This obese young woman with pseudotumor cerebri was misdiagnosed as a migraineur until fundus examination was performed, showing optic disc elevation, hemorrhages, and cotton-wool spots.

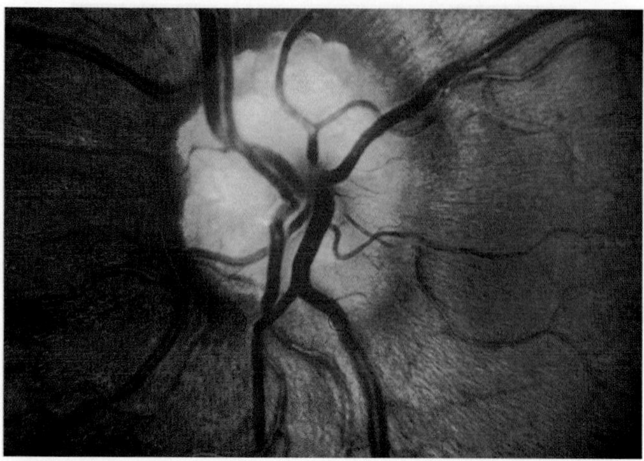

FIGURE 21-13
Optic disc drusen are calcified deposits of unknown etiology within the optic disc. They sometimes are confused with papilledema.

hemorrhage. Visual field testing shows enlarged blind spots and peripheral constriction (Fig. 21-3*F*). With unremitting papilledema, peripheral visual field loss progresses in an insidious fashion while the optic nerve develops atrophy. In this setting, reduction of optic disc swelling is an ominous sign of a dying nerve rather than an encouraging indication of resolving papilledema.

Evaluation of papilledema requires neuroimaging to exclude an intracranial lesion. MR angiography is appropriate in selected cases to search for a dural venous sinus occlusion or an arteriovenous shunt. If neuroradiologic studies are negative, the subarachnoid opening pressure should be measured by lumbar puncture. An elevated pressure, with normal cerebrospinal fluid, points by exclusion to the diagnosis of *pseudotumor cerebri* (idiopathic intracranial hypertension). The majority of patients are young, female, and obese. Treatment with a carbonic anhydrase inhibitor such as acetazolamide lowers intracranial pressure by reducing the production of cerebrospinal fluid. Weight reduction is vital but often unsuccessful. If acetazolamide and weight loss fail and visual field loss is progressive, a shunt should be performed without delay to prevent blindness. Occasionally, emergency surgery is required for sudden blindness caused by fulminant papilledema.

Optic disc drusen

These are refractile deposits within the substance of the optic nerve head (Fig. 21-13). They are unrelated to drusen of the retina, which occur in age-related macular degeneration. Optic disc drusen are most common in people of northern European descent. Their diagnosis is obvious when they are visible as glittering particles on the surface of the optic disc. However, in many patients they are hidden beneath the surface, producing pseudopapilledema. It is important to recognize optic disc drusen to avoid an unnecessary evaluation for papilledema. Ultrasound or CT scanning is sensitive for detection of buried optic disc drusen because they contain calcium. In most patients, optic disc drusen are an incidental, innocuous finding, but they can produce visual obscurations. On perimetry they give rise to enlarged blind spots and arcuate scotomas from damage to the optic disc. With increasing age, drusen tend to become more exposed on the disc surface as optic atrophy develops. Hemorrhage, choroidal neovascular membrane, and AION are more likely to occur in patients with optic disc drusen. No treatment is available.

Vitreous degeneration

This occurs in all individuals with advancing age, leading to visual symptoms. Opacities develop in the vitreous, casting annoying shadows on the retina. As the eye moves, these distracting "floaters" move synchronously, with a slight lag caused by inertia of the vitreous gel. Vitreous traction on the retina causes mechanical stimulation, resulting in perception of flashing lights. This photopsia is brief and is confined to one eye, in contrast to the bilateral, prolonged scintillations of cortical migraine. Contraction of the vitreous can result in sudden separation from the retina, heralded by an alarming shower of floaters and photopsia. This process, known as *vitreous detachment*, is a common involutional event in the elderly. It is not harmful unless it damages the retina. A careful examination of the dilated fundus is important in any patient complaining of floaters or photopsia to search for peripheral tears or holes. If such a lesion is found, laser application can forestall a retinal detachment. Occasionally a tear ruptures a retinal blood vessel, causing vitreous hemorrhage and sudden loss of vision. On attempted ophthalmoscopy the fundus is hidden by a dark red haze of blood. Ultrasound is required to examine the interior of the eye for a retinal tear or detachment. If the hemorrhage does not resolve spontaneously, the vitreous can be removed surgically. Vitreous hemorrhage also results from the fragile neovascular vessels that proliferate on the surface of the retina in diabetes, sickle cell anemia, and other ischemic ocular diseases.

Retinal detachment

This produces symptoms of floaters, flashing lights, and a scotoma in the peripheral visual field corresponding to the detachment (Fig. 21-14). If the detachment includes the fovea, there is an afferent pupil defect and the visual acuity is reduced. In most eyes, retinal detachment starts with a hole, flap, or tear in the peripheral retina (rhegmatogenous retinal detachment). Patients with peripheral retinal thinning (lattice degeneration) are particularly vulnerable to this process. Once a break has developed in the retina, liquefied vitreous is free to enter the subretinal space, separating the retina from the pigment epithelium. The combination of vitreous traction on the retinal surface and passage of fluid behind the retina leads inexorably to detachment. Patients with a history of myopia, trauma, or prior cataract extraction are at greatest risk for retinal detachment. The diagnosis is confirmed by ophthalmoscopic examination of the dilated eye.

Classic migraine

(See also Chap. 8) This usually occurs with a visual aura lasting about 20 min. In a typical attack, a small central disturbance in the field of vision marches toward the periphery, leaving a transient scotoma in its wake. The expanding border of migraine scotoma has a scintillating, dancing, or zigzag edge, resembling the bastions of a fortified city, hence the term *fortification spectra*. Patients' descriptions of fortification spectra vary widely and can be confused with amaurosis fugax. Migraine patterns usually last longer and are perceived in both eyes, whereas amaurosis fugax is briefer and occurs in only one eye. Migraine phenomena also remain visible in the dark or with the eyes closed. Generally they are confined to either the right or the left visual hemifield, but sometimes both fields are involved simultaneously. Patients often have a long history of stereotypic attacks. After the visual symptoms recede, headache develops in most patients.

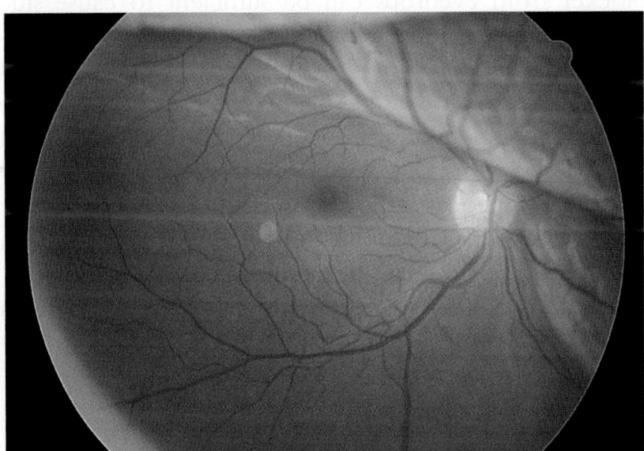

FIGURE 21-14
Retinal detachment appears as an elevated sheet of retinal tissue with folds. In this patient the fovea was spared, so acuity was normal, but a superior detachment produced an inferior scotoma.

Transient ischemic attacks

Vertebrobasilar insufficiency may result in acute homonymous visual symptoms. Many patients mistakenly describe symptoms in the left or right eye when in fact the symptoms are occurring in the left or right hemifield of both eyes. Interruption of blood supply to the visual cortex causes a sudden fogging or graying of vision, occasionally with flashing lights or other positive phenomena that mimic migraine. Cortical ischemic attacks are briefer in duration than migraine, occur in older patients, and are not followed by headache. There may be associated signs of brainstem ischemia, such as diplopia, vertigo, numbness, weakness, and dysarthria.

Stroke

Stroke occurs when interruption of blood supply from the posterior cerebral artery to the visual cortex is prolonged. The only finding on examination is a homonymous visual field defect that stops abruptly at the vertical meridian. Occipital lobe stroke usually is due to thrombotic occlusion of the vertebrobasilar system, embolus, or dissection. Lobar hemorrhage, tumor, abscess, and arteriovenous malformation are other common causes of hemianopic cortical visual loss.

Factitious (functional, nonorganic) visual loss

This is claimed by hysterics or malingerers. The latter account for the vast majority, seeking sympathy, special treatment, or financial gain by feigning loss of sight. The diagnosis is suspected when the history is atypical, physical findings are lacking or contradictory, inconsistencies emerge on testing, and a secondary motive can be identified. In our litigious society, the fraudulent pursuit of recompense has spawned an epidemic of factitious visual loss.

CHRONIC VISUAL LOSS

Cataract

Cataract is a clouding of the lens sufficient to reduce vision. Most cataracts develop slowly as a result of aging, leading to gradual impairment of vision. The formation of cataract occurs more rapidly in patients with a history of ocular trauma, uveitis, or diabetes mellitus. Cataracts are acquired in a variety of genetic diseases, such as myotonic dystrophy, neurofibromatosis type 2, and galactosemia. Radiation therapy and glucocorticoid treatment can induce cataract as a side effect. The cataracts associated with radiation or glucocorticoids have a typical posterior subcapsular location. Cataract can be detected by noting an impaired red reflex when viewing light reflected from the fundus with an ophthalmoscope or by examining the dilated eye with the slit lamp.

The only treatment for cataract is surgical extraction of the opacified lens. Over a million cataract operations are performed each year in the United States. The operation generally is done under local anesthesia on an outpatient basis. A plastic or silicone intraocular lens is placed within the empty lens capsule in the posterior chamber, substituting for the natural lens and leading to rapid recovery of sight. More than 95% of patients who undergo cataract extraction can expect an improvement in vision. In some patients, the lens capsule remaining in the eye after cataract extraction eventually turns cloudy, causing secondary loss of vision. A small opening is made in the lens capsule with a laser to restore clarity.

Glaucoma

Glaucoma is a slowly progressive, insidious optic neuropathy that usually is associated with chronic elevation of intraocular pressure. In African Americans it is the leading cause of blindness. The mechanism by which raised intraocular pressure injures the optic nerve is not understood. Axons entering the inferotemporal and superotemporal aspects of the optic disc are damaged first, producing typical nerve fiber bundle or arcuate scotomas on perimetric testing. As fibers are destroyed, the neural rim of the optic disc shrinks and the physiologic cup within the optic disc enlarges (Fig. 21-15). This process is referred to as pathologic "cupping." The cup-to-disc diameter is expressed as a ratio (e.g., 0.2/1). The cup-to-disc ratio ranges widely in normal individuals, making it difficult to diagnose glaucoma reliably simply by observing an unusually large or deep optic cup. Careful documentation of serial examinations is helpful. In a patient with physiologic cupping the large cup remains stable, whereas in a patient with glaucoma it expands relentlessly over the years. Detection of visual field loss by computerized perimetry also contributes to the diagnosis. Finally, most patients with glaucoma have raised intraocular pressure. However, many patients with typical glaucomatous cupping and visual field loss have intraocular pressures that apparently never exceed the normal limit of 20 mmHg (so-called low-tension glaucoma).

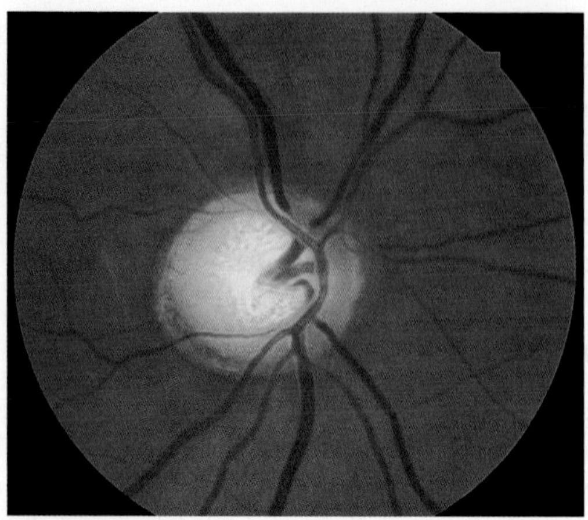

FIGURE 21-15
Glaucoma results in "cupping" as the neural rim is destroyed and the central cup becomes enlarged and excavated. The cup-to-disc ratio is about 0.7/1.0 in this patient.

In acute angle-closure glaucoma, the eye is red and painful due to abrupt, severe elevation of intraocular pressure. Such cases account for only a minority of glaucoma cases: most patients have open, anterior chamber angles. The cause of raised intraocular pressure in open angle glaucoma is unknown, but it is associated with gene mutations in the heritable forms.

Glaucoma is usually painless (except in angle-closure glaucoma). Foveal acuity is spared until end-stage disease is reached. For these reasons, severe and irreversible damage can occur before either the patient or the physician recognizes the diagnosis. Screening of patients for glaucoma by noting the cup-to-disc ratio on ophthalmoscopy and by measuring intraocular pressure is vital. Glaucoma is treated with topical adrenergic agonists, cholinergic agonists, beta blockers, and prostaglandin analogues. Occasionally, systemic absorption of beta blocker from eyedrops can be sufficient to cause side effects of bradycardia, hypotension, heart block, bronchospasm, or depression. Topical or oral carbonic anhydrase inhibitors are used to lower intraocular pressure by reducing aqueous production. Laser treatment of the trabecular meshwork in the anterior chamber angle improves aqueous outflow from the eye. If medical or laser treatments fail to halt optic nerve damage from glaucoma, a filter must be constructed surgically (trabeculectomy) or a valve placed to release aqueous from the eye in a controlled fashion.

Macular degeneration

This is a major cause of gradual, painless, bilateral central visual loss in the elderly. The old term, "senile macular degeneration," misinterpreted by many patients as an unflattering reference, has been replaced with "age-related macular degeneration." It occurs in a nonexudative (dry) form and an exudative (wet) form. Inflammation may be important in both forms of macular degeneration; recent genetic data indicate that susceptibility is associated with variants in the gene for complement factor H, an inhibitor of the alternative complement pathway. The nonexudative process begins with the accumulation of extracellular deposits called drusen underneath the retinal pigment epithelium. On ophthalmoscopy, they are pleomorphic but generally appear as small discrete yellow lesions clustered in the macula (Fig. 21-16). With time they become larger, more numerous, and confluent. The retinal pigment epithelium becomes focally detached and atrophic, causing visual loss by interfering with photoreceptor function. Treatment with vitamins C and E, beta-carotene, and zinc may retard dry macular degeneration.

Exudative macular degeneration, which develops in only a minority of patients, occurs when neovascular vessels from the choroid grow through defects in Bruch's membrane and proliferate underneath the retinal pigment epithelium or the retina. Leakage from these vessels produces elevation of the retina, with distortion (metamorphopsia) and blurring of vision. Although the onset of these symptoms is usually gradual, bleeding from a subretinal choroidal neovascular membrane sometimes causes acute visual loss. Neovascular membranes can be difficult to see on fundus examination because they are located beneath the retina. Fluorescein angiography and optical coherence tomography, a new technique for acquiring images of the retina in cross-section, are extremely useful for their detection. Major or repeated hemorrhage under the retina from neovascular membranes results in fibrosis, development of a round (disciform) macular scar, and permanent loss of central vision.

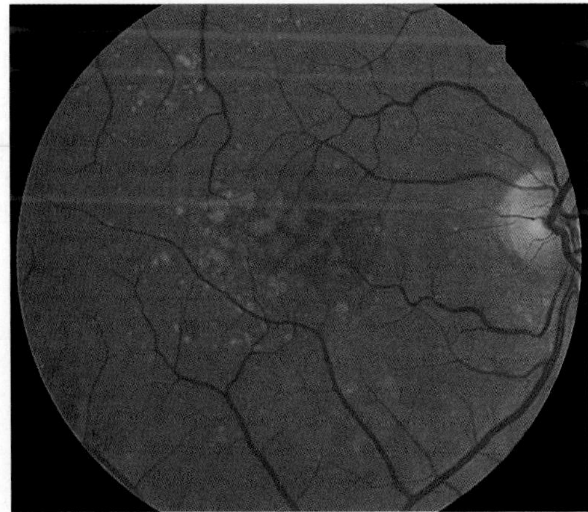

FIGURE 21-16

Age-related macular degeneration begins with the accumulation of drusen within the macula. They appear as scattered yellow subretinal deposits.

A major therapeutic advance has occurred recently with the discovery that exudative macular degeneration can be treated with intraocular injection of a vascular endothelial growth factor antagonist. Either bevacizumab or ranibizumab is administered by direct injection into the vitreous cavity, beginning on a monthly basis. These antibodies cause the regression of neovascular membranes by blocking the action of vascular endothelial growth factor, thereby improving visual acuity.

Central serous chorioretinopathy

This primarily affects males between the ages of 20 and 50. Leakage of serous fluid from the choroid causes small, localized detachment of the retinal pigment epithelium and the neurosensory retina. These detachments produce acute or chronic symptoms of metamorphopsia and blurred vision when the macula is involved. They are difficult to visualize with a direct ophthalmoscope because the detached retina is transparent and only slightly elevated. Diagnosis of central serous chorioretinopathy is made easily by fluorescein angiography, which shows dye streaming into the subretinal space. The cause of central serous chorioretinopathy is unknown. Symptoms may resolve spontaneously if the retina reattaches, but recurrent detachment is common. Laser photocoagulation has benefited some patients with this condition.

Diabetic retinopathy

A rare disease until 1921, when the discovery of insulin resulted in a dramatic improvement in life expectancy for patients with diabetes mellitus, diabetic retinopathy is now a leading cause of blindness in the United States. The retinopathy takes years to develop but eventually appears in nearly all cases. Regular surveillance of the dilated fundus is crucial for any patient with diabetes. In advanced diabetic retinopathy, the proliferation of neovascular vessels leads to blindness from vitreous hemorrhage, retinal detachment, and glaucoma. These complications can be avoided in most patients by administration of panretinal laser photocoagulation at the appropriate point in the evolution of the disease.

Retinitis pigmentosa

This is a general term for a disparate group of rod-cone dystrophies characterized by progressive night blindness, visual field constriction with a ring scotoma, loss of acuity, and an abnormal electroretinogram (ERG). It occurs sporadically or in an autosomal recessive, dominant, or X-linked pattern. Irregular black deposits of clumped pigment in the peripheral retina, called *bone*

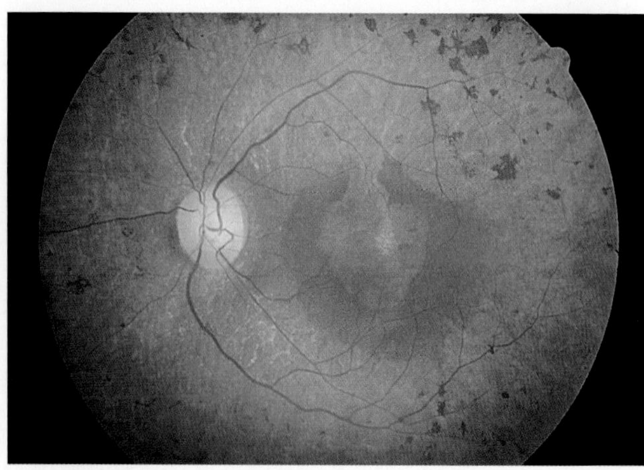

FIGURE 21-17
Retinitis pigmentosa with black clumps of pigment in the retinal periphery known as "bone spicules." There is also atrophy of the retinal pigment epithelium, making the vasculature of the choroid easily visible.

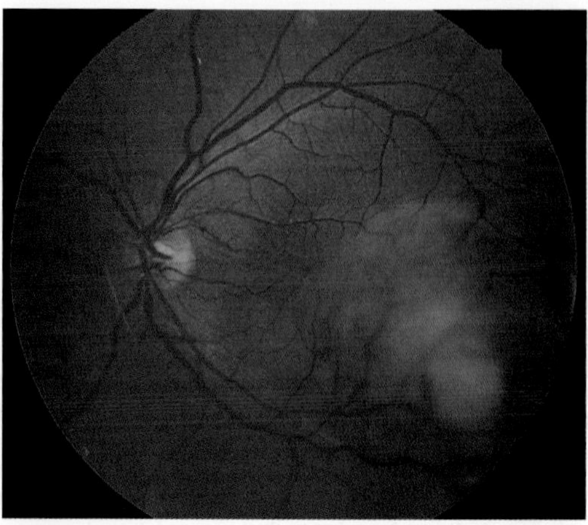

FIGURE 21-18
Melanoma of the choroid, appearing as an elevated dark mass in the inferior temporal fundus, just encroaching upon the fovea.

spicules because of their vague resemblance to the spicules of cancellous bone, give the disease its name (Fig. 21-17). The name is actually a misnomer because retinitis pigmentosa is not an inflammatory process. Most cases are due to a mutation in the gene for rhodopsin, the rod photopigment, or in the gene for peripherin, a glycoprotein located in photoreceptor outer segments. Vitamin A (15,000 IU/d) slightly retards the deterioration of the ERG in patients with retinitis pigmentosa but has no beneficial effect on visual acuity or fields.

Leber's congenital amaurosis, a rare cone dystrophy, has been treated by replacement of the missing RPE65 protein through gene therapy, resulting in modest improvement in visual function. Some forms of retinitis pigmentosa occur in association with rare, hereditary systemic diseases (olivopontocerebellar degeneration, Bassen-Kornzweig disease, Kearns-Sayre syndrome, Refsum's disease). Chronic treatment with chloroquine, hydroxychloroquine, and phenothiazines (especially thioridazine) can produce visual loss from a toxic retinopathy that resembles retinitis pigmentosa.

Epiretinal membrane

This is a fibrocellular tissue that grows across the inner surface of the retina, causing metamorphopsia and reduced visual acuity from distortion of the macula. A crinkled, cellophane-like membrane is visible on the retinal examination. Epiretinal membrane is most common in patients over 50 years of age and is usually unilateral. Most cases are idiopathic, but some occur as a result of hypertensive retinopathy, diabetes, retinal detachment, or trauma. When visual acuity is reduced to the level of about 6/24 (20/80), vitrectomy and surgical peeling of the membrane to relieve macular puckering are recommended. Contraction of an epiretinal membrane sometimes gives rise to a *macular hole*. Most macular holes, however, are caused by local vitreous traction within the fovea. Vitrectomy can improve acuity in selected cases.

Melanoma and other tumors

Melanoma is the most common primary tumor of the eye (Fig. 21-18). It causes photopsia, an enlarging scotoma, and loss of vision. A small melanoma is often difficult to differentiate from a benign choroidal nevus. Serial examinations are required to document a malignant pattern of growth. Treatment of melanoma is controversial. Options include enucleation, local resection, and irradiation. *Metastatic tumors* to the eye outnumber primary tumors. Breast and lung carcinomas have a special propensity to spread to the choroid or iris. Leukemia and lymphoma also commonly invade ocular tissues. Sometimes their only sign on eye examination is cellular debris in the vitreous, which can masquerade as a chronic posterior uveitis. *Retrobulbar tumor* of the optic nerve (meningioma, glioma) or *chiasmal tumor* (pituitary adenoma, meningioma) produces gradual visual loss with few objective findings except for optic disc pallor. Rarely, sudden expansion of a pituitary adenoma from infarction and bleeding (*pituitary apoplexy*) causes acute retrobulbar visual loss, with headache, nausea, and ocular motor nerve palsies. In any patient with visual field loss or optic atrophy, CT or MR scanning should be considered if the cause remains unknown after careful review of the history and thorough examination of the eye.

PROPTOSIS

When the globes appear asymmetric, the clinician must first decide which eye is abnormal. Is one eye recessed within the orbit (*enophthalmos*), or is the other eye protuberant (*exophthalmos*, or *proptosis*)? A small globe or a

Horner's syndrome can give the appearance of enophthalmos. True enophthalmos occurs commonly after trauma, from atrophy of retrobulbar fat, or from fracture of the orbital floor. The position of the eyes within the orbits is measured by using a Hertel exophthalmometer, a handheld instrument that records the position of the anterior corneal surface relative to the lateral orbital rim. If this instrument is not available, relative eye position can be judged by bending the patient's head forward and looking down upon the orbits. A proptosis of only 2 mm in one eye is detectable from this perspective. The development of proptosis implies a space-occupying lesion in the orbit and usually warrants CT or MR imaging.

Graves' ophthalmopathy

This is the leading cause of proptosis in adults. The proptosis is often asymmetric and can even appear to be unilateral. Orbital inflammation and engorgement of the extraocular muscles, particularly the medial rectus and the inferior rectus, account for the protrusion of the globe. Corneal exposure, lid retraction, conjunctival injection, restriction of gaze, diplopia, and visual loss from optic nerve compression are cardinal symptoms. Graves' ophthalmopathy is treated with oral prednisone (60 mg/d) for 1 month, followed by a taper over several months, topical lubricants, eyelid surgery, eye muscle surgery, or orbital decompression. Radiation therapy is not effective.

Orbital pseudotumor

This is an idiopathic, inflammatory orbital syndrome that frequently is confused with Graves' ophthalmopathy. Symptoms are pain, limited eye movements, proptosis, and congestion. Evaluation for sarcoidosis, granulomatosis with polyangiitis (Wegener's), and other types of orbital vasculitis or collagen-vascular disease is negative. Imaging often shows swollen eye muscles (orbital myositis) with enlarged tendons. By contrast, in Graves' ophthalmopathy the tendons of the eye muscles usually are spared. The Tolosa-Hunt syndrome may be regarded as an extension of orbital pseudotumor through the superior orbital fissure into the cavernous sinus. The diagnosis of orbital pseudotumor is difficult. Biopsy of the orbit frequently yields nonspecific evidence of fat infiltration by lymphocytes, plasma cells, and eosinophils. A dramatic response to a therapeutic trial of systemic glucocorticoids indirectly provides the best confirmation of the diagnosis.

Orbital cellulitis

This causes pain, lid erythema, proptosis, conjunctival chemosis, restricted motility, decreased acuity, afferent pupillary defect, fever, and leukocytosis. It often arises from the paranasal sinuses, especially by contiguous spread of infection from the ethmoid sinus through the lamina papyracea of the medial orbit. A history of recent upper respiratory tract infection, chronic sinusitis, thick mucus secretions, or dental disease is significant in any patient with suspected orbital cellulitis. Blood cultures should be obtained, but they are usually negative. Most patients respond to empirical therapy with broad-spectrum IV antibiotics. Occasionally, orbital cellulitis follows an overwhelming course, with massive proptosis, blindness, septic cavernous sinus thrombosis, and meningitis. To avert this disaster, orbital cellulitis should be managed aggressively in the early stages, with immediate imaging of the orbits and antibiotic therapy that includes coverage of methicillin-resistant *Staphylococcus aureus* (MRSA). Prompt surgical drainage of an orbital abscess or paranasal sinusitis is indicated if optic nerve function deteriorates despite antibiotics.

Tumors

Tumors of the orbit cause painless, progressive proptosis. The most common primary tumors are hemangioma, lymphangioma, neurofibroma, dermoid cyst, adenoid cystic carcinoma, optic nerve glioma, optic nerve meningioma, and benign mixed tumor of the lacrimal gland. Metastatic tumor to the orbit occurs frequently in breast carcinoma, lung carcinoma, and lymphoma. Diagnosis by fine-needle aspiration followed by urgent radiation therapy sometimes can preserve vision.

Carotid cavernous fistulas

With anterior drainage through the orbit these fistulas produce proptosis, diplopia, glaucoma, and corkscrew, arterialized conjunctival vessels. Direct fistulas usually result from trauma. They are easily diagnosed because of the prominent signs produced by high-flow, high-pressure shunting. Indirect fistulas, or dural arteriovenous malformations, are more likely to occur spontaneously, especially in older women. The signs are more subtle, and the diagnosis frequently is missed. The combination of slight proptosis, diplopia, enlarged muscles, and an injected eye often is mistaken for thyroid ophthalmopathy. A bruit heard upon auscultation of the head or reported by the patient is a valuable diagnostic clue. Imaging shows an enlarged superior ophthalmic vein in the orbits. Carotid cavernous shunts can be eliminated by intravascular embolization.

PTOSIS

Blepharoptosis

This is an abnormal drooping of the eyelid. Unilateral or bilateral ptosis can be congenital, from dysgenesis of the levator palpebrae superioris, or from abnormal insertion of its aponeurosis into the eyelid. Acquired ptosis can develop so gradually that the patient is unaware of the problem. Inspection of old photographs is helpful in dating the onset. A history of prior trauma, eye surgery, contact lens use, diplopia, systemic symptoms (e.g., dysphagia or peripheral muscle weakness), or a family history of ptosis should be sought. Fluctuating ptosis that worsens late in the day is typical of myasthenia gravis. Examination should focus on evidence for proptosis, eyelid masses or deformities, inflammation, pupil inequality, or limitation of motility. The width of the palpebral fissures is measured in primary gaze to quantitate the degree of ptosis. The ptosis will be underestimated if the patient compensates by lifting the brow with the frontalis muscle.

Mechanical ptosis

This occurs in many elderly patients from stretching and redundancy of eyelid skin and subcutaneous fat (dermatochalasis). The extra weight of these sagging tissues causes the lid to droop. Enlargement or deformation of the eyelid from infection, tumor, trauma, or inflammation also results in ptosis on a purely mechanical basis.

Aponeurotic ptosis

This is an acquired dehiscence or stretching of the aponeurotic tendon, which connects the levator muscle to the tarsal plate of the eyelid. It occurs commonly in older patients, presumably from loss of connective tissue elasticity. Aponeurotic ptosis is also a common sequela of eyelid swelling from infection or blunt trauma to the orbit, cataract surgery, or hard contact lens use.

Myogenic ptosis

The causes of *myogenic ptosis* include myasthenia gravis (Chap. 47) and a number of rare myopathies that manifest with ptosis. The term *chronic progressive external ophthalmoplegia* refers to a spectrum of systemic diseases caused by mutations of mitochondrial DNA. As the name implies, the most prominent findings are symmetric, slowly progressive ptosis and limitation of eye movements. In general, diplopia is a late symptom because all eye movements are reduced equally. In the *Kearns-Sayre* variant, retinal pigmentary changes and abnormalities of cardiac conduction develop. Peripheral muscle biopsy shows characteristic "ragged-red fibers." *Oculopharyngeal dystrophy* is a distinct autosomal dominant disease with onset in middle age, characterized by ptosis, limited eye movements, and trouble swallowing. *Myotonic dystrophy*, another autosomal dominant disorder, causes ptosis, ophthalmoparesis, cataract, and pigmentary retinopathy. Patients have muscle wasting, myotonia, frontal balding, and cardiac abnormalities.

Neurogenic ptosis

This results from a lesion affecting the innervation to either of the two muscles that open the eyelid: Müller's muscle or the levator palpebrae superioris. Examination of the pupil helps distinguish between these two possibilities. In Horner's syndrome, the eye with ptosis has a smaller pupil and the eye movements are full. In an oculomotor nerve palsy, the eye with the ptosis has a larger or a normal pupil. If the pupil is normal but there is limitation of adduction, elevation, and depression, a pupil-sparing oculomotor nerve palsy is likely (see next section). Rarely, a lesion affecting the small, central subnucleus of the oculomotor complex will cause bilateral ptosis with normal eye movements and pupils.

DOUBLE VISION (DIPLOPIA)

The first point to clarify is whether diplopia persists in either eye after the opposite eye is covered. If it does, the diagnosis is monocular diplopia. The cause is usually intrinsic to the eye and therefore has no dire implications for the patient. Corneal aberrations (e.g., keratoconus, pterygium), uncorrected refractive error, cataract, or foveal traction may give rise to monocular diplopia. Occasionally it is a symptom of malingering or psychiatric disease. Diplopia alleviated by covering one eye is binocular diplopia and is caused by disruption of ocular alignment. Inquiry should be made into the nature of the double vision (purely side-by-side versus partial vertical displacement of images), mode of onset, duration, intermittency, diurnal variation, and associated neurologic or systemic symptoms. If the patient has diplopia while being examined, motility testing should reveal a deficiency corresponding to the patient's symptoms. However, subtle limitation of ocular excursions is often difficult to detect. For example, a patient with a slight left abducens nerve paresis may appear to have full eye movements despite a complaint of horizontal diplopia upon looking to the left. In this situation, the cover test provides a more sensitive method for demonstrating the ocular misalignment. It should be conducted in primary gaze and then with the head turned and tilted in each direction. In the above example, a cover test with the head turned to the right will maximize the fixation shift evoked by the cover test.

Occasionally, a cover test performed in an asymptomatic patient during a routine examination will reveal an ocular deviation. If the eye movements are full and the ocular misalignment is equal in all directions of gaze (concomitant deviation), the diagnosis is strabismus. In this condition, which affects about 1% of the population, fusion is disrupted in infancy or early childhood. To avoid diplopia, vision is suppressed from the nonfixating eye. In some children, this leads to impaired vision (amblyopia, or "lazy" eye) in the deviated eye.

Binocular diplopia results from a wide range of processes: infectious, neoplastic, metabolic, degenerative, inflammatory, and vascular. One must decide whether the diplopia is neurogenic in origin or is due to restriction of globe rotation by local disease in the orbit. Orbital pseudotumor, myositis, infection, tumor, thyroid disease, and muscle entrapment (e.g., from a blowout fracture) cause restrictive diplopia. The diagnosis of restriction is usually made by recognizing other associated signs and symptoms of local orbital disease in conjunction with imaging.

Myasthenia gravis

(See also Chap. 47) This is a major cause of diplopia. The diplopia is often intermittent, variable, and not confined to any single ocular motor nerve distribution. The pupils are always normal. Fluctuating ptosis may be present. Many patients have a purely ocular form of the disease, with no evidence of systemic muscular weakness. The diagnosis can be confirmed by an IV edrophonium injection or by an assay for antiacetylcholine receptor antibodies. Negative results from these tests do not exclude the diagnosis. *Botulism* from food or wound poisoning can mimic ocular myasthenia.

After restrictive orbital disease and myasthenia gravis are excluded, a lesion of a cranial nerve supplying innervation to the extraocular muscles is the most likely cause of binocular diplopia.

Oculomotor nerve

The third cranial nerve innervates the medial, inferior, and superior recti; inferior oblique; levator palpebrae superioris; and the iris sphincter. Total palsy of the oculomotor nerve causes ptosis, results in a dilated pupil, and leaves the eye "down and out" because of the unopposed action of the lateral rectus and superior oblique. This combination of findings is obvious. More challenging is the diagnosis of early or partial oculomotor nerve palsy. In this setting, any combination of ptosis, pupil dilation, and weakness of the eye muscles supplied by the oculomotor nerve may be encountered. Frequent serial examinations during the evolving phase of the palsy help ensure that the diagnosis is not missed. The advent of an oculomotor nerve palsy with a pupil involvement, especially when accompanied by pain, suggests a compressive lesion, such as a tumor or circle of Willis aneurysm. Neuroimaging should be obtained, along with a CT or MR angiogram. Occasionally, a catheter arteriogram must be done to exclude an aneurysm.

A lesion of the oculomotor nucleus in the rostral midbrain produces signs that differ from those caused by a lesion of the nerve itself. There is bilateral ptosis because the levator muscle is innervated by a single central subnucleus. There is also weakness of the contralateral superior rectus, because it is supplied by the oculomotor nucleus on the other side. Occasionally both superior recti are weak. Isolated nuclear oculomotor palsy is rare. Usually neurologic examination reveals additional signs that suggest brainstem damage from infarction, hemorrhage, tumor, or infection.

Injury to structures surrounding fascicles of the oculomotor nerve descending through the midbrain has given rise to a number of classic eponymic designations. In *Nothnagel's syndrome*, injury to the superior cerebellar peduncle causes ipsilateral oculomotor palsy and contralateral cerebellar ataxia. In *Benedikt's syndrome*, injury to the red nucleus results in ipsilateral oculomotor palsy and contralateral tremor, chorea, and athetosis. *Claude's syndrome* incorporates features of both of these syndromes, by injury to both the red nucleus and the superior cerebellar peduncle. Finally, in *Weber's syndrome*, injury to the cerebral peduncle causes ipsilateral oculomotor palsy with contralateral hemiparesis.

In the subarachnoid space the oculomotor nerve is vulnerable to aneurysm, meningitis, tumor, infarction, and compression. In cerebral herniation the nerve becomes trapped between the edge of the tentorium and the uncus of the temporal lobe. Oculomotor palsy also can result from midbrain torsion and hemorrhages during herniation. In the cavernous sinus, oculomotor palsy arises from carotid aneurysm, carotid cavernous fistula, cavernous sinus thrombosis, tumor (pituitary adenoma, meningioma, metastasis), herpes zoster infection, and the Tolosa-Hunt syndrome.

The etiology of an isolated, pupil-sparing oculomotor palsy often remains an enigma even after neuroimaging and extensive laboratory testing. Most cases are thought to result from microvascular infarction of the nerve somewhere along its course from the brainstem to the orbit. Usually the patient complains of pain. Diabetes, hypertension, and vascular disease are major risk factors. Spontaneous recovery over a period of months is the rule. If this fails to occur or if new findings develop, the diagnosis of microvascular oculomotor nerve palsy should be reconsidered. Aberrant regeneration is common when the oculomotor nerve is injured by trauma or compression (tumor, aneurysm). Miswiring of sprouting fibers to the levator muscle and the rectus muscles results in elevation of the eyelid upon downgaze or adduction. The pupil also constricts upon attempted adduction, elevation, or depression of the globe. Aberrant regeneration is not seen after oculomotor palsy from microvascular infarct and hence vitiates that diagnosis.

Trochlear nerve

The fourth cranial nerve originates in the midbrain, just caudal to the oculomotor nerve complex. Fibers exit the brainstem dorsally and cross to innervate the contralateral superior oblique. The principal actions of this muscle are to depress and intort the globe. A palsy therefore results in hypertropia and excyclotorsion. The cyclotorsion seldom is noticed by patients. Instead, they complain of vertical diplopia, especially upon reading or looking down. The vertical diplopia also is exacerbated by tilting the head toward the side with the muscle palsy and alleviated by tilting it away. This "head tilt test" is a cardinal diagnostic feature.

Isolated trochlear nerve palsy results from all the causes listed earlier for the oculomotor nerve except aneurysm. The trochlear nerve is particularly apt to suffer injury after closed head trauma. The free edge of the tentorium is thought to impinge on the nerve during a concussive blow. Most isolated trochlear nerve palsies are idiopathic and hence are diagnosed by exclusion as "microvascular." Spontaneous improvement occurs over a period of months in most patients. A base-down prism (conveniently applied to the patient's glasses as a stick-on Fresnel lens) may serve as a temporary measure to alleviate diplopia. If the palsy does not resolve, the eyes can be realigned by weakening the inferior oblique muscle.

Abducens nerve

The sixth cranial nerve innervates the lateral rectus muscle. A palsy produces horizontal diplopia, worse on gaze to the side of the lesion. A nuclear lesion has different consequences, because the abducens nucleus contains interneurons that project via the medial longitudinal fasciculus to the medial rectus subnucleus of the contralateral oculomotor complex. Therefore, an abducens nuclear lesion produces a complete lateral gaze palsy from weakness of both the ipsilateral lateral rectus and the contralateral medial rectus. *Foville's syndrome* after dorsal pontine injury includes lateral gaze palsy, ipsilateral facial palsy, and contralateral hemiparesis incurred by damage to descending corticospinal fibers. *Millard-Gubler syndrome* from ventral pontine injury is similar except for the eye findings. There is lateral rectus weakness only, instead of gaze palsy, because the abducens fascicle is injured rather than the nucleus. Infarct, tumor, hemorrhage, vascular malformation, and multiple sclerosis are the most common etiologies of brainstem abducens palsy.

After leaving the ventral pons, the abducens nerve runs forward along the clivus to pierce the dura at the petrous apex, where it enters the cavernous sinus. Along its subarachnoid course it is susceptible to meningitis, tumor (meningioma, chordoma, carcinomatous meningitis), subarachnoid hemorrhage, trauma, and compression by aneurysm or dolichoectatic vessels. At the petrous apex, mastoiditis can produce deafness, pain, and ipsilateral abducens palsy (*Gradenigo's syndrome*). In the cavernous sinus, the nerve can be affected by carotid aneurysm, carotid cavernous fistula, tumor (pituitary adenoma, meningioma, nasopharyngeal carcinoma), herpes infection, and Tolosa-Hunt syndrome.

Unilateral or bilateral abducens palsy is a classic sign of raised intracranial pressure. The diagnosis can be confirmed if papilledema is observed on fundus examination. The mechanism is still debated but probably is related to rostral-caudal displacement of the brainstem. The same phenomenon accounts for abducens palsy from low intracranial pressure (e.g., after lumbar puncture, spinal anesthesia, or spontaneous dural cerebrospinal fluid leak).

Treatment of abducens palsy is aimed at prompt correction of the underlying cause. However, the cause remains obscure in many instances despite diligent evaluation. As was mentioned earlier for isolated trochlear or oculomotor palsy, most cases are assumed to represent microvascular infarcts because they often occur in the setting of diabetes or other vascular risk factors. Some cases may develop as a postinfectious mononeuritis (e.g., after a viral flu). Patching one eye or applying a temporary prism will provide relief of diplopia until the palsy resolves. If recovery is incomplete, eye muscle surgery nearly always can realign the eyes, at least in primary position. A patient with an abducens palsy that fails to improve should be reevaluated for an occult etiology (e.g., chordoma, carcinomatous meningitis, carotid cavernous fistula, myasthenia gravis). Skull base tumors are easily missed even on contrast-enhanced neuroimaging studies.

Multiple ocular motor nerve palsies

These should not be attributed to spontaneous microvascular events affecting more than one cranial nerve at a time. This remarkable coincidence does occur, especially in diabetic patients, but the diagnosis is made only in retrospect after all other diagnostic alternatives have been exhausted. Neuroimaging should focus on the cavernous sinus, superior orbital fissure, and orbital apex, where all three ocular motor nerves are in close proximity. In a diabetic or immunocompromised host, fungal infection (*Aspergillus*, Mucorales, *Cryptococcus*) is a common cause of multiple nerve palsies. In a patient with systemic malignancy, carcinomatous meningitis is a likely diagnosis. Cytologic examination may be negative despite repeated sampling of the cerebrospinal fluid. The cancer-associated Lambert-Eaton myasthenic syndrome also can produce ophthalmoplegia. Giant cell (temporal) arteritis occasionally manifests as diplopia from ischemic palsies of extraocular muscles. Fisher's syndrome, an ocular variant of Guillain-Barré, produces ophthalmoplegia with areflexia and ataxia. Often the ataxia is mild, and the reflexes are normal. Antiganglioside antibodies (GQ1b) can be detected in about 50% of cases.

Supranuclear disorders of gaze

These are often mistaken for multiple ocular motor nerve palsies. For example, Wernicke's encephalopathy can produce nystagmus and a partial deficit of horizontal and vertical gaze that mimics a combined abducens and oculomotor nerve palsy. The disorder occurs in malnourished or alcoholic patients and can be reversed by thiamine. Infarct, hemorrhage, tumor, multiple sclerosis, encephalitis, vasculitis, and Whipple's disease are other important causes of supranuclear gaze palsy. Disorders of vertical gaze, especially downward saccades, are an early feature of progressive supranuclear palsy. Smooth pursuit is affected later in the course of the disease. Parkinson's disease, Huntington's disease, and olivopontocerebellar degeneration also can affect vertical gaze.

The *frontal eye field* of the cerebral cortex is involved in generation of saccades to the contralateral side. After hemispheric stroke, the eyes usually deviate toward the lesioned side because of the unopposed action of the frontal eye field in the normal hemisphere. With time, this deficit resolves. Seizures generally have the opposite effect: the eyes deviate conjugately away from the irritative focus. *Parietal lesions* disrupt smooth pursuit of targets moving toward the side of the lesion. Bilateral parietal lesions produce *Bálint's syndrome,* which is characterized by impaired eye-hand coordination (optic ataxia), difficulty initiating voluntary eye movements (ocular apraxia), and visuospatial disorientation (simultanagnosia).

Horizontal gaze

Descending cortical inputs mediating horizontal gaze ultimately converge at the level of the pons. Neurons in the paramedian pontine reticular formation are responsible for controlling conjugate gaze toward the same side. They project directly to the ipsilateral abducens nucleus. A lesion of either the paramedian pontine reticular formation or the abducens nucleus causes an ipsilateral conjugate gaze palsy. Lesions at either locus produce nearly identical clinical syndromes, with the following exception: vestibular stimulation (oculocephalic maneuver or caloric irrigation) will succeed in driving the eyes conjugately to the side in a patient with a lesion of the paramedian pontine reticular formation but not in a patient with a lesion of the abducens nucleus.

Internuclear ophthalmoplegia

This results from damage to the medial longitudinal fasciculus ascending from the abducens nucleus in the pons to the oculomotor nucleus in the midbrain (hence, "internuclear"). Damage to fibers carrying the conjugate signal from abducens interneurons to the contralateral medial rectus motoneurons results in a failure of adduction on attempted lateral gaze. For example, a patient with a left internuclear ophthalmoplegia (INO) will have slowed or absent adducting movements of the left eye (Fig. 21-19). A patient with bilateral injury to the medial longitudinal fasciculus will have bilateral INO. Multiple sclerosis is the most common cause, although tumor, stroke, trauma, or any brainstem process may be responsible. *One-and-a-half syndrome* is due to a combined lesion of the medial longitudinal fasciculus and the abducens nucleus on the same side. The patient's only horizontal eye movement is abduction of the eye on the other side.

Vertical gaze

This is controlled at the level of the midbrain. The neuronal circuits affected in disorders of vertical gaze are not fully elucidated, but lesions of the rostral interstitial nucleus of the medial longitudinal fasciculus and the interstitial nucleus of Cajal cause supranuclear paresis of upgaze, downgaze, or all vertical eye movements. Distal basilar artery ischemia is the most common etiology. *Skew deviation* refers to a vertical misalignment of the eyes, usually constant in all positions of gaze. The finding has poor localizing value because skew deviation has been reported after lesions in widespread regions of the brainstem and cerebellum.

Parinaud's syndrome

Also known as dorsal midbrain syndrome, this is a distinct supranuclear vertical gaze disorder caused by damage to the posterior commissure. It is a classic sign of hydrocephalus from aqueductal stenosis. Pineal region tumors, cysticercosis, and stroke also cause Parinaud's syndrome. Features include loss of upgaze (and sometimes downgaze), convergence-retraction nystagmus on attempted upgaze, downward ocular deviation ("setting sun" sign), lid retraction (Collier's sign), skew deviation, pseudoabducens palsy, and light-near dissociation of the pupils.

Nystagmus

This is a rhythmic oscillation of the eyes, occurring physiologically from vestibular and optokinetic stimulation or pathologically in a wide variety of diseases (Chap. 11). Abnormalities of the eyes or optic nerves, present at birth or acquired in childhood, can produce a complex, searching nystagmus with irregular pendular

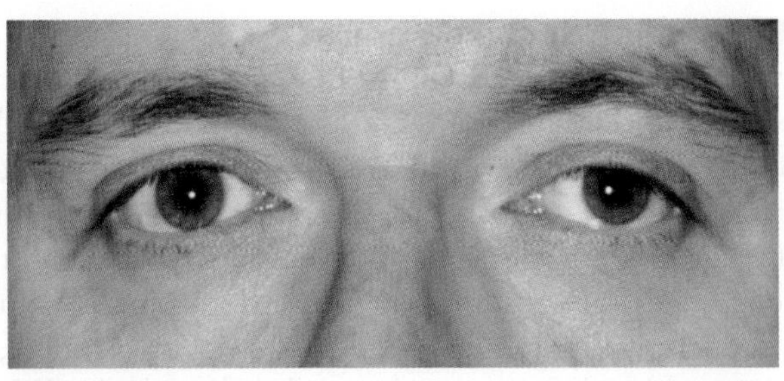

A

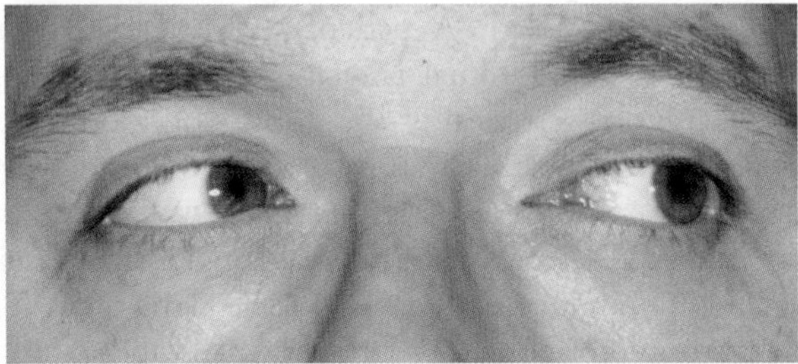

B

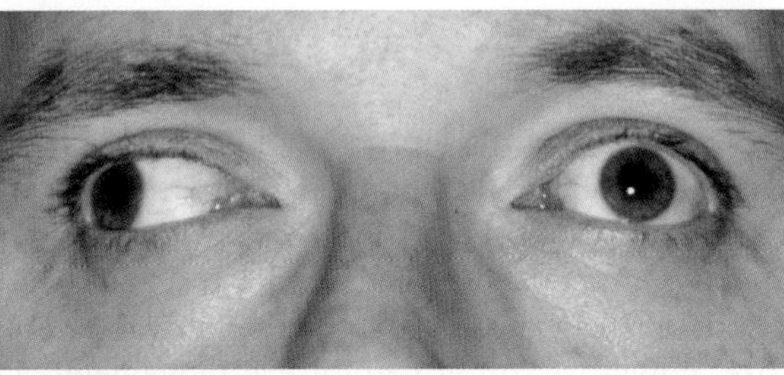

C

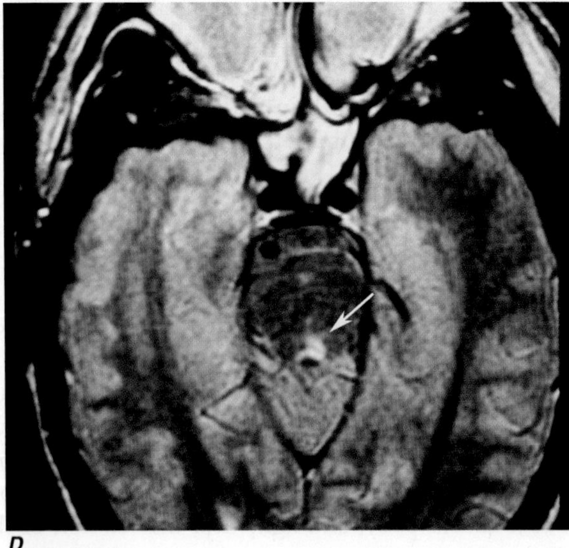

D

FIGURE 21-19

Left internuclear ophthalmoplegia (INO). ***A.*** In primary position of gaze the eyes appear normal. ***B.*** Horizontal gaze to the left is intact. ***C.*** On attempted horizontal gaze to the right, the left eye fails to adduct. In mildly affected patients the eye may adduct partially or more slowly than normal. Nystagmus is usually present in the abducted eye. ***D.*** T2-weighted axial MRI image through the pons showing a demyelinating plaque in the left medial longitudinal fasciculus (*arrow*).

(sinusoidal) and jerk features. This nystagmus is commonly referred to as *congenital sensory nystagmus*. This is a poor term because even in children with congenital lesions, the nystagmus does not appear until several months of age. *Congenital motor nystagmus*, which looks similar to congenital sensory nystagmus, develops in the absence of any abnormality of the sensory visual system. Visual acuity also is reduced in congenital motor nystagmus, probably by the nystagmus itself, but seldom below a level of 20/200.

Jerk nystagmus

This is characterized by a slow drift off the target, followed by a fast corrective saccade. By convention, the nystagmus is named after the quick phase. Jerk nystagmus can be downbeat, upbeat, horizontal (left or right), and torsional. The pattern of nystagmus may vary with gaze position. Some patients will be oblivious to their nystagmus. Others will complain of blurred vision or a subjective to-and-fro movement of the environment (oscillopsia) corresponding to the nystagmus. Fine nystagmus may be difficult to see on gross examination of the eyes. Observation of nystagmoid movements of the optic disc on ophthalmoscopy is a sensitive way to detect subtle nystagmus.

Gaze-evoked nystagmus

This is the most common form of jerk nystagmus. When the eyes are held eccentrically in the orbits, they have a natural tendency to drift back to primary position. The subject compensates by making a corrective saccade to maintain the deviated eye position. Many normal patients have mild gaze-evoked nystagmus. Exaggerated gaze-evoked nystagmus can be induced by drugs (sedatives, anticonvulsants, alcohol); muscle paresis; myasthenia gravis; demyelinating disease; and cerebellopontine angle, brainstem, and cerebellar lesions.

Vestibular nystagmus

Vestibular nystagmus results from dysfunction of the labyrinth (Ménière's disease), vestibular nerve, or vestibular nucleus in the brainstem. Peripheral vestibular nystagmus often occurs in discrete attacks, with symptoms of nausea and vertigo. There may be associated tinnitus and hearing loss. Sudden shifts in head position may provoke or exacerbate symptoms.

Downbeat nystagmus

Downbeat nystagmus results from lesions near the craniocervical junction (Chiari malformation, basilar invagination). It also has been reported in brainstem or cerebellar stroke, lithium or anticonvulsant intoxication, alcoholism, and multiple sclerosis. *Upbeat nystagmus* is associated with damage to the pontine tegmentum from stroke, demyelination, or tumor.

Opsoclonus

This rare, dramatic disorder of eye movements consists of bursts of consecutive saccades (saccadomania). When the saccades are confined to the horizontal plane, the term *ocular flutter* is preferred. It can result from viral encephalitis, trauma, or a paraneoplastic effect of neuroblastoma, breast carcinoma, and other malignancies. It has also been reported as a benign, transient phenomenon in otherwise healthy patients.

CHAPTER 22

VIDEO LIBRARY OF NEURO-OPHTHALMOLOGY

Shirley H. Wray

The proper control of eye movements requires the coordinated activity of many different anatomic structures in the peripheral and central nervous system, and in turn manifestations of a diverse array of neurological and medical disorders are revealed as disorders of eye movement. In this remarkable video collection, an introduction to distinctive eye movement disorders encountered in the context of neuromuscular, paraneoplastic, demyelinating, neurovascular, and neurodegenerative disorders is presented. Videos for this chapter can be accessed at the following link: http://www.mhprofessional.com/mediacenter/.

CHAPTER 23

DISORDERS OF SMELL AND TASTE

Richard L. Doty ■ Steven M. Bromley

All environmental chemicals necessary for life enter the body by the nose and mouth. The senses of smell (olfaction) and taste (gustation) monitor those chemicals, determine the flavor and palatability of foods and beverages, and warn of dangerous environmental conditions, including fire, air pollution, leaking natural gas, and bacteria-laden foodstuffs. These senses contribute significantly to quality of life and, when dysfunctional, can have untoward physical and psychological consequences. A basic understanding of these senses in health and disease is critical for the physician, since thousands of patients present to doctors' offices each year with complaints of chemosensory dysfunction. Among the more important developments in neurology has been the discovery that decreased smell function is perhaps the first sign of neurodegenerative diseases such as Alzheimer's disease (AD) and Parkinson's disease (PD), signifying their "presymptomatic" phase.

ANATOMY AND PHYSIOLOGY

Olfactory system

Odorous chemicals enter the nose during inhalation and active sniffing as well as during deglutition. After reaching the highest recesses of the nasal cavity, they dissolve in the olfactory mucus and diffuse or are actively transported to receptors on the cilia of olfactory receptor cells. The cilia, dendrites, cell bodies, and proximal axonal segments of these bipolar cells are situated within a specialized neuroepithelium that covers the cribriform plate, the superior nasal septum, the superior turbinate, and sectors of the middle turbinate (Fig. 23-1). Each of the ~6 million bipolar receptor cells expresses only one of ~450 receptor protein types, most of which respond to more than a single chemical. When damaged, the receptor cells can be replaced by stem cells near the basement membrane. Unfortunately, such replacement is often incomplete.

After coalescing into bundles surrounded by glia-like ensheathing cells (termed fila), the receptor cell axons pass through the cribriform plate to the olfactory bulbs, where they synapse with dendrites of other cell types within the glomeruli (Fig. 23-2). These spherical structures, which make up a distinct layer of the olfactory bulb, are a site of convergence of information, since many more fibers enter than leave them. Receptor cells that express the same type of receptor project to the same glomeruli, effectively making each glomerulus a functional unit. The major projection neurons of the olfactory system—the mitral and tufted cells—send primary dendrites into the glomeruli, connecting not only with the incoming receptor cell axons but with dendrites of periglomerular cells. The activity of the mitral/tufted cells is modulated by the periglomerular cells, secondary dendrites from other mitral/tufted cells, and granule cells, the most numerous cells of the bulb. The latter cells, which are largely GABAergic, receive inputs from central brain structures and modulate the output of the mitral/tufted cells. Interestingly, like the olfactory receptor cells, some cells within the bulb undergo replacement. Thus, neuroblasts formed within the anterior subventricular zone of the brain migrate along the rostral migratory stream, ultimately becoming granule and periglomerular cells.

The axons of the mitral and tufted cells synapse within the primary olfactory cortex (POC) (Fig. 23-3). The POC is defined as the cortical structures that receive direct projections from the olfactory bulb, most notably the piriform and entorhinal cortices. Although olfaction is unique in that its initial afferent projections bypass the thalamus, persons with damage to the thalamus can exhibit olfactory deficits, particularly ones of odor identification. Those deficits probably reflect the involvement of thalamic connections between the primary olfactory cortex and the orbitofrontal cortex (OFC), where odor identification occurs. The close anatomic ties between the olfactory system and the

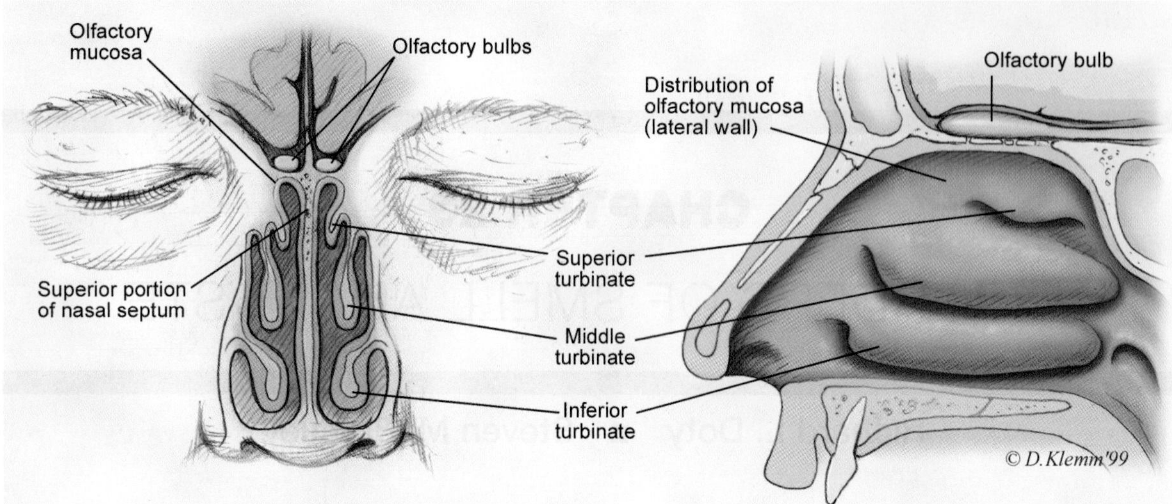

FIGURE 23-1

Anatomy of the olfactory neural pathways, showing the distribution of olfactory receptors in the roof of the nasal cavity. (*Copyright David Klemm, Faculty and Curriculum Support [FACS], Georgetown University Medical Center; used with permission*.)

amygdala, hippocampus, and hypothalamus help explain the intimate associations between odor perception and cognitive functions such as memory, motivation, arousal, autonomic activity, digestion, and sex.

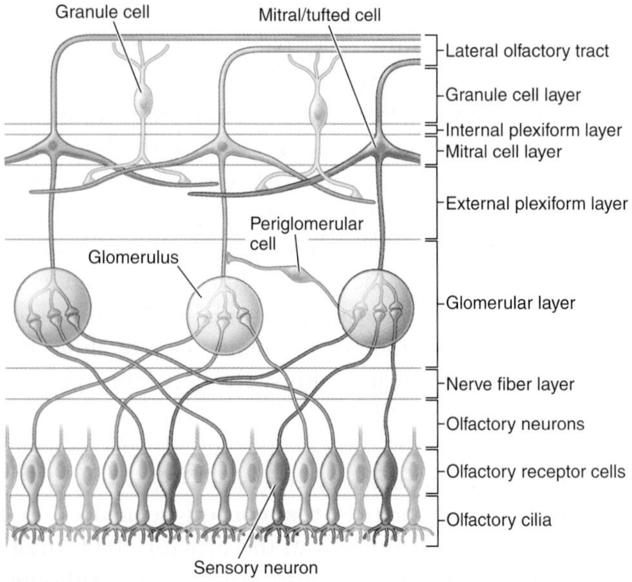

Granule cell
Mitral/tufted cell
Lateral olfactory tract
Granule cell layer
Internal plexiform layer
Mitral cell layer
External plexiform layer
Periglomerular cell
Glomerulus
Glomerular layer
Nerve fiber layer
Olfactory neurons
Olfactory receptor cells
Olfactory cilia
Sensory neuron

FIGURE 23-2

Schematic of the layers and wiring of the olfactory bulb. Each receptor type (red, green, blue) projects to a common glomerulus. The neural activity within each glomerulus is modulated by periglomerular cells. The activity of the primary projection cells, the mitral and tufted cells, is modulated by granule cells, periglomerular cells, and secondary dendrites from other mitral and tufted cells. (*From www.med.yale.edu/neurosurg/treloar/index.html*.)

Taste system

Tastants are sensed by specialized receptor cells present within taste buds: small grapefruit-like segmented structures on the lateral margins and dorsum of the tongue, the roof of the mouth, the pharynx, the larynx, and the superior esophagus (Fig. 23-4). Lingual taste buds are embedded in well-defined protuberances termed fungiform, foliate, and circumvallate papillae. After dissolving

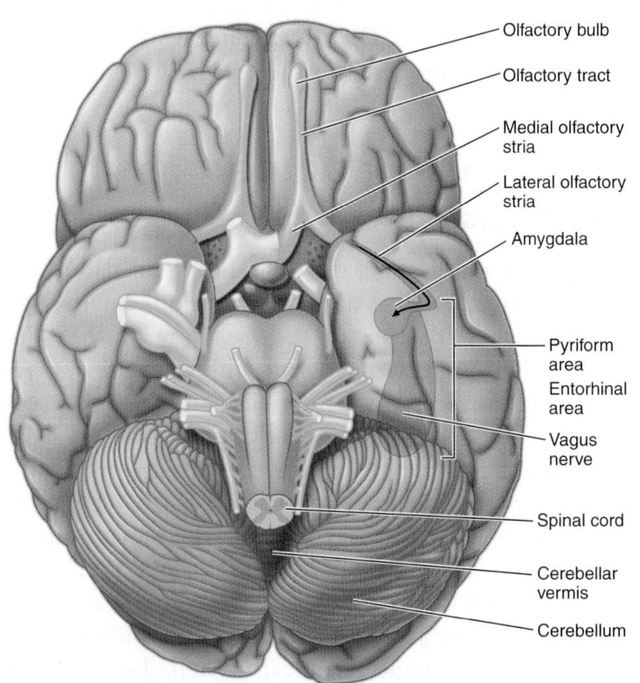

FIGURE 23-3

Anatomy of the base of the brain showing the primary olfactory cortex.

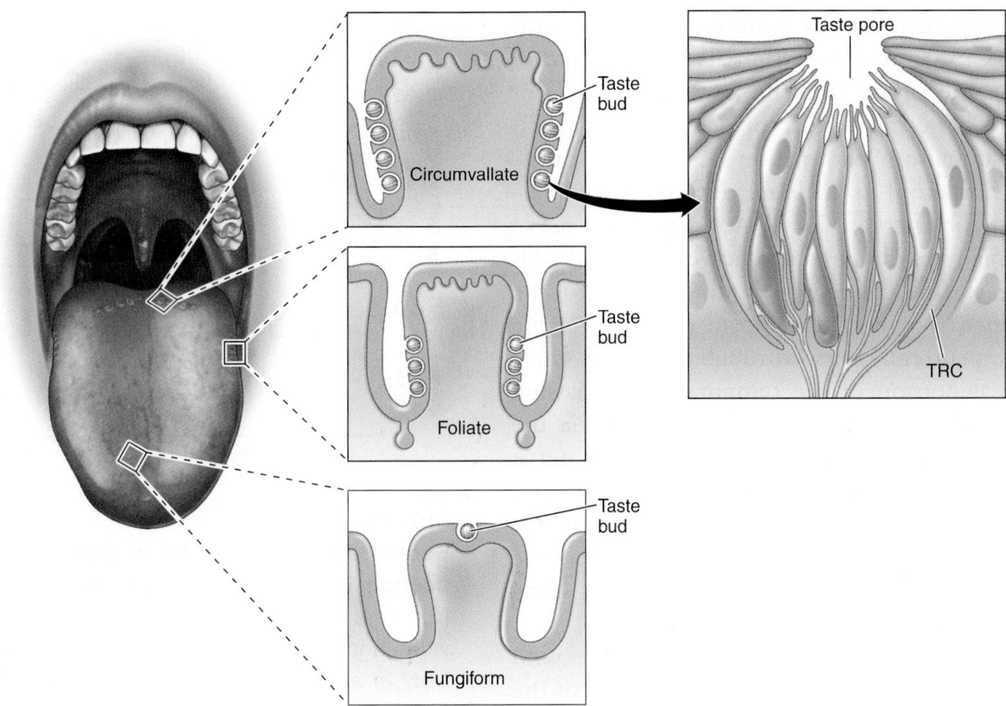

FIGURE 23-4

Schematic of the taste bud and its opening (pore), as well as the location of buds on the three major types of papillae: fungiform (anterior), foliate (lateral), and circumvallate (posterior). TRC, taste receptor cell.

in a liquid, tastants enter the opening of the taste bud—the taste pore—and bind to receptors on microvilli, small extensions of receptor cells within each taste bud. Such binding changes the electrical potential across the taste cell, resulting in neurotransmitter release onto the first-order taste neurons. Although humans have ~7500 taste buds, not all harbor taste-sensitive cells; some contain only one class of receptor (e.g., cells responsive only to sugars), whereas others contain cells sensitive to more than one class. The number of taste receptor cells per taste bud ranges from zero to well over 100. A small family of three G-protein-coupled receptors (GPCRs)—T1R1, T1R2, and T1R3—mediate sweet and umami taste sensations. Umami ("savory") refers to the flavors of meat, cheese, and broth due to glutamate and related compounds. Bitter sensations, in contrast, depend on T2R receptors, a family of ~30 GPCRs expressed on cells different from those which express the sweet and umami receptors. T2Rs sense a wide range of bitter substances but do not distinguish among them. Sour tastants are sensed by the PKD2L1 receptor, a member of the transient receptor potential protein (TRP) family. Perception of salty sensations, such as those induced by sodium chloride, arises from the entry of Na^+ ions into the cells via specialized membrane channels such as the amiloride-sensitive Na^+ channel.

Taste information is sent to the brain via three cranial nerves (CNs): CN VII (the *facial nerve,* which involves the intermediate nerve with its branches, the greater petrosal and chorda tympani nerves); CN IX (the *glossopharyngeal nerve*); and CN X (the *vagus nerve*) (Fig. 23-5). CN VII innervates the anterior tongue and

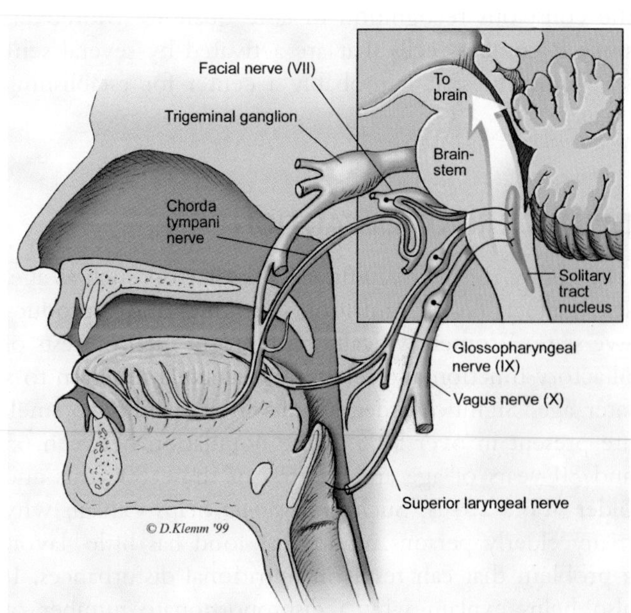

FIGURE 23-5

Schematic of the cranial nerves that mediate taste function, including the chorda tympani nerve (CN VII), the glossopharyngeal nerve (CN IX), and the vagus nerve (CN X). *(Copyright David Klemm, Faculty and Curriculum Support [FACS], Georgetown University Medical Center; used with permission.)*

all of the soft palate, CN IX innervates the posterior tongue, and CN X innervates the laryngeal surface of the epiglottis, the larynx, and the proximal portion of the esophagus. The mandibular branch of CN V (V_3) conveys somatosensory information (e.g., touch, burning, cooling, irritation) to the brain. Although not technically a gustatory nerve, CN V shares primary nerve routes with many of the gustatory nerve fibers and adds temperature, texture, pungency, and spiciness to the taste experience. The chorda tympani nerve is notable for taking a recurrent course through the facial canal in the petrosal portion of the temporal bone, passing through the middle ear, then exiting the skull via the petrotympanic fissure, where it joins the lingual nerve (a division of CN V) near the tongue. This nerve also carries parasympathetic fibers to the submandibular and sublingual glands, whereas the greater petrosal nerve supplies the palatine glands, thereby influencing saliva production.

The axons of the projection cells that synapse with taste buds enter the rostral portion of the nucleus of the solitary tract (NTS) within the medulla of the brainstem (Fig. 23-5). From the NTS, neurons then project to a division of the ventroposteromedial thalamic nucleus (VPM) via the medial lemniscus. From there projections are made to the rostral part of the frontal operculum and adjoining insula, a brain region considered the *primary taste cortex* (PTC). Projections from the primary taste cortex then go to the *secondary taste cortex*, namely, the caudolateral OFC. This brain region is involved in the conscious recognition of taste qualities. Moreover, since it contains cells that are activated by several sensory modalities, it is probably a center for establishing "flavor."

DISORDERS OF OLFACTION

The ability to smell is influenced by factors such as age, sex, general health, nutrition, smoking, and reproductive state. Women typically outperform men on tests of olfactory function and retain normal smell function to a later age. Significant decrements in the ability to smell are present in over 50% of the population between 65 and 80 years of age and in 75% of those 80 years and older (Fig. 23-6). Such *presbyosmia* helps explain why many elderly persons report that food has little flavor, a problem that can result in nutritional disturbances. It also helps explain why a disproportionate number of the elderly die in accidental gas poisonings. A relatively complete listing of conditions and disorders that have been associated with olfactory dysfunction is presented in Table 23-1.

Aside from aging, the three most common identifiable causes of long-lasting or permanent smell loss seen in the clinic are, in order of frequency, severe upper respiratory

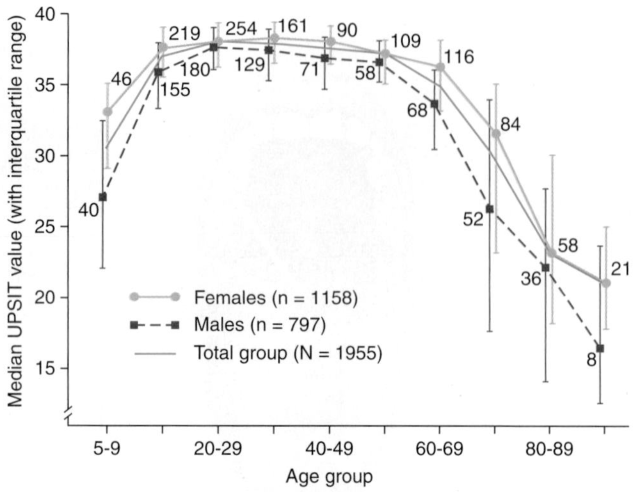

FIGURE 23-6

Scores on the University of Pennsylvania Smell Identification Test (UPSIT) as a function of subject age and sex. Numbers by each data point indicate sample sizes. Note that women identify odorants better than men at all ages. (*From Doty et al: Science 226:1421, 1984. Copyright 1984 American Association for the Advancement of Science.*)

infections, head trauma, and chronic rhinosinusitis. The physiologic basis for most head trauma–related losses is the shearing and subsequent scarring of the olfactory fila as they pass from the nasal cavity into the brain cavity. The cribriform plate does not have to be fractured or show pathology for smell loss to be present. Severity of trauma, as indexed by a poor Glasgow Coma Rating on presentation and the length of posttraumatic amnesia, is associated with higher risk of olfactory impairment. Fewer than 10% of posttraumatic anosmic patients recover age-related normal function over time. Upper respiratory infections, such as those associated with the common cold, influenza, pneumonia, or HIV, can directly and permanently harm the olfactory epithelium by decreasing receptor cell numbers, damaging cilia on remaining receptor cells, and inducing the replacement of sensory epithelium with respiratory epithelium. The smell loss associated with chronic rhinosinusitis is related to disease severity, with most loss occurring in cases in which rhinosinusitis and polyposis are both present. Although systemic glucocorticoid therapy usually can induce short-term functional improvement, it does not, on average, return smell test scores to normal, implying that chronic permanent neural loss is present and/or that short-term administration of systemic glucocorticoids does not mitigate the inflammation completely. It is well established that microinflammation in an otherwise seemingly normal epithelium can influence smell function.

A number of neurodegenerative diseases are accompanied by olfactory impairment, including AD, PD, Huntington's disease, Down syndrome, parkinsonism-dementia complex of Guam, dementia with Lewy bodies

TABLE 23-1

DISORDERS AND CONDITIONS ASSOCIATED WITH COMPROMISED OLFACTORY FUNCTION AS MEASURED BY OLFACTORY TESTING

22q11 deletion syndrome	Liver disease
AIDS/HIV infection	Lubag disease
Adenoid hypertrophy	Medications
Adrenal cortical insufficiency	Migraine
Age	Multiple sclerosis
Alcoholism	Multi-infarct dementia
Allergies	Narcolepsy with cataplexy
Alzheimer's disease	Neoplasms, cranial/nasal
Amyotrophic lateral sclerosis	Nutritional deficiencies
Anorexia nervosa	Obstructive pulmonary disease
Asperger's syndrome	Obesity
Ataxias	Obsessive-compulsive disorder
Attention deficit/hyperactivity disorder	Orthostatic tremor
Bardet-Biedl syndrome	Panic disorder
Chemical exposure	Parkinson's disease
Chronic obstructive pulmonary disease	Pick's disease
Congenital	Posttraumatic stress disorder
Cushing's syndrome	Pregnancy
Cystic fibrosis	Pseudohypoparathyroidism
Degenerative ataxias	Psychopathy
Diabetes	Radiation (therapeutic, cranial)
Down syndrome	REM behavior disorder
Epilepsy	Refsum disease
Facial paralysis	Renal failure/end-stage kidney disease
Frontotemporal lobe degeneration	Restless leg syndrome
Gonadal dysgenesis (Turner syndrome)	Rhinosinusitis/polyposis
Guamanian ALS/PD/dementia syndrome	Schizophrenia
Head trauma	Seasonal affective disorder
Herpes simplex encephalitis	Sjögren's syndrome
Hypothyroidism	Stroke
Huntington's disease	Tobacco smoking
Iatrogenesis	Toxic chemical exposure
Kallmann's syndrome	Upper respiratory infections
Korsakoff's psychosis	Usher syndrome
Leprosy	Vitamin B_{12} deficiency

(DLB), multiple system atrophy, vascular parkinsonism, corticobasal syndrome, frontotemporal dementia, multiple sclerosis (MS), and idiopathic rapid eye movement (REM) behavioral sleep disorder (iRBD). The olfactory disturbance of MS varies as a function of the plaque activity within the frontal and temporal lobes. In postmortem studies of patients with very mild "presymptomatic" signs of AD, poorer smell function has been associated with higher levels of AD-related pathology even after controlling for apolipoprotein E4 alleles and the level of episodic memory function present at the time of olfactory testing. Olfactory impairment in PD often predates the clinical diagnosis by at least 4 years. Studies of the sequence of Lewy body and abnormal α-synuclein development in staged PD cases, along with evidence that the smell loss presents early, is stable over time, and is not affected by PD medications, suggest that the olfactory bulbs may be, along with the dorsomotor nucleus of the vagus, the site of first neural damage in PD. Smell loss is more marked in patients with early clinical manifestations of DLB than in those with mild AD. Interestingly, smell loss is minimal or nonexistent in progressive supranuclear palsy and 1-methyl-4-phenyl-1,2,3,6-tetrahydropyridine (MPTP)-induced parkinsonism.

The smell loss seen in iRBD is of the same magnitude as that found in PD. This is of particular interest to clinicians since patients with iRBD frequently develop PD and hyposmia. iRBD may actually represent an early associated condition of PD. REM behavior disorder not only is seen in its idiopathic form but also can be associated with narcolepsy. This led to a study of narcoleptic patients with and without REM behavior disorder that demonstrated that narcolepsy, independent of REM behavior disorder, was associated with significant impairments in olfactory function. Orexin A, also known as hypocretin-1, is dramatically diminished or undetectable in the cerebrospinal fluid of patients with narcolepsy and cataplexy. The orexin-containing neurons in the hypothalamus project throughout the olfactory system (from the olfactory epithelium to the olfactory cortex), and damage to these orexin-containing projections may be one underlying mechanism for impaired olfactory performance in narcoleptic patients. The administration of intranasal orexin A (hypocretin-1) appears to result in improved olfactory function relative to a placebo, supporting the notion that mild olfactory impairment is not only a primary feature of narcolepsy with cataplexies but that CNS orexin deficiency may be a fundamental part of the mechanism for this loss.

DISORDERS OF TASTE

The majority of patients who present with complaints of taste dysfunction exhibit olfactory, not taste, loss. This is the case because most flavors attributed to taste actually depend on retronasal stimulation of the olfactory receptors during deglutition. As noted earlier, taste buds only mediate basic tastes such as sweet, sour, bitter, salty, and umami. Significant impairment of whole-mouth gustatory function is rare outside of generalized metabolic disturbances or systemic use of some medications, since taste bud regeneration occurs and peripheral damage alone would require the involvement of multiple cranial nerve pathways. Nonetheless, taste can be influenced by (1) the release of foul-tasting materials from the oral cavity from oral medical conditions and appliances (e.g., gingivitis, purulent sialadenitis), (2) transport problems of tastants to the taste buds (e.g., drying of the orolingual mucosa, infections, inflammatory conditions), (3) damage to the taste buds themselves (e.g., local trauma, invasive carcinomas), (4) damage to the neural pathways innervating the taste buds (e.g., middle ear infections), (5) damage to central structures (e.g., multiple sclerosis, tumor, epilepsy, stroke), and (6) systemic disturbances of metabolism (e.g., diabetes, thyroid disease, medications). Bell's palsy is among the most common causes of CN VII injury that results in taste disturbance. Unlike CN VII, CN IX is relatively protected along its path, although iatrogenic interventions such as tonsillectomy, bronchoscopy, laryngoscopy, and radiation therapy can result in selective injury. Migraine is associated on rare occasions with a gustatory prodrome or aura, and certain tastes may trigger a migraine. Although a number of disorders can affect CN IX, including tumors, trauma, vascular lesions, and infection, it remains unclear if noticeable taste disturbance can result from such factors.

Although both taste and smell can be adversely influenced by pharmacologic agents, drug-related taste alterations are more common. Indeed, over 250 medications have been reported to alter the ability to taste. Major offenders include antineoplastic agents, antirheumatic drugs, antibiotics, and blood pressure medications. Terbinafine, a commonly used antifungal, has been linked to taste disturbance lasting up to 3 years. In a controlled trial, nearly two-thirds of individuals taking eszopiclone (Lunesta) experienced a bitter dysgeusia which was stronger in women, systematically related to the time since drug administration, and positively correlated with both blood and saliva levels of the drug. Intranasal use of nasal gels and sprays containing zinc—common over-the-counter prophylactics for upper respiratory viral infections—has been implicated in loss of smell function. Whether their efficacy in preventing such infections, which are the most common cause of anosmia and hyposmia, outweighs their potential detriment to smell function requires study.

As with olfaction, a number of systemic disorders can affect taste. They include chronic renal failure, end-stage liver disease, vitamin and mineral deficiencies, diabetes, and hypothyroidism, to name a few. Psychiatric conditions can be associated with chemosensory alterations (e.g., depression, schizophrenia, bulimia). A review of tactile, gustatory, and olfactory hallucinations demonstrated that no one type of hallucinatory experience is pathognomonic to any specific diagnosis.

CLINICAL EVALUATION

In most cases, a careful clinical history will establish the probable etiology of a chemosensory problem, including questions about its nature, onset, duration, and pattern of fluctuations. *Sudden loss* suggests the possibility of head trauma, ischemia, infection, or a psychiatric condition.

Gradual loss can reflect the development of a progressive obstructive lesion. *Intermittent loss* suggests the likelihood of an inflammatory process. The patient should be asked about potential precipitating events, such as cold or flu infections before symptom onset, as they often are underappreciated. Information regarding head trauma, smoking habits, drug and alcohol abuse (e.g., intranasal cocaine, chronic alcoholism in the context of Wernicke's and Korsakoff's syndromes), exposures to pesticides and other toxic agents, and medical interventions are also informative. A determination of all the medications the patient was taking before and at the time of symptom onset is important, since many can cause chemosensory disturbances. Comorbid medical conditions associated with smell impairment, such as renal failure, liver disease, hypothyroidism, diabetes, and dementia, should be assessed. Delayed puberty in association with anosmia (with or without midline craniofacial abnormalities, deafness, and renal anomalies) suggests the possibility of Kallmann syndrome. Recollection of epistaxis, discharge (clear, purulent, or bloody), nasal obstruction, allergies, and somatic symptoms, including headache or irritation, may have localizing value. Questions related to memory, parkinsonian signs, and seizure activity (e.g., automatisms, occurrence of blackouts, auras, and déjàvu) should be posed. Pending litigation and the possibility of malingering should be considered.

Neurologic and otorhinolaryngologic (ORL) examinations, along with appropriate brain and nasosinus imaging, aid in the evaluation of patients with olfactory or gustatory complaints. The neural evaluation should focus on cranial nerve function, with particular attention to possible skull base and intracranial lesions. Visual acuity, field, and optic disc examinations aid in the detection of intracranial mass lesions that induce elevations in intracranial pressure (papilledema) and optic atrophy, especially when one is considering Foster Kennedy syndrome (ipsilateral optic nerve atrophy and contralateral papilledema usually due to a meningioma near the olfactory bulb or tract). The ORL examination should thoroughly assess the intranasal architecture and mucosal surfaces. Polyps, masses, and adhesions of the turbinates to the septum may compromise the flow of air to the olfactory receptors, since less than a fifth of the inspired air traverses the olfactory cleft in the unobstructed state. Blood serum tests may be helpful to identify conditions such as diabetes, infection, heavy metal exposure, nutritional deficiency (e.g., vitamins B_6 and B_{12}), allergy, and thyroid, liver, and kidney disease.

As with other sensory disorders, quantitative sensory testing is advised. Self-reports of patients can be misleading, and a number who complain of chemosensory dysfunction have normal function for their age and sex. Quantitative smell and taste testing provides valid information for worker's compensation and other legal claims as well as a way to assess treatment interventions accurately. A number of standardized olfactory and taste tests are commercially available. Most evaluate the ability of patients to detect and identify odors or tastes. For example, the most widely used of these tests, the 40-item University of Pennsylvania Smell Identification Test (UPSIT), employs norms based on nearly 4000 normal subjects. A determination is made of both absolute dysfunction (i.e., mild loss, moderate loss, severe loss, total loss, probable malingering) and relative dysfunction (percentile rank for age and sex). Although electrophysiologic testing is available at some smell and taste centers (e.g., odor event-related potentials), such tests require complex stimulus presentation and recording equipment and rarely provide additional diagnostic information. In addition to electrogustometers, commercial chemical taste tests are now available. Most employ filter paper strips impregnated with tastants, so no stimulus preparation is required. Like the UPSIT, these tests have published norms for establishing the degree of dysfunction.

TREATMENT AND MANAGEMENT

Because of the various mechanisms by which olfactory and gustatory disturbance can occur, management of patients tends to be condition-specific. For example, patients with hypothyroidism, diabetes, or infections need to be given specific treatments to correct the underlying process adversely influencing chemoreception. For most patients who present primarily with obstructive/transport loss affecting the nasal and paranasal regions (e.g., allergic rhinitis, polyposis, intranasal neoplasms, nasal deviations), medical and/or surgical intervention is often beneficial. Antifungal and antibiotic treatments may reverse taste problems secondary to candidiasis or other oral infections. Chlorohexidine mouthwash mitigates some salty or bitter dysgeusias, conceivably as a result of its strong positive charge. Excessive dryness of the oral mucosa is a problem with many medications and conditions, and artificial saliva (e.g., Xerolube) or oral pilocarpine treatments may prove beneficial. Other methods to improve salivary flow include the use of mints, lozenges, or sugarless gum. Flavor enhancers may make food more palatable (e.g., monosodium glutamate), but caution is advised to avoid overusing ingredients containing sodium or sugar, particularly in circumstances in which a patient also has underlying hypertension or diabetes. Medications that induce distortions of taste often can be discontinued and replaced with other types of medications or modes of therapy. As mentioned earlier, pharmacologic agents result in taste disturbances much more frequently than smell disturbances, and over 250 medications have been reported to alter the sense of taste. Many drug-related effects are long-lasting and are not reversed by short-term drug discontinuance.

A study of endoscopic sinus surgery in patients with chronic rhinosinusitis and hyposmia revealed that patients with severe olfactory dysfunction before the surgery had a more dramatic and sustained improvement over time compared with patients with more mild olfactory dysfunction before intervention. In the case of intranasal and sinus-related inflammatory conditions such as those seen with allergy, viruses, and traumas, the use of intranasal or systemic glucocorticoids may be helpful. One common approach is a short course of oral prednisone, typically 60 mg daily for 4 days and then tapered by 10 mg daily. The utility of restoring olfaction with either topical or systemic glucocorticoids has been studied. Topical intranasal glucocorticoids were less effective in general than systemic glucocorticoids; however, nasal steroid administration techniques were not analyzed. Intranasal glucocorticoids are more effective if administered in Moffett's position (head in the inverted position such as over the edge of the bed with the bridge of the nose perpendicular to the floor). After head trauma, an initial trial of glucocorticoids may help reduce local edema and the potential deleterious deposition of scar tissue around olfactory fila at the level of the cribriform plate.

Treatments are limited for patients with chemosensory loss or primary injury to neural pathways. Nonetheless, spontaneous recovery can occur. In a follow-up study of 542 patients presenting with smell loss from a variety of causes, modest improvement occurred over an average period of 4 years in about half the participants. However, only 11% of the anosmic and 23% of the hyposmic patients regained normal age-related function. Interestingly, the amount of dysfunction present at the time of presentation, not etiology, was the best predictor of prognosis. Other predictors were the patient's age and the time between the onset of dysfunction and initial testing.

A nonblinded study reported that patients with hyposmia may benefit from smelling strong odors (e.g., eucalyptol, citronella, eugenol, and phenyl ethyl alcohol) before going to bed and immediately upon awaking each day over the course of several months. The rationale for this approach comes from animal studies demonstrating that prolonged exposure to odorants can induce increased neural activity within the olfactory bulb. α-Lipoic acid (200 mg two or three times daily), an essential cofactor for many enzyme complexes with possible antioxidant effects, has been reported to be beneficial in mitigating smell loss after viral infection of the upper respiratory tract, although double-blind studies are needed to confirm this observation. This agent has also been suggested to be useful in some cases of hypogeusia and burning mouth syndrome.

The use of zinc and vitamin A in treating olfactory disturbances is controversial; not much benefit is obtained beyond replenishing established deficiencies. However, zinc improves taste function secondary to hepatic deficiencies, and retinoids (bioactive vitamin A derivatives) are known to play an essential role in the survival of olfactory neurons. One protocol in which zinc was infused with chemotherapy treatments suggested a possible protective effect against developing taste impairment. Diseases of the alimentary tract can not only influence chemoreceptive function but occasionally influence B_{12} absorption. This can result in a relative deficiency of B_{12}, theoretically contributing to olfactory nerve disturbance. B_2 (riboflavin) and magnesium supplements are reported in the alternative medicine literature to aid in the management of migraine headaches that may be associated with smell dysfunction.

A number of medicines have been reported to ameliorate olfactory symptoms, although strong scientific evidence for efficacy is generally lacking. A report that theophylline improved smell function was not double-blinded and lacked a control group, failing to take into account that some meaningful improvement occurs without treatment. Indeed, the percentage of patients reported to be responsive to the treatment was about the same as that noted by others to show spontaneous improvement over a similar time period (~50%). Antiepileptics and some antidepressants (e.g., amitriptyline) have been used to treat dysosmias and smell distortions, particularly after head trauma. Ironically, amitriptyline is also frequently on the list of medications that can ultimately distort smell and taste function, possibly from its anticholinergic effects. The use of donepezil (an acetylcholinesterase inhibitor) in AD may result in improvements in smell identification measures that correlate with overall clinician-based impressions of change scales (Clinician Interview Based Impression of Severity [CIBIC]-plus). Smell identification function could become a useful measure to assess overall treatment response with this medication.

A major and often overlooked element of therapy comes from chemosensory testing itself. Confirmation or lack of confirmation of loss is beneficial to patients who come to believe, in light of unsupportive family members and medical providers, that they may be "crazy." In cases in which the loss is minor, patients can be informed of the likelihood of a more positive prognosis. Importantly, quantitative testing places the patient's problem into overall perspective. Thus, it is often therapeutic for an older person to know that although his or her smell function is not what it used to be, it still falls above the average of his or her peer group. Without testing, many such patients are simply told they are getting old and nothing can be done for them, leading in some cases to depression and decreased self-esteem.

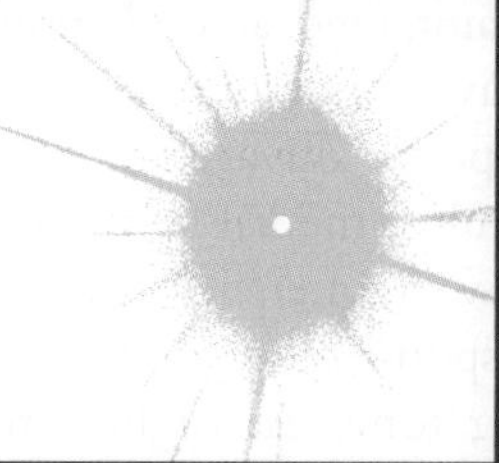

CHAPTER 24

DISORDERS OF HEARING

Anil K. Lalwani

Hearing loss is one of the most common sensory disorders in humans and can present at any age. Nearly 10% of the adult population has some hearing loss, and one-third of individuals age >65 years have a hearing loss of sufficient magnitude to require a hearing aid.

PHYSIOLOGY OF HEARING

The function of the external and middle ear is to amplify sound to facilitate conversion of the mechanical energy of the sound wave into an electrical signal by the inner ear hair cells, a process called mechanotransduction (Fig. 24-1). Sound waves enter the external auditory canal and set the tympanic membrane in motion, which in turn moves the malleus, incus, and stapes of the middle ear. Movement of the footplate of the stapes causes pressure changes in the fluid-filled inner ear, eliciting a traveling wave in the basilar membrane of the cochlea. The tympanic membrane and the ossicular chain in the middle ear serve as an impedance-matching mechanism, improving the efficiency of energy transfer from air to the fluid-filled inner ear.

Stereocilia of the hair cells of the organ of Corti, which rests on the basilar membrane, are in contact with the tectorial membrane and are deformed by the traveling wave. A point of maximal displacement of the basilar membrane is determined by the frequency of the stimulating tone. High-frequency tones cause maximal displacement of the basilar membrane near the base of the cochlea, whereas for low-frequency sounds, the point of maximal displacement is toward the apex of the cochlea.

The inner and outer hair cells of the organ of Corti have different innervation patterns, but both are mechanoreceptors. The afferent innervation relates principally to the inner hair cells, and the efferent innervation relates principally to outer hair cells. The motility of the outer hair cells alters the micromechanics of the inner

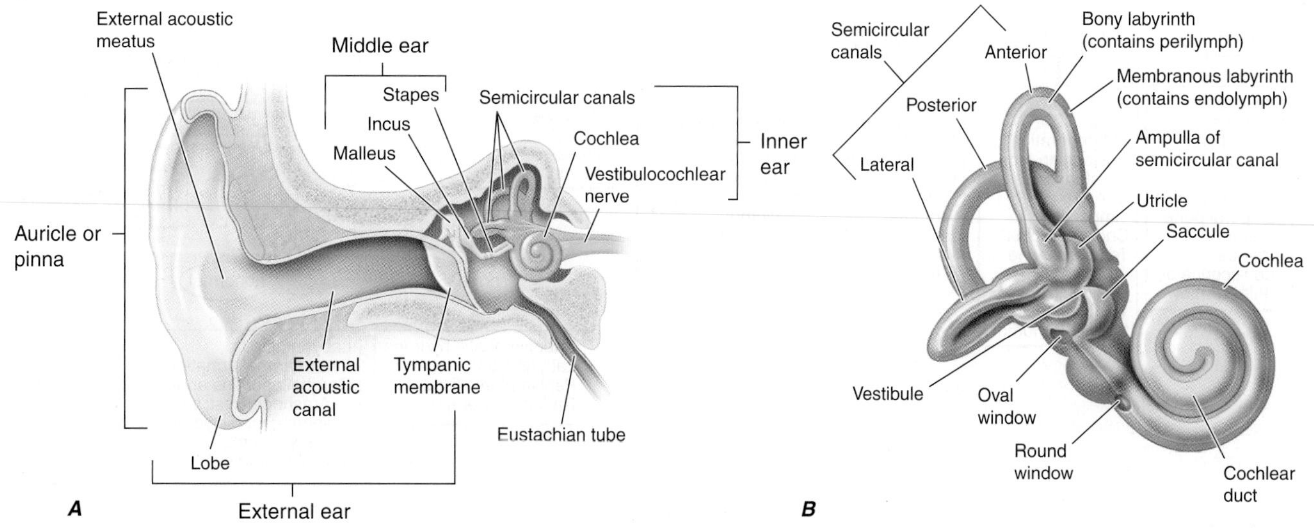

FIGURE 24-1
Ear anatomy. ***A.*** Drawing of modified coronal section through external ear and temporal bone, with structures of the middle and inner ear demonstrated. ***B.*** High-resolution view of inner ear.

hair cells, creating a cochlear amplifier, which explains the exquisite sensitivity and frequency selectivity of the cochlea.

Beginning in the cochlea, the frequency specificity is maintained at each point of the central auditory pathway: dorsal and ventral cochlear nuclei, trapezoid body, superior olivary complex, lateral lemniscus, inferior colliculus, medial geniculate body, and auditory cortex. At low frequencies, individual auditory nerve fibers can respond more or less synchronously with the stimulating tone. At higher frequencies, phase-locking occurs so that neurons alternate in response to particular phases of the cycle of the sound wave. Intensity is encoded by the amount of neural activity in individual neurons, the number of neurons that are active, and the specific neurons that are activated.

DISORDERS OF THE SENSE OF HEARING

Hearing loss can result from disorders of the auricle, external auditory canal, middle ear, inner ear, or central auditory pathways (Fig. 24-2). *In general, lesions in the auricle, external auditory canal, or middle ear that impede the transmission of sound from the external environment to the inner ear cause conductive hearing loss, whereas lesions that impair mechanotransduction in the inner ear or transmission of the electrical signal along the eighth nerve to the brain cause sensorineural hearing loss.*

Conductive hearing loss

The external ear, the external auditory canal, and the middle ear apparatus are designed to collect and amplify sound and efficiently transfer the mechanical energy of the sound wave to the fluid-filled cochlea. Factors that obstruct the transmission of sound or serve to dampen the acoustical energy result in conductive hearing loss. Conductive hearing loss can occur from obstruction of the external auditory canal by cerumen, debris, and foreign bodies; swelling of the lining of the canal; atresia or neoplasms of the canal; perforations of the tympanic membrane; disruption of the ossicular chain, as

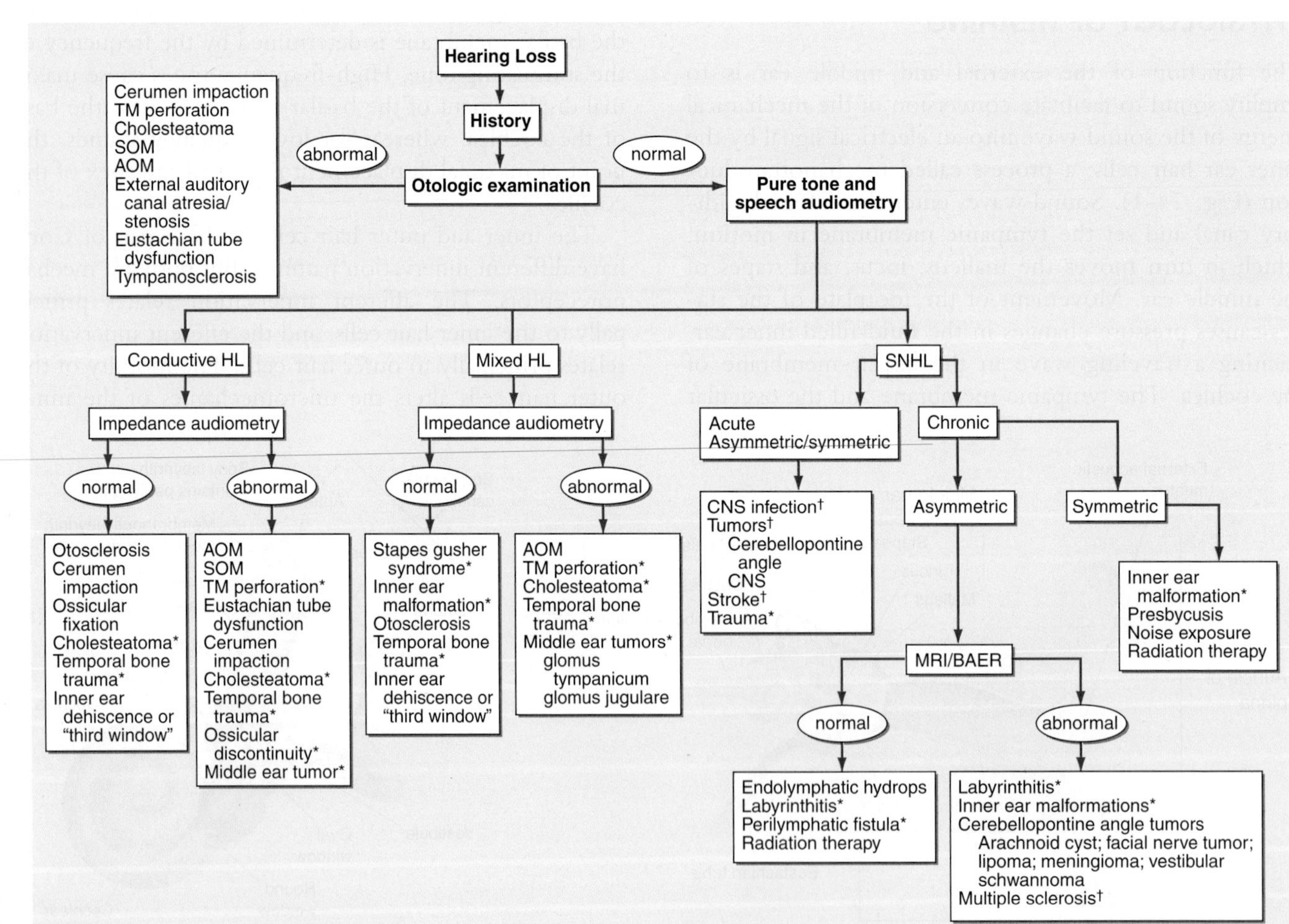

FIGURE 24-2

An algorithm for the approach to hearing loss. HL, hearing loss; SNHL, sensorineural hearing loss; TM, tympanic membrane; SOM, serous otitis media; AOM, acute otitis media; BAER, brainstem auditory evoked response; *CT scan of temporal bone; †MRI scan.

occurs with necrosis of the long process of the incus in trauma or infection; otosclerosis; or fluid, scarring, or neoplasms in the middle ear. Rarely, inner ear malformations or pathologies may also be associated with conductive hearing loss.

Eustachian tube dysfunction is extremely common in adults and may predispose to acute otitis media (AOM) or serous otitis media (SOM). Trauma, AOM, or chronic otitis media are the usual factors responsible for tympanic membrane perforation. While small perforations often heal spontaneously, larger defects usually require surgical intervention. Tympanoplasty is highly effective (>90%) in the repair of tympanic membrane perforations. Otoscopy is usually sufficient to diagnose AOM, SOM, chronic otitis media, cerumen impaction, tympanic membrane perforation, and eustachian tube dysfunction; tympanometry can be useful to confirm the clinical suspicion of these conditions.

Cholesteatoma, a benign tumor composed of stratified squamous epithelium in the middle ear or mastoid, occurs frequently in adults. This is a slowly growing lesion that destroys bone and normal ear tissue. Theories of pathogenesis include traumatic immigration and invasion of squamous epithelium through a retraction pocket, implantation of squamous epithelia in the middle ear through a perforation or surgery, and metaplasia following chronic infection and irritation. On examination, there is often a perforation of the tympanic membrane filled with cheesy white squamous debris. A chronically draining ear that fails to respond to appropriate antibiotic therapy should raise suspicion of a cholesteatoma. Conductive hearing loss secondary to ossicular erosion is common. Surgery is required to remove this destructive process.

Conductive hearing loss with a normal ear canal and intact tympanic membrane suggests either ossicular pathology or the presence of "third window" in the inner ear (see later). Fixation of the stapes from *otosclerosis* is a common cause of low-frequency conductive hearing loss. It occurs equally in men and women and is inherited as an autosomal dominant trait with incomplete penetrance; in some cases, it may be a manifestation of osteogenesis imperfecta. Hearing impairment usually presents between the late teens and the forties. In women, the otosclerotic process is accelerated during pregnancy, and the hearing loss is often first noticeable at this time. A hearing aid or a simple outpatient surgical procedure (stapedectomy) can provide adequate auditory rehabilitation. Extension of otosclerosis beyond the stapes footplate to involve the cochlea (cochlear otosclerosis) can lead to mixed or sensorineural hearing loss. Fluoride therapy to prevent hearing loss from cochlear otosclerosis is of uncertain value.

Disorders that lead to the formation of a pathologic "third window" in the inner ear can be associated with conductive hearing loss. There are normally two major openings, or windows, that connect the inner ear with the middle ear and serve as conduits for transmission of sound; these are, respectively, the oval and round windows. A third window is formed where the normally hard otic bone surrounding the inner ear is eroded; dissipation of the acoustic energy at the third window is responsible for the "inner ear conductive hearing loss." The superior semicircular canal dehiscence syndrome resulting from erosion of the otic bone over the superior circular canal can present with conductive hearing loss that mimics otosclerosis. A common symptom is vertigo evoked by loud sounds (Tullio phenomenon), by Valsalva maneuvers that change middle ear pressure, or by applying positive pressure on the tragus (the cartilage anterior to the external opening of the ear canal). Patients with this syndrome also complain of being able to hear the movement of their eyes and neck. A large jugular bulb or jugular bulb diverticulum can create a "third window" by eroding into the vestibular aqueduct or posterior semicircular canal; the symptoms are similar to those of the superior semicircular canal dehiscence syndrome.

Sensorineural hearing loss

Sensorineural hearing loss results from either damage to the mechanotransduction apparatus of the cochlea or disruption of the electrical conduction pathway from the inner ear to the brain. Thus, injury to hair cells, supporting cells, auditory neurons, or the central auditory pathway can cause sensorineural hearing loss. Damage to the hair cells of the organ of Corti may be caused by intense noise, viral infections, ototoxic drugs (e.g., salicylates, quinine and its synthetic analogues, aminoglycoside antibiotics, loop diuretics such as furosemide and ethacrynic acid, and cancer chemotherapeutic agents such as cisplatin), fractures of the temporal bone, meningitis, cochlear otosclerosis (see earlier), Ménière's disease, and aging. Congenital malformations of the inner ear may be the cause of hearing loss in some adults. Genetic predisposition alone or in concert with environmental exposures may also be responsible (see later).

Presbycusis (age-associated hearing loss) is the most common cause of sensorineural hearing loss in adults. In the early stages, it is characterized by symmetric, gentle to sharply sloping high-frequency hearing loss. With progression, the hearing loss involves all frequencies. More importantly, the hearing impairment is associated with significant loss in clarity. There is a loss of discrimination for phonemes, recruitment (abnormal growth of loudness), and particular difficulty in understanding speech in noisy environments such as at restaurants and social events. Hearing aids are helpful in enhancing the signal-to-noise ratio by amplifying sounds that are close to the listener. *Although hearing aids are able to amplify sounds, they cannot restore the clarity of hearing.* Thus, amplification with hearing aids may provide only limited rehabilitation once the word recognition score deteriorates below 50%. Cochlear implants are the treatment of choice when hearing aids prove inadequate, even when hearing loss is incomplete (see later).

Ménière's disease is characterized by episodic vertigo, fluctuating sensorineural hearing loss, tinnitus, and aural fullness. Tinnitus and/or deafness may be absent during the initial attacks of vertigo, but it invariably appears as the disease progresses and increases in severity during acute attacks. The annual incidence of Ménière's disease is 0.5–7.5 per 1000; onset is most frequently in the fifth decade of life but may also occur in young adults or the elderly. Histologically, there is distention of the endolymphatic system (endolymphatic hydrops) leading to degeneration of vestibular and cochlear hair cells. This may result from endolymphatic sac dysfunction secondary to infection, trauma, autoimmune disease, inflammatory causes, or tumor; an idiopathic etiology constitutes the largest category and is most accurately referred to as Ménière's disease. Although any pattern of hearing loss can be observed, typically, low-frequency, unilateral sensorineural hearing impairment is present. MRI should be obtained to exclude retrocochlear pathology such as a cerebellopontine angle tumor or demyelinating disorder. Therapy is directed toward the control of vertigo. A 2-g/d low-salt diet is the mainstay of treatment for control of rotatory vertigo. Diuretics, a short course of glucocorticoids, and intratympanic gentamicin may also be useful adjuncts in recalcitrant cases. Surgical therapy of vertigo is reserved for unresponsive cases and includes endolymphatic sac decompression, labyrinthectomy, and vestibular nerve section. Both labyrinthectomy and vestibular nerve section abolish rotatory vertigo in >90% of cases. Unfortunately, there is no effective therapy for hearing loss, tinnitus, or aural fullness from Ménière's disease.

Sensorineural hearing loss may also result from any neoplastic, vascular, demyelinating, infectious, or degenerative disease or trauma affecting the central auditory pathways. HIV leads to both peripheral and central auditory system pathology and is associated with sensorineural hearing impairment.

Primary diseases of the central nervous system can also present with hearing impairment. Characteristically, a reduction in clarity of hearing and speech comprehension is much greater than the loss of the ability to hear pure tone. Auditory testing is consistent with an auditory neuropathy; normal otoacoustic emissions (OAE) and an abnormal auditory brainstem response (ABR) are typical (see later). Hearing loss can accompany hereditary sensorimotor neuropathies and inherited disorders of myelin. Tumors of the cerebellopontine angle such as vestibular schwannoma and meningioma usually present with asymmetric sensorineural hearing loss with greater deterioration of speech understanding than pure tone hearing. Multiple sclerosis may present with acute unilateral or bilateral hearing loss; typically, pure tone testing remains relatively stable while speech understanding fluctuates. Isolated labyrinthine infarction can present with acute hearing loss and vertigo due to a cerebrovascular accident involving the posterior circulation, usually the anterior inferior cerebellar artery; it may also be the heralding sign of impending catastrophic basilar artery infarction (Chap. 27).

A finding of conductive and sensory hearing loss in combination is termed *mixed hearing loss*. Mixed hearing losses are due to pathology of both the middle and inner ear, as can occur in otosclerosis involving the ossicles and the cochlea, head trauma, chronic otitis media, cholesteatoma, middle ear tumors, and some inner ear malformations.

Trauma resulting in temporal bone fractures may be associated with conductive, sensorineural, or mixed hearing loss. If the fracture spares the inner ear, there may simply be conductive hearing loss due to rupture of the tympanic membrane or disruption of the ossicular chain. These abnormalities can be surgically corrected. Profound hearing loss and severe vertigo are associated with temporal bone fractures involving the inner ear. A perilymphatic fistula associated with leakage of inner ear fluid into the middle ear can occur and may require surgical repair. An associated facial nerve injury is not uncommon. CT is best suited to assess fracture of the traumatized temporal bone, evaluate the ear canal, and determine the integrity of the ossicular chain and the involvement of the inner ear. CSF leaks that accompany temporal bone fractures are usually self-limited; the value of prophylactic antibiotics is uncertain.

Tinnitus is defined as the perception of a sound when there is no sound in the environment. It may have a buzzing, roaring, or ringing quality and may be pulsatile (synchronous with the heartbeat). Tinnitus is often associated with either a conductive or sensorineural hearing loss. The pathophysiology of tinnitus is not well understood. The cause of the tinnitus can usually be determined by finding the cause of the associated hearing loss. Tinnitus may be the first symptom of a serious condition such as a vestibular schwannoma. Pulsatile tinnitus requires evaluation of the vascular system of the head to exclude vascular tumors such as glomus jugulare tumors, aneurysms, dural arteriovenous fistulas, and stenotic arterial lesions; it may also occur with SOM. It is most commonly associated with some abnormality of the jugular bulb such as a large jugular bulb or jugular bulb diverticulum.

GENETIC CAUSES OF HEARING LOSS

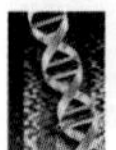

More than half of childhood hearing impairment is thought to be hereditary; hereditary hearing impairment (HHI) can also manifest later in life. HHI may be classified as either nonsyndromic, when hearing loss is the only clinical abnormality, or syndromic, when hearing loss is associated with anomalies in other organ systems. Nearly two-thirds of HHIs are nonsyndromic, and the remaining one-third are syndromic. Between 70 and 80% of nonsyndromic HHI is inherited in an autosomal recessive manner and designated DFNB; another 15–20% is autosomal dominant (DFNA). Less than 5% is X-linked or maternally inherited via the mitochondria.

Nearly 100 loci harboring genes for nonsyndromic HHI have been mapped, with equal numbers of dominant and recessive modes of inheritance; numerous genes have now been cloned (Table 24-1). The hearing genes fall into the categories of structural proteins (MYH9, MYO7A, MYO15, TECTA, DIAPH1), transcription factors (POU3F4, POU4F3), ion channels (KCNQ4, SLC26A4), and gap junction proteins (GJB2, GJB3, GJB6). Several of these genes, including GJB2, TECTA, and TMC1, cause both autosomal dominant and recessive forms of nonsyndromic HHI. In general,

TABLE 24-1

HEREDITARY HEARING IMPAIRMENT GENES

DESIGNATION	GENE	FUNCTION
Autosomal Dominant		
	CRYM	Thyroid hormone–binding protein
DFNA1	*DIAPH1*	Cytoskeletal protein
DFNA2A	*KCNQ4*	Potassium channel
DFNA2B	*GJB3 (Cx31)*	Gap junction
DFNA3A	*GJB2 (Cx26)*	Gap junction
DFNA3B	*GJB6 (Cx30)*	Gap junction
DFNA4	*MYH14*	Class II nonmuscle myosin
DFNA5	*DFNA5*	Unknown
DFNA6/14/38	*WFS1*	Transmembrane protein
DFNA8/12	*TECTA*	Tectorial membrane protein
DFNA9	*COCH*	Unknown
DFNA10	*EYA4*	Developmental gene
DFNA11	*MYO7A*	Cytoskeletal protein
DFNA13	*COL11A2*	Cytoskeletal protein
DFNA15	*POU4F3*	Transcription factor
DFNA17	*MYH9*	Cytoskeletal protein
DFNA20/26	*ACTG1*	Cytoskeletal protein
DFNA22	*MYO6*	Unconventional myosin
DFNA28	*TFCP2L3*	Transcription factor
DFNA36	*TMC1*	Transmembrane protein
DFNA44	*CCDC50*	Effector of EGF-mediated signaling
DFNA48	*MYO1A*	Unconventional myosin
DFNA50	*MIRN96*	MicroRNA
DFNA51	*TJP2*	Tight junction protein
Autosomal Recessive		
DFNB1A	*GJB2 (CX26)*	Gap junction
DFNB1B	*GJB6 (CX30)*	Gap junction
DFNB2	*MYO7A*	Cytoskeletal protein
DFNB3	*MYO15*	Cytoskeletal protein
DFNB4	*PDS (SLC26A4)*	Chloride/iodide transporter
DFNB6	*TMIE*	Transmembrane protein
DFNB7/B11	*TMC1*	Transmembrane protein
DFNB9	*OTOF*	Trafficking of membrane vesicles
DFNB8/10	*TMPRSS3*	Transmembrane serine protease
DFNB12	*CDH23*	Intercellular adherence protein
DFNB16	*STRC*	Stereocilia protein
DFNB18	*USH1C*	Unknown
DFNB21	*TECTA*	Tectorial membrane protein
DFNB22	*OTOA*	Gel attachment to nonsensory
DFNB23	*PCDH15*	Morphogenesis and cohesion
DFNB24	*RDX*	Cytoskeletal protein
DFNB25	*GRXCR1*	Reversible *S*-glutathionylation of proteins
DFNB28	*TRIOBP*	Cytoskeletal-organizing protein
DFNB29	*CLDN14*	Tight junctions
DFNB30	*MYO3A*	Hybrid motor-signaling myosin
DFNB31	*WHRN*	PDZ domain–containing protein
DFNB35	*ESRRB*	Estrogen-related receptor beta protein
DFNB36	*ESPN*	Ca-insensitive actin-bundling protein
DFNB37	*MYO6*	Unconventional myosin
DFNB39	*HFG*	Hepatocyte growth factor
DFNB49	*MARVELD2*	Tight junction protein
DFNB53	*COL11A2*	Collagen protein
DFNB59	*PJVK*	Zn-binding protein
DFNB61	*SLC26A5*	Motor protein
DFNB63	*LRTOMT/ COMT2*	Putative methyltransferase
DFNB66/67	*LHFPL5*	Tetraspan protein
DFNB77	*LOXHD1*	Stereociliary protein
DFNB79	*TPRN*	Unknown
DFNB82	*GPSM2*	G protein signaling modulator
DFNB84	*PTPRQ*	Type III receptor-like protein-tyrosine phosphatase family

the hearing loss associated with dominant genes has its onset in adolescence or adulthood and varies in severity, whereas the hearing loss associated with recessive inheritance is congenital and profound. Connexin 26, product of the GJB2 gene, is particularly important because it is responsible for nearly 20% of all cases of childhood deafness; half of genetic deafness in children is GJB2-related. Two frameshift mutations, 35delG and 167delT, account for >50% of the cases; however, screening for these two mutations alone is insufficient and sequencing of the entire gene is required to diagnose GJB2-related recessive deafness. The 167delT mutation is highly prevalent in Ashkenazi Jews; ~1 in 1765 individuals in this population are homozygous and affected. The hearing loss can also vary among the members of the same family, suggesting that other genes or factors influence the auditory phenotype.

In addition to GJB2, several other nonsyndromic genes are associated with hearing loss that progresses with age. The contribution of genetics to presbycusis is also becoming better understood. Sensitivity to aminoglycoside ototoxicity can be maternally transmitted through a mitochondrial mutation. Susceptibility to noise-induced hearing loss may also be genetically determined.

There are >400 syndromic forms of hearing loss. These include Usher syndrome (retinitis pigmentosa and hearing loss), Waardenburg syndrome (pigmentary abnormality and hearing loss), Pendred syndrome (thyroid organification defect and hearing loss), Alport syndrome (renal disease and hearing loss), Jervell and Lange-Nielsen syndrome (prolonged QT interval and hearing loss), neurofibromatosis type 2 (bilateral acoustic schwannoma), and mitochondrial disorders (mitochondrial encephalopathy, lactic acidosis, and stroke-like episodes [MELAS]; myoclonic epilepsy and ragged red fibers [MERRF]; progressive external ophthalmoplegia [PEO]) (**Table 24-2**).

TABLE 24-2

SYNDROMIC HEREDITARY HEARING IMPAIRMENT GENES

SYNDROME	GENE	FUNCTION
Alport syndrome	*COL4A3-5*	Cytoskeletal protein
BOR syndrome	*EYA1*	Developmental gene
	SIX5	Developmental gene
	SIX1	Developmental gene
Jervell and Lange-Nielsen syndrome	*KCNQ1*	Delayed rectifier K⁺ channel
	KCNE1	Delayed rectifier K⁺ channel
Norrie disease	*NDP*	Cell-cell interactions
Pendred syndrome	*SLC26A4*	Chloride/iodide transporter
	FOXI1	Transcriptional activator of *SLC26A4*
Treacher Collins	*TCOF1*	Nucleolar-cytoplasmic transport
Usher syndrome	*MYO7A*	Cytoskeletal protein
	USH1C	Unknown
	CDH23	Intercellular adherence protein
	PCDH15	Cell adhesion molecule
	SANS	Harmonin-associated protein
	USH2A	Cell adhesion molecule
	VLGR1	G protein–coupled receptor
	USH3	Unknown
	WHRN	PDZ domain–containing protein
WS type I, III	*PAX3*	Transcription factor
WS type II	*MITF*	Transcription factor
	SNAI2	Transcription factor
WS type IV	*EDNRB*	Endothelin B receptor
	EDN3	Endothelin B receptor ligand
	SOX10	Transcription factor

Abbreviations: BOR, branchio-oto-renal syndrome; WS, Waardenburg syndrome.

APPROACH TO THE PATIENT

Disorders of the Sense of Hearing

The goal in the evaluation of a patient with auditory complaints is to determine (1) the nature of the hearing impairment (conductive vs. sensorineural vs. mixed), (2) the severity of the impairment (mild, moderate, severe, profound), (3) the anatomy of the impairment (external ear, middle ear, inner ear, or central auditory pathway), and (4) the etiology. The history should elicit characteristics of the hearing loss, including the duration of deafness, unilateral vs. bilateral involvement, nature of onset (sudden vs. insidious), and rate of progression (rapid vs. slow). Symptoms of tinnitus, vertigo, imbalance, aural fullness, otorrhea, headache, facial nerve dysfunction, and head and neck paresthesias should be noted. Information regarding head trauma, exposure to ototoxins, occupational or recreational noise exposure, and family history of hearing impairment may also be important. A sudden onset of unilateral hearing loss, with or without tinnitus, may represent a viral infection of the inner ear or a stroke. Patients with unilateral hearing loss (sensory or conductive) usually complain of reduced hearing, poor sound localization, and difficulty hearing clearly with background noise. Gradual progression of a hearing deficit is common with otosclerosis, noise-induced hearing loss, vestibular schwannoma, or Ménière's disease. Small vestibular schwannomas typically present with asymmetric hearing impairment, tinnitus, and imbalance (rarely vertigo); cranial neuropathy, in particular of the trigeminal or facial nerve, may accompany larger tumors. In addition to hearing loss, Ménière's disease may be associated with episodic vertigo, tinnitus, and aural fullness. Hearing loss with otorrhea is most likely due to chronic otitis media or cholesteatoma.

Examination should include the auricle, external ear canal, and tympanic membrane. The external ear canal of the elderly is often dry and fragile; it is preferable to clean cerumen with wall-mounted suction or cerumen loops and to avoid irrigation. In examining the eardrum, the topography of the tympanic membrane is more important than the presence or absence of the light reflex. In addition to the pars tensa (the lower two-thirds of the eardrum), the pars flaccida above the short process of the malleus should also be examined for retraction pockets that may be evidence of chronic eustachian tube dysfunction or cholesteatoma. Insufflation of the ear canal is necessary to assess tympanic membrane mobility and compliance. Careful inspection of the nose, nasopharynx, and upper respiratory tract is indicated. Unilateral serous effusion should prompt a fiberoptic examination of the nasopharynx to exclude neoplasms. Cranial nerves should be evaluated with special attention to facial and trigeminal nerves, which are commonly affected with tumors involving the cerebellopontine angle.

The Rinne and Weber tuning fork tests, with a 512-Hz tuning fork, are used to screen for hearing loss, differentiate conductive from sensorineural hearing losses, and to confirm the findings of audiologic evaluation. Rinne's test compares the ability to hear by air conduction with the ability to hear by bone conduction. The tines of a vibrating tuning fork are held near the opening of the external auditory canal, and then the stem is placed on the mastoid process; for direct contact, it may be placed on teeth or dentures. The patient is asked to indicate whether the tone is louder by air conduction or bone conduction. Normally, and in the presence of sensorineural hearing loss, a tone is heard louder by air conduction than by bone conduction; however, with conductive hearing loss of ≥30 dB (see "Audiologic Assessment"), the bone-conduction stimulus is perceived as louder than the air-conduction stimulus. For the Weber test, the stem of a vibrating tuning fork is placed on the head in the midline and the patient asked whether the tone is heard in both ears or better in one ear than in the other. With a unilateral conductive hearing loss, the tone is perceived in the affected ear. With a unilateral sensorineural hearing loss, the tone is perceived in the unaffected ear. A 5-dB difference in hearing between the two ears is required for lateralization.

LABORATORY ASSESSMENT OF HEARING

Audiologic assessment

The minimum audiologic assessment for hearing loss should include the measurement of pure tone air-conduction and bone-conduction thresholds, speech reception threshold, word recognition score, tympanometry, acoustic reflexes, and acoustic-reflex decay. This test battery provides a screening evaluation of the entire auditory system and allows one to determine whether further differentiation of a sensory (cochlear) from a neural (retrocochlear) hearing loss is indicated.

Pure tone audiometry assesses hearing acuity for pure tones. The test is administered by an audiologist and is performed in a sound-attenuated chamber. The pure tone stimulus is delivered with an audiometer, an electronic device that allows the presentation of specific frequencies (generally between 250 and 8000 Hz) at specific intensities. Air- and bone-conduction thresholds are established for each ear. Air-conduction thresholds are determined by presenting the stimulus in air with the use of headphones. Bone-conduction thresholds are determined by placing the stem of a vibrating tuning fork or an oscillator of an audiometer in contact with the head. In the presence of a hearing loss, broad-spectrum noise is presented to the nontest ear for *masking* purposes so that responses are based on perception from the ear under test.

The responses are measured in decibels. An *audiogram* is a plot of intensity in decibels of hearing threshold versus frequency. A decibel (dB) is equal to 20 times the logarithm of the ratio of the sound pressure required to achieve threshold in the patient to the sound pressure required to achieve threshold in a normal hearing person. Therefore, a change of 6 dB represents doubling of sound pressure, and a change of 20 dB represents a tenfold change in sound pressure. Loudness, which depends on the frequency, intensity, and duration of a sound, doubles with approximately each 10-dB increase in sound pressure level. Pitch, on the other hand, does not directly correlate with frequency. The perception of pitch changes slowly in the low and high frequencies. In the middle tones, which are important for human speech, pitch varies more rapidly with changes in frequency.

Pure tone audiometry establishes the presence and severity of hearing impairment, unilateral vs. bilateral involvement, and the type of hearing loss. Conductive hearing losses with a large mass component, as is often seen in middle ear effusions, produce elevation of thresholds that predominate in the higher frequencies. Conductive hearing losses with a large stiffness component, as in fixation of the footplate of the stapes in early otosclerosis, produce threshold elevations in the lower frequencies. Often, the conductive hearing loss involves all frequencies, suggesting involvement of both stiffness and mass. In general, sensorineural hearing losses such as presbycusis affect higher frequencies more than lower frequencies. An exception is Ménière's disease, which is characteristically associated with low-frequency sensorineural hearing loss. Noise-induced hearing loss has an unusual pattern of hearing impairment in which the loss at 4000 Hz is greater than at higher frequencies. Vestibular schwannomas characteristically affect the higher frequencies, but any pattern of hearing loss can be observed.

Speech recognition requires greater synchronous neural firing than is necessary for appreciation of pure tones. *Speech audiometry* tests the clarity with which one hears. The *speech reception threshold* (SRT) is defined as the intensity at which speech is recognized as a meaningful symbol and is obtained by presenting two-syllable words with an equal accent on each syllable. The intensity at which the patient can repeat 50% of the words correctly is the SRT. Once the SRT is determined, discrimination or word recognition ability is tested by presenting one-syllable words at 25–40 dB above the SRT. The words are phonetically balanced in that the phonemes (speech sounds) occur in the list of words at the same frequency that they occur in ordinary conversational English. An individual with normal hearing or conductive hearing loss can repeat 88–100% of the phonetically balanced words correctly. Patients with a sensorineural hearing loss have variable loss of discrimination. As a general rule, neural lesions produce greater deficits in discrimination than do cochlear lesions. For example, in a patient with mild asymmetric sensorineural hearing loss, a clue to the diagnosis of vestibular schwannoma is the presence of greater than expected deterioration in discrimination ability. Deterioration in discrimination ability at higher intensities above the SRT also suggests a lesion in the eighth nerve or central auditory pathways.

Tympanometry measures the impedance of the middle ear to sound and is useful in diagnosis of middle-ear effusions. A *tympanogram* is the graphic representation of change in impedance or compliance as the pressure in the ear canal is changed. Normally, the middle ear is most compliant at atmospheric pressure, and the compliance decreases as the pressure is increased or decreased (type A); this pattern is seen with normal hearing or in the presence of sensorineural hearing loss. Compliance that does not change with change in pressure suggests middle-ear effusion (type B). With a negative pressure in the middle ear, as with eustachian tube obstruction, the point of maximal compliance occurs with negative pressure in the ear canal (type C). A tympanogram in which no point of maximal compliance can be obtained is most commonly seen with discontinuity of the ossicular chain (type A_d). A reduction in the maximal compliance peak can be seen in otosclerosis (type A_s).

During tympanometry, an intense tone elicits contraction of the stapedius muscle. The change in compliance of the middle ear with contraction of the stapedius muscle can be detected. The presence or absence of this *acoustic reflex* is important in determining the etiology of hearing loss as well as in the anatomic localization of facial nerve paralysis. The acoustic reflex can help differentiate between conductive hearing loss due to otosclerosis and that caused by an inner ear "third window": it is absent in otosclerosis and present in inner ear conductive hearing loss. Normal or elevated acoustic reflex thresholds in an individual with sensorineural hearing impairment suggests a cochlear hearing loss. An absent acoustic reflex in the setting of sensorineural hearing loss is not helpful in localizing the site of lesion. Assessment of *acoustic reflex decay* helps differentiate sensory from neural hearing losses. In neural hearing loss, the reflex adapts or decays with time.

Otoacoustic emissions (OAEs) generated by outer hair cells only can be measured with microphones inserted into the external auditory canal. The emissions may be spontaneous or evoked with sound stimulation. The presence of OAEs indicates that the outer hair cells of the organ of Corti are intact and can be used to assess auditory thresholds and to distinguish sensory from neural hearing losses.

Evoked responses

Electrocochleography measures the earliest evoked potentials generated in the cochlea and the auditory nerve. Receptor potentials recorded include the cochlear microphonic, generated by the outer hair cells of the organ of Corti, and the summating potential, generated by the inner hair cells in response to sound. The whole nerve action potential representing the composite firing of the first-order neurons can also be recorded during electrocochleography. Clinically, the test is useful in the diagnosis of Ménière's disease, where an elevation of the ratio of summating potential to action potential is seen.

Brainstem auditory evoked responses (BAERs), also known as *auditory brainstem responses* (ABRs), are useful in differentiating the site of sensorineural hearing loss. In response to sound, five distinct electrical potentials arising from different stations along the peripheral and central auditory pathway can be identified using computer averaging from scalp surface electrodes. BAERs are valuable in situations in which patients cannot or will not give reliable voluntary thresholds. They are also used to assess the integrity of the auditory nerve and brainstem in various clinical situations, including intraoperative monitoring and in determination of brain death.

The *vestibular-evoked myogenic potential (VEMP) test* elicits a vestibulocollic reflex whose afferent limb arises from acoustically sensitive cells in the saccule, with signals conducted via the inferior vestibular nerve. VEMP is a biphasic, short-latency response recorded from the tonically contracted sternocleidomastoid muscle in response to loud auditory clicks or tones. VEMPs may be diminished or absent in patients with early and late Ménière's disease, vestibular neuritis, benign paroxysmal positional vertigo, and vestibular schwannoma. On the other hand, the threshold for VEMPs may be lower in cases of superior canal dehiscence, other inner ear dehiscence, and perilymphatic fistula.

Imaging studies

The choice of radiologic tests is largely determined by whether the goal is to evaluate the bony anatomy of the external, middle, and inner ear or to image the auditory nerve and brain. Axial and coronal CT of the temporal bone with fine 0.3- to 0.6-mm cuts is ideal for determining the caliber of the external auditory canal, integrity of the ossicular chain, and presence of middle-ear or mastoid disease; it can also detect inner ear malformations. CT is also ideal for the detection of bone erosion with chronic otitis media and cholesteatoma. MRI is superior to CT for imaging of retrocochlear pathology such as vestibular schwannoma, meningioma, other lesions of the cerebellopontine angle, demyelinating lesions of the brainstem, and brain tumors. Both CT and MRI are equally capable of identifying inner ear malformations and assessing cochlear patency for preoperative evaluation of patients for cochlear implantation.

TREATMENT Disorders of the Sense of Hearing

In general, conductive hearing losses are amenable to surgical correction, while sensorineural hearing losses are more difficult to manage. Atresia of the ear canal can be surgically repaired, often with significant improvement in hearing. Tympanic membrane perforations due to chronic otitis media or trauma can be repaired with an outpatient tympanoplasty. Likewise, conductive hearing loss associated with otosclerosis can be treated by stapedectomy, which is successful in 90–95% of cases. Tympanostomy tubes allow the prompt return of normal hearing in individuals with middle ear effusions. Hearing aids are effective and well tolerated in patients with conductive hearing losses.

Patients with mild, moderate, and severe sensorineural hearing losses are regularly rehabilitated with hearing aids of varying configuration and strength. Hearing aids have been improved to provide greater fidelity and have been miniaturized. The current generation of hearing aids can be placed entirely within the ear canal, thus reducing any stigma associated with their use. In general, the more severe the hearing impairment, the larger the hearing aid required for auditory rehabilitation. Digital hearing aids lend themselves to individual programming, and multiple and directional microphones at the ear level may be helpful in noisy surroundings. Since all hearing aids amplify noise as well as speech, the only absolute solution to the problem of noise is to place the microphone closer to the speaker than the noise source. This arrangement is not possible with a self-contained, cosmetically acceptable device. A significant limitation of rehabilitation with a hearing aid is that while it is able to enhance detection of sound with amplification, it cannot restore clarity of hearing that is lost with presbycusis.

Patients with unilateral deafness have difficulty with sound localization and reduced clarity of hearing in background noise. They may benefit from a CROS (contralateral routing of signal) hearing aid in which a microphone is placed on the hearing-impaired side and the sound is transmitted to the receiver placed on the contralateral ear. The same result may be obtained with a bone-anchored hearing aid (BAHA), in which a hearing aid clamps to a screw osseointegrated into the skull on the hearing-impaired side. Like the CROS hearing aid, the BAHA transfers the acoustic signal to the contralateral hearing ear, but it does so by vibrating the skull. Patients with profound deafness on one side and some hearing loss in the better ear are candidates for a BICROS hearing aid; it differs from the CROS hearing aid in that the patient wears a hearing aid, and not simply a receiver, in the better ear. Unfortunately, CROS and BAHA devices are often judged by patients to be unsatisfactory.

In many situations, including lectures and the theater, hearing-impaired persons benefit from assistive devices that are based on the principle of having the speaker closer to the microphone than any source of noise. Assistive devices include infrared and frequency-modulated (FM) transmission as well as an electromagnetic loop around the room for transmission to the individual's hearing aid. Hearing aids with telecoils can also be used with properly equipped telephones in the same way.

In the event that the hearing aid provides inadequate rehabilitation, cochlear implants may be appropriate. Criteria for implantation include severe to profound hearing loss with open-set sentence cognition of ≤40% under best aided conditions. Worldwide, nearly 200,000 hearing impaired children and adults have received cochlear implants. Cochlear implants are neural prostheses that convert sound energy to electrical energy and can be used to stimulate the auditory division of the eighth nerve directly. In most cases of profound hearing impairment, the auditory hair cells are lost but the ganglionic cells of the auditory division of the eighth nerve are preserved. Cochlear implants consist of electrodes that are inserted into the cochlea through the round window, speech processors that extract acoustical elements of speech for conversion to electrical currents, and a means of transmitting the electrical energy through the skin. Patients with implants experience sound that helps with speech reading, allows open-set word recognition, and helps in modulating the person's own voice. Usually, within the first 3–6 months after implantation, adult patients can understand speech without visual cues. With the current generation of multichannel cochlear implants, nearly 75% of patients are able to converse on the telephone. For individuals who have had both eighth nerves destroyed by trauma or bilateral vestibular schwannomas (e.g., neurofibromatosis type 2), brainstem auditory implants placed near the cochlear nucleus may provide auditory rehabilitation.

Tinnitus often accompanies hearing loss. As for background noise, tinnitus can degrade speech comprehension in individuals with hearing impairment. Therapy for tinnitus is usually directed toward minimizing the appreciation of tinnitus. Relief of the tinnitus may be obtained by masking it with background music. Hearing aids are also helpful in tinnitus suppression, as are tinnitus maskers, devices that present a sound to the affected ear that is more pleasant to listen to than the tinnitus. The use of a tinnitus masker is often followed by several hours of inhibition of the tinnitus. Antidepressants have been shown to be beneficial in helping patients cope with tinnitus.

Hard-of-hearing individuals often benefit from a reduction in unnecessary noise in the environment (e.g., radio or television) to enhance the signal-to-noise ratio. Speech comprehension is aided by lip reading; therefore, the impaired listener should be seated so that the face of the speaker is well illuminated and easily seen. Although speech should be in a loud, clear voice, one should be aware that in sensorineural hearing losses in general and in hard-of-hearing elderly in particular, recruitment (abnormal perception of loud sounds) may be troublesome. Above all, optimal communication cannot take place without both parties giving it their full and undivided attention.

PREVENTION

Conductive hearing losses may be prevented by prompt antibiotic therapy of adequate duration for AOM and by ventilation of the middle ear with tympanostomy tubes in middle-ear effusions lasting ≥12 weeks. Loss of vestibular function and deafness due to aminoglycoside antibiotics can largely be prevented by careful monitoring of serum peak and trough levels.

Some 10 million Americans have noise-induced hearing loss, and 20 million are exposed to hazardous noise in their employment. Noise-induced hearing loss can be prevented by avoidance of exposure to loud noise or by regular use of ear plugs or fluid-filled ear muffs to attenuate intense sound. High-risk activities for noise-induced hearing loss include wood and metal working with electrical equipment and target practice and hunting with small firearms. All internal-combustion and electric engines, including snow and leaf blowers, snowmobiles, outboard motors, and chain saws, require protection of the user with hearing protectors. Virtually all noise-induced hearing loss is preventable through education, which should begin before the teenage years. Programs of industrial conservation of hearing are required by Occupational Safety and Health Administration (OSHA) when the exposure over an 8-h period averages 85 dB. OSHA mandates that workers in such noisy environments have hearing monitoring and protection programs that include a pre-employment screen, annual audiologic assessment, as well as the mandatory use of hearing protectors. Exposure to loud sounds above 85 dB in the work environment is restricted by OSHA, with halving of allowed exposure time for each increment of 5 dB above this threshold: for example 90 dB exposure is permitted for 8 h; 95 dB for 4 h, and 100 dB for 2 h.

SECTION III

DISEASES OF THE NERVOUS SYSTEM

CHAPTER 25

MECHANISMS OF NEUROLOGIC DISEASES

Stephen L. Hauser ■ M. Flint Beal

The human nervous system is the organ of consciousness, cognition, ethics, and behavior; as such, it is the most intricate structure known to exist. More than one-third of the 23,000 genes encoded in the human genome are expressed in the nervous system. Each mature brain is composed of 100 billion neurons, several million miles of axons and dendrites, and $>10^{15}$ synapses. Neurons exist within a dense parenchyma of multifunctional glial cells that synthesize myelin, preserve homeostasis, and regulate immune responses. Measured against this background of complexity, the achievements of molecular neuroscience have been extraordinary. This chapter reviews selected themes in neuroscience that provide a context for understanding fundamental mechanisms that underlie neurologic disorders.

NEUROGENETICS

The landscape of neurology has been transformed by modern molecular genetics. More than 350 different disease-causing genes have been identified, and >1000 neurologic disorders have been genetically mapped to various chromosomal locations. Several hundred neurologic and psychiatric disorders now can be diagnosed through genetic testing (*http://www.ncbi.nlm.nih.gov/sites/GeneTests/?db=GeneTests*). The vast majority of these disorders represent highly penetrant mutations that cause rare neurologic disorders; alternatively, they represent rare monogenic causes of common phenotypes. Examples of the latter include mutations of the amyloid precursor protein in familial Alzheimer's disease, the microtubule-associated protein tau (MAPT) in frontotemporal dementia, and α-synuclein in Parkinson's disease. These discoveries have been profoundly important because the mutated gene in a familial disorder often encodes a protein that is also pathogenetically involved (although not mutated) in the typical, sporadic form. The common mechanism involves disordered processing and, ultimately, aggregation of the protein, leading to cell death (see "Protein Aggregation and Neurodegeneration").

There is great optimism that complex genetic disorders that are caused by combinations of genetic and environmental factors have become tractable problems. Genome-wide association studies (GWAS) have been carried out in many complex neurologic disorders, with many hundreds of variants identified, nearly all of which confer only a small increment in disease risk (1.15–1.5 fold). GWAS are rooted in the "common disease, common variant" hypothesis, as they examine potential risk alleles that are relatively common (e.g., >5%) in the general population. More than 1000 GWAS have been carried out to date, with notable successes such as the identification of >50 risk alleles for multiple sclerosis. Furthermore, when bioinformatics tools are used, risk variants can be aligned in functional biologic pathways to identify novel pathogenic mechanisms as well as to reveal heterogeneity (e.g., different pathways in different individuals). Despite these successes, many experienced geneticists question the value of common disease-associated variants, particularly whether they are actually causative or merely mark the approximate locations of more important—truly causative—rare mutations.

This debate has set the stage for the next revolution in human genetics, made possible by the development of increasingly efficient and cost-effective high-throughput sequencing methodologies. It is currently possible to sequence an entire human genome in approximately an hour, at a cost of only $4000 for the entire coding sequence ("whole-exome") or $10,000 for the entire genome; it is certain that these costs will continue to decline. This makes it feasible to look for disease-causing sequence variations in individual patients with the possibility of identifying rare variants that cause disease. The utility of this approach was demonstrated by whole-genome sequencing in a patient with Charcot-Marie-Tooth neuropathy in which compound heterozygous mutations were identified in the *SH3TC2* gene that then were shown to co-segregate with the disease in other members of the family.

It is also increasingly recognized that not all genetic diseases or predispositions are caused by simple changes in the linear nucleotide sequence of genes. As the complex architecture of the human genome becomes better defined, many disorders that result from alterations in copy numbers of genes ("gene-dosage" effects) resulting from unequal crossing-over are likely to be identified. As much as 5–10% of the human genome consists of nonhomologous duplications and deletions, and these appear to occur with a much higher mutational rate than is the case for single base pair mutations. The first copy-number disorders to be recognized were Charcot-Marie-Tooth disease type 1A (CMT1A), caused by a duplication in the gene encoding the myelin protein PMP22, and the reciprocal deletion of the gene causing hereditary liability to pressure palsies (HNPP) (Chap. 45). Gene-dosage effects are causative in some cases of Parkinson's disease (α-synuclein), Alzheimer's disease (amyloid precursor protein), spinal muscular atrophy (survival motor neuron 2), the dysmyelinating disorder Pelizaeus-Merzbacher syndrome (proteolipid protein 1), late-onset leukodystrophy (lamin B1), and a variety of developmental neurologic disorders. It is now evident that copy-number variations contribute substantially to normal human genomic variation for numerous genes involved in neurologic function, regulation of cell growth, and regulation of metabolism. It is also already clear that gene-dosage effects will influence many behavioral phenotypes, learning disorders, and autism spectrum disorders. Deletions at ch1q and ch15q have been associated with schizophrenia, and deletions at 15q and 16p with autism. Interestingly, the 16p deletion also is associated with epilepsy. Duplications of the X-linked *MeCP2* gene cause autism in males and psychiatric disorders with anxiety in females, whereas point mutations in this gene produce the neurodevelopmental disorder Rett syndrome. The understanding of the role of copy-number variation in human disease is still in its infancy.

The role of splicing variation as a contributor to neurologic disease is another area of active investigation. *Alternative splicing* refers to the inclusion of different combinations of exons in mature mRNA, resulting in the potential for many different protein products encoded by a single gene. Alternative splicing represents a powerful mechanism for generation of complexity and variation, and this mechanism appears to be highly prevalent in the nervous system, affecting key processes such as neurotransmitter receptors and ion channels. Numerous diseases are known to result from abnormalities in alternative splicing. Increased inclusion of exon 10–containing transcripts of *MAPT* can cause frontotemporal dementia. Aberrant splicing also contributes to the pathogenesis of Duchenne's, myotonic, and fascioscapulohumeral muscular dystrophies; ataxia-telangiectasia; neurofibromatosis; some inherited ataxias; and fragile X syndrome, among other disorders. It is also likely that subtle variations of splicing will influence many genetically complex disorders. For example, a splicing variant of the interleukin 7 receptor α chain, resulting in production of more soluble and less membrane-bound receptor, was found to be associated with susceptibility to multiple sclerosis (MS) in multiple different populations.

Epigenetics refers to the mechanisms by which levels of gene expression can be exquisitely modulated not by variations in the primary genetic sequence of DNA but rather by postgenomic alterations in DNA and chromatin structure, which influence how, when, and where genes are expressed. DNA methylation and the methylation and acetylation of histone proteins that interact with nuclear DNA to form chromatin are key mediators of these events. Epigenetic processes appear to be dynamically active even in postmitotic neurons. *Imprinting* refers to an epigenetic feature, present for a subset of genes, in which the predominant expression of one allele is determined by its parent of origin. The distinctive neurodevelopmental disorders Prader-Willi syndrome (mild mental retardation and endocrine abnormalities) and Angelman syndrome (cortical atrophy, cerebellar dysmyelination, Purkinje cell loss) are classic examples of imprinting disorders whose distinctive features are determined by whether the paternal or maternal copy of chromosome of the critical genetic region 15q11-13 was responsible. In a study of discordant monozygotic twins for MS in which the entire DNA sequence, transcriptome (e.g., mRNA levels), and methylome were assessed genomewide, tantalizing allelic differences in the use of the paternal, compared to maternal, copy for a group of genes were identified. Preferential allelic expression, whether due to imprinting, resistance to X inactivation, or other mechanisms, is likely to play a major role in determining complex behaviors and susceptibility to many neurologic and psychiatric disorders.

Another advance is the development of transgenic mouse models of neurologic diseases, which has been particularly fruitful in producing models relevant to Alzheimer's disease, Parkinson's disease, Huntington's disease, and amyotrophic lateral sclerosis. These models are useful in both studying disease pathogenesis and developing and testing new therapies. Models in both *Caenorhabditis elegans* and *Drosophila* have also been extremely useful, particularly in studying genetic modifiers as well as therapeutic interventions.

ION CHANNELS AND CHANNELOPATHIES

The resting potential of neurons and the action potentials responsible for impulse conduction are generated by ion currents and ion channels. Most ion channels are gated, meaning that they can transition between conformations that are open or closed to ion conductance. Individual ion channels are distinguished by the specific ions they conduct; their kinetics; and whether they directly sense voltage, are linked to receptors for neurotransmitters or other ligands such as neurotrophins, or are activated by second messengers. The diverse characteristics of different ion channels provide a means by which neuronal excitability can be modulated exquisitely at both the cellular and subcellular levels. Disorders of ion channels—channelopathies—are responsible for a growing list of human neurologic diseases (Table 25-1). Most are caused by mutations in ion channel genes or by autoantibodies against ion channel proteins. One example is epilepsy, a syndrome of diverse causes characterized by repetitive, synchronous firing of neuronal action potentials. Action potentials normally are generated by the opening of sodium channels and the inward movement of sodium ions down the intracellular concentration gradient. Depolarization of the neuronal membrane opens potassium channels, resulting in outward movement of potassium ions, repolarization, closure of the sodium channel, and hyperpolarization. Sodium or potassium channel subunit genes have long been considered candidate disease genes in inherited epilepsy syndromes, and recently such mutations were identified. These mutations appear to alter the normal gating function of these channels, increasing the inherent excitability of neuronal membranes in regions where the abnormal channels are expressed.

Whereas the specific clinical manifestations of channelopathies are quite variable, one common feature is that manifestations tend to be intermittent or paroxysmal, as occurs in epilepsy, migraine, ataxia, myotonia, or periodic paralysis. Exceptions are clinically progressive channel disorders such as autosomal dominant hearing impairment. The genetic channelopathies identified to date are all uncommon disorders caused by obvious mutations in channel genes. As the full repertoire of human ion channels and related proteins is identified, it is likely that additional channelopathies will be discovered. In addition to rare disorders that result from obvious mutations, it is likely that less penetrant allelic variations in channel genes or their pattern of expression might underlie susceptibility to some apparently sporadic forms of epilepsy, migraine, or other disorders. For example, mutations in the potassium channel gene Kir2.6 have been found in many individuals with thyrotoxic hypokalemic periodic paralysis, a disorder similar

TABLE 25-1

EXAMPLES OF NEUROLOGIC CHANNELOPATHIES

CATEGORY	DISORDER	CHANNEL TYPE	MUTATED GENE	CHAP. REF.
Genetic				
Ataxias	Episodic ataxia-1	K	*KCNA1*	31
	Episodic ataxia-2	Ca	*CACNL1A*	
	Spinocerebellar ataxia-6	Ca	*CACNL1A*	
Migraine	Familial hemiplegic migraine 1	Ca	*CACNL1A*	8
	Familial hemiplegic migraine 3	Na	*SCN1A*	
Epilepsy	Benign neonatal familial convulsions	K	*KCNQ2, KCNQ3*	26
	Generalized epilepsy with febrile convulsions plus	Na	*SCN1B*	
Periodic paralysis	Hyperkalemic periodic paralysis	Na	*SCN4A*	48
	Hypokalemic periodic paralysis	Ca	*CACNL1A3*	
Myotonia	Myotonia congenita	Cl	*CLCN1*	48
	Paramyotonia congenita	Na	*SCN4A*	
Deafness	Jervell and Lange-Nielsen syndrome (deafness, prolonged QT interval, and arrhythmia)	K	*KCNQ1, KCNE1*	24
	Autosomal dominant progressive deafness	K	*KCNQ4*	
Autoimmune				
Paraneoplastic	Limbic encephalitis	Kv1	—	44
	Acquired neuromyotonia	Kv1	—	44
	Cerebellar ataxia	Ca (P/Q type)	—	44
	Lambert-Eaton syndrome	Ca (P/Q type)	—	44

to hypokalemic periodic paralysis but precipitated by stress from thyrotoxicosis or carbohydrate loading.

NEUROTRANSMITTERS AND NEUROTRANSMITTER RECEPTORS

Synaptic neurotransmission is the predominant means by which neurons communicate with each other. Classic neurotransmitters are synthesized in the presynaptic region of the nerve terminal; stored in vesicles; and released into the synaptic cleft, where they bind to receptors on the postsynaptic cell. Secreted neurotransmitters are eliminated by reuptake into the presynaptic neuron (or glia), diffusion away from the synaptic cleft, and/or specific inactivation. In addition to the classic neurotransmitters, many neuropeptides have been identified as definite or probable neurotransmitters; they include substance P, neurotensin, enkephalins, β-endorphin, histamine, vasoactive intestinal polypeptide, cholecystokinin, neuropeptide Y, and somatostatin. Peptide neurotransmitters are synthesized in the cell body rather than the nerve terminal and may colocalize with classic neurotransmitters in single neurons. A number of neuropeptides are important in pain modulation, including substance P and calcitonin gene-related peptide (CGRP), which causes migraine-like headaches in patients. As a consequence, CGRP receptor antagonists have been developed and shown to be effective in treating migraine headaches. Nitric oxide and carbon monoxide are gases that appear also to function as neurotransmitters, in part by signaling in a retrograde fashion from the postsynaptic to the presynaptic cell.

Neurotransmitters modulate the function of postsynaptic cells by binding to specific neurotransmitter receptors, of which there are two major types. *Ionotropic receptors* are direct ion channels that open after engagement by the neurotransmitter. *Metabotropic receptors* interact with G proteins, stimulating production of second messengers and activating protein kinases, which modulate a variety of cellular events. Ionotropic receptors are multiple-subunit structures, whereas metabotropic receptors are composed of single subunits only. One important difference between ionotropic and metabotropic receptors is that the kinetics of ionotropic receptor effects are fast (generally <1 ms) because neurotransmitter binding directly alters the electrical properties of the postsynaptic cell, whereas metabotropic receptors function over longer periods. These different properties contribute to the potential for selective and finely modulated signaling by neurotransmitters.

Neurotransmitter systems are perturbed in a large number of clinical disorders, examples of which are highlighted in **Table 25-2**. One example is the involvement of dopaminergic neurons originating in the substantia nigra of the midbrain and projecting to the striatum (nigrostriatal pathway) in Parkinson's disease and in heroin addicts after the ingestion of the toxin MPTP (1-methyl-4-phenyl-1,2,5,6-tetrahydropyridine).

A second important dopaminergic system arising in the midbrain is the mediocorticolimbic pathway, which is implicated in the pathogenesis of addictive behaviors including drug reward. Its key components include the midbrain ventral tegmental area (VTA), median forebrain bundle, and nucleus accumbens (see Fig. 53-1). The cholinergic pathway originating in the nucleus basalis of Meynert plays a role in memory function in Alzheimer's disease.

Addictive drugs share the property of increasing dopamine release in the nucleus accumbens. Amphetamine increases intracellular release of dopamine from vesicles and reverses transport of dopamine through the dopamine transporters. Patients prone to addiction show increased activation of the nucleus accumbens after administration of amphetamine. Cocaine binds to dopamine transporters and inhibits dopamine reuptake. Ethanol inhibits inhibitory neurons in the VTA, leading to increased dopamine release in the nucleus accumbens. Opioids also disinhibit these dopaminergic neurons by binding to μ receptors expressed by γ-aminobutyric acid (GABA)-containing interneurons in the VTA. Nicotine increases dopamine release by activating nicotinic acetylcholine receptors on cell bodies and nerve terminals of dopaminergic VTA neurons. Tetrahydrocannabinol, the active ingredient of cannabis, also increases dopamine levels in the nucleus accumbens. Blockade of dopamine in the nucleus accumbens can terminate the rewarding effects of addictive drugs.

Not all cell-to-cell communication in the nervous system occurs via neurotransmission. Gap junctions provide for direct neuron-neuron electrical conduction and also create openings for the diffusion of ions and metabolites between cells. In addition to neurons, gap junctions are widespread in glia, creating a syncytium that protects neurons by removing glutamate and potassium from the extracellular environment. Gap junctions consist of membrane-spanning proteins, termed *connexins*, that pair across adjacent cells. Mechanisms that involve gap junctions have been related to a variety of neurologic disorders. Mutations in connexin 32, a gap junction protein expressed by Schwann cells, are responsible for the X-linked form of CMT disease. Mutations in either of two gap junction proteins expressed in the inner ear—connexin 26 and connexin 31—result in autosomal dominant progressive hearing loss (Chap. 24). Glial calcium waves mediated through gap junctions also appear to explain the phenomenon of spreading depression associated with migraine auras and the march of epileptic discharges. Spreading depression is a neural response that follows a variety of

TABLE 25-2

PRINCIPAL CLASSIC NEUROTRANSMITTERS

NEUROTRANSMITTER	ANATOMY	CLINICAL ASPECTS
Acetylcholine (ACh) $CH_3—C(=O)—O—CH_2—N—(CH_3)_3$	Motor neurons in spinal cord → neuromuscular junction	Acetylcholinesterases (nerve gases) Myasthenia gravis (antibodies to ACh receptor) Congenital myasthenic syndromes (mutations in ACh receptor subunits) Lambert-Eaton syndrome (antibodies to Ca channels impair ACh release) Botulism (toxin disrupts ACh release by exocytosis)
	Basal forebrain → widespread cortex	Alzheimer's disease (selective cell death) Autosomal dominant frontal lobe epilepsy (mutations in CNS ACh receptor)
	Interneurons in striatum	Parkinson's disease (tremor)
	Autonomic nervous system (preganglionic and postganglionic parasympathetic; preganglionic sympathetic)	
Dopamine HO, HO—(ring)—$CH_2—CH_2—NH_3$	Substantia nigra → striatum (nigrostriatal pathway)	Parkinson's disease (selective cell death) MPTP parkinsonism (toxin transported into neurons)
	Substantia nigra → limbic system and widespread cortex	Addiction, behavioral disorders
	Arcuate nucleus of hypothalamus → anterior pituitary (via portal veins)	Inhibits prolactin secretion
Norepinephrine (NE) HO, HO—(ring)—$CH(OH)—CH_2—NH_2$	Locus coeruleus (pons) → limbic system, hypothalamus, cortex	Mood disorders (MAOA inhibitors and tricyclics increase NE and improve depression)
	Medulla → locus coeruleus, spinal cord	Anxiety
	Postganglionic neurons of sympathetic nervous system	Orthostatic tachycardia syndrome (mutations in NE transporter)
Serotonin HO—(indole ring, N–H)—$CH_2—CH_2—NH_2$	Pontine raphe nuclei → widespread projections	Mood disorders (SSRIs improve depression) Migraine pain pathway
	Medulla/pons → dorsal horn of spinal cord	Pain pathway
γ-Aminobutyric acid (GABA) $H_2N—CH_2—CH_2—CH_2—COOH$	Major inhibitory neurotransmitter in brain; widespread cortical interneurons and long projection pathways	Stiff-person syndrome (antibodies to glutamic acid decarboxylase, the biosynthetic enzyme for GABA) Epilepsy (gabapentin and valproic acid increase GABA)
Glycine $H_2N—CH_2—COOH$	Major inhibitory neurotransmitter in spinal cord	Spasticity Hyperekplexia (myoclonic startle syndrome) due to mutations in glycine receptor
Glutamate $H_2N—CH(COOH)—CH_2—CH_2—COOH$	Major excitatory neurotransmitter; located throughout CNS, including cortical pyramidal cells	Seizures due to ingestion of domoic acid (a glutamate analogue) Rasmussen's encephalitis (antibody against glutamate receptor 3) Excitotoxic cell death

Abbreviations: CNS, central nervous system; MAOA, monoamine oxidase A; MPTP, 1-methyl-4-phenyl-1,2,3,6-tetrahydropyridine; SSRI, selective serotonin reuptake inhibitor.

different stimuli and is characterized by a circumferentially expanding negative potential that propagates at a characteristic speed of 20 m/s and is associated with an increase in extracellular potassium.

SIGNALING PATHWAYS AND GENE TRANSCRIPTION

The fundamental issue of how memory, learning, and thinking are encoded in the nervous system is likely to be clarified by identification of the signaling pathways involved in neuronal differentiation, axon guidance, and synapse formation and by an understanding of how these pathways are modulated by experience. Many families of transcription factors, each consisting of multiple individual components, are expressed in the nervous system. Elucidation of these signaling pathways has begun to provide insights into the causes of a variety of neurologic disorders, including inherited disorders of cognition such as X-linked mental retardation. This problem affects ~1 in 500 males, and linkage studies in different families suggest that as many as 60 different X-chromosome-encoded genes may be responsible. Rett syndrome, a common cause of (dominant) X-linked progressive mental retardation in females, is due to a mutation in a gene (*MECP2*) that encodes a DNA-binding protein involved in transcriptional repression. As the X chromosome accounts for only ~3% of germ-line DNA, by extrapolation, the number of genes that potentially contribute to clinical disorders affecting intelligence in humans must be potentially very large. As discussed later in the chapter, there is increasing evidence that abnormal gene transcription may play a role in neurodegenerative diseases such as Huntington's disease, in which proteins with polyglutamine expansions bind to and sequester transcription factors. A critical transcription factor for neuronal survival is CREB (cyclic adenosine monophosphate responsive element-binding) protein, which also plays an important role in memory in the hippocampus.

MYELIN

Myelin is the multilayered insulating substance that surrounds axons and speeds impulse conduction by permitting action potentials to jump between naked regions of axons (nodes of Ranvier) and across myelinated segments. Molecular interactions between the myelin membrane and the axon are required to maintain the stability, function, and normal life span of both structures. A single oligodendrocyte usually ensheathes multiple axons in the central nervous system (CNS), whereas in the peripheral nervous system (PNS) each Schwann cell typically myelinates a single axon. Myelin is a lipid-rich material formed by a spiraling process of the membrane of the myelinating cell around the axon, creating multiple membrane bilayers that are tightly apposed (compact myelin) by charged protein interactions. Several inhibitors of axon growth are expressed on the innermost (periaxonal) lamellae of the myelin membrane (see "Stem Cells and Transplantation"). A number of clinically important neurologic disorders are caused by inherited mutations in myelin proteins of the CNS or PNS (Fig. 25-1). Constituents of myelin also have a propensity to be targeted as autoantigens in autoimmune demyelinating disorders (Fig. 25-2). Specification to oligodendrocyte

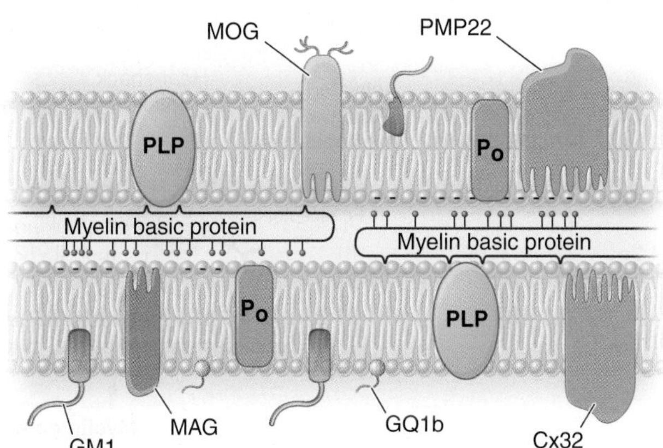

FIGURE 25-1

The molecular architecture of the myelin sheath illustrating the most important disease-related proteins. The illustration represents a composite of CNS and PNS myelin. Proteins restricted to CNS myelin are shown in green, proteins of PNS myelin are lavender, and proteins present in both CNS and PNS are red. In the CNS, the X-linked allelic disorders Pelizaeus-Merzbacher disease and one variant of familial spastic paraplegia are caused by mutations in the gene for proteolipid protein (PLP) that normally promotes extracellular compaction between adjacent myelin lamellae. The homologue of PLP in the PNS is the P_0 protein, mutations in which cause the neuropathy Charcot-Marie-Tooth disease (CMT) type 1B. The most common form of CMT is the 1A subtype caused by a duplication of the *PMP22* gene; deletions in *PMP22* are responsible for another inherited neuropathy termed *hereditary liability to pressure palsies* (Chap. 45).

In multiple sclerosis (MS), myelin basic protein (MBP) and the quantitatively minor CNS protein myelin oligodendrocyte glycoprotein (MOG) are probably T cell and B cell antigens, respectively (Chap. 39). The location of MOG at the outermost lamella of the CNS myelin membrane may facilitate its targeting by autoantibodies. In the PNS, autoantibodies against myelin gangliosides are implicated in a variety of disorders, including GQ1b in the Fisher variant of Guillain-Barré syndrome, GM1 in multifocal motor neuropathy, and sulfatide constituents of myelin-associated glycoprotein (MAG) in peripheral neuropathies associated with monoclonal gammopathies (Chap. 46).

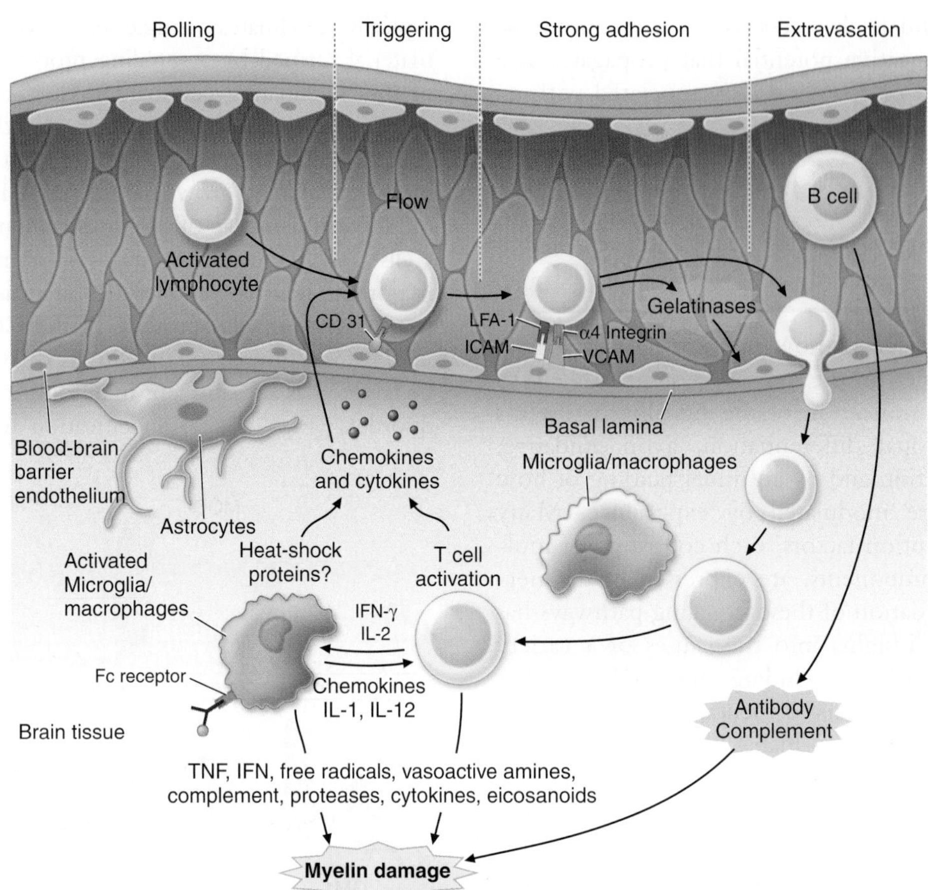

FIGURE 25-2

A model for experimental allergic encephalomyelitis (EAE). Crucial steps for disease initiation and progression include peripheral activation of preexisting autoreactive T cells; homing to the CNS and extravasation across the blood-brain barrier; reactivation of T cells by exposed autoantigens; secretion of cytokines; activation of microglia and astrocytes and recruitment of a secondary inflammatory wave; and immune-mediated myelin destruction. ICAM, intercellular adhesion molecule; LFA-1, lymphocyte function-associated antigen-1; VCAM, vascular cell adhesion molecule; IFN, interferon; IL, interleukin; TNF, tumor necrosis factor.

precursor cells (OPCs) is transcriptionally regulated by the *Olig 2* and *Yin Yang 1* genes, whereas myelination mediated by postmitotic oligodendrocytes depends on a different transcription factor, *myelin gene regulatory factor (MRF)*. It is noteworthy that in the normal adult brain large numbers of OPCs (expressing platelet-derived growth factor receptor alpha [PDGFR-α] and NG2) are widely distributed but do not myelinate axons, even in demyelinating environments such as lesions of MS. The characterization of these cells, including an understanding of their transcriptional regulation and functional roles, could result in novel approaches to remyelination and brain repair.

NEUROTROPHIC FACTORS

Neurotrophic factors (Table 25-3) are secreted proteins that modulate neuronal growth, differentiation, repair, and survival; some have additional functions, including roles in neurotransmission and in the synaptic reorganization involved in learning and memory. The neurotrophin (NT) family contains nerve growth factor (NGF), brain-derived neurotrophic factor (BDNF), NT3, and NT4/5. The neurotrophins act at TrK and p75 receptors to promote survival of neurons. Because

TABLE 25-3

NEUROTROPHIC FACTORS	
Neurotrophin family	Transforming growth factor β family
Nerve growth factor	Glial-derived neurotrophic family
Brain-derived neurotrophic factor	Neurturin
	Persephin
Neurotrophin-3	Fibroblast growth factor family
Neurotrophin-4	Hepatocyte growth factor
Neurotrophin-6	Insulin-like growth factor (IGF) family
Cytokine family	IGF-1
Ciliary neurotrophic factor	IGF-2
Leukemia inhibitory factor	
Interleukin 6	
Cardiotrophin-1	

of their survival-promoting and antiapoptotic effects, neurotrophic factors are in theory outstanding candidates for therapy for disorders characterized by premature death of neurons as occurs in amyotrophic lateral sclerosis (ALS) and other degenerative motor neuron disorders. Knockout mice lacking receptors for ciliary neurotrophic factor (CNTF) or BDNF show loss of motor neurons, and experimental motor neuron death can be rescued by treatment with various neurotrophic factors, including CNTF, BDNF, and vascular endothelial growth factor (VEGF). However, in phase 3 clinical trials, growth factors were ineffective in human ALS. The growth factor glial-derived neurotrophic factor (GDNF) is important for survival of dopaminergic neurons. Direct infusions of GDNF showed initial promise in Parkinson's disease (PD), but the benefits were not replicated in a larger clinical trial.

STEM CELLS AND TRANSPLANTATION

The nervous system is traditionally considered to be a nonmitotic organ, particularly with respect to neurons. These concepts have been challenged by the finding that neural progenitor or stem cells exist in the adult CNS that are capable of differentiation, migration over long distances, and extensive axonal arborization and synapse formation with appropriate targets. These capabilities also indicate that the repertoire of factors required for growth, survival, differentiation, and migration of these cells exists in the mature nervous system. In rodents, neural stem cells, defined as progenitor cells capable of differentiating into mature cells of neural or glial lineage, have been experimentally propagated from fetal CNS and neuroectodermal tissues and also from adult germinal matrix and ependyma regions. Human fetal CNS tissue is also capable of differentiation into cells with neuronal, astrocyte, and oligodendrocyte morphology when cultured in the presence of growth factors.

Once the repertoire of signals required for cell type specification is better understood, differentiation into specific neural or glial subpopulations could be directed in vitro; such cells also could be engineered to express therapeutic molecules. Another promising approach is to utilize growth factors such as BDNF to stimulate endogenous stem cells to proliferate and migrate to areas of neuronal damage. Administration of epidermal growth factor with fibroblast growth factor replenished up to 50% of hippocampal CA1 neurons a month after global ischemia in rats. The new neurons made connections and improved performance in a memory task.

A major advance has been the development of induced pluripotent stem cells. Using this technique, adult somatic cells such as skin fibroblasts are treated with four pluripotency factors (SOX2, KLF4, cMYC, and Oct4), and this generates induced pluripotent stem cells (iPSCs). These adult-derived stem cells sidestep the ethical issues of utilizing stem cells derived from human embryos. The development of these cells has tremendous promise for both studying disease mechanisms and testing therapeutics. There is no consensus on the best way to generate and differentiate iPSCs; however, techniques to avoid using viral vectors and the use of Cre-lox systems to remove reprogramming factors result in a better match of gene expression profiles with those of embryonic stem cells. Thus far, iPSC cells have been made from patients with all the major human neurodegenerative diseases, and studies utilizing them are under way.

Although stem cells hold tremendous promise for the treatment of debilitating neurologic diseases such as Parkinson's disease and spinal cord injury, it should be emphasized that medical application is in its infancy. Major obstacles are the generation of position- and neurotransmitter-defined subtypes of neurons and their isolation as pure populations of the desired cells. This is crucial to avoid persistence of undifferentiated embryonic stem (ES) cells, which can generate tumors. The establishment of appropriate neural connections and afferent control is also critical. For instance, human ES motor neurons will have to be introduced at multiple segments in the neuraxis, and then their axons will have to regenerate from the spinal cord to distal musculature.

Experimental transplantation of human fetal dopaminergic neurons in patients with Parkinson's disease has shown that these transplanted cells can survive within the host striatum; however, some patients developed disabling dyskinesias, and this approach is no longer in clinical development. Human ES cells can be differentiated into dopaminergic neurons, which reverse symptoms of Parkinson's disease in experimental animal models. Studies of transplantation for patients with Huntington's disease have reported encouraging, although very preliminary, results. Oligodendrocyte precursor cells transplanted into mice with a dysmyelinating disorder effectively migrated in the new environment, interacted with axons, and mediated myelination; such experiments raise hope that similar transplantation strategies may be feasible in human disorders of myelin such as MS. The promise of stem cells for treatment of both neurodegenerative diseases and neural injury is great, but development has been slowed by unresolved concerns over safety (including the theoretical risk of malignant transformation of transplanted cells), ethics (particularly with respect to use of fetal tissue), and efficacy.

In developing brain, the extracellular matrix provides stimulatory and inhibitory signals that promote neuronal migration, neurite outgrowth, and axonal extension.

After neuronal damage, reexpression of inhibitory molecules such as chondroitin sulfate proteoglycans may prevent tissue regeneration. Chondroitinase degraded these inhibitory molecules and enhanced axonal regeneration and motor recovery in a rat model of spinal cord injury. Several myelin proteins, specifically Nogo, oligodendrocyte myelin glycoprotein (OMGP), and myelin-associated glycoprotein (MAG), also may interfere with axon regeneration. Sialidase, which cleaves one class of receptors for MAG, enhances axonal outgrowth. Antibodies against Nogo promote regeneration after experimental focal ischemia or spinal cord injury. Nogo, OMGP, and MAG all bind to the same neural receptor, the Nogo receptor, which mediates its inhibitory function via the p75 neurotrophin receptor signaling.

CELL DEATH: EXCITOTOXICITY AND APOPTOSIS

Excitotoxicity refers to neuronal cell death caused by activation of excitatory amino acid receptors (Fig. 25-3). Compelling evidence for a role of excitotoxicity, especially in ischemic neuronal injury, is derived from experiments in animal models. Experimental models of stroke are associated with increased extracellular concentrations of the excitatory amino acid neurotransmitter glutamate, and neuronal damage is attenuated by denervation of glutamate-containing neurons or the administration of glutamate receptor antagonists. The distribution of cells sensitive to ischemia corresponds closely with that of *N*-methyl-D-aspartate (NMDA) receptors (except for cerebellar Purkinje cells, which are vulnerable to hypoxemia-ischemia but lack NMDA receptors), and competitive and noncompetitive NMDA antagonists are effective in preventing focal ischemia. In global cerebral ischemia, non-NMDA receptors (kainic acid and α-amino-3-hydroxyl-5-methyl-4-isoxazole-propionate [AMPA]) are activated, and antagonists to these receptors are protective. Experimental brain damage induced by hypoglycemia also is attenuated by NMDA antagonists.

Excitotoxicity is not a single event but rather a cascade of cell injury. Excitotoxicity causes influx of calcium into cells, and much of the calcium is sequestered in mitochondria rather than in the cytoplasm. Increased cytoplasmic calcium causes metabolic dysfunction and free radical generation; activates protein kinases, phospholipases, nitric oxide synthase, proteases, and endonucleases; and inhibits protein synthesis. Activation of nitric oxide synthase generates nitric oxide ($NO^{\bullet}$), which can react with superoxide ($O_2^{\bullet}$) to generate peroxynitrite ($ONOO^-$), which may play a direct role in neuronal injury. Another critical pathway is activation of poly-ADP-ribose polymerase, which occurs in response to free radical–mediated DNA damage. Experimentally, mice with knockout mutations of neuronal nitric oxide synthase or poly-ADP-ribose polymerase, or those which overexpress superoxide dismutase, are resistant to focal ischemia.

Another aspect of excitotoxicity is that it has been demonstrated that stimulation of extrasynaptic NMDA receptors mediates cell death, whereas stimulation of synaptic receptors is protective. This has been shown to play a role in excitotoxicity in transgenic mouse models of Huntington's disease, in which the use of low-dose memantine to selectively block the extrasynaptic receptors is beneficial.

Although excitotoxicity is clearly implicated in the pathogenesis of cell death in stroke, to date treatment with NMDA antagonists has not proved clinically useful. Transient receptor potentials (TRPs) are calcium channels that are activated by oxidative stress in parallel with excitotoxic signal pathways. In addition, glutamate-independent pathways of calcium influx via acid-sensing ion channels have been identified. These channels transport calcium in the setting of acidosis and substrate depletion, and pharmacologic blockade of these channels markedly attenuates stroke injury. These channels offer a potential new therapeutic target for stroke.

Apoptosis, or programmed cell death, plays an important role in both physiologic and pathologic conditions. During embryogenesis, apoptotic pathways operate to destroy neurons that fail to differentiate appropriately or reach their intended targets. There is mounting evidence for an increased rate of apoptotic cell death in a variety of acute and chronic neurologic diseases. Apoptosis is characterized by neuronal shrinkage, chromatin condensation, and DNA fragmentation, whereas necrotic cell death is associated with cytoplasmic and mitochondrial swelling followed by dissolution of the cell membrane. Apoptotic death and necrotic cell death can coexist or be sequential events, depending on the severity of the initiating insult. Cellular energy reserves appear to have an important role in these two forms of cell death, with apoptosis favored under conditions in which ATP levels are preserved. Evidence of DNA fragmentation has been found in a number of degenerative neurologic disorders, including Alzheimer's disease, Huntington's disease, and ALS. The best characterized genetic neurologic disorder related to apoptosis is infantile spinal muscular atrophy (Werdnig-Hoffmann disease), in which two genes thought to be involved in the apoptosis pathways are causative.

Mitochondria are essential in controlling specific apoptosis pathways. The redistribution of cytochrome *c*, as well as apoptosis-inducing factor (AIF), from mitochondria during apoptosis leads to the activation of a cascade of intracellular proteases known as *caspases*. Caspase-independent apoptosis occurs after DNA damage, activation of poly-ADP-ribose polymerase, and

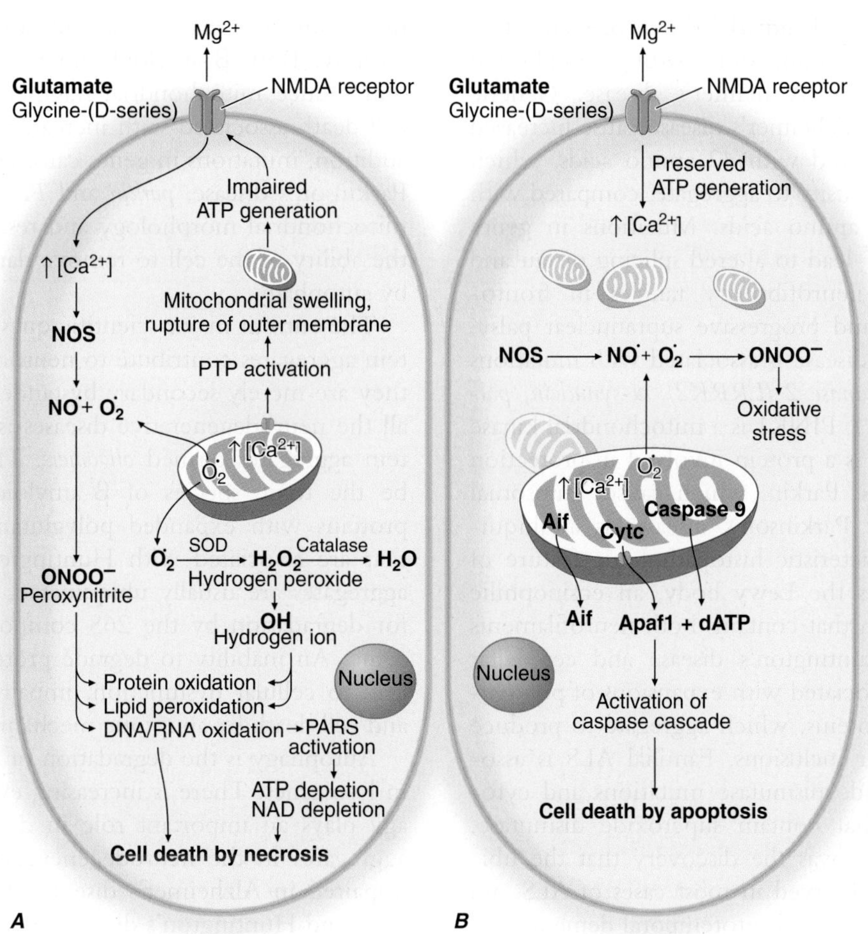

FIGURE 25-3

Involvement of mitochondria in cell death. A severe excitotoxic insult (***A***) results in cell death by necrosis, whereas a mild excitotoxic insult (***B***) results in apoptosis. After a severe insult (such as ischemia), there is a large increase in glutamate activation of NMDA receptors, an increase in intracellular Ca^{2+} concentrations, activation of nitric oxide synthase (NOS), and increased mitochondrial Ca^{2+} and superoxide generation followed by the formation of $ONOO^-$. This sequence results in damage to cellular macromolecules including DNA, leading to activation of poly-ADP-ribose polymerase (PARS). Both mitochondrial accumulation of Ca^{2+} and oxidative damage lead to activation of the permeability transition pore (PTP) that is linked to excitotoxic cell death. A mild excitotoxic insult can occur due either to an abnormality in an excitotoxicity amino acid receptor, allowing more Ca^{2+} flux, or to impaired functioning of other ionic channels or of energy production, which may allow the voltage-dependent NMDA receptor to be activated by ambient concentrations of glutamate. This event can then lead to increased mitochondrial Ca^{2+} and free radical production, yet relatively preserved ATP generation. The mitochondria may then release cytochrome *c* (Cytc), caspase 9, apoptosis-inducing factor (Aif), and perhaps other mediators that lead to apoptosis. The precise role of the PTP in this mode of cell death is still being clarified, but there does appear to be involvement of the adenine nucleotide transporter that is a key component of the PTP.

translocation of AIF into the nucleus. Redistribution of cytochrome *c* is prevented by overproduction of the apoptotic protein BCL2 and is promoted by the pro-apoptotic protein BAX. These pathways may be triggered by activation of a large pore in the mitochondrial inner membrane known as the *permeability transition pore*, although in other circumstances they occur independently. Recent studies suggest that blocking the mitochondrial pore reduces both hypoglycemic and ischemic cell death. Mice deficient in cyclophilin D, a key protein involved in opening the permeability transition pore, are resistant to necrosis produced by focal cerebral ischemia.

PROTEIN AGGREGATION AND NEURODEGENERATION

The possibility that protein aggregation plays a role in the pathogenesis of neurodegenerative diseases is a major focus of current research. Protein aggregation is a major histopathologic hallmark of neurodegenerative diseases. Deposition of β-amyloid is strongly implicated in the pathogenesis of Alzheimer's disease. Genetic mutations in familial Alzheimer's disease cause increased production of β-amyloid with 42 amino acids, which has an increased propensity to aggregate, compared with β-amyloid with 40 amino acids. Mutations in genes encoding the MAPT lead to altered splicing of tau and the production of neurofibrillary tangles in frontotemporal dementia and progressive supranuclear palsy. Familial Parkinson's disease is associated with mutations in *leucine-rich repeat kinase 2 (LRRK2), α-synuclein, parkin, PINK1,* and *DJ-1.* PINK1 is a mitochondrial kinase (see later), and DJ-1 is a protein involved in protection from oxidative stress. Parkin, which causes autosomal recessive early-onset Parkinson's disease, is a ubiquitin ligase. The characteristic histopathologic feature of Parkinson's disease is the Lewy body, an eosinophilic cytoplasmic inclusion that contains both neurofilaments and α-synuclein. Huntington's disease and cerebellar degenerations are associated with expansions of polyglutamine repeats in proteins, which aggregate to produce neuronal intranuclear inclusions. Familial ALS is associated with superoxide dismutase mutations and cytoplasmic inclusions that contain superoxide dismutase. An important finding was the discovery that the ubiquinated inclusions observed in most cases of ALS and the most common form of frontotemporal dementia are composed of TAR DNA binding protein 43 (TDP-43). Subsequently, mutations in the TDP-43 gene and in the fused in sarcoma gene (FUS) were found in familial ALS. These two proteins are involved in transcription regulation as well as RNA metabolism. In autosomal dominant neurohypophyseal diabetes insipidus, mutations in vasopressin result in abnormal protein processing, accumulation in the endoplasmic reticulum, and cell death.

Another key mechanism linked to cell death is mitochondrial dynamics, which refer to the processes involved in movement of mitochondria, as well as in mitochondrial fission and fusion, which play a critical role in mitochondrial turnover and in replenishment of damaged mitochondria. Mitochondrial dysfunction is strongly linked to the pathogenesis of a number of neurodegenerative diseases, such as Friedreich's ataxia, which is caused by mutations in an iron-binding protein that plays an important role in transferring iron to iron-sulfur clusters in aconitase and complex I and II of the electron transport chain. Mitochondrial fission is dependent on the dynamin-related proteins (Drp1), which bind to its receptor Fis, whereas mitofuscins 1 and 2 (MF 1/2) and optic atrophy protein 1 (Opa1) are responsible for fusion of the outer and inner mitochondrial membrane, respectively. Mutations in Mfn2 cause Charcot-Marie-Tooth neuropathy type 2A, and mutations in Opa1 cause autosomal dominant optic atrophy. Both β-amyloid and mutant huntingtin protein induce mitochondrial fragmentation and neuronal cell death associated with increased activity of Drp1. In addition, mutations in genes causing autosomal recessive Parkinson's disease, *parkin* and *PINK1,* cause abnormal mitochondrial morphology and result in impairment of the ability of the cell to remove damaged mitochondria by autophagy.

The current major scientific question is whether protein aggregates contribute to neuronal death or whether they are merely secondary bystanders. A major focus in all the neurodegenerative diseases is now on small protein aggregates termed *oligomers.* These aggregates may be the toxic species of β-amyloid, α-synuclein, and proteins with expanded polyglutamines such as those that are associated with Huntington's disease. Protein aggregates are usually ubiquinated, which targets them for degradation by the 26S component of the proteasome. An inability to degrade protein aggregates could lead to cellular dysfunction, impaired axonal transport, and cell death by apoptotic mechanisms.

Autophagy is the degradation of cystolic components in lysosomes. There is increasing evidence that autophagy plays an important role in degradation of protein aggregates in the neurodegenerative diseases, and it is impaired in Alzheimer's disease (AD), Parkinson's disease, and Huntington's disease (HD). Autophagy is particularly important to the health of neurons, and failure of autophagy contributes to cell death. In Huntington's disease, a failure of cargo recognition occurs, contributing to protein aggregates and cell death. Rapamycin, which induces autophagy, exerts beneficial therapeutic effects in transgenic mouse models of AD, PD, and HD.

In experimental models of Huntington's disease and cerebellar degeneration, protein aggregates are not well correlated with neuronal death and may be protective. A substantial body of evidence suggests that the mutant proteins with polyglutamine expansions in these diseases bind to transcription factors and that this contributes to disease pathogenesis. In Huntington's disease there is dysfunction of the transcriptional co-regulator PGC-1α, a key regulator of mitochondrial biogenesis. There is evidence that impaired function of PGC-1α is also important in both Parkinson's disease and Alzheimer's disease, making it an attractive target for treatments. Agents that upregulate gene transcription are neuroprotective in animal models of these diseases. A number of compounds have been developed to block β-amyloid production and/or aggregation, and these agents are being studied in early clinical trials in humans. Another approach under investigation is immunotherapy with antibodies that bind β-amyloid, tau, or α-synuclein.

Another emerging theme is the role of chronic inflammation, and in particular of activated microglia and innate immunity, in the pathogenesis of many neurodegenerative diseases. Activation of Toll-like receptors (TLR) in response to pattern-recognition signals from damaged or aging cells, including those mediated by heat shock proteins or aggregated proteins, can trigger or amplify pro-inflammatory responses. Familial frontotemporal degeneration (Chap. 29) is caused by mutations in the gene encoding progranulin, a growth factor that regulates inflammation via binding to tumor necrosis factor (TNF) receptors.

SYSTEMS NEUROSCIENCE

Systems neuroscience refers to study of the functions of neurocircuits and the way they relate to brain function, behavior, motor activity, and cognition. Brain imaging techniques, primarily functional MRI (fMRI) and positron emission tomography (PET), have made it possible to investigate cognitive processes such as perception, making judgments, paying attention, and thinking. This has allowed insights into how networks of neurons operate to produce behavior. Many of these studies at present are based on determining the connectivity of neural circuits and how they operate and how this can be modeled to produce improved understanding of physiologic processes. fMRI uses contrast mechanisms related to physiologic changes in tissue, and brain perfusion can be studied by observing the time course of changes in brain water signal as a bolus of injected paramagnetic gadolinium contrast moves through the brain. More recently, to study intrinsic contrast-related local changes in blood oxygenation with brain activity, blood-oxygen-level-dependent (BOLD) contrast has been used to provide a rapid noninvasive approach for functional assessment. These techniques have been used reliably in both behavioral and cognitive sciences. One example is the use of fMRI to demonstrate mirror neuron systems, imitative pathways activated when observing actions of others (Fig. 25-4). Mirror neurons are thought to be important for social conditioning and for many forms of learning, and abnormalities in mirror neurons may underlie some autism disorders. Data also suggest that enhancement of mirror neuron pathways might have potential for rehabilitation after stroke. Other examples of the use of fMRI include the study of memory. Recent studies have shown that not only is hippocampal activity correlated with declarative

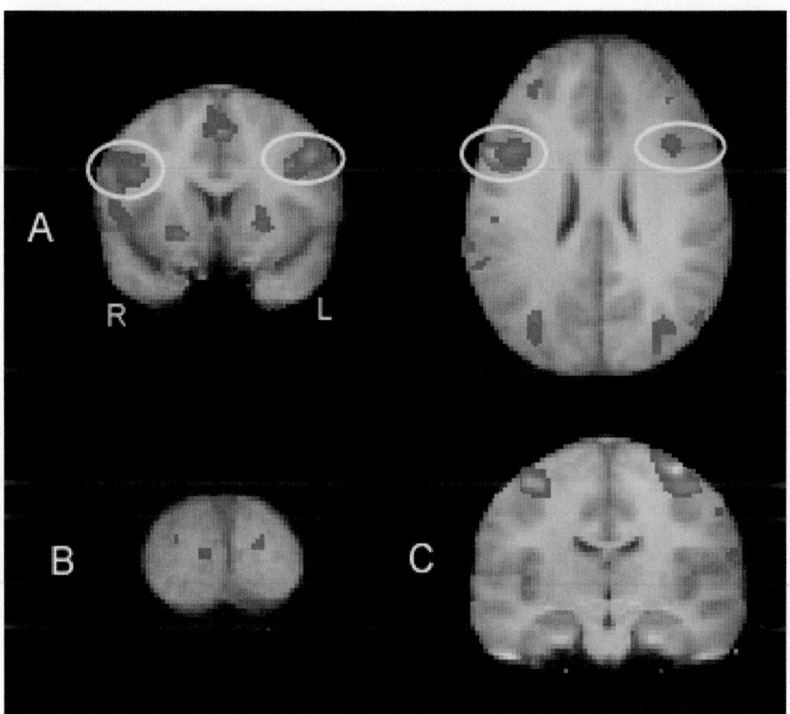

FIGURE 25-4

Mirror neuron systems are bilaterally activated during imitation. ***A.*** Bilateral activations (circled in yellow) in inferior frontal mirror neuron areas during imitation, as measured by BOLD fMRI signal changes. In red, activation during right hand imitation. In blue, activation during left hand imitation. ***B.*** In contrast, there is lateralized (contralateral) primary visual activation of the primary visual cortex for imitated actions presented to the right visual field (in red, left visual cortex) and to the left visual field (in blue, right visual cortex). ***C.*** Lateralized primary motor activation for hand actions imitated with the right hand (in red, left motor cortex) and with the left hand (in blue, right motor cortex). (*From L Aziz-Zadeh et al: J Neurosci 26:2964, 2006.*)

memory consolidation, it also involves activation in the ventral medial prefrontal cortex. Consolidation of memory over time results in decreased activity of the hippocampus and progressively stronger activation in the ventral medial prefrontal region associated with retrieval of consolidated memories. fMRI also has been utilized to identify sequences of brain activation involved in normal movements and alterations in their activation associated with both injury and recovery and to plan neurosurgical operations. Diffusion tensor imaging is a recently developed MRI technique that can measure macroscopic axonal organization in nervous system tissues; it appears to be useful in assessing myelin and axonal injuries as well as brain development. Advances in understanding neural processing have led to the development of the ability to demonstrate that humans have on-line voluntary control of human temporal lobe neurons.

A further advance that has far-reaching implications for the development of novel interventions for neurologic, including behavioral, conditions has been the development of deep-brain stimulation as a highly effective therapeutic intervention for treating excessively firing neurons in the subthalamic nucleus of patients with Parkinson's disease and the precingulate cortex in patients with depression.

CHAPTER 26

SEIZURES AND EPILEPSY

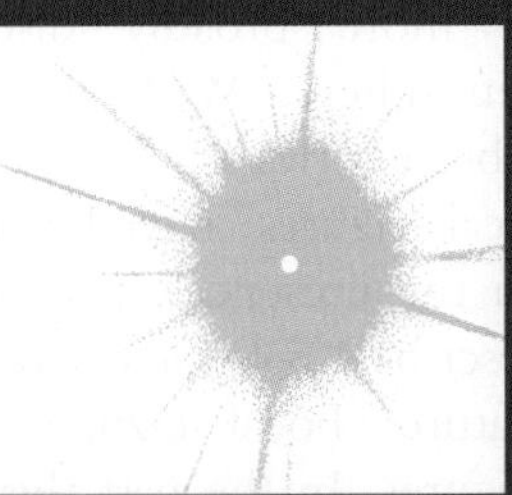

Daniel H. Lowenstein

A *seizure* (from the Latin *sacire*, "to take possession of") is a paroxysmal event due to abnormal excessive or synchronous neuronal activity in the brain. Depending on the distribution of discharges, this abnormal brain activity can have various manifestations, ranging from dramatic convulsive activity to experiential phenomena not readily discernible by an observer. Although a variety of factors influence the incidence and prevalence of seizures, ~5–10% of the population will have at least one seizure, with the highest incidence occurring in early childhood and late adulthood.

The meaning of the term *seizure* needs to be carefully distinguished from that of epilepsy. *Epilepsy* describes a condition in which a person has *recurrent* seizures due to a chronic, underlying process. This definition implies that a person with a single seizure, or recurrent seizures due to correctable or avoidable circumstances, does not necessarily have epilepsy. Epilepsy refers to a clinical phenomenon rather than a single disease entity, since there are many forms and causes of epilepsy. However, among the many causes of epilepsy there are various *epilepsy syndromes* in which the clinical and pathologic characteristics are distinctive and suggest a specific underlying etiology.

Using the definition of epilepsy as two or more unprovoked seizures, the incidence of epilepsy is ~0.3–0.5% in different populations throughout the world, and the prevalence of epilepsy has been estimated at 5–10 persons per 1000.

CLASSIFICATION OF SEIZURES

Determining the type of seizure that has occurred is essential for focusing the diagnostic approach on particular etiologies, selecting the appropriate therapy, and providing potentially vital information regarding prognosis. The International League against Epilepsy (ILAE) Commission on Classification and Terminology, 2005–2009 has provided an updated approach to classification of seizures (Table 26-1). This system is based on the clinical features of seizures and associated electroencephalographic findings. Other potentially distinctive features such as etiology or cellular substrate are not considered in this classification system, although this will undoubtedly change in the future as more is learned about the pathophysiologic mechanisms that underlie specific seizure types.

A fundamental principle is that seizures may be either focal or generalized. *Focal seizures* originate within networks limited to one cerebral hemisphere (note that the term *partial seizures* is no longer used). *Generalized seizures* arise within and rapidly engage networks distributed across both cerebral hemispheres. Focal seizures are usually associated with structural abnormalities of the brain. In contrast, generalized seizures may result from cellular, biochemical, or structural abnormalities that have a more widespread distribution. There are clear exceptions in both cases, however.

TABLE 26-1

CLASSIFICATION OF SEIZURES

1. **Focal seizures**
   (Can be further described as having motor, sensory, autonomic, cognitive, or other features)
2. **Generalized seizures**
   a. Absence
      Typical
      Atypical
   b. Tonic clonic
   c. Clonic
   d. Tonic
   e. Atonic
   f. Myoclonic
3. **May be focal, generalized, or unclear**
   Epileptic spasms

FOCAL SEIZURES

Focal seizures arise from a neuronal network either discretely localized within one cerebral hemisphere or more broadly distributed but still within the hemisphere. With the new classification system, the subcategories of "simple focal seizures" and "complex focal seizures" have been eliminated. Instead, depending on the presence of cognitive impairment, they can be described as focal seizures with or without dyscognitive features. Focal seizures can also evolve into generalized seizures. In the past this was referred to as *focal seizures with secondary generalization,* but the new system relies on specific descriptions of the type of generalized seizures that evolve from the focal seizure.

The routine interictal (i.e., between seizures) electroencephalogram (EEG) in patients with focal seizures is often normal or may show brief discharges termed *epileptiform spikes*, or *sharp waves*. Since focal seizures can arise from the medial temporal lobe or inferior frontal lobe (i.e., regions distant from the scalp), the EEG recorded during the seizure may be nonlocalizing. However, the seizure focus is often detected using sphenoidal or surgically placed intracranial electrodes.

Focal seizures without dyscognitive features

Focal seizures can cause motor, sensory, autonomic, or psychic symptoms without impairment of cognition. For example, a patient having a focal motor seizure arising from the right primary motor cortex near the area controlling hand movement will note the onset of involuntary movements of the contralateral, left hand. These movements are typically clonic (i.e., repetitive, flexion/extension movements) at a frequency of ~2–3 Hz; pure tonic posturing may be seen as well. Since the cortical region controlling hand movement is immediately adjacent to the region for facial expression, the seizure may also cause abnormal movements of the face synchronous with the movements of the hand. The EEG recorded with scalp electrodes during the seizure (i.e., an ictal EEG) may show abnormal discharges in a very limited region over the appropriate area of cerebral cortex if the seizure focus involves the cerebral convexity. Seizure activity occurring within deeper brain structures is often not recorded by the standard EEG, however, and may require intracranial electrodes for its detection.

Three additional features of focal motor seizures are worth noting. First, in some patients the abnormal motor movements may begin in a very restricted region such as the fingers and gradually progress (over seconds to minutes) to include a larger portion of the extremity. This phenomenon, described by Hughlings Jackson and known as a "Jacksonian march," represents the spread of seizure activity over a progressively larger region of motor cortex. Second, patients may experience a localized paresis (Todd's paralysis) for minutes to many hours in the involved region following the seizure. Third, in rare instances the seizure may continue for hours or days. This condition, termed *epilepsia partialis continua*, is often refractory to medical therapy.

Focal seizures may also manifest as changes in somatic sensation (e.g., paresthesias), vision (flashing lights or formed hallucinations), equilibrium (sensation of falling or vertigo), or autonomic function (flushing, sweating, piloerection). Focal seizures arising from the temporal or frontal cortex may also cause alterations in hearing, olfaction, or higher cortical function (psychic symptoms). This includes the sensation of unusual, intense odors (e.g., burning rubber or kerosene) or sounds (crude or highly complex sounds), or an epigastric sensation that rises from the stomach or chest to the head. Some patients describe odd, internal feelings such as fear, a sense of impending change, detachment, depersonalization, déjá vu, or illusions that objects are growing smaller (micropsia) or larger (macropsia). These subjective, "internal" events that are not directly observable by someone else are referred to as *auras*.

Focal seizures with dyscognitive features

Focal seizures may also be accompanied by a transient impairment of the patient's ability to maintain normal contact with the environment. The patient is unable to respond appropriately to visual or verbal commands during the seizure and has impaired recollection or awareness of the ictal phase. The seizures frequently begin with an aura (i.e., a focal seizure without cognitive disturbance) that is stereotypic for the patient. The start of the ictal phase is often a sudden behavioral arrest or motionless stare, which marks the onset of the period of impaired awareness. The behavioral arrest is usually accompanied by *automatisms*, which are involuntary, automatic behaviors that have a wide range of manifestations. Automatisms may consist of very basic behaviors such as chewing, lip smacking, swallowing, or "picking" movements of the hands, or more elaborate behaviors such as a display of emotion or running. The patient is typically confused following the seizure, and the transition to full recovery of consciousness may range from seconds up to an hour. Examination immediately following the seizure may show an anterograde amnesia or, in cases involving the dominant hemisphere, a postictal aphasia.

The range of potential clinical behaviors linked to focal seizures is so broad that extreme caution is advised before concluding that stereotypic episodes of bizarre or atypical behavior are not due to seizure activity. In such cases additional, detailed EEG studies may be helpful.

EVOLUTION OF FOCAL SEIZURES TO GENERALIZED SEIZURES

Focal seizures can spread to involve both cerebral hemispheres and produce a generalized seizure, usually of the tonic-clonic variety (discussed later). This evolution is observed frequently following focal seizures arising from a focus in the frontal lobe, but may also be associated with focal seizures occurring elsewhere in the brain. A focal seizure that evolves into a generalized seizure is often difficult to distinguish from a primary generalized-onset tonic-clonic seizure, since bystanders tend to emphasize the more dramatic, generalized convulsive phase of the seizure and overlook the more subtle, focal symptoms present at onset. In some cases, the focal onset of the seizure becomes apparent only when a careful history identifies a preceding aura. Often, however, the focal onset is not clinically evident and may be established only through careful EEG analysis. Nonetheless, distinguishing between these two entities is extremely important, as there may be substantial differences in the evaluation and treatment of epilepsies associated with focal versus generalized seizures.

GENERALIZED SEIZURES

Generalized seizures are thought to arise at some point in the brain but immediately and rapidly engage neuronal networks in both cerebral hemispheres. Several types of generalized seizures have features that place them in distinctive categories and facilitate clinical diagnosis.

Typical absence seizures

Typical absence seizures are characterized by sudden, brief lapses of consciousness without loss of postural control. The seizure typically lasts for only seconds, consciousness returns as suddenly as it was lost, and there is no postictal confusion. Although the brief loss of consciousness may be clinically inapparent or the sole manifestation of the seizure discharge, absence seizures are usually accompanied by subtle, bilateral motor signs such as rapid blinking of the eyelids, chewing movements, or small-amplitude, clonic movements of the hands.

Typical absence seizures are associated with a group of genetically determined epilepsies with onset usually in childhood (ages 4–8 years) or early adolescence and are the main seizure type in 15–20% of children with epilepsy. The seizures can occur hundreds of times per day, but the child may be unaware of or unable to convey their existence. Since the clinical signs of the seizures are subtle, especially to parents who may not have had previous experience with seizures, it is not surprising that the first clue to absence epilepsy is often unexplained "daydreaming" and a decline in school performance recognized by a teacher.

The electrophysiologic hallmark of typical absence seizures is a generalized, symmetric, 3-Hz spike-and-wave discharge that begins and ends suddenly, superimposed on a normal EEG background. Periods of spike-and-wave discharges lasting more than a few seconds usually correlate with clinical signs, but the EEG often shows many more brief bursts of abnormal cortical activity than were suspected clinically. Hyperventilation tends to provoke these electrographic discharges and even the seizures themselves and is routinely used when recording the EEG.

Atypical absence seizures

Atypical absence seizures have features that deviate both clinically and electrophysiologically from typical absence seizures. For example, the lapse of consciousness is usually of longer duration and less abrupt in onset and cessation, and the seizure is accompanied by more obvious motor signs that may include focal or lateralizing features. The EEG shows a generalized, slow spike-and-wave pattern with a frequency of ≤2.5 per second, as well as other abnormal activity. Atypical absence seizures are usually associated with diffuse or multifocal structural abnormalities of the brain and therefore may accompany other signs of neurologic dysfunction such as mental retardation. Furthermore, the seizures are less responsive to anticonvulsants compared to typical absence seizures.

Generalized, tonic-clonic seizures

Generalized-onset tonic-clonic seizures are the main seizure type in ~10% of all persons with epilepsy. They are also the most common seizure type resulting from metabolic derangements and are therefore frequently encountered in many different clinical settings. The seizure usually begins abruptly without warning, although some patients describe vague premonitory symptoms in the hours leading up to the seizure. This prodrome is distinct from the stereotypic auras associated with focal seizures that generalize. The initial phase of the seizure is usually tonic contraction of muscles throughout the body, accounting for a number of the classic features of the event. Tonic contraction of the muscles of expiration and the larynx at the onset will produce a loud moan or "ictal cry." Respirations are impaired, secretions pool in the oropharynx, and cyanosis develops. Contraction of the jaw muscles may cause biting of the tongue.

A marked enhancement of sympathetic tone leads to increases in heart rate, blood pressure, and pupillary size. After 10–20 s, the tonic phase of the seizure typically evolves into the clonic phase, produced by the superimposition of periods of muscle relaxation on the tonic muscle contraction. The periods of relaxation progressively increase until the end of the ictal phase, which usually lasts no more than 1 min. The postictal phase is characterized by unresponsiveness, muscular flaccidity, and excessive salivation that can cause stridorous breathing and partial airway obstruction. Bladder or bowel incontinence may occur at this point. Patients gradually regain consciousness over minutes to hours, and during this transition there is typically a period of postictal confusion. Patients subsequently complain of headache, fatigue, and muscle ache that can last for many hours. The duration of impaired consciousness in the postictal phase can be extremely long (i.e., many hours) in patients with prolonged seizures or underlying central nervous system (CNS) diseases such as alcoholic cerebral atrophy.

The EEG during the tonic phase of the seizure shows a progressive increase in generalized low-voltage fast activity, followed by generalized high-amplitude, polyspike discharges. In the clonic phase, the high-amplitude activity is typically interrupted by slow waves to create a spike-and-wave pattern. The postictal EEG shows diffuse slowing that gradually recovers as the patient awakens.

There are a number of variants of the generalized tonic-clonic seizure, including pure tonic and pure clonic seizures. Brief tonic seizures lasting only a few seconds are especially noteworthy since they are usually associated with specific epileptic syndromes having mixed seizure phenotypes, such as the Lennox-Gastaut syndrome (discussed later).

Atonic seizures

Atonic seizures are characterized by sudden loss of postural muscle tone lasting 1–2 s. Consciousness is briefly impaired, but there is usually no postictal confusion. A very brief seizure may cause only a quick head drop or nodding movement, while a longer seizure will cause the patient to collapse. This can be extremely dangerous, since there is a substantial risk of direct head injury with the fall. The EEG shows brief, generalized spike-and-wave discharges followed immediately by diffuse slow waves that correlate with the loss of muscle tone. Similar to pure tonic seizures, atonic seizures are usually seen in association with known epilepsy syndromes.

Myoclonic seizures

Myoclonus is a sudden and brief muscle contraction that may involve one part of the body or the entire body. A normal, common physiologic form of myoclonus is the sudden jerking movement observed while falling asleep. Pathologic myoclonus is most commonly seen in association with metabolic disorders, degenerative CNS diseases, or anoxic brain injury (Chap. 28). Although the distinction from other forms of myoclonus is imprecise, myoclonic seizures are considered to be true epileptic events since they are caused by cortical (versus subcortical or spinal) dysfunction. The EEG may show bilaterally synchronous spike-and-wave discharges synchronized with the myoclonus, although these can be obscured by movement artifact. Myoclonic seizures usually coexist with other forms of generalized seizures but are the predominant feature of juvenile myoclonic epilepsy (discussed later).

CURRENTLY UNCLASSIFIABLE SEIZURES

Not all seizure types can be designated as focal or generalized, and they should therefore be labeled as "unclassifiable" until additional evidence allows a valid classification. *Epileptic spasms* are such an example. These are characterized by a briefly sustained flexion or extension of predominantly proximal muscles, including truncal muscles. The EEG in these patients usually shows hypsarrhythmias, which consist of diffuse, giant slow waves with a chaotic background of irregular, multifocal spikes and sharp waves. During the clinical spasm, there is a marked suppression of the EEG background (the "electrodecremental response"). The electromyogram (EMG) also reveals a characteristic rhomboid pattern that may help distinguish spasms from brief tonic and myoclonic seizures. Epileptic spasms occur predominantly in infants and likely result from differences in neuronal function and connectivity in the immature versus mature CNS.

EPILEPSY SYNDROMES

Epilepsy syndromes are disorders in which epilepsy is a predominant feature, and there is sufficient evidence (e.g., through clinical, EEG, radiologic, or genetic observations) to suggest a common underlying mechanism. Three important epilepsy syndromes are listed next; additional examples with a known genetic basis are shown in Table 26-2.

JUVENILE MYOCLONIC EPILEPSY

Juvenile myoclonic epilepsy (JME) is a generalized seizure disorder of unknown cause that appears in early adolescence and is usually characterized by bilateral myoclonic jerks that may be single or repetitive. The myoclonic seizures are most frequent in the morning after awakening

TABLE 26-2

EXAMPLES OF GENES ASSOCIATED WITH EPILEPSY SYNDROMES[a]

GENE (LOCUS)	FUNCTION OF GENE	CLINICAL SYNDROME	COMMENTS
CHRNA4 (20q13.2)	Nicotinic acetylcholine receptor subunit; mutations cause alterations in Ca^{2+} flux through the receptor; this may reduce amount of GABA release in presynaptic terminals	Autosomal dominant nocturnal frontal lobe epilepsy (ADNFLE); childhood onset; brief, nighttime seizures with prominent motor movements; often misdiagnosed as primary sleep disorder	Rare; first identified in a large Australian family; other families found to have mutations in CHRNA2 or CHRNB2, and some families appear to have mutations at other loci
KCNQ2 (20q13.3)	Voltage-gated potassium channel subunits; mutation in pore regions may cause a 20–40% reduction of potassium currents, which will lead to impaired repolarization	Benign familial neonatal convulsions (BFNC); autosomal dominant inheritance; onset in 1st week of life in infants who are otherwise normal; remission usually within weeks to months; long-term epilepsy in 10–15%	Rare; other families found to have mutations in KCNQ3; sequence and functional homology to KCNQ1, mutations of which cause long QT syndrome and a cardiac-auditory syndrome
SCN1B (19q12.1)	β-Subunit of a voltage-gated sodium channel; mutation disrupts disulfide bridge that is crucial for structure of extracellular domain; mutated β-subunit leads to slower sodium channel inactivation	Generalized epilepsy with febrile seizures plus (GEFS+); autosomal dominant inheritance; presents with febrile seizures at median 1 year, which may persist >6 years, then variable seizure types not associated with fever	Incidence uncertain; GEFS+ identified in other families with mutations in other sodium channel subunits (SCN1A and SCN2A) and GABAA receptor subunit (GABRG2 and GABRA1); significant phenotypic heterogeneity within same family, including members with febrile seizures only
LGI1 (10q24)	Leucine-rich glioma-inactivated 1 gene; previous evidence for role in glial tumor progression; protein homology suggests a possible role in nervous system development	Autosomal dominant partial epilepsy with auditory features (ADPEAF); a form of idiopathic lateral temporal lobe epilepsy with auditory symptoms or aphasia as a major simple partial seizure manifestation; age of onset usually between 10 and 25 years	Mutations found in approximately 50% of families containing two or more subjects with idiopathic localization-related epilepsy with ictal auditory symptoms, suggesting that at least one other gene may underlie this syndrome. *LGI1* is the only gene identified so far in temporal lobe epilepsy
CSTB (21q22.3)	Cystatin B, a noncaspase cysteine protease inhibitor; normal protein may block neuronal apoptosis by inhibiting caspases directly or indirectly (via cathepsins), or controlling proteolysis	Progressive myoclonus epilepsy (PME) (Unverricht-Lundborg disease); autosomal recessive inheritance; age of onset between 6 and 15 years, myoclonic seizures, ataxia, and progressive cognitive decline; brain shows neuronal degeneration	Overall rare, but relatively common in Finland and Western Mediterranean (>1 in 20,000); precise role of cystatin B in human disease unknown, although mice with null mutations of cystatin B have similar syndrome
EPM2A (6q24)	Laforin, a protein tyrosine phosphatase (PTP); involved in glycogen metabolism and may have antiapoptotic activity	Progressive myoclonus epilepsy (Lafora's disease); autosomal recessive inheritance; onset age 6–19 years, death within 10 years; brain degeneration associated with polyglucosan intracellular inclusion bodies in numerous organs	Most common PME in Southern Europe, Middle East, Northern Africa, and Indian subcontinent; genetic heterogeneity; unknown whether seizure phenotype due to degeneration or direct effects of abnormal laforin expression
Doublecortin (Xq21-24)	Doublecortin, expressed primarily in frontal lobes; directly regulates microtubule polymerization and bundling	Classic lissencephaly associated with severe mental retardation and seizures in males; subcortical band heterotopia with more subtle findings in females (presumably due to random X-inactivation); X-linked dominant	Relatively rare but of uncertain incidence, recent increased ascertainment due to improved imaging techniques; relationship between migration defect and seizure phenotype unknown

[a]The first four syndromes listed in the table (ADNFLE, BFNC, GEFS+, and ADPEAF) are examples of idiopathic epilepsies associated with identified gene mutations. The last three syndromes are examples of the numerous Mendelian disorders in which seizures are one part of the phenotype.
Abbreviations: GABA, γ-aminobutyric acid; PME, progressive myoclonus epilepsy.

and can be provoked by sleep deprivation. Consciousness is preserved unless the myoclonus is especially severe. Many patients also experience generalized tonic-clonic seizures, and up to one-third have absence seizures. Although complete remission is relatively uncommon, the seizures respond well to appropriate anticonvulsant medication. There is often a family history of epilepsy, and genetic linkage studies suggest a polygenic cause.

LENNOX-GASTAUT SYNDROME

Lennox-Gastaut syndrome occurs in children and is defined by the following triad: (1) multiple seizure types (usually including generalized tonic-clonic, atonic, and atypical absence seizures); (2) an EEG showing slow (<3 Hz) spike-and-wave discharges and a variety of other abnormalities; and (3) impaired cognitive function in most but not all cases. Lennox-Gastaut syndrome is associated with CNS disease or dysfunction from a variety of causes, including developmental abnormalities, perinatal hypoxia/ischemia, trauma, infection, and other acquired lesions. The multifactorial nature of this syndrome suggests that it is a nonspecific response of the brain to diffuse neural injury. Unfortunately, many patients have a poor prognosis due to the underlying CNS disease and the physical and psychosocial consequences of severe, poorly controlled epilepsy.

MESIAL TEMPORAL LOBE EPILEPSY SYNDROME

Mesial temporal lobe epilepsy (MTLE) is the most common syndrome associated with focal seizures with dyscognitive features and is an example of an epilepsy syndrome with distinctive clinical, electroencephalographic, and pathologic features (Table 26-3). High-resolution MRI can detect the characteristic hippocampal sclerosis that appears to be essential in the pathophysiology of MTLE for many patients (Fig. 26-1). Recognition of this syndrome is especially important because it tends to be refractory to treatment with anticonvulsants but responds extremely well to surgical intervention. Advances in the understanding of basic mechanisms of epilepsy have come through studies of experimental models of MTLE, discussed next.

TABLE 26-3

CHARACTERISTICS OF THE MESIAL TEMPORAL LOBE EPILEPSY SYNDROME

History	
History of febrile seizures Family history of epilepsy Early onset	Rare generalized seizures Seizures may remit and reappear Seizures often intractable
Clinical Observations	
Aura common Behavioral arrest/stare Complex automatisms Unilateral posturing	Postictal disorientation Memory loss Dysphasia (with focus in dominant hemisphere)
Laboratory Studies	
Unilateral or bilateral anterior temporal spikes on EEG	
Hypometabolism on interictal PET	
Hypoperfusion on interictal SPECT	
Material-specific memory deficits on intracranial amobarbital (Wada) test	
MRI Findings	
Small hippocampus with increased signal on T2-weighted sequences	
Small temporal lobe	
Enlarged temporal horn	
Pathologic Findings	
Highly selective loss of specific cell populations within hippocampus in most cases	

Abbreviations: EEG, electroencephalogram; PET, positron emission tomography; SPECT, single-photon emission computed tomography.

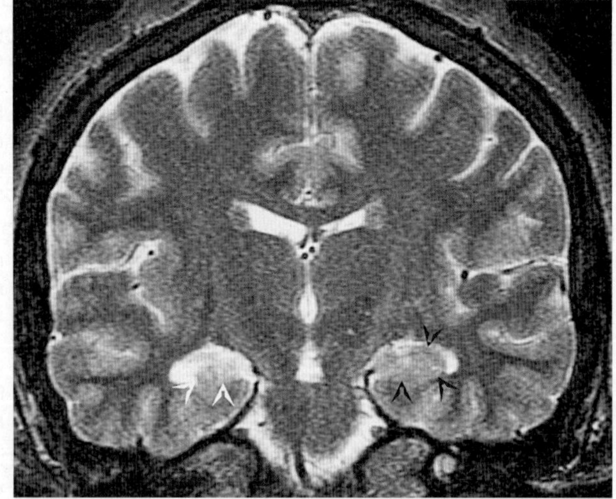

FIGURE 26-1

Mesial temporal lobe epilepsy. The EEG suggested a right temporal lobe focus. Coronal high-resolution T2-weighted fast spin echo magnetic resonance image obtained through the body of the hippocampus demonstrates abnormal high-signal intensity in the right hippocampus (*white arrows*; compare with the normal hippocampus on the left, *black arrows*) consistent with mesial temporal sclerosis.

THE CAUSES OF SEIZURES AND EPILEPSY

Seizures are a result of a shift in the normal balance of excitation and inhibition within the CNS. Given the numerous properties that control neuronal excitability, it is not surprising that there are many different ways to perturb this normal balance, and therefore many different causes of both seizures and epilepsy. Three clinical observations emphasize how a variety of factors determine why certain conditions may cause seizures or epilepsy in a given patient.

1. *The normal brain is capable of having a seizure under the appropriate circumstances, and there are differences between individuals in the susceptibility or threshold for seizures.* For example, seizures may be induced by high fevers in children who are otherwise normal and who never develop other neurologic problems, including epilepsy. However, febrile seizures occur only in a relatively small proportion of children. This implies there are various underlying *endogenous factors* that influence the threshold for having a seizure. Some of these factors are clearly genetic, as it has been shown that a family history of epilepsy will influence the likelihood of seizures occurring in otherwise normal individuals. Normal development also plays an important role, since the brain appears to have different seizure thresholds at different maturational stages.
2. *There are a variety of conditions that have an extremely high likelihood of resulting in a chronic seizure disorder.* One of the best examples of this is severe, penetrating head trauma, which is associated with up to a 45% risk of subsequent epilepsy. The high propensity for severe traumatic brain injury to lead to epilepsy suggests that the injury results in a long-lasting pathologic change in the CNS that transforms a presumably normal neural network into one that is abnormally hyperexcitable. This process is known as *epileptogenesis*, and the specific changes that result in a lowered seizure threshold can be considered *epileptogenic factors*. Other processes associated with epileptogenesis include stroke, infections, and abnormalities of CNS development. Likewise, the genetic abnormalities associated with epilepsy likely involve processes that trigger the appearance of specific sets of epileptogenic factors.
3. *Seizures are episodic.* Patients with epilepsy have seizures intermittently and, depending on the underlying cause, many patients are completely normal for months or even years between seizures. This implies there are important provocative or *precipitating factors* that induce seizures in patients with epilepsy. Similarly, precipitating factors are responsible for causing the single seizure in someone without epilepsy. Precipitants include those due to intrinsic physiologic processes such as psychological or physical stress, sleep deprivation, or hormonal changes associated with the menstrual cycle. They also include exogenous factors such as exposure to toxic substances and certain medications.

These observations emphasize the concept that the many causes of seizures and epilepsy result from a dynamic interplay between endogenous factors, epileptogenic factors, and precipitating factors. The potential role of each needs to be carefully considered when determining the appropriate management of a patient with seizures. For example, the identification of predisposing factors (e.g., family history of epilepsy) in a patient with febrile seizures may increase the necessity for closer follow-up and a more aggressive diagnostic evaluation. Finding an epileptogenic lesion may help in the estimation of seizure recurrence and duration of therapy. Finally, removal or modification of a precipitating factor may be an effective and safer method for preventing further seizures than the prophylactic use of anticonvulsant drugs.

CAUSES ACCORDING TO AGE

In practice, it is useful to consider the etiologies of seizures based on the age of the patient, as age is one of the most important factors determining both the incidence and the likely causes of seizures or epilepsy (Table 26-4). During the *neonatal period and early infancy*, potential causes include hypoxic-ischemic encephalopathy, trauma, CNS infection, congenital CNS abnormalities, and metabolic disorders. Babies born to mothers using neurotoxic drugs such as cocaine, heroin, or ethanol are susceptible to drug-withdrawal seizures in the first few days after delivery. Hypoglycemia and hypocalcemia, which can occur as secondary complications of perinatal injury, are also causes of seizures early after delivery. Seizures due to inborn errors of metabolism usually present once regular feeding begins, typically 2–3 days after birth. Pyridoxine (vitamin B_6) deficiency, an important cause of neonatal seizures, can be effectively treated with pyridoxine replacement. The idiopathic or inherited forms of benign neonatal convulsions are also seen during this time period.

The most common seizures arising in *late infancy and early childhood* are febrile seizures, which are seizures associated with fevers but without evidence of CNS infection or other defined causes. The overall prevalence is 3–5% and even higher in some parts of the world such as Asia. Patients often have a family history of febrile seizures or epilepsy. Febrile seizures usually occur between 3 months and 5 years of age and have a peak incidence between 18 and 24 months. The typical scenario is a child who has a generalized, tonic-clonic seizure during a febrile illness in the setting of a common childhood infection such as otitis media, respiratory infection, or gastroenteritis. The seizure is likely to occur during the rising phase of the temperature curve (i.e., during the first day) rather than

TABLE 26-4

CAUSES OF SEIZURES	
Neonates (<1 month)	Perinatal hypoxia and ischemia Intracranial hemorrhage and trauma Acute CNS infection Metabolic disturbances (hypoglycemia, hypocalcemia, hypomagnesemia, pyridoxine deficiency) Drug withdrawal Developmental disorders Genetic disorders
Infants and children (>1 month and <12 years)	Febrile seizures Genetic disorders (metabolic, degenerative, primary epilepsy syndromes) CNS infection Developmental disorders Trauma Idiopathic
Adolescents (12–18 years)	Trauma Genetic disorders Infection Brain tumor Illicit drug use Idiopathic
Young adults (18–35 years)	Trauma Alcohol withdrawal Illicit drug use Brain tumor Idiopathic
Older adults (>35 years)	Cerebrovascular disease Brain tumor Alcohol withdrawal Metabolic disorders (uremia, hepatic failure, electrolyte abnormalities, hypoglycemia, hyperglycemia) Alzheimer's disease and other degenerative CNS diseases Idiopathic

Abbreviation: CNS, central nervous system.

well into the course of the illness. A *simple* febrile seizure is a single, isolated event, brief, and symmetric in appearance. *Complex* febrile seizures are characterized by repeated seizure activity, duration >15 min, or by focal features. Approximately one-third of patients with febrile seizures will have a recurrence, but <10% have three or more episodes. Recurrences are much more likely when the febrile seizure occurs in the first year of life. Simple febrile seizures are not associated with an increase in the risk of developing epilepsy, while complex febrile seizures have a risk of 2–5%; other risk factors include the presence of preexisting neurologic deficits and a family history of nonfebrile seizures.

Childhood marks the age at which many of the well-defined epilepsy syndromes present. Some children who are otherwise normal develop idiopathic, generalized tonic-clonic seizures without other features that fit into specific syndromes. Temporal lobe epilepsy usually presents in childhood and may be related to mesial temporal lobe sclerosis (as part of the MTLE syndrome) or other focal abnormalities such as cortical dysgenesis. Other types of focal seizures, including those that evolve into generalized seizures, may be the relatively late manifestation of a developmental disorder, an acquired lesion such as head trauma, CNS infection (especially viral encephalitis), or very rarely a CNS tumor.

The period of *adolescence and early adulthood* is one of transition during which the idiopathic or genetically based epilepsy syndromes, including JME and juvenile absence epilepsy, become less common, while epilepsies secondary to acquired CNS lesions begin to predominate. Seizures that begin in patients in this age range may be associated with head trauma, CNS infections (including parasitic infections such as cysticercosis), brain tumors, congenital CNS abnormalities, illicit drug use, or alcohol withdrawal.

Head trauma is a common cause of epilepsy in adolescents and adults. The head injury can be caused by a variety of mechanisms, and the likelihood of developing epilepsy is strongly correlated with the severity of the injury. A patient with a penetrating head wound, depressed skull fracture, intracranial hemorrhage, or prolonged posttraumatic coma or amnesia has a 40–50% risk of developing epilepsy, while a patient with a closed head injury and cerebral contusion has a 5–25% risk. Recurrent seizures usually develop within 1 year after head trauma, although intervals of ≥10 years are well known. In controlled studies, mild head injury, defined as a concussion with amnesia or loss of consciousness of <30 min, was found to be associated with only a slightly increased likelihood of epilepsy. Nonetheless, most epileptologists know of patients who have focal seizures within hours or days of a mild head injury and subsequently develop chronic seizures of the same type; such cases may represent rare examples of chronic epilepsy resulting from mild head injury.

The causes of seizures in *older adults* include cerebrovascular disease, trauma (including subdural hematoma), CNS tumors, and degenerative diseases. Cerebrovascular disease may account for ~50% of new cases of epilepsy in patients older than age 65. Acute seizures (i.e., occurring at the time of the stroke) are seen more often with embolic rather than hemorrhagic or thrombotic stroke. Chronic seizures typically appear months to years after the initial event and are associated with all forms of stroke.

TABLE 26-5

DRUGS AND OTHER SUBSTANCES THAT CAN CAUSE SEIZURES

Alkylating agents (e.g., busulfan, chlorambucil)	**Psychotropics**
Antimalarials (chloroquine, mefloquine)	Antidepressants
Antimicrobials/antivirals	Antipsychotics
β-lactam and related compounds	Lithium
Quinolones	**Radiographic contrast agents**
Acyclovir	Theophylline
Isoniazid	**Sedative-hypnotic drug withdrawal**
Ganciclovir	Alcohol
Anesthetics and analgesics	Barbiturates (short-acting)
Meperidine	Benzodiazepines (short-acting)
Tramadol	**Drugs of abuse**
Local anesthetics	Amphetamine
Dietary supplements	Cocaine
Ephedra (ma huang)	Phencyclidine
Gingko	Methylphenidate
Immunomodulatory drugs	**Flumazenil**[a]
Cyclosporine	
OKT3 (monoclonal antibodies to T cells)	
Tacrolimus	
Interferons	

[a]In benzodiazepine-dependent patients.

Metabolic disturbances such as electrolyte imbalance, hypo- or hyperglycemia, renal failure, and hepatic failure may cause seizures at any age. Similarly, endocrine disorders, hematologic disorders, vasculitides, and many other systemic diseases may cause seizures over a broad age range. A wide variety of medications and abused substances are known to precipitate seizures as well (Table 26-5).

BASIC MECHANISMS

MECHANISMS OF SEIZURE INITIATION AND PROPAGATION

Focal seizure activity can begin in a very discrete region of cortex and then spread to neighboring regions, i.e., there is a *seizure initiation* phase and a *seizure propagation* phase. The initiation phase is characterized by two concurrent events in an aggregate of neurons: (1) high-frequency bursts of action potentials and (2) hypersynchronization. The bursting activity is caused by a relatively long-lasting depolarization of the neuronal membrane due to influx of extracellular calcium (Ca^{2+}), which leads to the opening of voltage-dependent sodium (Na^+) channels, influx of Na^+, and generation of repetitive action potentials. This is followed by a hyperpolarizing afterpotential mediated by γ-aminobutyric acid (GABA) receptors or potassium (K^+) channels, depending on the cell type. The synchronized bursts from a sufficient number of neurons result in a so-called spike discharge on the EEG.

Normally, the spread of bursting activity is prevented by intact hyperpolarization and a region of "surround" inhibition created by inhibitory neurons. With sufficient activation there is a recruitment of surrounding neurons via a number of synaptic and nonsynaptic mechanisms, including: (1) an increase in extracellular K^+, which blunts hyperpolarization and depolarizes neighboring neurons; (2) accumulation of Ca^{2+} in presynaptic terminals, leading to enhanced neurotransmitter release; and (3) depolarization-induced activation of the *N*-methyl-D-aspartate (NMDA) subtype of the excitatory amino acid receptor, which causes additional Ca^{2+} influx and neuronal activation; and (4) ephaptic interactions related to changes in tissue osmolarity and cell swelling. The recruitment of a sufficient number of neurons leads to the propagation of seizure activity into contiguous areas via local cortical connections, and to more distant areas via long commissural pathways such as the corpus callosum.

Many factors control neuronal excitability, and thus there are many potential mechanisms for altering a neuron's propensity to have bursting activity. Mechanisms *intrinsic* to the neuron include changes in the conductance of ion channels, response characteristics of membrane receptors, cytoplasmic buffering, second-messenger systems, and protein expression as determined by gene transcription, translation, and posttranslational modification. Mechanisms *extrinsic* to the neuron include changes in the amount or type of neurotransmitters present at the synapse, modulation of receptors by extracellular ions and other molecules, and temporal and spatial properties of synaptic and nonsynaptic input. Nonneural cells such as astrocytes and oligodendrocytes, have an important role in many of these mechanisms as well.

Certain recognized causes of seizures are explained by these mechanisms. For example, accidental ingestion of domoic acid, which is an analogue of glutamate (the principal excitatory neurotransmitter in the brain), causes profound seizures via direct activation of excitatory amino acid receptors throughout the CNS. Penicillin, which can lower the seizure threshold in humans and is a potent convulsant in experimental models, reduces inhibition by antagonizing the effects of GABA at its receptor. The basic mechanisms of other precipitating factors of seizures such as sleep deprivation, fever, alcohol withdrawal, hypoxia, and infection, are not as well understood but presumably involve analogous perturbations in neuronal excitability. Similarly, the endogenous factors that determine an individual's seizure threshold may relate to these properties as well.

Knowledge of the mechanisms responsible for initiation and propagation of most generalized seizures (including tonic-clonic, myoclonic, and atonic types) remains rudimentary and reflects the limited understanding of the connectivity of the brain at a systems level. Much more is understood about the origin of generalized spike-and-wave discharges in absence seizures. These appear to be related to oscillatory rhythms normally generated during sleep by circuits connecting the thalamus and cortex. This oscillatory behavior involves an interaction between $GABA_B$ receptors, T-type Ca^{2+} channels, and K^+ channels located within the thalamus. Pharmacologic studies indicate that modulation of these receptors and channels can induce absence seizures, and there is good evidence that the genetic forms of absence epilepsy may be associated with mutations of components of this system.

MECHANISMS OF EPILEPTOGENESIS

Epileptogenesis refers to the transformation of a normal neuronal network into one that is chronically hyperexcitable. There is often a delay of months to years between an initial CNS injury such as trauma, stroke, or infection and the first seizure. The injury appears to initiate a process that gradually lowers the seizure threshold in the affected region until a spontaneous seizure occurs. In many genetic and idiopathic forms of epilepsy, epileptogenesis is presumably determined by developmentally regulated events.

Pathologic studies of the hippocampus from patients with temporal lobe epilepsy have led to the suggestion that some forms of epileptogenesis are related to *structural changes in neuronal networks*. For example, many patients with MTLE have a highly selective loss of neurons that may contribute to inhibition of the main excitatory neurons within the dentate gyrus. There is also evidence that, in response to the loss of neurons, there is reorganization or "sprouting" of surviving neurons in a way that affects the excitability of the network. Some of these changes can be seen in experimental models of prolonged electrical seizures or traumatic brain injury. Thus, an initial injury such as head injury may lead to a very focal, confined region of structural change that causes local hyperexcitability. The local hyperexcitability leads to further structural changes that evolve over time until the focal lesion produces clinically evident seizures. Similar models have provided strong evidence for long-term alterations in *intrinsic, biochemical properties of cells* within the network such as chronic changes in glutamate or GABA receptor function. Recent work has suggested that induction of inflammatory cascades may be a critical factor in these processes as well.

GENETIC CAUSES OF EPILEPSY

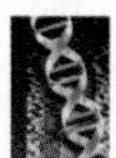

The most important recent progress in epilepsy research has been the identification of genetic mutations associated with a variety of epilepsy syndromes (Table 26-2). Although all of the mutations identified to date cause rare forms of epilepsy, their discovery has led to extremely important conceptual advances. For example, it appears that many of the inherited, idiopathic epilepsies (i.e., the relatively "pure" forms of epilepsy in which seizures are the phenotypic abnormality and brain structure and function are otherwise normal) are due to mutations affecting ion channel function. These syndromes are therefore part of the larger group of channelopathies causing paroxysmal disorders such as cardiac arrhythmias, episodic ataxia, periodic weakness, and familial hemiplegic migraine. In contrast, gene mutations observed in symptomatic epilepsies (i.e., disorders in which other neurologic abnormalities such as cognitive impairment, coexist with seizures) are proving to be associated with pathways influencing CNS development or neuronal homeostasis. A current challenge is to identify the multiple susceptibility genes that underlie the more common forms of idiopathic epilepsies. Recent studies suggest that ion channel mutations and chromosomal microdeletions may be the cause of epilepsy in a subset of these patients.

MECHANISMS OF ACTION OF ANTIEPILEPTIC DRUGS

Antiepileptic drugs appear to act primarily by blocking the initiation or spread of seizures. This occurs through a variety of mechanisms that modify the activity of ion channels or neurotransmitters, and in most cases the drugs have pleiotropic effects. The mechanisms include inhibition of Na^+-dependent action potentials in a frequency-dependent manner (e.g., phenytoin, carbamazepine, lamotrigine, topiramate, zonisamide, lacosamide, rufinamide), inhibition of voltage-gated Ca^{2+} channels (phenytoin, gabapentin, pregabalin), attenuation of glutamate activity (lamotrigine, topiramate, felbamate), potentiation of GABA receptor function (benzodiazepines and barbiturates), increase in the availability of GABA (valproic acid, gabapentin, tiagabine), and modulation of release of synaptic vesicles (levetiracetam). The two most effective drugs for absence seizures, ethosuximide and valproic acid, probably act by inhibiting T-type Ca^{2+} channels in thalamic neurons.

In contrast to the relatively large number of antiepileptic drugs that can attenuate seizure activity, there are currently no drugs known to prevent the formation of a seizure focus following CNS injury. The eventual development of such "antiepileptogenic" drugs will provide an important means of preventing the emergence of epilepsy following injuries such as head trauma, stroke, and CNS infection.

APPROACH TO THE PATIENT Seizure

When a patient presents shortly after a seizure, the first priorities are attention to vital signs, respiratory and cardiovascular support, and treatment of seizures if they resume (see "Treatment: Seizures and Epilepsy"). Life-threatening conditions such as CNS infection, metabolic derangement, or drug toxicity must be recognized and managed appropriately.

When the patient is not acutely ill, the evaluation will initially focus on whether there is a history of earlier seizures (Fig. 26-2). If this is the first seizure, then the emphasis will be to: (1) establish whether the reported episode was a seizure rather than another paroxysmal event, (2) determine the cause of the seizure by identifying risk factors and precipitating events, and (3) decide whether anticonvulsant therapy is required in addition to treatment for any underlying illness.

In the patient with prior seizures or a known history of epilepsy, the evaluation is directed toward (1) identification of the underlying cause and precipitating factors, and (2) determination of the adequacy of the patient's current therapy.

HISTORY AND EXAMINATION

The first goal is to determine whether the event was truly a seizure. An in-depth history is essential, for *in many cases the diagnosis of a seizure is based solely on clinical grounds—the examination and laboratory studies are often normal.* Questions should focus on the symptoms before, during, and after the episode in order to differentiate a seizure from other paroxysmal events (see "Differential Diagnosis of Seizures"). Seizures frequently occur out-of-hospital, and the patient may be unaware of the ictal and immediate postictal phases; thus, witnesses to the event should be interviewed carefully.

The history should also focus on risk factors and predisposing events. Clues for a predisposition to seizures include a history of febrile seizures, earlier auras or brief seizures not recognized as such, and a family history of seizures. Epileptogenic factors such as prior head trauma, stroke, tumor, or infection of the nervous system should be identified. In children, a careful assessment of developmental milestones may provide evidence for underlying CNS disease. Precipitating factors such as sleep deprivation, systemic diseases, electrolyte or metabolic derangements, acute infection, drugs that lower the seizure threshold (Table 26-5), or alcohol or illicit drug use should also be identified.

The general physical examination includes a search for signs of infection or systemic illness. Careful examination of the skin may reveal signs of neurocutaneous disorders such as tuberous sclerosis or neurofibromatosis, or chronic liver or renal disease. A finding of organomegaly may indicate a metabolic storage disease, and limb asymmetry may provide a clue to brain injury early in development. Signs of head trauma and use of alcohol or illicit drugs should be sought. Auscultation of the heart and carotid arteries may identify an abnormality that predisposes to cerebrovascular disease.

All patients require a complete neurologic examination, with particular emphasis on eliciting signs of cerebral hemispheric disease (Chap. 1). Careful assessment of mental status (including memory, language function, and abstract thinking) may suggest lesions in the anterior frontal, parietal, or temporal lobes. Testing of visual fields will help screen for lesions in the optic pathways and occipital lobes. Screening tests of motor function such as pronator drift, deep tendon reflexes, gait, and coordination may suggest lesions in motor (frontal) cortex, and cortical sensory testing (e.g., double simultaneous stimulation) may detect lesions in the parietal cortex.

LABORATORY STUDIES

Routine blood studies are indicated to identify the more common metabolic causes of seizures such as abnormalities in electrolytes, glucose, calcium, or magnesium, and hepatic or renal disease. A screen for toxins in blood and urine should also be obtained from all patients in appropriate risk groups, especially when no clear precipitating factor has been identified. A lumbar puncture is indicated if there is any suspicion of meningitis or encephalitis, and it is mandatory in all patients infected with HIV, even in the absence of symptoms or signs suggesting infection.

ELECTROPHYSIOLOGIC STUDIES

All patients who have a possible seizure disorder should be evaluated with an EEG as soon as possible. Details about the EEG are covered in Chap. 5.

In the evaluation of a patient with suspected epilepsy, the presence of *electrographic seizure activity* during the clinically evident event (i.e., abnormal, repetitive, rhythmic activity having a discrete onset and termination) clearly establishes the diagnosis. The absence of electrographic seizure activity does not exclude a seizure

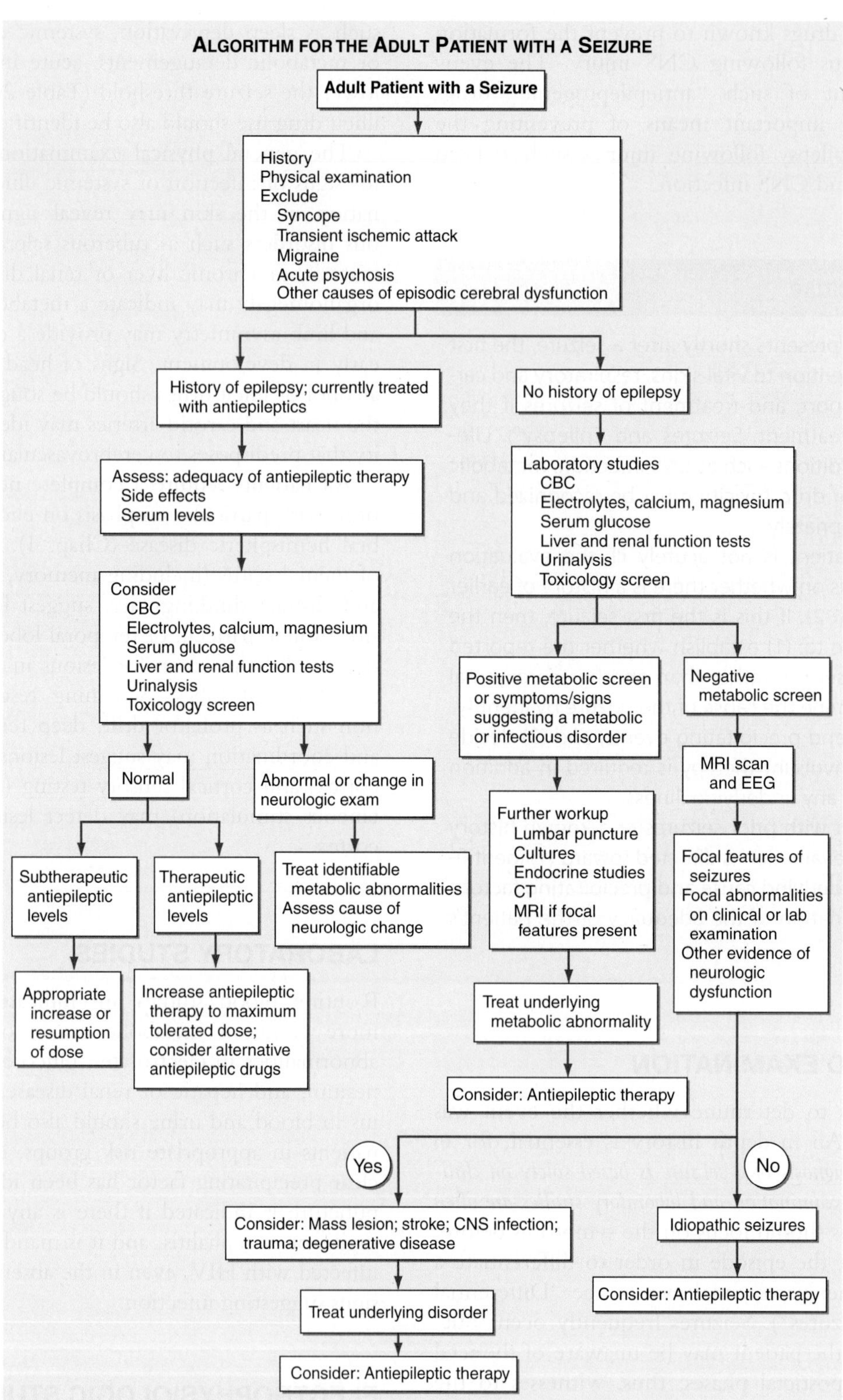

FIGURE 26-2

Evaluation of the adult patient with a seizure. CBC, complete blood count; CNS, central nervous system; CT, computed tomography; EEG, electroencephalogram; MRI, magnetic resonance imaging.

disorder, however, because focal seizures may originate from a region of the cortex that cannot be detected by standard scalp electrodes. The EEG is always abnormal during generalized tonic-clonic seizures. Since seizures are typically infrequent and unpredictable, it is often not possible to obtain the EEG during a clinical event. Continuous monitoring for prolonged periods in video-EEG telemetry units for hospitalized patients or the use of portable equipment to record the EEG continuously on cassettes for ≥24 h in ambulatory patients has made it easier to capture the electrophysiologic accompaniments of clinical events. In particular, video-EEG telemetry is now a routine approach for the accurate diagnosis of epilepsy in patients with poorly characterized events or seizures that are difficult to control.

The EEG may also be helpful in the interictal period by showing certain abnormalities that are highly supportive of the diagnosis of epilepsy. Such *epileptiform activity* consists of bursts of abnormal discharges containing spikes or sharp waves. The presence of epileptiform activity is not specific for epilepsy, but it has a much greater prevalence in patients with epilepsy than in normal individuals. However, even in an individual who is known to have epilepsy, the initial routine interictal EEG may be normal up to 60% of the time. Thus, the EEG cannot establish the diagnosis of epilepsy in many cases.

The EEG is also used for classifying seizure disorders and aiding in the selection of anticonvulsant medications. For example, episodic generalized spike-wave activity is usually seen in patients with typical absence epilepsy and may be seen with other generalized epilepsy syndromes. Focal interictal epileptiform discharges would support the diagnosis of a focal seizure disorder such as temporal lobe epilepsy or frontal lobe seizures, depending on the location of the discharges.

The routine scalp-recorded EEG may also be used to assess the prognosis of seizure disorders; in general, a normal EEG implies a better prognosis, whereas an abnormal background or profuse epileptiform activity suggests a poor outlook. Unfortunately, the EEG has not proved to be useful in predicting which patients with predisposing conditions such as head injury or brain tumor, will go on to develop epilepsy, because in such circumstances epileptiform activity is commonly encountered regardless of whether seizures occur.

Magnetoencephalography (MEG) provides another way of looking noninvasively at cortical activity. Instead of measuring electrical activity of the brain, it measures the small magnetic fields that are generated by this activity. Epileptiform activity seen on the MEG can be analyzed, and its source in the brain can be estimated using a variety of mathematical techniques. These source estimates can then be plotted on an anatomic image of the brain such as an MRI (discussed next), to generate a magnetic source image (MSI). MSI can be useful to localize potential seizure foci.

BRAIN IMAGING

Almost all patients with new-onset seizures should have a brain imaging study to determine whether there is an underlying structural abnormality that is responsible. The only potential exception to this rule is children who have an unambiguous history and examination suggestive of a benign, generalized seizure disorder such as absence epilepsy. MRI has been shown to be superior to CT for the detection of cerebral lesions associated with epilepsy. In some cases MRI will identify lesions such as tumors, vascular malformations, or other pathologies that need immediate therapy. The use of newer MRI methods such as 3-Tesla scanners, multichannel head coils, three-dimensional structural imaging at submillimeter resolution, and new pulse sequences including fluid-attenuated inversion recovery (FLAIR), has increased the sensitivity for detection of abnormalities of cortical architecture, including hippocampal atrophy associated with mesial temporal sclerosis, as well as abnormalities of cortical neuronal migration. In such cases the findings may not lead to immediate therapy, but they do provide an explanation for the patient's seizures and point to the need for chronic anticonvulsant therapy or possible surgical resection.

In the patient with a suspected CNS infection or mass lesion, CT scanning should be performed emergently when MRI is not immediately available. Otherwise, it is usually appropriate to obtain an MRI study within a few days of the initial evaluation. Functional imaging procedures such as positron emission tomography (PET) and single-photon emission computed tomography (SPECT) are also used to evaluate certain patients with medically refractory seizures (discussed later).

DIFFERENTIAL DIAGNOSIS OF SEIZURES

Disorders that may mimic seizures are listed in Table 26-6. In most cases seizures can be distinguished from other conditions by meticulous attention to the history and relevant laboratory studies. On occasion, additional studies such as video-EEG monitoring, sleep studies, tilt-table analysis, or cardiac electrophysiology, may be required to reach a correct diagnosis. Two of the more common nonepileptic syndromes in the differential diagnosis are detailed next.

SYNCOPE

(See also Chap. 10) The diagnostic dilemma encountered most frequently is the distinction between a generalized seizure and syncope. Observations by the patient and bystanders that can help differentiate between the two are listed in Table 26-7. Characteristics of a seizure include the presence of an aura, cyanosis, unconsciousness, motor manifestations lasting >15 s, postictal disorientation, muscle soreness, and sleepiness. In contrast, a syncopal episode is more likely if the event was provoked by acute pain or anxiety or occurred immediately after arising

TABLE 26-6

DIFFERENTIAL DIAGNOSIS OF SEIZURES	
Syncope	**Transient ischemic attack (TIA)**
Vasovagal syncope	Basilar artery TIA
Cardiac arrhythmia	**Sleep disorders**
Valvular heart disease	Narcolepsy/cataplexy
Cardiac failure	Benign sleep myoclonus
Orthostatic hypotension	**Movement disorders**
Psychological disorders	Tics
Psychogenic seizure	Nonepileptic myoclonus
Hyperventilation	Paroxysmal choreoathetosis
Panic attack	**Special considerations in children**
Metabolic disturbances	Breath-holding spells
Alcoholic blackouts	Migraine with recurrent abdominal pain and cyclic vomiting
Delirium tremens	Benign paroxysmal vertigo
Hypoglycemia	Apnea
Hypoxia	Night terrors
Psychoactive drugs (e.g., hallucinogens)	Sleepwalking
Migraine	
Confusional migraine	
Basilar migraine	

from the lying or sitting position. Patients with syncope often describe a stereotyped transition from consciousness to unconsciousness that includes tiredness, sweating, nausea, and tunneling of vision, and they experience a relatively brief loss of consciousness. Headache or incontinence usually suggests a seizure but may on occasion also occur with syncope. A brief period (i.e., 1–10 s) of convulsive motor activity is frequently seen immediately at the onset of a syncopal episode, especially if the patient remains in an upright posture after fainting (e.g., in a dentist's chair) and therefore has a sustained decrease in cerebral perfusion. Rarely, a syncopal episode can induce a full tonic-clonic seizure. In such cases the evaluation must focus on both the cause of the syncopal event as well as the possibility that the patient has a propensity for recurrent seizures.

TABLE 26-7

FEATURES THAT DISTINGUISH GENERALIZED TONIC-CLONIC SEIZURE FROM SYNCOPE

FEATURES	SEIZURE	SYNCOPE
Immediate precipitating factors	Usually none	Emotional stress, Valsalva, orthostatic hypotension, cardiac etiologies
Premonitory symptoms	None or aura (e.g., odd odor)	Tiredness, nausea, diaphoresis, tunneling of vision
Posture at onset	Variable	Usually erect
Transition to unconsciousness	Often immediate	Gradual over seconds[a]
Duration of unconsciousness	Minutes	Seconds
Duration of tonic or clonic movements	30–60 s	Never more than 15 s
Facial appearance during event	Cyanosis, frothing at mouth	Pallor
Disorientation and sleepiness after event	Many minutes to hours	<5 min
Aching of muscles after event	Often	Sometimes
Biting of tongue	Sometimes	Rarely
Incontinence	Sometimes	Sometimes
Headache	Sometimes	Rarely

[a]May be sudden with certain cardiac arrhythmias.

PSYCHOGENIC SEIZURES

Psychogenic seizures are nonepileptic behaviors that resemble seizures. They are often part of a conversion reaction precipitated by underlying psychological distress. Certain behaviors such as side-to-side turning of the head, asymmetric and large-amplitude shaking movements of the limbs, twitching of all four extremities without loss of consciousness, and pelvic thrusting are more commonly associated with psychogenic rather than epileptic seizures. Psychogenic seizures often last longer than epileptic seizures and may wax and wane over minutes to hours. However, the distinction is sometimes difficult on clinical grounds alone, and there are many examples of diagnostic errors made by experienced epileptologists. This is especially true for psychogenic seizures that resemble focal seizures with dyscognitive features, since the behavioral manifestations of focal seizures (especially of frontal lobe origin) can be extremely unusual, and in both cases the routine surface EEG may be normal. Video-EEG monitoring is very useful when historic features are nondiagnostic. Generalized tonic-clonic seizures always produce marked EEG abnormalities during and after the seizure. For suspected focal seizures of temporal lobe origin, the use of additional electrodes beyond the standard scalp locations (e.g., sphenoidal electrodes) may be required to localize a seizure focus. Measurement of serum prolactin levels may also help to distinguish between organic and psychogenic seizures, since most generalized seizures and some focal seizures are accompanied by rises in serum prolactin (during the immediate 30-min postictal period), whereas psychogenic seizures are not. The diagnosis of psychogenic seizures does not exclude a concurrent diagnosis of epilepsy, since the two often coexist.

TREATMENT Seizures and Epilepsy

Therapy for a patient with a seizure disorder is almost always multimodal and includes treatment of underlying conditions that cause or contribute to the seizures, avoidance of precipitating factors, suppression of recurrent seizures by prophylactic therapy with antiepileptic medications or surgery, and addressing a variety of psychological and social issues. Treatment plans must be individualized, given the many different types and causes of seizures as well as the differences in efficacy and toxicity of antiepileptic medications for each patient. In almost all cases a neurologist with experience in the treatment of epilepsy should design and oversee implementation of the treatment strategy. Furthermore, patients with refractory epilepsy or those who require polypharmacy with antiepileptic drugs should remain under the regular care of a neurologist.

TREATMENT OF UNDERLYING CONDITIONS If the sole cause of a seizure is a metabolic disturbance such as an abnormality of serum electrolytes or glucose, then treatment is aimed at reversing the metabolic problem and preventing its recurrence. Therapy with antiepileptic drugs is usually unnecessary unless the metabolic disorder cannot be corrected promptly and the patient is at risk of having further seizures. If the apparent cause of a seizure was a medication (e.g., theophylline) or illicit drug use (e.g., cocaine), then appropriate therapy is avoidance of the drug; there is usually no need for antiepileptic medications unless subsequent seizures occur in the absence of these precipitants.

Seizures caused by a structural CNS lesion such as a brain tumor, vascular malformation, or brain abscess may not recur after appropriate treatment of the underlying lesion. However, despite removal of the structural lesion, there is a risk that the seizure focus will remain in the surrounding tissue or develop de novo as a result of gliosis and other processes induced by surgery, radiation, or other therapies. Most patients are therefore maintained on an antiepileptic medication for at least 1 year, and an attempt is made to withdraw medications only if the patient has been completely seizure free. If seizures are refractory to medication, the patient may benefit from surgical removal of the epileptic brain region (see later).

AVOIDANCE OF PRECIPITATING FACTORS Unfortunately, little is known about the specific factors that determine precisely when a seizure will occur in a patient with epilepsy. Some patients can identify particular situations that appear to lower their seizure threshold; these situations should be avoided. For example, a patient who has seizures in the setting of sleep deprivation should obviously be advised to maintain a normal sleep schedule. Many patients note an association between alcohol intake and seizures, and they should be encouraged to modify their drinking habits accordingly. There are also relatively rare cases of patients with seizures that are induced by highly specific stimuli such as a video game monitor, music, or an individual's voice ("reflex epilepsy"). If there is an association between stress and seizures, stress reduction techniques such as physical exercise, meditation, or counseling may be helpful.

ANTIEPILEPTIC DRUG THERAPY Antiepileptic drug therapy is the mainstay of treatment for most patients with epilepsy. The overall goal is to completely prevent seizures without causing any untoward side effects, preferably with a single medication and a dosing schedule that is easy for the patient to follow. Seizure classification is an important element in designing the treatment plan, since some antiepileptic drugs have different activities against various seizure types. However, there is considerable overlap between many antiepileptic drugs such that the choice of therapy is often determined more by the patient's specific needs, especially his or her assessment of side effects.

When to Initiate Antiepileptic Drug Therapy Antiepileptic drug therapy should be started in any patient with recurrent seizures of unknown etiology or a known cause that cannot be reversed. Whether to initiate therapy in a patient with a single seizure is controversial. Patients with a single seizure due to an identified lesion such as a CNS tumor, infection, or trauma, in which there is strong evidence that the lesion is epileptogenic, should be treated. The risk of seizure recurrence in a patient with an apparently unprovoked or idiopathic seizure is uncertain, with estimates ranging from 31 to 71% in the first 12 months after the initial seizure. This uncertainty arises from differences in the underlying seizure types and etiologies in various published epidemiologic studies. Generally accepted risk factors associated with recurrent seizures include the following: (1) an abnormal neurologic examination, (2) seizures presenting as status epilepticus, (3) postictal Todd's paralysis, (4) a strong family history of seizures, or (5) an abnormal EEG. Most patients with one or more of these risk factors should be treated. Issues such as employment or driving may influence the decision whether to start medications as well. For example, a patient with a single, idiopathic seizure whose job depends on driving may prefer taking antiepileptic drugs rather than risk a seizure recurrence and the potential loss of driving privileges.

Selection of Antiepileptic Drugs Antiepileptic drugs available in the United States are shown in

Table 26-8, and the main pharmacologic characteristics of commonly used drugs are listed in Table 26-9. Worldwide, older medications such as phenytoin, valproic acid, carbamazepine, phenobarbital, and ethosuximide are generally used as first-line therapy for most seizure disorders since, overall, they are as effective as recently marketed drugs and significantly less expensive. Most of the new drugs that have become available in the past decade are used as add-on or alternative therapy, although some are now being used as first-line monotherapy.

In addition to efficacy, factors influencing the choice of an initial medication include the convenience of dosing (e.g., once daily versus three or four times daily) and potential side effects. In this regard, a number of the newer drugs have the advantage of a relative lack of drug-drug interactions and easier dosing. Almost all of the commonly used antiepileptic drugs can cause similar, dose-related side effects such as sedation, ataxia, and diplopia. Long-term use of some agents in adults, especially the elderly, can lead to osteoporosis. Close follow-up is required to ensure these side effects are promptly recognized and reversed. Most of the older drugs and some of the newer ones can also cause idiosyncratic toxicity such as rash, bone marrow suppression, or hepatotoxicity. Although rare, these side effects should be considered during drug selection, and patients must be instructed about symptoms or signs that should signal the need to alert their health care provider. For some drugs, laboratory tests (e.g., complete blood count and liver function tests) are recommended prior to the institution of therapy (to establish baseline values) and during initial dosing and titration of the agent. Importantly, recent studies have shown that Asian individuals carrying the human leukocyte antigen allele, HLA-B*1502, are at particularly high risk of developing serious skin reactions from carbamazepine and phenytoin, so racial background and genotype are additional factors to consider in drug selection.

Antiepileptic Drug Selection for Focal Seizures Carbamazepine (or a related drug, oxcarbazepine), lamotrigine, and phenytoin are currently the drugs of choice approved for the initial treatment of focal seizures, including those that evolve into generalized seizures. Overall they have very similar efficacy, but differences in pharmacokinetics and toxicity are the main determinants for use in a given patient. For example, an advantage of carbamazepine (which is also available in an extended-release form) is that its metabolism follows first-order pharmacokinetics, and the relationship between drug dose, serum levels, and toxicity is linear. Carbamazepine can cause leukopenia, aplastic anemia, or hepatotoxicity and would therefore be contraindicated in patients with predispositions to these problems. Oxcarbazepine has the advantage of being metabolized in a way that avoids an intermediate metabolite associated with some of the side effects of carbamazepine. Oxcarbazepine also has fewer drug interactions than carbamazepine. Lamotrigine tends to be well tolerated in terms of side effects. However, patients need to be particularly vigilant about the possibility of a skin rash during the initiation of therapy. This can be extremely severe and lead to Stevens-Johnson syndrome if unrecognized and if the medication is not discontinued immediately. This risk can be reduced by slow introduction and titration. Lamotrigine must be started slowly when used as add-on therapy with valproic acid, since valproic acid inhibits lamotrigine metabolism, thereby substantially prolonging its half-life. Phenytoin has a relatively long half-life and offers the advantage of once or twice daily dosing compared to two or three times daily dosing for many of the other drugs. However, phenytoin shows properties of saturation kinetics, such that small increases in phenytoin doses above a standard maintenance dose can precipitate marked side effects. This is one of the main causes of acute phenytoin toxicity. Long-term use of phenytoin is associated with untoward cosmetic effects (e.g., hirsutism, coarsening of facial features, and gingival hypertrophy), and effects on bone metabolism, so it is often avoided in young patients who are likely to require the drug for many years. Topiramate can be used for both focal and generalized seizures. Similar to some of the other antiepileptic drugs, topiramate can cause significant psychomotor slowing and other cognitive

TABLE 26-8

SELECTION OF ANTIEPILEPTIC DRUGS

GENERALIZED-ONSET TONIC-CLONIC	FOCAL	TYPICAL ABSENCE	ATYPICAL ABSENCE, MYOCLONIC, ATONIC
First-Line			
Valproic acid	Lamotrigine	Valproic acid	Valproic acid
Lamotrigine	Carbamazepine	Ethosuximide	Lamotrigine
Topiramate	Oxcarbazepine		Topiramate
	Phenytoin		
	Levetiracetam		
Alternatives			
Zonisamide[a]	Topiramate	Lamotrigine	Clonazepam
Phenytoin	Zonisamide[a]	Clonazepam	Felbamate
Carbamazepine	Valproic acid		
Oxcarbazepine	Tiagabine[a]		
Phenobarbital	Gabapentin[a]		
Primidone	Lacosamide[a]		
Felbamate	Phenobarbital		
	Primidone		
	Felbamate		

[a]As adjunctive therapy.

TABLE 26-9

DOSAGE AND ADVERSE EFFECTS OF COMMONLY USED ANTIEPILEPTIC DRUGS

GENERIC NAME	TRADE NAME	PRINCIPAL USES	TYPICAL DOSE; DOSE INTERVAL	HALF-LIFE	THERAPEUTIC RANGE	ADVERSE EFFECTS		DRUG INTERACTIONS
						NEUROLOGIC	SYSTEMIC	
Phenytoin (diphenylhydantoin	Dilantin	Tonic-clonic Focal-onset	300–400 mg/d (3–6 mg/kg, adult; 4–8 mg/kg, child); qd-bid	24 h (wide variation, dose-dependent)	10–20 μg/mL	Dizziness Diplopia Ataxia Incoordination Confusion	Gum hyperplasia Lymphadenopathy Hirsutism Osteomalacia Facial coarsening Skin rash	Level increased by isoniazid, sulfonamides, fluoxetine Level decreased by enzyme-inducing drugs[a] Altered folate metabolism
Carbamazepine	Tegretol[b] Carbatrol	Tonic-clonic Focal-onset	600–1800 mg/d (15–35 mg/kg, child); bid-qid	10–17 h	6–12 μg/mL	Ataxia Dizziness Diplopia Vertigo	Aplastic anemia Leukopenia Gastrointestinal irritation Hepatotoxicity Hyponatremia	Level decreased by enzyme-inducing drugs[a] Level increased by erythromycin, propoxyphene, isoniazid, cimetidine, fluoxetine
Valproic acid	Depakene Depakote[b]	Tonic-clonic Absence Atypical absence Myoclonic Focal-onset Atonic	750–2000 mg/d (20–60 mg/kg); bid-qid	15 h	50–125 μg/mL	Ataxia Sedation Tremor	Hepatotoxicity Thrombocytopenia Gastrointestinal irritation Weight gain Transient alopecia Hyperammonemia	Level decreased by enzyme-inducing drugs[a]
Lamotrigine	Lamictal[b]	Focal-onset Tonic-clonic Atypical absence Myoclonic Lennox-Gastaut syndrome	150–500 mg/d; bid	25 h 14 h (with enzyme-inducers) 59 h (with valproic acid)	Not established	Dizziness Diplopia Sedation Ataxia Headache	Skin rash Stevens-Johnson syndrome	Level decreased by enzyme-inducing drugs[a] and oral contraceptives Level increased by valproic acid
Ethosuximide	Zarontin	Absence	750–1250 mg/d (20–40 mg/kg); qd-bid	60 h, adult 30 h, child	40–100 μg/mL	Ataxia Lethargy Headache	Gastrointestinal irritation Skin rash Bone marrow suppression	Level decreased by enzyme-inducing drugs[a] Level increased by valproic acid

(continued)

TABLE 26-9

DOSAGE AND ADVERSE EFFECTS OF COMMONLY USED ANTIEPILEPTIC DRUGS (*CONTINUED*)

GENERIC NAME	TRADE NAME	PRINCIPAL USES	TYPICAL DOSE; DOSE INTERVAL	HALF-LIFE	THERAPEUTIC RANGE	ADVERSE EFFECTS: NEUROLOGIC	ADVERSE EFFECTS: SYSTEMIC	DRUG INTERACTIONS
Gabapentin	Neurontin	Focal-onset	900–2400 mg/d; tid-qid	5–9 h	Not established	Sedation Dizziness Ataxia Fatigue	Gastrointestinal irritation Weight gain Edema	No known significant interactions
Topiramate	Topamax	Focal-onset Tonic-clonic Lennox-Gastaut syndrome	200–400 mg/d; bid	20–30 h	Not established	Psychomotor slowing Sedation Speech or language problems Fatigue Paresthesias	Renal stones (avoid use with other carbonic anhydrase inhibitors) Glaucoma Weight loss Hypohidrosis	Level decreased by enzyme-inducing drugs[a]
Tiagabine	Gabitril	Focal-onset	32–56 mg/d; bid-qid	7–9 h	Not established	Confusion Sedation Depression Dizziness Speech or language problems Paresthesias Psychosis	Gastrointestinal irritation	Level decreased by enzyme-inducing drugs[a]
Phenobarbital	Luminol	Tonic-clonic Focal-onset	60–180 mg/d; qd	90 h	10–40 μg/mL	Sedation Ataxia Confusion Dizziness Decreased libido Depression	Skin rash	Level increased by valproic acid, phenytoin
Primidone	Mysoline	Tonic-clonic Focal-onset	750–1000 mg/d; bid-tid	Primidone, 8–15 h Phenobarbital, 90 h	Primidone, 4–12 μg/mL Phenobarbital, 10–40 μg/mL	Same as phenobarbital		Level increased by valproic acid, phenytoin
Clonazepam	Klonopin	Absence Atypical absence Myoclonic	1–12 mg/d; qd-tid	24–48 h	10–70 ng/mL	Ataxia Sedation Lethargy	Anorexia	Level decreased by enzyme-inducing drugs[a]

Felbamate	Felbatol	Focal-onset Lennox-Gastaut syndrome Tonic-clonic	2400–3600 mg/d, tid-qid	16–22 h	Not established	Insomnia Dizziness Sedation Headache	Aplastic anemia Hepatic failure Weight loss Gastrointestinal irritation	Increases phenytoin, valproic acid, active carbamazepine metabolite
Levetiracetam	Keppra[b]	Focal-onset	1000–3000 mg/d; qd-bid	6–8 h	Not established	Sedation Fatigue Incoordination Mood changes	Anemia Leukopenia	No known significant interactions
Zonisamide	Zonegran	Focal-onset Tonic-clonic	200–400 mg/d; qd-bid	50–68 h	Not established	Sedation Dizziness Confusion Headache Psychosis	Anorexia Renal stones Hypohidrosis	Level decreased by enzyme-inducing drugs[a]
Oxcarbazepine	Trileptal	Focal-onset Tonic-clonic	900–2400 mg/d (30–45 mg/kg, child); bid	10–17 h (for active metabolite)	Not established	Fatigue Ataxia Dizziness Diplopia Vertigo Headache	See carbamazepine	Level decreased by enzyme-inducing drugs[a] May increase phenytoin
Lacosamide	Vimpat	Focal-onset	200–400 mg/d; bid	13 h	Not established	Dizziness Ataxia Diplopia Vertigo	GI irritation Cardiac conduction (PR interval prolongation)	Level decreased by enzyme-inducing drugs[a]
Rufinamide	Banzel	Lennox-Gastaut syndrome	3200 mg/d (45 mg/kg, child); bid	6–10 h	Not established	Sedation Fatigue Dizziness Ataxia Headache Diplopia	GI irritation Leukopenia Cardiac conduction (QT interval prolongation)	Level decreased by enzyme-inducing drugs[a] Level increased by valproic acid May increase phenytoin

[a]Phenytoin, carbamazepine, phenobarbital.
[b]Extended-release product available.

problems, and it should not be used in patients at risk for the development of glaucoma or renal stones.

Valproic acid is an effective alternative for some patients with focal seizures, especially when the seizures generalize. Gastrointestinal side effects are fewer when using the valproate semisodium formulation (Depakote). Valproic acid also rarely causes reversible bone marrow suppression and hepatotoxicity, and laboratory testing is required to monitor toxicity. This drug should generally be avoided in patients with preexisting bone marrow or liver disease. Irreversible, fatal hepatic failure appearing as an idiosyncratic rather than dose-related side effect is a relatively rare complication; its risk is highest in children <2 years old, especially those taking other antiepileptic drugs or with inborn errors of metabolism.

Levetiracetam, zonisamide, tiagabine, gabapentin, and lacosamide are additional drugs currently used for the treatment of focal seizures with or without evolution into generalized seizures. Phenobarbital and other barbiturate compounds were commonly used in the past as first-line therapy for many forms of epilepsy. However, the barbiturates frequently cause sedation in adults, hyperactivity in children, and other more subtle cognitive changes; thus, their use should be limited to situations in which no other suitable treatment alternatives exist.

Antiepileptic Drug Selection for Generalized Seizures Valproic acid and lamotrigine are currently considered the best initial choice for the treatment of primary generalized, tonic-clonic seizures. Topiramate, zonisamide, phenytoin, and carbamazepine are suitable alternatives. Valproic acid is also particularly effective in absence, myoclonic, and atonic seizures and is therefore the drug of choice in patients with generalized epilepsy syndromes having mixed seizure types. Importantly, carbamazepine, oxcarbazepine, and phenytoin can worsen certain types of generalized seizures, including absence, myoclonic, tonic, and atonic seizures. Ethosuximide is a particularly effective drug for the treatment of uncomplicated absence seizures, but it is not useful for tonic-clonic or focal seizures. Ethosuximide rarely causes bone marrow suppression, so that periodic monitoring of blood cell counts is required. Lamotrigine appears to be particularly effective in epilepsy syndromes with mixed, generalized seizure types such as JME and Lennox-Gastaut syndrome. Topiramate, zonisamide, and felbamate may have similar broad efficacy.

Initiation and Monitoring of Therapy Because the response to any antiepileptic drug is unpredictable, patients should be carefully educated about the approach to therapy. The goal is to prevent seizures and minimize the side effects of therapy; determination of the optimal dose is often a matter of trial and error. This process may take months or longer if the baseline seizure frequency is low. Most anticonvulsant drugs need to be introduced relatively slowly to minimize side effects, and patients should expect that minor side effects such as mild sedation, slight changes in cognition, or imbalance will typically resolve within a few days. Starting doses are usually the lowest value listed under the dosage column in Table 26-9. Subsequent increases should be made only after achieving a steady state with the previous dose (i.e., after an interval of five or more half-lives).

Monitoring of serum antiepileptic drug levels can be very useful for establishing the initial dosing schedule. However, the published therapeutic ranges of serum drug concentrations are only an approximate guide for determining the proper dose for a given patient. The key determinants are the clinical measures of seizure frequency and presence of side effects, not the laboratory values. Conventional assays of serum drug levels measure the total drug (i.e., both free and protein bound). However, it is the concentration of free drug that reflects extracellular levels in the brain and correlates best with efficacy. Thus, patients with decreased levels of serum proteins (e.g., decreased serum albumin due to impaired liver or renal function) may have an increased ratio of free to bound drug, yet the concentration of free drug may be adequate for seizure control. These patients may have a "subtherapeutic" drug level, but the dose should be changed only if seizures remain uncontrolled, not just to achieve a "therapeutic" level. It is also useful to monitor free drug levels in such patients. In practice, other than during the initiation or modification of therapy, monitoring of antiepileptic drug levels is most useful for documenting compliance.

If seizures continue despite gradual increases to the maximum tolerated dose and documented compliance, then it becomes necessary to switch to another antiepileptic drug. This is usually done by maintaining the patient on the first drug while a second drug is added. The dose of the second drug should be adjusted to decrease seizure frequency without causing toxicity. Once this is achieved, the first drug can be gradually withdrawn (usually over weeks unless there is significant toxicity). The dose of the second drug is then further optimized based on seizure response and side effects. Monotherapy should be the goal whenever possible.

When to Discontinue Therapy Overall, about 70% of children and 60% of adults who have their seizures completely controlled with antiepileptic drugs can eventually discontinue therapy. The following patient profile yields the greatest chance of remaining seizure free after drug withdrawal: (1) complete medical control of seizures for 1–5 years; (2) single seizure type, either focal or generalized; (3) normal neurologic examination, including intelligence; and (4) normal EEG. The appropriate seizure-free interval is unknown and undoubtedly varies for different forms of epilepsy. However, it seems reasonable to attempt withdrawal of therapy after 2 years in a patient who meets all of the above criteria, is motivated to discontinue the medication, and clearly understands the potential risks and benefits. In most cases it is preferable to reduce the dose of the drug gradually over 2–3 months. Most recurrences occur in the first 3 months after discontinuing therapy, and patients should be advised to avoid potentially dangerous situations such as driving or swimming during this period.

Treatment of Refractory Epilepsy Approximately one-third of patients with epilepsy do not respond to treatment with a single antiepileptic drug, and it becomes necessary to try a combination of drugs to control seizures. Patients who have focal epilepsy related to an underlying structural lesion or those with multiple seizure types and developmental delay are particularly likely to require multiple drugs. There are currently no clear guidelines for rational polypharmacy, although in theory a combination of drugs with different mechanisms of action may be most useful. In most cases the initial combination therapy combines first-line drugs (i.e., carbamazepine, oxcarbazepine, lamotrigine, valproic acid, and phenytoin). If these drugs are unsuccessful, then the addition of a newer drug such as levetiracetam, topiramate, and zonisamide is indicated. Patients with myoclonic seizures resistant to valproic acid may benefit from the addition of clonazepam, and those with absence seizures may respond to a combination of valproic acid and ethosuximide. The same principles concerning the monitoring of therapeutic response, toxicity, and serum levels for monotherapy apply to polypharmacy, and potential drug interactions need to be recognized. If there is no improvement, a third drug can be added while the first two are maintained. If there is a response, the less effective or less well tolerated of the first two drugs should be gradually withdrawn.

SURGICAL TREATMENT OF REFRACTORY EPILEPSY Approximately 20–30% of patients with epilepsy continue to have seizures despite efforts to find an effective combination of antiepileptic drugs. For some, surgery can be extremely effective in substantially reducing seizure frequency and even providing complete seizure control. Understanding the potential value of surgery is especially important when a patient's seizures are not controlled with initial treatment, as such patients often fail to respond to subsequent medication trials. Rather than submitting the patient to years of unsuccessful medical therapy and the psychosocial trauma and increased mortality associated with ongoing seizures, the patient should have an efficient but relatively brief attempt at medical therapy and then be referred for surgical evaluation.

The most common surgical procedure for patients with temporal lobe epilepsy involves resection of the anteromedial temporal lobe (temporal lobectomy) or a more limited removal of the underlying hippocampus and amygdala (amygdalohippocampectomy). Focal seizures arising from extratemporal regions may be abolished by a focal neocortical resection with precise removal of an identified lesion (lesionectomy). When the cortical region cannot be removed, multiple subpial transection, which disrupts intracortical connections, is sometimes used to prevent seizure spread. Hemispherectomy or multilobar resection is useful for some patients with severe seizures due to hemispheric abnormalities such as hemimegalencephaly or other dysplastic abnormalities, and corpus callosotomy has been shown to be effective for disabling tonic or atonic seizures, usually when they are part of a mixed-seizure syndrome (e.g., Lennox-Gastaut syndrome).

Presurgical evaluation is designed to identify the functional and structural basis of the patient's seizure disorder. Inpatient video-EEG monitoring is used to define the anatomic location of the seizure focus and to correlate the abnormal electrophysiologic activity with behavioral manifestations of the seizure. Routine scalp or scalp-sphenoidal recordings are usually sufficient for localization, and advances in neuroimaging have made the use of invasive electrophysiologic monitoring such as implanted depth electrodes or subdural electrodes less common. A high-resolution MRI scan is routinely used to identify structural lesions, and this is sometimes augmented with MEG. Functional imaging studies such as SPECT and PET are adjunctive tests that may help verify the localization of an apparent epileptogenic region. Once the presumed location of the seizure onset is identified, additional studies, including neuropsychological testing and the intracarotid amobarbital test (Wada test) may be used to assess language and memory localization and to determine the possible functional consequences of surgical removal of the epileptogenic region. In some cases, the exact extent of the resection to be undertaken is determined by performing cortical mapping at the time of the surgical procedure, allowing for a tailored resection. This involves electrocorticographic recordings made with electrodes on the surface of the brain to identify the extent of epileptiform disturbances. If the region to be resected is within or near brain regions suspected of having sensorimotor or language function, electrical cortical stimulation mapping is performed on the awake patient to determine the function of cortical regions in question in order to avoid resection of so-called eloquent cortex and thereby minimize postsurgical deficits.

Advances in presurgical evaluation and microsurgical techniques have led to a steady increase in the success of epilepsy surgery. Clinically significant complications of surgery are <5%, and the use of functional mapping procedures has markedly reduced the neurologic sequelae due to removal or sectioning of brain tissue. For example, about 70% of patients treated with temporal lobectomy will become seizure free, and another 15–25% will have at least a 90% reduction in seizure frequency. Marked improvement is also usually seen in patients treated with hemispherectomy for catastrophic seizure disorders due to large hemispheric abnormalities. Postoperatively, patients generally need to remain on antiepileptic drug therapy, but the marked reduction of seizures following resective surgery can have a very beneficial effect on quality of life.

Not all medically refractory patients are suitable candidates for resective surgery. For example, some patients have seizures arising from more than one site, making the risk of ongoing seizures or potential harm from the surgery unacceptably high. Vagus nerve stimulation (VNS) may be useful in some of these cases, although the benefit for most patients seems to be very limited (i.e., the efficacy of VNS appears to be no greater than trying another drug, which rarely works if a patient has proved to be refractory to the first two to three drugs). The precise mechanism of action of VNS is unknown, although experimental studies have shown that stimulation of vagal nuclei leads to widespread activation of cortical and subcortical pathways and an associated increased seizure threshold. Adverse effects of the surgery are rare, and stimulation-induced side effects, including transient hoarseness, cough, and dyspnea, are usually mild.

Although still in development, there are some additional therapies that will likely be of benefit to patients with medically refractory epilepsy. Preliminary studies suggest that stereotactic radiosurgery may be effective in certain focal seizure disorders. There has also been great interest in the development of implantable devices that can detect the onset of a seizure (in some instances, before the seizure becomes clinically apparent) and deliver either an electrical stimulation or drug directly to the seizure focus to abort the event.

STATUS EPILEPTICUS

Status epilepticus refers to continuous seizures or repetitive, discrete seizures with impaired consciousness in the interictal period. Status epilepticus has numerous subtypes, including generalized convulsive status epilepticus (GCSE) (e.g., persistent, generalized electrographic seizures, coma, and tonic-clonic movements) and nonconvulsive status epilepticus (e.g., persistent absence seizures or focal seizures, confusion or partially impaired consciousness, and minimal motor abnormalities). The duration of seizure activity sufficient to meet the definition of status epilepticus has traditionally been specified as 15–30 min. However, a more practical definition is to consider status epilepticus as a situation in which the duration of seizures prompts the acute use of anticonvulsant therapy. For GCSE, this is typically when seizures last beyond 5 min.

GCSE is an emergency and must be treated immediately, since cardiorespiratory dysfunction, hyperthermia, and metabolic derangements can develop as a consequence of prolonged seizures, and these can lead to irreversible neuronal injury. Furthermore, CNS injury can occur even when the patient is paralyzed with neuromuscular blockade but continues to have electrographic seizures. The most common causes of GCSE are anticonvulsant withdrawal or noncompliance, metabolic disturbances, drug toxicity, CNS infection, CNS tumors, refractory epilepsy, and head trauma.

GCSE is obvious when the patient is having overt convulsions. However, after 30–45 min of uninterrupted seizures, the signs may become increasingly subtle. Patients may have mild clonic movements of only the fingers or fine, rapid movements of the eyes. There may be paroxysmal episodes of tachycardia, hypertension, and pupillary dilation. In such cases, the EEG may be the only method of establishing the diagnosis. Thus, if the patient stops having overt seizures, yet remains comatose, an EEG should be performed to rule out ongoing status epilepticus. This is obviously also essential when a patient with GCSE has been paralyzed with neuromuscular blockade in the process of protecting the airway.

The first steps in the management of a patient in GCSE are to attend to any acute cardiorespiratory problems or hyperthermia, perform a brief medical and neurologic examination, establish venous access, and send samples for laboratory studies to identify metabolic abnormalities. Anticonvulsant therapy should then begin without delay; a treatment approach is shown in Fig. 26-3.

The treatment of nonconvulsive status epilepticus is thought to be less urgent than GCSE, since the ongoing seizures are not accompanied by the severe metabolic disturbances seen with GCSE. However, evidence suggests that nonconvulsive status epilepticus, especially that caused by ongoing, focal seizure activity, is associated with cellular injury in the region of the seizure focus; therefore this condition should be treated as promptly as possible using the general approach described for GCSE.

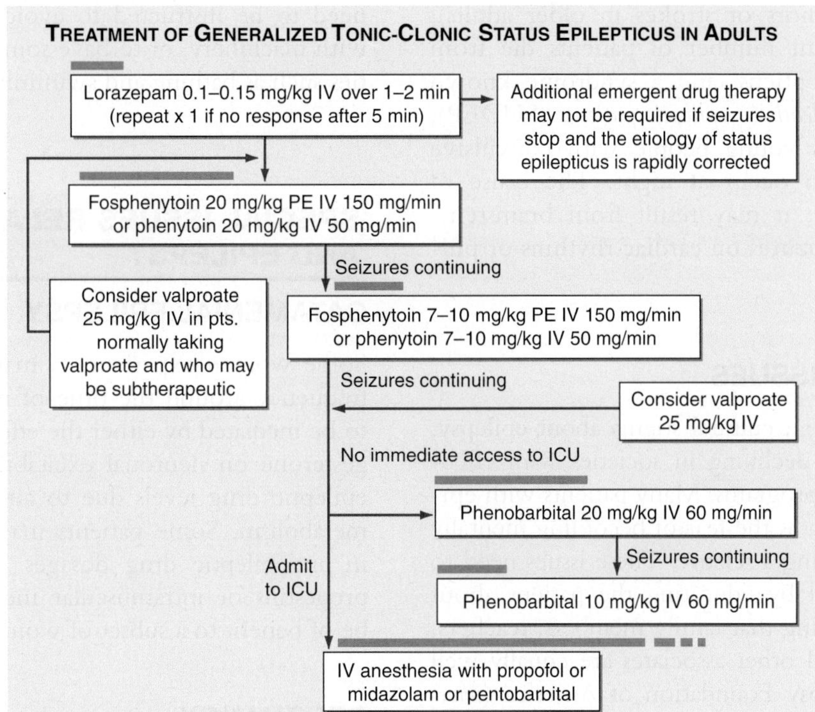

FIGURE 26-3

Pharmacologic treatment of generalized tonic-clonic status epilepticus in adults. The horizontal bars indicate the approximate duration of drug infusions. IV, intravenous; PE, phenytoin equivalents.

BEYOND SEIZURES: OTHER MANAGEMENT ISSUES

INTERICTAL BEHAVIOR

The adverse effects of epilepsy often go beyond the occurrence of clinical seizures, and the extent of these effects largely depends on the etiology of the seizure disorder, the degree to which the seizures are controlled, and the presence of side effects from antiepileptic therapy. Many patients with epilepsy are completely normal between seizures and able to live highly successful and productive lives. In contrast, patients with seizures secondary to developmental abnormalities or acquired brain injury may have impaired cognitive function and other neurologic deficits. Frequent interictal EEG abnormalities have been shown to be associated with subtle dysfunction of memory and attention. Patients with many seizures, especially those emanating from the temporal lobe, often note an impairment of short-term memory that may progress over time.

Patients with epilepsy are at risk of developing a variety of psychiatric problems, including depression, anxiety, and psychosis. This risk varies considerably depending on many factors, including the etiology, frequency, and severity of seizures and the patient's age and previous history. Depression occurs in ~20% of patients, and the incidence of suicide is higher in epileptic patients than in the general population. Depression should be treated through counseling or medication. The selective serotonin reuptake inhibitors (SSRIs) typically have no effect on seizures, while high doses of tricyclic antidepressants may lower the seizure threshold. Anxiety can appear as a manifestation of a seizure, and anxious or psychotic behavior can sometimes be observed as part of a postictal delirium. Postictal psychosis is a rare phenomenon that typically occurs after a period of increased seizure frequency. There is usually a brief lucid interval lasting up to a week, followed by days to weeks of agitated, psychotic behavior. The psychosis will usually resolve spontaneously but frequently will require short-term treatment with antipsychotic or anxiolytic medications.

There is ongoing controversy as to whether some patients with epilepsy (especially temporal lobe epilepsy) have a stereotypical "interictal personality." The predominant view is that the unusual or abnormal personality traits observed in such patients are, in most cases, not due to epilepsy but result from an underlying structural brain lesion, the effects of antiepileptic drugs, or psychosocial factors related to suffering from a chronic disease.

MORTALITY OF EPILEPSY

Patients with epilepsy have a risk of death that is roughly two to three times greater than expected in a matched population without epilepsy. Most of the increased mortality is due to the underlying etiology of epilepsy (e.g., tumors or strokes in older adults). However, a significant number of patients die from accidents, status epilepticus, and a syndrome known as *sudden unexpected death in epileptic patients* (SUDEP), which usually affects young people with convulsive seizures and tends to occur at night. The cause of SUDEP is unknown; it may result from brainstem-mediated effects of seizures on cardiac rhythms or pulmonary function.

PSYCHOSOCIAL ISSUES

There continues to be a cultural stigma about epilepsy, although it is slowly declining in societies with effective health education programs. Many patients with epilepsy harbor fears such as the fear of becoming mentally retarded or dying during a seizure. These issues need to be carefully addressed by educating the patient about epilepsy and by ensuring that family members, teachers, fellow employees, and other associates are equally well informed. The Epilepsy Foundation of America (*www.epilepsyfoundation.org*) is a patient advocacy organization and a useful source of educational material, as is the Web site *www.epilepsy.com*.

EMPLOYMENT, DRIVING, AND OTHER ACTIVITIES

Many patients with epilepsy face difficulty in obtaining or maintaining employment, even when their seizures are well controlled. Federal and state legislation is designed to prevent employers from discriminating against patients with epilepsy, and patients should be encouraged to understand and claim their legal rights. Patients in these circumstances also benefit greatly from the assistance of health providers who act as strong patient advocates.

Loss of driving privileges is one of the most disruptive social consequences of epilepsy. Physicians should be very clear about local regulations concerning driving and epilepsy, since the laws vary considerably among states and countries. In all cases, it is the physician's responsibility to warn patients of the danger imposed on themselves and others while driving if their seizures are uncontrolled (unless the seizures are not associated with impairment of consciousness or motor control). In general, most states allow patients to drive after a seizure-free interval (on or off medications) of between 3 months and 2 years.

Patients with incompletely controlled seizures must also contend with the risk of being in situations where an impairment of consciousness or loss of motor control could lead to major injury or death. Thus, depending on the type and frequency of seizures, many patients need to be instructed to avoid working at heights or with machinery, or to have someone close by for activities such as bathing and swimming.

SPECIAL ISSUES RELATED TO WOMEN AND EPILEPSY

CATAMENIAL EPILEPSY

Some women experience a marked increase in seizure frequency around the time of menses. This is believed to be mediated by either the effects of estrogen and progesterone on neuronal excitability or changes in antiepileptic drug levels due to altered protein binding or metabolism. Some patients may benefit from increases in antiepileptic drug dosages during menses. Natural progestins or intramuscular medroxyprogesterone may be of benefit to a subset of women.

PREGNANCY

Most women with epilepsy who become pregnant will have an uncomplicated gestation and deliver a normal baby. However, epilepsy poses some important risks to a pregnancy. Seizure frequency during pregnancy will remain unchanged in ~50% of women, increase in 30%, and decrease in 20%. Changes in seizure frequency are attributed to endocrine effects on the CNS, variations in antiepileptic drug pharmacokinetics (such as acceleration of hepatic drug metabolism or effects on plasma protein binding), and changes in medication compliance. It is useful to see patients at frequent intervals during pregnancy and monitor serum antiepileptic drug levels. Measurement of the unbound drug concentrations may be useful if there is an increase in seizure frequency or worsening of side effects of antiepileptic drugs.

The overall incidence of fetal abnormalities in children born to mothers with epilepsy is 5–6%, compared to 2–3% in healthy women. Part of the higher incidence is due to teratogenic effects of antiepileptic drugs, and the risk increases with the number of medications used (e.g., 10–20% risk of malformations with three drugs) and possibly with higher doses. A recent meta-analysis of published pregnancy registries and cohorts found that the most common malformations were defects in the cardiovascular and musculoskeletal system (1.4–1.8%). Valproic acid is strongly associated with an increased risk of adverse fetal outcomes (7–20%). Little is currently known about the safety of newer drugs, although reports suggest a higher than expected incidence of cleft lip or palate with the use of lamotrigine during pregnancy.

Since the potential harm of uncontrolled convulsive seizures on the mother and fetus is considered greater than the teratogenic effects of antiepileptic drugs, it is currently recommended that pregnant women be maintained on effective drug therapy. When possible, it seems prudent to have the patient on monotherapy at the lowest effective dose, especially during the first trimester. For some women, however, the type and frequency of their seizures may allow for them to safely wean off antiepileptic drugs prior to conception. Patients should also take folate (1–4 mg/d), since the antifolate effects of anticonvulsants are thought to play a role in the development of neural tube defects, although the benefits of this treatment remain unproved in this setting.

Enzyme-inducing drugs such as phenytoin, carbamazepine, oxcarbazepine, topiramate, phenobarbital, and primidone cause a transient and reversible deficiency of vitamin K–dependent clotting factors in ~50% of newborn infants. Although neonatal hemorrhage is uncommon, the mother should be treated with oral vitamin K (20 mg/d, phylloquinone) in the last 2 weeks of pregnancy, and the infant should receive intramuscular vitamin K (1 mg) at birth.

CONTRACEPTION

Special care should be taken when prescribing antiepileptic medications for women who are taking oral contraceptive agents. Drugs such as carbamazepine, phenytoin, phenobarbital, and topiramate can significantly decrease the efficacy of oral contraceptives via enzyme induction and other mechanisms. Patients should be advised to consider alternative forms of contraception, or their contraceptive medications should be modified to offset the effects of the antiepileptic medications.

BREAST-FEEDING

Antiepileptic medications are excreted into breast milk to a variable degree. The ratio of drug concentration in breast milk relative to serum ranges from ~5% (valproic acid) to 300% (levetiracetam). Given the overall benefits of breast-feeding and the lack of evidence for long-term harm to the infant by being exposed to antiepileptic drugs, mothers with epilepsy can be encouraged to breast-feed. This should be reconsidered, however, if there is any evidence of drug effects on the infant such as lethargy or poor feeding.

CHAPTER 27

CEREBROVASCULAR DISEASES

Wade S. Smith ■ Joey D. English ■ S. Claiborne Johnston

Cerebrovascular diseases include some of the most common and devastating disorders: ischemic stroke, hemorrhagic stroke, and cerebrovascular anomalies such as intracranial aneurysms and arteriovenous malformations (AVMs). They cause ~200,000 deaths each year in the United States and are a major cause of disability. The incidence of cerebrovascular diseases increases with age, and the number of strokes is projected to increase as the elderly population grows, with a doubling in stroke deaths in the United States by 2030. Most cerebrovascular diseases are manifest by the abrupt onset of a focal neurologic deficit, as if the patient was "struck by the hand of God." A stroke, or cerebrovascular accident, is defined by this abrupt onset of a neurologic deficit that is attributable to a focal vascular cause. Thus, the definition of stroke is clinical, and laboratory studies including brain imaging are used to support the diagnosis. The clinical manifestations of stroke are highly variable because of the complex anatomy of the brain and its vasculature. *Cerebral ischemia* is caused by a reduction in blood flow that lasts longer than several seconds. Neurologic symptoms are manifest within seconds because neurons lack glycogen, so energy failure is rapid. If the cessation of flow lasts for more than a few minutes, *infarction* or death of brain tissue results. When blood flow is quickly restored, brain tissue can recover fully and the patient's symptoms are only transient: This is called a *transient ischemic attack* (TIA). The standard definition of TIA requires that all neurologic signs and symptoms resolve within 24 h regardless of whether there is imaging evidence of new permanent brain injury; stroke has occurred if the neurologic signs and symptoms last for >24 h. However, a newly proposed definition classifies those with new brain infarction as ischemic strokes regardless of whether symptoms persist. A generalized reduction in cerebral blood flow due to systemic hypotension (e.g., cardiac arrhythmia, myocardial infarction, or hemorrhagic shock) usually produces syncope (Chap. 10). If low cerebral blood flow persists for a longer duration, then infarction in the border zones between the major cerebral artery distributions may develop. In more severe instances, *global hypoxia-ischemia* causes widespread brain injury; the constellation of cognitive sequelae that ensues is called *hypoxic-ischemic encephalopathy* (Chap. 28). *Focal ischemia* or infarction, conversely, is usually caused by thrombosis of the cerebral vessels themselves or by emboli from a proximal arterial source or the heart. *Intracranial hemorrhage* is caused by bleeding directly into or around the brain; it produces neurologic symptoms by producing a mass effect on neural structures, from the toxic effects of blood itself, or by increasing intracranial pressure.

APPROACH TO THE PATIENT: Cerebrovascular Disease

Rapid evaluation is essential for use of time-sensitive treatments such as thrombolysis. However, patients with acute stroke often do not seek medical assistance on their own, both because they are rarely in pain, as well as because they may lose the appreciation that something is wrong (anosognosia); it is often a family member or a bystander who calls for help. Therefore, patients and their family members should be counseled to call emergency medical services immediately if they experience or witness the sudden onset of any of the following: loss of sensory and/or motor function on one side of the body (nearly 85% of ischemic stroke patients have hemiparesis); change in vision, gait, or ability to speak or understand; or if they experience a sudden, severe headache.

There are several common causes of sudden-onset neurologic symptoms that may mimic stroke, including seizure, intracranial tumor, migraine, and metabolic encephalopathy. An adequate history from an observer that no convulsive activity occurred at the onset reasonably excludes seizure; however, ongoing complex partial seizures without tonic-clonic activity may mimic stroke. Tumors may present with acute neurologic symptoms due to hemorrhage, seizure, or hydrocephalus. Surprisingly, migraine can mimic stroke, even in patients without a significant migraine history. When it develops without head pain (*acephalgic migraine*), the diagnosis may remain elusive. Patients without any prior history of migraine may develop acephalgic migraine even after age 65. A sensory disturbance is often prominent, and the sensory deficit, as well as any motor deficits, tends to migrate slowly across a limb over minutes rather than seconds as with stroke. The diagnosis of migraine becomes more secure as the cortical disturbance begins to cross vascular boundaries or if typical visual symptoms are present such as scintillating scotomata (Chap. 8). At times it may be difficult to make the diagnosis until multiple episodes have occurred leaving behind no residual symptoms and with a normal MRI study of the brain. Classically, metabolic encephalopathies produce fluctuating mental status without focal neurologic findings. However, in the setting of prior stroke or brain injury, a patient with fever or sepsis may manifest hemiparesis, which clears rapidly when the infection is remedied. The metabolic process serves to "unmask" a prior deficit.

Once the diagnosis of stroke is made, a brain imaging study is necessary to determine if the cause of stroke is ischemia or hemorrhage (Fig. 27-1). CT imaging of the brain is the standard imaging modality to detect the presence or absence of intracranial hemorrhage (see "Imaging Studies"). If the stroke is ischemic, administration of recombinant tissue plasminogen activator (rtPA) or endovascular mechanical thrombectomy may be beneficial in restoring cerebral perfusion (see "Treatment: Acute Ischemic Stroke"). Medical management to reduce the risk of complications becomes the next priority, followed by plans for secondary prevention. For ischemic stroke, several strategies can reduce the risk of subsequent stroke in all patients, while other strategies are effective for patients with specific causes of stroke such as cardiac embolus and carotid atherosclerosis. For hemorrhagic stroke, aneurysmal subarachnoid hemorrhage (SAH) and hypertensive intracranial hemorrhage are two important causes. The treatment and prevention of hypertensive intracranial hemorrhage are discussed later in this chapter. SAH is discussed in Chap. 28.

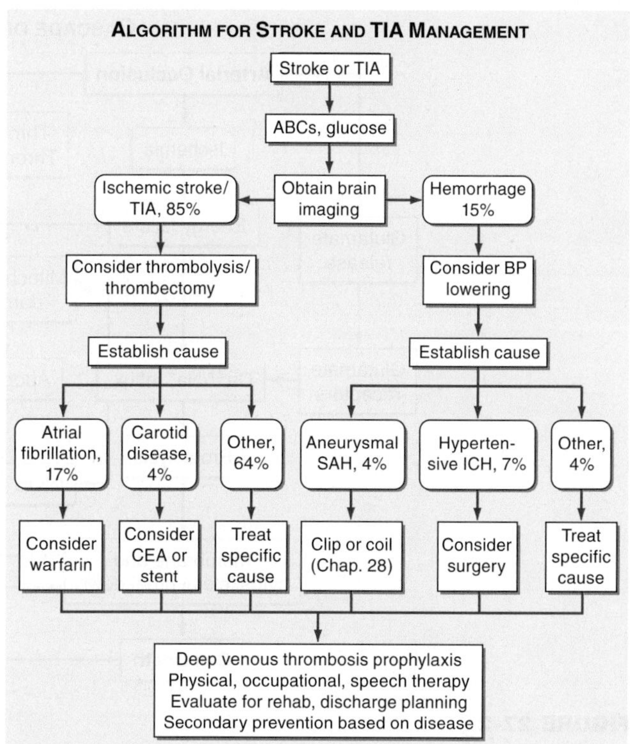

FIGURE 27-1
Medical management of stroke and TIA. Rounded boxes are diagnoses; rectangles are interventions. Numbers are percentages of stroke overall. ABCs, airway, breathing, circulation; BP, blood pressure; CEA, carotid endarterectomy; ICH, intracerebral hemorrhage; SAH, subarachnoid hemorrhage; TIA, transient ischemic attack.

ISCHEMIC STROKE

PATHOPHYSIOLOGY OF ISCHEMIC STROKE

Acute occlusion of an intracranial vessel causes reduction in blood flow to the brain region it supplies. The magnitude of flow reduction is a function of collateral blood flow and this depends on individual vascular anatomy, the site of occlusion, and likely systemic blood pressure. A decrease in cerebral blood flow to zero causes death of brain tissue within 4–10 min; values <16–18 mL/100 g tissue per minute cause infarction within an hour; and values <20 mL/100 g tissue per minute cause ischemia without infarction unless prolonged for several hours or days. If blood flow is restored prior to a significant amount of cell death, the patient may experience only transient symptoms, and the clinical syndrome is called a TIA. Tissue surrounding the core region of infarction is ischemic but reversibly dysfunctional and is referred to as the *ischemic penumbra.* The penumbra may be imaged by using perfusion-diffusion imaging with MRI or CT (see later and Figs. 27-15 and 27-16). The ischemic penumbra will eventually infarct if no change in flow occurs, and hence saving the ischemic penumbra is the goal of revascularization therapies.

Focal cerebral infarction occurs via two distinct pathways (Fig. 27-2): (1) a necrotic pathway in which cellular cytoskeletal breakdown is rapid, due principally to energy failure of the cell; and (2) an apoptotic pathway in which cells become programmed to die. Ischemia produces necrosis by starving neurons of glucose and oxygen, which in turn results in failure of mitochondria

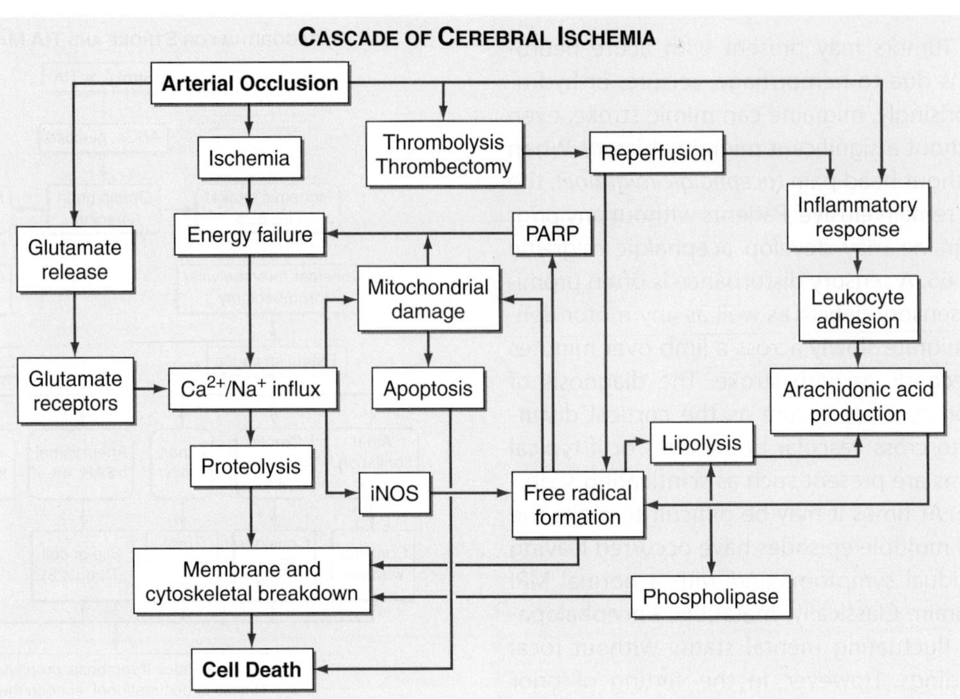

FIGURE 27-2

Major steps in the cascade of cerebral ischemia. See text for details. iNOS, inducible nitric oxide synthase; PARP, poly-A ribose polymerase.

to produce ATP. Without ATP, membrane ion pumps stop functioning and neurons depolarize, allowing intracellular calcium to rise. Cellular depolarization also causes glutamate release from synaptic terminals; excess extracellular glutamate produces neurotoxicity by activating postsynaptic glutamate receptors that increase neuronal calcium influx. Free radicals are produced by membrane lipid degradation and mitochondrial dysfunction. Free radicals cause catalytic destruction of membranes and likely damage other vital functions of cells. Lesser degrees of ischemia, as are seen within the ischemic penumbra, favor apoptotic cellular death causing cells to die days to weeks later. Fever dramatically worsens brain injury during ischemia, as does hyperglycemia (glucose >11.1 mmol/L [200 mg/dL]), so it is reasonable to suppress fever and prevent hyperglycemia as much as possible. Induced moderate hypothermia to mitigate stroke is the subject of continuing clinical research.

TREATMENT Acute Ischemic Stroke

After the clinical diagnosis of stroke is made, an orderly process of evaluation and treatment should follow (Fig. 27-1). The first goal is to prevent or reverse brain injury. Attend to the patient's airway, breathing, and circulation (ABC's), and treat hypoglycemia or hyperglycemia if identified. Perform an emergency noncontrast head CT scan to differentiate between ischemic stroke and hemorrhagic stroke; there are no reliable clinical findings that conclusively separate ischemia from hemorrhage, although a more depressed level of consciousness, higher initial blood pressure, or worsening of symptoms after onset favor hemorrhage, and a deficit that is maximal at onset, or remits, suggests ischemia. Treatments designed to reverse or lessen the amount of tissue infarction and improve clinical outcome fall within six categories: (1) medical support, (2) IV thrombolysis, (3) endovascular techniques, (4) antithrombotic treatment, (5) neuroprotection, and (6) stroke centers and rehabilitation.

MEDICAL SUPPORT When ischemic stroke occurs, the immediate goal is to optimize cerebral perfusion in the surrounding ischemic penumbra. Attention is also directed toward preventing the common complications of bedridden patients—infections (pneumonia, urinary, and skin) and deep venous thrombosis (DVT) with pulmonary embolism. Many physicians use pneumatic compression stockings to prevent DVT; subcutaneous heparin (unfractionated and low-molecular weight) is safe and more effective and can be used concomitantly.

Because collateral blood flow within the ischemic brain is blood pressure dependent, there is controversy about whether blood pressure should be lowered acutely. Blood pressure should be lowered if there is malignant hypertension or concomitant myocardial ischemia or if blood pressure is >185/110 mmHg and thrombolytic therapy is anticipated. When faced with the competing demands of myocardium and brain, lowering the heart rate with a β_1-adrenergic blocker (such as esmolol) can be a first step to decrease cardiac work and maintain blood pressure. Fever is detrimental and should be treated with antipyretics and surface cooling. Serum glucose should be monitored and kept at <6.1 mmol/L (110 mg/dL) using an insulin infusion if necessary.

Between 5 and 10% of patients develop enough cerebral edema to cause obtundation or brain herniation. Edema peaks on the second or third day but can cause mass effect for ~10 days. The larger the infarct, the greater the likelihood that clinically significant edema will develop. Water restriction and IV mannitol may be used to raise the serum osmolarity, but hypovolemia should be avoided as this may contribute to hypotension and worsening infarction. Combined analysis of three randomized European trials of hemicraniectomy (craniotomy and temporary removal of part of the skull) shows that hemicraniectomy markedly reduces mortality, and the clinical outcomes of survivors are acceptable.

Special vigilance is warranted for patients with cerebellar infarction. Such strokes may mimic labyrinthitis because of prominent vertigo and vomiting; the presence of head or neck pain should alert the physician to consider cerebellar stroke from vertebral artery dissection. Even small amounts of cerebellar edema can acutely increase intracranial pressure (ICP) or directly compress the brainstem. The resulting brainstem compression can result in coma and respiratory arrest and require emergency surgical decompression. Prophylactic suboccipital decompression of large cerebellar infarcts before brainstem compression, although not tested rigorously in a clinical trial, is practiced at most stroke centers.

INTRAVENOUS THROMBOLYSIS The National Institute of Neurological Disorders and Stroke (NINDS) recombinant tPA (rtPA) Stroke Study showed a clear benefit for IV rtPA in selected patients with acute stroke. The NINDS study used IV rtPA (0.9 mg/kg to a 90-mg max; 10% as a bolus, then the remainder over 60 min) versus placebo in patients with ischemic stroke within 3 h of onset. One-half of the patients were treated within 90 min. Symptomatic intracerebral hemorrhage occurred in 6.4% of patients on rtPA and 0.6% on placebo. There was a nonsignificant 4% reduction in mortality in patients on rtPA (21% on placebo and 17% on rtPA); there was a significant 12% absolute increase in the number of patients with only minimal disability (32% on placebo and 44% on rtPA). Thus, despite an increased incidence of symptomatic intracerebral hemorrhage, treatment with IV rtPA within 3 h of the onset of ischemic stroke improved clinical outcome.

Three subsequent trials of IV rtPA did not confirm this benefit, perhaps because of the dose of rtPA used, the timing of its delivery, and small sample size. When data from all randomized IV rtPA trails were combined, however, efficacy was confirmed in the <3-h time window, and efficacy likely extended to 4.5 h if not 6 h. Based on these combined results, the European Cooperative Acute Stroke Study (ECASS) III study explored the safety and efficacy of rtPA in the 3- to 4.5-h time window. Unlike the NINDS study, patients older than 85 years of age and diabetic patients were excluded. In this 821-patient, randomized study efficacy was again confirmed, although less robust than in the 0–3 h time window. In the rtPA group, 52.4% achieved a good outcome while 45.2% of the placebo group had a good outcome at 90 days (OR 1.34, $p = 0.04$). The symptomatic intracranial hemorrhage rate was 2.4% in the rtPA group and 0.2% in the placebo group ($p = 0.008$).

Based on these data, rtPA is being reviewed for approval in the 3–4.5-h window in Europe, but is only approved for 0–3 h in the United States and Canada. Use of IV tPA is now considered a central component of primary stroke centers (see later) as the first treatment proven to improve clinical outcomes in ischemic stroke and is cost-effective and cost-saving. One may be able to select patients beyond the 4.5-h window, who will benefit from thrombolysis using advanced neuroimaging (see neuroimaging section), but this is currently investigational. The time of stroke onset is defined as the time the patient's symptoms began or the time the patient was last seen as normal. Patients who awaken with stroke have the onset defined as when they went to bed. Table 27-1 summarizes eligibility criteria and instructions for administration of IV rtPA.

ENDOVASCULAR TECHNIQUES Ischemic stroke from large-vessel intracranial occlusion results in high rates of mortality and morbidity. Occlusions in such large vessels (middle cerebral artery [MCA], internal carotid artery, and the basilar artery) generally involve a large clot volume and often fail to open with IV rtPA alone. Therefore, there is growing interest in using thrombolytics via an intraarterial route to increase the concentration of drug at the clot and minimize systemic bleeding complications. The Prolyse in Acute Cerebral Thromboembolism (PROACT) II trial found benefit for intraarterial pro urokinase for acute MCA occlusions up to the sixth hour following onset of stroke. Intraarterial treatment of basilar artery occlusions may also be beneficial for selected patients. Intraarterial administration of a thrombolytic agent for acute ischemic stroke (AIS) is not approved by the U.S. Food and Drug Administration

TABLE 27-1

ADMINISTRATION OF INTRAVENOUS RECOMBINANT TISSUE PLASMINOGEN ACTIVATOR (rtPA) FOR ACUTE ISCHEMIC STROKE (AIS)[a]

INDICATION	CONTRAINDICATION
Clinical diagnosis of stroke	Sustained BP >185/110 mmHg despite treatment
Onset of symptoms to time of drug administration ≤3 h	Platelets <100,000; HCT <25%; glucose <50 or >400 mg/dL
CT scan showing no hemorrhage or edema of >1/3 of the MCA territory	Use of heparin within 48 h and prolonged PTT, or elevated INR
Age ≥18 years	Rapidly improving symptoms
Consent by patient or surrogate	Prior stroke or head injury within 3 months; prior intracranial hemorrhage
	Major surgery in preceding 14 days
	Minor stroke symptoms
	Gastrointestinal bleeding in preceding 21 days
	Recent myocardial infarction
	Coma or stupor

Administration of rtPA

Intravenous access with two peripheral IV lines (avoid arterial or central line placement)

Review eligibility for rtPA

Administer 0.9 mg/kg IV (maximum 90 mg) IV as 10% of total dose by bolus, followed by remainder of total dose over 1 h

Frequent cuff blood pressure monitoring

No other antithrombotic treatment for 24 h

For decline in neurologic status or uncontrolled blood pressure, stop infusion, give cryoprecipitate, and reimage brain emergently

Avoid urethral catheterization for ≥2 h

[a]See Activase (tissue plasminogen activator) package insert for complete list of contraindications and dosing.

Abbreviations: BP, blood pressure; HCT, hematocrit; INR, international normalized ratio; MCA, middle cerebral artery; PTT, partial thromboplastin time.

(FDA); however, many stroke centers offer this treatment based on these data.

Endovascular mechanical thrombectomy has recently shown promise as an alternative or adjunctive treatment of acute stroke in patients who are ineligible for, or have contraindications to, thrombolytics or in those who have failed to have vascular recanalization with IV thrombolytics (see Fig. 27-15). The Mechanical Embolus Removal in Cerebral Ischemia (MERCI) and multi-MERCI single-arm trials investigated the ability of a novel endovascular thrombectomy device to restore patency of occluded intracranial vessels within 8 h of ischemic stroke symptoms. Recanalization of the target vessel occurred in 48–58% of treated patients and in 60–69% following use of adjuvant endovascular methods, and successful recanalization at 90 days correlated well with favorable outcomes. Based upon these nonrandomized data, the FDA approved this device as the first device for revascularization of occluded vessels in acute ischemic stroke even if the patient has been given rtPA and that therapy has failed. The Penumbra Pivotal Stroke trial tested another mechanical device that showed even higher rates of recanalization and led to FDA clearance of the tested device as well. Because use of endovascular devices in combination with rtPA appears safe, primary stroke centers may administer rtPA to eligible patients, and then rapidly refer such patients to comprehensive stroke centers that have endovascular capability for further intervention. Such a design allows centralization of resource-intensive endovascular centers in order to serve larger populations of patients. Use of mechanical techniques to restore blood flow have not as yet been studied in a randomized trial so the clinical efficacy of these treatments remain unproven and the focus of active investigation.

ANTITHROMBOTIC TREATMENT

Platelet Inhibition Aspirin is the only antiplatelet agent that has been proven effective for the acute treatment of ischemic stroke; there are several antiplatelet agents proven for the secondary prevention of stroke (see later). Two large trials, the International Stroke Trial (IST) and the Chinese Acute Stroke Trial (CAST), found that the use of aspirin within 48 h of stroke onset reduced both stroke recurrence risk and mortality minimally. Among 19,435 patients in IST, those allocated to aspirin, 300 mg/d, had slightly fewer deaths within 14 days (9.0 versus 9.4%), significantly fewer recurrent ischemic strokes (2.8 versus 3.9%), no excess of hemorrhagic strokes (0.9 versus 0.8%), and a trend toward a reduction in death or dependence at 6 months (61.2 versus 63.5%). In CAST, 21,106 patients with ischemic stroke received 160 mg/d of aspirin or a placebo for up to 4 weeks. There were very small reductions in the aspirin group in early mortality (3.3 versus 3.9%), recurrent ischemic strokes (1.6 versus 2.1%), and dependency at discharge or death (30.5 versus 31.6%). These trials demonstrate that the use of aspirin in the treatment of AIS is safe and produces a small net benefit. For every 1000 acute strokes treated with aspirin, about 9 deaths or nonfatal stroke recurrences will be prevented in the first few weeks and ~13 fewer patients will be dead or dependent at 6 months.

The glycoprotein IIb/IIIa receptor inhibitor abciximab was found to cause excess intracranial hemorrhage and should be avoided in acute stroke. Clopidogrel is being tested as a way to prevent stroke following TIA and minor ischemic stroke.

Anticoagulation Numerous clinical trials have failed to demonstrate any benefit of anticoagulation in the primary treatment of atherothrombotic cerebral ischemia. Several trials have investigated antiplatelet versus anticoagulant medications given within 12–24 h of the initial event. The U.S. Trial of Organon 10172 in Acute Stroke Treatment (TOAST), an investigational low-molecular-weight heparin (LMWH), failed to show any benefit over aspirin. Use of SC unfractionated heparin versus aspirin was tested in IST. Heparin given SC afforded no additional benefit over aspirin and increased bleeding rates. Several trials of LMWHs have also shown no consistent benefit in AIS. Furthermore, trials generally have shown an excess risk of brain and systemic hemorrhage with acute anticoagulation. Therefore, trials do not support the routine use of heparin or other anticoagulants for patients with atherothrombotic stroke.

NEUROPROTECTION Neuroprotection is the concept of providing a treatment that prolongs the brain's tolerance to ischemia. Drugs that block the excitatory amino acid pathways have been shown to protect neurons and glia in animals, but despite multiple human trials, they have not yet been proven to be beneficial. Hypothermia is a powerful neuroprotective treatment in patients with cardiac arrest (Chap. 28) and is neuroprotective in animal models of stroke, but it has not been adequately studied in patients with ischemic stroke.

STROKE CENTERS AND REHABILITATION Patient care in comprehensive stroke units followed by rehabilitation services improves neurologic outcomes and reduces mortality. Use of clinical pathways and staff dedicated to the stroke patient can improve care. Stroke teams that provide emergency 24-h evaluation of acute stroke patients for acute medical management and consideration of thrombolysis or endovascular treatments are essential components of primary and comprehensive stroke centers, respectively.

Proper rehabilitation of the stroke patient includes early physical, occupational, and speech therapy. It is directed toward educating the patient and family about the patient's neurologic deficit, preventing the complications of immobility (e.g., pneumonia, DVT and pulmonary embolism, pressure sores of the skin, and muscle contractures), and providing encouragement and instruction in overcoming the deficit. The goal of rehabilitation is to return the patient to home and to maximize recovery by providing a safe, progressive regimen suited to the individual patient. Additionally, the use of restraint therapy (immobilizing the unaffected side) has been shown to improve hemiparesis following stroke, even years following the stroke, suggesting that physical therapy can recruit unused neural pathways. This finding suggests that the human nervous system is more adaptable than originally thought and has stimulated active research into physical and pharmacologic strategies that can enhance long-term neural recovery.

ETIOLOGY OF ISCHEMIC STROKE

(Figs. 27-1 and 27-3 and Table 27-2) Although the initial management of AIS often does not depend on the etiology, establishing a cause is essential in reducing the risk of recurrence. Particular focus should be on atrial fibrillation and carotid atherosclerosis, as these etiologies have proven secondary prevention strategies. The clinical presentation and examination findings often establish the cause of stroke or narrow the possibilities to a few. Judicious use of laboratory testing and imaging studies completes the initial evaluation. Nevertheless, nearly 30% of strokes remain unexplained despite extensive evaluation.

Clinical examination should focus on the peripheral and cervical vascular system (carotid auscultation for bruits, blood pressure, and pressure comparison between arms), the heart (dysrhythmia, murmurs), extremities (peripheral emboli), and retina (effects of hypertension and cholesterol emboli [Hollenhorst plaques]). A complete neurologic examination is performed to localize the site of stroke. An imaging study of the brain is nearly always indicated and is required for patients being considered for thrombolysis; it may be combined with CT- or MRI-based angiography to interrogate the neck and intracranial vessels (see "Imaging Studies"). A chest x-ray, electrocardiogram (ECG), urinalysis, complete blood count, erythrocyte sedimentation rate (ESR), serum electrolytes, blood urea nitrogen (BUN), creatinine, blood sugar, serologic test for syphilis, serum lipid profile, prothrombin time (PT), and partial thromboplastin time (PTT) are often useful and should be considered in all patients. An ECG may demonstrate arrhythmias or reveal evidence of recent myocardial infarction (MI).

Cardioembolic stroke

Cardioembolism is responsible for ~20% of all ischemic strokes. Stroke caused by heart disease is primarily due

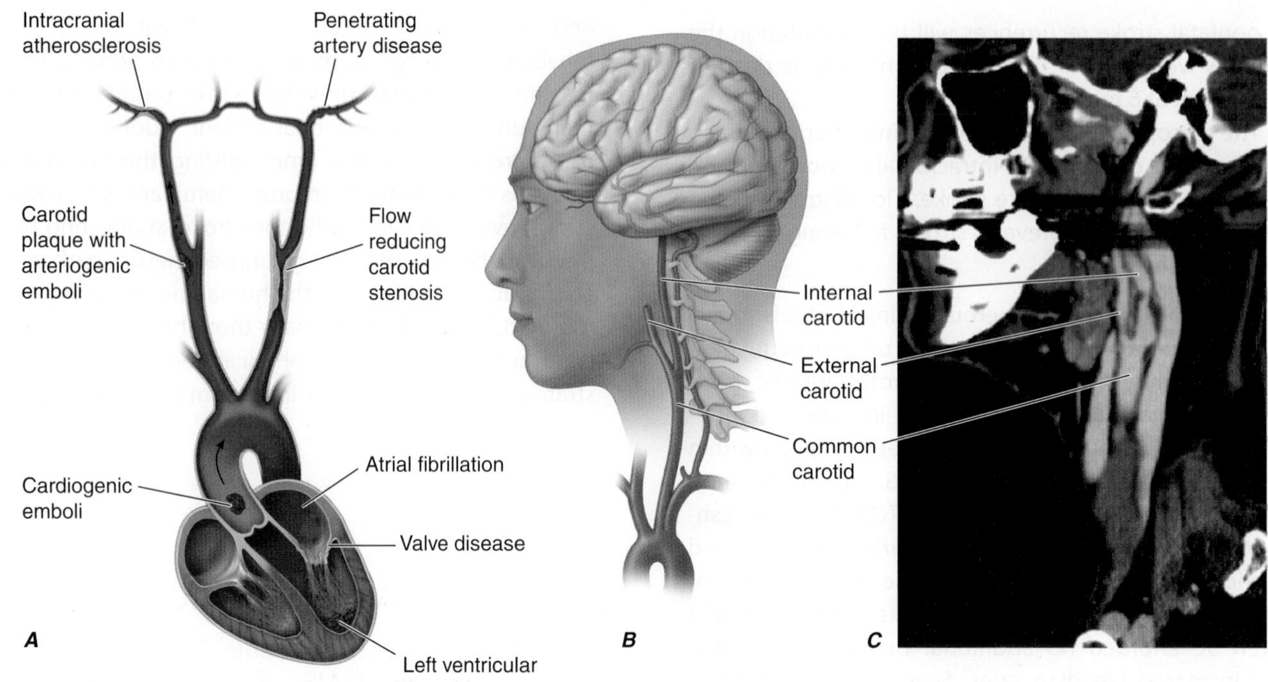

FIGURE 27-3

Pathophysiology of ischemic stroke. ***A.*** Diagram illustrating the three major mechanisms that underlie ischemic stroke: (1) occlusion of an intracranial vessel by an embolus that arises at a distant site (e.g., cardiogenic sources such as atrial fibrillation or artery-to-artery emboli from carotid atherosclerotic plaque), often affecting the large intracranial vessels; (2) in situ thrombosis of an intracranial vessel, typically affecting the small penetrating arteries that arise from the major intracranial arteries; and (3) hypoperfusion caused by flow-limiting stenosis of a major extracranial (e.g., internal carotid) or intracranial vessel, often producing "watershed" ischemia. ***B*** and ***C.*** Diagram and reformatted CT angiogram of the common, internal, and external carotid arteries. High-grade stenosis of the internal carotid artery, which may be associated with either cerebral emboli or flow-limiting ischemia, was identified in this patient.

to embolism of thrombotic material forming on the atrial or ventricular wall or the left heart valves. These thrombi then detach and embolize into the arterial circulation. The thrombus may fragment or lyse quickly, producing only a TIA. Alternatively, the arterial occlusion may last longer, producing stroke. Embolic strokes tend to be sudden in onset, with maximum neurologic deficit at once. With reperfusion following more prolonged ischemia, petechial hemorrhage can occur within the ischemic territory. This is usually of no clinical significance and should be distinguished from frank intracranial hemorrhage into a region of ischemic stroke where the mass effect from the hemorrhage can cause a decline in neurologic function.

Emboli from the heart most often lodge in the MCA, the posterior cerebral artery (PCA), or one of their branches; infrequently, the anterior cerebral artery (ACA) territory is involved. Emboli large enough to occlude the stem of the MCA (3–4 mm) lead to large infarcts that involve both deep gray and white matter and some portions of the cortical surface and its underlying white matter. A smaller embolus may occlude a small cortical or penetrating arterial branch. The location and size of an infarct within a vascular territory depend on the extent of the collateral circulation.

The most significant causes of cardioembolic stroke in most of the world are nonrheumatic (often called nonvalvular) atrial fibrillation, MI, prosthetic valves, rheumatic heart disease, and ischemic cardiomyopathy (Table 27-2). Cardiac disorders causing brain embolism are discussed in the respective chapters on heart diseases. A few pertinent aspects are highlighted here.

Nonrheumatic atrial fibrillation is the most common cause of cerebral embolism overall. The presumed stroke mechanism is thrombus formation in the fibrillating atrium or atrial appendage, with subsequent embolization. Patients with atrial fibrillation have an average annual risk of stroke of ~5%. The risk of stroke can be estimated by calculating the CHADS2 score (see Table 27-3). Left atrial enlargement is an additional risk factor for formation of atrial thrombi. Rheumatic heart disease usually causes ischemic stroke when there is prominent mitral stenosis or atrial fibrillation. Recent MI may be a source of emboli, especially when transmural and involving the anteroapical ventricular wall, and prophylactic anticoagulation following MI has been shown to

TABLE 27-2

CAUSES OF ISCHEMIC STROKE

COMMON CAUSES	UNCOMMON CAUSES
Thrombosis	Hypercoagulable disorders
Lacunar stroke (small vessel)	Protein C deficiency
Large vessel thrombosis	Protein S deficiency
Dehydration	Antithrombin III deficiency
Embolic occlusion	Antiphospholipid syndrome
Artery-to-artery	Factor V Leiden mutation[a]
Carotid bifurcation	Prothrombin G20210 mutation[a]
Aortic arch	Systemic malignancy
Arterial dissection	Sickle cell anemia
Cardioembolic	β-Thalassemia
Atrial fibrillation	Polycythemia vera
Mural thrombus	Systemic lupus erythematosus
Myocardial infarction	Homocysteinemia
Dilated cardiomyopathy	Thrombotic thrombocytopenic purpura
Valvular lesions	Disseminated intravascular coagulation
Mitral stenosis	Dysproteinemias
Mechanical valve	Nephrotic syndrome
Bacterial endocarditis	Inflammatory bowel disease
Paradoxical embolus	Oral contraceptives
Atrial septal defect	Venous sinus thrombosis[b]
Patent foramen ovale	Fibromuscular dysplasia
Atrial septal aneurysm	Vasculitis
Spontaneous echo contrast	Systemic vasculitis (PAN, granulomatosis with polyangiitis [Wegener's], Takayasu's, giant cell arteritis)
	Primary CNS vasculitis
	Meningitis (syphilis, tuberculosis, fungal, bacterial, zoster)
	Cardiogenic
	Mitral valve calcification
	Atrial myxoma
	Intracardiac tumor
	Marantic endocarditis
	Libman-Sacks endocarditis
	Subarachnoid hemorrhage vasospasm
	Drugs: cocaine, amphetamine
	Moyamoya disease
	Eclampsia

[a]Chiefly cause venous sinus thrombosis.

[b]May be associated with any hypercoagulable disorder.

Abbreviations: CNS, central nervous system; PAN, polyarteritis nodosa.

reduce stroke risk. Mitral valve prolapse is not usually a source of emboli unless the prolapse is severe.

Paradoxical embolization occurs when venous thrombi migrate to the arterial circulation, usually via a patent foramen ovale or atrial septal defect. Bubble-contrast echocardiography (IV injection of agitated saline coupled with either transthoracic or transesophageal echocardiography) can demonstrate a right-to-left cardiac shunt, revealing the conduit for paradoxical embolization. Alternatively, a right-to-left shunt is implied if immediately following IV injection of agitated saline, the ultrasound signature of bubbles is observed during transcranial Doppler insonation of the MCA; pulmonary AVMs should be considered if this test is positive yet an echocardiogram fails to reveal an intracardiac shunt. Both techniques are highly sensitive for detection of right-to-left shunts. Besides venous clot, fat and tumor emboli, bacterial endocarditis, IV air, and amniotic fluid emboli at childbirth may occasionally be responsible for paradoxical embolization. The importance of right-to-left shunt as a cause of stroke is debated, particularly because such shunts are present in ~15% of the general population. Some studies have suggested that the risk is only elevated in the presence of a coexisting atrial septal aneurysm. The presence of a venous source of embolus, most commonly a deep venous thrombus, may provide confirmation of the importance of a right-to-left shunt in a particular case.

Bacterial endocarditis can cause valvular vegetations that can give rise to septic emboli. The appearance of multifocal symptoms and signs in a patient with stroke makes bacterial endocarditis more likely. Infarcts of microscopic size occur, and large septic infarcts may evolve into brain abscesses or cause hemorrhage into the infarct, which generally precludes use of anticoagulation or thrombolytics. Mycotic aneurysms caused by septic emboli give rise to SAH or intracerebral hemorrhage.

Artery-to-artery embolic stroke

Thrombus formation on atherosclerotic plaques may embolize to intracranial arteries producing an artery-to-artery embolic stroke. Less commonly, a diseased vessel may acutely thrombose. Unlike the myocardial vessels, artery-to-artery embolism, rather than local thrombosis, appears to be the dominant vascular mechanism causing brain ischemia. Any diseased vessel may be an embolic source, including the aortic arch, common carotid, internal carotid, vertebral, and basilar arteries. Carotid bifurcation atherosclerosis is the most common source of artery-to-artery embolus, and specific treatments have proven efficacy in reducing risk.

Carotid atherosclerosis

Atherosclerosis within the carotid artery occurs most frequently within the common carotid bifurcation and proximal internal carotid artery. Additionally, the carotid siphon (portion within the cavernous sinus) is

TABLE 27-3

RECOMMENDATIONS ON CHRONIC USE OF ANTITHROMBOTICS FOR VARIOUS CARDIAC CONDITIONS

CONDITION	RECOMMENDATION
Nonvalvular atrial fibrillation	Calculate CHADS2[a] score
• CHADS2 score 0	Aspirin or no antithrombotic
• CHADS2 score 1	Aspirin or VKA
• CHADS2 score >1	VKA
Rheumatic mitral valve disease	
• With atrial fibrillation, previous embolization, or atrial appendage thrombus, or left atrial diameter >55 mm	VKA
• Embolization or appendage clot despite INR 2–3	VKA plus aspirin
Mitral valve prolapse	
• Asymptomatic	No therapy
• With otherwise cryptogenic stroke or TIA	Aspirin
• Atrial fibrillation	VKA
Mitral annular calcification	
• Without atrial fibrillation but systemic embolization, or otherwise cryptogenic stroke or TIA	Aspirin
• Recurrent embolization despite aspirin	VKA
• With atrial fibrillation	VKA
Aortic valve calcification	
• Asymptomatic	No therapy
• Otherwise cryptogenic stroke or TIA	Aspirin
Aortic arch mobile atheroma	
• Otherwise cryptogenic stroke or TIA	Aspirin or VKA
Patent foramen ovale	
• Otherwise cryptogenic ischemic stroke or TIA	Aspirin
• Indication for VKA (deep venous thrombosis or hypercoagulable state)	VKA
Mechanical heart value	
• Aortic position, bileaflet or Medtronic Hall tilting disk with normal left atrial size and sinus rhythm	VKA INR 2.5, range 2–3
• Mitral position tilting disk or bileaflet valve	VKA INR 3.0, range 2.5–3.5
• Mitral or aortic position, anterior-apical myocardial infarct or left atrial enlargement	VKA INR 3.0, range 2.5–3.5
• Mitral or aortic position, with atrial fibrillation, or hypercoagulable state, or low ejection fraction, or atherosclerotic vascular disease	Aspirin plus VKA INR 3.0, range 2.5–3.5
• Systemic embolization despite target INR	Add aspirin and/or increase INR: prior target was 2.5 increase to 3.0, range 2.5–3.5; prior target was 3.0 increase to 3.5, range 3–4
Bioprosthetic valve	
• No other indication for VKA therapy	Aspirin
Infective endocarditis	Avoid antithrombotic agents
Nonbacterial thrombotic endocarditis	
• With systemic embolization	Full-dose unfractionated heparin or SC LMWH

[a]CHADS2 score calculated as follows: 1 point for age >75 years, 1 point for hypertension, 1 point for congestive heart failure, 1 point for diabetes, and 2 points for stroke or TIA; sum of points is the total CHADS2 score.

Abbreviations: Dose of aspirin is 50–325 mg/d; target INR for VKA is 2.5 unless otherwise specified. INR, international normalized ratio; LMWH, low-molecular-weight heparin; TIA, transient ischemic attack; VKA, vitamin K antagonist.

Sources: Modified from DE Singer et al: Chest 133:546S, 2008; DN Salem et al: Chest 133:593S, 2008.

also vulnerable to atherosclerosis. Male gender, older age, smoking, hypertension, diabetes, and hypercholesterolemia are risk factors for carotid disease, as they are for stroke in general (Table 27-4). Carotid atherosclerosis produces an estimated 10% of ischemic stroke.

Carotid disease can be classified by whether the stenosis is symptomatic or asymptomatic and by the degree of stenosis (percent narrowing of the narrowest segment compared to a more distal internal carotid segment). Symptomatic carotid disease implies that the patient has experienced a stroke or TIA within the vascular distribution of the artery, and it is associated with a greater risk of subsequent stroke than asymptomatic stenosis, in which the patient is symptom free and the stenosis is detected through screening. Greater degrees of arterial narrowing are generally associated with a greater risk of stroke, except that those with near occlusions are at lower risk of stroke.

Other causes of artery-to-artery embolic stroke

Intracranial atherosclerosis produces stroke either by an embolic mechanism or by in situ thrombosis of a diseased vessel. It is more common in patients of Asian and African-American descent. Recurrent stroke risk is ~15% per year, similar to symptomatic untreated carotid atherosclerosis.

Dissection of the internal carotid or vertebral arteries or even vessels beyond the circle of Willis is a common source of embolic stroke in young (age <60 years) patients. The dissection is usually painful and precedes the stroke by several hours or days. Extracranial dissections do not cause hemorrhage because of the tough adventitia of these vessels. Intracranial dissections, conversely, may produce SAH because the adventitia of intracranial vessels is thin and pseudoaneurysms may form, requiring urgent treatment to prevent rerupture. Treating asymptomatic pseudoaneurysms following dissection is controversial. The cause of dissection is usually unknown and recurrence is rare. Ehlers-Danlos type IV, Marfan's disease, cystic medial necrosis, and fibromuscular dysplasia are associated with dissections. Trauma (usually a motor vehicle accident or a sports injury) can cause carotid and vertebral artery dissections. Spinal manipulative therapy is independently associated with vertebral artery dissection and stroke. Most dissections heal spontaneously, and stroke or TIA is uncommon beyond 2 weeks. Although there are no trials comparing anticoagulation to antiplatelet agents, many physicians treat acutely with anticoagulants then convert to antiplatelet therapy after demonstration of satisfactory vascular recanalization.

SMALL-VESSEL STROKE

The term *lacunar infarction* refers to infarction following atherothrombotic or lipohyalinotic occlusion of a small artery (30–300 μm) in the brain. The term *small-vessel stroke* denotes occlusion of such a small penetrating artery and is now the preferred term. Small-vessel strokes account for ~20% of all strokes.

Pathophysiology

The MCA stem, the arteries comprising the circle of Willis (A1 segment, anterior and posterior communicating arteries, and P1 segment), and the basilar and vertebral arteries all give rise to 30- to 300-μm branches that penetrate the deep gray and white matter of the cerebrum or brainstem (Fig. 27-4). Each of these small branches can occlude either by atherothrombotic disease at its origin or by the development of

TABLE 27-4

RISK FACTORS FOR STROKE

RISK FACTOR	RELATIVE RISK	RELATIVE RISK REDUCTION WITH TREATMENT	NUMBER NEEDED TO TREAT[a]: PRIMARY PREVENTION	NUMBER NEEDED TO TREAT[a]: SECONDARY PREVENTION
Hypertension	2–5	38%	100–300	50–100
Atrial fibrillation	1.8–2.9	68% warfarin, 21% aspirin	20–83	13
Diabetes	1.8–6	No proven effect		
Smoking	1.8	50% at 1 year, baseline risk at 5 years' postcessation		
Hyperlipidemia	1.8–2.6	16–30%	560	230
Asymptomatic carotid stenosis	2.0	53%	85	N/A
Symptomatic carotid stenosis (70–99%)		65% at 2 years	N/A	12
Symptomatic carotid stenosis (50–69%)		29% at 5 years	N/A	77

[a]Number needed to treat to prevent one stroke annually. Prevention of other cardiovascular outcomes is not considered here.
Abbreviation: N/A, not applicable.

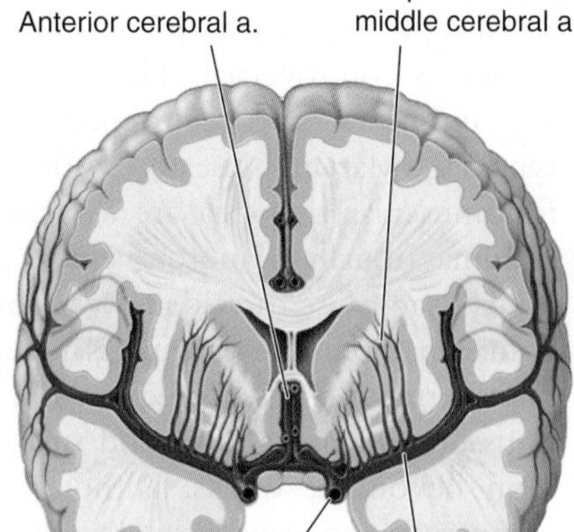

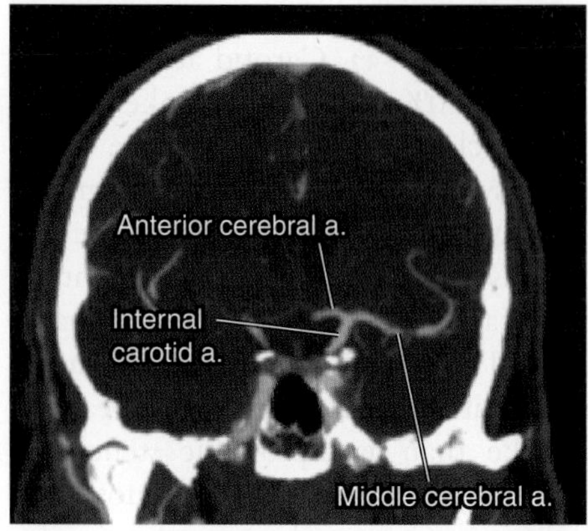

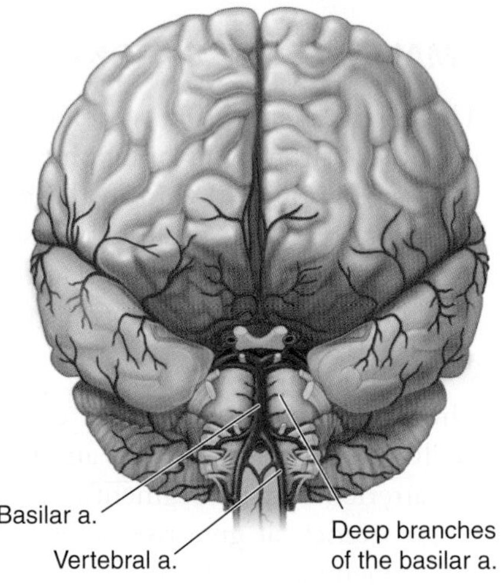

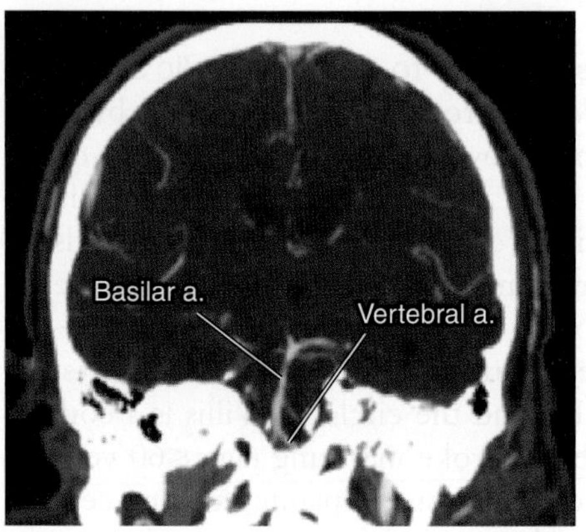

FIGURE 27-4

Diagrams and reformatted CT angiograms in the coronal section illustrating the deep penetrating arteries involved in small-vessel strokes. In the anterior circulation, small penetrating arteries called *lenticulostriates* arise from the proximal portion of the anterior and middle cerebral arteries and supply deep subcortical structures (***upper panels***). In the posterior circulation, similar arteries arise directly from the vertebral and basilar arteries to supply the brainstem (***lower panels***). Occlusion of a single penetrating artery gives rise to a discrete area of infarct (pathologically termed a "lacune," or lake). Note that these vessels are too small to be visualized on CT angiography.

lipohyalinotic thickening. Thrombosis of these vessels causes small infarcts that are referred to as *lacunes* (Latin for "lake" of fluid noted at autopsy). These infarcts range in size from 3 mm to 2 cm in diameter. Hypertension and age are the principal risk factors.

Clinical manifestations

The most common *lacunar syndromes* are the following: (1) *pure motor hemiparesis* from an infarct in the posterior limb of the internal capsule or basis pontis; the face, arm, and leg are almost always involved; (2) *pure sensory stroke* from an infarct in the ventral thalamus; (3) *ataxic hemiparesis* from an infarct in the ventral pons or internal capsule; and (4) *dysarthria and a clumsy hand* or arm due to infarction in the ventral pons or in the genu of the internal capsule.

Transient symptoms (small-vessel TIAs) may herald a small-vessel infarct; they may occur several times a day and last only a few minutes. Recovery from small-vessel strokes tends to be more rapid and complete than recovery from large-vessel strokes; in some cases, however, there is severe permanent disability. Often, institution of combined antithrombotic treatments does not prevent eventual stroke in "stuttering lacunes."

A large-vessel source (either thrombosis or embolism) may manifest initially as a lacunar syndrome with small-vessel infarction. Therefore, the search for embolic sources (carotid and heart) should not be completely abandoned in the evaluation of these patients. Secondary prevention of lacunar stroke involves risk factor modification, specifically reduction in blood pressure (see "Primary and Secondary Prevention of Stroke and TIA").

LESS COMMON CAUSES OF STROKE

(Table 27-2) *Hypercoagulable disorders* primarily cause increased risk of venous thrombosis and therefore may cause venous sinus thrombosis. Protein S deficiency and homocysteinemia may cause arterial thromboses as well. Systemic lupus erythematosus with Libman-Sacks endocarditis can be a cause of embolic stroke. These conditions overlap with the antiphospholipid syndrome, which probably requires long-term anticoagulation to prevent further stroke.

Venous sinus thrombosis of the lateral or sagittal sinus or of small cortical veins (cortical vein thrombosis) occurs as a complication of oral contraceptive use, pregnancy and the postpartum period, inflammatory bowel disease, intracranial infections (meningitis), and dehydration. It is also seen with increased incidence in patients with laboratory-confirmed thrombophilia (Table 27-2) including polycythemia, sickle cell anemia, deficiencies of proteins C and S, factor V Leiden mutation (resistance to activated protein C), antithrombin III deficiency, homocysteinemia, and the prothrombin G20210 mutation. Women who take oral contraceptives and have the prothrombin G20210 mutation may be at particularly high risk for sinus thrombosis. Patients present with headache and may also have focal neurologic signs (especially paraparesis) and seizures. Often, CT imaging is normal unless an intracranial venous hemorrhage has occurred, but the venous sinus occlusion is readily visualized using MR- or CT-venography or conventional x-ray angiography. With greater degrees of sinus thrombosis, the patient may develop signs of increased ICP and coma. Intravenous heparin, regardless of the presence of intracranial hemorrhage, has been shown to reduce morbidity and mortality, and the long-term outcome is generally good. Heparin prevents further thrombosis and reduces venous hypertension and ischemia. If an underlying hypercoagulable state is not found, many physicians treat with vitamin K antagonists (VKAs) for 3–6 months then convert to aspirin, depending on the degree of resolution of the venous sinus thrombus. Anticoagulation is often continued indefinitely if thrombophilia is diagnosed.

Sickle cell anemia (SS disease) is a common cause of stroke in children. A subset of homozygous carriers of this hemoglobin mutation develop stroke in childhood, and this may be predicted by documenting high-velocity blood flow within the MCAs using transcranial Doppler ultrasonography. In children who are identified to have high velocities, treatment with aggressive exchange transfusion dramatically reduces risk of stroke, and if exchange transfusion is ceased, their stroke rate increases again along with MCA velocities.

Fibromuscular dysplasia affects the cervical arteries and occurs mainly in women. The carotid or vertebral arteries show multiple rings of segmental narrowing alternating with dilatation. Occlusion is usually incomplete. The process is often asymptomatic but occasionally is associated with an audible bruit, TIAs, or stroke. Involvement of the renal arteries is common and may cause hypertension. The cause and natural history of fibromuscular dysplasia are unknown. TIA or stroke generally occurs only when the artery is severely narrowed or dissects. Anticoagulation or antiplatelet therapy may be helpful.

Temporal (giant cell) arteritis is a relatively common affliction of elderly persons in which the external carotid system, particularly the temporal arteries, undergo subacute granulomatous inflammation with giant cells. Occlusion of posterior ciliary arteries derived from the ophthalmic artery results in blindness in one or both eyes and can be prevented with glucocorticoids. It rarely causes stroke as the internal carotid artery is usually not inflamed. Idiopathic giant cell arteritis involving the great vessels arising from the aortic arch (*Takayasu's arteritis*) may cause carotid or vertebral thrombosis; it is rare in the Western hemisphere.

Necrotizing (or granulomatous) arteritis, occurring alone or in association with generalized polyarteritis nodosa or granulomatosis with polyangiitis (Wegener's), involves the distal small branches (<2 mm diameter) of the main intracranial arteries and produces small ischemic infarcts in the brain, optic nerve, and spinal cord. The cerebrospinal fluid (CSF) often shows pleocytosis, and the protein level is elevated. *Primary central nervous system vasculitis* is rare; small or medium-sized vessels are usually affected, without apparent systemic vasculitis. The differential diagnosis includes other inflammatory causes of vascular caliber change including infection (tubercular, fungal), sarcoidosis, angiocentric lymphoma, carcinomatous meningitis, as well as noninflammatory causes such as atherosclerosis, emboli, connective tissue disease, vasospasm, migraine-associated vasculopathy, and drug-associated causes. Some cases follow the postpartum period and are self-limited.

Patients with any form of vasculopathy may present with insidious progression of combined white and gray matter infarctions, prominent headache, and cognitive decline. Brain biopsy or high-resolution conventional x-ray angiography is usually required to make the diagnosis (Fig. 27-5). An inflammatory profile found on lumbar puncture favors an inflammatory cause. In cases where inflammation is confirmed, aggressive immunosuppression with glucocorticoids, and often cyclophosphamide, is usually necessary to prevent progression; a diligent investigation for infectious causes such

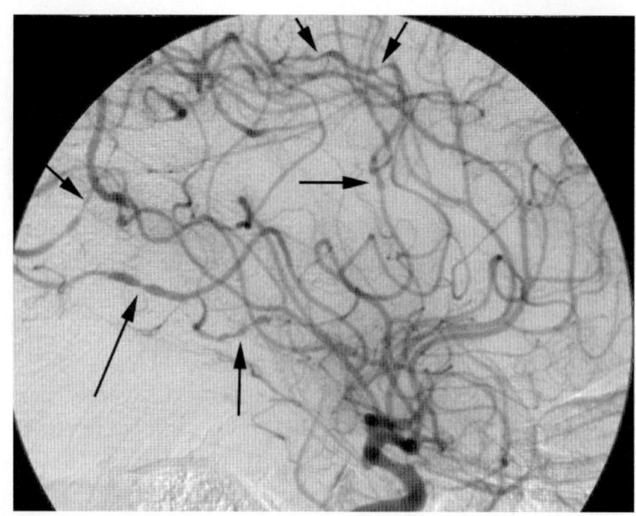

FIGURE 27-5
Cerebral angiogram from a 32-year-old male with central nervous system vasculopathy. Dramatic beading (*arrows*) typical of vasculopathy is seen.

as tuberculosis is essential prior to immunosuppression. With prompt recognition and treatment, many patients can make an excellent recovery.

Drugs, in particular amphetamines and perhaps cocaine, may cause stroke on the basis of acute hypertension or drug-induced vasculopathy. No data exist on the value of any treatment. Phenylpropanolamine has been linked with intracranial hemorrhage, as has cocaine and methamphetamine, perhaps related to a drug-induced vasculopathy. *Moyamoya disease* is a poorly understood occlusive disease involving large intracranial arteries, especially the distal internal carotid artery and the stem of the MCA and ACA. Vascular inflammation is absent. The lenticulostriate arteries develop a rich collateral circulation around the occlusive lesion, which gives the impression of a "puff of smoke" (*moyamoya* in Japanese) on conventional x-ray angiography. Other collaterals include transdural anastomoses between the cortical surface branches of the meningeal and scalp arteries. The disease occurs mainly in Asian children or young adults, but the appearance may be identical in adults who have atherosclerosis, particularly in association with diabetes. Because of the occurrence of intracranial hemorrhage from rupture of the transdural and pial anastomotic channels, anticoagulation is risky. Breakdown of dilated lenticulostriate arteries may produce parenchymal hemorrhage, and progressive occlusion of large surface arteries can occur, producing large-artery distribution strokes. Surgical bypass of extracranial carotid arteries to the dura or MCAs may prevent stroke and hemorrhage.

Reversible posterior leukoencephalopathy can occur in head injury, seizure, migraine, sympathomimetic drug use, eclampsia, and the postpartum period. The pathophysiology is uncertain but likely involves widespread cerebral segmental vasoconstriction and cerebral edema. Patients complain of headache and manifest fluctuating neurologic symptoms and signs, especially visual symptoms. Sometimes cerebral infarction ensues, but typically the clinical and imaging findings suggest that ischemia reverses completely. MRI findings are characteristic, and conventional x-ray angiography may also be helpful in establishing the diagnosis.

Leukoaraiosis, or *periventricular white matter disease,* is the result of multiple small-vessel infarcts within the subcortical white matter. It is readily seen on CT or MRI scans as areas of white matter injury surrounding the ventricles and within the corona radiata. Areas of lacunar infarction are often seen also. The pathophysiologic basis of the disease is lipohyalinosis of small penetrating arteries within the white matter, likely produced by chronic hypertension. Patients with periventricular white matter disease may develop a subcortical dementia syndrome, depending on the amount of white matter infarction, and it is likely that this common form of dementia may be delayed or prevented with antihypertensive medications (Chap. 29).

CADASIL (cerebral autosomal dominant arteriopathy with subcortical infarcts and leukoencephalopathy) is an inherited disorder that presents as small-vessel strokes, progressive dementia, and extensive symmetric white matter changes visualized by MRI. Approximately 40% of patients have migraine with aura, often manifest as transient motor or sensory deficits. Onset is usually in the fourth or fifth decade of life. This autosomal dominant condition is caused by one of several mutations in Notch-3, a member of a highly conserved gene family characterized by epidermal growth factor repeats in its extracellular domain. Other monogenic ischemic stroke syndromes include cerebral autosomal recessive arteriopathy with subcortical infarcts and leukoencephalopathy (CARASIL) and hereditary endotheliopathy, retinopathy, nephropathy, and stroke (HERNS). Fabry's disease also produces both large-vessel arteriopathy and small-vessel infarcts by an unknown mechanism.

TRANSIENT ISCHEMIC ATTACKS

TIAs are episodes of stroke symptoms that last only briefly; the standard definition of duration is <24 h, but most TIAs last <1 h. The causes of TIA are similar to the causes of ischemic stroke, but because TIAs may herald stroke they are an important risk factor that should be considered separately. TIAs may arise from emboli to the brain or from in situ thrombosis of an intracranial vessel. With a TIA, the occluded blood vessel reopens and neurologic function is restored. However, infarcts of the brain do occur in 15–50% of TIAs even though neurologic signs and symptoms are absent. Newer definitions of TIA categorize those with new infarct as having ischemic stroke rather than TIA regardless of symptom duration, but the vast majority of studies have used the standard, time-based definition.

In addition to the stroke syndromes discussed later, one specific TIA symptom should receive special notice. *Amaurosis fugax*, or transient monocular blindness, occurs from emboli to the central retinal artery of one eye. This may indicate carotid stenosis as the cause or local ophthalmic artery disease.

The risk of stroke after a TIA is ~10–15% in the first 3 months, with most events occurring in the first 2 days. This risk can be directly estimated using the well-validated ABCD^2 method (Table 27-5). Therefore, urgent evaluation and treatment are justified. Since etiologies for stroke and TIA are identical, evaluation for TIA should parallel that of stroke (Figs. 27-1 and 27-3). The improvement characteristic of TIA is a contraindication to thrombolysis. However, since the risk of subsequent stroke in the first few days after a TIA is high, the opportunity to give rtPA rapidly if a stroke occurs probably justifies hospital admission for most patients. Acute antiplatelet therapy has not been tested specifically after TIA but is likely to be effective and is recommended. A large-scale trial of acute antithrombotic treatment to prevent stroke following TIA is ongoing.

TABLE 27-5

RISK OF STROKE FOLLOWING TIA: THE ABCD^2 SCORE

CLINICAL FACTOR	SCORE
A: Age ≥60 years	1
B: SBP >140 mmHg or DBP >90 mmHg	1
C: Clinical symptoms	
Unilateral weakness	2
Speech disturbance without weakness	1
D: Duration	
>60 min	2
10–59 min	1
D: Diabetes (oral medications or insulin)	1
Total Score	**Sum Each Category**
ABCD^2 Score Total	3-Month Rate of Stroke (%)[a]
0	0
1	2
2	3
3	3
4	8
5	12
6	17
7	22

[a]Data ranges are from 5 cohorts.

Abbreviations: DBP, diastolic blood pressure; SBP, systolic blood pressure.

Source: SC Johnston et al: Validation and refinement of score to predict very early stroke risk after transient ischaemic attack. Lancet 369: 283, 2007.

TREATMENT Primary and Secondary Prevention of Stroke and TIA

GENERAL PRINCIPLES A number of medical and surgical interventions, as well as lifestyle modifications, are available for preventing stroke. Some of these can be widely applied because of their low cost and minimal risk; others are expensive and carry substantial risk but may be valuable for selected high-risk patients. Identification and control of modifiable risk factors is the best strategy to reduce the burden of stroke, and the total number of strokes could be reduced substantially by these means (Table 27-4).

ATHEROSCLEROSIS RISK FACTORS Older age, family history of thrombotic stroke, diabetes mellitus, hypertension, tobacco smoking, abnormal blood cholesterol (particularly, low high-density lipoprotein [HDL] and/or high low-density lipoprotein [LDL]), and other factors are either proven or probable risk factors for ischemic stroke, largely by their link to atherosclerosis. Risk of stroke is much greater in those with prior stroke or TIA. Many cardiac conditions predispose to stroke, including atrial fibrillation and recent MI. Oral contraceptives and hormone replacement therapy increase stroke risk, and certain inherited and acquired hypercoagulable states predispose to stroke. Hypertension is the most significant of the risk factors; in general, all hypertension should be treated. The presence of known cerebrovascular disease is not a contraindication to treatment aimed at achieving normotension. Also, the value of treating systolic hypertension in older patients has been clearly established. Lowering blood pressure to levels below those traditionally defining hypertension appears to reduce the risk of stroke even further. Data are particularly strong in support of thiazide diuretics and angiotensin-converting enzyme inhibitors.

Several trials have confirmed that statin drugs reduce the risk of stroke even in patients without elevated LDL or low HDL. The Stroke Prevention by Aggressive Reduction in Cholesterol Levels (SPARCL) trial showed benefit in secondary stroke reduction for patients with recent stroke or TIA, who were prescribed atorvastatin, 80 mg/d. The primary prevention trial, Justification for the Use of Statins in Prevention: An Intervention Trial Evaluating Rosuvastatin (JUPITER), found that patients with low LDL (<130 mg/dL) caused by elevated C-reactive protein benefitted by daily use of this statin. Primary stroke occurrence was reduced by 51% (hazard ratio 0.49, $p = 0.004$) and there was no increase in the rates of intracranial hemorrhage. Therefore, a statin should be considered in all patients with prior ischemic stroke. Tobacco smoking should be discouraged in all patients. Tight control of blood sugar in patients with type 2 diabetes lowers stroke risk MI and death of any cause, but no trial sufficiently powered to detect a significant reduction in stroke has yet been performed. Statins, more aggressive blood pressure control, and pioglitazone (an agonist of peroxisome proliferator-activated receptor gamma) are effective.

ANTIPLATELET AGENTS *Platelet antiaggregation agents* can prevent atherothrombotic events, including TIA and stroke, by inhibiting the formation of intraarterial platelet aggregates. These can form on diseased arteries, induce thrombus formation, and occlude the artery or embolize into the distal circulation. Aspirin, clopidogrel, and the combination of aspirin plus extended-release dipyridamole are the antiplatelet agents most commonly used for this purpose. Ticlopidine has been largely abandoned because of its adverse effects but may be used as an alternative to clopidogrel.

Aspirin is the most widely studied antiplatelet agent. Aspirin acetylates platelet cyclooxygenase, which irreversibly inhibits the formation in platelets of thromboxane A_2, a platelet aggregating and vasoconstricting prostaglandin. This effect is permanent and lasts for the usual 8-day life of the platelet. Paradoxically, aspirin also inhibits the formation in endothelial cells of prostacyclin, an antiaggregating and vasodilating prostaglandin. This effect is transient. As soon as aspirin is cleared from the blood, the nucleated endothelial cells again produce prostacyclin. Aspirin in low doses given once daily inhibits the production of thromboxane A_2 in platelets without substantially inhibiting prostacyclin formation. Higher doses of aspirin have not been proven to be more effective than lower doses, and 50–325 mg/d of aspirin is generally recommended for stroke prevention.

Ticlopidine and clopidogrel block the adenosine diphosphate (ADP) receptor on platelets and thus prevent the cascade resulting in activation of the glycoprotein IIb/IIIa receptor that leads to fibrinogen binding to the platelet and consequent platelet aggregation. Ticlopidine is more effective than aspirin; however, it has the disadvantage of causing diarrhea, skin rash, and, in rare instances, neutropenia and thrombotic thrombocytopenic purpura (TTP). Clopidogrel rarely causes TTP but does not cause neutropenia. The Clopidogrel versus Aspirin in Patients at Risk of Ischemic Events (CAPRIE) trial, which led to FDA approval, found that it was only marginally more effective than aspirin in reducing risk of stroke. The Management of Atherothrombosis with Clopidogrel in High-Risk Patients (MATCH) trial was a large multicenter, randomized double-blind study that compared clopidogrel in combination with aspirin to clopidogrel alone in the secondary prevention of TIA or stroke. The MATCH trial found no difference in TIA or stroke prevention with this combination, but did show a small but significant increase in major bleeding complications (3% versus 1%). In the Clopidogrel for High Atherothrombotic Risk and Ischemic Stabilization, Management, and Avoidance (CHARISMA) trial, which included a subgroup of patients with prior stroke or TIA along with other groups at high risk of cardiovascular events, there was no benefit of clopidogrel combined with aspirin compared to aspirin alone. Thus, the use of clopidogrel in combination with aspirin is not recommended for stroke prevention. However, these trials did not enroll patients immediately after the stroke or TIA, and the benefits of combination therapy were greater among those treated earlier, so it is possible that clopidogrel combined with aspirin may be beneficial in this acute period. Ongoing studies are currently addressing this question.

Dipyridamole is an antiplatelet agent that inhibits the uptake of adenosine by a variety of cells, including those of the vascular endothelium. The accumulated adenosine is an inhibitor of aggregation. At least in part through its effects on platelet and vessel wall phosphodiesterases, dipyridamole also potentiates the antiaggregatory effects of prostacyclin and nitric oxide produced by the endothelium and acts by inhibiting platelet phosphodiesterase, which is responsible for the breakdown of cyclic AMP. The resulting elevation in cyclic AMP inhibits aggregation of platelets. Dipyridamole is erratically absorbed depending on stomach pH, but a newer formulation combines timed-release dipyridamole, 200 mg, with aspirin, 25 mg, and has better oral bioavailability. This combination drug was studied in three trials. The European Stroke Prevention Study (ESPS) II showed efficacy of both 50 mg/d of aspirin and extended-release dipyridamole in preventing stroke, and a significantly better risk reduction when the two agents were combined. The ESPRIT (European/Australasian Stroke Prevention in Reversible Ischaemia Trial) trial confirmed the ESPS-II results. This was an open-label, academic trial in which 2739 patients with stroke or TIA treated with aspirin were randomized to dipyridamole, 200 mg twice daily, or no dipyridamole. Primary outcome was the composite of death from all vascular causes, nonfatal stroke, nonfatal MI, or major bleeding complication. After 3.5 years of follow-up, 13% of patients on aspirin and dipyridamole and 16% on aspirin alone (hazard ratio 0.80, 95% confidence index [CI] 0.66–0.98) met the primary outcome. In the Prevention Regimen for Effectively Avoiding Second Strokes (PRoFESS) trial, the combination of extended-release dipyridamole and aspirin was compared directly with clopidogrel with and without the angiotensin receptor blocker telmisartan in a study of 20,332 patients. There were no differences in the rates of second stroke (9% each) or degree of disability in patients with median follow-up of 2.4 years. Telmisartan also had no effect on these outcomes. This suggests that these antiplatelet regimens are similar, and also raises questions about default prescription of agents to block the angiotensin pathway in all stroke patients. The principal side effect of dipyridamole is headache. The combination capsule of extended-release dipyridamole and aspirin is approved for prevention of stroke.

Many large clinical trials have demonstrated clearly that most antiplatelet agents reduce the risk of all important vascular atherothrombotic events (i.e., ischemic stroke, MI, and death due to all vascular causes) in patients at risk for these events. The overall *relative* reduction in risk of nonfatal stroke is about 25–30% and of all vascular events is about 25%. The *absolute* reduction varies considerably, depending on the particular patient's risk. Individuals at very low risk for stroke seem to experience the same relative reduction, but their risks may be so low that the "benefit" is meaningless. Conversely, individuals with a 10–15% risk of vascular events per year experience a reduction to about 7.5–11%.

Aspirin is inexpensive, can be given in low doses, and could be recommended for all adults to prevent both stroke and MI. However, it causes epigastric discomfort, gastric ulceration, and gastrointestinal hemorrhage, which may be asymptomatic or life threatening. Consequently, not every 40- or 50-year-old should be advised to take aspirin regularly because the risk of atherothrombotic stroke is extremely low and is outweighed by the risk of adverse side effects. Conversely, every patient who has experienced an atherothrombotic stroke or TIA and has no contraindication should be taking an antiplatelet agent regularly because the average annual risk of another stroke is 8–10%; another few percent will experience an MI or vascular death. Clearly, the likelihood of benefit far outweighs the risks of treatment.

The choice of antiplatelet agent and dose must balance the risk of stroke, the expected benefit, and the risk and cost of treatment. However, there are no definitive data, and opinions vary. Many authorities believe low-dose (30–75 mg/d) and high-dose (650–1300 mg/d) aspirin are about equally effective. Some advocate very low doses to avoid adverse effects, and still others advocate very high doses to be sure the benefit is maximal. Most physicians in North America recommend 81–325 mg/d, while most Europeans recommend 50–100 mg. Clopidogrel or extended-release dipyridamole plus aspirin are being increasingly recommended as first-line drugs for secondary prevention. Similarly, the choice of aspirin, clopidogrel, or dipyridamole plus aspirin must balance the fact that the latter are more effective than aspirin but the cost is higher, and this is likely to affect long-term patient adherence. The use of platelet aggregation studies in individual patients taking aspirin is controversial because of limited data.

ANTICOAGULATION THERAPY AND EMBOLIC STROKE Several trials have shown that anticoagulation (INR range, 2–3) in patients with chronic nonvalvular (nonrheumatic) atrial fibrillation prevents cerebral embolism and is safe. For primary prevention and for patients who have experienced stroke or TIA, anticoagulation with a VKA reduces the risk by about 67%, which clearly outweighs the 1–3% risk per year of a major bleeding complication. A recent randomized trial compared the new oral thrombin inhibitor dabigatran to VKAs in a noninferiority trial to prevent stroke or systemic embolization in nonvalvular atrial fibrillation. Two doses of dabigatran were used: 110 mg/d and 150 mg/d. Both dose tiers of dabigatran were noninferior to VKAs in preventing second stroke and systemic embolization, and the higher dose tier was superior (relative risk 0.66; 95% CI, 0.53 to 0.82; $P < 0.001$) and the rate of major bleeding was lower in the lower dose tier of dabigatran compared to VKAs. This drug is likely more convenient to take as no blood monitoring is required to titrate the dose and its effect is independent of oral intake of vitamin K. For patients who cannot take anticoagulant medications, clopidogrel plus aspirin was compared to aspirin alone in the Atrial Fibrillation Clopidogrel Trial with Irbesartan for Prevention of Vascular Events (ACTIVE-A). Clopidogrel combined with aspirin was more effective than aspirin alone in preventing vascular events, principally stroke, but increases the risk of major bleeding (relative risk 1.57, $P < 0.001$).

The decision to use anticoagulation for primary prevention is based primarily on risk factors (Table 27-3). The history of a TIA or stroke tips the balance in favor of anticoagulation regardless of other risk factors. Since this risk factor is so important, many clinicians are performing extended ambulatory monitoring to detect intermittent atrial fibrillation in otherwise cryptogenic stroke since its detection would shift toward prescription of oral anticoagulation long term.

Because of the high annual stroke risk in untreated rheumatic heart disease with atrial fibrillation, primary prophylaxis against stroke has not been studied in a double-blind fashion. These patients generally should receive long-term anticoagulation.

Anticoagulation also reduces the risk of embolism in acute MI. Most clinicians recommend a 3-month course of anticoagulation when there is anterior Q-wave infarction, substantial left ventricular dysfunction, congestive heart failure, mural thrombosis, or atrial fibrillation. VKAs are recommended long-term if atrial fibrillation persists.

Stroke secondary to thromboembolism is one of the most serious complications of prosthetic heart valve implantation. The intensity of anticoagulation and/or antiplatelet therapy is dictated by the type of prosthetic valve and its location.

If the embolic source cannot be eliminated, anticoagulation should in most cases be continued indefinitely. Many neurologists recommend combining antiplatelet agents with anticoagulants for patients who "fail" anticoagulation (i.e., have another stroke or TIA).

ANTICOAGULATION THERAPY AND NONCARDIOGENIC STROKE Data do not support the use of long-term VKAs for preventing atherothrombotic stroke for either intracranial or extracranial cerebrovascular disease. The Warfarin-Aspirin Reinfarction Stroke Study (WARSS) study found no benefit of warfarin sodium (INR, 1.4–2.8) over aspirin, 325 mg, for secondary prevention of stroke but did find a slightly higher bleeding rate in the warfarin group. A recent European study confirmed this finding. The Warfarin-Aspirin Symptomatic Intracranial Disease (WASID) study (see later) demonstrated no benefit of warfarin (INR, 2–3) over aspirin in patients with symptomatic intracranial atherosclerosis, and also found higher bleeding complications.

TREATMENT Carotid Atherosclerosis

Carotid atherosclerosis can be removed surgically (endarterectomy) or mitigated with endovascular stenting with or without balloon angioplasty. Anticoagulation has not been directly compared with antiplatelet therapy for carotid disease.

SURGICAL THERAPY *Symptomatic carotid stenosis* was studied in the North American Symptomatic Carotid Endarterectomy Trial (NASCET) and the European Carotid Surgery Trial (ECST). Both showed a substantial benefit for surgery in patients with a stenosis of ≥70%. In NASCET, the average cumulative ipsilateral stroke risk at 2 years was 26% for patients treated medically and 9% for those receiving the same medical treatment plus a carotid endarterectomy. This 17% *absolute* reduction in the surgical group is a 65% *relative* risk reduction favoring surgery (Table 27-4). NASCET also showed a significant, although less robust, benefit for patients with 50–70% stenosis. ECST found harm for patients with stenosis <30% treated surgically.

A patient's risk of stroke and possible benefit from surgery are related to the presence of retinal versus hemispheric symptoms, degree of arterial stenosis, extent of associated medical conditions (of note, NASCET and ECST excluded "high-risk" patients with significant cardiac, pulmonary, or renal disease), institutional surgical morbidity and mortality, timing of surgery relative to symptoms, and other factors. A recent meta-analysis of the NASCET and ECST trials demonstrated that endarterectomy is most beneficial when performed within 2 weeks of symptom onset. In addition, benefit is more pronounced in patients >75 years, and men appear to benefit more than women.

In summary, a patient with recent symptomatic hemispheric ischemia, high-grade stenosis in the appropriate internal carotid artery, and an institutional perioperative morbidity and mortality rate of ≤6% generally should undergo carotid endarterectomy. If the perioperative stroke rate is >6% for any particular surgeon, however, the benefits of carotid endarterectomy are questionable.

The indications for surgical treatment of *asymptomatic carotid disease* have been clarified by the results of the Asymptomatic Carotid Atherosclerosis Study (ACAS) and the Asymptomatic Carotid Surgery Trial (ACST). ACAS randomized asymptomatic patients with ≥60% stenosis to medical treatment with aspirin or the same medical treatment plus carotid endarterectomy. The surgical group had a risk over 5 years for ipsilateral stroke (and any perioperative stroke or death) of 5.1%, compared to a risk in the medical group of 11%. While this demonstrates a 53% *relative* risk reduction, the *absolute* risk reduction is only 5.9% over 5 years, or 1.2% annually (Table 27-4). Nearly one-half of the strokes in the surgery group were caused by preoperative angiograms. The recently published ACST randomized 3120 asymptomatic patients with >60% carotid stenosis to endarterectomy or medical therapy. The 5-year risk of stroke in the surgical group (including perioperative stroke or death) was 6.4%, compared to 11.8% in the medically treated group (46% relative risk reduction and 5.4% absolute risk reduction).

In both ACAS and ACST, the perioperative complication rate was higher in women, perhaps negating any benefit in the reduction of stroke risk within 5 years. It is possible that with longer follow-up, a clear benefit in women will emerge. At present, carotid endarterectomy in asymptomatic women remains particularly controversial.

In summary, the natural history of asymptomatic stenosis is a ~2% per year stroke rate, while symptomatic patients experience a 13% per year risk of stroke. Whether to recommend carotid revascularization for an asymptomatic patient is somewhat controversial and depends on many factors, including patient preference, degree of stenosis, age, gender, and comorbidities. Medical therapy for reduction of atherosclerosis risk factors, including cholesterol-lowering agents and antiplatelet medications, is generally recommended for patients with asymptomatic carotid stenosis. As with atrial fibrillation, it is imperative to counsel the patient about TIAs so that therapy can be revised if symptoms develop.

ENDOVASCULAR THERAPY Balloon angioplasty coupled with stenting is being used with increasing frequency to open stenotic carotid arteries and maintain their patency. These techniques can treat carotid stenosis not only at the bifurcation but also near the skull base and in the intracranial segments. The Stenting and Angioplasty with Protection in Patients at High Risk for Endarterectomy (SAPPHIRE) trial randomized high-risk patients (defined as patients with clinically significant coronary or pulmonary disease, contralateral carotid occlusion, restenosis after endarterectomy, contralateral laryngeal-nerve palsy, prior radical neck surgery or radiation, or age >80) with symptomatic carotid stenosis >50% or asymptomatic stenosis >80% to either stenting combined with a distal emboli-protection device or endarterectomy. The risk of death, stroke, or MI within 30 days and ipsilateral stroke or death within 1 year was 12.2% in the stenting group and 20.1% in the endarterectomy group ($p = .055$), suggesting that stenting is at the very least comparable to endarterectomy as a treatment option for this patient group at high risk of surgery. However, the outcomes with both interventions may not have been better than leaving the carotid stenoses untreated, particularly for the asymptomatic patients, and much of the benefit seen in the stenting group was due to a reduction in periprocedure MI. In 2010, the results of two randomized trials comparing stents to endarterectomy in low-risk patients were published. The Carotid Revascularization Endarterectomy versus Stenting Trial (CREST) enrolled 2502 patients with either asymptomatic or symptomatic stenosis. The 30-day risk of stroke was 4.1% in the stent group and 2.3% in the surgical group, but the 30-day risk of MI was 1.1% in the stent group and 2.3% in the surgery group, suggesting relative equivalence of risk between the procedures. At median follow-up of 2.5 years, the combined endpoint of stroke, MI, and death was the same (7.2% stent versus 6.8% surgery). The International Carotid Stenting (ICSS) trial randomized 1713 symptomatic patients to stents versus endarterectomy and found a different result: At 120 days, the incidence of stroke, MI, or death was 8.5% in the stenting group versus 5.2% in the endarterectomy group ($p = 0.006$), and longer term follow-up is currently under way. Differences between trial designs, selection of stent, and operator experience may explain these important differences. Until more data are available on both trials, there remains controversy as to who should receive a stent or have endarterectomy; it is likely that the procedures carry similar risks if performed by experienced physicians.

BYPASS SURGERY Extracranial-to-intracranial (EC-IC) bypass surgery has been proven ineffective for atherosclerotic stenoses that are inaccessible to conventional carotid endarterectomy. However, a trial is under way to evaluate whether patients with decreased brain perfusion based on positron emission tomography (PET) imaging will benefit from EC-IC bypass.

INTRACRANIAL ATHEROSCLEROSIS The WASID trial randomized patients with symptomatic stenosis (50–99%) of a major intracranial vessel to either high-dose aspirin (1300 mg/d) or warfarin (target INR, 2.0–3.0), with a combined primary endpoint of ischemic stroke, brain hemorrhage, or death from vascular cause other than stroke. The trial was terminated early because of an increased risk of adverse events related to warfarin anticoagulation. With a mean follow-up of 1.8 years, the primary endpoint was seen in 22.1% in the aspirin group and 21.8% of the warfarin group. Death from any cause was seen in 4.3% of the aspirin group and 9.7% of the warfarin group; 3.2% of patients on aspirin experienced major hemorrhage, compared to 8.3% of patients taking warfarin.

Given the worrisome natural history of symptomatic intracranial atherosclerosis (in the aspirin arm of the WASID trial, 15% of patients experienced a stroke within the first year, despite current standard aggressive medical therapy), some centers treat symptomatic lesions with intracranial angioplasty and stenting. This intervention is currently being compared to aspirin therapy in a prospective, randomized trial. It is unclear whether EC-IC bypass, or other grafting procedures of extracranial blood supply to the pial arteries, are of value in such patients.

Dural Sinus Thrombosis Limited evidence exists to support short-term usage of anticoagulants, regardless of the presence of intracranial hemorrhage, for venous infarction following sinus thrombosis.

STROKE SYNDROMES

A careful history and neurologic examination can often localize the region of brain dysfunction; if this region corresponds to a particular arterial distribution, the possible causes responsible for the syndrome can be narrowed. This is of particular importance when the patient presents with a TIA and a normal examination. For example, if a patient develops language loss and a right homonymous hemianopia, a search for causes of left middle cerebral emboli should be performed. A finding of an isolated stenosis of the right internal carotid artery in that patient, for example, suggests an asymptomatic carotid stenosis, and the search for other causes of stroke should continue. The following sections describe the clinical findings of cerebral ischemia associated with cerebral vascular territories depicted in Figs. 27-4, and 27-6 through 27-14. Stroke syndromes are divided into: (1) large-vessel stroke within the anterior circulation, (2) large-vessel stroke within the posterior circulation, and (3) small-vessel disease of either vascular bed.

Stroke within the anterior circulation

The internal carotid artery and its branches comprise the anterior circulation of the brain. These vessels can be occluded by intrinsic disease of the vessel (e.g., atherosclerosis or dissection) or by embolic occlusion from a proximal source as discussed earlier. Occlusion of each major intracranial vessel has distinct clinical manifestations.

Middle cerebral artery

Occlusion of the proximal MCA or one of its major branches is most often due to an embolus (artery-to-artery, cardiac, or of unknown source) rather than intracranial atherothrombosis. Atherosclerosis of the proximal MCA may cause distal emboli to the middle cerebral territory or, less commonly, may produce low-flow TIAs. Collateral formation via leptomeningeal vessels often prevents MCA stenosis from becoming symptomatic.

The cortical branches of the MCA supply the lateral surface of the hemisphere except for (1) the frontal pole and a strip along the superomedial border of the frontal and parietal lobes supplied by the ACA, and (2) the lower temporal and occipital pole convolutions supplied by the PCA (Figs. 27-6, 27-7, 27-8, and 27-9).

The proximal MCA (M1 segment) gives rise to penetrating branches (termed *lenticulostriate arteries*) that supply the putamen, outer globus pallidus, posterior limb of the internal capsule, the adjacent corona radiata, and most of the caudate nucleus (Fig. 27-6). In the sylvian fissure, the MCA in most patients divides into *superior* and *inferior* divisions (M2 branches). Branches of the inferior division supply the inferior parietal and temporal cortex, and those from the superior division supply the frontal and superior parietal cortex (Fig. 27-7).

If the entire MCA is occluded at its origin (blocking both its penetrating and cortical branches) and the distal collaterals are limited, the clinical findings are contralateral hemiplegia, hemianesthesia, homonymous hemianopia, and a day or two of gaze preference to the ipsilateral side. Dysarthria is common because of facial weakness. When the dominant hemisphere is involved,

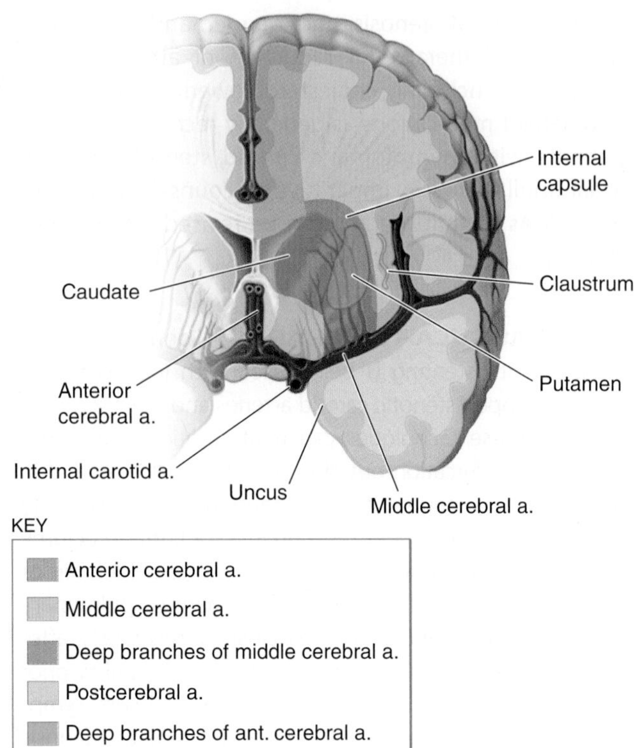

FIGURE 27-6

Diagram of a cerebral hemisphere in coronal section showing the territories of the major cerebral vessels that branch from the internal carotid arteries.

global aphasia is present also, and when the nondominant hemisphere is affected, anosognosia, constructional apraxia, and neglect are found (Chap. 18).

Complete MCA syndromes occur most often when an embolus occludes the stem of the artery. Cortical collateral blood flow and differing arterial configurations are probably responsible for the development of many partial syndromes. Partial syndromes may also be due to emboli that enter the proximal MCA without complete occlusion, occlude distal MCA branches, or fragment and move distally.

Partial syndromes due to embolic occlusion of a single branch include hand, or arm and hand, weakness alone (brachial syndrome) or facial weakness with nonfluent (Broca) aphasia (Chap. 18), with or without arm weakness (frontal opercular syndrome). A combination of sensory disturbance, motor weakness, and nonfluent aphasia suggests that an embolus has occluded the proximal superior division and infarcted large portions of the frontal and parietal cortices (Fig. 27-7). If a fluent (Wernicke's) aphasia occurs without weakness, the inferior division of the MCA supplying the posterior part (temporal cortex) of the dominant hemisphere is probably involved. Jargon speech and an inability to comprehend written and spoken language are prominent features, often accompanied by a contralateral, homonymous superior quadrantanopia. Hemineglect or spatial agnosia without weakness indicates that the inferior

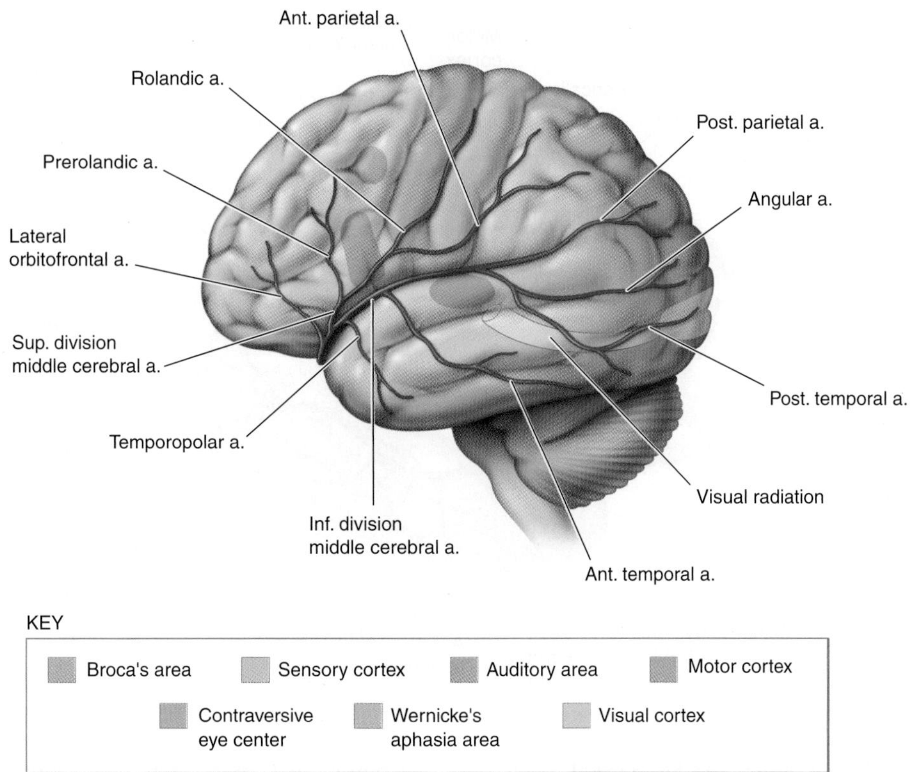

FIGURE 27-7

Diagram of a cerebral hemisphere, lateral aspect, showing the branches and distribution of the middle cerebral artery and the principal regions of cerebral localization. Note the bifurcation of the middle cerebral artery into a superior and inferior division.

Signs and symptoms: *Structures involved*

Paralysis of the contralateral face, arm, and leg; sensory impairment over the same area (pinprick, cotton touch, vibration, position, two-point discrimination, stereognosis, tactile localization, barognosis, cutaneographia): *Somatic motor area for face and arm and the fibers descending from the leg area to enter the corona radiata and corresponding somatic sensory system*

Motor aphasia: *Motor speech area of the dominant hemisphere*

Central aphasia, word deafness, anomia, jargon speech, sensory agraphia, acalculia, alexia, finger agnosia, right-left confusion (the last four comprise the Gerstmann syndrome): *Central, suprasylvian speech area and parietooccipital cortex of the dominant hemisphere*

Conduction aphasia: *Central speech area (parietal operculum)*

Apractagnosia of the nondominant hemisphere, anosognosia, hemiasomatognosia, unilateral neglect, agnosia for the left half of external space, dressing "apraxia," constructional "apraxia," distortion of visual coordinates, inaccurate localization in the half field, impaired ability to judge distance, upside-down reading, visual illusions (e.g., it may appear that another person walks through a table): *Nondominant parietal lobe (area corresponding to speech area in dominant hemisphere); loss of topographic memory is usually due to a nondominant lesion, occasionally to a dominant one*

Homonymous hemianopia (often homonymous inferior quadrantanopia): *Optic radiation deep to second temporal convolution*

Paralysis of conjugate gaze to the opposite side: *Frontal contraversive eye field or projecting fibers*

division of the MCA in the nondominant hemisphere is involved.

Occlusion of a lenticulostriate vessel produces small-vessel (lacunar) stroke within the internal capsule (Fig. 27-6). This produces pure motor stroke or sensory-motor stroke contralateral to the lesion. Ischemia within the genu of the internal capsule causes primarily facial weakness followed by arm then leg weakness as the ischemia moves posterior within the capsule. Alternatively, the contralateral hand may become ataxic and dysarthria will be prominent (clumsy hand, dysarthria lacunar syndrome). Lacunar infarction affecting the globus pallidus and putamen often has few clinical signs, but parkinsonism and hemiballismus have been reported.

Anterior cerebral artery

The ACA is divided into two segments: the precommunal (A1) circle of Willis, or stem, which connects the internal carotid artery to the anterior communicating

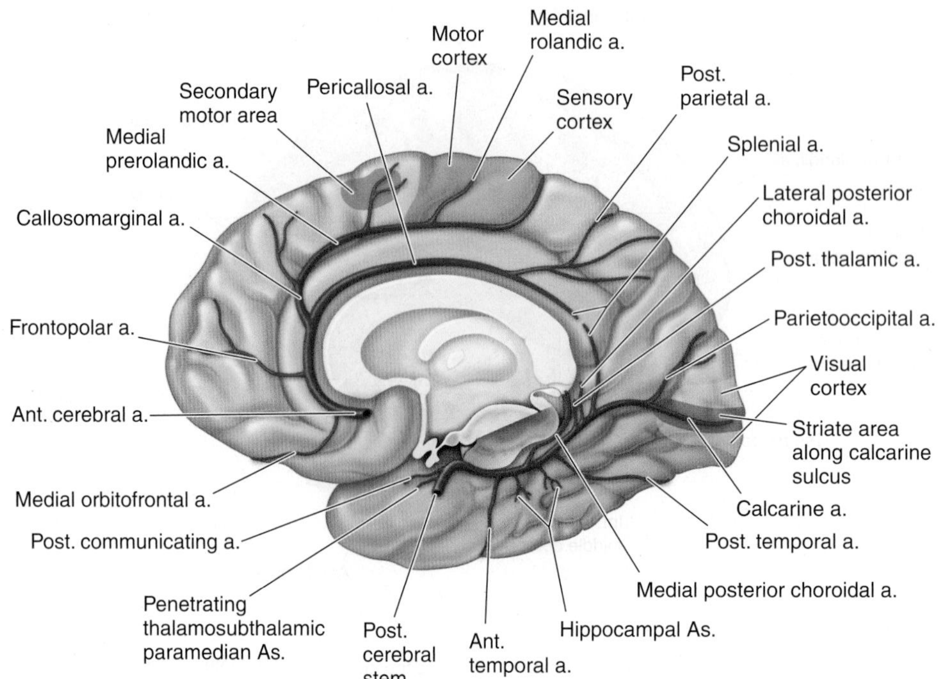

FIGURE 27-8

Diagram of a cerebral hemisphere, medial aspect, showing the branches and distribution of the anterior cerebral artery and the principal regions of cerebral localization.

Signs and symptoms: *Structures involved*

Paralysis of opposite foot and leg: *Motor leg area*

A lesser degree of paresis of opposite arm: *Arm area of cortex or fibers descending to corona radiata*

Cortical sensory loss over toes, foot, and leg: *Sensory area for foot and leg*

Urinary incontinence: *Sensorimotor area in paracentral lobule*

Contralateral grasp reflex, sucking reflex, gegenhalten (paratonic rigidity): *Medial surface of the posterior frontal lobe; likely supplemental motor area*

Abulia (akinetic mutism), slowness, delay, intermittent interruption, lack of spontaneity, whispering, reflex distraction to sights and sounds: *Uncertain localization—probably cingulate gyrus and medial inferior portion of frontal, parietal, and temporal lobes*

Impairment of gait and stance (gait apraxia): *Frontal cortex near leg motor area*

Dyspraxia of left limbs, tactile aphasia in left limbs: *Corpus callosum*

artery, and the postcommunal (A2) segment distal to the anterior communicating artery (Figs. 27-4, 27-6, and 27-8). The A1 segment gives rise to several deep penetrating branches that supply the anterior limb of the internal capsule, the anterior perforate substance, amygdala, anterior hypothalamus, and the inferior part of the head of the caudate nucleus (Fig. 27-6).

Occlusion of the proximal ACA is usually well tolerated because of collateral flow through the anterior communicating artery and collaterals through the MCA and PCA. Occlusion of a single A2 segment results in the contralateral symptoms noted in Fig. 27-8. If both A2 segments arise from a single anterior cerebral stem (contralateral A1 segment atresia), the occlusion may affect both hemispheres. Profound abulia (a delay in verbal and motor response) and bilateral pyramidal signs with paraparesis or quadriparesis and urinary incontinence result.

Anterior choroidal artery

This artery arises from the internal carotid artery and supplies the posterior limb of the internal capsule and the white matter posterolateral to it, through which pass some of the geniculocalcarine fibers (Fig. 27-9). The complete syndrome of anterior choroidal artery occlusion consists of contralateral hemiplegia, hemianesthesia (hypesthesia), and homonymous hemianopia. However, because this territory is also supplied by penetrating vessels of the proximal MCA and the posterior communicating and posterior choroidal arteries, minimal deficits may occur, and patients frequently recover substantially. Anterior choroidal strokes are usually the result of in situ thrombosis of the vessel, and the vessel is particularly vulnerable to iatrogenic occlusion during surgical clipping of aneurysms arising from the internal carotid artery.

Internal carotid artery

The clinical picture of internal carotid occlusion varies depending on whether the cause of ischemia is propagated thrombus, embolism, or low flow. The cortex supplied by the MCA territory is affected most often. With a competent circle of Willis, occlusion may go

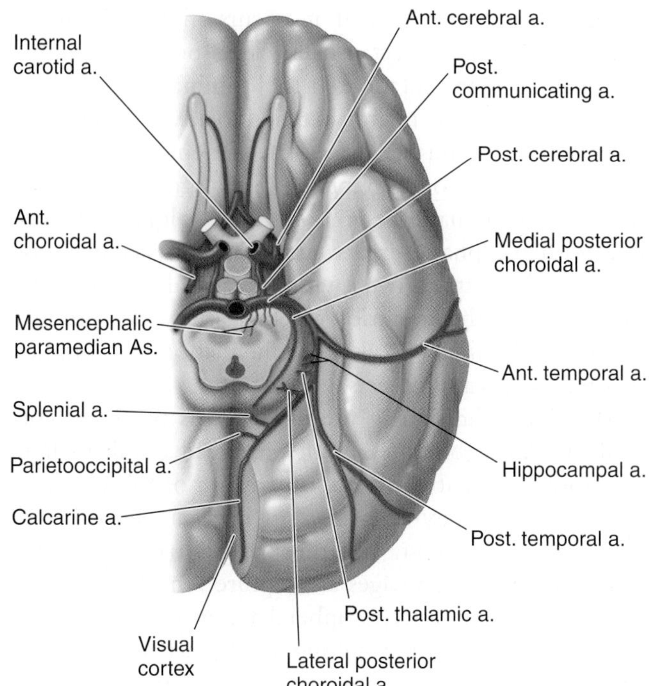

FIGURE 27-9
Inferior aspect of the brain with the branches and distribution of the posterior cerebral artery and the principal anatomic structures shown.

Signs and symptoms: *Structures involved*

Peripheral territory (see also Fig. 27-12). Homonymous hemianopia (often upper quadrantic): *Calcarine cortex or optic radiation nearby*. Bilateral homonymous hemianopia, cortical blindness, awareness or denial of blindness; tactile naming, achromatopia (color blindness), failure to see to-and-fro movements, inability to perceive objects not centrally located, apraxia of ocular movements, inability to count or enumerate objects, tendency to run into things that the patient sees and tries to avoid: *Bilateral occipital lobe with possibly the parietal lobe involved*. Verbal dyslexia without agraphia, color anomia: *Dominant calcarine lesion and posterior part of corpus callosum*. Memory defect: *Hippocampal lesion bilaterally or on the dominant side only*. Topographic disorientation and prosopagnosia: *Usually with lesions of nondominant, calcarine, and lingual gyrus*. Simultanagnosia, hemivisual neglect: *Dominant visual cortex, contralateral hemisphere*. Unformed visual hallucinations, peduncular hallucinosis, metamorphopsia, teleopsia, illusory visual spread, palinopsia, distortion of outlines, central photophobia: *Calcarine cortex*. Complex hallucinations: *Usually nondominant hemisphere*.

Central territory. Thalamic syndrome: sensory loss (all modalities), spontaneous pain and dysesthesias, choreoathetosis, intention tremor, spasms of hand, mild hemiparesis: *Posteroventral nucleus of thalamus; involvement of the adjacent subthalamus body or its afferent tracts*. Thalamoperforate syndrome: crossed cerebellar ataxia with ipsilateral third nerve palsy (Claude's syndrome): *Dentatothalamic tract and issuing third nerve*. Weber's syndrome: third nerve palsy and contralateral hemiplegia: *Third nerve and cerebral peduncle*. Contralateral hemiplegia: *Cerebral peduncle*. Paralysis or paresis of vertical eye movement, skew deviation, sluggish pupillary responses to light, slight miosis and ptosis (retraction nystagmus and "tucking" of the eyelids may be associated): *Supranuclear fibers to third nerve, interstitial nucleus of Cajal, nucleus of Darkschewitsch, and posterior commissure*. Contralateral rhythmic, ataxic action tremor; rhythmic postural or "holding" tremor (rubral tremor): *Dentatothalamic tract*.

unnoticed. If the thrombus propagates up the internal carotid artery into the MCA or embolizes it, symptoms are identical to proximal MCA occlusion (see earlier). Sometimes there is massive infarction of the entire deep white matter and cortical surface. When the origins of both the ACA and MCA are occluded at the top of the carotid artery, abulia or stupor occurs with hemiplegia, hemianesthesia, and aphasia or anosognosia. When the PCA arises from the internal carotid artery (a configuration called a *fetal posterior cerebral artery*), it may also become occluded and give rise to symptoms referable to its peripheral territory (Figs. 27-8 and 27-9).

In addition to supplying the ipsilateral brain, the internal carotid artery perfuses the optic nerve and retina via the ophthalmic artery. In ~25% of symptomatic internal carotid disease, recurrent transient monocular blindness (amaurosis fugax) warns of the lesion. Patients typically describe a horizontal shade that sweeps down or up across the field of vision. They may also complain that their vision was blurred in that eye or that the upper or lower half of vision disappeared. In most cases, these symptoms last only a few minutes. Rarely, ischemia or infarction of the ophthalmic artery or central retinal arteries occurs at the time of cerebral TIA or infarction.

A high-pitched prolonged carotid bruit fading into diastole is often associated with tightly stenotic lesions. As the stenosis grows tighter and flow distal to the stenosis becomes reduced, the bruit becomes fainter and may disappear when occlusion is imminent.

Common carotid artery

All symptoms and signs of internal carotid occlusion may also be present with occlusion of the common carotid artery. Jaw claudication may result from low flow in the external carotid branches. Bilateral common carotid artery occlusions at their origin may occur in Takayasu's arteritis.

Stroke within the posterior circulation

The posterior circulation is composed of the paired vertebral arteries, the basilar artery, and the paired posterior cerebral arteries. The vertebral arteries join to form the basilar artery at the pontomedullary junction. The basilar artery divides into two posterior cerebral arteries in the interpeduncular fossa (Figs. 27-4, 27-8, and 27-9). These major arteries give rise to long and short circumferential branches and to smaller deep penetrating branches that supply the cerebellum, medulla, pons, midbrain, subthalamus, thalamus, hippocampus, and medial temporal and occipital lobes. Occlusion of each vessel produces its own distinctive syndrome.

Posterior cerebral artery

In 75% of cases, both PCAs arise from the bifurcation of the basilar artery; in 20%, one has its origin from the ipsilateral internal carotid artery via the posterior communicating artery; in 5%, both originate from the respective ipsilateral internal carotid arteries (Figs. 27-8 and 27-9). The precommunal, or P1, segment of the true posterior cerebral artery is atretic in such cases.

PCA syndromes usually result from atheroma formation or emboli that lodge at the top of the basilar artery; posterior circulation disease may also be caused by dissection of either vertebral artery and fibromuscular dysplasia.

Two clinical syndromes are commonly observed with occlusion of the PCA: (1) *P1 syndrome*: midbrain, subthalamic, and thalamic signs, which are due to disease of the proximal P1 segment of the PCA or its penetrating branches (thalamogeniculate, Percheron, and posterior choroidal arteries); and (2) *P2 syndrome*: cortical temporal and occipital lobe signs, due to occlusion of the P2 segment distal to the junction of the PCA with the posterior communicating artery.

P1 syndromes

Infarction usually occurs in the ipsilateral subthalamus and medial thalamus and in the ipsilateral cerebral peduncle and midbrain (Figs. 27-9 and 27-14). A third nerve palsy with contralateral ataxia (Claude's syndrome) or with contralateral hemiplegia (Weber's syndrome) may result. The ataxia indicates involvement of the red nucleus or dentatorubrothalamic tract; the hemiplegia is localized to the cerebral peduncle (Fig. 27-14). If the subthalamic nucleus is involved, contralateral hemiballismus may occur. Occlusion of the artery of Percheron produces paresis of upward gaze and drowsiness, and often abulia. Extensive infarction in the midbrain and subthalamus occurring with bilateral proximal PCA occlusion presents as coma, unreactive pupils, bilateral pyramidal signs, and decerebrate rigidity.

Occlusion of the penetrating branches of thalamic and thalamogeniculate arteries produces less extensive thalamic and thalamocapsular lacunar syndromes. The *thalamic Déjérine-Roussy syndrome* consists of contralateral hemisensory loss followed later by an agonizing, searing or burning pain in the affected areas. It is persistent and responds poorly to analgesics. Anticonvulsants (carbamazepine or gabapentin) or tricyclic antidepressants may be beneficial.

P2 syndromes

(See also Figs. 27-8 and 27-9.) Occlusion of the distal PCA causes infarction of the medial temporal and occipital lobes. Contralateral homonymous hemianopia with macula sparing is the usual manifestation. Occasionally, only the upper quadrant of visual field is involved. If the visual association areas are spared and only the calcarine cortex is involved, the patient may be aware of visual defects. Medial temporal lobe and hippocampal involvement may cause an acute disturbance in memory, particularly if it occurs in the dominant hemisphere. The defect usually clears because memory has bilateral representation. If the dominant hemisphere is affected and the infarct extends to involve the splenium of the corpus callosum, the patient may demonstrate alexia without agraphia. Visual agnosia for faces, objects, mathematical symbols, and colors and anomia with paraphasic errors (amnestic aphasia) may also occur in this setting, even without callosal involvement. Occlusion of the posterior cerebral artery can produce *peduncular hallucinosis* (visual hallucinations of brightly colored scenes and objects).

Bilateral infarction in the distal PCAs produces cortical blindness (blindness with preserved pupillary light reaction). The patient is often unaware of the blindness or may even deny it (*Anton's syndrome*). Tiny islands of vision may persist, and the patient may report that vision fluctuates as images are captured in the preserved portions. Rarely, only peripheral vision is lost and central vision is spared, resulting in "gun-barrel" vision. Bilateral visual association area lesions may result in *Balint's syndrome*, a disorder of the orderly visual scanning of the environment (Chap. 18), usually resulting from infarctions secondary to low flow in the "watershed" between the distal PCA and MCA territories, as occurs after cardiac arrest. Patients may experience persistence of a visual image for several minutes despite gazing at another scene (*palinopsia*) or an inability to synthesize the whole of an image (*asimultanagnosia*). Embolic occlusion of the top of the basilar artery can produce any or all of the central or peripheral territory symptoms. The hallmark is the sudden onset of bilateral signs, including ptosis, pupillary asymmetry or lack of reaction to light, and somnolence.

Vertebral and posterior inferior cerebellar arteries

The vertebral artery, which arises from the innominate artery on the right and the subclavian artery on the left, consists of four segments. The first (V1) extends from its origin to its entrance into the sixth or fifth transverse vertebral foramen. The second segment (V2) traverses the vertebral foramina from C6 to C2. The third (V3) passes through the transverse foramen and circles around the arch of the atlas to pierce the dura at the foramen magnum. The fourth (V4) segment courses upward to join the other vertebral artery to form the basilar artery; only the fourth segment gives rise to branches that supply the brainstem and cerebellum. The posterior inferior cerebellar artery (PICA) in its proximal segment supplies the lateral medulla and, in its distal branches, the inferior surface of the cerebellum.

Atherothrombotic lesions have a predilection for V1 and V4 segments of the vertebral artery. The first segment may become diseased at the origin of the vessel and may produce posterior circulation emboli;

collateral flow from the contralateral vertebral artery or the ascending cervical, thyrocervical, or occipital arteries is usually sufficient to prevent low-flow TIAs or stroke. When one vertebral artery is atretic and an atherothrombotic lesion threatens the origin of the other, the collateral circulation, which may also include retrograde flow down the basilar artery, is often insufficient (Figs. 27-4 and 27-9). In this setting, low-flow TIAs may occur, consisting of syncope, vertigo, and alternating hemiplegia; this state also sets the stage for thrombosis. Disease of the distal fourth segment of the vertebral artery can promote thrombus formation manifest as embolism or with propagation as basilar artery thrombosis. Stenosis proximal to the origin of the PICA can threaten the lateral medulla and posterior inferior surface of the cerebellum.

If the subclavian artery is occluded proximal to the origin of the vertebral artery, there is a reversal in the direction of blood flow in the ipsilateral vertebral artery. Exercise of the ipsilateral arm may increase demand on vertebral flow, producing posterior circulation TIAs, or "subclavian steal."

Although atheromatous disease rarely narrows the second and third segments of the vertebral artery, this region is subject to dissection, fibromuscular dysplasia, and, rarely, encroachment by osteophytic spurs within the vertebral foramina.

Embolic occlusion or thrombosis of a V4 segment causes ischemia of the lateral medulla. The constellation of vertigo, numbness of the ipsilateral face and contralateral limbs, diplopia, hoarseness, dysarthria, dysphagia, and ipsilateral Horner's syndrome is called the *lateral medullary (or Wallenberg's) syndrome* (Fig. 27-10). Most cases result from ipsilateral vertebral artery occlusion; in the remainder, PICA occlusion is responsible. Occlusion of the medullary penetrating branches of the vertebral artery or PICA results in partial syndromes. *Hemiparesis is not a feature of vertebral artery occlusion; however, quadriparesis may result from occlusion of the anterior spinal artery.*

Rarely, a *medial medullary syndrome* occurs with infarction of the pyramid and contralateral hemiparesis of the arm and leg, sparing the face. If the medial lemniscus and emerging hypoglossal nerve fibers are involved, contralateral loss of joint position sense and ipsilateral tongue weakness occur.

Cerebellar infarction with edema can lead to *sudden respiratory arrest* due to raised ICP in the posterior fossa. Drowsiness, Babinski signs, dysarthria, and bifacial weakness may be absent, or present only briefly, before respiratory arrest ensues. Gait unsteadiness, headache, dizziness, nausea, and vomiting may be the only early symptoms and signs and should arouse suspicion of this impending complication, which may require neurosurgical decompression, often with an excellent outcome. Separating these symptoms from those of viral labyrinthitis can be a challenge, but headache, neck stiffness, and unilateral dysmetria favor stroke.

Basilar artery

Branches of the basilar artery supply the base of the pons and superior cerebellum and fall into three groups: (1) paramedian, 7–10 in number, which supply a wedge of pons on either side of the midline; (2) short circumferential, 5–7 in number, that supply the lateral two-thirds of the pons and middle and superior cerebellar peduncles; and (3) bilateral long circumferential (superior cerebellar and anterior inferior cerebellar arteries), which course around the pons to supply the cerebellar hemispheres.

Atheromatous lesions can occur anywhere along the basilar trunk but are most frequent in the proximal basilar and distal vertebral segments. Typically, lesions occlude either the proximal basilar and one or both vertebral arteries. The clinical picture varies depending on the availability of retrograde collateral flow from the posterior communicating arteries. Rarely, dissection of a vertebral artery may involve the basilar artery and, depending on the location of true and false lumen, may produce multiple penetrating artery strokes.

Although atherothrombosis occasionally occludes the distal portion of the basilar artery, emboli from the heart or proximal vertebral or basilar segments are more commonly responsible for "top of the basilar" syndromes.

Because the brainstem contains many structures in close apposition, a diversity of clinical syndromes may emerge with ischemia, reflecting involvement of the corticospinal and corticobulbar tracts, ascending sensory tracts, and cranial nerve nuclei (Figs. 27-11, 27-12, 27-13, and 27-14).

The symptoms of transient ischemia or infarction in the territory of the basilar artery often do not indicate whether the basilar artery itself or one of its branches is diseased, yet this distinction has important implications for therapy. *The picture of complete basilar occlusion, however, is easy to recognize as a constellation of bilateral long tract signs (sensory and motor) with signs of cranial nerve and cerebellar dysfunction.* A "locked-in" state of preserved consciousness with quadriplegia and cranial nerve signs suggests complete pontine and lower midbrain infarction. The therapeutic goal is to identify *impending* basilar occlusion before devastating infarction occurs. A series of TIAs and a slowly progressive, fluctuating stroke are extremely significant, as they often herald an atherothrombotic occlusion of the distal vertebral or proximal basilar artery.

TIAs in the proximal basilar distribution may produce vertigo (often described by patients as "swimming," "swaying," "moving," "unsteadiness," or "light-headedness"). Other symptoms that warn of basilar thrombosis include diplopia, dysarthria, facial or circumoral numbness,

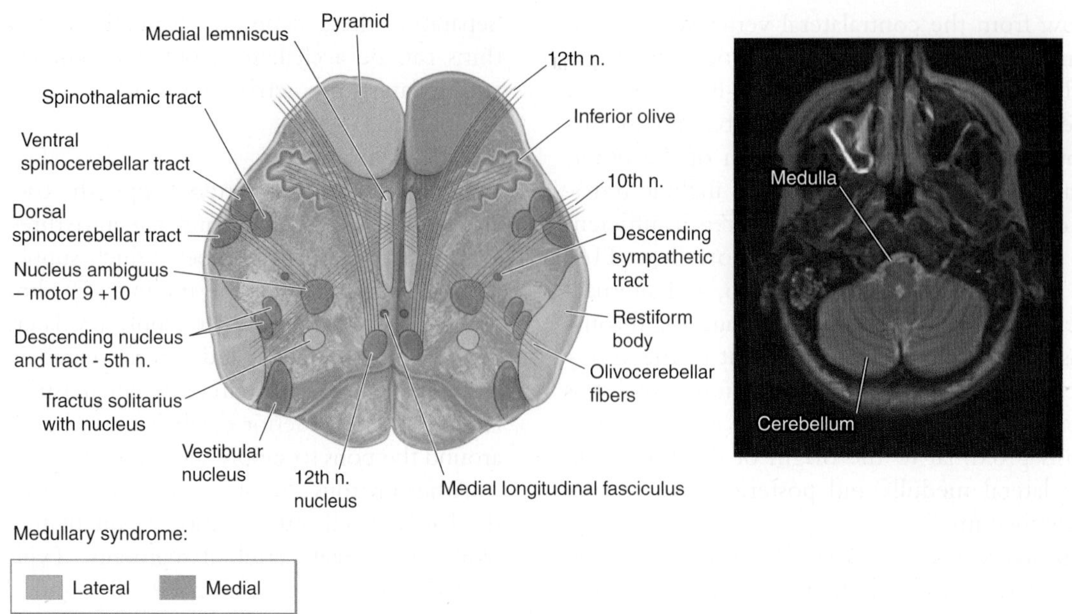

FIGURE 27-10

Axial section at the level of the medulla, depicted schematically on the left, with a corresponding MR image on the right. Note that in Figs. 27-10 through 27-14, all drawings are oriented with the dorsal surface at the bottom, matching the orientation of the brainstem that is commonly seen in all modern neuroimaging studies. Approximate regions involved in medial and lateral medullary stroke syndromes are shown.

Signs and symptoms: *Structures involved*

1. Medial medullary syndrome (occlusion of vertebral artery or of branch of vertebral or lower basilar artery)
   On side of lesion
      Paralysis with atrophy of one-half half the tongue: *Ipsilateral twelfth nerve*
   On side opposite lesion
      Paralysis of arm and leg, sparing face; impaired tactile and proprioceptive sense over one-half the body: *Contralateral pyramidal tract and medial lemniscus*
2. Lateral medullary syndrome (occlusion of any of five vessels may be responsible—vertebral, posterior inferior cerebellar, superior, middle, or inferior lateral medullary arteries)
   On side of lesion
      Pain, numbness, impaired sensation over one-half the face: *Descending tract and nucleus fifth nerve*
      Ataxia of limbs, falling to side of lesion: *Uncertain—restiform body, cerebellar hemisphere, cerebellar fibers, spinocerebellar tract (?)*
      Nystagmus, diplopia, oscillopsia, vertigo, nausea, vomiting: *Vestibular nucleus*
      Horner's syndrome (miosis, ptosis, decreased sweating): *Descending sympathetic tract*
      Dysphagia, hoarseness, paralysis of palate, paralysis of vocal cord, diminished gag reflex: *Issuing fibers ninth and tenth nerves*
      Loss of taste: *Nucleus and tractus solitarius*
      Numbness of ipsilateral arm, trunk, or leg: *Cuneate and gracile nuclei*
      Weakness of lower face: *Genuflected upper motor neuron fibers to ipsilateral facial nucleus*
   On side opposite lesion
      Impaired pain and thermal sense over half the body, sometimes face: *Spinothalamic tract*
3. Total unilateral medullary syndrome (occlusion of vertebral artery): Combination of medial and lateral syndromes
4. Lateral pontomedullary syndrome (occlusion of vertebral artery): Combination of lateral medullary and lateral inferior pontine syndrome
5. Basilar artery syndrome (the syndrome of the lone vertebral artery is equivalent): A combination of the various brainstem syndromes plus those arising in the posterior cerebral artery distribution.
   Bilateral long tract signs (sensory and motor; cerebellar and peripheral cranial nerve abnormalities): *Bilateral long tract; cerebellar and peripheral cranial nerves*
   Paralysis or weakness of all extremities, plus all bulbar musculature: *Corticobulbar and corticospinal tracts bilaterally*

and hemisensory symptoms. In general, symptoms of basilar branch TIAs affect one side of the brainstem, whereas symptoms of basilar artery TIAs usually affect both sides, although a "herald" hemiparesis has been emphasized as an initial symptom of basilar occlusion. Most often TIAs, whether due to impending occlusion of the basilar artery or a basilar branch, are short lived (5–30 min) and repetitive, occurring several times a day. The pattern suggests

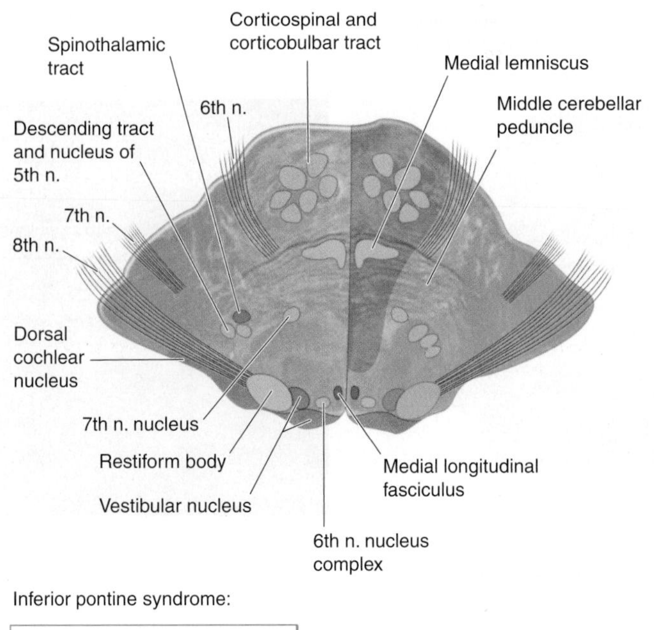

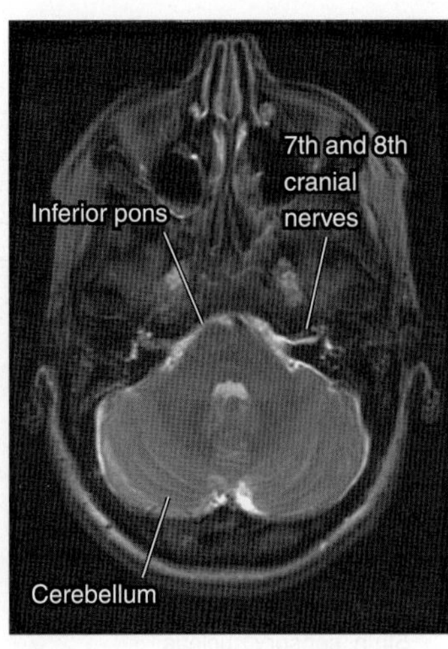

FIGURE 27-11
Axial section at the level of the inferior pons, depicted schematically on the left, with a corresponding MR image on the right. Approximate regions involved in medial and lateral inferior pontine stroke syndromes are shown.

Signs and symptoms: *Structures involved*

1. Medial inferior pontine syndrome (occlusion of paramedian branch of basilar artery)
   - On side of lesion
     - Paralysis of conjugate gaze to side of lesion (preservation of convergence): *Center for conjugate lateral gaze*
     - Nystagmus: *Vestibular nucleus*
     - Ataxia of limbs and gait: Likely *middle cerebellar peduncle*
     - Diplopia on lateral gaze: *Abducens nerve*
   - On side opposite lesion
     - Paralysis of face, arm, and leg: *Corticobulbar and corticospinal tract in lower pons*
     - Impaired tactile and proprioceptive sense over one-half of the body: *Medial lemniscus*
2. Lateral inferior pontine syndrome (occlusion of anterior inferior cerebellar artery)
   - On side of lesion
     - Horizontal and vertical nystagmus, vertigo, nausea, vomiting, oscillopsia: *Vestibular nerve or nucleus*
     - Facial paralysis: *Seventh nerve*
     - Paralysis of conjugate gaze to side of lesion: *Center for conjugate lateral gaze*
     - Deafness, tinnitus: *Auditory nerve or cochlear nucleus*
     - Ataxia: *Middle cerebellar peduncle and cerebellar hemisphere*
     - Impaired sensation over face: *Descending tract and nucleus fifth nerve*
   - On side opposite lesion
     - Impaired pain and thermal sense over one-half the body (may include face): *Spinothalamic tract*

intermittent reduction of flow. Many neurologists treat with heparin to prevent clot propagation.

Atherothrombotic occlusion of the basilar artery with infarction usually causes *bilateral* brainstem signs. A gaze paresis or internuclear ophthalmoplegia associated with ipsilateral hemiparesis may be the only manifestation of bilateral brainstem ischemia. More often, unequivocal signs of bilateral pontine disease are present. Complete basilar thrombosis carries a high mortality.

Occlusion of a branch of the basilar artery usually causes *unilateral* symptoms and signs involving motor, sensory, and cranial nerves. As long as symptoms remain unilateral, concern over pending basilar occlusion should be reduced.

Occlusion of the superior cerebellar artery results in severe ipsilateral cerebellar ataxia, nausea and vomiting, dysarthria, and contralateral loss of pain and temperature sensation over the extremities, body, and face (spino- and trigeminothalamic tracts). Partial deafness, ataxic

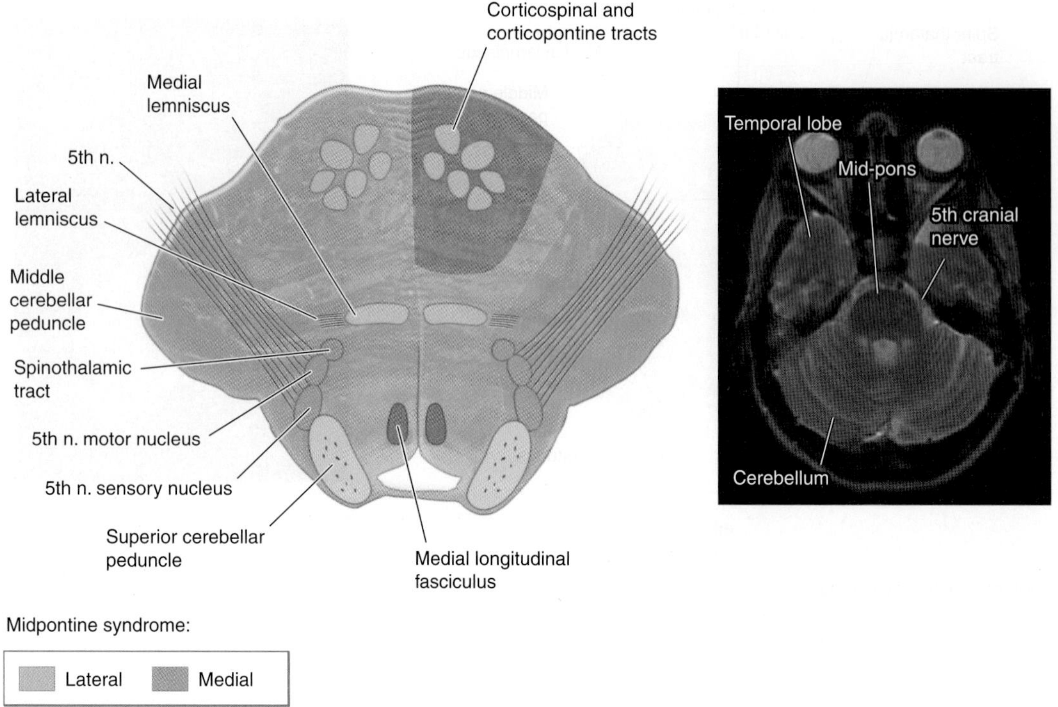

FIGURE 27-12
Axial section at the level of the midpons, depicted schematically on the left, with a corresponding MR image on the right. Approximate regions involved in medial and lateral midpontine stroke syndromes are shown.

Signs and symptoms: *Structures involved*

1. Medial midpontine syndrome (paramedian branch of midbasilar artery)
   - On side of lesion
     - Ataxia of limbs and gait (more prominent in bilateral involvement): *Pontine nuclei*
   - On side opposite lesion
     - Paralysis of face, arm, and leg: *Corticobulbar and corticospinal tract*
     - Variable impaired touch and proprioception when lesion extends posteriorly: *Medial lemniscus*
2. Lateral midpontine syndrome (short circumferential artery)
   - On side of lesion
     - Ataxia of limbs: *Middle cerebellar peduncle*
     - Paralysis of muscles of mastication: *Motor fibers or nucleus of fifth nerve*
     - Impaired sensation over side of face: *Sensory fibers or nucleus of fifth nerve*
   - On side opposite lesion
     - Impaired pain and thermal sense on limbs and trunk: *Spinothalamic tract*

tremor of the ipsilateral upper extremity, Horner's syndrome, and palatal myoclonus may occur rarely. Partial syndromes occur frequently (Fig. 27-13). With large strokes, swelling and mass effects may compress the midbrain or produce hydrocephalus; these symptoms may evolve rapidly. Neurosurgical intervention may be lifesaving in such cases.

Occlusion of the anterior inferior cerebellar artery produces variable degrees of infarction because the size of this artery and the territory it supplies vary inversely with those of the PICA. The principal symptoms include: (1) ipsilateral deafness, facial weakness, vertigo, nausea and vomiting, nystagmus, tinnitus, cerebellar ataxia, Horner's syndrome, and paresis of conjugate lateral gaze; and (2) contralateral loss of pain and temperature sensation. An occlusion close to the origin of the artery may cause corticospinal tract signs (Fig. 27-11).

Occlusion of one of the short circumferential branches of the basilar artery affects the lateral two-thirds of the pons and middle or superior cerebellar peduncle, whereas occlusion of one of the paramedian branches affects a wedge-shaped area on either side of the medial pons (Figs. 27-11 through 27-13).

IMAGING STUDIES

See also Chap. 4.

CT scans

CT radiographic images identify or exclude hemorrhage as the cause of stroke, and they identify extraparenchymal hemorrhages, neoplasms, abscesses, and other conditions masquerading as stroke. Brain CT scans obtained

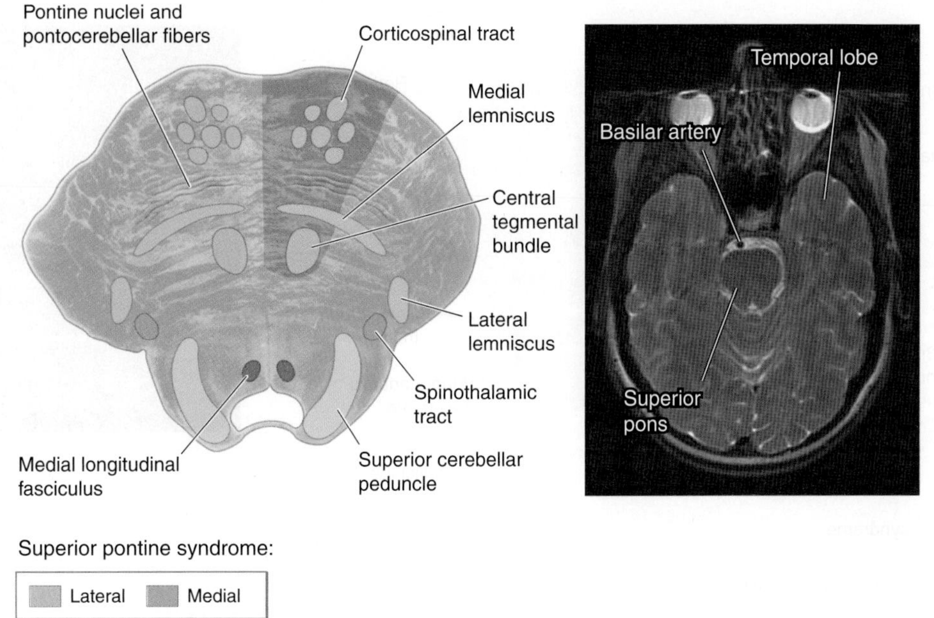

FIGURE 27-13

Axial section at the level of the superior pons, depicted schematically on the left, with a corresponding MR image on the right. Approximate regions involved in medial and lateral superior pontine stroke syndromes are shown.

Signs and symptoms: *Structures involved*

1. Medial superior pontine syndrome (paramedian branches of upper basilar artery)
   - On side of lesion
     - Cerebellar ataxia (probably): *Superior and/or middle cerebellar peduncle*
     - Internuclear ophthalmoplegia: *Medial longitudinal fasciculus*
     - Myoclonic syndrome, palate, pharynx, vocal cords, respiratory apparatus, face, oculomotor apparatus, etc.: *Localization uncertain—central tegmental bundle, dentate projection, inferior olivary nucleus*
   - On side opposite lesion
     - Paralysis of face, arm, and leg: *Corticobulbar and corticospinal tract*
     - Rarely touch, vibration, and position are affected: *Medial lemniscus*
2. Lateral superior pontine syndrome (syndrome of superior cerebellar artery)
   - On side of lesion
     - Ataxia of limbs and gait, falling to side of lesion: *Middle and superior cerebellar peduncles, superior surface of cerebellum, dentate nucleus*
     - Dizziness, nausea, vomiting; horizontal nystagmus: *Vestibular nucleus*
     - Paresis of conjugate gaze (ipsilateral): *Pontine contralateral gaze*
     - Skew deviation: *Uncertain*
     - Miosis, ptosis, decreased sweating over face (Horner's syndrome): *Descending sympathetic fibers*
     - Tremor: Localization unclear—*Dentate nucleus, superior cerebellar peduncle*
   - On side opposite lesion
     - Impaired pain and thermal sense on face, limbs, and trunk: *Spinothalamic tract*
     - Impaired touch, vibration, and position sense, more in leg than arm (there is a tendency to incongruity of pain and touch deficits): *Medial lemniscus (lateral portion)*

in the first several hours after an infarction generally show no abnormality, and the infarct may not be seen reliably for 24–48 h. CT may fail to show small ischemic strokes in the posterior fossa because of bone artifact; small infarcts on the cortical surface may also be missed.

Contrast-enhanced CT scans add specificity by showing contrast enhancement of subacute infarcts and allow visualization of venous structures. Coupled with newer generation multidetector scanners, CT angiography (CTA) can be performed with administration of IV iodinated contrast allowing visualization of the cervical and intracranial arteries, intracranial veins, aortic arch, and even the coronary arteries in one imaging session. Carotid disease and intracranial vascular occlusions are readily identified with this method (Fig. 27-3). After an IV bolus of contrast, deficits in brain perfusion produced by vascular occlusion can also be demonstrated (Fig. 27-15) and used to predict the region of infarcted brain and the brain at risk of further infarction (i.e., the ischemic penumbra, see "Pathophysiology of Ischemic Stroke"). CT imaging is also sensitive for detecting SAH (though by itself does not rule it out), and CTA can readily identify intracranial aneurysms (Chap. 28).

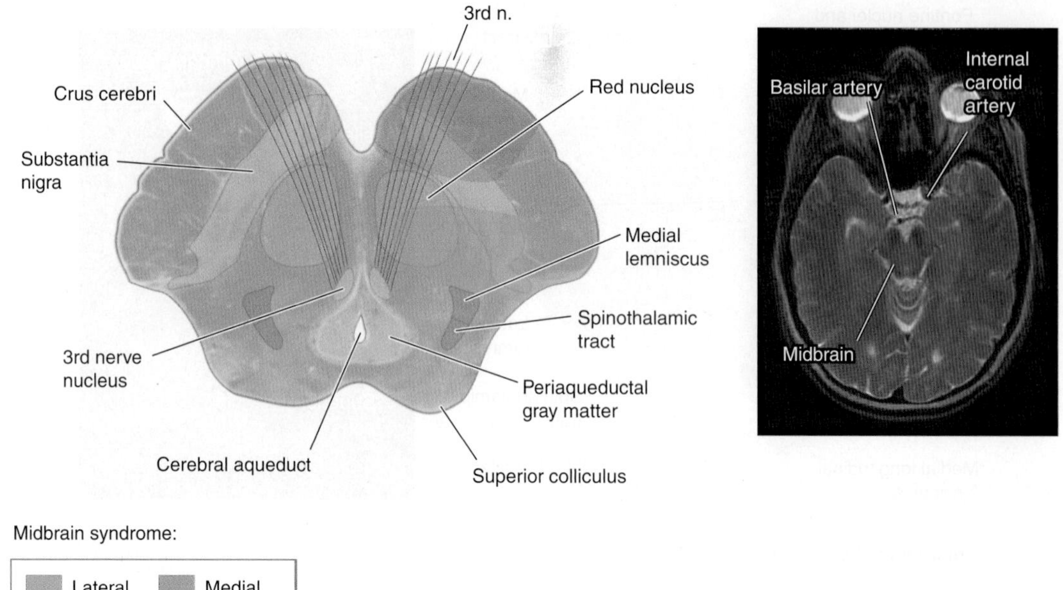

FIGURE 27-14

Axial section at the level of the midbrain, depicted schematically on the left, with a corresponding MR image on the right. Approximate regions involved in medial and lateral midbrain stroke syndromes are shown.

Signs and symptoms: *Structures involved*

1. Medial midbrain syndrome (paramedian branches of upper basilar and proximal posterior cerebral arteries)
   On side of lesion
   Eye "down and out" secondary to unopposed action of fourth and sixth cranial nerves, with dilated and unresponsive pupil: *Third nerve fibers*
   On side opposite lesion
   Paralysis of face, arm, and leg: *Corticobulbar and corticospinal tract descending in crus cerebri*
2. Lateral midbrain syndrome (syndrome of small penetrating arteries arising from posterior cerebral artery)
   On side of lesion
   Eye "down and out" secondary to unopposed action of fourth and sixth cranial nerves, with dilated and unresponsive pupil: *Third nerve fibers and/or third nerve nucleus*
   On side opposite lesion
   Hemiataxia, hyperkinesias, tremor: *Red nucleus, dentatorubrothalamic pathway*

Because of its speed and wide availability, noncontrast head CT is the imaging modality of choice in patients with acute stroke (Fig. 27-1), and CTA and CT perfusion imaging may also be useful and convenient adjuncts.

MRI

MRI reliably documents the extent and location of infarction in all areas of the brain, including the posterior fossa and cortical surface. It also identifies intracranial hemorrhage and other abnormalities but is less sensitive than CT for detecting acute blood. MRI scanners with magnets of higher field strength produce more reliable and precise images. Diffusion-weighted imaging is more sensitive for early brain infarction than standard MR sequences or CT (Fig. 27-16), as is fluid-attenuated inversion recovery (FLAIR) imaging (Chap. 4). Using IV administration of gadolinium contrast, MR perfusion studies can be performed. Brain regions showing poor perfusion but no abnormality on diffusion are equivalent measure of the ischemic penumbra (see "Pathophysiology of Ischemic Stroke" and Fig. 27-16), and patients showing large regions of mismatch may be better candidates for acute revascularization. MR angiography is highly sensitive for stenosis of extracranial internal carotid arteries and of large intracranial vessels. With higher degrees of stenosis, MR angiography tends to overestimate the degree of stenosis when compared to conventional x-ray angiography. MRI with fat saturation is an imaging sequence used to visualize extra or intracranial arterial dissection. This sensitive technique images clotted blood within the dissected vessel wall.

MRI is less sensitive for acute blood products than CT and is more expensive and time consuming and less readily available. Claustrophobia also limits its application. Most acute stroke protocols use CT because of these limitations. However, MRI is useful outside the acute period by more clearly defining the extent of tissue injury and discriminating new from old regions of brain infarction. MRI may have particular utility in patients with

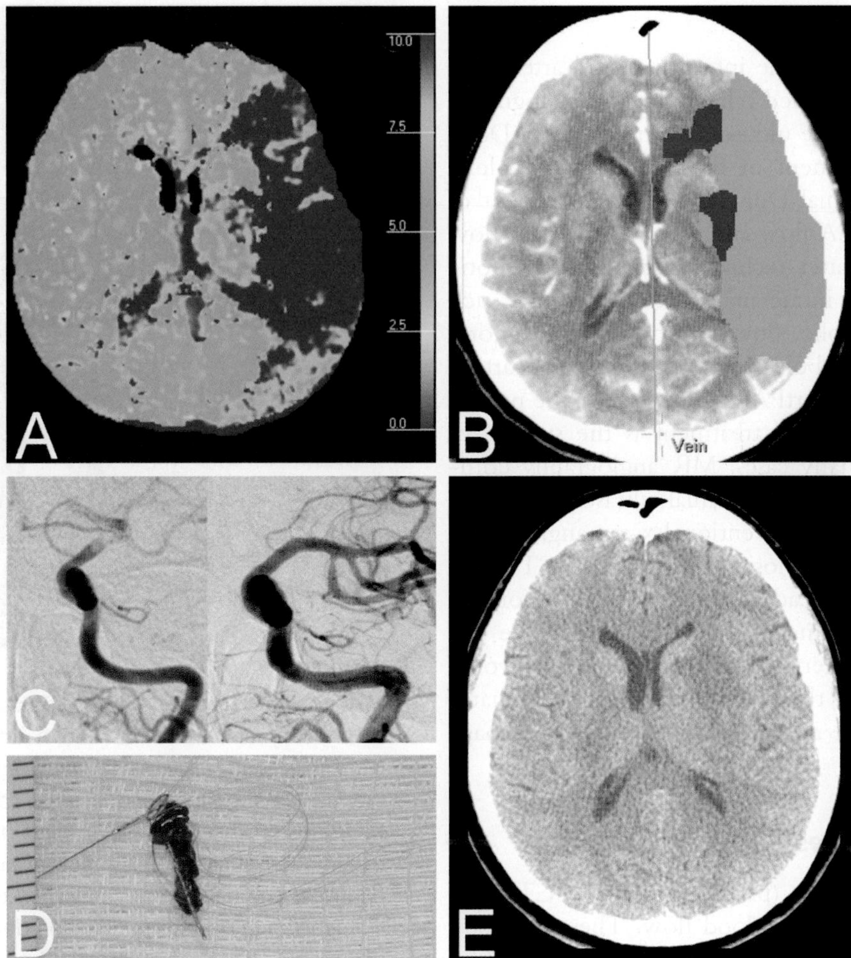

FIGURE 27-15

Acute left middle cerebral artery (MCA) stroke with right hemiplegia but preserved language. ***A.*** CT perfusion mean-transit time map showing delayed perfusion of the left MCA distribution (*blue*). ***B.*** Predicted region of infarct (*red*) and penumbra (*green*) based on CT perfusion data. ***C.*** Conventional angiogram showing occlusion of the left internal carotid–MCA bifurcation (*left panel*), and revascularization of the vessels following successful thrombectomy 8 h after stroke symptom onset (*right panel*). ***D.*** The clot removed with a thrombectomy device (L5, Concentric Medical, Inc.). ***E.*** CT scan of the brain 2 days later; note infarction in the region predicted in ***B*** but preservation of the penumbral region by successful revascularization.

TIA. It is also more likely to identify new infarction, which is a strong predictor of subsequent stroke.

Cerebral angiography

Conventional x-ray cerebral angiography is the gold standard for identifying and quantifying atherosclerotic stenoses of the cerebral arteries and for identifying and characterizing other pathologies, including aneurysms, vasospasm, intraluminal thrombi, fibromuscular dysplasia, arteriovenous fistula, vasculitis, and collateral channels of blood flow. Endovascular techniques, which are evolving rapidly, can be used to deploy stents within delicate intracranial vessels, to perform balloon angioplasty of stenotic lesions, to treat intracranial aneurysms by embolization, and to open occluded vessels in acute stroke with mechanical thrombectomy devices. Randomized trials support use of thrombolytic agents delivered intraarterially in patients with acute MCA stroke by showing that vessels are effectively recanalized and clinical outcomes are improved at 90 days. Cerebral angiography coupled with endovascular techniques for cerebral revascularization are becoming routine in the United States and Europe and likely soon in Japan. Centers capable of these techniques are termed *comprehensive stroke centers* to distinguish them from primary stroke centers that can administer IV rtPA but not perform endovascular therapy. Conventional angiography carries risks of arterial damage, groin hemorrhage, embolic stroke, and renal failure from contrast nephropathy, so it should be reserved for situations where less invasive means are inadequate.

Ultrasound techniques

Stenosis at the origin of the internal carotid artery can be identified and quantified reliably by ultrasonography that combines a B-mode ultrasound image with a Doppler ultrasound assessment of flow velocity ("duplex" ultrasound). Transcranial Doppler (TCD) assessment of MCA, ACA, and PCA flow and of vertebrobasilar flow is also useful. This latter technique can detect stenotic lesions in the large intracranial arteries because such lesions increase systolic flow velocity. Furthermore, TCD can assist thrombolysis and improve large artery recanalization following rtPA administration; the potential clinical benefit of this treatment is the subject of ongoing study. In many cases, MR angiography combined with carotid and transcranial ultrasound studies eliminates the need for conventional x-ray angiography in evaluating vascular stenosis. Alternatively, CT angiography of the entire head and neck can be performed during the initial imaging of acute stroke. Because this images the entire arterial system relevant to stroke, with the exception of the heart, much of the clinician's stroke workup can be completed with this single imaging study.

Perfusion techniques

Both xenon techniques (principally xenon-CT) and PET can quantify cerebral blood flow. These tools are generally used for research (Chap.4) but can be useful for determining the significance of arterial stenosis and planning for revascularization surgery. Single-photon emission computed tomography (SPECT) and MR perfusion techniques report relative cerebral blood flow. Since CT imaging is used as the initial imaging modality for acute stroke, some centers combine both CT angiography and CT perfusion imaging together with the noncontrast CT scan. CT perfusion imaging increases the sensitivity for detecting ischemia, and can measure the ischemic penumbra (Fig. 27-15). Alternatively, MR perfusion can be combined with MR diffusion imaging to identify the ischemic penumbra as the mismatch between these two imaging sequences (Fig. 27-16). The ability to image the ischemic penumbra allows more judicious selection of patients who may or may not benefit from acute interventions such as thrombolysis, thrombectomy, or investigational neuroprotective strategies.

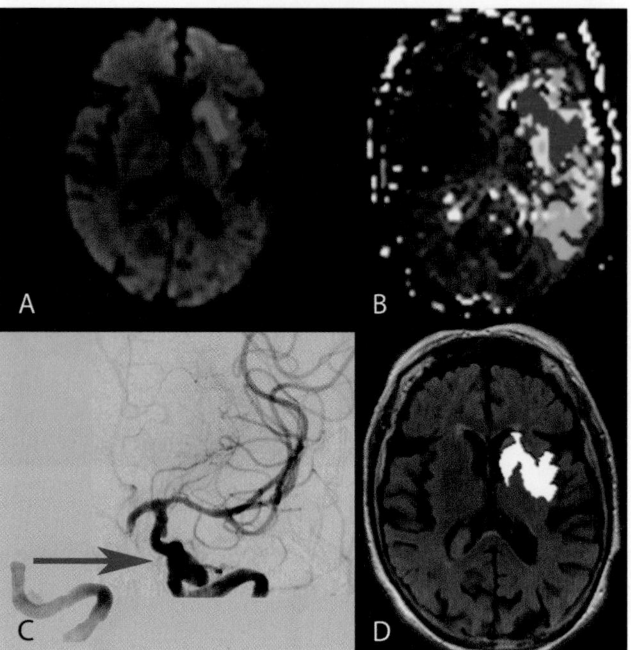

FIGURE 27-16

MRI of acute stroke. *A.* MRI diffusion-weighted image (DWI) of an 82-year-old woman 2.5 h after onset of right-sided weakness and aphasia reveals restricted diffusion within the left basal ganglia and internal capsule (*colored regions*). ***B.*** Perfusion defect within the left hemisphere (*colored signal*) imaged after administration of an IV bolus of gadolinium contrast. The discrepancy between the region of poor perfusion shown in ***B*** and the diffusion deficit shown in ***A*** is called *diffusion-perfusion mismatch* and provides an estimate of the ischemic penumbra. Without specific therapy the region of infarction will expand into much or all of the perfusion deficit. ***C.*** Cerebral angiogram of the left internal carotid artery in this patient before (*left*) and after (*right*) successful endovascular embolectomy. The occlusion is within the carotid terminus. ***D.*** FLAIR image obtained 3 days later showing a region of infarction (*coded as white*) that corresponds to the initial DWI image in ***A,*** but not the entire area at risk shown in ***B,*** suggesting that successful embolectomy saved a large region of brain tissue from infarction. (*Courtesy of Gregory Albers, MD, Stanford University; with permission.*)

INTRACRANIAL HEMORRHAGE

Hemorrhages are classified by their location and the underlying vascular pathology. Bleeding into subdural and epidural spaces is principally produced by trauma. SAHs are produced by trauma and rupture of intracranial aneurysms (Chap. 28). Intraparenchymal and intraventricular hemorrhage will be considered here.

DIAGNOSIS

Intracranial hemorrhage is often discovered on noncontrast CT imaging of the brain during the acute evaluation of stroke. Since CT is more sensitive than routine MRI for acute blood, CT imaging is the preferred method for acute stroke evaluation (Fig. 27-1). The location of the hemorrhage narrows the differential diagnosis to a few entities. Table 27-6 lists the causes and anatomic spaces involved in hemorrhages.

TABLE 27-6

CAUSES OF INTRACRANIAL HEMORRHAGE

CAUSE	LOCATION	COMMENTS
Head trauma	Intraparenchymal: frontal lobes, anterior temporal lobes; subarachnoid	Coup and contrecoup injury during brain deceleration
Hypertensive hemorrhage	Putamen, globus pallidus, thalamus, cerebellar hemisphere, pons	Chronic hypertension produces hemorrhage from small (~100 μm) vessels in these regions
Transformation of prior ischemic infarction	Basal ganglion, subcortical regions, lobar	Occurs in 1–6% of ischemic strokes with predilection for large hemispheric infarctions
Metastatic brain tumor	Lobar	Lung, choriocarcinoma, melanoma, renal cell carcinoma, thyroid, atrial myxoma
Coagulopathy	Any	Uncommon cause; often associated with prior stroke or underlying vascular anomaly
Drug	Lobar, subarachnoid	Cocaine, amphetamine, phenylpropanolamine
Arteriovenous malformation	Lobar, intraventricular, subarachnoid	Risk is ~2–4% per year for bleeding
Aneurysm	Subarachnoid, intraparenchymal, rarely subdural	Mycotic and nonmycotic forms of aneurysms
Amyloid angiopathy	Lobar	Degenerative disease of intracranial vessels; linkage to Alzheimer's disease, rare in patients <60 years
Cavernous angioma	Intraparenchymal	Multiple cavernous angiomas linked to mutations in KRIT1, CCM2, and PDCD10 genes
Dural arteriovenous fistula	Lobar, subarachnoid	Produces bleeding by venous hypertension
Capillary telangiectasias	Usually brainstem	Rare cause of hemorrhage

EMERGENCY MANAGEMENT

Close attention should be paid to airway management since a reduction in the level of consciousness is common and often progressive. The initial blood pressure should be maintained until the results of the CT scan are reviewed. Expansion of hemorrhage volume is associated with elevated blood pressure, but it remains unclear if lowering of blood pressure reduces hematoma growth. A recent feasibility trial of 60 patients showed that blood pressure could be safely lowered in acute spontaneous intraparenchymal (intracerebral) hemorrhage (ICH) using nicardipine and forms the basis for a planned pivotal trial powered for detecting improved clinical outcome. Another trial (Intensive Blood Pressure Reduction in Acute Cerebral Hemorrhage Trial [INTERACT]) randomized hypertensive, spontaneous ICH patients to maintain systolic blood pressure (SBP) <180 mmHg versus SBP <140 mmHg using IV antihypertensives. There was a statistical decrease in hematoma growth and a reduction in perihematoma edema in the patients assigned to the lower blood pressure goal. Whether these reductions in hematoma growth will translate to clinical benefit is unclear. Until more results are available it is recommended to keep mean arterial pressure (MAP) <130 mmHg, unless an increase in ICP is suspected. In patients who have ICP monitors in place, current recommendations are to keep the cerebral perfusion pressure (MAP-ICP) above 60 mmHg (i.e., one should lower MAP to this target if blood pressure is elevated). Blood pressure should be lowered with nonvasodilating IV drugs such as nicardipine, labetalol, or esmolol. Patients with cerebellar hemorrhages or with depressed mental status and radiographic evidence of hydrocephalus should undergo urgent neurosurgical evaluation. Based on the clinical examination and CT findings, further imaging studies may be necessary, including MRI or conventional x-ray angiography. Stuporous or comatose patients generally are treated presumptively for elevated ICP, with tracheal intubation and hyperventilation, mannitol administration, and elevation of the head of the bed while surgical consultation is obtained (Chap. 28).

ICH is the most common type of intracranial hemorrhage. It accounts for ~10% of all strokes and is associated with a 50% case fatality rate. Incidence rates are particularly high in Asians and blacks. Hypertension, trauma, and cerebral amyloid angiopathy cause the majority of these hemorrhages. Advanced age and heavy alcohol consumption increase the risk, and cocaine and methamphetamine use is one of the most important causes in the young.

Hypertensive intraparenchymal hemorrhage

Pathophysiology

Hypertensive intraparenchymal hemorrhage (hypertensive hemorrhage or hypertensive intracerebral hemorrhage) usually results from spontaneous rupture of a small penetrating artery deep in the brain. The most common sites are the basal ganglia (especially the putamen), thalamus, cerebellum, and pons. When hemorrhages occur in other brain areas or in nonhypertensive patients, greater consideration should be given to hemorrhagic disorders, neoplasms, vascular malformations, and other causes. The small arteries in these areas seem most prone to hypertension-induced vascular injury. The hemorrhage may be small or a large clot may form and compress adjacent tissue, causing herniation and death. Blood may dissect into the ventricular space, which substantially increases morbidity and may cause hydrocephalus.

Most hypertensive intraparenchymal hemorrhages develop over 30–90 min, whereas those associated with anticoagulant therapy may evolve for as long as 24–48 h. Within 48 h macrophages begin to phagocytize the hemorrhage at its outer surface. After 1–6 months, the hemorrhage is generally resolved to a slitlike orange cavity lined with glial scar and hemosiderin-laden macrophages.

Clinical manifestations

Although not particularly associated with exertion, ICHs almost always occur while the patient is awake and sometimes when stressed. The hemorrhage generally presents as the abrupt onset of focal neurologic deficit. Seizures are uncommon. The focal deficit typically worsens steadily over 30–90 min and is associated with a diminishing level of consciousness and signs of increased ICP such as headache and vomiting.

The putamen is the most common site for hypertensive hemorrhage, and the adjacent internal capsule is usually damaged (Fig. 27-17). Contralateral hemiparesis is therefore the sentinel sign. When mild, the face sags on one side over 5–30 min, speech becomes slurred, the arm and leg gradually weaken, and the eyes deviate away from the side of the hemiparesis. The

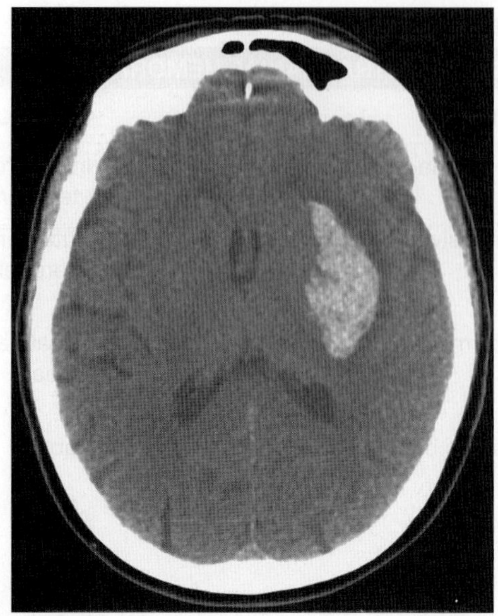

FIGURE 27-17
Hypertensive hemorrhage. Transaxial noncontrast CT scan through the region of the basal ganglia reveals a hematoma involving the left putamen in a patient with rapidly progressive onset of right hemiparesis.

paralysis may worsen until the affected limbs become flaccid or extend rigidly. When hemorrhages are large, drowsiness gives way to stupor as signs of upper brainstem compression appear. Coma ensues, accompanied by deep, irregular, or intermittent respiration, a dilated and fixed ipsilateral pupil, and decerebrate rigidity. In milder cases, edema in adjacent brain tissue may cause progressive deterioration over 12–72 h.

Thalamic hemorrhages also produce a contralateral hemiplegia or hemiparesis from pressure on, or dissection into, the adjacent internal capsule. A prominent sensory deficit involving all modalities is usually present. Aphasia, often with preserved verbal repetition, may occur after hemorrhage into the dominant thalamus, and constructional apraxia or mutism occurs in some cases of nondominant hemorrhage. There may also be a homonymous visual field defect. Thalamic hemorrhages cause several typical ocular disturbances by virtue of extension inferiorly into the upper midbrain. These include deviation of the eyes downward and inward so that they appear to be looking at the nose, unequal pupils with absence of light reaction, skew deviation with the eye opposite the hemorrhage displaced downward and medially, ipsilateral Horner's syndrome, absence of convergence, paralysis of vertical gaze, and retraction nystagmus. Patients may later develop a chronic, contralateral pain syndrome (Déjérine-Roussy syndrome).

In pontine hemorrhages, deep coma with quadriplegia usually occurs over a few minutes. There is often prominent decerebrate rigidity and "pinpoint" (1 mm) pupils that react to light. There is impairment of reflex horizontal eye movements evoked by head turning (doll's-head or oculocephalic maneuver) or by irrigation of the ears with ice water (Chap. 17). Hyperpnea, severe hypertension, and hyperhidrosis are common. Death often occurs within a few hours, but small hemorrhages are compatible with survival.

Cerebellar hemorrhages usually develop over several hours and are characterized by occipital headache, repeated vomiting, and ataxia of gait. In mild cases there may be no other neurologic signs other than gait ataxia. Dizziness or vertigo may be prominent. There is often paresis of conjugate lateral gaze toward the side of the hemorrhage, forced deviation of the eyes to the opposite side, or an ipsilateral sixth nerve palsy. Less frequent ocular signs include blepharospasm, involuntary closure of one eye, ocular bobbing, and skew deviation. Dysarthria and dysphagia may occur. As the hours pass, the patient often becomes stuporous and then comatose from brainstem compression or obstructive hydrocephalus; immediate surgical evacuation before brainstem compression occurs may be lifesaving. Hydrocephalus from fourth ventricle compression can be relieved by external ventricular drainage, but definitive hematoma evacuation is essential for survival. If the deep cerebellar nuclei are spared, full recovery is common.

Lobar hemorrhage

Symptoms and signs appear over several minutes. Most lobar hemorrhages are small and cause a restricted clinical syndrome that simulates an embolus to an artery supplying one lobe. For example, the major neurologic deficit with an occipital hemorrhage is hemianopia; with a left temporal hemorrhage, aphasia and delirium; with a parietal hemorrhage, hemisensory loss; and with frontal hemorrhage, arm weakness. Large hemorrhages may be associated with stupor or coma if they compress the thalamus or midbrain. Most patients with lobar hemorrhages have focal headaches, and more than one-half vomit or are drowsy. Stiff neck and seizures are uncommon.

Other causes of intracerebral hemorrhage

Cerebral amyloid angiopathy is a disease of the elderly in which arteriolar degeneration occurs and amyloid is deposited in the walls of the cerebral arteries. Amyloid angiopathy causes both single and recurrent lobar hemorrhages and is probably the most common cause of lobar hemorrhage in the elderly. It accounts for some intracranial hemorrhages associated with IV thrombolysis given for MI. This disorder can be suspected in patients who present with multiple hemorrhages (and infarcts) over several months or years, or in patients with "micro-bleeds" seen on brain MRI sequences sensitive for hemosiderin, but it is definitively diagnosed by pathologic demonstration of Congo red staining of amyloid in cerebral vessels. The ε2 and ε4 allelic variations of the apolipoprotein E gene are associated with increased risk of recurrent lobar hemorrhage and may therefore be markers of amyloid angiopathy. Currently, there is no specific therapy, although antiplatelet and anticoagulating agents are typically avoided.

Cocaine and methamphetamine are frequent causes of stroke in young (age <45 years) patients. ICH, ischemic stroke, and SAH are all associated with stimulant use. Angiographic findings vary from completely normal arteries to large-vessel occlusion or stenosis, vasospasm, or changes consistent with vasculopathy. The mechanism of sympathomimetic-related stroke is not known, but cocaine enhances sympathetic activity causing acute, sometimes severe, hypertension, and this may lead to hemorrhage. Slightly more than one-half of stimulant-related intracranial hemorrhages are intracerebral, and the rest are subarachnoid. In cases of SAH, a saccular aneurysm is usually identified. Presumably, acute hypertension causes aneurysmal rupture.

Head injury often causes intracranial bleeding. The common sites are intracerebral (especially temporal and inferior frontal lobes) and into the subarachnoid, subdural, and epidural spaces. Trauma must be considered in any patient with an unexplained acute neurologic deficit (hemiparesis, stupor, or confusion), particularly if the deficit occurred in the context of a fall (Chap. 36).

Intracranial hemorrhages associated with *anticoagulant therapy* can occur at any location; they are often lobar or subdural. Anticoagulant-related ICHs may evolve slowly, over 24–48 h. Coagulopathy and thrombocytopenia should be reversed rapidly, as discussed later. ICH associated with *hematologic disorders* (leukemia, aplastic anemia, thrombocytopenic purpura) can occur at any site and may present as multiple ICHs. Skin and mucous membrane bleeding is usually evident and offers a diagnostic clue.

Hemorrhage into a *brain tumor* may be the first manifestation of neoplasm. Choriocarcinoma, malignant melanoma, renal cell carcinoma, and bronchogenic carcinoma are among the most common metastatic tumors associated with ICH. Glioblastoma multiforme in adults and medulloblastoma in children may also have areas of ICH.

Hypertensive encephalopathy is a complication of malignant hypertension. In this acute syndrome, severe hypertension is associated with headache, nausea, vomiting, convulsions, confusion, stupor, and coma. Focal or lateralizing neurologic signs, either transitory or permanent, may occur but are infrequent and therefore suggest some other vascular disease (hemorrhage, embolism, or atherosclerotic thrombosis). There are retinal hemorrhages, exudates, papilledema (hypertensive retinopathy), and evidence of renal and cardiac disease.

In most cases ICP and CSF protein levels are elevated. MRI brain imaging shows a pattern of typically posterior (occipital > frontal) brain edema that is reversible and termed *reversible posterior leukoencephalopathy*. The hypertension may be essential or due to chronic renal disease, acute glomerulonephritis, acute toxemia of pregnancy, pheochromocytoma, or other causes. Lowering the blood pressure reverses the process, but stroke can occur, especially if blood pressure is lowered too rapidly. Neuropathologic examination reveals multifocal to diffuse cerebral edema and hemorrhages of various sizes from petechial to massive. Microscopically, there are necrosis of arterioles, minute cerebral infarcts, and hemorrhages. The term *hypertensive encephalopathy* should be reserved for this syndrome and not for chronic recurrent headaches, dizziness, recurrent TIAs, or small strokes that often occur in association with high blood pressure.

Primary intraventricular hemorrhage is rare. It usually begins within the substance of the brain and dissects into the ventricular system without leaving signs of intraparenchymal hemorrhage. Alternatively, bleeding can arise from periependymal veins. Vasculitis, usually polyarteritis nodosa or lupus erythematosus, can produce hemorrhage in any region of the central nervous system; most hemorrhages are associated with hypertension, but the arteritis itself may cause bleeding by disrupting the vessel wall. Nearly one-half of patients with primary intraventricular hemorrhage have identifiable bleeding sources seen using conventional angiography. *Sepsis* can cause small petechial hemorrhages throughout the cerebral white matter. *Moyamoya disease*, mainly an occlusive arterial disease that causes ischemic symptoms, may on occasion produce intraparenchymal hemorrhage, particularly in the young. Hemorrhages into the spinal cord are usually the result of an AVM, cavernous malformation, or metastatic tumor. *Epidural spinal hemorrhage* produces a rapidly evolving syndrome of spinal cord or nerve root compression (Chap. 35). Spinal hemorrhages usually present with sudden back pain and some manifestation of myelopathy.

Laboratory and imaging evaluation

Patients should have routine blood chemistries and hematologic studies. Specific attention to the platelet count and PT/PTT are important to identify coagulopathy. CT imaging reliably detects acute focal hemorrhages in the supratentorial space. Small pontine hemorrhages may not be identified because of motion and bone-induced artifact that obscure structures in the posterior fossa. After the first 2 weeks, x-ray attenuation values of clotted blood diminish until they become isodense with surrounding brain. Mass effect and edema may remain. In some cases, a surrounding rim of contrast enhancement appears after 2–4 weeks and may persist for months. MRI, although more sensitive for delineating posterior fossa lesions, is generally not necessary in most instances. Images of flowing blood on MRI scan may identify AVMs as the cause of the hemorrhage. MRI, CT angiography, and conventional x-ray angiography are used when the cause of intracranial hemorrhage is uncertain, particularly if the patient is young or not hypertensive and the hematoma is not in one of the four usual sites for hypertensive hemorrhage. Postcontrast CT imaging may reveal acute hematoma enhancement signifying bleeding at the time of imaging; this "dot-sign" portends increased mortality. Some centers routinely perform CT and CT angiography with postcontrast CT imaging in one sitting to rapidly identify any macrovascular etiology of the hemorrhage and provide prognostic information at the same time. Since patients typically have focal neurologic signs and obtundation, and often show signs of increased ICP, a lumbar puncture should be avoided as it may induce cerebral herniation.

TREATMENT Intracerebral Hemorrhage

ACUTE MANAGEMENT Nearly 50% of patients with a hypertensive ICH die, but others have a good to complete recovery if they survive the initial hemorrhage. The ICH scoring system (Table 27-7) is a validated metric that is useful for prediction of mortality and clinical outcomes. Any identified coagulopathy should be reversed as soon as possible. For patients taking VKAs, rapid reversal of coagulopathy can be achieved by infusing prothrombin complex concentrates which can be administered quickly, followed by fresh-frozen plasma and vitamin K. When ICH is associated with thrombocytopenia (platelet count <50,000/μL), transfusion of fresh platelets is indicated. The role of urgent platelet inhibition assays in the decision to transfuse platelets remains unclear.

At present, little can be done about the hemorrhage itself. Hematomas may expand for several hours following the initial hemorrhage, so treating severe hypertension seems reasonable to prevent hematoma progression. A phase 3 trial of treatment with recombinant factor VIIa reduced hematoma expansion; however, clinical outcomes were not improved, so use of this drug cannot be advocated at present.

Evacuation of supratentorial hematomas does not appear to improve outcome. The International Surgical Trial in Intracerebral Haemorrhage (STICH) randomized 1033 patients with supratentorial ICH to either early surgical evacuation or initial medical management. No benefit was found in the early surgery arm, although analysis was complicated by the fact that 26% of

TABLE 27-7

PROGNOSIS AND CLINICAL OUTCOMES IN INTRACEREBRAL HEMORRHAGE

CLINICAL OR IMAGING FACTOR	POINT SCORE
Age	
<80 years	0
≥80 years	1
Hematoma Volume	
<30 cc	0
≥30 cc	1
Intraventricular Hemorrhage Present	
No	0
Yes	1
Infratentorial Origin of Hemorrhage	
No	0
Yes	1
Glasgow Coma Scale Score	
13–15	0
5–12	1
3–4	2
Total Score	Sum of each category above

ICH SCORE TOTAL	OBSERVED MORTALITY AT 30 DAYS (%)	WALK INDEPENDENTLY AT 12 MONTHS (%)
0	0	70
1	13	60
2	26	33
3	72	3
4	97	8
5	100	None

Although a score of 6 is possible with the scale, no patient was observed to present with this combination of findings, and it is considered highly likely to be fatal.

Abbreviation: ICH, intracerebral hemorrhage.

Sources: JC Hemphill et al: Stroke 32:891, 2001; JC Hemphill et al: Neurology 73:1088, 2009.

patients in the initial medical management group ultimately had surgery for neurologic deterioration. Overall, these data do not support routine surgical evacuation of supratentorial hemorrhages; however, many centers operate on patients with progressive neurologic deterioration. Surgical techniques continue to evolve, and minimally invasive endoscopic hematoma evacuation may prove beneficial in future trials.

For cerebellar hemorrhages, a neurosurgeon should be consulted immediately to assist with the evaluation; most cerebellar hematomas >3 cm in diameter will require surgical evacuation. If the patient is alert without focal brainstem signs and if the hematoma is <1 cm in diameter, surgical removal is usually unnecessary. Patients with hematomas between 1 and 3 cm require careful observation for signs of impaired consciousness and precipitous respiratory failure.

Tissue surrounding hematomas is displaced and compressed but not necessarily infarcted. Hence, in survivors, major improvement commonly occurs as the hematoma is reabsorbed and the adjacent tissue regains its function. Careful management of the patient during the acute phase of the hemorrhage can lead to considerable recovery.

Surprisingly, ICP is often normal even with large intraparenchymal hemorrhages. However, if the hematoma causes marked midline shift of structures with consequent obtundation, coma, or hydrocephalus, osmotic agents coupled with induced hyperventilation can be instituted to lower ICP (Chap. 28). These maneuvers will provide enough time to place a ventriculostomy or ICP monitor. Once ICP is recorded, further hyperventilation and osmotic therapy can be tailored to the individual patient to keep cerebral perfusion pressure (MAP-ICP) above 60 mmHg. For example, if ICP is found to be high, CSF can be drained from the ventricular space and osmotic therapy continued; persistent or progressive elevation in ICP may prompt surgical evacuation of the clot or withdrawal of support. Alternately, if ICP is normal or only mildly elevated, induced hyperventilation can be reversed and osmotic therapy tapered. Since hyperventilation may actually produce ischemia by cerebral vasoconstriction, induced hyperventilation should be limited to acute resuscitation of the patient with presumptive high ICP and eliminated once other treatments (osmotic therapy or surgical treatments) have been instituted. Glucocorticoids are not helpful for the edema from intracerebral hematoma.

PREVENTION Hypertension is the leading cause of primary ICH. Prevention is aimed at reducing hypertension, eliminating excessive alcohol use, and discontinuing use of illicit drugs such as cocaine and amphetamines. Patients with amyloid angiopathy should avoid antithrombotic agents.

VASCULAR ANOMALIES

Vascular anomalies can be divided into congenital vascular malformations and acquired vascular lesions.

CONGENITAL VASCULAR MALFORMATIONS

True *arteriovenous malformations* (AVMs), venous anomalies, and capillary telangiectasias are lesions that usually remain clinically silent through life. AVMs are probably congenital but cases of acquired lesions have been reported.

True AVMs are congenital shunts between the arterial and venous systems that may present as headache, seizures, and intracranial hemorrhage. AVMs consist of a tangle of abnormal vessels across the cortical surface or deep within the brain substance. AVMs vary in size from a small blemish a few millimeters in diameter to a large mass of tortuous channels composing an arteriovenous shunt of sufficient magnitude to raise cardiac output and precipitate heart failure. Blood vessels forming the tangle interposed between arteries and veins are usually abnormally thin and histologically resemble both arteries and veins. AVMs occur in all parts of the cerebral hemispheres, brainstem, and spinal cord, but the largest ones are most frequently in the posterior half of the hemispheres, commonly forming a wedge-shaped lesion extending from the cortex to the ventricle.

Bleeding, headache, or seizures are most common between the ages of 10 and 30, occasionally as late as the fifties. AVMs are more frequent in men, and rare familial cases have been described. Familial AVM may be a part of the autosomal dominant syndrome of hereditary hemorrhagic telangiectasia (Osler-Rendu-Weber) syndrome due to mutations in endoglin (chromosome 9) or activin receptor-like kinase 1 (chromosome 12).

Headache (without bleeding) may be hemicranial and throbbing, like migraine, or diffuse. Focal seizures, with or without generalization, occur in ~30% of cases. One-half of AVMs become evident as ICHs. In most, the hemorrhage is mainly intraparenchymal with extension into the subarachnoid space in some cases. Blood is usually not deposited in the basal cisterns, and symptomatic cerebral vasospasm is rare. The risk of rerupture is ~2–4% per year and is particularly high in the first few weeks. Hemorrhages may be massive, leading to death, or may be as small as 1 cm in diameter, leading to minor focal symptoms or no deficit. The AVM may be large enough to steal blood away from adjacent normal brain tissue or to increase venous pressure significantly to produce venous ischemia locally and in remote areas of the brain. This is seen most often with large AVMs in the territory of the MCA.

Large AVMs of the anterior circulation may be associated with a systolic and diastolic bruit (sometimes self-audible) over the eye, forehead, or neck and a bounding carotid pulse. Headache at the onset of AVM rupture is not generally as explosive as with aneurysmal rupture. MRI is better than CT for diagnosis, although noncontrast CT scanning sometimes detects calcification of the AVM and contrast may demonstrate the abnormal blood vessels. Once identified, conventional x-ray angiography is the gold standard for evaluating the precise anatomy of the AVM.

Surgical treatment of symptomatic AVMs, often with preoperative embolization to reduce operative bleeding, is usually indicated for accessible lesions. Stereotaxic radiation, an alternative to surgery, can produce a slow sclerosis of the AVM over 2–3 years.

Patients with asymptomatic AVMs have about an ~2–4% per year risk for hemorrhage. Several angiographic features can be used to help predict future bleeding risk. Paradoxically, smaller lesions seem to have a higher hemorrhage rate. The impact of recurrent hemorrhage on disability is relatively modest, so the indication for surgery in asymptomatic AVMs is debated. A large-scale randomized trial is currently addressing this question.

Venous anomalies are the result of development of anomalous cerebral, cerebellar, or brainstem venous drainage. These structures, unlike AVMs, are functional venous channels. They are of little clinical significance and should be ignored if found incidentally on brain imaging studies. Surgical resection of these anomalies may result in venous infarction and hemorrhage. Venous anomalies may be associated with cavernous malformations (see later), which do carry some bleeding risk. If resection of a cavernous malformation is attempted, the venous anomaly should not be disturbed.

Capillary telangiectasias are true capillary malformations that often form extensive vascular networks through an otherwise normal brain structure. The pons and deep cerebral white matter are typical locations, and these capillary malformations can be seen in patients with hereditary hemorrhagic telangiectasia (Osler-Rendu-Weber) syndrome. If bleeding does occur, it rarely produces mass effect or significant symptoms. No treatment options exist.

ACQUIRED VASCULAR LESIONS

Cavernous angiomas are tufts of capillary sinusoids that form within the deep hemispheric white matter and brainstem with no normal intervening neural structures. The pathogenesis is unclear. Familial cavernous angiomas have been mapped to several different chromosomal loci: KRIT1 (7q21-q22), CCM2 (7p13), and PDCD10 (3q26.1). Both KRIT1 and CCM2 have roles in blood vessel formation while PDCD10 is an apoptotic gene. Cavernous angiomas are typically <1 cm in diameter and are often associated with a venous anomaly. Bleeding is usually of small volume, causing slight mass effect only. The bleeding risk for single cavernous malformations is 0.7–1.5% per year and may be higher for patients with prior clinical hemorrhage or multiple malformations. Seizures may occur if the malformation is located near the cerebral cortex. Surgical resection eliminates bleeding risk and may reduce seizure risk, but it is reserved for those malformations that form near the brain surface. Radiation treatment has not been shown to be of benefit.

Dural arteriovenous fistulas are acquired connections usually from a dural artery to a dural sinus. Patients may complain of a pulse-synchronous cephalic bruit ("pulsatile tinnitus") and headache. Depending on the magnitude of the shunt, venous pressures may rise high enough to cause cortical ischemia or venous hypertension and hemorrhage, particularly subarachnoid hemorrhage. Surgical and endovascular techniques are usually curative. These fistulas may form because of trauma, but most are idiopathic. There is an association between fistulas and dural sinus thrombosis. Fistulas have been observed to appear months to years following venous sinus thrombosis, suggesting that angiogenesis factors elaborated from the thrombotic process may cause these anomalous connections to form. Alternatively, dural arteriovenous fistulas can produce venous sinus occlusion over time, perhaps from the high pressure and high flow through a venous structure.

CHAPTER 28

NEUROLOGIC CRITICAL CARE, INCLUDING HYPOXIC-ISCHEMIC ENCEPHALOPATHY, AND SUBARACHNOID HEMORRHAGE

J. Claude Hemphill, III ■ Wade S. Smith ■ Daryl R. Gress

Life-threatening neurologic illness may be caused by a primary disorder affecting any region of the neuraxis or may occur as a consequence of a systemic disorder such as hepatic failure, multisystem organ failure, or cardiac arrest (Table 28-1). Neurologic critical care focuses on preservation of neurologic tissue and prevention of secondary brain injury caused by ischemia, edema, and elevated intracranial pressure (ICP). Management of other organ systems proceeds concurrently and may need to be modified in order to maintain the overall focus on neurologic issues.

PATHOPHYSIOLOGY

Brain edema

Swelling, or edema, of brain tissue occurs with many types of brain injury. The two principal types of edema are vasogenic and cytotoxic. *Vasogenic edema* refers to the influx of fluid and solutes into the brain through an incompetent blood-brain barrier (BBB). In the normal cerebral vasculature, endothelial tight junctions associated with astrocytes create an impermeable barrier (the BBB), through which access into the brain interstitium is dependent upon specific transport mechanisms. The BBB may be compromised in ischemia, trauma, infection, and metabolic derangements. Typically, vasogenic edema develops rapidly following injury. *Cytotoxic edema* refers to cellular swelling and occurs in a variety of settings, including brain ischemia and trauma. Early astrocytic swelling is a hallmark of ischemia. Brain edema that is clinically significant usually represents a combination of vasogenic and cellular components. Edema can lead to increased ICP as well as tissue shifts and brain displacement from focal processes (Chap. 17). These tissue shifts can cause injury by mechanical distention and compression in addition to the ischemia of impaired perfusion consequent to the elevated ICP.

Ischemic cascade and cellular injury

When delivery of substrates, principally oxygen and glucose, is inadequate to sustain cellular function, a series of interrelated biochemical reactions known as the *ischemic cascade* is initiated (see Fig. 27-2). The release of excitatory amino acids, especially glutamate, leads to influx of calcium and sodium ions, which disrupt cellular homeostasis. An increased intracellular calcium concentration may activate proteases and lipases, which then lead to lipid peroxidation and free radical–mediated cell membrane injury. Cytotoxic edema ensues, and ultimately necrotic cell death and tissue infarction occur. This pathway to irreversible cell death is common to ischemic stroke, global cerebral ischemia, and traumatic brain injury. *Penumbra* refers to areas of ischemic brain tissue that have not yet undergone irreversible infarction, implying that these regions are potentially salvageable if ischemia can be reversed. Factors that may exacerbate ischemic brain injury include systemic hypotension and hypoxia, which further reduce substrate delivery to vulnerable brain tissue, and fever, seizures, and hyperglycemia, which can increase cellular metabolism, outstripping compensatory processes. Clinically, these events are known as *secondary brain insults* because they lead to exacerbation of the primary brain injury. Prevention, identification, and

TABLE 28-1

NEUROLOGIC DISORDERS IN CRITICAL ILLNESS

LOCALIZATION ALONG NEUROAXIS	SYNDROME
Central Nervous System	
Brain: Cerebral hemispheres	Global encephalopathy
	Delirium
	Sepsis
	Organ failure—hepatic, renal
	Medication related—sedatives, hypnotics, analgesics, H_2 blockers, antihypertensives
	Drug overdose
	Electrolyte disturbance—hyponatremia, hypoglycemia
	Hypotension/hypoperfusion
	Hypoxia
	Meningitis
	Subarachnoid hemorrhage
	Wernicke's disease
	Seizure—postictal or nonconvulsive status
	Hypertensive encephalopathy
	Hypothyroidism—myxedema
	Focal deficits
	Ischemic stroke
	Tumor
	Abscess, subdural empyema
	Subdural/epidural hematoma
Brainstem	Mass effect and compression
	Ischemic stroke, intraparenchymal hemorrhage
	Hypoxia
Spinal cord	Mass effect and compression
	Disk herniation
	Epidural hematoma
	Ischemia—hypotension/embolic
	Epidural abscess
	Trauma, central cord syndrome
Peripheral Nervous System	
Peripheral nerve	
Axonal	Critical illness polyneuropathy
	Possible neuromuscular blocking agent complication
	Metabolic disturbances, uremia, hyperglycemia
	Medication effects—chemotherapeutic, antiretroviral
Demyelinating	Guillain-Barré syndrome
	Chronic inflammatory demyelinating polyneuropathy
Neuromuscular junction	Prolonged effect of neuromuscular blockade
	Medication effects—aminoglycosides
	Myasthenia gravis, Lambert-Eaton sydrome
Muscle	Critical illness myopathy
	Septic myopathy
	Cachectic myopathy—with or without disuse atrophy
	Electrolyte distubances—hypokalemia/hyperkalemia, hypophosphatemia
	Acute quadriplegic myopathy

treatment of secondary brain insults are fundamental goals of management.

An alternative pathway of cellular injury is *apoptosis*. This process implies programmed cell death, which may occur in the setting of ischemic stroke, global cerebral ischemia, traumatic brain injury, and possibly intracerebral hemorrhage. Apoptotic cell death can be distinguished histologically from the necrotic cell death of ischemia and is mediated through a different set of biochemical pathways. At present, interventions for prevention and treatment of apoptotic cell death remain less well defined than those for ischemia. Excitotoxicity and mechanisms of cell death are discussed in more detail in Chap. 25.

Cerebral perfusion and autoregulation

Brain tissue requires constant perfusion in order to ensure adequate delivery of substrate. The hemodynamic response of the brain has the capacity to preserve perfusion across a wide range of systemic blood pressures. Cerebral perfusion pressure (CPP), defined as the mean systemic arterial pressure (MAP) minus the ICP, provides the driving force for circulation across the capillary beds of the brain. *Autoregulation* refers to the physiologic response whereby cerebral blood flow (CBF) is regulated via alterations in cerebrovascular resistance in order to maintain perfusion over wide physiologic changes such as neuronal activation or changes in hemodynamic function. If systemic blood pressure drops, cerebral perfusion is preserved through vasodilation of arterioles in the brain; likewise, arteriolar vasoconstriction occurs at high systemic pressures to prevent hyperperfusion, resulting in fairly constant perfusion across a wide range of systemic blood pressures (Fig. 28-1). At the extreme limits of MAP or CPP (high or low), flow becomes directly related to perfusion pressure. These autoregulatory changes occur in the microcirculation and are mediated by vessels below the resolution of those seen on angiography. CBF is also strongly influenced by pH and $Paco_2$. CBF increases with hypercapnia and acidosis and decreases with hypocapnia and alkalosis. This forms the basis for the use of hyperventilation to lower ICP, and this effect on ICP is mediated through a decrease in intracranial blood volume. Cerebral autoregulation is a complex process critical to the normal homeostatic functioning of the brain, and this process may be disordered focally and unpredictably in disease states such as traumatic brain injury and severe focal cerebral ischemia.

Cerebrospinal fluid and intracranial pressure

The cranial contents consist essentially of brain, cerebrospinal fluid (CSF), and blood. CSF is produced principally in the choroid plexus of each lateral

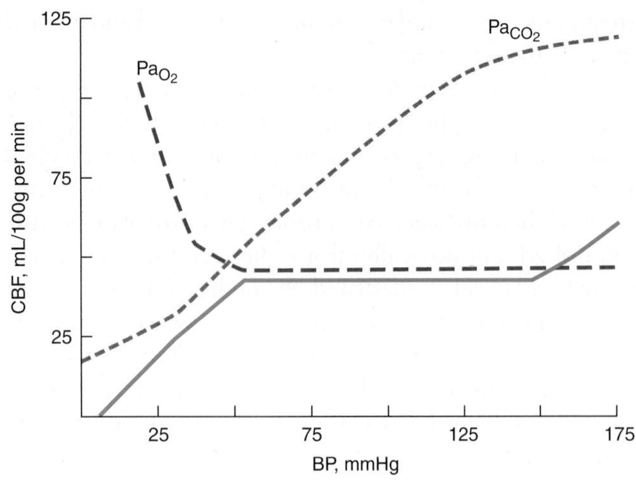

FIGURE 28-1

Autoregulation of cerebral blood flow (*solid line*). Cerebral perfusion is constant over a wide range of systemic blood pressure. Perfusion is increased in the setting of hypoxia or hypercarbia. BP, blood pressure; CBF, cerebral blood flow. (*Reprinted with permission from HM Shapiro: Anesthesiology 43:447, 1975. Copyright 1975, Lippincott Company.*)

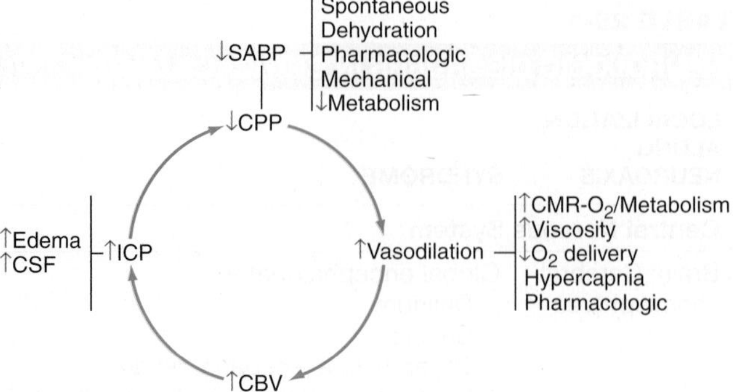

FIGURE 28-2

Ischemia and vasodilatation. Reduced cerebral perfusion pressure (CPP) leads to increased ischemia, vasodilation, increased intracranial pressure (ICP), and further reductions in CPP, a cycle leading to further neurologic injury. CBV, cerebral blood volume; CMR, cerebral metabolic rate; CSF, cerebrospinal fluid; SABP, systolic arterial blood pressure. (*Adapted from MJ Rosner et al: J Neurosurg 83:949, 1995; with permission.*)

ventricle, exits the brain via the foramens of Luschka and Magendi, and flows over the cortex to be absorbed into the venous system along the superior sagittal sinus. Approximately 150 mL of CSF are contained within the ventricles and surrounding the brain and spinal cord; the cerebral blood volume is also ~150 mL. The bony skull offers excellent protection for the brain but allows little tolerance for additional volume. Significant increases in volume eventually result in increased ICP. Obstruction of CSF outflow, edema of cerebral tissue, or increases in volume from tumor or hematoma may increase ICP. Elevated ICP diminishes cerebral perfusion and can lead to tissue ischemia. Ischemia in turn may lead to vasodilation via autoregulatory mechanisms designed to restore cerebral perfusion. However, vasodilation also increases cerebral blood volume, which in turn then increases ICP, lowers CPP, and provokes further ischemia (Fig. 28-2). This vicious cycle is commonly seen in traumatic brain injury, massive intracerebral hemorrhage, and large hemispheric infarcts with significant tissue shifts.

APPROACH TO THE PATIENT Severe CNS Dysfunction

Critically ill patients with severe central nervous system dysfunction require rapid evaluation and intervention in order to limit primary and secondary brain injury. Initial neurologic evaluation should be performed concurrent with stabilization of basic respiratory, cardiac, and hemodynamic parameters. Significant barriers may exist to neurologic assessment in the critical care unit, including endotracheal intubation and the use of sedative or paralytic agents to facilitate procedures.

An impaired level of consciousness is common in critically ill patients. The essential first task in assessment is to determine whether the cause of dysfunction is related to a diffuse, usually metabolic, process or whether a focal, usually structural, process is implicated. Examples of diffuse processes include metabolic encephalopathies related to organ failure, drug overdose, or hypoxia-ischemia. Focal processes include ischemic and hemorrhagic stroke and traumatic brain injury, especially with intracranial hematomas. Since these two categories of disorders have fundamentally different causes, treatments, and prognoses, the initial focus is on making this distinction rapidly and accurately. The approach to the comatose patient is discussed in Chap. 17; etiologies are listed in Table 17-1.

Minor focal deficits may be present on the neurologic examination in patients with metabolic encephalopathies. However, the finding of prominent focal signs such as pupillary asymmetry, hemiparesis, gaze palsy, or paraplegia should suggest the possibility of a structural lesion. All patients with a decreased level of consciousness associated with focal findings should undergo an urgent neuroimaging procedure, as should all patients with coma of unknown etiology. CT scanning is usually the most appropriate initial study because it can be performed quickly in critically ill patients and demonstrates hemorrhage, hydrocephalus, and intracranial tissue shifts well. MRI may provide more specific information in some situations, such as acute ischemic stroke (diffusion-weighted imaging, DWI) and cerebral venous sinus thrombosis (magnetic resonance venography, MRV). Any suggestion of trauma from the history or examination should alert the examiner to the possibility of cervical spine injury and prompt an imaging evaluation using plain x-rays, CT, or MRI.

Other diagnostic studies are best utilized in specific circumstances, usually when neuroimaging studies fail to reveal a structural lesion and the etiology of the altered mental state remains uncertain. Electroencephalography (EEG) can be important in the evaluation of critically ill patients with severe brain dysfunction. The EEG of metabolic encephalopathy typically reveals generalized slowing. One of the most important uses of EEG is to help exclude inapparent seizures, especially nonconvulsive status epilepticus. Untreated continuous or frequently recurrent seizures may cause neuronal injury, making the diagnosis and treatment of seizures crucial in this patient group. Lumbar puncture (LP) may be necessary to exclude infectious processes, and an elevated opening pressure may be an important clue to cerebral venous sinus thrombosis. In patients with coma or profound encephalopathy, it is preferable to perform a neuroimaging study prior to LP. If bacterial meningitis is suspected, an LP may be performed first or antibiotics may be empirically administered before the diagnostic studies are completed. Standard laboratory evaluation of critically ill patients should include assessment of serum electrolytes (especially sodium and calcium), glucose, renal and hepatic function, complete blood count, and coagulation. Serum or urine toxicology screens should be performed in patients with encephalopathy of unknown cause. EEG, LP, and other specific laboratory tests are most useful when the mechanism of the altered level of consciousness is uncertain; they are not routinely performed in clear-cut cases of stroke or traumatic brain injury.

Monitoring of ICP can be an important tool in selected patients. In general, patients who should be considered for ICP monitoring are those with primary neurologic disorders, such as stroke or traumatic brain injury, who are at significant risk for secondary brain injury due to elevated ICP and decreased CPP. Included are patients with the following: severe traumatic brain injury (Glasgow Coma Scale [GCS] score ≤ 8 [Table 36-2]); large tissue shifts from supratentorial ischemic or hemorrhagic stroke; or hydrocephalus from subarachnoid hemorrhage (SAH), intraventricular hemorrhage, or posterior fossa stroke. An additional disorder in which ICP monitoring can add important information is fulminant hepatic failure, in which elevated ICP may be treated with barbiturates or, eventually, liver transplantation. In general, ventriculostomy is preferable to ICP monitoring devices that are placed in the brain parenchyma, because ventriculostomy allows CSF drainage as a method of treating elevated ICP. However, parenchymal ICP monitoring is most appropriate for patients with diffuse edema and small ventricles (which may make ventriculostomy placement more difficult) or any degree of coagulopathy (in which ventriculostomy carries a higher risk of hemorrhagic complications) (Fig 28-3).

Treatment of Elevated ICP Elevated ICP may occur in a wide range of disorders, including head trauma, intracerebral hemorrhage, SAH with hydrocephalus, and fulminant hepatic failure. Because CSF and blood volume can be redistributed initially, by the time elevated ICP occurs, intracranial compliance is severely impaired. At this point, any small increase in the volume of CSF, intravascular blood, edema, or a mass lesion may result in a significant increase in ICP and a decrease in cerebral perfusion. This is a fundamental mechanism of secondary ischemic brain injury and constitutes an emergency that requires immediate attention. In general, ICP should be maintained at <20 mmHg and CPP should be maintained at ≥60 mmHg.

Interventions to lower ICP are ideally based on the underlying mechanism responsible for the elevated ICP (Table 28-2). For example, in hydrocephalus from SAH, the principal cause of elevated ICP is impairment of CSF drainage. In this setting, ventricular drainage of CSF is likely to be sufficient and most appropriate. In head trauma and stroke, cytotoxic edema may be most responsible, and the use of osmotic agents such as

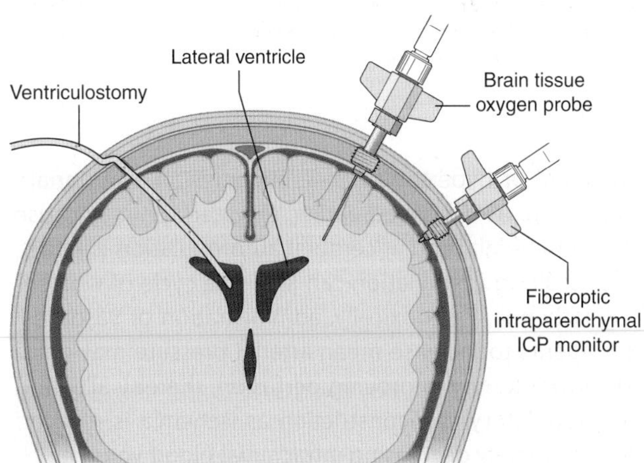

FIGURE 28-3
Intracranial pressure and brain tissue oxygen monitoring. A ventriculostomy allows for drainage of cerebrospinal fluid to treat elevated intracranial pressure (ICP). Fiberoptic ICP and brain tissue oxygen monitors are usually secured using a screwlike skull bolt. Cerebral blood flow and microdialysis probes (not shown) may be placed in a manner similar to the brain tissue oxygen probe.

TABLE 28-2

STEPWISE APPROACH TO TREATMENT OF ELEVATED INTRACRANIAL PRESSURE[a]

Insert ICP monitor—ventriculostomy versus parenchymal device

General goals: maintain ICP <20 mmHg and CPP ≥60 mmHg

For ICP >20–25 mmHg for >5 min:

1. Drain CSF via ventriculostomy (if in place)
2. Elevate head of the bed; midline head position
3. Osmotherapy—mannitol 25–100 g q4h as needed (maintain serum osmolality <320 mosmol) or hypertonic saline (30 mL, 23.4% NaCl bolus)
4. Glucocorticoids—dexamethasone 4 mg q6h for vasogenic edema from tumor, abscess (avoid glucocorticoids in head trauma, ischemic and hemorrhagic stroke)
5. Sedation (e.g., morphine, propofol, or midazolam); add neuromuscular paralysis if necessary (patient will require endotracheal intubation and mechanical ventilation at this point, if not before)
6. Hyperventilation—to $Paco_2$ 30–35 mmHg
7. Pressor therapy—phenylephrine, dopamine, or norepinephrine to maintain adequate MAP to ensure CPP ≥60 mmHg (maintain euvolemia to minimize deleterious systemic effects of pressors)
8. Consider second-tier therapies for refractory elevated ICP
   a. High-dose barbiturate therapy ("pentobarb coma")
   b. Aggressive hyperventilation to $Paco_2$ <30 mmHg
   c. Hypothermia
   d. Hemicraniectomy

[a]Throughout ICP treatment algorithm, consider repeat head CT to identify mass lesions amenable to surgical evacuation.

Abbreviations: CPP, cerebral perfusion pressure; CSF, cerebrospinal fluid; MAP, mean arterial pressure; $Paco_2$, arterial partial pressure of carbon dioxide.

mannitol or hypertonic saline becomes an appropriate early step. As described earlier, elevated ICP may cause tissue ischemia, and, if cerebral autoregulation is intact, the resulting vasodilation can lead to a cycle of worsening ischemia. Paradoxically, administration of vasopressor agents to increase mean arterial pressure may actually lower ICP by improving perfusion, thereby allowing autoregulatory vasoconstriction as ischemia is relieved and ultimately decreasing intracranial blood volume.

Early signs of elevated ICP include drowsiness and a diminished level of consciousness. Neuroimaging studies may reveal evidence of edema and mass effect. Hypotonic IV fluids should be avoided, and elevation of the head of the bed is recommended. Patients must be carefully observed for risk of aspiration and compromise of the airway as the level of alertness declines. Coma and unilateral pupillary changes are late signs and require immediate intervention. Emergent treatment of elevated ICP is most quickly achieved by intubation and hyperventilation, which causes vasoconstriction and reduces cerebral blood volume. In order to avoid provoking or worsening cerebral ischemia, hyperventilation is best used for short periods of time until a more definitive treatment can be instituted. Furthermore, the effects of hyperventilation on ICP are short-lived, often lasting only for several hours because of the buffering capacity of the cerebral interstitium, and rebound elevations of ICP may accompany abrupt discontinuation of hyperventilation. As the level of consciousness declines to coma, the ability to follow the neurologic status of the patient by examination deteriorates and measurement of ICP assumes greater importance. If a ventriculostomy device is in place, direct drainage of CSF to reduce ICP is possible. Finally, high-dose barbiturates, decompressive hemicraniectomy, or hypothermia are sometimes used for refractory elevations of ICP, although these have significant side effects and have not been proven to improve outcome.

Secondary Brain Insults Patients with primary brain injuries, whether due to trauma or stroke, are at risk for ongoing secondary ischemic brain injury. Because secondary brain injury can be a major determinant of a poor outcome, strategies for minimizing secondary brain insults are an integral part of the critical care of all patients. While elevated ICP may lead to secondary ischemia, most secondary brain injury is mediated through other clinical events that exacerbate the ischemic cascade already initiated by the primary brain injury. Episodes of secondary brain insults are usually not associated with apparent neurologic worsening. Rather, they lead to cumulative injury limiting eventual recovery, which manifests as higher mortality rate or worsened long-term functional outcome. Thus, close monitoring of vital signs is important, as is early intervention to prevent secondary ischemia. Avoiding hypotension and hypoxia is critical, as significant hypotensive events (systolic blood pressure <90 mmHg) as short as 10 min in duration have been shown to adversely influence outcome after traumatic brain injury. Even in patients with stroke or head trauma who do not require ICP monitoring, close attention to adequate cerebral perfusion is warranted. Hypoxia (pulse oximetry saturation <90%), particularly in combination with hypotension, also leads to secondary brain injury. Likewise, fever and hyperglycemia both worsen experimental ischemia and have been associated with worsened clinical outcome after stroke and head trauma. Aggressive control of fever with a goal of normothermia is warranted but may be difficult to achieve with antipyretic medications and cooling blankets. The value of newer surface or intravascular temperature control devices for the management of refractory fever is under investigation. The use of IV insulin infusion is encouraged for control of hyperglycemia as this allows better regulation of serum glucose levels than SC insulin. A reasonable goal is to maintain the serum glucose level at <7.8 mmol/L (<140 mg/dL), although episodes of hypoglycemia appear equally detrimental and the optimal targets remain uncertain. New cerebral monitoring tools that allow continuous evaluation of brain tissue oxygen tension, CBF, and metabolism (via microdialysis) may further improve the management of secondary brain injury.

CRITICAL CARE DISORDERS OF THE CENTRAL NERVOUS SYSTEM

HYPOXIC-ISCHEMIC ENCEPHALOPATHY

This occurs from lack of delivery of oxygen to the brain because of hypotension or respiratory failure. Causes include myocardial infarction, cardiac arrest, shock, asphyxiation, paralysis of respiration, and carbon monoxide or cyanide poisoning. In some circumstances, hypoxia may predominate. Carbon monoxide and cyanide poisoning are termed *histotoxic hypoxia* since they cause a direct impairment of the respiratory chain.

Clinical manifestations

Mild degrees of pure hypoxia, such as occur at high altitudes, cause impaired judgment, inattentiveness, motor incoordination, and, at times, euphoria. However, with hypoxia-ischemia, such as occurs with circulatory arrest, consciousness is lost within seconds. If circulation is restored within 3–5 min, full recovery may occur, but if hypoxia-ischemia lasts beyond 3–5 min, some degree of permanent cerebral damage usually results. Except in extreme cases, it may be difficult to judge the precise degree of hypoxia-ischemia, and some patients make a relatively full recovery after even 8–10 min of global cerebral ischemia. The distinction between pure hypoxia and hypoxia-ischemia is important, since a $Pa{O_2}$ as low as 20 mmHg (2.7 kPa) can be well tolerated if it develops gradually and normal blood pressure is maintained, but short durations of very low or absent cerebral circulation may result in permanent impairment.

Clinical examination at different time points after a hypoxic-ischemic insult (especially cardiac arrest) is useful in assessing prognosis for long-term neurologic outcome. The prognosis is better for patients with intact brainstem function, as indicated by normal pupillary light responses and intact oculocephalic (doll's eyes), oculovestibular (caloric), and corneal reflexes (Fig. 28-4). Absence of these reflexes and the presence of persistently dilated pupils that do not react to light

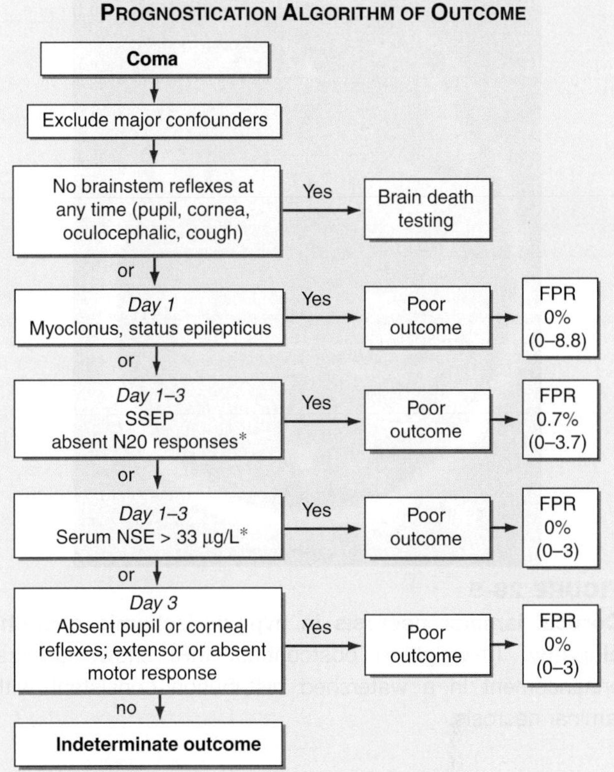

FIGURE 28-4

Prognostication of outcome in comatose survivors of cardiopulmonary resuscitation. Numbers in parentheses are 95% confidence intervals. Confounders could include use of sedatives or neuromuscular blocking agents, hypothermia therapy, organ failure, or shock. Tests denoted with an asterisk (*) may not be available in a timely and standardized manner. SSEP, somatosensory evoked potentials; NSE, neuron-specific enolase; FPR, false-positive rate. *(From EFM Wijdicks et al: Neurology 67:203, 2006; with permission.)*

are grave prognostic signs. A uniformly dismal prognosis from hypoxic-ischemic coma is conveyed by an absent pupillary light reflex or extensor or absent motor response to pain on day 3 following the injury. Electrophysiologically, the bilateral absence of the N20 component of the somatosensory evoked potential (SSEP) in the first several days also conveys a poor prognosis. A very elevated serum level (>33 μg/L) of the biochemical marker neuron-specific enolase (NSE) is indicative of brain damage after resuscitation from cardiac arrest and predicts a poor outcome. However, at present, SSEPs and NSE levels may be difficult to obtain in a timely fashion, with SSEP testing requiring substantial expertise in interpretation and NSE measurements not yet standardized. Whether administration of mild hypothermia after cardiac arrest (see "Treatment") will alter the usefulness of these clinical and electrophysiologic predictors is unknown. Long-term consequences of hypoxic-ischemic encephalopathy include persistent coma or a vegetative state (Chap. 17), dementia, visual agnosia (Chap. 18), parkinsonism, choreoathetosis,

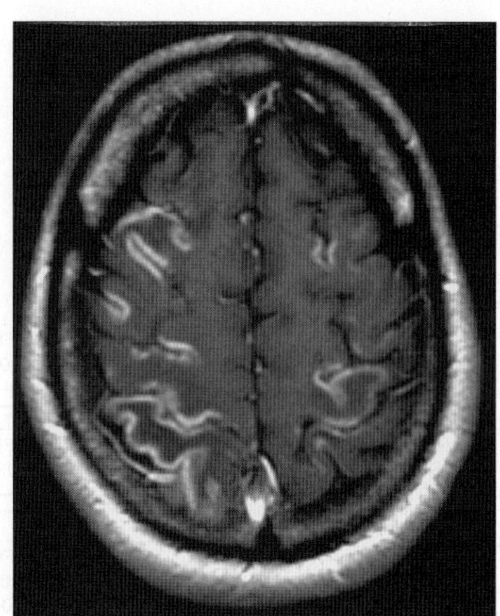

FIGURE 28-5
Cortical laminar necrosis in hypoxic-ischemic encephalopathy. T1-weighted postcontrast MRI shows cortical enhancement in a watershed distribution consistent with laminar necrosis.

cerebellar ataxia, myoclonus, seizures, and an amnestic state, which may be a consequence of selective damage to the hippocampus.

Pathology

Principal histologic findings are extensive multifocal or diffuse laminar cortical necrosis (Fig. 28-5), with almost invariable involvement of the hippocampus. The hippocampal CA1 neurons are vulnerable to even brief episodes of hypoxia-ischemia, perhaps explaining why selective persistent memory deficits may occur after brief cardiac arrest. Scattered small areas of infarction or neuronal loss may be present in the basal ganglia, hypothalamus, or brainstem. In some cases, extensive bilateral thalamic scarring may affect pathways that mediate arousal, and this pathology may be responsible for the persistent vegetative state. A specific form of hypoxic-ischemic encephalopathy, so-called watershed infarcts, occurs at the distal territories between the major cerebral arteries and can cause cognitive deficits, including visual agnosia, and weakness that is greater in proximal than in distal muscle groups.

Diagnosis

Diagnosis is based upon the history of a hypoxic-ischemic event such as cardiac arrest. Blood pressure <70 mmHg systolic or Pao_2 <40 mmHg is usually necessary, although both absolute levels as well as duration of exposure are important determinants of cellular injury. Carbon monoxide intoxication can be confirmed by measurement of carboxyhemoglobin and is suggested by a cherry red color of the skin, although the latter is an inconsistent clinical finding.

TREATMENT Hypoxic-Ischemic Encephalopathy

Treatment should be directed at restoration of normal cardiorespiratory function. This includes securing a clear airway, ensuring adequate oxygenation and ventilation, and restoring cerebral perfusion, whether by cardiopulmonary resuscitation, fluid, pressors, or cardiac pacing. Hypothermia may target the neuronal cell injury cascade and has substantial neuroprotective properties in experimental models of brain injury. In two trials, mild hypothermia (33°C) improved functional outcome in patients who remained comatose after resuscitation from a cardiac arrest. Treatment was initiated within minutes of cardiac resuscitation and continued for 12 h in one study and 24 h in the other. Potential complications of hypothermia include coagulopathy and an increased risk of infection. Based upon these studies, the International Liaison Committee on Resuscitation issued the following advisory statement in 2003: "Unconscious adult patients with spontaneous circulation after out-of-hospital cardiac arrest should be cooled to 32°–34°C for 12–24 h when the initial rhythm was ventricular fibrillation."

Severe carbon monoxide intoxication may be treated with hyperbaric oxygen. Anticonvulsants may be needed to control seizures, although these are not usually given prophylactically. Posthypoxic myoclonus may respond to oral administration of clonazepam at doses of 1.5–10 mg daily or valproate at doses of 300–1200 mg daily in divided doses. Myoclonic status epilepticus within 24 h after a primary circulatory arrest generally portends a very poor prognosis, even if seizures are controlled.

Carbon monoxide and cyanide intoxication can also cause a delayed encephalopathy. Little clinical impairment is evident when the patient first regains consciousness, but a parkinsonian syndrome characterized by akinesia and rigidity without tremor may develop. Symptoms can worsen over months, accompanied by increasing evidence of damage in the basal ganglia as seen on both CT and MRI.

METABOLIC ENCEPHALOPATHIES

Altered mental states, variously described as confusion, delirium, disorientation, and encephalopathy, are present in many patients with severe illness in an intensive care unit (ICU). Older patients are particularly vulnerable to delirium, a confusional state characterized by disordered perception, frequent hallucinations, delusions, and sleep disturbance. This is often attributed to medication effects, sleep deprivation, pain, and anxiety. The presence of delirium is associated with worsened outcome in critically ill patients, even in those without an identifiable central nervous system pathology such as stroke or brain trauma. In these patients, the cause of delirium is often multifactorial, resulting from organ dysfunction, sepsis, and especially the use of medications given to treat pain, agitation, or anxiety. Critically ill patients are often treated with a variety of sedative and analgesic medications, including opiates, benzodiazepines, neuroleptics, and sedative-anesthetic medications, such as propofol. Recent studies suggest that in critically ill patients requiring sedation, the use of the centrally acting α_2 agonist dexmedetomidine reduces delirium and shortens the duration of mechanical ventilation compared to the use of benzodiazepines such as lorazepam or midazolam. The presence of family members in the ICU may also help to calm and orient agitated patients, and in severe cases, low doses of neuroleptics (e.g., haloperidol 0.5–1 mg) can be useful. Current strategies focus on limiting the use of sedative medications when this can be done safely.

In the ICU setting, several metabolic causes of an altered level of consciousness predominate. Hypercarbic encephalopathy can present with headache, confusion, stupor, or coma. Hypoventilation syndrome occurs most frequently in patients with a history of chronic CO_2 retention who are receiving oxygen therapy for emphysema or chronic pulmonary disease. The elevated $Paco_2$ leading to CO_2 narcosis may have a direct anesthetic effect, and cerebral vasodilation from increased $Paco_2$ can lead to increased ICP. Hepatic encephalopathy is suggested by asterixis and can occur in chronic liver failure or acute fulminant hepatic failure. Both hyperglycemia and hypoglycemia can cause encephalopathy, as can hypernatremia and hyponatremia. Confusion, impairment of eye movements, and gait ataxia are the hallmarks of acute Wernicke's disease (see later).

SEPSIS-ASSOCIATED ENCEPHALOPATHY

Pathogenesis

In patients with sepsis, the systemic response to infectious agents leads to the release of circulating inflammatory mediators that appear to contribute to encephalopathy. Critical illness, in association with the systemic inflammatory response syndrome (SIRS), can lead to multisystem organ failure. This syndrome can occur in the setting of apparent sepsis, severe burns, or trauma, even without clear identification of an infectious agent. Many patients with critical illness, sepsis, or SIRS develop encephalopathy without obvious explanation. This condition is broadly termed *sepsis-associated encephalopathy*. While the specific mediators leading to neurologic dysfunction remain uncertain, it is clear that the encephalopathy is not simply the result of metabolic derangements of multiorgan failure. The cytokines tumor necrosis factor, interleukin (IL)-1, IL-2, and IL-6 are thought to play a role in this syndrome.

Diagnosis

Sepsis-associated encephalopathy presents clinically as a diffuse dysfunction of the brain without prominent focal findings. Confusion, disorientation, agitation, and fluctuations in level of alertness are typical. In more profound cases, especially with hemodynamic compromise, the decrease in level of alertness can be more prominent, at times resulting in coma. Hyperreflexia and frontal release signs such as a grasp or snout reflex (Chap. 18) can be seen. Abnormal movements such as myoclonus, tremor, or asterixis can occur. Sepsis-associated encephalopathy is quite common, occurring in the majority of patients with sepsis and multisystem organ failure. Diagnosis is often difficult because of the multiple potential causes of neurologic dysfunction in critically ill patients and requires exclusion of structural, metabolic, toxic, and infectious (e.g., meningitis or encephalitis) causes. The mortality rate of patients with sepsis-associated encephalopathy severe enough to produce coma approaches 50%, although this principally reflects the severity of the underlying critical illness and is not a direct result of the encephalopathy. Patients dying from severe sepsis or septic shock may have elevated levels of the serum brain injury biomarker S-100β and neuropathologic findings of neuronal apoptosis and cerebral ischemic injury. However, successful treatment of the underlying critical illness almost always results in complete resolution of the encephalopathy, with profound long-term cognitive disability being uncommon.

CENTRAL PONTINE MYELINOLYSIS

This disorder typically presents in a devastating fashion as quadriplegia and pseudobulbar palsy. Predisposing factors include severe underlying medical illness or nutritional deficiency; most cases are associated with rapid correction of hyponatremia or with hyperosmolar states. The pathology consists of demyelination without inflammation in the base of the pons, with relative sparing of axons and nerve cells. MRI is useful in establishing the diagnosis (Fig. 28-6) and may also identify partial forms that present as confusion, dysarthria, and/or disturbances of conjugate gaze without quadriplegia. Occasional cases present with lesions outside of the brainstem. Therapeutic guidelines for the restoration of severe hyponatremia should aim for gradual correction, i.e., by ≤10 mmol/L (10 meq/L) within 24 h and 20 mmol/L (20 meq/L) within 48 h.

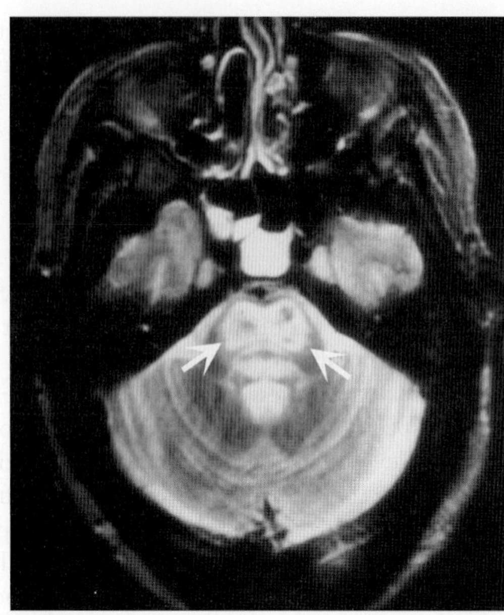

FIGURE 28-6
Central pontine myelinolysis. Axial T2-weighted MR scan through the pons reveals a symmetric area of abnormal high signal intensity within the basis pontis (*arrows*).

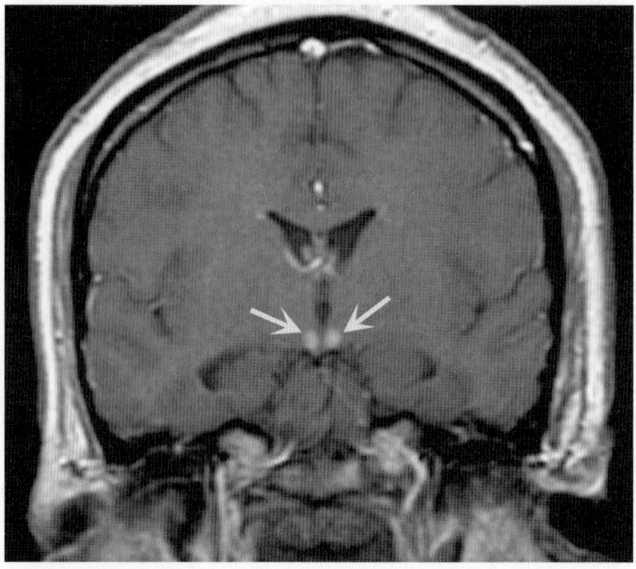

FIGURE 28-7
Wernicke's disease. Coronal T1-weighted postcontrast MRI reveals abnormal enhancement of the mammillary bodies (*arrows*), typical of acute Wernicke's encephalopathy.

WERNICKE'S DISEASE

Wernicke's disease is a common and preventable disorder due to a deficiency of thiamine. In the United States, alcoholics account for most cases, but patients with malnutrition due to hyperemesis, starvation, renal dialysis, cancer, AIDS, or rarely gastric surgery are also at risk. The characteristic clinical triad is that of ophthalmoplegia, ataxia, and global confusion. However, only one-third of patients with acute Wernicke's disease present with the classic clinical triad. Most patients are profoundly disoriented, indifferent, and inattentive, although rarely they have an agitated delirium related to ethanol withdrawal. If the disease is not treated, stupor, coma, and death may ensue. Ocular motor abnormalities include horizontal nystagmus on lateral gaze, lateral rectus palsy (usually bilateral), conjugate gaze palsies, and rarely ptosis. Gait ataxia probably results from a combination of polyneuropathy, cerebellar involvement, and vestibular paresis. The pupils are usually spared, but they may become miotic with advanced disease.

Wernicke's disease is usually associated with other manifestations of nutritional disease, such as polyneuropathy. Rarely, amblyopia or myelopathy occurs. Tachycardia and postural hypotension may be related to impaired function of the autonomic nervous system or to the coexistence of cardiovascular beriberi. Patients who recover show improvement in ocular palsies within hours after the administration of thiamine, but horizontal nystagmus may persist. Ataxia improves more slowly than the ocular motor abnormalities. Approximately half recover incompletely and are left with a slow, shuffling, wide-based gait and an inability to tandem walk. Apathy, drowsiness, and confusion improve more gradually. As these symptoms recede, an amnestic state with impairment in recent memory and learning may become more apparent (*Korsakoff's psychosis*). Korsakoff's psychosis is frequently persistent; the residual mental state is characterized by gaps in memory, confabulation, and disordered temporal sequencing.

Pathology

Periventricular lesions surround the third ventricle, aqueduct, and fourth ventricle, with petechial hemorrhages in occasional acute cases and atrophy of the mamillary bodies in most chronic cases. There is frequently endothelial proliferation, demyelination, and some neuronal loss. These changes may be detected by MRI scanning (Fig. 28-7). The amnestic defect is related to lesions in the dorsal medial nuclei of the thalamus.

Pathogenesis

Thiamine is a cofactor of several enzymes, including transketolase, pyruvate dehydrogenase, and α-ketoglutarate dehydrogenase. Thiamine deficiency produces a diffuse decrease in cerebral glucose utilization and results in mitochondrial damage. Glutamate accumulates owing to impairment of α-ketoglutarate dehydrogenase activity and, in combination with the energy deficiency, may result in excitotoxic cell damage.

TREATMENT Wernicke's Disease

Wernicke's disease is a medical emergency and requires immediate administration of thiamine, in a dose of 100 mg either IV or IM. The dose should be given daily until the patient resumes a normal diet and should be begun prior to treatment with IV glucose solutions. Glucose infusions may precipitate Wernicke's disease in a previously unaffected patient or cause a rapid worsening of an early form of the disease. For this reason, thiamine should be administered to all alcoholic patients requiring parenteral glucose.

CRITICAL CARE DISORDERS OF THE PERIPHERAL NERVOUS SYSTEM

Critical illness with disorders of the peripheral nervous system (PNS) arises in two contexts: (1) primary neurologic diseases that require critical care interventions such as intubation and mechanical ventilation, and (2) secondary PNS manifestations of systemic critical illness, often involving multisystem organ failure. The former include acute polyneuropathies such as Guillain-Barré syndrome (Chap. 46), neuromuscular junction disorders including myasthenia gravis (Chap. 47) and botulism, and primary muscle disorders such as polymyositis (Chap. 49). The latter result either from the systemic disease itself or as a consequence of interventions.

General principles of respiratory evaluation in patients with PNS involvement, regardless of cause, include assessment of pulmonary mechanics, such as maximal inspiratory force (MIF) and vital capacity (VC), and evaluation of strength of bulbar muscles. Regardless of the cause of weakness, endotracheal intubation should be considered when the MIF falls to <-25 cmH_2O or the VC is <1 L. Also, patients with severe palatal weakness may require endotracheal intubation in order to prevent acute upper airway obstruction or recurrent aspiration. Arterial blood gases and oxygen saturation from pulse oximetry are used to follow patients with potential respiratory compromise from PNS dysfunction. However, intubation and mechanical ventilation should be undertaken based on clinical assessment rather than waiting until oxygen saturation drops or CO_2 retention develops from hypoventilation. Noninvasive mechanical ventilation may be considered initially in lieu of endotracheal intubation but is generally insufficient in patients with severe bulbar weakness or ventilatory failure with hypercarbia.

NEUROPATHY

While encephalopathy may be the most obvious neurologic dysfunction in critically ill patients, dysfunction of the PNS is also quite common. It is typically present in patients with prolonged critical illnesses lasting several weeks and involving sepsis; clinical suspicion is aroused when there is failure to wean from mechanical ventilation despite improvement of the underlying sepsis and critical illness. *Critical illness polyneuropathy* refers to the most common PNS complication related to critical illness; it is seen in the setting of prolonged critical illness, sepsis, and multisystem organ failure. Neurologic findings include diffuse weakness, decreased reflexes, and distal sensory loss. Electrophysiologic studies demonstrate a diffuse, symmetric, distal axonal sensorimotor neuropathy, and pathologic studies have confirmed axonal degeneration. The precise mechanism of critical illness polyneuropathy remains unclear, but circulating factors such as cytokines, which are associated with sepsis and SIRS, are thought to play a role. It has been reported that up to 70% of patients with the sepsis syndrome have some degree of neuropathy, although far fewer have a clinical syndrome profound enough to cause severe respiratory muscle weakness requiring prolonged mechanical ventilation or resulting in failure to wean. Aggressive glycemic control with insulin infusions appears to decrease the risk of critical illness polyneuropathy. Treatment is otherwise supportive, with specific intervention directed at treating the underlying illness. While spontaneous recovery is usually seen, the time course may extend over weeks to months and necessitate long-term ventilatory support and care even after the underlying critical illness has resolved.

DISORDERS OF NEUROMUSCULAR TRANSMISSION

A defect in neuromuscular transmission may be a source of weakness in critically ill patients. Myasthenia gravis may be a consideration; however, persistent weakness secondary to impaired neuromuscular junction transmission is almost always due to administration of drugs. A number of medications impair neuromuscular transmission; these include antibiotics, especially aminoglycosides, and beta-blocking agents. In the ICU, the nondepolarizing neuromuscular blocking agents (nd-NMBAs), also known as muscle relaxants, are most commonly responsible. Included in this group of drugs are such agents as pancuronium, vecuronium, rocuronium, and atracurium. They are often used to facilitate mechanical ventilation or other critical care procedures, but with prolonged use persistent neuromuscular blockade may result in weakness even after discontinuation of these agents hours or days earlier. Risk factors for this prolonged action of neuromuscular blocking agents include female sex, metabolic acidosis, and renal failure.

Prolonged neuromuscular blockade does not appear to produce permanent damage to the PNS. Once the offending medications are discontinued, full strength is restored, although this may take days. In general, the lowest dose of neuromuscular blocking agent should be used to achieve the desired result and, when these agents are used in the ICU, a peripheral nerve stimulator should be used to monitor neuromuscular junction function.

MYOPATHY

Critically ill patients, especially those with sepsis, frequently develop muscle wasting, often in the face of seemingly adequate nutritional support. The assumption has been that this represents a catabolic myopathy brought about as a result of multiple factors, including elevated cortisol and catecholamine release and other circulating factors induced by the SIRS. In this syndrome, known as *cachectic myopathy*, serum creatine kinase levels and electromyography (EMG) are normal. Muscle biopsy shows type II fiber atrophy. Panfascicular muscle fiber necrosis may also occur in the setting of profound sepsis. This so-called *septic myopathy* is characterized clinically by weakness progressing to a profound level over just a few days. There may be associated elevations in serum creatine kinase and urine myoglobin. Both EMG and muscle biopsy may be normal initially but eventually show abnormal spontaneous activity and panfascicular necrosis with an accompanying inflammatory reaction. Both of these myopathic syndromes may be considered under the broader heading of *critical illness myopathy*.

Acute quadriplegic myopathy describes a clinical syndrome of severe weakness seen in the setting of glucocorticoid and nd-NMBA use. The most frequent scenario in which this is encountered is the asthmatic patient who requires high-dose glucocorticoids and nd-NMBA to facilitate mechanical ventilation. This muscle disorder is not due to prolonged action of nd-NMBAs at the neuromuscular junction but, rather, is an actual myopathy with muscle damage; it has occasionally been described with high-dose glucocorticoid use alone. Clinically this syndrome is most often recognized when a patient fails to wean from mechanical ventilation despite resolution of the primary pulmonary process. Pathologically, there may be vacuolar changes in both type I and type II muscle fibers with evidence of regeneration. Acute quadriplegic myopathy has a good prognosis. If patients survive their underlying critical illness, the myopathy invariably improves and most patients return to normal. However, because this syndrome is a result of true muscle damage, not just prolonged blockade at the neuromuscular junction, this process may take weeks or months, and tracheotomy with prolonged ventilatory support may be necessary. Some patients do have residual long-term weakness, with atrophy and fatigue limiting ambulation. At present, it is unclear how to prevent this myopathic complication, except by avoiding use of nd-NMBAs, a strategy not always possible. Monitoring with a peripheral nerve stimulator can help to avoid the overuse of these agents. However, this is more likely to prevent the complication of prolonged neuromuscular junction blockade than it is to prevent this myopathy.

SUBARACHNOID HEMORRHAGE

Subarachnoid hemorrhage (SAH) renders the brain critically ill from both primary and secondary brain insults. Excluding head trauma, the most common cause of SAH is rupture of a saccular aneurysm. Other causes include bleeding from a vascular malformation (arteriovenous malformation or dural arterial-venous fistula) and extension into the subarachnoid space from a primary intracerebral hemorrhage. Some idiopathic SAHs are localized to the perimesencephalic cisterns and are benign; they probably have a venous or capillary source, and angiography is unrevealing.

Saccular ("berry") aneurysm

Autopsy and angiography studies have found that about 2% of adults harbor intracranial aneurysms, for a prevalence of 4 million persons in the United States; the aneurysm will rupture, producing SAH, in 25,000–30,000 cases per year. For patients who arrive alive at hospital, the mortality rate over the next month is about 45%. Of those who survive, more than half are left with major neurologic deficits as a result of the initial hemorrhage, cerebral vasospasm with infarction, or hydrocephalus. If the patient survives but the aneurysm is not obliterated, the rate of rebleeding is about 20% in the first 2 weeks, 30% in the first month, and about 3% per year afterwards. Given these alarming figures, the major therapeutic emphasis is on preventing the predictable early complications of the SAH.

Unruptured, asymptomatic aneurysms are much less dangerous than a recently ruptured aneurysm. The annual risk of rupture for aneurysms <10 mm in size is ~0.1%, and for aneurysms ≥10 mm in size is ~0.5–1%; the surgical morbidity rate far exceeds these percentages. Because of the longer length of exposure to risk of rupture, younger patients with aneurysms >10 mm in size may benefit from prophylactic treatment. As with the treatment of asymptomatic carotid stenosis, this risk-benefit strongly depends on the complication rate of treatment.

Giant aneurysms, those >2.5 cm in diameter, occur at the same sites (see later) as small aneurysms and account for 5% of cases. The three most common locations are the terminal internal carotid artery, middle cerebral artery (MCA) bifurcation, and top of the basilar artery. Their risk of rupture is ~6% in the first year after identification and may remain high indefinitely. They often cause symptoms by compressing the adjacent brain or cranial nerves.

Mycotic aneurysms are usually located distal to the first bifurcation of major arteries of the circle of Willis. Most result from infected emboli due to bacterial endocarditis causing septic degeneration of arteries and subsequent dilation and rupture. Whether these lesions should be sought and repaired prior to rupture or left to heal spontaneously is controversial.

Pathophysiology

Saccular aneurysms occur at the bifurcations of the large- to medium-sized intracranial arteries; rupture is into the subarachnoid space in the basal cisterns and often into the parenchyma of the adjacent brain. Approximately 85% of aneurysms occur in the anterior circulation, mostly on the circle of Willis. About 20% of patients have multiple aneurysms, many at mirror sites bilaterally. As an aneurysm develops, it typically forms a neck with a dome. The length of the neck and the size of the dome vary greatly and are important factors in planning neurosurgical obliteration or endovascular embolization. The arterial internal elastic lamina disappears at the base of the neck. The media thins, and connective tissue replaces smooth-muscle cells. At the site of rupture (most often the dome) the wall thins, and the tear that allows bleeding is often ≤0.5 mm long. Aneurysm size and site are important in predicting risk of rupture. Those >7 mm in diameter and those at the top of the basilar artery and at the origin of the posterior communicating artery are at greater risk of rupture.

Clinical manifestations

Most unruptured intracranial aneurysms are completely asymptomatic. Symptoms are usually due to rupture and resultant SAH, although some unruptured aneurysms present with mass effect on cranial nerves or brain parenchyma. At the moment of aneurysmal rupture with major SAH, the ICP suddenly rises. This may account for the sudden transient loss of consciousness that occurs in nearly half of patients. Sudden loss of consciousness may be preceded by a brief moment of excruciating headache, but most patients first complain of headache upon regaining consciousness. In 10% of cases, aneurysmal bleeding is severe enough to cause loss of consciousness for several days. In ~45% of cases, severe headache associated with exertion is the presenting complaint. The patient often calls the headache "the worst headache of my life"; however, the most important characteristic is sudden onset. Occasionally, these ruptures may present as headache of only moderate intensity or as a change in the patient's usual headache pattern. The headache is usually generalized, often with neck stiffness, and vomiting is common.

Although sudden headache in the absence of focal neurologic symptoms is the hallmark of aneurysmal rupture, focal neurologic deficits may occur. Anterior communicating artery or MCA bifurcation aneurysms may rupture into the adjacent brain or subdural space and form a hematoma large enough to produce mass effect. The deficits that result can include hemiparesis, aphasia, and abulia.

Occasionally, prodromal symptoms suggest the location of a progressively enlarging unruptured aneurysm. A third cranial nerve palsy, particularly when associated with pupillary dilation, loss of ipsilateral (but retained contralateral) light reflex, and focal pain above or behind the eye, may occur with an expanding aneurysm at the junction of the posterior communicating artery and the internal carotid artery. A sixth nerve palsy may indicate an aneurysm in the cavernous sinus, and visual field defects can occur with an expanding supraclinoid carotid or anterior cerebral artery aneurysm. Occipital and posterior cervical pain may signal a posterior inferior cerebellar artery or anterior inferior cerebellar artery aneurysm (Chap. 27). Pain in or behind the eye and in the low temple can occur with an expanding MCA aneurysm. Thunderclap headache is a variant of migraine that simulates an SAH. Before concluding that a patient with sudden, severe headache has thunderclap migraine, a definitive workup for aneurysm or other intracranial pathology is required.

Aneurysms can undergo small ruptures and leaks of blood into the subarachnoid space, so-called *sentinel bleeds*. Sudden unexplained headache at any location should raise suspicion of SAH and be investigated, because a major hemorrhage may be imminent.

The initial clinical manifestations of SAH can be graded using the Hunt-Hess or World Federation of Neurosurgical Societies classification schemes (Table 28-3). For ruptured aneurysms, prognosis for good outcomes falls as the grade increases. For example, it is unusual for a Hunt-Hess grade 1 patient to die if the aneurysm is treated, but the mortality rate for grade 4 and 5 patients may be as high as 80%.

Delayed neurologic deficits

There are four major causes of delayed neurologic deficits: rerupture, hydrocephalus, vasospasm, and hyponatremia.

1. *Rerupture*. The incidence of rerupture of an untreated aneurysm in the first month following SAH is ~30%, with the peak in the first 7 days. Rerupture is associated with a 60% mortality rate and poor outcome.

TABLE 28-3

GRADING SCALES FOR SUBARACHNOID HEMORRHAGE

GRADE	HUNT-HESS SCALE	WORLD FEDERATION OF NEUROSURGICAL SOCIETIES (WFNS) SCALE
1	Mild headache, normal mental status, no cranial nerve or motor findings	GCS[a] score 15, no motor deficits
2	Severe headache, normal mental status, may have cranial nerve deficit	GCS score 13–14, no motor deficits
3	Somnolent, confused, may have cranial nerve or mild motor deficit	GCS score 13–14, with motor deficits
4	Stupor, moderate to severe motor deficit, may have intermittent reflex posturing	GCS score 7–12, with or without motor deficits
5	Coma, reflex posturing or flaccid	GCS score 3–6, with or without motor deficits

[a]Glasgow Coma Scale: See Table 36-2.

Early treatment eliminates this risk.

2. *Hydrocephalus.* Acute hydrocephalus can cause stupor and coma and can be mitigated by placement of an external ventricular drain. More often, subacute hydrocephalus may develop over a few days or weeks and causes progressive drowsiness or slowed mentation (abulia) with incontinence. Hydrocephalus is differentiated from cerebral vasospasm with a CT scan, CT angiogram, transcranial Doppler (TCD) ultrasound, or conventional x-ray angiography. Hydrocephalus may clear spontaneously or require temporary ventricular drainage. Chronic hydrocephalus may develop weeks to months after SAH and manifest as gait difficulty, incontinence, or impaired mentation. Subtle signs may be a lack of initiative in conversation or a failure to recover independence.
3. *Vasospasm.* Narrowing of the arteries at the base of the brain following SAH causes symptomatic ischemia and infarction in ~30% of patients and is the major cause of delayed morbidity and death. Signs of ischemia appear 4–14 days after the hemorrhage, most often at 7 days. The severity and distribution of vasospasm determine whether infarction will occur.

   Delayed vasospasm is believed to result from direct effects of clotted blood and its breakdown products on the arteries within the subarachnoid space. In general, the more blood that surrounds the arteries, the greater the chance of symptomatic vasospasm. Spasm of major arteries produces symptoms referable to the appropriate vascular territory (Chap. 27). All of these focal symptoms may present abruptly, fluctuate, or develop over a few days. In most cases, focal spasm is preceded by a decline in mental status.

   Vasospasm can be detected reliably with conventional x-ray angiography, but this invasive procedure is expensive and carries the risk of stroke and other complications. TCD ultrasound is based on the principle that the velocity of blood flow within an artery will rise as the lumen diameter is narrowed. By directing the probe along the MCA and proximal anterior cerebral artery (ACA), carotid terminus, and vertebral and basilar arteries on a daily or every-other-day basis, vasospasm can be reliably detected and treatments initiated to prevent cerebral ischemia (see later). CT angiography is another method that can detect vasospasm.

   Severe cerebral edema in patients with infarction from vasospasm may increase the ICP enough to reduce cerebral perfusion pressure. Treatment may include mannitol, hyperventilation, and hemicraniectomy; moderate hypothermia may have a role as well.
4. *Hyponatremia.* Hyponatremia may be profound and can develop quickly in the first 2 weeks following SAH. There is both natriuresis and volume depletion with SAH, so that patients become both hyponatremic and hypovolemic. Both atrial natriuretic peptide and brain natriuretic peptide have a role in producing this "cerebral salt-wasting syndrome." Typically, it clears over the course of 1–2 weeks and, in the setting of SAH, should not be treated with free-water restriction as this may increase the risk of stroke (see later).

Laboratory evaluation and imaging

(Fig. 28-8) The hallmark of aneurysmal rupture is blood in the CSF. More than 95% of cases have enough blood to be visualized on a high-quality noncontrast CT scan obtained within 72 h. If the scan fails to establish the diagnosis of SAH and no mass lesion or obstructive hydrocephalus is found, a lumbar puncture should be performed to establish the presence of subarachnoid blood. Lysis of the red blood cells and subsequent conversion of hemoglobin to bilirubin stains the spinal fluid yellow within 6–12 h. This xanthochromic spinal fluid peaks in intensity at 48 h and lasts for 1–4 weeks, depending on the amount of subarachnoid blood.

The extent and location of subarachnoid blood on noncontrast CT scan help locate the underlying aneurysm, identify the cause of any neurologic deficit, and predict delayed vasospasm. A high incidence of symptomatic vasospasm in the MCA and ACA has been found when early CT scans show subarachnoid clots >5 × 3 mm in the basal cisterns or layers of blood >1 mm

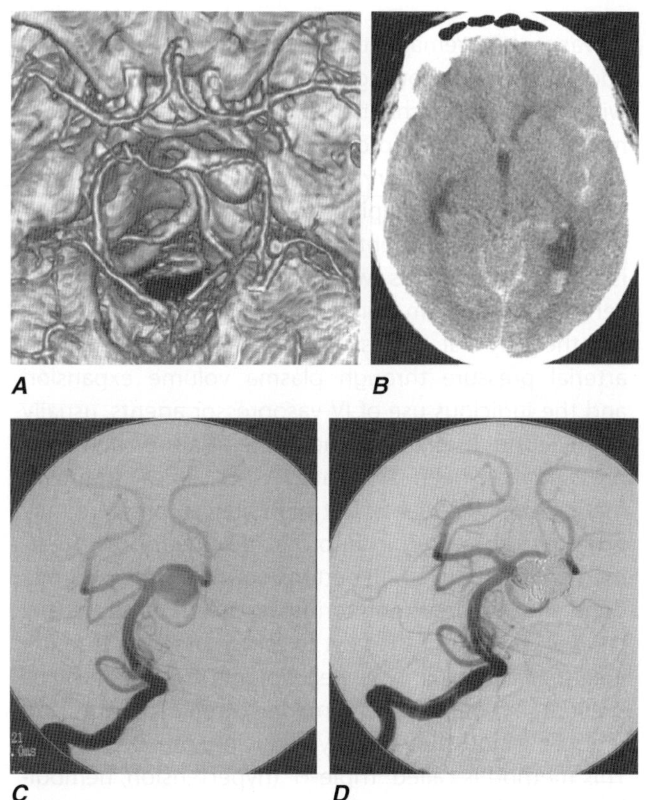

FIGURE 28-8

Subarachnoid hemorrhage. *A.* CT angiography revealing an aneurysm of the left superior cerebellar artery. ***B.*** Noncontrast CT scan at the level of the third ventricle revealing subarachnoid blood (*bright*) in the left sylvian fissure and within the left lateral ventricle. ***C.*** Conventional anteroposterior x-ray angiogram of the right vertebral and basilar artery showing the large aneurysm. ***D.*** Conventional angiogram following coil embolization of the aneurysm, whereby the aneurysm body is filled with platinum coils delivered through a microcatheter navigated from the femoral artery into the aneurysm neck.

thick in the cerebral fissures. CT scans less reliably predict vasospasm in the vertebral, basilar, or posterior cerebral arteries.

Lumbar puncture prior to an imaging procedure is indicated only if a CT scan is not available at the time of the suspected SAH. Once the diagnosis of hemorrhage from a ruptured saccular aneurysm is suspected, four-vessel conventional x-ray angiography (both carotids and both vertebrals) is generally performed to localize and define the anatomic details of the aneurysm and to determine if other unruptured aneurysms exist (Fig. 28-8*C*). At some centers, the ruptured aneurysm can be treated using endovascular techniques at the time of the initial angiogram as a way to expedite treatment and minimize the number of invasive procedures. CT angiography is an alternative method for locating the aneurysm and may be sufficient to plan definitive therapy.

Close monitoring (daily or twice daily) of electrolytes is important because hyponatremia can occur precipitously during the first 2 weeks following SAH (see earlier).

The electrocardiogram (ECG) frequently shows ST-segment and T-wave changes similar to those associated with cardiac ischemia. Prolonged QRS complex, increased QT interval, and prominent "peaked" or deeply inverted symmetric T waves are usually secondary to the intracranial hemorrhage. There is evidence that structural myocardial lesions produced by circulating catecholamines and excessive discharge of sympathetic neurons may occur after SAH, causing these ECG changes and a reversible cardiomyopathy sufficient to cause shock or congestive heart failure. Echocardiography reveals a pattern of regional wall motion abnormalities that follow the distribution of sympathetic nerves rather than the major coronary arteries, with relative sparing of the ventricular wall apex. The sympathetic nerves themselves appear to be injured by direct toxicity from the excessive catecholamine release. An asymptomatic troponin elevation is common. Serious ventricular dysrhythmias are unusual.

TREATMENT Subarachnoid Hemorrhage

Early aneurysm repair prevents rerupture and allows the safe application of techniques to improve blood flow (e.g., induced hypertension and hypervolemia) should symptomatic vasospasm develop. An aneurysm can be "clipped" by a neurosurgeon or "coiled" by an endovascular surgeon. Surgical repair involves placing a metal clip across the aneurysm neck, thereby immediately eliminating the risk of rebleeding. This approach requires craniotomy and brain retraction, which is associated with neurologic morbidity. Endovascular techniques involve placing platinum coils, or other embolic material, within the aneurysm via a catheter that is passed from the femoral artery. The aneurysm is packed tightly to enhance thrombosis and over time is walled off from the circulation (Fig. 28-8*D*). The only prospective randomized trial of surgery versus endovascular treatment for ruptured aneurysm, the International Subarachnoid Aneurysm Trial (ISAT), was terminated early when 24% of patients treated with endovascular therapy were dead or dependent at 1 year compared to 31% treated with surgery, a significant 23% relative reduction. After 5 years, risk of death was lower in the coiling group, although the proportion of survivors who were independent was the same in both groups. Risk of rebleeding was low, but more common in the coiling group. Also, because some aneurysms have a morphology that is not amenable to endovascular treatment, surgery remains an important treatment option. Centers that combine both endovascular and neurosurgical expertise likely offer the best outcomes for patients, and there are reliable data showing that centers that specialize in aneurysm treatment have improved mortality rates.

The medical management of SAH focuses on protecting the airway, managing blood pressure before and after aneurysm treatment, preventing rebleeding prior to treatment, managing vasospasm, treating hydrocephalus, treating hyponatremia, and preventing pulmonary embolus.

Intracranial hypertension following aneurysmal rupture occurs secondary to subarachnoid blood, parenchymal hematoma, acute hydrocephalus, or loss of vascular autoregulation. Patients who are stuporous should undergo emergent ventriculostomy to measure ICP and to treat high ICP in order to prevent cerebral ischemia. Medical therapies designed to combat raised ICP (e.g., mild hyperventilation, mannitol, and sedation) can also be used as needed. High ICP refractory to treatment is a poor prognostic sign.

Prior to definitive treatment of the ruptured aneurysm, care is required to maintain adequate cerebral perfusion pressure while avoiding excessive elevation of arterial pressure. If the patient is alert, it is reasonable to lower the blood pressure to normal using nicardipine, labetolol, or esmolol. If the patient has a depressed level of consciousness, ICP should be measured and the cerebral perfusion pressure targeted to 60–70 mmHg. If headache or neck pain is severe, mild sedation and analgesia are prescribed. Extreme sedation is avoided because it can obscure changes in neurologic status. Adequate hydration is necessary to avoid a decrease in blood volume predisposing to brain ischemia.

Seizures are uncommon at the onset of aneurysmal rupture. The quivering, jerking, and extensor posturing that often accompany loss of consciousness with SAH are probably related to the sharp rise in ICP rather than seizure. However, anticonvulsants are sometimes given as prophylactic therapy since a seizure could theoretically promote rebleeding.

Glucocorticoids may help reduce the head and neck ache caused by the irritative effect of the subarachnoid blood. There is no good evidence that they reduce cerebral edema, are neuroprotective, or reduce vascular injury, and their routine use therefore is not recommended.

Antifibrinolytic agents are not routinely prescribed but may be considered in patients in whom aneurysm treatment cannot proceed immediately. They are associated with a reduced incidence of aneurysmal rerupture but may also increase the risk of delayed cerebral infarction and deep-vein thrombosis (DVT).

Vasospasm remains the leading cause of morbidity and mortality following aneurysmal SAH. Treatment with the calcium channel antagonist nimodipine (60 mg PO every 4 h) improves outcome, perhaps by preventing ischemic injury rather than reducing the risk of vasospasm. Nimodipine can cause significant hypotension in some patients, which may worsen cerebral ischemia in patients with vasospasm. Symptomatic cerebral vasospasm can also be treated by increasing the cerebral perfusion pressure by raising mean arterial pressure through plasma volume expansion and the judicious use of IV vasopressor agents, usually phenylephrine or norepinephrine. Raised perfusion pressure has been associated with clinical improvement in many patients, but high arterial pressure may promote rebleeding in unprotected aneurysms. Treatment with induced hypertension and hypervolemia generally requires monitoring of arterial and central venous pressures; it is best to infuse pressors through a central venous line as well. Volume expansion helps prevent hypotension, augments cardiac output, and reduces blood viscosity by reducing the hematocrit. This method is called "triple-H" (hypertension, hemodilution, and hypervolemic) therapy.

If symptomatic vasospasm persists despite optimal medical therapy, intraarterial vasodilators and percutaneous transluminal angioplasty are considered. Vasodilatation by direct angioplasty appears to be permanent, allowing triple-H therapy to be tapered sooner. The pharmacologic vasodilators (verapamil and nicardipine) do not last more than about 24 h, and therefore multiple treatments may be required until the subarachnoid blood is reabsorbed. Although intraarterial papaverine is an effective vasodilator, there is evidence that papaverine may be neurotoxic, so its use should generally be avoided.

Acute hydrocephalus can cause stupor or coma. It may clear spontaneously or require temporary ventricular drainage. When chronic hydrocephalus develops, ventricular shunting is the treatment of choice.

Free-water restriction is contraindicated in patients with SAH at risk for vasospasm because hypovolemia and hypotension may occur and precipitate cerebral ischemia. Many patients continue to experience a decline in serum sodium despite receiving parenteral fluids containing normal saline. Frequently, supplemental oral salt coupled with normal saline will mitigate hyponatremia, but often patients also require hypertonic saline. Care must be taken not to correct serum sodium too quickly in patients with marked hyponatremia of several days' duration, as central pontine myelinolysis may occur.

All patients should have pneumatic compression stockings applied to prevent pulmonary embolism.

Unfractionated heparin administered subcutaneously for DVT prophylaxis can be initiated immediately following endovascular treatment and within days following craniotomy and surgical clipping and is a useful adjunct to pneumatic compression stockings. Treatment of pulmonary embolus depends on whether the aneurysm has been treated and whether or not the patient has had a craniotomy. Systemic anticoagulation with heparin is contraindicated in patients with ruptured and untreated aneurysms. It is a relative contraindication following craniotomy for several days, and it may delay thrombosis of a coiled aneurysm. Following craniotomy, use of inferior vena cava filters is preferred to prevent further pulmonary emboli, while systemic anticoagulation with heparin is preferred following successful endovascular treatment.

CHAPTER 29

ALZHEIMER'S DISEASE AND OTHER DEMENTIAS

William W. Seeley ■ Bruce L. Miller

Dementia, a syndrome with many causes, affects >4 million Americans and results in a total health care cost of >$100 billion annually. It is defined as an acquired deterioration in cognitive abilities that impairs the successful performance of activities of daily living. Memory is the most common cognitive ability lost with dementia; 10% of persons >70 and 20–40% of individuals >85 have clinically identifiable memory loss. In addition to memory, other mental faculties may be affected; these include language, visuospatial ability, calculation, judgment, and problem solving. Neuropsychiatric and social deficits also arise in many dementia syndromes, resulting in depression, apathy, hallucinations, delusions, agitation, insomnia, and disinhibition. The most common forms of dementia are progressive, but some are static and unchanging or fluctuate from day to day or even minute to minute. Most patients with Alzheimer's disease (AD), the most prevalent form of dementia, begin with memory impairment, although in other dementias, such as frontotemporal dementia, memory loss is not a presenting feature. Focal cerebral disorders are discussed in Chap. 18 and illustrated in a video library in Chap. 19.

FUNCTIONAL ANATOMY OF THE DEMENTIAS

Dementia syndromes result from the disruption of specific large-scale neuronal networks; the location and severity of synaptic and neuronal loss combine to produce the clinical features (Chap. 18). Behavior and mood are modulated by noradrenergic, serotonergic, and dopaminergic pathways, whereas cholinergic signaling is critical for attention and memory functions. The dementias differ in the relative neurotransmitter deficit profiles; accordingly, accurate diagnosis guides effective pharmacotherapy.

AD begins in the transentorhinal region, spreads to the hippocampus, and then moves to lateral and posterior temporal and parietal neocortex, eventually causing a more widespread degeneration. *Vascular dementia* is associated with focal damage in a random patchwork of cortical and subcortical regions or white matter tracts that disconnect nodes within distributed networks. In keeping with the anatomy, AD typically presents with memory loss accompanied later by aphasia or navigational problems. In contrast, patients with dementias that begin in frontal or subcortical regions such as *frontotemporal dementia* (FTD) or *Huntington's disease* (HD) are less likely to begin with memory problems and more likely to have difficulties with judgment, mood, and behavior.

Lesions of cortical-striatal pathways produce specific effects on behavior. The dorsolateral prefrontal cortex bears connections with a central band of the caudate. Lesions of either node or connecting white matter pathways result in poor organization and planning, decreased cognitive flexibility, and impaired working memory. The lateral orbital frontal cortex connects with the ventromedial caudate. Lesions of this system cause impulsiveness, distractibility, and disinhibition. The anterior cingulate cortex projects to the nucleus accumbens, and interruption of these connections produces apathy, poverty of speech, or even akinetic mutism. All corticostriatal systems also include topographically organized projections through the pallidum and thalamus, and damage to these nodes can likewise reproduce the clinical syndrome of corticostriatal damage.

THE CAUSES OF DEMENTIA

The single strongest risk factor for dementia is increasing age. The prevalence of disabling memory loss increases with each decade over age 50 and is usually associated with the microscopic changes of AD at autopsy. Yet some centenarians have intact memory function and no evidence of clinically significant dementia. Whether dementia is an inevitable consequence of normal human aging remains controversial.

The many causes of dementia are listed in Table 29-1. The frequency of each condition depends on the age group under study, the access of the group to medical care, the country of origin, and perhaps racial or ethnic background. AD is the most common cause of dementia in Western countries, accounting for more than half of all patients. Vascular disease is considered the second most frequent cause for dementia and is particularly common in elderly patients or populations with limited access to medical care, where vascular risk factors are undertreated. Often, vascular disease is mixed with other neurodegenerative disorders, making it difficult, even for the neuropathologist, to estimate the contribution of cerebrovascular disease to the cognitive disorder in an individual patient. Dementias related to Parkinson's disease (PD) are extremely common, and temporally can follow a parkinsonian disorder as seen with PD-related dementia (PDD) or can occur concurrently with or preceding the motor syndrome as with dementia with Lewy bodies (DLB). In patients under the age of 65, FTD rivals AD as the most common cause of dementia. Chronic intoxications, including those resulting from alcohol and prescription drugs, are an important and often treatable cause of dementia. Other disorders listed in the table are uncommon but important because many are reversible. The classification of dementing illnesses into reversible and irreversible disorders is a useful approach to differential diagnosis. When effective treatments for the neurodegenerative conditions emerge, this dichotomy will become obsolete.

In a study of 1000 persons attending a memory disorders clinic, 19% had a potentially reversible cause of the cognitive impairment and 23% had a potentially reversible concomitant condition. The three most common potentially reversible diagnoses were depression, hydrocephalus, and alcohol dependence (Table 29-1).

Subtle cumulative decline in episodic memory is a natural part of aging. This frustrating experience, often the source of jokes and humor, is referred to as *benign forgetfulness of the elderly. Benign* means that it is not so progressive or serious that it impairs reasonably successful and productive daily functioning, although the distinction between benign and more significant memory loss can be difficult to make. At age 85, the average person is able to learn and recall approximately one-half the number of items (e.g., words on a list) that he or she could at age 18. A measurable cognitive problem that does not disrupt daily activities is often referred to as *mild cognitive impairment* (MCI). Factors that predict progression from

TABLE 29-1

DIFFERENTIAL DIAGNOSIS OF DEMENTIA

Most Common Causes of Dementia	
Alzheimer's disease *Vascular dementia* Multi-infarct Diffuse white matter disease (Binswanger's)	Alcoholism[a] Parkinson's disease Drug/medication intoxication[a]

Less Common Causes of Dementia	
Vitamin deficiencies Thiamine (B_1): Wernicke's encephalopathy[a] B_{12} (subacute combined degeneration)[a] Nicotinic acid (pellagra)[a]	Toxic disorders Drug, medication, and narcotic poisoning[a] Heavy metal intoxication[a] Dialysis dementia (aluminum) Organic toxins
Endocrine and other organ failure Hypothyroidism[a] Adrenal insufficiency and Cushing's syndrome[a] Hypo- and hyperparathyroidism[a] Renal failure[a] Liver failure[a] Pulmonary failure[a]	Psychiatric Depression (pseudodementia)[a] Schizophrenia[a] Conversion reaction[a]
Chronic infections HIV Neurosyphilis[a] Papovavirus (JC virus) (progressive multifocal leukoencephalopathy) Tuberculosis, fungal, and protozoal[a] Whipple's disease[a]	Degenerative disorders Huntington's disease Dementia with Lewy bodies Progressive supranuclear palsy Multisystem atrophy Hereditary ataxias (some forms) Motor neuron disease (amyotrophic lateral sclerosis [ALS]; some forms) Frontotemporal dementia Corticobasal degeneration Multiple sclerosis Adult Down syndrome with Alzheimer's disease ALS Parkinson's dementia complex of Guam Prion (Creutzfeldt-Jakob and Gerstmann-Sträussler-Scheinker diseases)
Head trauma and diffuse brain damage Dementia pugilistica Chronic subdural hematoma[a] Postanoxia Postencephalitis Normal-pressure hydrocephalus[a]	Miscellaneous Sarcoidosis[a] Vasculitis[a] CADASIL, etc. Acute intermittent porphyria[a] Recurrent nonconvulsive seizures[a]
Neoplastic Primary brain tumor[a] Metastatic brain tumor[a] Paraneoplastic limbic encephalitis	Additional conditions in children or adolescents Pantothenate kinase-associated neurodegeneration Subacute sclerosing panencephalitis Metabolic disorders (e.g., Wilson's and Leigh's diseases, leukodystrophies, lipid storage diseases, mitochondrial mutations)

[a]Potentially reversible dementia.

Abbreviation: CADASIL, cerebral autosomal dominant arteriopathy with subcortical infarcts and leukoencephalopathy.

TABLE 29-2

THE MOLECULAR BASIS FOR DEGENERATIVE DEMENTIA

DEMENTIA	MOLECULAR BASIS	CAUSAL GENES AND (CHROMOSOME)	SUSCEPTIBILITY GENES	PATHOLOGY
AD	Aβ	<2% carry these mutations. *APP* (21), *PS*-1 (14), *PS*-2 (1) (most mutations are in *PS*-1)	*Apo ε4* (19)	Amyloid plaques, neurofibrillary tangles
FTD	Tau	Tau exon and intron mutations (17) (about 10% of familial cases) Progranulin (17) (10% of familial cases)	H1 tau haplotypes	Tau inclusions, Pick bodies, neurofibrillary tangles
	TDP-43 FUS			TDP-43 inclusions FUS inclusions
DLB	α-synuclein	Very rare α-synuclein (4) (dominant)	Unknown	α-synuclein inclusions (Lewy bodies)
CJD	PrP^{SC} proteins	Prion (20) (up to 15% of cases carry these dominant mutations)	Codon 129 homozygosity for methionine or valine	Tau inclusions, spongiform changes, gliosis

Abbreviations: AD, Alzheimer's disease; CJD, Creutzfeldt-Jakob disease; DLB, dementia with Lewy bodies; FTD, frontotemporal dementia.

MCI to AD include a prominent memory deficit, family history of dementia, presence of an apolipoprotein ε4 (Apo ε4) allele, small hippocampal volumes, and AD-like signature of cortical atrophy, low cerebrospinal fluid Aβ and elevated tau or positive amyloid imaging with Pittsburgh Compound-B (PiB), although the latter remains an experimental approach not yet available for routine clinical use.

The major degenerative dementias include AD, DLB, FTD and related disorders, HD, and prion diseases, including Creutzfeldt-Jakob disease (CJD). These disorders are all associated with the abnormal aggregation of a specific protein: $A\beta_{42}$ and tau in AD; α-synuclein in DLB; tau, TAR DNA-binding protein of 43kDa (TDP-43), or *fu*sed in *s*arcoma (FUS) in FTD; huntingtin in HD; and misfolded prion protein (PrP^{sc}) in CJD (Table 29-2).

APPROACH TO THE PATIENT **Dementias**

Three major issues should be kept at the forefront: (1) What is the most accurate diagnosis? (2) Is there a treatable or reversible component to the dementia? (3) Can the physician help to alleviate the burden on caregivers? A broad overview of the approach to dementia is shown in Table 29-3. The major degenerative dementias can usually be distinguished by the initial symptoms; neuropsychological, neuropsychiatric, and neurologic findings; and neuroimaging features (Table 29-4).

HISTORY The history should concentrate on the onset, duration, and tempo of progression. An acute or subacute onset of confusion may represent delirium and should trigger the search for intoxication, infection, or metabolic derangement. An elderly person with slowly progressive memory loss over several years is likely to suffer from AD. Nearly 75% of patients with AD begin with memory symptoms, but other early symptoms include difficulty with managing money, driving, shopping, following instructions, finding words, or navigating. A personality change, disinhibition, and weight gain or compulsive eating suggest FTD, not AD. FTD is also suggested by prominent apathy, compulsivity, or progressive loss of speech fluency or word comprehension, and by a relative sparing of memory or visuospatial abilities. The diagnosis of DLB is suggested by early visual hallucinations; parkinsonism; brittle proneness to delirium or sensitivity to psychoactive medications; REM behavior disorder (RBD, the loss of skeletal muscle paralysis during dreaming); or Capgras' syndrome, the delusion that a familiar person has been replaced by an impostor.

A history of stroke with irregular stepwise progression suggests vascular dementia. Vascular dementia is also commonly seen in the setting of hypertension, atrial fibrillation, peripheral vascular disease, and diabetes. In patients suffering from cerebrovascular disease, it can be difficult to determine whether the dementia is due to AD, vascular disease, or a mixture of the two as many of the risk factors for vascular dementia, including diabetes, high cholesterol, elevated homocysteine,

TABLE 29-3

EVALUATION OF THE PATIENT WITH DEMENTIA

ROUTINE EVALUATION	OPTIONAL FOCUSED TESTS	OCCASIONALLY HELPFUL TESTS
History	Psychometric testing	EEG
Physical examination	Chest x-ray	Parathyroid function
Laboratory tests	Lumbar puncture	Adrenal function
Thyroid function (TSH)	Liver function	Urine heavy metals
Vitamin B_{12}	Renal function	RBC sedimentation rate
Complete blood count	Urine toxin screen	Angiogram
Electrolytes	HIV	Brain biopsy
CT/MRI	Apolipoprotein E	SPECT
	RPR or VDRL	PET

Diagnostic Categories

REVERSIBLE CAUSES	IRREVERSIBLE/DEGENERATIVE DEMENTIAS	PSYCHIATRIC DISORDERS
Examples	Examples	Depression
Hypothyroidism	Alzheimer's	Schizophrenia
Thiamine deficiency	Frontotemporal dementia	Conversion reaction
Vitamin B_{12} deficiency	Huntington's	
Normal-pressure hydrocephalus	Dementia with Lewy bodies	
Subdural hematoma	Vascular	
Chronic infection	Leukoencephalopathies	
Brain tumor	Parkinson's	
Drug intoxication		

Associated Treatable Conditions

Depression	Agitation
Seizures	Caregiver "burnout"
Insomnia	Drug side effects

Abbreviations: PET, positron emission tomography; RPR, rapid plasma reagin (test); SPECT, single-photon emission CT; VDRL, Venereal Disease Research Laboratory (test for syphilis).

and low exercise, are also risk factors for AD. Rapid progression with motor rigidity and myoclonus suggests CJD. Seizures may indicate strokes or neoplasm but also occur in AD, particularly early age of onset AD. Gait disturbance is common in vascular dementia, PD/DLB, or normal-pressure hydrocephalus (NPH). A prior history of high-risk sexual behaviors or intravenous drug use should trigger a search for central nervous system (CNS) infection, especially for HIV or syphilis. A history of recurrent head trauma could indicate chronic subdural hematoma, dementia pugilistica, or NPH. Subacute onset of severe amnesia and psychosis with mesial temporal T2 hyperintensities on MRI should raise concern for paraneoplastic limbic encephalitis, especially in a long-term smoker or other patients at risk for cancer. Related nonparaneoplastic autoimmune conditions can present with a similar tempo and imaging signature. Alcoholism creates risk for malnutrition and thiamine deficiency. Veganism, bowel irradiation, an autoimmune diathesis, or a remote history of gastric surgery can result in B_{12} deficiency. Certain occupations, such as working in a battery or chemical factory, might indicate heavy metal intoxication. Careful review of medication intake, especially for sedatives and analgesics, may raise the issue of chronic drug intoxication. An autosomal dominant family history is found in HD and in familial forms of AD, FTD, DLB, or prion disorders. The recent death of a loved one, or depressive signs such as insomnia or weight loss, raises the possibility of depression-related cognitive impairments.

PHYSICAL AND NEUROLOGIC EXAMINATION A thorough general and neurologic examination is essential to document dementia, to look for other signs of nervous system involvement, and to search for clues suggesting a systemic disease that might be responsible for the cognitive disorder. Typical AD does not affect

TABLE 29-4

CLINICAL DIFFERENTIATION OF THE MAJOR DEMENTIAS

DISEASE	FIRST SYMPTOM	MENTAL STATUS	NEUROPSYCHIATRY	NEUROLOGY	IMAGING
AD	Memory loss	Episodic memory loss	Initially normal	Initially normal	Entorhinal cortex and hippocampal atrophy
FTD	Apathy; poor judgment/insight, speech/language; hyperorality	Frontal/executive, language; spares drawing	Apathy, disinhibition, hyperorality, euphoria, depression	May have vertical gaze palsy, axial rigidity, dystonia, alien hand, or MND	Frontal, insular, and/or temporal atrophy; spares posterior parietal lobe
DLB	Visual hallucinations, REM sleep disorder, delirium, Capgras' syndrome, parkinsonism	Drawing and frontal/executive; spares memory; delirium prone	Visual hallucinations, depression, sleep disorder, delusions	Parkinsonism	Posterior parietal atrophy; hippocampi larger than in AD
CJD	Dementia, mood, anxiety, movement disorders	Variable, frontal/executive, focal cortical, memory	Depression, anxiety	Myoclonus, rigidity, parkinsonism	Cortical ribboning and basal ganglia or thalamus hyperintensity on diffusion/FLAIR MRI
Vascular	Often but not always sudden; variable; apathy, falls, focal weakness	Frontal/executive, cognitive slowing; can spare memory	Apathy, delusions, anxiety	Usually motor slowing, spasticity; can be normal	Cortical and/or subcortical infarctions, confluent white matter disease

Abbreviations: AD, Alzheimer's disease; CBD, cortical basal degeneration; CJD, Creutzfeldt-Jakob disease; DLB, dementia with Lewy bodies; FTD, frontotemporal dementia; MND, motor neuron disease; PSP, progressive supranuclear palsy.

motor systems until later in the course. In contrast, FTD patients often develop axial rigidity, supranuclear gaze palsy, or a motor neuron disease reminiscent of amyotrophic lateral sclerosis (ALS). In DLB, the initial symptoms may include the new onset of a parkinsonian syndrome (resting tremor, cogwheel rigidity, bradykinesia, festinating gait) but often starts with visual hallucinations or dementia. Symptoms referable to the lower brainstem (RBD, gastrointestinal or autonomic problems) may arise years before parkinsonism or dementia. Corticobasal syndrome (CBS) features asymmetric akinesia and rigidity, dystonia, myoclonus, alien limb phenomena, and pyramidal or cortical sensory deficits. Associated cognitive features include nonfluent aphasia with or without motor speech impairment, executive dysfunction, apraxia, or a behavioral disorder. Progressive supranuclear palsy (PSP) is associated with unexplained falls, axial rigidity, dysphagia, and vertical gaze deficits. CJD is suggested by the presence of diffuse rigidity, an akinetic-mute state, and prominent, often startle-sensitive myoclonus.

Hemiparesis or other focal neurologic deficits suggest vascular dementia or brain tumor. Dementia with a myelopathy and peripheral neuropathy suggests vitamin B_{12} deficiency. Peripheral neuropathy could also indicate another vitamin deficiency, heavy metal intoxication, thyroid dysfunction, Lyme disease, or vasculitis. Dry, cool skin, hair loss, and bradycardia suggest hypothyroidism. Fluctuating confusion associated with repetitive stereotyped movements may indicate ongoing limbic, temporal, or frontal seizures. Hearing impairment or visual loss may produce confusion and disorientation misinterpreted as dementia. Such sensory deficits are common in the elderly but can be a manifestation of mitochondrial disorders.

COGNITIVE AND NEUROPSYCHIATRIC EXAMINATION Brief screening tools such as the mini-mental status examination (MMSE) help to confirm the presence of cognitive impairment and to follow the progression of dementia (Table 29-5). The MMSE, a simple 30-point test of cognitive function, contains tests of orientation, working memory (e.g., spell *world* backwards), episodic memory (orientation and 3-word recall), language comprehension, naming, and figure copying. In most patients with MCI and some with clinically apparent AD, the MMSE may be normal and a more rigorous set of neuropsychological tests will be required. When the etiology for the dementia syndrome remains in doubt, a specially tailored evaluation should be performed that includes tasks of working and episodic memory,

TABLE 29-5

THE MINI-MENTAL STATUS EXAMINATION

	POINTS
Orientation	
Name: season/date/day/month/ year	5 (1 for each name)
Name: hospital/floor/town/state/ country	5 (1 for each name)
Registration	
Identify three objects by name and ask patient to repeat	3 (1 for each object)
Attention and calculation	
Serial 7s; subtract from 100 (e.g., 93–86–79–72–65)	5 (1 for each subtraction)
Recall	
Recall the three objects presented earlier	3 (1 for each object)
Language	
Name pencil and watch	2 (1 for each object)
Repeat "No ifs, ands, or buts"	1
Follow a 3-step command (e.g., "Take this paper, fold it in half, and place it on the table")	3 (1 for each command)
Write "close your eyes" and ask patient to obey written command	1
Ask patient to write a sentence	1
Ask patient to copy a design (e.g., intersecting pentagons)	1
Total	30

executive function, language, and visuospatial and perceptual abilities. In AD the early deficits involve episodic memory, category generation ("name as many animals as you can in one minute"), and visuoconstructive ability. Usually deficits in verbal or visual episodic memory are the first neuropsychological abnormalities detected, and tasks that require the patient to recall a long list of words or a series of pictures after a predetermined delay will demonstrate deficits in most patients. In FTD, the earliest deficits on cognitive testing involve executive or language (speech or naming) function. DLB patients have more severe deficits in visuospatial function but do better on episodic memory tasks than patients with AD. Patients with vascular dementia often demonstrate a mixture of executive and visuospatial deficits, with prominent psychomotor slowing. In delirium, the most prominent deficits involve attention, working memory, and executive function, making the assessment of other cognitive domains challenging and often uninformative.

A functional assessment should also be performed. The physician should determine the day-to-day impact of the disorder on the patient's memory, community affairs, hobbies, judgment, dressing, and eating. Knowledge of the patient's day-to-day function will help the clinician and the family to organize a therapeutic approach.

Neuropsychiatric assessment is important for diagnosis, prognosis, and treatment. In the early stages of AD, mild depressive features, social withdrawal, and irritability or anxiety are the most prominent psychiatric changes, but patients often maintain core social skills into the middle or late stages, when delusions, agitation, and sleep disturbance may emerge. In FTD, dramatic personality change featuring apathy, overeating, compulsions, disinhibition, euphoria, and loss of empathy are early and common. DLB is associated with visual hallucinations, delusions related to person or place identity, RBD, and excessive daytime sleepiness. Dramatic fluctuations occur not only in cognition but also in primary arousal, such that caregivers may seek emergency room evaluation for suspected stroke. Vascular dementia can present with psychiatric symptoms such as depression, anxiety, delusions, disinhibition, or apathy.

LABORATORY TESTS The choice of laboratory tests in the evaluation of dementia is complex. The physician must take measures to avoid missing a reversible or treatable cause, yet no single treatable etiology is common; thus, a screen must employ multiple tests, each of which has a low yield. Cost/benefit ratios are difficult to assess, and many laboratory screening algorithms for dementia discourage multiple tests. Nevertheless, even a test with only a 1–2% positive rate is probably worth undertaking if the alternative is missing a treatable cause of dementia. Table 29-3 lists most screening tests for dementia. The American Academy of Neurology recommends the routine measurement of thyroid function, a vitamin B_{12} level, and a neuroimaging study (CT or MRI).

Neuroimaging studies help to rule out primary and metastatic neoplasms, locate areas of infarction, detect subdural hematomas, and suggest NPH or diffuse white matter disease. They also help to establish a regional pattern of atrophy. Support for the diagnosis of AD includes hippocampal atrophy in addition to posterior-predominant cortical atrophy. Focal frontal and/or anterior temporal atrophy suggests FTD. DLB often features less prominent atrophy, with greater involvement of amygdala than hippocampus. In CJD, MR diffusion-weighted imaging reveals abnormalities in the cortical ribbon and basal ganglia in the majority of patients. Extensive white matter abnormalities correlate with a vascular etiology for dementia. The role of functional-metabolic imaging in the diagnosis of dementia is still under study, although the Federal Drug Administration has approved the use of positron emission tomography (PET) in dementia differential diagnosis. Single-photon emission computed tomography (SPECT) and PET scanning show temporal-parietal hypoperfusion or hypometabolism in AD and frontotemporal deficits in FTD, but these changes often reflect atrophy and can therefore be detected with MRI alone in many patients. Recently, amyloid imaging has shown promise for the diagnosis of AD, and Pittsburgh Compound-B (PiB) and ^{18}F-AV-45 appear to be reliable radioligands for detecting brain amyloid associated with amyloid angiopathy or neuritic plaques (Fig. 29-1). Because these abnormalities can be seen in cognitively normal older persons, however, amyloid imaging may detect preclinical or incidental AD in patients lacking an AD-like dementia syndrome. Once powerful disease-modifying therapies become available, use of these biomarkers may help to identify treatment candidates before irreversible brain injury has occurred. In the meantime, however, the significance of detecting brain amyloid in an asymptomatic elder remains a topic of vigorous investigation. Similarly, MRI perfusion and functional connectivity methods are being explored as potential treatment-monitoring strategies.

Lumbar puncture need not be done routinely in the evaluation of dementia, but it is indicated when CNS infection or inflammation are credible diagnostic possibilities. Cerebrospinal fluid (CSF) levels of tau protein and $A\beta_{42}$ show differing patterns with the various dementias; however, the sensitivity and specificity of these measures are not yet sufficiently high to warrant routine use. Formal psychometric testing, although not necessary in every patient with dementia, helps to document the severity of cognitive disturbance, suggest psychogenic causes, and provide a more formal method for following the disease course. Electroencephalogram (EEG) is rarely helpful except to suggest CJD (repetitive bursts of diffuse high-amplitude sharp waves, or "periodic complexes") or an underlying nonconvulsive seizure disorder (epileptiform discharges). Brain biopsy (including meninges) is not advised except to diagnose vasculitis, potentially treatable neoplasms, or unusual infections when the diagnosis is uncertain. Systemic disorders with CNS manifestations, such as sarcoidosis, can usually be confirmed through biopsy of lymph node or solid organ rather than brain. Angiography should be considered when cerebral vasculitis or cerebral venous thrombosis is a possible cause of the dementia.

ALZHEIMER'S DISEASE

Approximately 10% of all persons over the age of 70 have significant memory loss, and in more than half the cause is AD. It is estimated that the annual total cost of caring for a single AD patient in an advanced stage of the disease is >$50,000. The disease also exacts a heavy emotional toll on family members and caregivers. AD can occur in any decade of adulthood, but it is the most common cause of dementia in the elderly. AD most often presents with an insidious onset of memory loss followed by a slowly progressive dementia over several years. Pathologically, atrophy is distributed throughout the medial temporal lobes, as well as lateral and medial parietal lobes and lateral frontal cortex. Microscopically, there are neuritic plaques containing Aβ, neurofibrillary tangles (NFTs) composed of hyperphosphorylated tau filaments, and accumulation of amyloid in blood vessel walls in cortex and leptomeninges (see "Pathology"). The identification of four different susceptibility genes for AD has provided a foundation for rapid progress in understanding the biologic basis of the disorder.

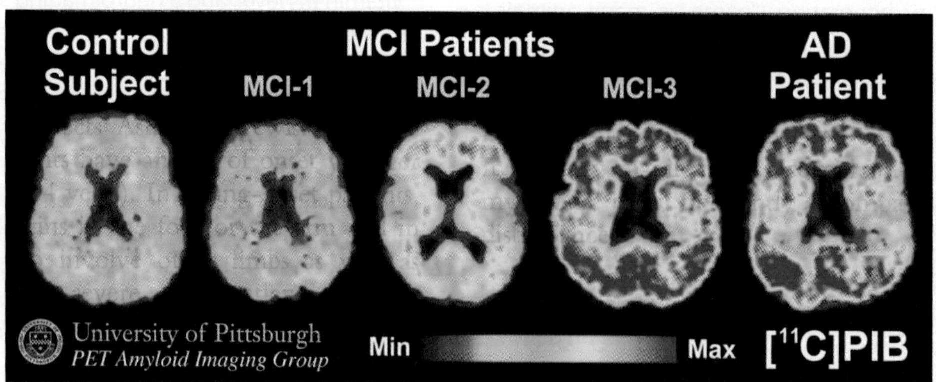

FIGURE 29-1

PET images obtained with the amyloid-imaging agent Pittsburgh Compound-B ([^{11}C]PIB) in a normal control (*left*); three different patients with mild cognitive impairment (MCI, *center*); and a mild AD patient (*right*). Some MCI patients have control-like levels of amyloid, some have AD-like levels of amyloid, and some have intermediate levels. AD, Alzheimer's disease; MCI, mild cognitive impairment; PET, positron emission tomography.

CLINICAL MANIFESTATIONS

The cognitive changes of AD tend to follow a characteristic pattern, beginning with memory impairment and spreading to language and visuospatial deficits. Yet, approximately 20% of patients with AD present with nonmemory complaints such as word-finding, organizational, or navigational difficulty. In the early stages of the disease, the memory loss may go unrecognized or be ascribed to benign forgetfulness. Once the memory loss becomes noticeable to the patient and spouse and falls 1.5 standard deviations below normal on standardized memory tests, the term MCI is applied. This construct provides useful prognostic information, because approximately 50% of patients with MCI (roughly 12% per year) will progress to AD over 4 years. Slowly the cognitive problems begin to interfere with daily activities, such as keeping track of finances, following instructions on the job, driving, shopping, and housekeeping. Some patients are unaware of these difficulties (*anosognosia*), while others remain acutely attuned to their deficits. Changes in environment (such as vacations or hospital stays) may be disorienting, and the patient may become lost on walks or while driving. In the middle stages of AD, the patient is unable to work, is easily lost and confused, and requires daily supervision. Social graces, routine behavior, and superficial conversation may be surprisingly intact. Language becomes impaired—first naming, then comprehension, and finally fluency. In some patients, *aphasia* is an early and prominent feature. Word-finding difficulties and circumlocution may be a problem even when formal testing demonstrates intact naming and fluency. *Apraxia* emerges, and patients have trouble performing learned sequential motor tasks. Visuospatial deficits begin to interfere with dressing, eating, or even walking, and patients fail to solve simple puzzles or copy geometric figures. Simple calculations and clock reading become difficult in parallel.

In the late stages of the disease, some persons remain ambulatory but wander aimlessly. Loss of judgment and reasoning is inevitable. Delusions are common and usually simple, with common themes of theft, infidelity, or misidentification. Approximately 10% of AD patients develop *Capgras' syndrome*, believing that a caregiver has been replaced by an impostor. In contrast to DLB, where Capgras' syndrome is an early feature, in AD this syndrome emerges later. Loss of inhibitions and aggression may occur and alternate with passivity and withdrawal. Sleep-wake patterns are disrupted, and nighttime wandering becomes disturbing to the household. Some patients develop a shuffling gait with generalized muscle rigidity associated with slowness and awkwardness of movement. Patients often look parkinsonian (Chap. 30) but rarely have a high-amplitude, rhythmic, resting tremor. In end-stage AD, patients become rigid, mute, incontinent, and bedridden. Help is needed with eating, dressing, and toileting. Hyperactive tendon reflexes and myoclonic jerks (sudden brief contractions of various muscles or the whole body) may occur spontaneously or in response to physical or auditory stimulation. Generalized seizures may also occur. Often death results from malnutrition, secondary infections, pulmonary emboli, heart disease, or, most commonly, aspiration. The typical duration of AD is 8–10 years, but the course can range from 1 to 25 years. For unknown reasons, some AD patients show a steady decline in function, while others have prolonged plateaus without major deterioration.

DIFFERENTIAL DIAGNOSIS

Early in the disease course, other etiologies of dementia should be excluded (Table 29-1). Neuroimaging studies (CT and MRI) do not show a single specific pattern with AD and may be normal early in the course of the disease. As AD progresses, more distributed but usually posterior-predominant cortical atrophy becomes apparent, along with atrophy of the medial temporal memory structures (Fig. 29-2*A*, *B*). The main purpose of imaging is to exclude other disorders, such as primary and secondary neoplasms, vascular dementia, diffuse white matter disease, and NPH; it also helps to distinguish AD from other degenerative disorders with distinctive imaging patterns such as FTD or CJD. Functional imaging studies in AD reveal hypoperfusion or hypometabolism in the posterior temporal-parietal cortex (Fig. 29-2*C*,*D*). The EEG in AD is normal or shows nonspecific slowing. Routine spinal fluid examination is also normal. CSF $A\beta_{42}$ levels are reduced, whereas levels of hyperphosphorylated tau protein are elevated, but the considerable overlap of these levels with those of the normal aged population limits the usefulness of these measurements in diagnosis. The use of blood ApoE genotyping is discussed under "Pathology." *Slowly progressive decline in memory and orientation, normal results on laboratory tests, and an MRI or CT scan showing only distributed or posteriorly predominant cortical and hippocampal atrophy is highly suggestive of AD.* A clinical diagnosis of AD reached after careful evaluation is confirmed at autopsy about 90% of the time, with misdiagnosed cases usually representing one of the other dementing disorders described later in this chapter, a mixture of AD with vascular pathology, or DLB.

Simple clinical clues are useful in the differential diagnosis. Early prominent gait disturbance with only mild memory loss suggests vascular dementia or, rarely, NPH (see later). Resting tremor with stooped posture, bradykinesia, and masked facies suggest PD (Chap. 30). When dementia occurs after a well-established diagnosis of PD, PDD is usually the correct diagnosis. The early appearance of parkinsonian features in association with fluctuating alertness, visual hallucinations, or delusional misidentification suggests DLB. Chronic alcoholism should

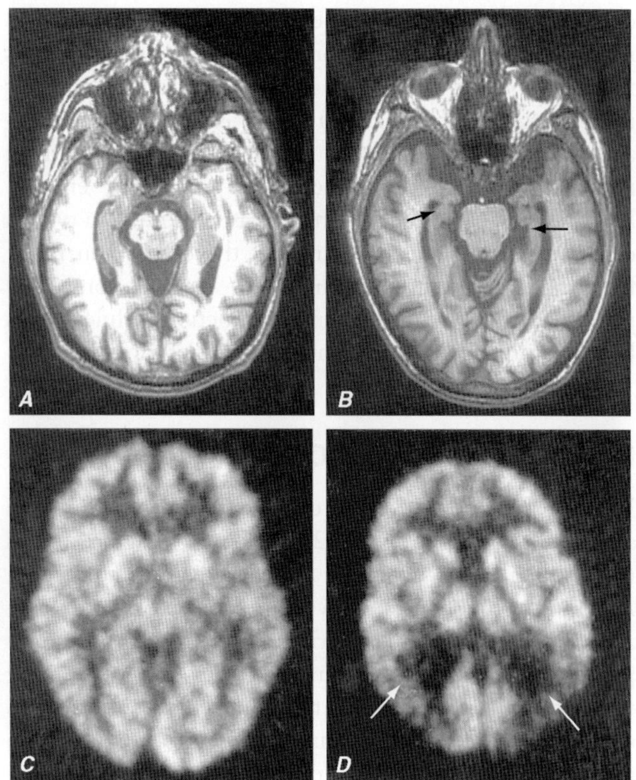

FIGURE 29-2

Alzheimer's disease. Axial T1-weighted MR images through the midbrain of a normal 86-year-old athlete (***A***) and a 77-year-old man with AD (***B***). Note that both individuals have mild sulcal widening and slight dilation of the temporal horns of the lateral ventricles. However, there is a reduction in hippocampal volume in the patient with AD (*arrows*) compared with the volume of the normal-for-age hippocampus (***A***). Fluorodeoxyglucose PET scans of a normal control (***C***) and a patient with AD (***D***). Note that the patient with AD shows decreased glucose metabolism in the posterior temporoparietal regions bilaterally (*arrows*), a typical finding in this condition. AD, Alzheimer's disease; PET, positron emission tomography. (*Images courtesy of TF Budinger, University of California.*)

prompt the search for vitamin deficiency. Loss of sensibility to position and vibration stimuli accompanied by Babinski responses suggests vitamin B_{12} deficiency (Chap. 35). Early onset of a focal seizure suggests a metastatic or primary brain neoplasm (Chap. 37). Previous or ongoing depression raises suspicion for depression-related cognitive impairment, although AD can feature a depressive prodrome. A history of treatment for insomnia, anxiety, psychiatric disturbance, or epilepsy suggests chronic drug intoxication. Rapid progression over a few weeks or months associated with rigidity and myoclonus suggests CJD (Chap. 43). Prominent behavioral changes with intact navigation and focal anterior-predominant atrophy on brain imaging are typical of FTD. A positive family history of dementia suggests either one of the familial forms of AD or one of the other genetic disorders associated with dementia, such as HD (see later), FTD (see later), prion disease (Chap. 43), or rare hereditary ataxias (Chap. 31).

EPIDEMIOLOGY

The most important risk factors for AD are old age and a positive family history. The frequency of AD increases with each decade of adult life, reaching 20–40% of the population over the age of 85. A positive family history of dementia suggests a genetic cause of AD, although autosomal dominant inheritance occurs in only 2% of patients with AD. Female sex may also be a risk factor independent of the greater longevity of women. Some AD patients have a past history of head trauma with concussion. AD is more common in groups with low educational attainment, but education influences test-taking ability, and it is clear that AD can affect persons of all intellectual levels. One study found that the capacity to express complex written language in early adulthood correlated with a decreased risk for AD. Numerous environmental factors, including aluminum, mercury, and viruses, have been proposed as causes of AD, but none has been demonstrated to play a significant role. Similarly, several studies suggest that the use of nonsteroidal anti-inflammatory agents is associated with a decreased risk of AD, but this has not been confirmed in large prospective studies. Vascular disease, and stroke in particular, seems to lower the threshold for the clinical expression of AD. Also, in many patients with AD, amyloid angiopathy can lead to microhemorrhages, large lobar hemorrhages, or ischemic infarctions. Diabetes increases the risk of AD threefold. Elevated homocysteine and cholesterol levels; hypertension; diminished serum levels of folic acid; low dietary intake of fruits, vegetables, and red wine; and low levels of exercise are all being explored as potential risk factors for AD.

PATHOLOGY

At autopsy, the earliest and most severe degeneration is usually found in the medial temporal lobe (entorhinal/perirhinal cortex and hippocampus), lateral temporal cortex, and nucleus basalis of Meynert. The characteristic microscopic findings are neuritic plaques and NFTs. These lesions accumulate in small numbers during normal brain aging but dominate the picture in AD. Increasing evidence suggests that soluble amyloid species called *oligomers* may cause cellular dysfunction and represent the early toxic molecule in AD. Eventually, further amyloid polymerization and fibril formation lead to neuritic plaques (Fig. 29-3), which contain a central amyloid core, proteoglycans, Apo ε4, α-antichymotrypsin, and other proteins. Aβ is a protein of 39–42 amino acids that is derived proteolytically from a larger transmembrane protein, *amyloid precursor protein* (APP), when APP

SECTION III Diseases of the Nervous System

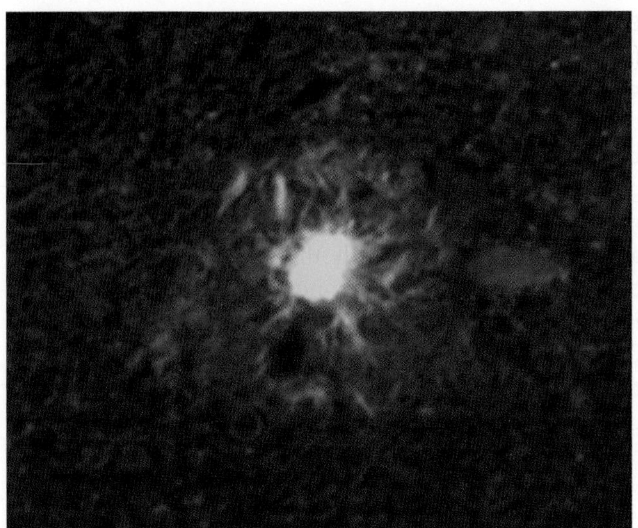

FIGURE 29-3
Mature neuritic plaque with a dense central amyloid core surrounded by dystrophic neurites (thioflavin S stain). (*Image courtesy of S. DeArmond, University of California; with permission.*)

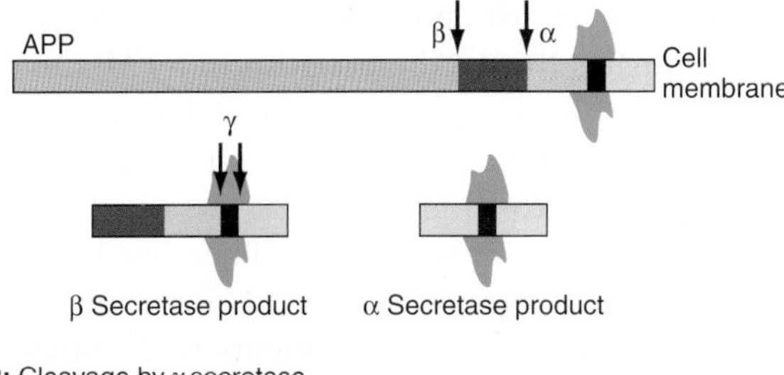

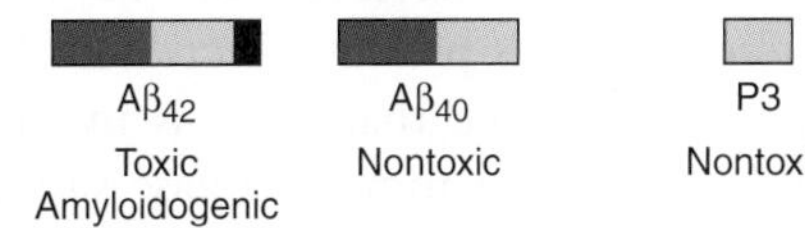

FIGURE 29-4
Amyloid precursor protein (APP) is catabolized by α, β, and γ secretases. A key initial step is the digestion by either β secretase (BASE) or α secretase (ADAM10 or ADAM17 [TACE]), producing smaller nontoxic products. Cleavage of the β secretase product by γ secretase (Step 2) results in either the toxic $A\beta_{42}$ or the nontoxic $A\beta_{40}$ peptide; cleavage of the α secretase product by γ secretase produces the nontoxic P3 peptide. Excess production of $A\beta_{42}$ is a key initiator of cellular damage in Alzheimer's disease. Current AD research is focused on developing therapies designed to reduce accumulation of $A\beta_{42}$ by antagonizing β or γ secretases, promoting α secretase, or clearing $A\beta_{42}$ that has already formed by use of specific antibodies.

is cleaved by β and γ secretases. The normal function of Aβ is unknown. APP has neurotrophic and neuroprotective properties. The plaque core is surrounded by a halo, which contains dystrophic, tau-immunoreactive neurites and activated microglia. The accumulation of Aβ in cerebral arterioles is termed *amyloid angiopathy*. NFTs are composed of silver-staining neuronal cytoplasmic fibrils composed of abnormally phosphorylated tau (τ) protein; they appear as paired helical filaments by electron microscopy. Tau binds to and stabilizes microtubules, supporting axonal transport of organelles, glycoproteins, neurotransmitters, and other important cargoes throughout the neuron. Once hyperphosphorylated, tau can no longer bind properly to microtubules and its functions are disrupted. Finally, patients with AD often show comorbid DLB and vascular pathology.

Biochemically, AD is associated with a decrease in the cortical levels of several proteins and neurotransmitters, especially acetylcholine, its synthetic enzyme choline acetyltransferase, and nicotinic cholinergic receptors. Reduction of acetylcholine may be related in part to degeneration of cholinergic neurons in the nucleus basalis of Meynert that project throughout the cortex. There is also noradrenergic and serotonergic depletion due to degeneration of brainstem nuclei such as the locus coeruleus and dorsal raphe.

GENETIC CONSIDERATIONS

Several genes play important pathogenic roles in at least some patients with AD. One is the *APP* gene on chromosome 21. Adults with trisomy 21 (Down syndrome) consistently develop the typical neuropathologic hallmarks of AD if they survive beyond age 40. Many develop a progressive dementia superimposed on their baseline mental retardation. APP is a membrane-spanning protein that is subsequently processed into smaller units, including Aβ, which is deposited in neuritic plaques. Aβ peptide results from cleavage of APP by β and γ secretases (Fig. 29-4). Presumably, the extra dose of the *APP* gene on chromosome 21 is the initiating cause of AD in adult Down syndrome and results in excess cerebral amyloid. Furthermore, a few families with early-onset familial Alzheimer's disease (FAD) have been discovered to have point mutations in the *APP* gene. Although very rare, these families were the first examples of single-gene autosomal dominant transmission of AD.

Investigation of large families with multigenerational FAD led to the discovery of two additional AD genes, the *presenilins*. Presenilin-1 (*PS-1*) is on chromosome 14 and encodes a protein called S182. Mutations in this gene cause an early-onset AD (onset before age 60 and often before age 50) transmitted in an autosomal dominant, highly penetrant fashion. More than 100 different mutations have been found in the *PS-1* gene in families from a wide range of ethnic backgrounds. Presenilin-2 (*PS-2*) is on chromosome 1 and encodes a protein called STM2. A mutation in the *PS-2* gene was first found in a group of American families with Volga German ethnic background. Mutations in *PS-1* are much more common than those in *PS-2*. The presenilins are highly homologous and encode similar proteins that at first appeared to have seven transmembrane domains (hence the designation *STM*), but subsequent studies have suggested eight such domains, with a ninth submembrane region. Both S182 and STM2 are cytoplasmic neuronal proteins that are widely expressed throughout the nervous system. They are homologous to a cell-trafficking protein, sel 12, found in the nematode *Caenorhabditis elegans*. Patients with mutations in these genes have elevated plasma levels of $A\beta_{42}$, and *PS-1* mutations in cell cultures produce increased $A\beta_{42}$ in the media. There is evidence that *PS-1* is involved in the cleavage of APP at the gamma secretase site and mutations in either gene (*PS-1* or *APP*) may disturb this function. Mutations in *PS-1* have thus far proved to be the most common cause of early-age-of-onset FAD, representing perhaps 40–70% of this relatively rare syndrome. Mutations in *PS-1* tend to produce AD with an earlier age of onset (mean onset 45 years) and a shorter, more rapidly progressive course (mean duration 6–7 years) than the disease caused by mutations in *PS-2* (mean onset 53 years; duration 11 years). Although some carriers of uncommon *PS-2* mutations have had onset of dementia after the age of 70, mutations in the presenilins are rarely involved in the more common sporadic cases of late-onset AD occurring in the general population. Genetic testing for these uncommon mutations is now commercially available. This diagnostic avenue is likely to be revealing only in early-age-of-onset familial AD and should be performed in the context of formal genetic counseling, especially when there are asymptomatic persons at risk.

A discovery of great importance has been that the *Apo* ε gene on chromosome 19 is involved in the pathogenesis of late-onset familial and sporadic forms of AD. *Apo* ε participates in cholesterol transport and has three alleles: ε2, ε3, and ε4. The Apo ε4 allele confers increased risk of AD in the general population, including sporadic and late-age-of-onset familial forms. Approximately 24–30% of the nondemented white population has at least one ε4 allele (12–15% allele frequency), and about 2% are ε4/4 homozygotes. Among patients with AD, 40–65% have at least one ε4 allele, a highly significant difference compared with controls. Conversely, many AD patients have no ε4 allele, and ε4 carriers may never develop AD. Therefore, ε4 is neither necessary nor sufficient to cause AD. Nevertheless, the Apo ε4 allele, especially in the homozygous state, represents the most important genetic risk factor for AD and acts as a dose-dependent disease modifier, with the earliest age of onset associated with the ε4 homozygosity. Precise mechanisms through which Apo ε4 confers AD risk or hastens onset remain unclear, but ε4 may produce less efficient amyloid clearance. Apo ε can be identified in neuritic plaques and may also be involved in neurofibrillary tangle formation, because it binds to tau protein. Apo ε4 decreases neurite outgrowth in dorsal root ganglion neuronal cultures, perhaps indicating a deleterious role in the brain's response to injury. Some evidence suggests that the ε2 allele may reduce AD risk, but the issue remains to be clarified. Use of Apo ε testing in AD diagnosis remains controversial. It is not indicated as a predictive test in normal persons because its precise predictive value is unclear, and many individuals with the ε4 allele never develop dementia. Many cognitively normal ε4 heterozygotes and homozygotes show decreased cerebral cortical metabolic function with PET, suggesting presymptomatic abnormalities due to AD or an inherited vulnerability of the AD target network. In demented persons who meet clinical criteria for AD, finding an ε4 allele increases the reliability of diagnosis however, the absence of an ε4 allele cannot be considered evidence against AD. Furthermore, all patients with dementia, including those with an ε4 allele, require a search for reversible causes of their cognitive impairment. Nevertheless, Apo ε4 remains the single most important biologic marker associated with AD risk, and studies of ε4's functional role and diagnostic utility are progressing rapidly. The ε4 allele is not associated with risk for FTD, DLB, or CJD, although some evidence suggests that ε4 may exacerbate the phenotype of non-AD degenerative disorders. Additional genes are also likely to be involved in AD, especially as minor risk alleles for sporadic forms of the disease. Recent genome-wide association studies have implicated the clusterin (*CLU*), phosphatidylinositol-binding clathrin assembly protein (*PICALM*), and complement component (3b/4b) receptor 1 (*CR1*) *genes*, and researchers are now working to understand the potential role of these genes in AD pathogenesis. CLU may play a role in synapse turnover, PICALM participates in clathrin-mediated endocytosis, and CR1 may be involved in amyloid clearance through the complement pathway.

TREATMENT Alzheimer's Disease

The management of AD is challenging and gratifying, despite the absence of a cure or a robust pharmacologic treatment. The primary focus is on long-term amelioration of associated behavioral and neurologic problems, as well as providing caregiver support.

Building rapport with the patient, family members, and other caregivers is essential to successful management. In the early stages of AD, memory aids such as notebooks and posted daily reminders can be helpful. Family members should emphasize activities that are pleasant and curtail those that are unpleasant. In other words, practicing skills that have become difficult, such as through memory games and puzzles, will often frustrate and depress the patient without proven benefits.

Kitchens, bathrooms, stairways, and bedrooms need to be made safe, and eventually patients must stop driving. Loss of independence and change of environment may worsen confusion, agitation, and anger. Communication and repeated calm reassurance are necessary. Caregiver "burnout" is common, often resulting in nursing home placement of the patient or new health problems for the caregiver, and respite breaks for the caregiver help to maintain a successful long-term therapeutic milieu. Use of adult day care centers can be helpful. Local and national support groups, such as the Alzheimer's Association and the Family Caregiver Alliance, are valuable resources. Internet access to these resources has become available to clinicians and families in recent years.

Donepezil (target dose, 10 mg daily), rivastigmine (target dose, 6 mg twice daily or 9.5-mg patch daily), galantamine (target dose 24 mg daily, extended-release), memantine (target dose, 10 mg twice daily), and tacrine are the drugs presently approved by the Food and Drug Administration (FDA) for treatment of AD. Due to hepatotoxicity, tacrine is no longer used. Dose escalations for each of these medications must be carried out over 4–6 weeks to minimize side effects. The pharmacologic action of donepezil, rivastigmine, and galantamine is inhibition of the cholinesterases, primarily acetylcholinesterase, with a resulting increase in cerebral acetylcholine levels. Memantine appears to act by blocking overexcited *N*-methyl-D-aspartate (NMDA) glutamate receptors. Double-blind, placebo-controlled, crossover studies with cholinesterase inhibitors and memantine have shown them to be associated with improved caregiver ratings of patients' functioning and with an apparent decreased rate of decline in cognitive test scores over periods of up to 3 years. The average patient on an anticholinesterase compound maintains his or her MMSE score for close to a year, whereas a placebo-treated patient declines 2–3 points over the same time period. Memantine, used in conjunction with cholinesterase inhibitors or by itself, slows cognitive deterioration and decreases caregiver burden for patients with moderate to severe AD but is not approved for mild AD. Each of these compounds has only modest efficacy for AD. Cholinesterase inhibitors are relatively easy to administer, and their major side effects are gastrointestinal symptoms (nausea, diarrhea, cramps), altered sleep with unpleasant or vivid dreams, bradycardia (usually benign), and muscle cramps.

In a prospective observational study, the use of estrogen replacement therapy appeared to protect—by about 50%—against development of AD in women. This study seemed to confirm the results of two earlier case-controlled studies. Sadly, a prospective placebo-controlled study of a combined estrogen-progesterone therapy for asymptomatic postmenopausal women increased, rather than decreased, the prevalence of dementia. This study markedly dampened enthusiasm for hormonal treatments to prevent dementia. Additionally, no benefit has been found in the treatment of AD with estrogen alone.

A randomized, double-blind, placebo-controlled trial of an extract of *Ginkgo biloba* found modest improvement in cognitive function in subjects with AD and vascular dementia. Unfortunately, a comprehensive 6-year multicenter prevention study using *Ginkgo biloba* found no slowing of progression to dementia in the treated group.

Vaccination against $A\beta_{42}$ has proved highly efficacious in mouse models of AD, helping clear brain amyloid and preventing further amyloid accumulation. In human trials, this approach led to life-threatening complications, including meningoencephalitis, but modifications of the vaccine approach using passive immunization with monoclonal antibodies are currently being evaluated in phase 3 trials. Another experimental approach to AD treatment has been the use of β and γ secretase inhibitors that diminish the production of $A\beta_{42}$, but the first two placebo-controlled trials of γ secretase inhibitors, tarenflurbil and semagacestat, were negative, and semagacestat may have accelerated cognitive decline compared to placebo. Medications that modify tau phosphorylation and aggregation are beginning to be studied as possible treatments for both AD and non-AD tau-related disorders including FTD and PSP.

Several retrospective studies suggest that nonsteroidal anti-inflammatory agents and 3-hydroxy-3-methylglutaryl-coenzyme A (HMG-CoA) reductase inhibitors (statins) may have a protective effect on dementia, and controlled prospective studies are being conducted. Similarly, prospective studies with the goal of lowering serum homocysteine are underway to slow the progression to dementia, following an association of elevated homocysteine with dementia progression in epidemiologic studies. Finally, there is now a strong interest in the relationship between diabetes and AD, and insulin-regulating studies are being conducted.

Mild to moderate depression is common in the early stages of AD and may respond to antidepressants or cholinesterase inhibitors. Selective serotonin reuptake inhibitors (SSRIs) are commonly used due to their low anticholinergic side effects (escitalopram 5–10 mg daily). Generalized seizures should be treated with an appropriate anticonvulsant, such as phenytoin or carbamazepine. Agitation, insomnia, hallucinations, and belligerence are especially troublesome characteristics of some AD patients, and these behaviors can lead to nursing home placement. The newer generation of atypical antipsychotics, such as risperidone, quetiapine, and olanzapine, are being used in low doses to treat these neuropsychiatric symptoms. The few controlled studies comparing drugs against behavioral intervention in the treatment of agitation suggest mild efficacy with significant side effects related to sleep, gait, and cardiovascular complications, including an increased risk of death. All antipsychotics carry a black-box FDA warning and should be used with caution in the demented elderly; however, careful, daily, nonpharmacologic behavior management is often not available, rendering medications necessary for some patients. Finally, medications with strong anticholinergic effects should be vigilantly avoided, including prescription and over-the-counter sleep aids (e.g., diphenhydramine) or incontinence therapies (e.g., oxybutynin).

VASCULAR DEMENTIA

Dementia associated with cerebrovascular disease can be divided into two general categories: multi-infarct dementia and diffuse white matter disease (also called *leukoaraiosis*, *subcortical arteriosclerotic leukoencephalopathy*, or *Binswanger's disease*). Cerebrovascular disease appears to be a more common cause of dementia in Asia than in Europe and North America, perhaps due to the increased prevalence of intracranial atherosclerosis. Individuals who have had several strokes may develop chronic cognitive deficits, commonly called *multi-infarct dementia*. The strokes may be large or small (sometimes lacunar) and usually involve several different brain regions. The occurrence of dementia depends partly on the total volume of damaged cortex, but it is also more common in individuals with left-hemisphere lesions, independent of any language disturbance. Patients typically report previous discrete episodes of sudden neurologic deterioration. Many patients with multi-infarct dementia have a history of hypertension, diabetes, coronary artery disease, or other manifestations of widespread atherosclerosis. Physical examination usually shows focal neurologic deficits such as hemiparesis, a unilateral Babinski sign, a visual field defect, or pseudobulbar palsy. Recurrent strokes result in a stepwise disease progression. Neuroimaging reveals multiple areas of infarction. Thus, the history and neuroimaging findings differentiate this condition from AD; however, both AD and multiple infarctions are common and sometimes co-occur. With normal aging, there is also an accumulation of amyloid in cerebral blood vessels, leading to a condition called *cerebral amyloid angiopathy* (without dementia), which predisposes older persons to lobar hemorrhage and brain microhemorrhages. AD patients appear to be at increased risk for amyloid angiopathy, and this may explain some of the observed association between AD and stroke.

Some individuals with dementia are discovered on MRI to have bilateral abnormalities of subcortical white matter, termed *diffuse white matter disease*, often occurring in association with lacunar infarctions (Fig. 29-5). The dementia may be insidious in onset and progress slowly, features that distinguish it from multi-infarct dementia, but other patients show a stepwise deterioration more typical of multi-infarct dementia. Early symptoms are mild confusion, apathy, anxiety, psychosis, and memory, spatial, or executive deficits. Marked difficulties in judgment and orientation and dependence on others for daily activities develop later. Euphoria, elation, depression, or aggressive behaviors are common as the disease progresses. Both pyramidal and cerebellar signs may be present. A gait disorder is present in at least half of these patients. With advanced disease, urinary incontinence and dysarthria with or without other pseudobulbar features (e.g., dysphagia, emotional lability) are frequent. Seizures and myoclonic jerks appear in a minority of patients. This disorder appears to result from chronic ischemia due to occlusive disease of small, penetrating cerebral arteries and arterioles (microangiopathy). Any disease-causing stenosis of small cerebral vessels may be the critical underlying factor, although hypertension is the major cause. The term *Binswanger's disease* should be used with caution, because it does not clearly identify a single entity.

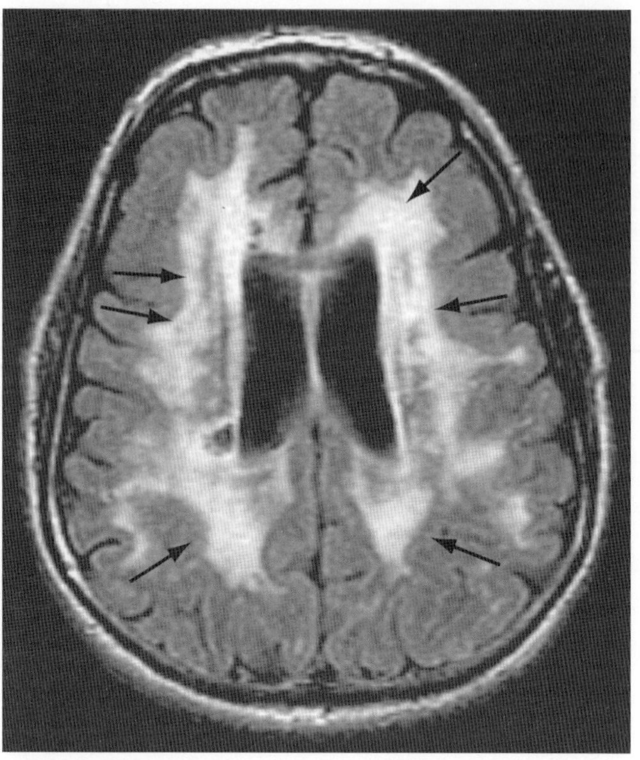

FIGURE 29-5
Diffuse white matter disease. Axial fluid-attenuated inversion recovery (FLAIR) MR image through the lateral ventricles reveals multiple areas of hyperintensity involving the periventricular white matter as well as the corona radiata and striatum (*arrows*). While seen in some individuals with normal cognition, this appearance is more pronounced in patients with dementia of a vascular etiology.

Other rare causes of white matter disease also present with dementia, such as adult metachromatic leukodystrophy (arylsulfatase A deficiency) and progressive multifocal leukoencephalopathy (JC virus infection). A dominantly inherited form of diffuse white matter disease is known as *cerebral autosomal dominant arteriopathy with subcortical infarcts and leukoencephalopathy* (CADASIL). Clinically, there is a progressive dementia developing in the fifth to seventh decades in multiple family members who may also have a history of migraine and recurrent lacunar stroke without hypertension. Skin biopsy may show pathognomonic osmophilic granules in the media of arterioles. The disease is caused by mutations in the *Notch 3* gene, and genetic testing is commercially available. The frequency of this disorder is unknown, and there are no effective treatments.

Mitochondrial disorders can present with stroke-like episodes and can selectively injure basal ganglia or cortex. Many such patients show other findings suggestive of a neurologic or systemic disorder such as ophthalmoplegia, retinal degeneration, deafness, myopathy, neuropathy, or diabetes. Diagnosis is difficult, but serum or (especially) CSF levels of lactate and pyruvate may be abnormal, and biopsy of affected tissue, preferably muscle, may be diagnostic.

Treatment of vascular dementia must be focused on preventing new ischemic injury by stabilizing or removing the underlying causes, such as hypertension, diabetes, smoking, or lack of exercise. Recovery of lost cognitive function is not likely, although fluctuations with periods of improvement are common.

FRONTOTEMPORAL DEMENTIA, PROGRESSIVE SUPRANUCLEAR PALSY, AND CORTICOBASAL DEGENERATION

Frontotemporal dementia (FTD) often begins in the fifth to seventh decades, and in this age group it is nearly as prevalent as AD. Early studies suggested that FTD may be more common in men than women, although more recent reports cast some doubt on this finding. *Unlike in AD, behavioral symptoms predominate in the early stages of FTD.* Although a family history of dementia is common, autosomal dominant inheritance is seen in about 10% of all FTD cases. The clinical heterogeneity in familial and sporadic forms of FTD is remarkable, with patients demonstrating variable mixtures of behavioral, language, movement, and motor neuron symptoms. The most common autosomal dominantly inherited mutations causing FTD involve the *MAPT* or *GRN* genes, both on chromosome 17. *MAPT* mutations lead to a change in the alternate splicing of tau or cause loss of function in the tau molecule. With *GRN*, mutations in the coding sequence of the gene encoding progranulin protein result in mRNA degradation due to nonsense-mediated decay. Progranulin appears to be a rare example of an autosomal dominant mutation that leads to haploinsufficiency, resulting in around one-half the normal level of progranulin protein. Progranulin is a growth factor that binds to tumor necrosis factor (TNF) receptors. How progranulin mutations lead to FTD is unknown. Both *MAPT* and *GRN* mutations are associated with parkinsonian features, while ALS is rare with these mutations. In contrast, familial FTD with ALS has been linked to chromosome 9. Mutations in the valosin-containing protein (chromosome 9) and the charged multivesicular body protein 2b (CHMP2b) genes (chromosome 3) also lead to rare autosomal dominant forms of familial FTD. Mutations in the TDP-43 and FUS genes (see later) cause familial ALS, sometimes in association with an FTD syndrome, although a few patients presenting with FTD alone have been reported.

In FTD, early symptoms are divided among behavioral, language, and sometimes motor abnormalities, reflecting degeneration of the anterior insular, frontal, and temporal regions, basal ganglia, and motor neurons. Cognitive testing typically reveals spared memory but impaired planning, judgment, or language. Poor business decisions and difficulty organizing work tasks are common, and speech and language deficits often emerge. Patients with FTD often show an absence of insight into their condition. Common behavioral features include apathy, disinhibition, weight gain, food fetishes, compulsions, and emotional distance or loss of empathy.

Findings at the bedside are dictated by the anatomic localization of the disorder. Asymmetric left frontal cases present with nonfluent aphasia, while left anterior temporal degeneration is characterized by loss of word meaning (semantic dementia). Nonfluent patients quickly progress to mutism, while those with semantic dementia develop features of a multimodal associative agnosia, losing the ability to recognize faces, objects, words, and the emotions of others. Visuoconstructive ability, arithmetic calculations, and navigation often remain normal late into the illness. Recently it has become apparent that many patients with nonfluent aphasia progress to clinical syndromes that overlap with PSP and corticobasal degeneration (CBD) and show these pathologies at autopsy. This left hemisphere presentation of FTD has been called *primary progressive aphasia with nonfluent and semantic variants.* In contrast, right frontal or temporal cases show profound alterations in social conduct, with loss of empathy, disinhibition, and antisocial behaviors predominating. There is a striking overlap among FTD, PSP, CBD, and motor neuron disease; ophthalmoplegia, dystonia, swallowing symptoms, and fasciculations are common at presentation of FTD or emerge during the course of the illness.

The distinguishing anatomic hallmark of FTD is a focal atrophy of frontal, insular, and/or temporal cortex, which can be visualized with neuroimaging studies and is often profound at autopsy (Figs. 29-6 and 29-7). Despite the appearance of advanced FTD, however, the atrophy often begins focally in one hemisphere before spreading to anatomically interconnected regions, including basal ganglia. Microscopic findings seen across

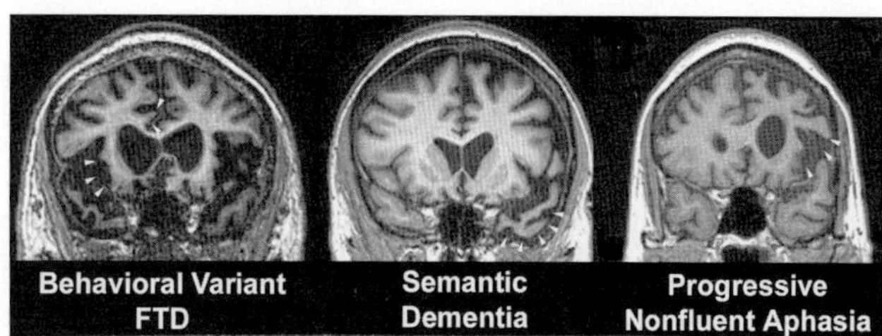

FIGURE 29-6
Frontotemporal dementia (FTD). Coronal MRI sections from representative patients with behavioral variant FTD (***left***), semantic dementia (***center***), and progressive nonfluent aphasia (***right***). Areas of early and severe atrophy in each syndrome are highlighted (*white arrowheads*). The behavioral variant features anterior cingulate and frontoinsular atrophy, spreading to orbital and dorsolateral prefrontal cortex. Semantic dementia shows prominent temporopolar atrophy, more often on the left. Progressive nonfluent aphasia is associated with dominant frontal opercular and dorsal insula degeneration.

all patients with FTD include gliosis, microvacuolation, and neuronal loss, but the disease is subtyped according to the protein composition of neuronal and glial inclusions, which contain either tau or TDP-43 in at least 90% of patients, with the remaining 10% showing inclusions containing FUS (Fig. 29-8).

A toxic gain of function related to tau underlies the pathogenesis of many familial cases and is presumed to be a factor in sporadic tauopathies, although loss of tau microtubule stabilizing function may also play a role.

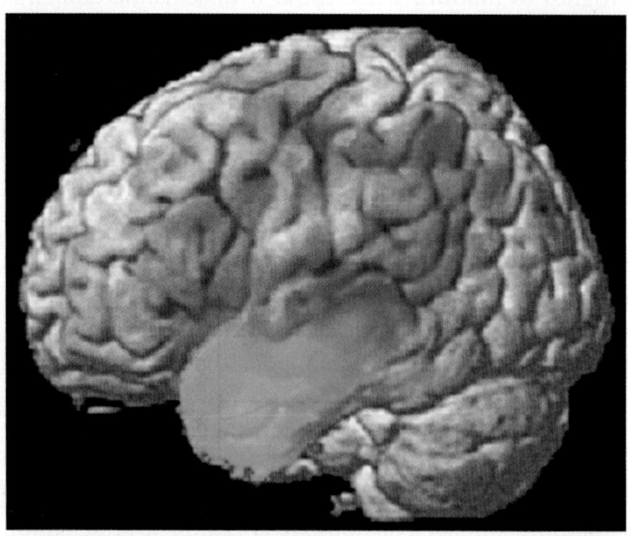

FIGURE 29-7
Voxel-based morphometry analysis showing differing patterns of brain atrophy in three variants of progressive aphasia, including nonfluent (*red*), semantic (*green*), and logopedic subtypes (*blue*). Voxel-based morphometry allows comparison of MRI gray matter volumes between patient groups and control subjects, as shown here. (*Image courtesy of M Gorno-Tempini, University of California at San Francisco; with permission.*)

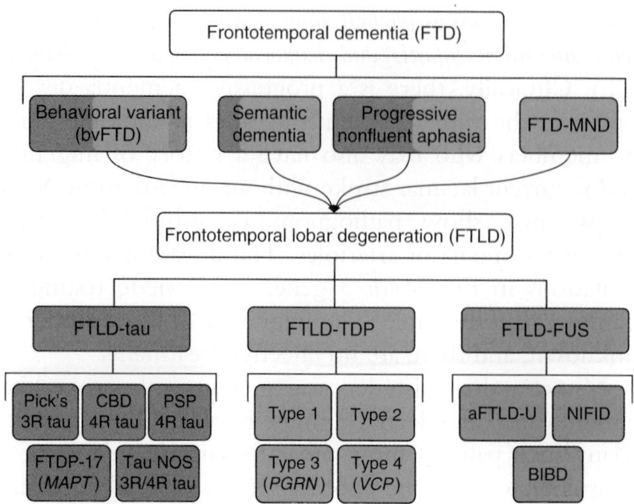

FIGURE 29-8
Frontotemporal dementia syndromes are united by underlying frontotemporal lobar degeneration pathology, which can be divided according to the presence of tau, TPD-43, or fused in sarcoma (FUS) inclusions in neurons and glia. Correlations between clinical syndrome and major molecular category are shown with colored shading.

TDP-43 and FUS, in contrast, are RNA/DNA binding proteins whose roles in neuronal function are still being actively investigated. Loss of cortical serotonergic innervation is seen in many patients. In contrast to AD, the cholinergic system is relatively spared in FTD.

Historically, *Pick's disease* was described as a progressive degenerative disorder characterized by selective involvement of the anterior frontal and temporal neocortex and pathologically by intraneuronal cytoplasmic inclusions (*Pick bodies*). Classical Pick bodies are argyrophilic, staining positively with the Bielschowsky silver method and also with immunostaining for tau (Fig. 29-9). Subsequent pathologic studies revealed a significant subset of patients with silver-negative, tau-negative inclusions, which have since been shown mainly to contain TDP-43, although a minority stain only for FUS. Although the nomenclature used to describe these patients has continued to evolve, the term *FTD* is increasingly used to refer to the clinical syndromes, while *frontotemporal lobar degeneration (FTLD)* refers to the underlying pathology, with three major subtypes recognized: FTLD-tau, FTLD-TDP, and FTLD-FUS. Despite significant progress, available data do not yet allow a reliable prediction of underlying pathology based on clinical features. Accordingly researchers continue to seek serum, CSF, or neuroimaging biomarkers that will afford greater diagnostic accuracy, defined as concordance with neuropathology.

The burden on caregivers of patients with FTD is extremely high because the illness disrupts core emotional and personality functions of the loved one. Treatment is symptomatic, and there are currently no therapies known to slow progression or improve symptoms. Many

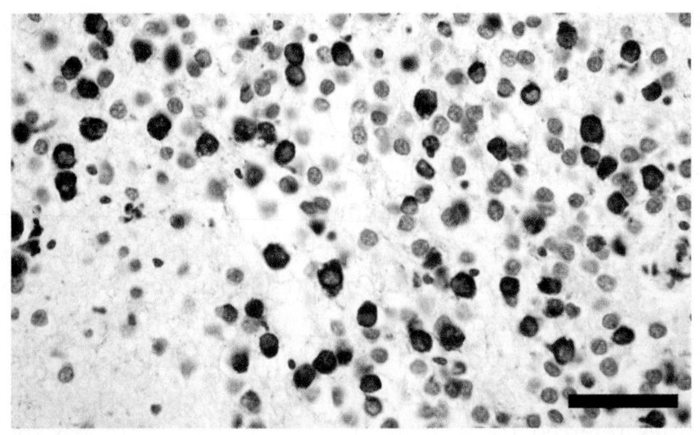

FIGURE 29-9

Pick's disease, a subtype of frontotemporal lobar degeneration (FTLD)-tau. Pick bodies, shown here in the dentate gyrus of a patient with advanced bvFTD, consist of loosely arranged paired helical and straight filaments and stain positively for hyperphosphorylated tau. Classical Pick's disease is seen in only 10–20% of patients with frontotemporal dementia. Scale bar represents 50 microns. *(CP-13 antibody courtesy of P. Davies.)*

of the behaviors that accompany FTD, such as depression, hyperorality, compulsions, and irritability, can be ameliorated with antidepressants, especially SSRIs. The co-association with motor disorders such as parkinsonism necessitates the careful use of antipsychotics, which can exacerbate this problem.

Progressive supranuclear palsy (PSP) is a degenerative disease that involves the brainstem, basal ganglia, limbic structures, and selected areas of cortex. Clinically, this disorder begins with falls and executive or subtle personality changes (such as mental rigidity, impulsivity, or apathy). Shortly thereafter, a progressive oculomotor syndrome ensues that begins with square wave jerks, followed by slowed saccades (vertical worse than horizontal) before resulting in progressive supranuclear ophthalmoparesis. Dysarthria, dysphagia, and symmetric axial rigidity can be prominent features that emerge at any point in the illness. A stiff, unstable posture with hyperextension of the neck and a slow, jerky, toppling gait is characteristic. Frequent unexplained and sometimes spectacular falls are common secondary to a combination of axial rigidity, inability to look down, and bad judgment. Even once patients have severely limited voluntary eye movements, they retain oculocephalic reflexes (demonstrated using a vertical doll's head maneuver); thus, the oculomotor disorder is supranuclear. The dementia overlaps with FTD, featuring apathy, frontal-executive dysfunction, poor judgment, slowed thought processes, impaired verbal fluency, and difficulty with sequential actions and with shifting from one task to another. These features are common at presentation and often precede the motor syndrome. Some patients begin with a nonfluent aphasia or motor speech disorder and progress to classical PSP. Response to L-dopa is limited or absent; no other treatments exist. Death occurs within 5–10 years of onset. At autopsy, accumulation of hyperphosphorylated tau is seen within neurons and glia. Neuronal inclusions often take the form of neurofibrillary tangles (NFTs), which may be large, spherical, and coarse when found in brainstem oculomotor control system neurons. These characteristic tau inclusions are called globose tangles, and may be found in multiple subcortical structures (including the subthalamic nucleus, globus pallidus, substantia nigra, locus coeruleus, periaqueductal gray, superior colliculi, oculomotor nuclei, and dentate nucleus). Neocortical NFTs, like those in AD, often take on a more flame-shaped morphology, but on electron microscopy PSP tangles can be shown to consist of straight tubules rather than the paired helical filaments found in AD. Furthermore, PSP is associated with prominent tau-positive glial pathomorphologies, such as tufted and thorny astrocytes.

In addition to its overlap with FTD and CBD (see later), PSP is often confused with idiopathic *Parkinson's disease* (PD). Although elderly patients with PD may have restricted upgaze, they do not develop downgaze paresis or other abnormalities of voluntary eye movements typical of PSP. Dementia occurs in ~20% of patients with PD, often due to the emergence of a full-blown DLB syndrome. Furthermore, the behavioral syndromes seen with DLB differ from PSP (see later). Dementia in PD becomes more likely with increasing age, increasing severity of extrapyramidal signs, a long disease duration, and the presence of depression. Patients with PD who develop dementia also show cortical atrophy on brain imaging. Neuropathologically, there may be Alzheimer's disease–related changes in the cortex, DLB-related α-synuclein inclusions in both the limbic system and cortex, or no specific microscopic changes other than gliosis and neuronal loss. Parkinson's disease is discussed in detail in Chap. 30.

Corticobasal degeneration (CBD) is a slowly progressive dementing illness associated with severe gliosis and neuronal loss in both the cortex and basal ganglia (substantia nigra and striatopallidum). Some patients present with a unilateral onset with rigidity, dystonia, and apraxia of one arm and hand, sometimes called the *alien limb* when it begins to exhibit unintended motor actions, while in other instances the disease presents as a progressive behavioral, executive, or language syndrome or as progressive symmetric parkinsonism. Some patients begin with a progressive nonfluent aphasia or a progressive motor speech disorder. Eventually CBD becomes bilateral and leads to dysarthria, slow gait, action tremor, and dementia. The microscopic features include ballooned, achromatic, tau-positive neurons with astrocytic plaques and other dystrophic glial tau pathomorphologies that overlap with those seen in PSP. Most specifically, CBD features a severe tauopathy burden in the subcortical white matter, consisting of threads and oligodendroglial coiled bodies. The condition is rarely familial, the cause is unknown, and there is no specific treatment.

PARKINSON'S DISEASE DEMENTIA AND DEMENTIA WITH LEWY BODIES

The parkinsonian dementia syndromes are under increasing study, with many cases unified by Lewy body and Lewy neurite pathology that ascends from the low brainstem up through the substantia nigra, limbic system, and cortex. The DLB clinical syndrome is characterized by visual hallucinations, parkinsonism, fluctuating alertness, falls, and often RBD. Dementia can precede or follow the appearance of parkinsonism. Hence, one pathway occurs in patients with long-standing PD without cognitive impairment, who slowly develop a dementia that is associated with visual hallucinations and fluctuating alertness. When this occurs after an established diagnosis of PD, many use the term *Parkinson's disease dementia* (PDD). In others, the dementia and neuropsychiatric syndrome precede the parkinsonism, and this constellation is referred to as DLB. Both PDD and DLB may be accompanied or preceded by symptoms referable to brainstem pathology below the substantia nigra, and many researchers conceptualize these disorders as points on a spectrum of α-synuclein pathology.

Patients with PDD and DLB are highly sensitive to metabolic perturbations, and in some patients the first manifestation of illness is a delirium, often precipitated by an infection, new medicine, or other systemic disturbance. A hallucinatory delirium induced by L-dopa, prescribed for parkinsonian symptoms attributed to PD may likewise provide the initial clue to a PDD diagnosis. Conversely, patients with mild cognitive deficits and hallucinations may receive typical or atypical antipsychotic medications, which induce profound parkinsonism at low doses due to a subclinical DLB-related nigral dopaminergic neuron loss. Even without an underlying precipitant, fluctuations can be marked in DLB, with episodic confusion or even stupor admixed with lucid intervals. However, despite the fluctuating pattern, the clinical features persist over a long period, unlike delirium, which resolves following correction of the inciting factor. Cognitively, DLB features relative preservation of memory but more severe visuospatial and executive deficits than patients with early AD.

The key neuropathologic feature in DLB is the presence of Lewy bodies and Lewy neurites throughout specific brainstem nuclei, substantia nigra, amygdala, cingulate gyrus, and, ultimately, the neocortex. Lewy bodies are intraneuronal cytoplasmic inclusions that stain with periodic acid–Schiff (PAS) and ubiquitin but are now identified with antibodies to the presynaptic protein, α-synuclein. They are composed of straight neurofilaments 7–20 nm long with surrounding amorphous material and contain epitopes recognized by antibodies against phosphorylated and nonphosphorylated neurofilament proteins, ubiquitin, and α-synuclein. Lewy bodies are typically found in the substantia nigra of patients with idiopathic PD, where they can be readily seen with hematoxylin-and-eosin staining. A profound cholinergic deficit, owing to basal forebrain and pedunculopontine nucleus involvement, is present in many patients with DLB and may be a factor responsible for the fluctuations, inattention, and visual hallucinations. In patients without other pathologic features, the condition is sometimes referred to as *diffuse Lewy body disease*. In patients whose brains also contain a substantial burden of amyloid plaques and NFTs, the condition is sometimes called the *Lewy body variant of Alzheimer's disease*.

Due to the overlap with AD and the cholinergic deficit in DLB, cholinesterase inhibitors often provide significant benefit, reducing hallucinosis, stabilizing delusional symptoms, and even helping with RBD in some patients. Exercise programs maximize motor function and protect against fall-related injury. Antidepressants are often necessary. Atypical antipsychotics may be required for psychosis but can worsen extrapyramidal syndromes, even at low doses, and increase risk of death. As noted earlier, patients with DLB are extremely sensitive to dopaminergic medications, which must be carefully titrated; tolerability may be improved by concomitant use of a cholinesterase inhibitor.

OTHER CAUSES OF DEMENTIA

Prion diseases such as *Creutzfeldt-Jakob disease* (CJD) are rare neurodegenerative conditions (prevalence ~1 per million) that produce dementia. CJD is a rapidly progressive disorder associated with dementia, focal cortical signs, rigidity, and myoclonus, causing death <1 year after first symptoms appear. The rapidity of progression seen with CJD is uncommon in AD so that the distinction between the two disorders is usually straightforward. CBD and DLB, more rapid degenerative dementias with prominent movement abnormalities, are more likely to be mistaken for CJD. The differential diagnosis for CJD includes other rapidly progressive dementing conditions such as viral or bacterial encephalitides, Hashimoto's encephalopathy, CNS vasculitis, lymphoma, or paraneoplastic syndromes. The markedly abnormal periodic complexes on EEG and cortical ribbon and basal ganglia hyperintensities on MR diffusion-weighted imaging are highly specific diagnostic features of CJD, although rarely prolonged focal or generalized seizures can produce a similar imaging appearance. Prion diseases are discussed in detail in Chap. 43.

Huntington's disease (HD) (Chap. 30) is an autosomal dominant, degenerative brain disorder. HD clinical hallmarks include chorea, behavioral disturbance, and executive impairment. Symptoms typically begin in the fourth or fifth decade, but there is a wide range, from childhood to >70 years. Memory is frequently not impaired until late in the disease, but attention, judgment, awareness, and executive functions are often deficient at an early stage. Depression, apathy, social withdrawal, irritability, and intermittent disinhibition are common. Delusions and obsessive-compulsive behavior may occur. Disease duration is typically around 15 years but is quite variable.

Normal-pressure hydrocephalus (NPH) is a relatively uncommon but treatable syndrome. The clinical, physiologic, and neuroimaging characteristics of NPH must be carefully distinguished from those of other dementias associated with gait impairment. Historically, many patients treated for NPH have suffered from other dementias, particularly AD, vascular dementia, DLB, and PSP. For NPH, the clinical triad includes an abnormal gait (ataxic or apractic), dementia (usually mild to moderate, with an emphasis on executive impairment), and urinary urgency or incontinence. Neuroimaging reveals enlarged lateral ventricles (hydrocephalus) with little or no cortical atrophy, although the sylvian fissures may appear propped open (so-called "boxcarring"), which can be mistaken for perisylvian atrophy. This syndrome is a communicating hydrocephalus with a patent aqueduct of Sylvius (Fig. 29-10), in contrast to aqueductal stenosis, in which the aqueduct is small. Lumbar puncture opening pressure falls in the high normal range, and the CSF protein, glucose, and cell counts are normal. NPH may be caused by obstruction to normal CSF flow over the cerebral convexities and delayed resorption into the venous system. The indolent nature of the process results in enlarged lateral ventricles with relatively little increase in CSF pressure. Presumed stretching and distortion of subfrontal white matter tracts may lead to clinical symptoms, but the precise underlying pathophysiology remains unclear. Some patients provide a history of conditions that produce meningeal scarring (blocking CSF resorption) such as previous meningitis, subarachnoid hemorrhage, or head trauma. Others with long-standing but asymptomatic congenital hydrocephalus may have adult-onset deterioration in gait or memory that is confused with NPH. In contrast to AD, the patient with NPH complains of an early and prominent gait disturbance without cortical atrophy on CTor MRI.

Numerous attempts to improve NPH diagnosis with various special studies and predict the success of ventricular shunting have been undertaken. These tests include radionuclide cisternography (showing a delay in CSF absorption over the convexity) and various efforts to monitor and alter CSF flow dynamics, including a constant-pressure infusion test. None has proven to be specific or consistently useful. A transient improvement in gait or cognition may follow lumbar puncture (or serial punctures) with removal of 30–50 mL of CSF, but this finding has also not proved to be consistently predictive of postshunt improvement. Perhaps the most reliable strategy is a period of close inpatient evaluation before,

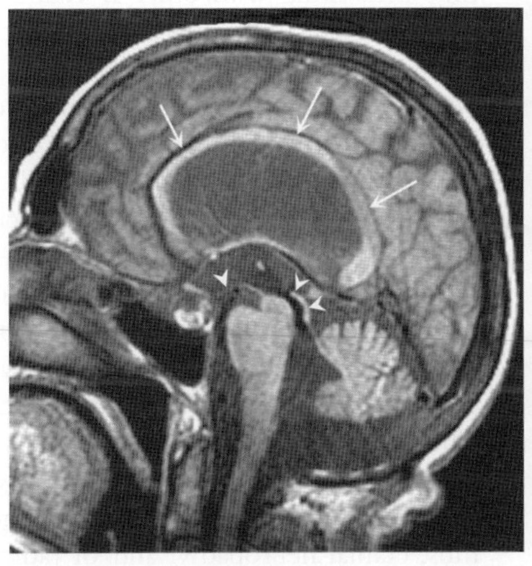
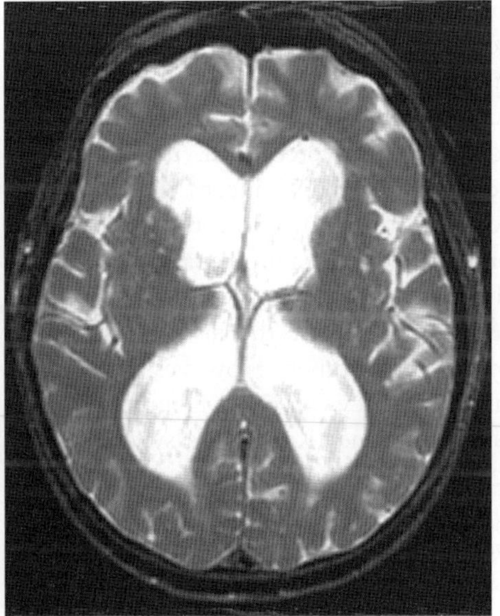

A *B*

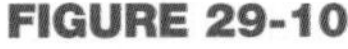

FIGURE 29-10

Normal-pressure hydrocephalus. ***A.*** Sagittal T1-weighted MR image demonstrates dilation of the lateral ventricle and stretching of the corpus callosum (*arrows*), depression of the floor of the third ventricle (*single arrowhead*), and enlargement of the aqueduct (*double arrowheads*). Note the diffuse dilation of the lateral, third, and fourth ventricles with a patent aqueduct, typical of communicating hydrocephalus. ***B.*** Axial T2-weighted MR images demonstrate dilation of the lateral ventricles. This patient underwent successful ventriculoperitoneal shunting.

during, and after lumbar CSF drainage. Occasionally, when a patient with AD presents with gait impairment (at times due to comorbid subfrontal vascular injury) and absent or only mild cortical atrophy on CT or MRI, distinguishing NPH from AD can be challenging. Hippocampal atrophy on MRI favors AD, whereas a characteristic "magnetic" gait with external hip rotation, low foot clearance and short strides, along with prominent truncal sway or instability, favors NPH. The diagnosis of NPH should be avoided when hydrocephalus is not detected on imaging studies, even if the symptoms otherwise fit. Thirty to fifty percent of patients identified by careful diagnosis as having NPH will improve with ventricular shunting. Gait may improve more than cognition, but many reported failures to improve cognitively may have resulted from comorbid AD. Short-lasting improvement is common. Patients should be carefully selected for shunting, because subdural hematoma, infection, and shunt failure are known complications and can be a cause for early nursing home placement in an elderly patient with previously mild dementia.

Dementia can accompany *chronic alcoholism* (Chap. 56) and may result from associated malnutrition, especially of B vitamins, particularly thiamine. Other poorly defined aspects of chronic alcoholism may, however, also produce cerebral damage. A rare idiopathic syndrome of dementia and seizures with degeneration of the corpus callosum has been reported primarily in male Italian red wine drinkers (Marchiafava-Bignami disease).

Thiamine (vitamin B_1) deficiency causes Wernicke's encephalopathy (Chap. 28). The clinical presentation features a malnourished patient (frequently but not necessarily alcoholic) with confusion, ataxia, and diplopia resulting from inflammation and necrosis of periventricular midline structures, including dorsomedial thalamus, mammillary bodies, midline cerebellum, periaqueductal gray matter, and trochlear and abducens nuclei. Damage to the dorsomedial thalamus correlates most closely with the memory loss. Prompt administration of parenteral thiamine (100 mg intravenously for 3 days followed by daily oral dosage) may reverse the disease if given in the first days of symptom onset. However, prolonged untreated thiamine deficiency can result in an irreversible dementia/amnestic syndrome (Korsakoff's syndrome) or even death.

In *Korsakoff's syndrome*, the patient is unable to recall new information despite normal immediate memory, attention span, and level of consciousness. Memory for new events is seriously impaired, whereas knowledge acquired prior to the illness remains relatively intact. Patients are easily confused, disoriented, and cannot store information for more than a few minutes. Superficially, they may be conversant, engaging, and able to perform simple tasks and follow immediate commands. Confabulation is common, although not always present. There is no specific treatment because the previous thiamine deficiency has produced irreversible damage to the medial thalamic nuclei and mammillary bodies. Mammillary body atrophy may be visible on MRI in the chronic phase (Fig. 28-7).

Vitamin B_{12} deficiency, as can occur in pernicious anemia, causes a megaloblastic anemia and may also damage the nervous system (Chap. 35). Neurologically, it most commonly produces a spinal cord syndrome (myelopathy) affecting the posterior columns (loss of vibration and position sense) and corticospinal tracts (hyperactive tendon reflexes with Babinski signs); it also damages peripheral nerves (neuropathy), resulting in sensory loss with depressed tendon reflexes. Damage to myelinated axons may also cause dementia. The mechanism of neurologic damage is unclear but may be related to a deficiency of *S*-adenosyl methionine (required for methylation of myelin phospholipids) due to reduced methionine synthase activity or accumulation of methylmalonate, homocysteine, and propionate, providing abnormal substrates for fatty acid synthesis in myelin. The neurologic sequelae of vitamin B_{12} deficiency may occur in the absence of hematologic manifestations, making it critical to avoid using the CBC and blood smear as a substitute for measuring B_{12} blood levels. Treatment with parenteral vitamin B_{12} (1000 μg intramuscularly daily for a week, weekly for a month, and monthly for life for pernicious anemia) stops progression of the disease if instituted promptly, but complete reversal of advanced nervous system damage will not occur.

Deficiency of nicotinic acid (*pellagra*) is associated with skin rash over sun-exposed areas, glossitis, and angular stomatitis. Severe dietary deficiency of nicotinic acid along with other B vitamins such as pyridoxine may result in spastic paraparesis, peripheral neuropathy, fatigue, irritability, and dementia. This syndrome has been seen in prisoners of war and in concentration camps but should be considered in any malnourished individual. Low serum folate levels appear to be a rough index of malnutrition, but isolated folate deficiency has not been proved as a specific cause of dementia.

CNS infections usually cause delirium and other acute neurologic syndromes. However, some chronic CNS infections, particularly those associated with chronic meningitis (Chap. 41), may produce a dementing illness. The possibility of chronic infectious meningitis should be suspected in patients presenting with a dementia or behavioral syndrome, who also have headache, meningismus, cranial neuropathy, and/or radiculopathy. Between 20 and 30% of patients in the advanced stages of HIV infection become demented (Chap. 42). Cardinal features include psychomotor retardation, apathy, and impaired memory. This syndrome may result from secondary opportunistic infections but can also be caused by direct infection of CNS neurons with HIV. Neurosyphilis was a common cause of dementia in the preantibiotic era; it is now uncommon but can still be encountered in patients with multiple sex partners, particularly among patients with HIV. Characteristic CSF changes consist of pleocytosis, increased protein, and a positive Venereal Disease Research Laboratory (VDRL) test.

Primary and metastatic *neoplasms of the CNS* (Chap. 37) usually produce focal neurologic findings and seizures rather than dementia, but if tumor growth begins in the frontal or temporal lobes, the initial manifestations may be memory loss or behavioral changes. A paraneoplastic syndrome of dementia associated with occult carcinoma (often small cell lung cancer) is termed *limbic encephalitis*. In this syndrome, confusion, agitation, seizures, poor memory, emotional changes, and frank dementia may occur. Paraneoplastic *encephalitis associated with NMDA receptor antibodies* presents as a progressive psychiatric disorder with memory loss and seizures; affected patients are often young women with ovarian teratoma (Chap. 44).

A *nonconvulsive seizure disorder* may underlie a syndrome of confusion, clouding of consciousness, and garbled speech. Often, psychiatric disease is suspected, but an EEG demonstrates the epileptic nature of the illness. If recurrent or persistent, the condition may be termed *complex partial status epilepticus*. The cognitive disturbance often responds to anticonvulsant therapy. The etiology may be previous small strokes or head trauma; some cases are idiopathic.

It is important to recognize *systemic diseases* that indirectly affect the brain and produce chronic confusion or dementia. Such conditions include hypothyroidism; vasculitis; and hepatic, renal, or pulmonary disease. Hepatic encephalopathy may begin with irritability and confusion and slowly progress to agitation, lethargy, and coma.

Isolated vasculitis of the CNS (CNS granulomatous angiitis) (Chap. 27) occasionally causes a chronic encephalopathy associated with confusion, disorientation, and clouding of consciousness. Headache is common, and strokes and cranial neuropathies may occur. Brain imaging studies may be normal or nonspecifically abnormal. CSF analysis reveals a mild pleocytosis or protein elevation. Cerebral angiography can show multifocal stenoses involving medium-caliber vessels, but some patients have only small-vessel disease that is not revealed on angiography. The angiographic appearance is not specific and may be mimicked by atherosclerosis, infection, or other causes of vascular disease. Brain or meningeal biopsy demonstrates endothelial cell proliferation and mononuclear infiltrates within blood vessel walls. The prognosis is often poor, although the disorder may remit spontaneously. Some patients respond to glucocorticoids or chemotherapy.

Chronic metal exposure represents a rare cause of dementia. The key to diagnosis is to elicit a history of exposure at work or home. Chronic lead poisoning from inadequately fire-glazed pottery has been reported. Fatigue, depression, and confusion may be associated with episodic abdominal pain and peripheral neuropathy. Gray lead lines appear in the gums, usually accompanied by an anemia with basophilic stippling of red blood cells. The clinical presentation can resemble that of acute intermittent porphyria, including elevated levels of urine porphyrins as a result of the inhibition of δ-aminolevulinic acid dehydrase. The treatment is chelation therapy with agents such as ethylenediamine tetraacetic acid (EDTA). Chronic mercury poisoning produces dementia, peripheral neuropathy, ataxia, and tremulousness that may progress to a cerebellar intention tremor or choreoathetosis. The confusion and memory loss of chronic arsenic intoxication is also associated with nausea, weight loss, peripheral neuropathy, pigmentation and scaling of the skin, and transverse white lines of the fingernails (Mees' lines). Treatment is chelation therapy with dimercaprol (BAL). Aluminum poisoning is rare but was documented with the dialysis dementia syndrome, in which water used during renal dialysis was contaminated with excessive amounts of aluminum. This poisoning resulted in a progressive encephalopathy associated with confusion, nonfluent aphasia, memory loss, agitation, and, later, lethargy and stupor. Speech arrest and myoclonic jerks were common and associated with severe and generalized EEG changes. The condition has been eliminated by the use of deionized water for dialysis.

Recurrent head trauma in professional boxers may lead to a dementia sometimes called the "punch-drunk" syndrome, or *dementia pugilistica*. The symptoms can be progressive, beginning late in a boxer's career or even long after retirement. The severity of the syndrome correlates with the length of the boxing career and number of bouts. Early in the condition, a personality change associated with social instability and sometimes paranoia and delusions occurs. Later, memory loss progresses to full-blown dementia, often associated with parkinsonian signs and ataxia or intention tremor. At autopsy, the cerebral cortex may show changes similar to AD, although NFTs are usually more prominent than amyloid plaques (which are usually diffuse rather than neuritic). Superficial layer NFT aggregates have been reported to differentiate these patients from those with more typical AD. Also, there may be loss of neurons in the substantia nigra. Chronic subdural hematoma (Chap. 36) is also occasionally associated with dementia, often in the context of underlying cortical atrophy from conditions such as AD or HD.

Transient global amnesia (TGA) is characterized by the sudden onset of a severe episodic memory deficit, usually occurring in persons over the age of 50 years. Often the amnesia occurs in the setting of an emotional stimulus or physical exertion. During the attack, the individual is alert and communicative, general cognition seems intact, and there are no other neurologic signs or symptoms. The patient may seem confused and repeatedly ask about his or her location in place and time. The ability to form new memories returns after a period of hours, and the individual returns to normal with no recall for the period of the attack. Frequently no cause is determined, but cerebrovascular disease, epilepsy (7% in one study), migraine, or cardiac arrhythmias have all been implicated. A Mayo Clinic review of 277 patients with TGA found a history of migraine in 14% and cerebrovascular disease in 11%, but these conditions were not temporally related to the TGA episodes. Approximately one-quarter of the patients had recurrent attacks, but they were not at increased risk for subsequent stroke. Rare instances of permanent memory loss after sudden onset have been reported, usually representing ischemic infarction of the hippocampus or medial thalamic nucleus bilaterally.

The *ALS/parkinsonian/dementia complex of Guam* is a rare degenerative disease that has occurred in the Chamorro natives on the island of Guam. Individuals may have any combination of parkinsonian features, dementia, and motor neuron disease. The most characteristic pathologic features are the presence of NFTs in degenerating neurons of the cortex and substantia nigra and loss of motor neurons in the spinal cord, although recent reanalysis has shown that some patients with this illness also show coexisting TDP-43 pathology. Epidemiologic evidence supports a possible environmental cause, such as exposure to a neurotoxin or an infectious agent with a long latency period. One interesting but unproven candidate neurotoxin occurs in the seed of the false palm tree, which Guamanians traditionally used to make flour. The ALS syndrome is no longer present in Guam, but a dementing illness with rigidity continues to be seen.

Rarely, adult-onset leukodystrophies, lysosomal storage diseases, and other genetic disorders can present as a dementia in middle to late life. Metachromatic leukodystrophy (MLD) causes a progressive psychiatric or dementia syndrome associated with extensive, confluent frontal white matter abnormality. MLD is diagnosed by measuring arylsulfatase A enzyme activity in white blood cells. Adult-onset presentations of adrenoleukodystrophy have been reported in female carriers, and these patients often feature spinal cord and posterior white matter involvement. Adrenoleukodystrophy is diagnosed with measurement of plasma very long chain fatty acids. CADASIL is another genetic syndrome associated with white matter disease, often frontally and temporally predominant. Diagnosis is made with skin biopsy, which shows osmophilic granules in arterioles, or, increasingly, through genetic testing for mutations in Notch 3 (see earlier). The neuronal ceroid lipofuscinoses are a genetically heterogeneous group of disorders associated with myoclonus, seizures, and progressive dementia. Diagnosis is made by finding curvilinear inclusions within white blood cells or neuronal tissue.

Psychogenic amnesia for personally important memories can be seen. Whether this results from deliberate avoidance of unpleasant memories, outright malingering, or from unconscious repression remains unknown and probably depends on the patient. Event-specific amnesia is more likely to occur after violent crimes such as homicide of a close relative or friend or sexual abuse. It may develop in association with severe drug or alcohol intoxication and sometimes with schizophrenia. More prolonged psychogenic amnesia occurs in fugue states that also commonly follow severe emotional stress. The patient with a fugue state suffers from a sudden loss of personal identity and may be found wandering far from home. *In contrast to neurologic amnesia, fugue states are associated with amnesia for personal identity and events closely associated with the personal past.* At the same time, memory for other recent events and the ability to learn and use new information are preserved. The episodes usually last hours or days and occasionally weeks or months while the patient takes on a new identity. On recovery, there is a residual amnesia gap for the period of the fugue. Very rarely does selective loss of autobiographic information reflect a focal injury to the brain areas involved with these functions.

Psychiatric diseases may mimic dementia. Severely depressed or anxious individuals may appear demented, a phenomenon sometimes called *pseudodementia.* Memory and language are usually intact when carefully tested, and a significant memory disturbance usually suggests an underlying dementia, even if the patient is depressed. Patients in this condition may feel confused and unable to accomplish routine tasks. Vegetative symptoms, such as insomnia, lack of energy, poor appetite, and concern with bowel function, are common. Onset is often more abrupt, and the psychosocial milieu may suggest prominent reasons for depression. Such patients respond to treatment of the underlying psychiatric illness. Schizophrenia is usually not difficult to distinguish from dementia, but occasionally the distinction can be problematic. Schizophrenia generally has a much earlier age of onset (second and third decades) than most dementing illnesses, and is associated with intact memory. The delusions and hallucinations of schizophrenia are usually more complex and bizarre than those of dementia. Some chronic schizophrenics develop an unexplained progressive dementia late in life that is not related to AD. Conversely, FTD, HD, vascular dementia, DLB, AD, or leukoencephalopathy can begin with schizophrenia-like features, leading to the misdiagnosis of a psychiatric condition. Later age of onset, significant deficits on cognitive testing, or the presence of abnormal neuroimaging point toward a degenerative condition. Memory loss may also be part of a conversion disorder. In this situation, patients commonly complain bitterly of memory loss, but careful cognitive testing either does not confirm the deficits or demonstrates inconsistent or unusual patterns of cognitive problems. The patient's behavior and "wrong" answers to questions often indicate that he or she understands the question and knows the correct answer.

Clouding of cognition by *chronic drug or medication use*, often prescribed by physicians, is an important cause of dementia. Sedatives, tranquilizers, and analgesics used to treat insomnia, pain, anxiety, or agitation may cause confusion, memory loss, and lethargy, especially in the elderly. Discontinuation of the offending medication often improves mentation.

TREATMENT Dementia

The major goals of dementia management are to treat correctable causes and to provide comfort and support to the patient and caregivers. Treatment of underlying causes might include thyroid replacement for hypothyroidism; vitamin therapy for thiamine or B_{12} deficiency or for elevated serum homocysteine; antimicrobials for opportunistic infections or antiretrovirals for HIV; ventricular shunting for NPH; or appropriate surgical, radiation, and/or chemotherapeutic treatment for CNS neoplasms. Removal of cognition-impairing drugs or medications is the most frequently useful approach employed in a dementia clinic. If the patient's cognitive complaints stem from a psychiatric disorder, vigorous treatment of this condition should seek to eliminate the cognitive complaint or confirm that it persists despite adequate resolution of the mood or anxiety symptoms. Patients with degenerative diseases may also be depressed or anxious, and those aspects of their condition may respond to therapy. Antidepressants, such as SSRIs (Chap. 54), which feature anxiolytic properties but few cognitive side effects provide the mainstay of treatment when necessary. Anticonvulsants are used to control seizures.

Agitation, hallucinations, delusions, and confusion are difficult to treat. These behavioral problems represent major causes for nursing home placement and institutionalization. Before treating these behaviors with medications, the clinician should aggressively seek out modifiable environmental or metabolic factors. Hunger, lack of exercise, toothache, constipation, urinary tract infection, or drug toxicity all represent easily correctable causes that can be remedied without psychoactive drugs. Drugs such as phenothiazines and benzodiazepines may ameliorate the behavior problems but have untoward side effects such as sedation, rigidity, dyskinesia, and occasionally paradoxical disinhibition (benzodiazepines). Despite their unfavorable side-effect profile, second-generation antipsychotics such as quetiapine (starting dose, 12.5–25 mg daily) can be used for patients with agitation, aggression, and psychosis, although the risk profile for these compounds is significant. When patients do not respond to treatment, it is usually a mistake to advance to higher doses or to use anticholinergics or sedatives (such as barbiturates or benzodiazepines). It is important to recognize and treat depression; treatment can begin with a low dose of an SSRI (e.g., escitalopram 5–10 mg daily) while monitoring for efficacy and toxicity. Sometimes apathy, visual hallucinations, depression, and other psychiatric symptoms respond to the cholinesterase inhibitors, especially in DLB, obviating the need for other more toxic therapies.

Cholinesterase inhibitors are being used to treat AD (donepezil, rivastigmine, galantamine) and PDD (rivastigmine). Other compounds, such as anti-inflammatory agents, are being investigated in the treatment or prevention of AD. These approaches are reviewed in the treatment sections for individual disorders earlier in this chapter. Memantine proves useful when treating some patients with moderate to severe AD; its major benefit relates to decreasing caregiver burden, most likely by decreasing resistance to dressing and grooming support.

A proactive strategy has been shown to reduce the occurrence of delirium in hospitalized patients. This strategy includes frequent orientation, cognitive activities, sleep-enhancement measures, vision and hearing aids, and correction of dehydration.

Nondrug behavior therapy has an important place in dementia management. The primary goals are to make the patient's life comfortable, uncomplicated, and safe. Preparing lists, schedules, calendars, and labels can be helpful in the early stages. It is also useful to stress familiar routines, short-term tasks, walks, and simple physical exercises. For many demented patients, memory for events is worse than for routine activities, and they may still be able to take part in physical activities such as walking, bowling, dancing, and golf. Demented patients usually object to losing control over familiar tasks such as driving, cooking, and handling finances. Attempts to help or take over may be greeted with complaints, depression, or anger. Hostile responses on the part of the caretaker are useless and sometimes harmful. Explanation, reassurance, distraction, and calm positive statements are more productive in this setting. Eventually, tasks such as finances and driving must be assumed by others, and the patient will conform and adjust. Safety is an important issue that includes not only driving but controlling the kitchen, bathroom, and sleeping area environments, as well as stairways. These areas need to be monitored, supervised, and made as safe as possible. A move to a retirement home, assisted-living center, or nursing home can initially increase confusion and agitation. Repeated reassurance, reorientation, and careful introduction to the new personnel will help to smooth the process. Providing activities that are known to be enjoyable to the patient can be of considerable benefit. The clinician must pay special attention to frustration and depression among family members and caregivers. Caregiver guilt and burnout are common. Family members often feel overwhelmed and helpless and may vent their frustrations on the patient, each other, and health care providers. Caregivers should be encouraged to take advantage of day-care facilities and respite breaks. Education and counseling about dementia are important. Local and national support groups, such as the Alzheimer's Association (*www.alz.org*), can provide considerable help.

CHAPTER 30

PARKINSON'S DISEASE AND OTHER EXTRAPYRAMIDAL MOVEMENT DISORDERS

C. Warren Olanow ■ Anthony H.V. Schapira

PARKINSON'S DISEASE AND RELATED DISORDERS

Parkinson's disease (PD) is the second commonest neurodegenerative disease, exceeded only by Alzheimer's disease (AD). It is estimated that approximately 1 million persons in the United States and 5 million persons in the world suffer from this disorder. PD affects men and women of all races, all occupations, and all countries. The mean age of onset is about 60 years, but cases can be seen in patients in their 20s, and even younger. The frequency of PD increases with aging, and based on projected population demographics, it is estimated that the prevalence will dramatically increase in future decades.

Clinically, PD is characterized by rest tremor, rigidity, bradykinesia, and gait impairment, known as the "cardinal features" of the disease. Additional features can include freezing of gait, postural instability, speech difficulty, autonomic disturbances, sensory alterations, mood disorders, sleep dysfunction, cognitive impairment, and dementia (Table 30-1), all known as nondopaminergic features because they do not fully respond to dopaminergic therapy.

Pathologically, the hallmark features of PD are degeneration of dopaminergic neurons in the substantia nigra pars compacta (SNc), reduced striatal dopamine, and intracytoplasmic proteinaceous inclusions known as Lewy bodies (Fig. 30-1). While interest has primarily focused on the dopamine system, neuronal degeneration with inclusion body formation can also affect cholinergic neurons of the nucleus basalis of Meynert (NBM), norepinephrine neurons of the locus coeruleus (LC), serotonin neurons in the raphe nuclei of the brainstem, and neurons of the olfactory system, cerebral hemispheres, spinal cord, and peripheral autonomic nervous system. This "nondopaminergic" pathology is likely responsible for the nondopaminergic clinical features listed in Table 30-1. Indeed, there is evidence that pathology begins in the peripheral autonomic nervous system, olfactory system, and dorsal motor nucleus of the vagus nerve in the lower brainstem, and then spreads in a sequential manner to affect the upper brainstem and cerebral hemispheres. These studies suggest that dopamine neurons are affected in midstage disease. Indeed, several studies suggest that symptoms reflecting nondopaminergic degeneration such as constipation, anosmia, rapid eye movement (REM) behavior sleep disorder, and cardiac denervation precede the onset of the classic motor features of the illness.

DIFFERENTIAL DIAGNOSIS

Parkinsonism is a general term that is used to define a symptom complex manifest by bradykinesia with rigidity and/or tremor. It has a wide differential diagnosis (Table 30-2) and can reflect damage to different components of the basal ganglia. The basal ganglia comprise a group of subcortical nuclei that include the striatum (putamen and caudate nucleus), subthalamic nucleus (STN), globus pallidus pars externa (GPe), globus pallidus pars interna (GPi), and the SNc (Fig. 30-2). The basal ganglia play an important role in regulating normal motor behavior. It is now appreciated that basal ganglia also play a role in modulating emotional and cognitive functions. Among the different forms of parkinsonism, PD is the most common (approximately 75% of cases). Historically, PD was diagnosed based on the presence of two of three parkinsonian features (tremor, rigidity, bradykinesia). However, postmortem studies found a 24% error rate when these criteria were used. Clinicopathologic correlation studies subsequently determined that parkinsonism associated with rest tremor, asymmetry, and a good response to levodopa was more likely to predict the correct

TABLE 30-1

CLINICAL FEATURES OF PARKINSON'S DISEASE

CARDINAL FEATURES	OTHER MOTOR FEATURES	NONMOTOR FEATURES

Bradykinesia
Rest tremor
Rigidity
Gait disturbance/postural instability
	Micrographia
	Masked facies (hypomimia) equalize
	Reduced eye blink
	Soft voice (hypophonia)
	Dysphagia
	Freezing
		Anosmia
		Sensory disturbances (e.g., pain)
		Mood disorders (e.g., depression)
		Sleep disturbances
		Autonomic disturbances
		  Orthostatic hypotension
		  Gastrointestinal disturbances
		  Genitourinal disturbances
		  Sexual dysfunction
		Cognitive impairment/dementia

pathologic diagnosis. With these revised criteria (known as the U.K. brain bank criteria), the clinical diagnosis of PD is confirmed pathologically in 99% of cases.

Imaging of the brain dopamine system in PD with positron emission tomography (PET) or single-photon emission computed tomography (SPECT) shows reduced uptake of striatal dopaminergic markers, particularly in the posterior putamen (Fig. 30-3). Imaging can be useful in difficult cases or research studies but is rarely necessary in routine practice, as the diagnosis can usually be established on clinical criteria alone. This may change in the future when there is a disease-modifying therapy and it is important to make the diagnosis at as early a time point as possible. Genetic testing is not generally employed at present, but it can be helpful for identifying at-risk individuals in a research setting. Mutations of the *LRRK2* gene (see later) have attracted particular interest as they are the commonest cause of familial PD and are responsible for approximately 1% of typical sporadic cases of the disease. Mutations in *LRRK2* are particularly common causes of PD in Ashkenazi Jews and North African Berber Arabs. The penetrance of the most common *LRRK2* mutation ranges from 28 to 74%, depending on age. Mutations in the *parkin* gene

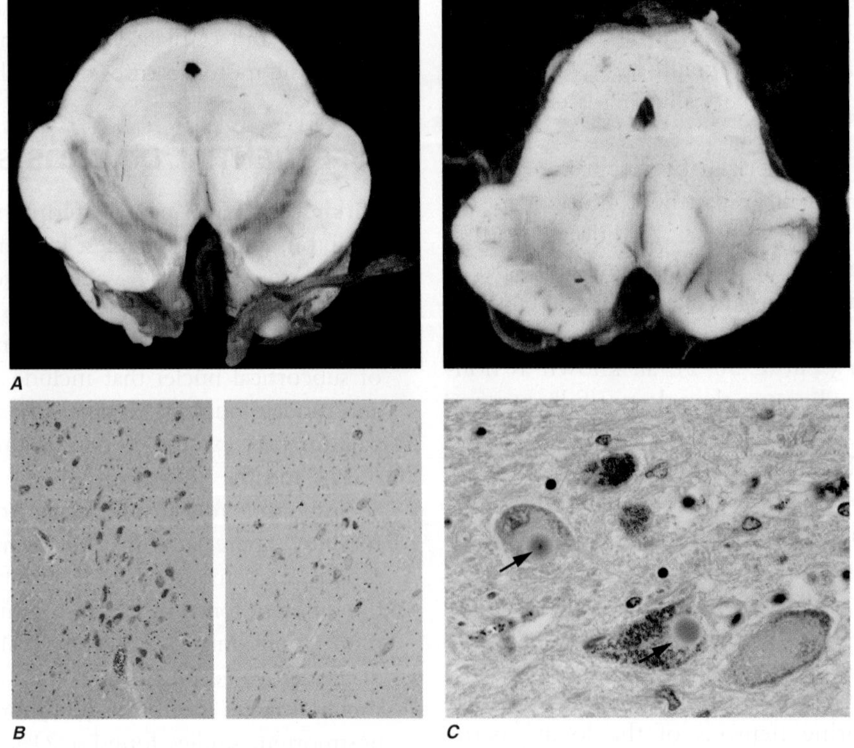

FIGURE 30-1

Pathologic specimens from a patient with Parkinson's disease (PD) compared to a normal control demonstrating (***A***) reduction of pigment in SNc in PD (*right*) vs control (*left*), (***B***) reduced numbers of cells in SNc in PD (*right*) compared to control (*left*), and (***C***) Lewy bodies (*arrows*) within melanized dopamine neurons in PD. SNc, substantia nigra pars compacta.

TABLE 30-2

DIFFERENTIAL DIAGNOSIS OF PARKINSONISM

Parkinson's Disease	Atypical Parkinsonisms	Secondary Parkinsonism	Other Neurodegenerative Disorders
Genetic	Multiple-system atrophy	Drug-induced	Wilson's disease
Sporadic	Cerebellar type (MSA-c)	Tumor	Huntington's disease
Dementia with Lewy bodies	Parkinson type (MSA-p)	Infection	Neurodegeneration with brain iron accumulation
	Progressive supranuclear palsy	Vascular	SCA 3 (spinocerebellar ataxia)
	Corticobasal ganglionic degeneration	Normal-pressure hydrocephalus	Fragile X–associated ataxia-tremor-parkinsonism
	Frontotemporal dementia	Trauma	Prion disease
		Liver failure	Dystonia-parkinsonism (DYT3)
		Toxins (e.g., carbon monoxide, manganese, MPTP, cyanide, hexane, methanol, carbon disulfide)	Alzheimer's disease with parkinsonism

should be considered in patients with disease onset prior to 40 years.

Atypical and secondary parkinsonism

Atypical parkinsonism refers to a group of neurodegenerative conditions that usually are associated with more widespread neurodegeneration than is found in PD (often involvement of SNc and striatum and/or pallidum). As a group, they present with a parkinsonism (rigidity and bradykinesia) but typically have a slightly different clinical picture than PD, reflecting differences in underlying pathology. Parkinsonism in these conditions is often characterized by early speech and gait impairment, absence of rest tremor, no asymmetry, poor or no response to levodopa, and an aggressive clinical course. In the early stages, they may show some modest benefit from levodopa and be difficult to distinguish from PD. Neuroimaging of the dopamine system is usually not helpful, as several atypical parkinsonisms also have degeneration of dopamine neurons. Pathologically, neurodegeneration occurs without Lewy bodies (see later for individual conditions). Metabolic imaging of the basal ganglia/thalamus network may be helpful, reflecting a pattern of decreased activity in the GPi with increased activity in the thalamus, the reverse of what is seen in PD.

Multiple-system atrophy (MSA) manifests as a combination of parkinsonian, cerebellar, and autonomic features and can be divided into a predominant parkinsonian (MSA-p) or cerebellar (MSA-c) form. Clinically, MSA is suspected when a patient presents with atypical parkinsonism in conjunction with cerebellar signs and/or early and prominent autonomic dysfunction, usually orthostatic hypotension (Chap. 33). Pathologically, MSA is characterized by degeneration of the SNc, striatum, cerebellum, and inferior olivary nuclei coupled with characteristic glial cytoplasmic inclusions (GCIs) that stain for α-synuclein. MRI can show pathologic iron accumulation in the striatum on T2-weighted

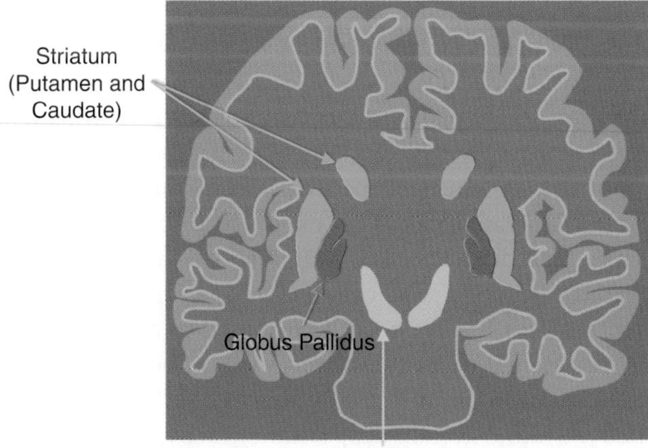

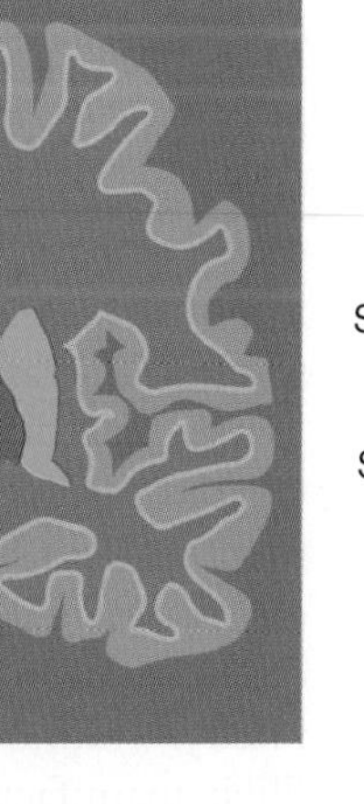

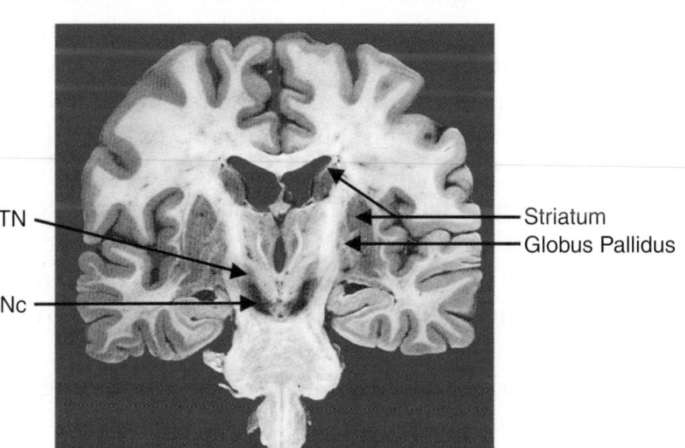

FIGURE 30-2

Basal ganglia nuclei. Schematic (***A***) and postmortem (***B***) coronal sections illustrating the various components of the basal ganglia. SNc, substantia nigra pars compacta; STN, subthalamic nucleus.

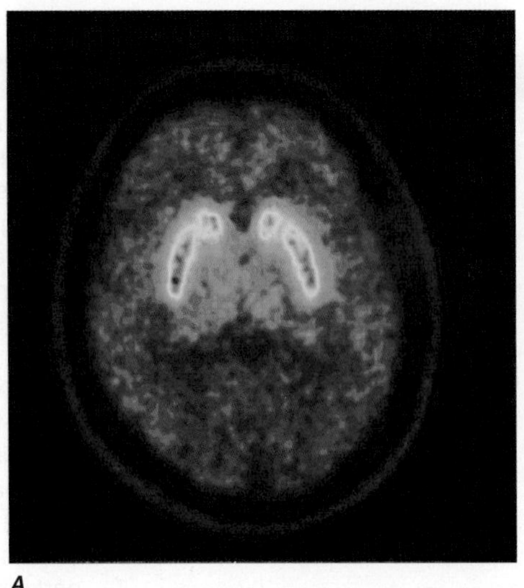

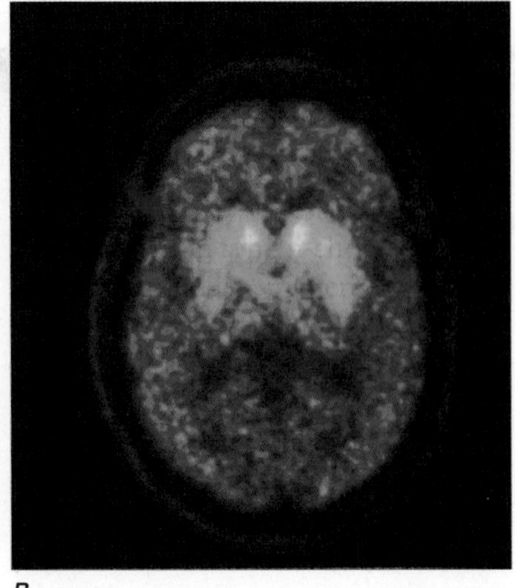

FIGURE 30-3
[^{11}C]dihydrotetrabenazine PET (a marker of VMAT2) in healthy control (*A*) and PD (*B*) patient. Note the reduced striatal uptake of tracer which is most pronounced in the posterior putamen and tends to be asymmetric. (*Courtesy of Dr. Jon Stoessl.*)

scans, high signal change in the region of the external surface of the putamen (putaminal rim) in MSA-p, or cerebellar and brainstem atrophy (the pontine "hot cross buns" sign [Fig. 33-2]) in MSA-c.

Progressive supranuclear palsy (PSP) is a form of atypical parkinsonism that is characterized by slow ocular saccades, eyelid apraxia, and restricted eye movements with particular impairment of downward gaze. Patients frequently experience hyperextension of the neck with early gait disturbance and falls. In later stages, speech and swallowing difficulty and dementia become evident. MRI may reveal a characteristic atrophy of the midbrain with relative preservation of the pons (the "hummingbird sign" on midsagittal images). Pathologically, PSP is characterized by degeneration of the SNc and pallidum along with neurofibrillary tangles and GCIs that stain for tau.

Corticobasal ganglionic degeneration is less common and is usually manifest by asymmetric dystonic contractions and clumsiness of one hand coupled with cortical sensory disturbances manifest as apraxia, agnosia, focal myoclonus, or alien limb phenomenon (where the limb assumes a position in space without the patient being aware of it). Dementia may occur at any stage of the disease. MRI frequently shows asymmetric cortical atrophy. Pathologic findings include achromatic neuronal degeneration with tau deposits similar to those found in PSP.

Secondary parkinsonism can be associated with drugs, stroke, tumor, infection, or exposure to toxins such as carbon monoxide or manganese. Dopamine-blocking agents such as the neuroleptics are the commonest cause of secondary parkinsonism. These drugs are most widely used in psychiatry, but physicians should be aware that drugs such as metoclopramide and chlorperazine, which are primarily used to treat gastrointestinal problems, are also neuroleptic agents and common causes of secondary parkinsonism and tardive dyskinesia. Other drugs that can cause secondary parkinsonism include tetrabenazine, amiodarone, and lithium.

Finally, parkinsonism can be seen as a feature of other degenerative disorders such as Wilson's disease, Huntington's disease (especially the juvenile form known as Westphal variant), dopa-responsive dystonia, and neurodegenerative disorders with brain iron accumulation such as pantothenate kinase (PANK)–associated neurodegeneration (formerly known as Hallervorden-Spatz disease).

Some features that suggest parkinsonism might be due to a condition other than PD are shown in Table 30-3.

ETIOLOGY AND PATHOGENESIS

Most PD cases occur sporadically (~85–90%) and are of unknown cause. Twin studies suggest that environmental factors likely play the more important role in patients older than 50 years, with genetic factors being more important in younger patients. Epidemiologic studies suggest increased risk with exposure to pesticides, rural living, and drinking well water and reduced risk with cigarette smoking and caffeine. However, no environmental factor has yet been determined to cause PD. The environmental hypothesis received a boost with the demonstration in the 1980s that MPTP (1-methyl-4-phenyl-1,2,5,6-tetrahydropyridine), a byproduct of the illicit manufacture of a heroin-like drug, caused a PD-like syndrome in addicts in northern California. MPTP is transported to the central nervous system, where it is metabolized to form MPP^+, a mitochondrial toxin that

TABLE 30-3

FEATURES SUGGESTING ALTERNATE DIAGNOSIS THAN PD

SYMPTOMS/SIGNS	ALTERNATE DIAGNOSIS TO CONSIDER
History	
Early speech and gait impairment	Atypical parkinsonism
Exposure to neuroleptics	Drug-induced parkinsonism
Onset prior to age 40	Genetic form of PD
Liver disease	Wilson's disease, non-Wilsonian hepatolenticular degeneration
Early hallucinations	Dementia with Lewy bodies
Diplopia	PSP
Poor or no response to an adequate trial of levodopa	Atypical or secondary parkinsonism
Physical Exam	
Dementia as first symptom	Dementia with Lewy bodies
Prominent orthostatic hypotension	MSA-p
Prominent cerebellar signs	MSA-c
Impairment of down gaze	PSP
High-frequency (8–10 Hz) symmetric postural tremor with a prominent kinetic component	Essential tremor

Abbreviations: MSA-c, multiple-system atrophy–cerebellar type; MSA-p, multiple-system atrophy–Parkinson type; PSP, progressive supranuclear palsy.

is selectively taken up by, and damages, dopamine neurons. However, MPTP or MPTP-like compounds have not been linked to sporadic PD. MPTP has, however, proved useful for generating an animal model of the disease. About 10–15% of cases are familial in origin, and multiple specific mutations and gene associations have been identified (Table 30-4). It has been proposed that most cases of PD are due to a "double hit" involving an interaction between a gene mutation that induces susceptibility coupled with exposure to a toxic environmental factor. In this scenario, both factors are required for PD to ensue, while the presence of either one alone is not sufficient to cause the disease.

Factors that have been implicated in the pathogenesis of cell death include oxidative stress, intracellular calcium accumulation with excitotoxicity, inflammation, mitochondrial dysfunction, and proteolytic stress. Whatever the pathogenic mechanism, cell death appears to occur, at least in part, by way of a signal-mediated apoptotic or "suicidal" process. Each of these mechanisms offer potential targets for neuroprotective

TABLE 30-4

GENETIC CAUSES OF PD

NAME	CHROMOSOME	LOCUS	GENE	INHERITANCE
Park 1	Chr 4	q21-23	α-Synuclein	AD
Park 2	Chr 6	q25-27	Parkin	AR
Park 3	Chr 2	p13	Unknown	AD
Park 4	Chr 4	q21-23	α-Synuclein	AD
Park 5	Chr 4	p14	UCHL-1	AD
Park 6	Chr 1	p35-36	PINK-1	AR
Park 7	Chr 1	p36	DJ-1	AR
Park 8	Chr 12	p11-q13	LRRK2	AR/Sp
Park 9	Chr 1	p36	ATP13A2	AR
Park 10	Chr 1	p32	Unknown	Sp
Park 11	Chr 2	q36-37	GIGYF2	AD
Park 12	Chr X	q21-25	Unknown	Sp
Park 13	Chr 2	p13	Omi/HtrA2	AD
Park 14	Chr 22	q13	PLA2G6	AR
Park 15	Chr 22	q12-13	FBX07	AR
Park 16	Chr 1	q32	Unknown	SP

Abbreviations: AD, autosomal dominant; AR, autosomal recessive; SP, sporadic.

drugs. However, it is not clear which of these factors is primary, if the cause is the same in each case, or if one or all merely represent epiphenomena unrelated to the true cause of cell death that remains undiscovered (Fig. 30-4).

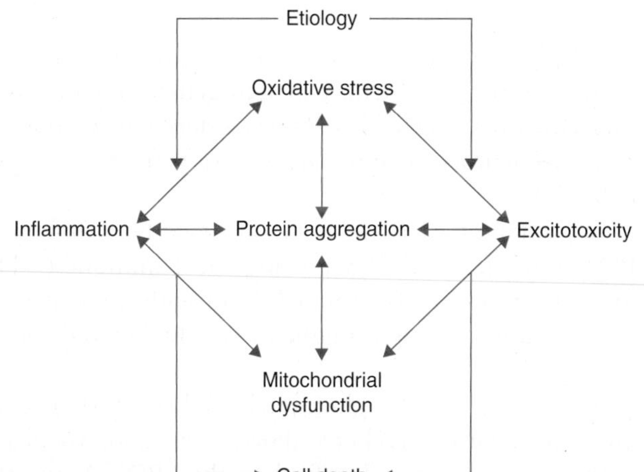

FIGURE 30-4

Schematic representation of how pathogenetic factors implicated in PD interact in a network manner, ultimately leading to cell death. This figure illustrates how interference with any one of these factors may not necessarily stop the cell death cascade. (*Adapted from CW Olanow: Movement Disorders 22:S-335, 2007.*)

Gene mutations discovered to date have been helpful in pointing to specific pathogenic mechanisms as being central to the neurodegenerative process. The most significant of these mechanisms appear to be protein misfolding and accumulation and mitochondrial dysfunction. The idea that proteins are involved in the pathogenesis of PD is not surprising, given that PD is characterized by Lewy bodies and Lewy neurites, which are composed of misfolded and aggregated proteins (Fig. 30-1). Protein accumulation could result from either increased formation or impaired clearance of proteins. Mutations in α-synuclein promote misfolding of the protein and the formation of oligomers and aggregates thought to be involved in the cell death process. Importantly, duplication or triplication of the wild-type α-synuclein gene can itself cause PD, indicating that increased production of even the normal protein can cause PD. Increased levels of unwanted proteins could also result from impaired clearance. Proteins are normally cleared by the ubiquitin proteasome system or the autophagy/lysosome pathway. These pathways are defective in patients with sporadic PD, and interestingly α-synuclein is a prominent component of Lewy bodies in these cases. Further, mutations in parkin (a ubiquitin ligase that attaches ubiquitin to misfolded proteins to promote their transport to the proteasome for degradation) and UCH-L1 (which cleaves ubiquitin from misfolded proteins to permit their entry into the proteasome) are causative in other cases of familial PD. Collectively, these findings implicate abnormal protein accumulation in the etiology of PD. Indeed, in laboratory models both overexpression of α-synuclein or impairment of proteasomal clearance mechanisms leads to degeneration of dopamine neurons with inclusion body formation.

Mitochondrial dysfunction has also been implicated in familial PD. Several causative genes (*parkin*, *PINK1*, and *DJ1*) either localize to mitochondria and/or cause mitochondrial dysfunction in transgenic animals. Postmortem studies have also shown a defect in complex I of the respiratory chain in the SNc of patients with sporadic PD.

Six different *LRRK2* mutations have been linked to PD, with the Gly2019Ser being the commonest. The mechanism responsible for cell death with this mutation is not known but is thought to involve altered kinase activity.

Mutations in the glucocerebrosidase (GBA) gene associated with Gaucher's disease are also associated with an increased risk of idiopathic PD. Again the mechanism is not precisely known, but it is noteworthy that it is associated with altered autophagy and lysosomal function, suggesting that mutations in this gene might also impair protein clearance leading to PD.

Whole-genome association studies have provided conflicting results. Most recently, linkage to mutations in human leukocyte antigen (HLA) genes were identified in PD patients, suggesting that altered immunity or inflammation may be a causative or contributory factor.

While gene mutations account for only a small percentage of cases of PD, it is hoped that better understanding of the mechanisms whereby they cause cell death will provide insight into the nature of the cell death process in the more common sporadic form of the disease. These mutations could also permit the development of more relevant animal models of PD in which to test putative neuroprotective drugs.

PATHOPHYSIOLOGY OF PD

The classic model of basal ganglia functional organization in the normal and PD states is provided in Fig. 30-5. A series of neuronal loops link the basal ganglia nuclei with corresponding cortical motor regions in a somatotopic manner to help regulate motor function. The striatum is the major input region of the basal ganglia, while the GPi and SNr are the major output regions. The input and output regions are connected via direct and indirect pathways that have reciprocal effects on the output pathway. The output of the basal ganglia provides inhibitory tone to thalamic and brainstem neurons that in turn connect to motor systems in the cerebral cortex and spinal cord to regulate motor function. Dopaminergic projections from SNc neurons serve to modulate neuronal firing and to stabilize the basal ganglia network.

In PD, dopamine denervation leads to increased firing of neurons in the STN and GPi, resulting in excessive inhibition of the thalamus, reduced activation of cortical motor systems, and the development of parkinsonian features (Fig. 30-5). The current role of surgery in the treatment of PD is based upon this model, which predicted that lesions or high-frequency stimulation of the STN or GPi might reduce this neuronal overactivity and improve PD features.

TREATMENT Parkinson's Disease

LEVODOPA Since its introduction in the late 1960s, levodopa has been the mainstay of therapy for PD. Experiments in the late 1950s by Carlsson demonstrated that blocking dopamine uptake with reserpine caused rabbits to become parkinsonian; this could be reversed with the dopamine precursor, levodopa. Subsequently, Hornykiewicz demonstrated a dopamine deficiency in the striatum of PD patients and suggested the potential benefit of dopaminergic replacement therapy. Dopamine does not cross the blood-brain barrier (BBB), so clinical trials were initiated with levodopa, a precursor of

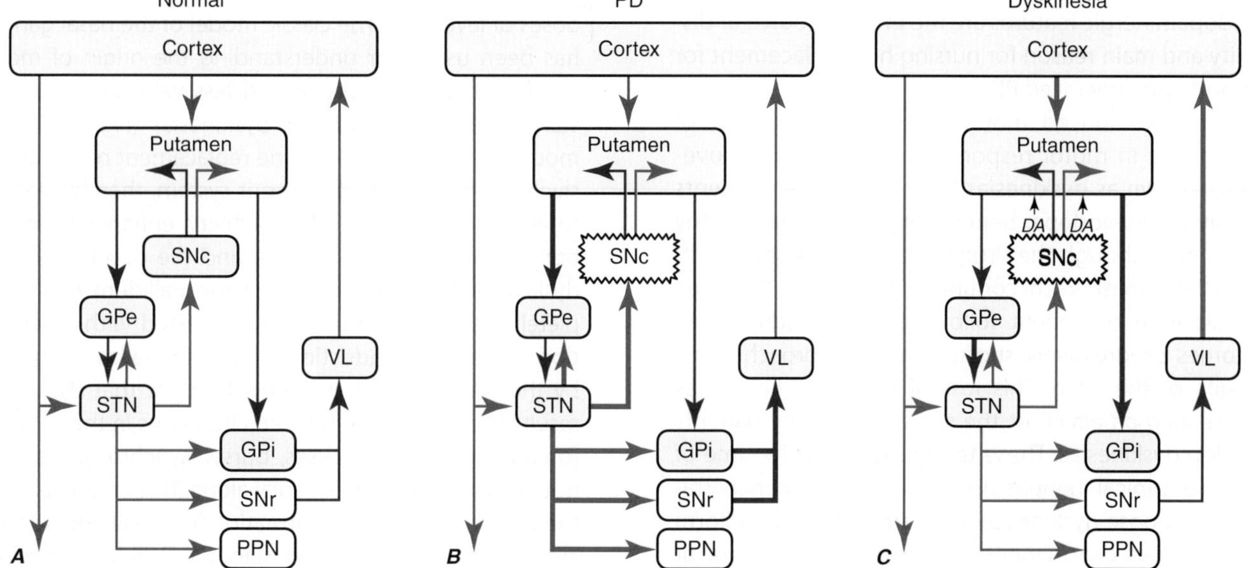

FIGURE 30-5

Basal ganglia organization. Classic model of the organization of the basal ganglia in the normal, PD, and levodopa-induced dyskinesia state. Inhibitory connections are shown as blue arrows and excitatory connections as red arrows. The striatum is the major input region and receives its major input from the cortex. The GPi and SNr are the major output regions and they project to the thalamocortical and brainstem motor regions. The striatum and GPi/SNr are connected by direct and indirect pathways. This model predicts that parkinsonism results from increased neuronal firing in the STN and GPi and that lesions or DBS of these targets might provide benefit. This concept led to the rationale for surgical therapies for PD. The model also predicts that dyskinesia results from decreased firing of the output regions, resulting in excessive cortical activation by the thalamus. This component of the model is not completely correct as lesions of the GPi ameliorate rather than increase dyskinesia in PD, suggesting that firing frequency is just one of the components that lead to the development of dyskinesia. DBS, deep brain stimulation; GPe, external segment of the globus pallidus; GPi, internal segment of the globus pallidus; SNr, substantia nigra, pars reticulata; SNc, substantia nigra, pars compacta; STN, subthalamic nucleus; VL, ventrolateral thalamus; PPN, pedunculopontine nucleus. (*Derived from JA Obeso et al: Trends Neurosci 23:S8, 2000.*)

dopamine. Studies over the course of the next decade confirmed the value of levodopa and revolutionized the treatment of PD.

Levodopa is routinely administered in combination with a peripheral decarboxylase inhibitor to prevent its peripheral metabolism to dopamine and the development of nausea and vomiting due to activation of dopamine receptors in the area postrema that are not protected by the BBB. In the United States, levodopa is combined with the decarboxylase inhibitor carbidopa (Sinemet), while in many other countries it is combined with benserazide (Madopar). Levodopa is also available in controlled-release formulations as well as in combination with a COMT inhibitor (see later). Levodopa remains the most effective symptomatic treatment for PD and the gold standard against which new therapies are compared. No current medical or surgical treatment provides antiparkinsonian benefits superior to what can be achieved with levodopa. Levodopa benefits the classic motor features of PD, prolongs independence and employability, improves quality of life, and increases life span. Almost all PD patients experience improvement, and failure to respond to an adequate trial should cause the diagnosis to be questioned.

There are, however, important limitations of levodopa therapy. Acute dopaminergic side effects include nausea, vomiting, and orthostatic hypotension. These are usually transient and can generally be avoided by gradual titration. If they persist, they can be treated with additional doses of a peripheral decarboxylase inhibitor (e.g., carbidopa) or a peripheral dopamine-blocking agent such as domperidone (not available in the United States). More important are motor complications (see later) that develop in the majority of patients treated long-term with levodopa therapy. In addition, features such as falling, freezing, autonomic dysfunction, sleep disorders, and dementia may emerge that are not adequately controlled by levodopa. Indeed, these nondopaminergic features are the primary source of disability and main reason for nursing home placement for patients with advanced PD.

Levodopa-induced motor complications consist of fluctuations in motor response and involuntary movements known as dyskinesias (Fig. 30-6). When patients initially take levodopa, benefits are long-lasting (many hours) even though the drug has a relatively short half-life (60–90 min). With continued treatment, however, the duration of benefit following an individual dose becomes progressively shorter until it approaches the half-life of the drug. This loss of benefit is known as the *wearing-off effect*. At the same time, many patients develop dyskinesias. These tend to occur at the time of maximal clinical benefit and peak plasma concentration (peak-dose dyskinesia). They are usually choreiform in nature but can manifest as dystonia, myoclonus, or other movement disorders. They are not troublesome when mild, but can be disabling when severe and can limit the ability to fully utilize levodopa to control PD features. In more advanced states, patients may cycle between "on" periods complicated by disabling dyskinesias and "off" periods in which they suffer severe parkinsonism. Patients may also experience "diphasic dyskinesias," which occur as the levodopa dose begins to take effect and again as it wears off. These dyskinesias typically consist of transient, stereotypic, rhythmic movements that predominantly involve the lower extremities and are frequently associated with parkinsonism in other body regions. They can be relieved by increasing the dose of levodopa, although higher doses may induce more severe peak-dose dyskinesia.

The cause of levodopa-induced motor complications is not precisely known. They are more likely to occur in young individuals with severe disease and with higher doses of levodopa. The classic model of the basal ganglia has been useful for understanding the origin of motor features in PD, but has proved less valuable for understanding levodopa-induced dyskinesias (Fig. 30-5). The model predicts that dopamine replacement might excessively inhibit the pallidal output system, thereby leading to increased thalamocortical activity, enhanced stimulation of cortical motor regions, and the development of dyskinesia. However, lesions of the pallidum that completely destroy its output are associated with amelioration rather than induction of dyskinesia as suggested by the classic model. It is now thought that dyskinesia results from levodopa-induced alterations in the GPi neuronal firing pattern (pauses, bursts, synchrony, etc.) and not simply the firing frequency alone. This in turn leads to the transmission of misinformation from pallidum to thalamus/cortex, resulting in dyskinesia. Pallidotomy might thus ameliorate dyskinesia by blocking this abnormal firing pattern and preventing the transfer of misinformation to motor systems.

Current information suggests that altered neuronal firing patterns and motor complications relate to nonphysiologic levodopa replacement. Striatal dopamine levels are normally maintained at a relatively constant level. In the PD state, dopamine neurons degenerate and striatal dopamine is dependent on peripheral availability of levodopa. Intermittent doses of short-acting levodopa do not restore dopamine in a physiologic manner and cause dopamine receptors to be exposed to alternating high and low concentrations of dopamine. This intermittent or pulsatile stimulation of dopamine receptors induces molecular changes in striatal neurons and neurophysiologic changes in pallidal neurons, leading to the development of motor complications. It has been hypothesized that more continuous

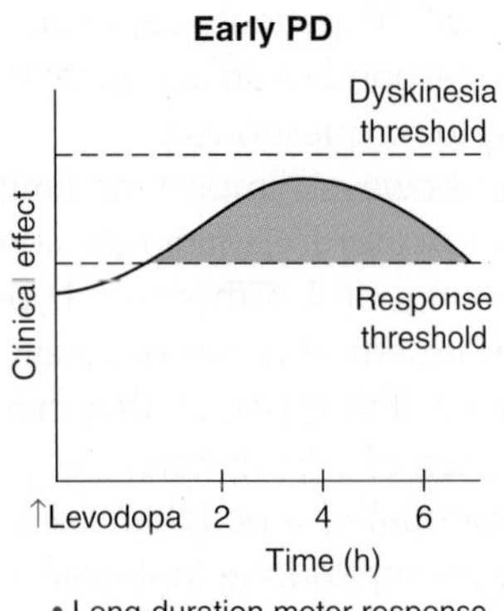

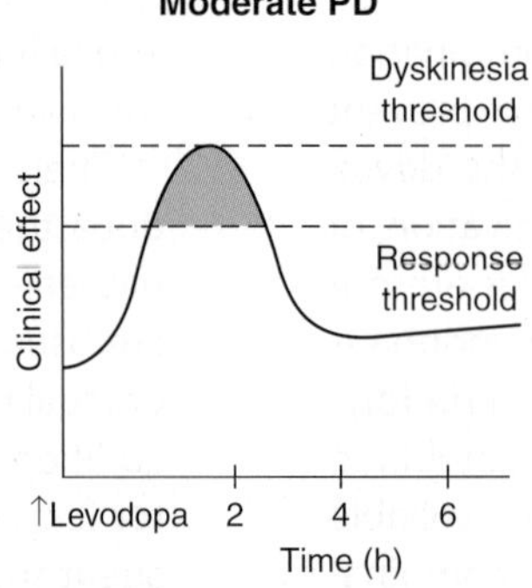

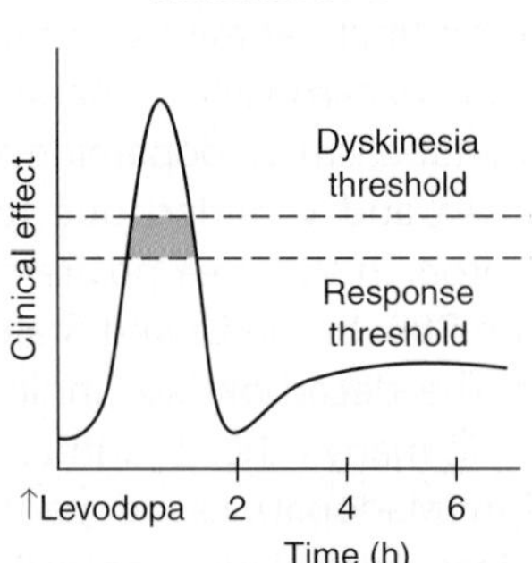

FIGURE 30-6

Changes in motor response associated with chronic levodopa treatment. Levodopa-induced motor complications. Schematic illustration of the gradual shortening of the duration of a beneficial motor response to levodopa (wearing off) and the appearance of dyskinesias complicating "on" time.

delivery of levodopa might prevent the development of motor complications. Indeed, continuous levodopa infusion is associated with improvement in both "off" time and dyskinesia in advanced PD patients, but this approach has not yet been proved to prevent dyskinesia in clinical trials.

Behavioral alterations can be encountered in levodopa-treated patients. A dopamine dysregulation syndrome has been described where patients have a craving for levodopa and take frequent and unnecessary doses of the drug in an addictive manner. PD patients taking high doses of levodopa can also have purposeless, stereotyped behaviors such as the meaningless assembly and disassembly or collection and sorting of objects. This is known as punding, a term taken from the Swedish description of the meaningless behaviors seen in chronic amphetamine users. Hypersexuality and other impulse-control disorders are occasionally encountered with levodopa, although these are more commonly seen with dopamine agonists.

DOPAMINE AGONISTS Dopamine agonists are a diverse group of drugs that act directly on dopamine receptors. Unlike levodopa, they do not require metabolism to an active product and do not undergo oxidative metabolism. Initial dopamine agonists were ergot derivatives (e.g., bromocriptine, pergolide, cabergoline) and were associated with ergot-related side effects, including cardiac valvular damage. They have largely been replaced by a second generation of non-ergot dopamine agonists (e.g., pramipexole, ropinirole, rotigotine). In general, dopamine agonists do not have comparable efficacy to levodopa. They were initially introduced as adjuncts to levodopa to enhance motor function and reduce "off" time in fluctuating patients. Subsequently, it was shown that dopamine agonists, possibly because they are relatively long-acting, are less prone than levodopa to induce dyskinesia. For this reason, many physicians initiate therapy with a dopamine agonist, although supplemental levodopa is eventually required in virtually all patients. Both ropinirole and pramipexole are available as orally administered immediate (tid) and extended-release (qd) formulations. Rotigotine is administered as a once-daily transdermal patch. Apomorphine is a dopamine agonist with efficacy comparable to levodopa, but it must be administered parenterally and has a very short half-life and duration of activity (45 min). It is generally administered SC as a rescue agent for the treatment of severe "off" episodes. Apomorphine can also be administered by continuous infusion and has been demonstrated to reduce both "off" time and dyskinesia in advanced patients. However, infusions are cumbersome, and this approach has not been approved in the United States.

Acute side effects of dopamine agonists include nausea, vomiting, and orthostatic hypotension. As with levodopa, these can usually be avoided by slow titration. Hallucinations and cognitive impairment are more common with dopamine agonists than with levodopa. Sedation with sudden unintended episodes of falling asleep while driving a motor vehicle have been reported. Patients should be informed about this potential problem and should not drive when tired. Injections of apomorphine and patch delivery of rotigotine can be complicated by development of skin lesions at sites of administration. Recently, it has become appreciated that dopamine agonists are associated with impulse-control disorders, including pathologic gambling, hypersexuality, and compulsive eating and shopping. The precise cause of these problems, and why they appear to occur more frequently with dopamine agonists than levodopa, remains to be resolved, but reward systems associated with dopamine and alterations in the ventral striatum have been implicated.

MAO-B INHIBITORS Inhibitors of monoamine oxidase type B (MAO-B) block central dopamine metabolism and increase synaptic concentrations of the neurotransmitter. Selegiline and rasagiline are relatively selective suicide inhibitors of the MAO-B enzyme. Clinically, MAO-B inhibitors provide modest antiparkinsonian benefits when used as monotherapy in early disease, and reduced "off" time when used as an adjunct to levodopa in patients with motor fluctuations. MAO-B inhibitors are generally safe and well tolerated. They may increase dyskinesia in levodopa-treated patients but this can usually be controlled by down-titrating the dose of levodopa. Inhibition of the MAO-A isoform prevents metabolism of tyramine in the gut, leading to a potentially fatal hypertensive reaction known as a "cheese effect" as it can be precipitated by foods rich in tyramine such as some cheeses, aged meats, and red wine. Selegiline and rasagiline do not functionally inhibit MAO-A in doses employed in clinical practice and are not associated with a cheese effect. There are theoretical risks of a serotonin reaction in patients receiving concomitant SSRI antidepressants, but these are rarely encountered.

Interest in MAO-B inhibitors has also focused on their potential to have disease-modifying effects. MPTP toxicity can be prevented by coadministration of a MAO-B inhibitor that blocks its conversion to the toxic pyridinium ion MPP^+. MAO-B inhibitors also have the potential to block the oxidative metabolism of dopamine and prevent oxidative stress. In addition, both selegiline and rasagiline incorporate a propargyl ring within their molecular structure that provides antiapoptotic effects in laboratory models. The DATATOP study showed that selegiline significantly delayed the time until the emergence of disability, necessitating the introduction of levodopa in untreated PD patients. However, it could not be determined whether this was due to a neuroprotective effect that slowed disease progression or a symptomatic effect that merely masked ongoing neurodegeneration. More recently, the ADAGIO study demonstrated that early treatment with rasagiline 1 mg/d but not 2 mg/d provided benefits that could not be achieved with delayed treatment with the same drug, consistent with a disease-modifying effect; however, the long-term significance of these findings is uncertain.

COMT INHIBITORS When levodopa is administered with a decarboxylase inhibitor, it is primarily metabolized by catechol-*O*-methyltransferase (COMT). Inhibitors of COMT increase the elimination half-life of levodopa and enhance its brain availability. Combining levodopa with a COMT inhibitor reduces "off" time and prolongs "on" time in fluctuating patients while enhancing motor scores. Two COMT inhibitors have been approved, tolcapone and entacapone. There is also a combination tablet of levodopa, carbidopa, and entacapone (Stalevo).

Side effects of COMT inhibitors are primarily dopaminergic (nausea, vomiting, increased dyskinesia) and can usually be controlled by down-titrating the dose of levodopa by 20–30%. Severe diarrhea has been described with tolcapone, and to a lesser degree with entacapone, and necessitates stopping the medication in 5–10% of individuals. Cases of fatal hepatic toxicity have been reported with tolcapone, and periodic monitoring of liver function is required. This problem has not been encountered with entacapone. Discoloration of urine can be seen with both COMT inhibitors due to accumulation of a metabolite, but it is of no clinical concern.

It has been proposed that initiating levodopa in combination with a COMT inhibitor to enhance its elimination half-life will provide more continuous levodopa delivery and reduce the risk of motor complications. While this result has been demonstrated in parkinsonian monkeys, and continuous infusion reduces "off" time and dyskinesia in advanced patients, no benefit of initiating levodopa with a COMT inhibitor compared to levodopa alone was detected in early PD patients in the STRIDE-PD study, and the main value of COMT inhibitors for now continues to be in patients who experience motor fluctuations.

OTHER MEDICAL THERAPIES Central-acting anticholinergic drugs such as trihexyphenidyl and benztropine were used historically for the treatment for PD, but they lost favor with the introduction of dopaminergic agents. Their major clinical effect is on tremor, although it is not certain that this is superior to what can be obtained with agents such as levodopa and dopamine agonists. Still, they can be helpful in individual patients. Their use is limited particularly in the elderly, due to their propensity to induce a variety of side effects including urinary dysfunction, glaucoma, and particularly cognitive impairment.

Amantadine also has historical importance. Originally introduced as an antiviral agent, it was appreciated to also have antiparkinsonian effects that are now thought to be due to NMDA-receptor antagonism. While some physicians use amantadine in patients with early disease for its mild symptomatic effects, it is most widely used as an antidyskinesia agent in patients with advanced PD. Indeed, it is the only oral agent that has been demonstrated in controlled studies to reduce dyskinesia while improving parkinsonian features, although benefits may be relatively transient. Side effects include livido reticularis, weight gain, and impaired cognitive function. Amantadine should always be discontinued gradually as patients can experience withdrawal symptoms.

A list of the major drugs and available dosage strengths is provided in Table 30-5.

NEUROPROTECTION Despite the many therapeutic agents available for the treatment of PD, patients can still experience intolerable disability due to disease progression and the emergence of features such as falling and dementia that are not controlled with dopaminergic therapies. Trials of several promising agents such as rasagiline, selegiline, coenzyme Q10, pramipexole, and ropinirole have had positive results in clinical trials consistent with disease-modifying effects. However, it is not possible to determine if the positive results are due to neuroprotection with slowed disease progression or confounding symptomatic or pharmacologic effects that mask ongoing progression. If it could be determined that a drug slowed disease progression, this would be a major advance in the treatment of PD.

SURGICAL TREATMENT Surgical treatments for PD have been employed for more than a century. Lesions placed in the motor cortex improved tremor, but were associated with motor deficits and this approach was abandoned. Subsequently, it was appreciated that lesions placed into the VIM nucleus of the thalamus reduced contralateral tremor without inducing hemiparesis, but these lesions did not meaningfully help other more disabling features of PD. Lesions placed in the GPi improved rigidity and bradykinesia as well as tremor, particularly if placed in the posteroventral portion of the nucleus. Importantly, pallidotomy was also associated with marked improvement in contralateral dyskinesia. This procedure gained favor with greater understanding of the pathophysiology of PD

TABLE 30-5

DRUGS COMMONLY USED FOR TREATMENT OF PD[a]

AGENT	AVAILABLE DOSAGES	TYPICAL DOSING
Levodopa[a]		
Carbidopa/levodopa	10/100, 25/100, 25/250	200–1000 mg levodopa/d 2–4 times/d
Benserazide/levodopa	25/100, 50/200	
Carbidopa/levodopa CR	25/100, 50/200	
Benserazide/levodopa MDS	25/200, 25/250	
Parcopa	10/100, 25/100, 25/250	
Carbidopa/levodopa/entacapone	12.5/50/200, 18.75/75/200, 25/100/200, 31.25/125/200, 37.5/150/200, 50/200/200	
Dopamine agonists		
Pramipexole	0.125, 0.25, 0.5, 1.0, 1.5 mg	0.25–1.0 mg tid
Pramipexole ER	0.375, 0.75, 1.5. 3.0, 4.5 mg	1–3 mg/d
Ropinirole	0.25, 0.5, 1.0, 3.0 mg	6–24 mg/d
Ropinirole XL	2, 4, 6, 8	6–24 mg/d
Rotigotine patch	2-, 4-, 6-mg patches	4–10 mg/d
Apomorphine SC		2–8 mg
COMT inhibitors		
Entacapone	200 mg	200 mg with each levodopa dose
Tolcapone	100, 200 mg	100–200 mg tid
MAO-B inhibitors		
Selegiline	5 mg	5 mg bid
Rasagiline	0.5, 1.0 mg	1.0 mg QAM

[a]Treatment should be individualized. Generally, drugs should be started in low doses and titrated to optimal dose.
Note: Drugs should not be withdrawn abruptly but should be gradually lowered or removed as appropriate.
Abbreviations: COMT, catechol-*O*-methyltransferase; MAO-B, monoamine oxidase type B.

(see earlier). However, this procedure is not optimal for patients with bilateral disease, as bilateral lesions are associated with side effects such as dysphagia, dysarthria, and impaired cognition.

Most surgical procedures for PD performed today utilize deep brain stimulation (DBS). Here, an electrode is placed into the target area and connected to a stimulator inserted SC over the chest wall. DBS simulates the effects of a lesion without necessitating a brain lesion. The stimulation variables can be adjusted with respect to electrode configuration, voltage, frequency, and pulse duration in order to maximize benefit and minimize adverse side effects. In cases with intolerable side effects, stimulation can be stopped and the system removed. The procedure has the advantage that it does not require making a lesion in the brain and is thus suitable for performing bilateral procedures with relative safety.

DBS for PD primarily targets the STN or the GPi. It provides dramatic results, particularly with respect to "off" time and dyskinesias, but does not improve features that fail to respond to levodopa and does not prevent the development or progression of nondopaminergic features such as freezing, falling, and dementia. The procedure is thus primarily indicated for patients who suffer disability resulting from levodopa-induced motor complications that cannot be satisfactorily controlled with drug manipulation. Side effects can be seen with respect to the surgical procedure (hemorrhage, infarction, infection), the DBS system (infection, lead break, lead displacement, skin ulceration), or stimulation (ocular and speech abnormalities, muscle twitches, paresthesias, depression, and rarely suicide). Recent studies indicate that benefits following DBS of the STN and GPi are comparable, but that GPi stimulation may be associated with a reduced frequency of depression. While not all PD patients are candidates, the procedure is profoundly beneficial for many. Research studies are currently examining additional targets that might benefit gait dysfunction, depression, and cognitive impairment in PD patients.

EXPERIMENTAL SURGICAL THERAPIES FOR PD There has been considerable scientific and public interest in a number of novel therapies as possible treatments for PD. These include cell-based therapies (such as transplantation of fetal nigral dopamine cells or dopamine neurons derived from stem cells), gene therapies, and trophic factors. Transplant strategies are based on implanting dopaminergic cells into the striatum to replace degenerating SNc dopamine neurons. Fetal nigral mesencephalic cells have been demonstrated to survive implantation, reinnervate the striatum in an organotypic manner, and restore motor function in PD models. Several open-label studies reported positive results. However, two double-blind, sham surgery–controlled studies failed to show significant benefit of fetal nigral transplantation in comparison to a sham operation with respect to their primary endpoints. Post hoc analyses showed possible benefits in patients aged <60 years and in those with milder disease. It is now appreciated that grafting of fetal nigral cells is associated with a previously unrecognized form of dyskinesia that persists even after lowering or stopping levodopa. In addition, there is evidence that after many years, transplanted healthy embryonic dopamine neurons from unrelated donors can develop PD pathology, suggesting that they somehow became affected by the disease process. Most importantly, it is not clear how replacing dopamine cells alone will improve nondopaminergic features such as falling and dementia, which are the major sources of disability for patients with advanced disease. These same concerns apply to dopamine neurons derived from stem cells, which have not yet been tested in PD patients, and bear the additional theoretical concern of unanticipated side effects such as tumors. The short-term future for this technology as a treatment for PD, at least in its current state, is therefore not promising.

Gene therapy involves viral vector delivery of the DNA of a therapeutic protein to specific target regions. The DNA of the therapeutic protein can then be incorporated into the genome of host cells and thereby, in principle, provide continuous and long-lasting delivery of the therapeutic molecule. The AAV2 virus has been most often used as the viral vector because it does not promote an inflammatory response, is not incorporated into the host genome, and is associated with long-lasting transgene expression. Studies performed to date in PD have delivered aromatic amino acid decarboxylase with or without tyrosine hydroxylase to the striatum to facilitate dopamine production; glutamic acid decarboxylase to the STN to inhibit overactive neuronal firing in this nucleus; and trophic factors such as GDNF (glial-derived neurotrophic factor) and neurturin to the striatum to enhance and protect residual dopamine neurons in the SNc by way of retrograde transmission. Positive results have been reported with open-label studies, but these have not yet been confirmed in double-blind trials. While gene delivery technology has great potential, this approach also carries the risk of possible unanticipated side effects, and current approaches also do not address the nondopaminergic features of the illness.

MANAGEMENT OF THE NONMOTOR AND NONDOPAMINERGIC FEATURES OF PD While most attention has focused on the dopaminergic features of PD, management of the nondopaminergic features of the illness should not be ignored. Some nonmotor features, while not thought to reflect dopaminergic pathology, nonetheless benefit from dopaminergic drugs. For example, problems such as anxiety, panic attacks, depression, sweating, sensory problems, freezing, and constipation all tend to be worse during "off" periods, and they improve with better dopaminergic control of the underlying PD state. Approximately 50% of PD patients suffer depression during the course of the disease that is frequently underdiagnosed and undertreated. Antiparkinsonian agents can help, but antidepressants should not be withheld, particularly for patients with major depression. Serotonin syndromes have been a theoretical concern with the combined use of selective serotonin reuptake inhibitors (SSRIs) and MAO-B inhibitors, but are rarely encountered. Anxiety can be treated with short-acting benzodiazepines.

Psychosis can be a major problem in PD. In contrast to AD, hallucinations are typically visual, formed, and nonthreatening and can limit the use of dopaminergic agents to adequately control PD features. Psychosis in PD often responds to low doses of atypical neuroleptics. Clozapine is the most effective, but it can be associated with agranulocytosis, and regular monitoring is required. For this reason, many physicians start with quetiapine even though it is not as effective as clozapine in controlled trials. Hallucinations in PD patients are often a harbinger of a developing dementia.

Dementia in PD (PDD) is common, affecting as many as 80% of patients. Its frequency increases with aging and, in contrast to AD, primarily affects executive functions and attention, with relative sparing of language, memory, and calculations. PDD is the commonest cause of nursing home placement for PD patients. When dementia precedes, or develops within 1 year after, the onset of motor dysfunction, it is by convention referred to as dementia with Lewy bodies (DLB; Chap. 29). These patients are particularly prone to have hallucinations and diurnal fluctuations. Pathologically, DLB is characterized by Lewy bodies distributed throughout the cerebral cortex (especially the hippocampus and amygdala). It is likely that DLB and PDD represent a PD spectrum rather than separate disease entities. Levodopa and other dopaminergic drugs can aggravate cognitive function in demented patients and should be stopped or reduced to try and provide a compromise between antiparkinsonian benefit and preserved cognitive function. Drugs are usually discontinued in the following sequence: anticholinergics, amantadine, dopamine agonists, COMT inhibitors, and MAO-B inhibitors. Eventually, patients with cognitive impairment should be managed with the lowest dose of standard levodopa that provides meaningful antiparkinsonian effects and does not aggravate mental function. Anticholinesterase agents such as rivastigmine and donepezil reduce the rate of deterioration of measures of cognitive function in controlled studies and can improve attention. Memantine, an antiglutamatergic agent, may also provide benefit for some PDD patients.

Autonomic disturbances are common and frequently require attention. Orthostatic hypotension can be problematic and contribute to falling. Initial treatment should include adding salt to the diet and elevating the head of the bed to prevent overnight sodium natriuresis. Low doses of fludrocortisol (Florinef) or midodrine control most cases. Vasopressin, erythropoietin, and the norepinephrine precursor 3-0-methylDOPS can be used in severe cases. If orthostatic hypotension is prominent in early disease, MSA should be considered. Sexual dysfunction can be helped with sildenafil or tadalafil. Urinary problems, especially in males, should be treated in consultation with a urologist to exclude prostate problems. Anticholinergic agents, such as Ditropan, may be helpful. Constipation can be a very important problem for PD patients. Mild laxatives can be useful, but physicians should first ensure that patients are drinking adequate amounts of fluid and consuming a diet rich in bulk with green leafy vegetables and bran. Agents that promote GI motility can also be helpful.

Sleep disturbances are common in PD patients, with many experiencing fragmented sleep with excess daytime sleepiness. Restless leg syndrome, sleep apnea, and other sleep disorders should be treated as appropriate. REM behavior disorder (RBD) may precede the onset of motor features. This syndrome is composed of violent movements and vocalizations during REM sleep, possibly representing acting out of dreams due to a failure of the normal inhibition of motor movements that typically accompanies REM sleep. Low doses of clonazepam are usually effective in controlling this problem. Consultation with a sleep specialist and polysomnography may be necessary to identify and optimally treat sleep problems.

NONPHARMACOLOGIC THERAPY Gait dysfunction with falling is an important cause of disability in PD. Dopaminergic therapies can help patients whose gait is worse in "off" time, but there are currently no specific therapies available. Canes and walkers may become necessary.

Freezing episodes, where patients freeze in place for seconds to minutes, are another cause of falling. Freezing during "off" periods may respond to dopaminergic therapies, but there are no specific treatments for "on" period freezing. Some patients will respond to sensory cues such as marching in place, singing a song, or stepping over an imaginary line.

Exercise, with a full range of active and passive movements, has been shown to improve and maintain function for PD patients. It is less clear that formal physical therapy is necessary, unless there is a specific indication. It is important for patients to maintain social and intellectual activities to the extent possible. Education, assistance with financial planning, social services, and attention to home safety are important elements of the overall care plan. Information is available through numerous PD foundations and on the web, but should be reviewed with physicians to ensure accuracy. The needs of the caregiver should not be neglected. Caring for a person with PD involves a substantial work effort and there is an increased incidence of depression among caregivers. Support groups for patients and caregivers may be useful.

CURRENT MANAGEMENT OF PD The management of PD should be tailored to the needs of the individual patient, and there is no single treatment approach that is universally accepted. Clearly, if an agent could be demonstrated to have disease-modifying effects, it should be initiated at the time of diagnosis. Indeed, constipation, REM behavior disorder, and anosmia may represent pre-motor features of PD and could permit the initiation of a disease-modifying therapy even prior to onset of the classical motor features of the disease. However, no therapy has yet been proved to be disease-modifying. For now, physicians must use their judgment in deciding whether or not to introduce rasagiline (see earlier) or other drugs for their possible disease-modifying effects.

The next important issue to address is when to initiate symptomatic therapy. Several studies now suggest that it may be best to start therapy at the time of diagnosis in order to preserve beneficial compensatory mechanisms and possibly provide functional benefits even in the early stage of the disease. Levodopa remains the most effective symptomatic therapy for PD, and some recommend starting it immediately using relatively low doses, but many others prefer to delay levodopa treatment, particularly in younger patients, in order to reduce the risk of motor complications. Another approach is to begin with an MAO-B inhibitor and/or a dopamine agonist, and reserve levodopa for later stages when these drugs can no longer provide satisfactory control. In making this decision, the age, degree of disability, and side-effect profile of the drug must all be considered. In patients with more severe disability, the elderly, those with cognitive impairment, or where the diagnosis is uncertain, most physicians would initiate therapy with levodopa. Regardless of initial choice, it is important not to deny patients levodopa when they cannot be adequately controlled with alternative medications.

If motor complications develop, they can initially be treated by manipulating the frequency and dose of levodopa or by combining lower doses of levodopa with a dopamine agonist, a COMT inhibitor, or an MAO-B inhibitor. Amantadine is the only drug that has been demonstrated to treat dyskinesia without worsening parkinsonism, but benefits may be short-lasting and there are important side effects. In severe cases, it is usually necessary to consider a surgical therapy such as DBS if the patient is a suitable candidate, but as described above, these procedures have their own set of complications. There are ongoing efforts aimed at developing a long-acting oral or transdermal formulation of levodopa that mirrors the pharmacokinetic properties of a levodopa infusion. Such a formulation might provide all of the benefits of levodopa without motor complications and avoid the need for polypharmacy and surgical intervention.

A decision tree that considers the various treatment options and decision points for the management of PD is provided in Fig. 30-7.

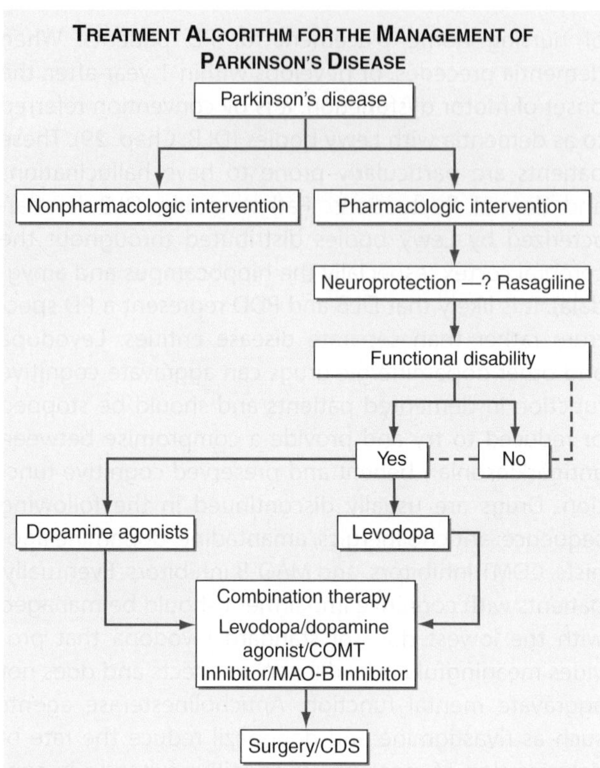

FIGURE 30-7

Treatment options for the management of PD. Decision points include:

a. Introduction of a neuroprotective therapy: No drug has been established to have or is currently approved for neuroprotection or disease modification, but there are several agents that have this potential based on laboratory and preliminary clinical studies (e.g., rasagiline 1 mg/d, coenzyme Q10 1200 mg/d, the dopamine agonists ropinirole and pramipexole).

b. When to initiate symptomatic therapy: There is a trend toward initiating therapy at the time of diagnosis or early in the course of the disease because patients may have some disability even at an early stage, and there is the possibility that early treatment may preserve beneficial compensatory mechanisms; however, some experts recommend waiting until there is functional disability before initiating therapy.

c. What therapy to initiate: Many experts favor starting with an MAO-B inhibitor in mildly affected patients because of the potential for a disease-modifying effect; dopamine agonists for younger patients with functionally significant disability to reduce the risk of motor complications; and levodopa for patients with more advanced disease, the elderly, or those with cognitive impairment.

d. Management of motor complications: Motor complications are typically approached with combination therapy to try and reduce dyskinesia and enhance the "on" time. When medical therapies cannot provide satisfactory control, surgical therapies can be considered.

e. Nonpharmacologic approaches: Interventions such as exercise, education, and support should be considered throughout the course of the disease.

Source: Adapted from CW Olanow et al: Neurology 72:S1, 2009.

HYPERKINETIC MOVEMENT DISORDERS

Hyperkinetic movement disorders are characterized by involuntary movements that may occur in isolation or in combination (Table 30-6). The major hyperkinetic movement disorders and the diseases with which they are associated are considered in this section.

TABLE 30-6

HYPERKINETIC MOVEMENT DISORDERS	
Tremor	Rhythmic oscillation of a body part due to intermittent muscle contractions
Dystonia	Involuntary patterned sustained or repeated muscle contractions often associated with twisting movements and abnormal posture
Athetosis	Slow, distal, writhing, involuntary movements with a propensity to affect the arms and hands
Chorea	Rapid, semipurposeful, graceful, dance-like nonpatterned involuntary movements involving distal or proximal muscle groups
Myoclonus	Sudden, brief (<100 ms), jerk-like, arrhythmic muscle twitches
Tic	Brief, repeated, stereotyped muscle contractions that are often suppressible. Can be simple and involve a single muscle group or complex and affect a range of motor activities

TREMOR

CLINICAL FEATURES

Tremor consists of alternating contractions of agonist and antagonist muscles in an oscillating, rhythmic manner. It can be most prominent at rest (rest tremor), on assuming a posture (postural tremor), or on actively reaching for a target (kinetic tremor). Tremor is also assessed based on distribution, frequency, and related neurologic dysfunction.

PD is characterized by a resting tremor, essential tremor (ET) by a postural tremor, and cerebellar disease by an intention or kinetic tremor. Normal individuals can have a physiologic tremor that typically manifests as a mild, high-frequency, postural or action tremor that is usually of no clinical consequence and often is only appreciated with an accelerometer. An enhanced physiologic tremor (EPT) can be seen in up to 10% of the population, often in association with anxiety, fatigue, underlying metabolic disturbance (e.g., hyperthyroidism, electrolyte abnormalities), drugs (e.g., valproate, lithium), or toxins (e.g., alcohol). Treatment is initially directed to the control of any underlying disorder and, if necessary, can often be improved with a β blocker.

ET is the commonest movement disorder, affecting approximately 5–10 million persons in the United States. It can present in childhood, but dramatically increases in prevalence over the age of 70 years. ET is characterized by a high-frequency tremor (up to 11 Hz) that predominantly affects the upper extremities. The tremor is most often manifest as a postural or kinetic tremor. It is typically bilateral and symmetric, but may begin on one side and remain asymmetric. Patients with severe ET can have an intention tremor with overshoot and slowness of movement. Tremor involves the head in ~30% of cases, voice in ~20%, tongue in ~20%, face/jaw in ~10%, and lower limbs in ~10%. The tremor is characteristically improved by alcohol and worsened by stress. Subtle impairment of coordination or tandem walking may be present. Disturbances of hearing, cognition, and even olfaction have been described, but usually the neurologic examination is normal aside from tremor. The major differential is a dystonic tremor (see later) or PD. PD can usually be differentiated from ET based on the presence of bradykinesia, rigidity, micrographia, and other parkinsonian features. However, the examiner should be aware that PD patients may have a postural tremor and ET patients may develop a rest tremor. These typically begin after a latency of a few seconds (emergent tremor). The examiner must take care to differentiate the effect of tremor on measurement of tone in ET from the cog-wheel rigidity found in PD.

ETIOLOGY AND PATHOPHYSIOLOGY

The etiology and pathophysiology of ET are not known. Approximately 50% of cases have a positive family history with an autosomal dominant pattern of inheritance. Linkage studies have detected loci at chromosomes 3q13 (ETM-1), 2p22-25 (ETM-2), and 6p23 (ETM-3). Recent genomewide studies demonstrate an association with the *LINGO1* gene, particularly in patients with young-onset ET, and it is likely that there are many other undiscovered loci. Candidate genes include the dopamine D3 receptor and proteins that map to the cerebellum. The cerebellum and inferior olives have been implicated as possible sites of a "tremor pacemaker" based on the presence of cerebellar signs and increased metabolic activity and blood flow in these regions in some patients. Recent pathologic studies have described cerebellar pathology with a loss of Purkinje's cells and axonal torpedoes. However, the precise pathologic correlate of ET remains to be defined.

TREATMENT

Many cases are mild and require no treatment other than reassurance. Occasionally, tremor can be severe and interfere with eating, writing, and activities of daily living. This is more likely to occur as the patient ages and is often associated with a reduction in tremor frequency. β Blockers or primidone are the standard drug therapies for ET and help in about 50% of cases. Propranolol (20–80 mg daily, given in divided doses) is usually effective at relatively low doses, but higher doses may be effective in some patients. The drug is contraindicated in patients with bradycardia or asthma. Hand tremor tends to be most improved, while head tremor is often refractory. Primidone can be helpful, but should be started at low doses (12.5 mg) and gradually increased (125–250 tid) to avoid sedation. Benefits have been reported with gabapentin and topiramate. Botulinum toxin injections may be helpful for limb or voice tremor, but treatment can be associated with secondary muscle weakness. Surgical therapies targeting the VIM nucleus of the thalamus can be very effective for severe and drug-resistant cases.

DYSTONIA

CLINICAL FEATURES

Dystonia is a disorder characterized by sustained or repetitive involuntary muscle contractions frequently associated with twisting or repetitive movements and abnormal postures. Dystonia can range from minor contractions in an individual muscle group to severe and disabling involvement of multiple muscle groups. The frequency is estimated at 300,000 cases in the United States, but is likely much higher as many cases may not be recognized. Dystonia is often brought out by voluntary movements (action dystonia) and can become sustained and extend to involve other body regions. It can be aggravated by stress and fatigue, and attenuated by relaxation and sensory tricks such as touching the affected body part (geste antagoniste). Dystonia can be classified according to age of onset (childhood vs adult), distribution (focal, multifocal, segmental, or generalized), or etiology (primary or secondary).

PRIMARY DYSTONIAS

Several gene mutations are associated with dystonia. Idiopathic torsion dystonia (ITD) or Oppenheim's dystonia is predominantly a childhood-onset form of dystonia with an autosomal dominant pattern of inheritance that primarily affects Ashkenazi Jewish families. The majority of patients have an age of onset younger than 26 years (mean 14 years). In young-onset patients, dystonia typically begins in the foot or the arm and in 60–70% progresses to involve other limbs as well as the head and neck. In severe cases, patients can suffer disabling postural deformities that compromise mobility. Severity can vary within a family, with some affected relatives having severe disability and others a mild dystonia that may not even be appreciated. Most childhood-onset cases are linked to a mutation in the DYT1 gene located on chromosome 9q34 resulting in a trinucleotide GAG deletion with loss of one of a pair of glutamic acid residues in the protein torsin A. DYT1 mutations are found in 90% of Ashkenazi Jewish patients with ITD and probably relate to a founder effect that occurred about 350 years ago. There is variable penetrance, with only about 30% of gene carriers expressing a clinical phenotype. Why some gene carriers express dystonia and others do not is not known. The function of torsin A is unknown, but it is a member of the AAA^+ (ATPase) family that resembles heat-shock proteins and may be related to protein regulation. The precise pathology responsible for dystonia is not known.

Dopa responsive dystonia (DRD) or the Segawa variant (DYT5) is a dominantly inherited form of childhood-onset dystonia due to a mutation in the gene that encodes for GTP cyclohydrolase-I, the rate-limiting enzyme for the synthesis of tetrahydrobiopterin. This mutation leads to a defect in the biochemical synthesis of tyrosine hydroxylase, the rate-limiting enzyme in the formation of dopamine. DRD typically presents in early childhood (1–12 years), and is characterized by foot dystonia that interferes with walking. Patients often experience diurnal fluctuations, with worsening of gait as the day progresses and improvement with sleep. DRD is typified by an excellent and sustained response to small doses of levodopa. Some patients may present with parkinsonian features, but can be differentiated from juvenile PD by normal striatal fluorodopa uptake on positron emission tomography and the absence of levodopa-induced dyskinesias. DRD may occasionally be confused with cerebral palsy because patients appear to have spasticity, increased reflexes, and Babinski responses (which likely reflect a dystonic contraction rather than an upper motor neuron lesion). Any patient suspected of having a childhood-onset dystonia should receive a trial of levodopa to exclude this condition.

Mutations in the *THAP1* gene (DYT6) on chromosome 8p21q22 have been identified in Amish families and are the cause of as many as 25% of cases of non-DYT1 young-onset primary torsion dystonia. Patients are more likely to have dystonia beginning in the brachial and cervical muscles, which later can become generalized and associated with speech impairment. Myoclonic dystonia (DYT11) results from a mutation in the epsilon-sarcoglycan gene on chromosome 7q21. It typically manifests as a combination of dystonia and myoclonic jerks, frequently accompanied by psychiatric disturbances.

FOCAL DYSTONIAS

These are the most common forms of dystonia. They typically present in the fourth to sixth decades and affect women more than men. The major types are (1) *blepharospasm*—dystonic contractions of the eyelids with increased blinking that can interfere with reading, watching TV, and driving. This can sometimes be so severe as to cause functional blindness. (2) *Oromandibular dystonia* (OMD)—contractions of muscles of the lower face, lips, tongue, and jaw (opening or closing). Meige syndrome is a combination of OMD and blepharospasm that predominantly affects women older than age 60 years. (3) *Spasmodic dysphonia*—dystonic contractions of the vocal cords during phonation, causing impaired speech. Most cases affect the adductor muscles and cause speech to have a choking or strained quality. Less commonly, the abductors are affected, leading to speech with a breathy or whispering quality. (4) *Cervical dystonia*—dystonic contractions of neck muscles causing the head to deviate to one side (*torticollis*), in a forward direction (*anterocollis*), or in a backward direction (*retrocollis*). Muscle contractions can be painful, and associated with a secondary cervical radiculopathy. (5) *Limb dystonias*—These can be present in either arms or legs and are often brought out by task-specific activities such as handwriting (writer's cramp), playing a musical instrument (musician's cramp), or putting (the yips). Focal dystonias can extend to involve other body regions (about 30% of cases), and are frequently misdiagnosed as psychiatric or orthopedic in origin. Their cause is not known, but genetic factors, autoimmunity, and trauma have been suggested. Focal dystonias are often associated with a high-frequency tremor that resembles ET. Dystonic tremor can usually be distinguished from ET because it tends to occur in conjunction with the dystonic contraction and disappears when the dystonia is relieved.

SECONDARY DYSTONIAS

These develop as a consequence of drugs or other neurologic disorders. Drug-induced dystonia is most commonly seen with neuroleptic drugs or after chronic levodopa treatment in PD patients. Secondary dystonia can also be observed following discrete lesions in the striatum, pallidum, thalamus, cortex, and brainstem due to infarction, anoxia, trauma, tumor, infection, or toxins such as manganese or carbon monoxide. In these cases, dystonia often assumes a segmental distribution. More rarely, dystonia can develop following peripheral nerve injury and be associated with features of chronic regional pain syndrome.

DYSTONIA PLUS SYNDROMES

Dystonia may occur as a part of neurodegenerative conditions such as HD, PD, Wilson's disease, CBGD, PSP, the Lubag form of dystonia-parkinsonism (DYT3), and mitochondrial encephalopathies. In contrast to the primary dystonias, dystonia is usually not the dominant neurologic feature in these conditions.

PATHOPHYSIOLOGY OF DYSTONIA

The pathophysiologic basis of dystonia is not known. The phenomenon is characterized by co-contracting synchronous bursts of agonist and antagonist muscle groups. This is associated with a loss of inhibition at multiple levels of the nervous system as well as increased cortical excitability and reorganization. Attention has focused on the basal ganglia as the site of origin of at least some types of dystonia as there are alterations in blood flow and metabolism in basal ganglia structures. Further, ablation or stimulation of the globus pallidus can both induce and ameliorate dystonia. The dopamine system has also been implicated, as dopaminergic therapies can both induce and treat some forms of dystonia.

TREATMENT Dystonia

Treatment of dystonia is for the most part symptomatic except in rare cases where treatment of a primary underlying condition is available. Wilson's disease should be ruled out in young patients with dystonia. Levodopa should be tried in all cases of childhood-onset dystonia to rule out DRD. High-dose anticholinergics (e.g., trihexyphenidyl 20–120 mg/d) may be beneficial in children, but adults can rarely tolerate high doses because of cognitive impairment with hallucinations. Oral baclofen (20–120 mg) may be helpful, but benefits if present are usually modest and side effects of sedation, weakness, and memory loss can be problematic. Intrathecal infusion of baclofen is more likely to be helpful particularly with leg and trunk dystonia, but benefits are frequently not sustained and complications can be serious and include infection, seizures, and coma. Tetrabenazine (the usual starting dose is 12.5 mg/d and the average treating dose is 25–75 mg/d) may be helpful in some patients, but use may be limited by sedation and the development of parkinsonism. Neuroleptics can improve as well as induce dystonia, but they are typically not recommended because of their potential to induce extrapyramidal side effects, including tardive dystonia. Clonazepam and diazepam are rarely effective.

Botulinum toxin has become the preferred treatment for patients with focal dystonia, particularly where involvement is limited to small muscle groups such as in blepharospasm, torticollis, and spasmodic dysphonia. Botulinum toxin acts by blocking the release of acetylcholine at the neuromuscular junction, leading to muscle weakness and reduced dystonia, but excessive weakness may ensue and can be troublesome particularly if it involves neck and swallowing muscles. Two serotypes of botulinum toxin are available (A and B). Both are effective, and it is not clear that there are advantages of one over the other. No systemic side effects are encountered with the doses typically employed, but benefits are transient and repeat injections are required at 2- to 5-month intervals. Some patients fail to respond after having experienced an initial benefit. This has been attributed to antibody formation, but improper muscle selection, injection technique, and inadequate dose should be excluded.

Surgical therapy is an alternative for patients with severe dystonia who are not responsive to other treatments. Peripheral procedures such as rhizotomy and myotomy were used in the past to treat cervical dystonia, but are now rarely employed. DBS of the pallidum can provide dramatic benefits for patients with primary DYT1 dystonia. This represents a major therapeutic advance as previously there was no consistently effective therapy, especially for these patients who had severe disability. Benefits tend to be obtained with a lower frequency of stimulation and often occur after a relatively long latency (weeks) in comparison to PD. Better results are typically obtained in younger patients. Recent studies suggest that DBS may also be valuable for patients with focal and secondary dystonias, although results are less consistent. Supportive treatments such as physical therapy and education are important and should be a part of the treatment regimen.

Physicians should be aware of dystonic storm, a rare but potentially fatal condition that can occur in response to a stress situation such as surgery in patients with preexisting dystonia. It consists of the acute onset of generalized and persistent dystonic contractions that can involve the vocal cords or laryngeal muscles, leading to airway obstruction. Patients may experience rhabdomyolysis with renal failure. Patients should be managed in an ICU with protection of airway if required. Treatment can be instituted with one or a combination of anticholinergics, diphenhydramine, baclofen, benzodiazepines, and dopamine agonists/antagonists. Spasms may be difficult to control, and anesthesia with muscle paralysis may be required.

CHOREAS

HUNTINGTON'S DISEASE (HD)

HD is a progressive, fatal, highly penetrant autosomal dominant disorder characterized by motor, behavioral, and cognitive dysfunction. The disease is named for George Huntington, a family physician who described cases on Long Island, New York, in the nineteenth century. Onset is typically between the ages of 25 and 45 years (range, 3–70 years) with a prevalence of 2–8 cases per 100,000 and an average age at death of 60 years. It is prevalent in Europe, North and South America, and Australia but is rare in African blacks and Asians. HD is characterized by rapid, nonpatterned, semipurposeful, involuntary choreiform movements. In the early stages, the chorea tends to be focal or segmental, but progresses over time to involve multiple body regions. Dysarthria, gait disturbance, and oculomotor abnormalities are common features. With advancing disease, there may be a reduction in chorea and emergence of dystonia, rigidity, bradykinesia, myoclonus, and spasticity. Functional decline is often predicted by progressive weight loss despite adequate calorie intake. In younger patients (about 10% of cases), HD can present as an akinetic-rigid or parkinsonian syndrome (Westphal variant). HD patients eventually develop behavioral and cognitive disturbances, and the majority progress to dementia. Depression with suicidal tendencies, aggressive behavior, and psychosis can be prominent features. HD patients may also develop non-insulin-dependent diabetes mellitus and neuroendocrine abnormalities, e.g., hypothalamic dysfunction. A clinical diagnosis of HD can be strongly suspected in cases of chorea with a positive family history. The disease predominantly strikes the striatum. Progressive atrophy of the caudate nuclei, which form the lateral margins of the lateral ventricles, can be visualized by MRI (Fig. 30-8). More diffuse cortical atrophy is seen in the middle and late stages of the disease. Supportive studies include reduced metabolic activity in the caudate nucleus and putamen. Genetic testing can be used to confirm the diagnosis and to detect at-risk individuals in the family, but this must be performed with caution and in conjunction with trained counselors, as positive results can worsen depression and generate suicidal reactions. The neuropathology of HD consists of prominent neuronal loss and gliosis in the caudate nucleus and putamen; similar changes are also widespread in the cerebral cortex. Intraneuronal inclusions containing aggregates of ubiquitin and the mutant protein huntingtin are found in the nuclei of affected neurons.

ETIOLOGY

HD is caused by an increase in the number of polyglutamine (CAG) repeats (>40) in the coding sequence of the huntingtin gene located on the short arm of chromosome 4. The larger the number of repeats, the earlier the disease is manifest. Acceleration of the process tends to occur, particularly in males, with subsequent generations having larger numbers of repeats and earlier age of disease onset, a phenomenon referred to as anticipation. The gene encodes the highly conserved cytoplasmic protein huntingtin, which is widely distributed clean in neurons throughout the CNS, but whose function is not known. Models of HD with striatal

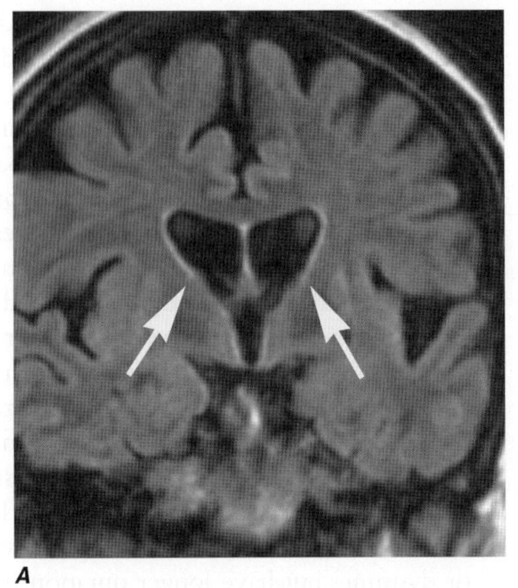
A

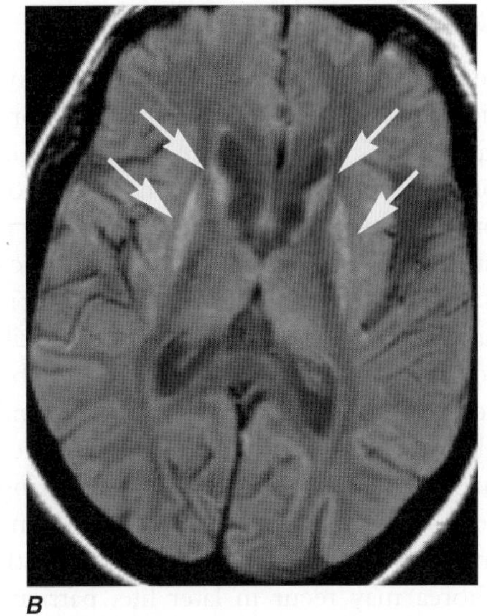
B

FIGURE 30-8

Huntington's disease. *A.* Coronal FLAIR MRI shows enlargement of the lateral ventricles reflecting typical atrophy (*arrows*). ***B.*** Axial FLAIR image demonstrates abnormal high signal in the caudate and putamen (*arrows*).

pathology can be induced by excitotoxic agents such as kainic acid and 3-nitropoprionic acid, which promote calcium entry into the cell and cytotoxicity. Mitochondrial dysfunction has been demonstrated in the striatum and skeletal muscle of symptomatic and presymptomatic individuals. Fragments of the mutant huntingtin protein can be toxic, possibly by translocating into the nucleus and interfering with transcriptional upregulation of regulatory proteins. Neuronal inclusions found in affected regions in HD may represent a protective mechanism aimed at segregating and facilitating the clearance of these toxic proteins.

TREATMENT Huntington's Disease

Treatment involves a multidisciplinary approach, with medical, neuropsychiatric, social, and genetic counseling for patients and their families. Dopamine-blocking agents may control the chorea. Tetrabenazine has recently been approved for the treatment of chorea in the United States, but it may cause secondary parkinsonism. Neuroleptics are generally not recommended because of their potential to induce other more troubling movement disorders and because HD chorea tends to be self-limited and is usually not disabling. Depression and anxiety can be greater problems, and patients should be treated with appropriate antidepressant and antianxiety drugs and monitored for mania and suicidal ideations. Psychosis can be treated with atypical neuroleptics such as clozapine (50–600 mg/d), quetiapine (50–600 mg/d), and risperidone (2–8 mg/d). There is no adequate treatment for the cognitive or motor decline. A neuroprotective therapy that slows or stops disease progression is the major unmet medical need in HD. Promitochondrial agents such as ubiquinone and creatine are being tested as possible disease-modifying therapies. Antiglutamate agents, caspase inhibitors, inhibitors of protein aggregation, neurotrophic factors, and transplantation of fetal striatal cells are areas of active research, but none has as yet been demonstrated to have a disease-modifying effect.

HUNTINGTON'S DISEASE–LIKE 1 (HDL1), HUNTINGTON'S DISEASE–LIKE 2 (HDL2)

HDL1 is a rare inherited disorder due to mutations of the protein located at 20p12. Patients exhibit onset of personality change in the third or fourth decade, followed by chorea, rigidity, myoclonus, ataxia, and epilepsy. HDL2 is an autosomal dominantly inherited disorder manifesting in the third or fourth decade with a variety of movement disorders, including chorea, dystonia, or parkinsonism and dementia. Most patients are of African descent. Acanthocytosis can sometimes be seen in these patients, and they must be differentiated from neuroacanthocytosis. HDL2 is caused by an abnormally expanded CTG/CAG trinucleotide repeat expansion in the *junctophilin-3* (*JPH3*) gene on chromosome 16q24.3. The pathology of HDL2 also demonstrates intranuclear inclusions immunoreactive for ubiquitin and expanded polyglutamine repeats.

OTHER CHOREAS

Chorea can be seen in a number of disorders. Sydenham's chorea (originally called St. Vitus' dance) is more common in females and is typically seen in childhood (5–15 years). It often develops in association with prior exposure to group A streptococcal infection and is thought to be autoimmune in nature. With the reduction in the incidence of rheumatic fever, the incidence of Sydenham's chorea has fallen, but it can still be seen in developing countries. It is characterized by the acute onset of choreiform movements, behavioral disturbances, and occasionally other motor dysfunctions. Chorea generally responds to dopamine-blocking agents, valproic acid, and carbamazepine, but is self-limited and treatment is generally restricted to those with severe chorea. Chorea may recur in later life, particularly in association with pregnancy (chorea gravidarum) or treatment with sex hormones.

Chorea-acanthocytosis (neuroacanthocytosis) is a progressive and typically fatal autosomal recessive disorder that is characterized by chorea coupled with red cell abnormalities on peripheral blood smear (acanthocytes). The chorea can be severe and associated with self-mutilating behavior, dystonia, tics, seizures, and a polyneuropathy. Mutations in the *VPS13A* gene on chromosome 9q21 encoding chorein have been described. A phenotypically similar X-linked form of the disorder has been described in older individuals who have reactivity with Kell blood group antigens (McLeod syndrome). A benign hereditary chorea of childhood (BHC1) due to mutations in the gene for thyroid transcription factor 1 and a late-onset benign senile chorea (BHC2) have also been described. It is important to ensure that patients with these types of choreas do not have HD.

A range of neurodegenerative diseases with brain iron accumulation (NBIA) manifesting with chorea and dystonia have been described including autosomal dominant neuroferritinopathy, autosomal recessive pantothenate-kinase-associated neurodegeneration (PKAN; Hallervorden-Spatz disease), and aceruloplasminemia. These disorders have excess iron accumulation on MRI and a characteristic "eye of the tiger" appearance in the globus pallidus due to iron accumulation.

Chorea may also occur in association with vascular diseases, hypo- and hyperglycemia, and a variety of infections and degenerative disorders. Systemic lupus erythematosus is the most common systemic disorder that causes chorea; the chorea can last for days to years. Choreas can also be seen with hyperthyroidism, autoimmune disorders including Sjögren's syndrome, infectious disorders including HIV disease, metabolic alterations, polycythemia rubra vera (following open-heart surgery in the pediatric population), and in association with many medications (especially anticonvulsants, cocaine, CNS stimulants, estrogens, lithium). Chorea can also be seen in paraneoplastic syndromes associated with anti-CRMP-5 or anti-Hu antibodies.

Paroxysmal dyskinesias are a group of rare disorders characterized by episodic, brief involuntary movements that can include chorea, dystonia, and ballismus. Paroxysmal kinesigenic dyskinesia (PKD) is a familial childhood-onset disorder in which chorea or chorea-dystonia is precipitated by sudden movement or running. Attacks may affect one side of the body, last seconds to minutes at a time, and recur several times a day. Prognosis is usually good, with spontaneous remission in later life. Low-dose anticonvulsant therapy (e.g., carbamazepine) is usually effective if required. Paroxysmal nonkinesigenic dyskinesia (PNKD) involves attacks of dyskinesia precipitated by alcohol, caffeine, stress, or fatigue. Like PKD, it is familial and childhood in onset and the episodes are often choreic or dystonic, but have longer duration (minutes to hours) and are less frequent (1–3/d).

TREATMENT Paroxysmal Nonkinesigenic Dyskinesia

Diagnosis and treatment of the underlying condition, where possible, are the first priority. Tetrabenazine, neuroleptics, dopamine-blocking agents, propranolol, clonazepam, and baclofen may be helpful. Treatment is not indicated if the condition is mild and self-limited. Most patients with PKND do not benefit from anticonvulsant drugs but some may respond to clonazepam.

HEMIBALLISMUS

Hemiballismus is a violent form of chorea composed of wild, flinging, large-amplitude movements on one side of the body. Proximal limb muscles tend to be predominantly affected. The movements may be so severe as to cause exhaustion, dehydration, local injury, and in extreme cases, death. The most common cause is a partial lesion (infarct or hemorrhage) in the subthalamic nucleus (STN), but rare cases can also be seen with lesions in the putamen. Fortunately, hemiballismus is usually self-limiting and tends to resolve spontaneously after weeks or months. Dopamine-blocking drugs can be helpful but can themselves lead to movement disorders. In extreme cases, pallidotomy can be very effective. Interestingly, surgically induced lesions or DBS of the STN in PD are usually not associated with hemiballismus.

TICS

TOURETTE'S SYNDROME (TS)

TS is a neurobehavioral disorder named after the French neurologist Georges Gilles de la Tourette. It predominantly affects males, and prevalence is estimated to be

0.03–1.6%, but it is likely that many mild cases do not come to medical attention. TS is characterized by multiple motor tics often accompanied by vocalizations (phonic tics). A *tic* is a brief, rapid, recurrent, and seemingly purposeless stereotyped motor contraction. Motor tics can be simple, with movement only affecting an individual muscle group (e.g., blinking, twitching of the nose, jerking of the neck), or complex, with coordinated involvement of multiple muscle groups (e.g., jumping, sniffing, head banging, and echopraxia [mimicking movements]). Vocal tics can also be simple (e.g., grunting) or complex (e.g., echolalia [repeating other people's words], palilalia [repeating one's own words], and coprolalia [expression of obscene words]). Patients may also experience sensory tics, composed of unpleasant focal sensations in the face, head, or neck. Patients characteristically can voluntarily suppress tics for short periods of time, but then experience an irresistible urge to express them. Tics vary in intensity and may be absent for days or weeks only to recur, occasionally in a different pattern. Tics tend to present between ages 2 and 15 years (mean 7 years) and often lessen or even disappear in adulthood. Associated behavioral disturbances include anxiety, depression, attention deficit hyperactivity disorder, and obsessive-compulsive disorder. Patients may experience personality disorders, self-destructive behaviors, difficulties in school, and impaired interpersonal relationships. Tics may present in adulthood and can be seen in association with a variety of other disorders, including PD, HD, trauma, dystonia, drugs (e.g., levodopa, neuroleptics), and toxins.

ETIOLOGY AND PATHOPHYSIOLOGY

TS is thought to be a genetic disorder, but no specific gene mutation has been identified. Current evidence supports a complex inheritance pattern, with one or more major genes, multiple loci, low penetrance, and environmental influences. The risk of a family with one affected child having a second is about 25%. The pathophysiology of TS is not known, but alterations in dopamine neurotransmission, opioids, and second-messenger systems have been proposed. Some cases of TS may be the consequence of an autoimmune response to β-hemolytic streptococcal infection (pediatric autoimmune neuropsychiatric disorder associated with streptococcal infection [PANDAS]); however, this remains controversial.

TREATMENT Tourette's Syndrome

Patients with mild disease often only require education and counseling (for themselves and family members). Drug treatment is indicated when the tics are disabling and interfere with quality of life. Therapy is generally initiated with the α-agonist clonidine, starting at low doses and gradually increasing the dose and frequency until satisfactory control is achieved. Guanfacine (0.5–2 mg/d) is an α-agonist that is preferred by many clinicians because it only requires once-a-day dosing. If these agents are not effective, antipsychotics can be employed. Atypical neuroleptics (risperidone, olanzapine, ziprasidone) are preferred as they are thought to be associated with a reduced risk of extrapyramidal side effects. If they are not effective, low doses of classical neuroleptics such as haloperidol, fluphenazine, or pimozide can be tried. Botulinum toxin injections can be effective in controlling focal tics that involve small muscle groups. Behavioral features, and particularly anxiety and compulsions, can be a disabling feature of TS and should be treated. The potential value of DBS targeting the anterior portion of the internal capsule is currently being explored.

MYOCLONUS

Myoclonus is a brief, rapid (<100 ms) shock-like, jerky movement consisting of single or repetitive muscle discharges. Myoclonic jerks can be focal, multifocal, segmental, or generalized and can occur spontaneously, in association with voluntary movement (action myoclonus) or in response to an external stimulus (reflex or startle myoclonus). Negative myoclonus consists of a twitch due to a brief loss of muscle activity (e.g., asterixis in hepatic failure). Myoclonic jerks differ from tics in that they interfere with normal movement and are not suppressible. They can be seen in association with pathology in cortical, subcortical, or spinal cord regions and associated with hypoxemic damage (especially following cardiac arrest), encephalopathy, and neurodegeneration. Reversible myoclonus can be seen with metabolic disturbances (renal failure, electrolyte imbalance, hypocalcemia), toxins, and many medications. Essential myoclonus is a relatively benign familial condition characterized by multifocal lightning-like movements. Myoclonic jerks can be disabling when they interfere with normal movement. They can also be innocent and are commonly observed in normal people when waking up or falling asleep (hypnogogic jerks).

TREATMENT Myoclonus

Treatment primarily consists of treating the underlying condition or removing an offending agent. Pharmacologic therapy involves one or a combination of GABAergic agents such as valproic acid (800–3000 mg/d), piracetam (8–20 g/d), clonazepam (2–15 mg/d), or primidone (500–1000 mg/d). Recent studies suggest that levetiracetam may be particularly effective.

DRUG-INDUCED MOVEMENT DISORDERS

This important group of movement disorders is primarily associated with drugs that block dopamine receptors (neuroleptics) or central dopaminergic transmission. These drugs are primarily used in psychiatry, but it is important to appreciate that drugs used in the treatment of nausea or vomiting (e.g., Compazine) or gastroesophageal disorders (e.g., metoclopramide) are neuroleptic agents. Hyperkinetic movement disorders secondary to neuroleptic drugs can be divided into those that present acutely, subacutely, or after prolonged exposure (tardive syndromes). Dopamine-blocking drugs can also be associated with a reversible parkinsonian syndrome for which anticholinergics are often concomitantly prescribed, but there is concern that this may increase the risk of developing a tardive syndrome.

ACUTE

Dystonia is the most common acute hyperkinetic drug reaction. It is typically generalized in children and focal in adults (e.g., blepharospasm, torticollis, or oromandibular dystonia). The reaction can develop within minutes of exposure, and can be successfully treated in most cases with parenteral administration of anticholinergics (benztropine or diphenhydramine) or benzodiazepines (lorazepam or diazepam). Choreas, stereotypic behaviors, and tics may also be seen, particularly following acute exposure to CNS stimulants such as methylphenidate, cocaine, or amphetamines.

SUBACUTE

Akathisia is the commonest reaction in this category. It consists of motor restlessness with a need to move that is alleviated by movement. Therapy consists of removing the offending agent. When this is not possible, symptoms may be ameliorated with benzodiazepines, anticholinergics, β blockers, or dopamine agonists.

TARDIVE SYNDROMES

These disorders develop months to years after initiation of neuroleptic treatment. Tardive dyskinesia (TD) is the commonest and is typically composed of choreiform movements involving the mouth, lips, and tongue. In severe cases, the trunk, limbs, and respiratory muscles may also be affected. In approximately one-third of patients, TD remits within 3 months of stopping the drug, and most patients gradually improve over the course of several years. In contrast, abnormal movements may develop after stopping the offending agent. The movements are often mild and more upsetting to the family than to the patient, but they can be severe and disabling, particularly in the context of an underlying psychiatric disorder. Atypical antipsychotics (e.g., clozapine, risperidone, olanzapine, quetiapine, ziprasidone, and aripiprazole) are associated with a significantly lower risk of TD in comparison to traditional antipsychotics. Younger patients have a lower risk of developing neuroleptic-induced TD, whereas the elderly, females, and those with underlying organic cerebral dysfunction have been reported to be at greater risk. In addition, chronic use is associated with increased risk, and specifically, the FDA has warned that use of metoclopramide for more than 12 weeks increases the risk of TD. Since TD can be permanent and resistant to treatment, antipsychotics should be used judiciously, atypical neuroleptics should be the preferred agent whenever possible, and the need for their continued use should be regularly monitored.

Treatment primarily consists of stopping the offending agent. If the patient is receiving a traditional antipsychotic and withdrawal is not possible, replacement with an atypical antipsychotic should be tried. Abrupt cessation of a neuroleptic should be avoided as acute withdrawal can induce worsening. TD can persist after withdrawal of antipsychotics and can be difficult to treat. Benefits may be achieved with valproic acid, anticholinergics, or botulinum toxin injections. In refractory cases, catecholamine depleters such as tetrabenazine may be helpful. Tetrabenazine can be associated with dose-dependent sedation and orthostatic hypotension. Other approaches include baclofen (40–80 mg/d), clonazepam (1–8 mg/d), or valproic acid (750–3000 mg/d).

Chronic neuroleptic exposure can also be associated with tardive dystonia with preferential involvement of axial muscles and characteristic rocking movements of the trunk and pelvis. Tardive dystonia frequently persists despite stopping medication and patients are often refractory to medical therapy. Valproic acid, anticholinergics, and botulinum toxin may occasionally be beneficial. Tardive akathisia, tardive Tourette, and tardive tremor syndromes are rare but may also occur after chronic neuroleptic exposure.

Neuroleptic medications can also be associated with a neuroleptic malignant syndrome (NMS). NMS is characterized by muscle rigidity, elevated temperature, altered mental status, hyperthermia, tachycardia, labile blood pressure, renal failure, and markedly elevated creatine kinase levels. Symptoms typically evolve within days or weeks after initiating the drug. NMS can also be precipitated by the abrupt withdrawal of antiparkinsonian medications in PD patients. Treatment involves immediate cessation of the offending antipsychotic drug and the introduction of a dopaminergic agent (e.g., a dopamine agonist or levodopa), dantrolene, or a benzodiazepine. Treatment may need to be undertaken in an intensive care setting and includes supportive measures such as control of body temperature (antipyretics and cooling blankets), hydration, electrolyte replacement, and control of renal function and blood pressure.

Drugs that have serotonin-like activity (tryptophan, MDMA or "ecstasy," meperidine) or that block serotonin reuptake can induce a rare, but potentially fatal, serotonin syndrome that is characterized by confusion, hyperthermia, tachycardia, and coma as well as rigidity, ataxia, and tremor. Myoclonus is often a prominent feature, in contrast to NMS, which it resembles. Patients can be managed with propranolol, diazepam, diphenhydramine, chlorpromazine, or cyproheptadine as well as supportive measures.

A variety of drugs can also be associated with parkinsonism (see earlier) and hyperkinetic movement disorders. Some examples include phenytoin (chorea, dystonia, tremor, myoclonus), carbamazepine (tics and dystonia), tricyclic antidepressants (dyskinesias, tremor, myoclonus), fluoxetine (myoclonus, chorea, dystonia), oral contraceptives (dyskinesia), β adrenergics (tremor), buspirone (akathisia, dyskinesias, myoclonus), and digoxin, cimetidine, diazoxide, lithium, methadone, and fentanyl (dyskinesias).

RESTLESS LEGS SYNDROME

Restless legs syndrome (RLS) is a neurologic disorder that affects approximately 10% of the adult population (it is rare in Asians) and can cause significant morbidity in some. It was first described in the seventeenth century by an English physician (Thomas Willis), but has only recently been recognized as being a bona fide movement disorder. The four core symptoms required for diagnosis are as follows: an urge to move the legs, usually caused or accompanied by an unpleasant sensation in the legs; symptoms begin or worsen with rest; partial or complete relief by movement; and worsening during the evening or night.

Symptoms most commonly begin in the legs, but can spread to or even begin in the upper limbs. The unpleasant sensation is often described as a creepy-crawly feeling, paresthesia, or burning. In about 80% of patients, RLS is associated with periodic leg movements (PLMs) during sleep and occasionally while awake. These involuntary movements are usually brief, lasting no more than a few seconds, and recur every 5–90 s. The restlessness and PLMs are a major cause of sleep disturbance in patients, leading to poor-quality sleep and daytime sleepiness.

RLS is a heterogeneous condition. Primary RLS is genetic, and several loci have been found with an autosomal dominant pattern of inheritance, although penetrance may be variable. The mean age of onset in genetic forms is 27 years, although pediatric cases are recognized. The severity of symptoms is variable. Secondary RLS may be associated with pregnancy or a range of underlying disorders, including anemia, ferritin deficiency, renal failure, and peripheral neuropathy. The pathogenesis probably involves disordered dopamine function, which may be peripheral or central, in association with an abnormality of iron metabolism. Diagnosis is made on clinical grounds but can be supported by polysomnography and the demonstration of PLMs. The neurologic examination is normal. Secondary RLS should be excluded and ferritin levels, glucose, and renal function should be measured.

Most RLS sufferers have mild symptoms that do not require specific treatment. General measures to improve sleep hygiene and quality should be attempted first. If symptoms remain intrusive, low doses of dopamine agonists, e.g., pramipexole (0.25–0.5 mg) and ropinirole (1–2 mg), are given 1–2 h before bedtime. Levodopa can be effective but is frequently associated with augmentation (spread and worsening of restlessness and its appearance earlier in the day) or rebound (reappearance sometimes with worsening of symptoms at a time compatible with the drug's short half-life). Other drugs that can be effective include anticonvulsants, analgesics, and even opiates. Management of secondary RLS should be directed to correcting the underlying disorder; for example, iron replacement for anemia. Iron infusion may also be helpful for severe primary RLS but requires expert supervision.

DISORDERS THAT PRESENT WITH PARKINSONISM AND HYPERKINETIC MOVEMENTS

WILSON'S DISEASE

Wilson's disease (WD) is an autosomal recessive inherited disorder of copper metabolism that may manifest with neurologic, psychiatric, and liver disorders, alone or in combination. It is caused by mutations in the gene encoding a P-type ATPase. The disease was first comprehensively described by the English neurologist Kinnear Wilson at the beginning of the twentieth century, although at around the same time the German physicians Kayser and Fleischer separately noted the characteristic association of corneal pigmentation with hepatic and neurologic features. WD has a worldwide prevalence of approximately 1 in 30,000, with a gene carrier frequency of 1 in 90. About half of WD patients (especially younger patients) manifest with liver abnormalities. The remainder present with neurologic disease (with or without underlying liver abnormalities), and a small proportion have hematologic or psychiatric problems at disease onset.

Neurologic onset usually manifests in the second decade with tremor and rigidity. The tremor is usually in the upper limbs, bilateral, and asymmetric. Tremor can be on intention or occasionally resting and, in advanced disease, can take on a wing-beating characteristic. Other features include parkinsonism with bradykinesia, dystonia (particularly facial grimacing), dysarthria, and dysphagia. More than half of those with neurologic features have a history of psychiatric disturbances, including depression, mood swings, and overt psychosis. Kayser-Fleischer (KF) rings are seen in 80% of those with hepatic presentations and virtually all with neurologic features. KF rings represent the deposition of copper in Descemet's membrane around the cornea. They consist of a characteristic grayish rim or circle at the limbus of the cornea and are best detected by slit-lamp examination. Neuropathologic examination is characterized by neurodegeneration and astrogliosis, particularly in the basal ganglia.

WD should always be considered in the differential diagnosis of a movement disorder in a child. Low levels of blood copper and ceruloplasmin and high levels of urinary copper may be present, but normal levels do not exclude the diagnosis. CT brain scan usually reveals generalized atrophy in established cases and ~50% have hypointensity in the caudate head, globus pallidum, substantia nigra, and red nucleus. MRI shows symmetric hyperintensity on T2-weighted images in the putamen, caudate, and pallidum. However, correlation of imaging changes with clinical features is not good. It is very rare for WD patients with neurologic features not to have KF rings. Nevertheless, liver biopsy with demonstration of high copper levels remains the gold standard for the diagnosis.

In the absence of treatment, the course is progressive and leads to severe neurologic dysfunction and early death. Treatment is directed at reducing tissue copper levels and maintenance therapy to prevent reaccumulation. There is no clear consensus on treatment and all patients should be managed in a unit with expertise in WD. Penicillamine is frequently used to increase copper excretion, but it may lead to a worsening of symptoms in the initial stages of therapy. Side effects are common and can to some degree be attenuated by coadministration of pyridoxine. Tetrathiomolybdate blocks the absorption of copper and is used instead of penicillamine in many centers. Trientine and zinc are useful drugs for maintenance therapy. Effective treatment can reverse the neurologic features in most patients, particularly when started early. Some patients stabilize and a few may still progress, especially those with hepatocerebral disease. KF rings tend to decrease after 3–6 months and disappear by 2 years. Adherence to maintenance therapy is a major challenge in long-term care.

OTHER DISORDERS

Pantothenate kinase (PANK)-associated neurodegeneration, acanthocytosis, and Huntington's disease can also present with parkinsonism associated with involuntary movements.

PSYCHOGENIC DISORDERS

Virtually all movement disorders including tremor, tics, dystonia, myoclonus, chorea, ballism, and parkinsonism can be psychogenic in origin. Tremor affecting the upper limbs is the most common psychogenic movement disorder. Psychogenic movements can result from a somatoform or conversion disorder, malingering (e.g., seeking financial gain), or a factitious disorder (e.g., seeking psychological gain). Psychogenic movement disorders are common (estimated 2–3% of patients in a movement disorder clinic), more frequent in women, disabling for the patient and family, and expensive for society (estimated $20 billion annually). Clinical features suggesting a psychogenic movement disorder include an acute onset and a pattern of abnormal movement that is inconsistent with a known movement disorder. Diagnosis is based on the nonorganic quality of the movement, the absence of findings of an organic disease process, and positive features that specifically point to a psychogenic illness such as variability and distractibility. For example, the magnitude of a psychogenic tremor is increased with attention and diminishes or even disappears when the patient is distracted by being asked to perform a different task or is unaware that he or she is being observed. Other positive features suggesting a psychogenic problem include a tremor frequency that is variable or that entrains with the frequency of movement in the contralateral limb, and a positive response to placebo medication. Associated features can include nonanatomic sensory findings, give-way weakness, and astasia-abasia (an odd, gyrating gait; Chap. 13). Comorbid psychiatric problems such as anxiety, depression, and emotional trauma may be present, but are not necessary for the diagnosis of a psychogenic movement disorder to be made. Psychogenic movement disorders can occur as an isolated entity or in association with an underlying organic problem. The diagnosis can often be made based on clinical features alone and unnecessary tests or medications avoided. Underlying psychiatric problems may be present and should be identified and treated, but many patients with psychogenic movement disorders have no obvious psychiatric pathology. Psychotherapy and hypnosis may be of value for patients with conversion reaction, and cognitive behavioral therapy may be helpful for patients with somatoform disorders. Patients with hypochondriasis, factitious disorders, and malingering have a poor prognosis.

CHAPTER 31

ATAXIC DISORDERS

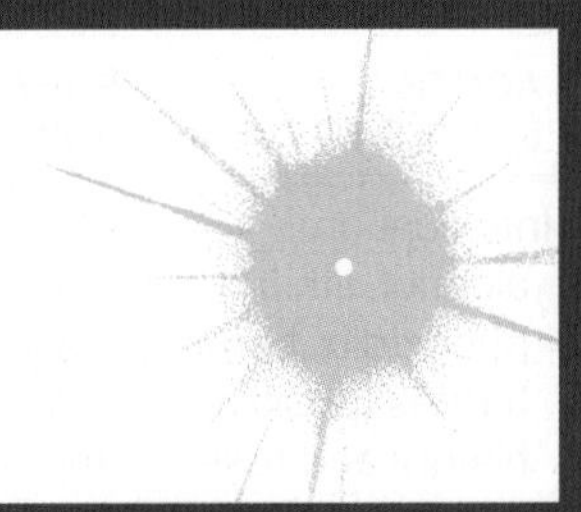

Roger N. Rosenberg

APPROACH TO THE PATIENT Ataxic Disorders

Symptoms and signs of ataxia consist of gait impairment, unclear ("scanning") speech, visual blurring due to nystagmus, hand incoordination, and tremor with movement. These result from the involvement of the cerebellum and its afferent and efferent pathways, including the spinocerebellar pathways, and the frontopontocerebellar pathway originating in the rostral frontal lobe. True cerebellar ataxia must be distinguished from ataxia associated with vestibular nerve or labyrinthine disease, as the latter results in a disorder of gait associated with a significant degree of dizziness, lightheadedness, or the perception of movement (Chap. 11). True cerebellar ataxia is devoid of these vertiginous complaints and is clearly an unsteady gait due to imbalance. Sensory disturbances can also on occasion simulate the imbalance of cerebellar disease; with sensory ataxia, imbalance dramatically worsens when visual input is removed (Romberg sign). Rarely, weakness of proximal leg muscles mimics cerebellar disease. In the patient who presents with ataxia, the rate and pattern of the development of cerebellar symptoms help to narrow the diagnostic possibilities (Table 31-1). A gradual and progressive increase in symptoms with bilateral and symmetric involvement suggests a genetic, metabolic, immune, or toxic etiology. Conversely, focal, unilateral symptoms with headache and impaired level of consciousness accompanied by ipsilateral cranial nerve palsies and contralateral weakness imply a space-occupying cerebellar lesion.

SYMMETRIC ATAXIA Progressive and symmetric ataxia can be classified with respect to onset as acute (over hours or days), subacute (weeks or months), or chronic (months to years). Acute and reversible ataxias include those caused by intoxication with alcohol, phenytoin, lithium, barbiturates, and other drugs. Intoxication caused by toluene exposure, gasoline sniffing, glue sniffing, spray painting, or exposure to methyl mercury or bismuth are additional causes of acute or subacute ataxia, as is treatment with cytotoxic chemotherapeutic drugs such as fluorouracil and paclitaxel. Patients with a postinfectious syndrome (especially after varicella) may develop gait ataxia and mild dysarthria, both of which are reversible (Chap. 39). Rare infectious causes of acquired ataxia include poliovirus, coxsackievirus, echovirus, Epstein-Barr virus, toxoplasmosis, *Legionella*, and Lyme disease.

The subacute development of ataxia of gait over weeks to months (degeneration of the cerebellar vermis) may be due to the combined effects of alcoholism and malnutrition, particularly with deficiencies of vitamins B_1 and B_{12}. Hyponatremia has also been associated with ataxia. Paraneoplastic cerebellar ataxia is associated with a number of different tumors (and autoantibodies) such as breast and ovarian cancers (anti-Yo), small cell lung cancer (anti-PQ type voltage-gated calcium channel), and Hodgkin's disease (anti-Tr) (Chap. 44). Another paraneoplastic syndrome associated with myoclonus and opsoclonus occurs with breast (anti-Ri) and lung cancers and neuroblastoma. Elevated serum anti–glutamic acid decarboxylase (GAD) antibodies have been associated with a progressive ataxic syndrome affecting speech and gait. For all of these paraneoplastic ataxias, the neurologic syndrome may be the presenting symptom of the cancer. Another immune-mediated progressive ataxia is associated with anti-gliadin (and anti-endomysium) antibodies and the human leukocyte antigen (HLA) DQB1*0201 haplotype; in some affected patients, biopsy of the small intestine reveals villus atrophy consistent with gluten-sensitive enteropathy. Finally, subacute progressive ataxia may be caused by a prion disorder, especially when an infectious etiology, such as transmission from contaminated human growth hormone, is responsible (Chap. 43).

Chronic symmetric gait ataxia suggests an inherited ataxia (discussed later), a metabolic disorder, or a

TABLE 31-1

ETIOLOGY OF CEREBELLAR ATAXIA

SYMMETRIC AND PROGRESSIVE SIGNS			FOCAL AND IPSILATERAL CEREBELLAR SIGNS		
ACUTE (HOURS TO DAYS)	**SUBACUTE (DAYS TO WEEKS)**	**CHRONIC (MONTHS TO YEARS)**	**ACUTE (HOURS TO DAYS)**	**SUBACUTE (DAYS TO WEEKS)**	**CHRONIC (MONTHS TO YEARS)**
Intoxication: alcohol, lithium, phenytoin, barbiturates (positive history and toxicology screen)	Intoxication: mercury, solvents, gasoline, glue; cytotoxic chemotherapeutic, hemotherapeutic drugs	Paraneoplastic syndrome Anti-gliadin antibody syndrome Hypothyroidism	Vascular: cerebellar infarction, hemorrhage, or subdural hematoma Infectious: cerebellar abscess (mass lesion on MRI/CT, history in support of lesion)	Neoplastic: cerebellar glioma or metastatic tumor (positive for neoplasm on MRI/CT) Demyelinating: multiple sclerosis (history, CSF, and MRI are consistent)	Stable gliosis secondary to vascular lesion or demyelinating plaque (stable lesion on MRI/CT older than several months)
Acute viral cerebellitis (CSF supportive of acute viral infection) Postinfection syndrome	Alcoholic-nutritional (vitamin B_1 and B_{12} deficiency) Lyme disease	Inherited diseases Tabes dorsalis (tertiary syphilis) Phenytoin toxicity Amiodarone		AIDS-related multifocal leukoencephalopathy (positive HIV test and CD4+ cell count for AIDS)	Congenital lesion: Chiari or Dandy-Walker malformations (malformation noted on MRI/CT)

Abbreviations: CSF, cerebrospinal fluid; CT, computed tomography; MRI, magnetic resonance imaging.

chronic infection. Hypothyroidism must always be considered as a readily treatable and reversible form of gait ataxia. Infectious diseases that can present with ataxia are meningovascular syphilis and tabes dorsalis due to degeneration of the posterior columns and spinocerebellar pathways in the spinal cord.

FOCAL ATAXIA Acute focal ataxia commonly results from cerebrovascular disease, usually ischemic infarction or cerebellar hemorrhage. These lesions typically produce cerebellar symptoms ipsilateral to the injured cerebellum and may be associated with an impaired level of consciousness due to brainstem compression and increased intracranial pressure; ipsilateral pontine signs, including sixth and seventh nerve palsies, may be present. Focal and worsening signs of acute ataxia should also prompt consideration of a posterior fossa subdural hematoma, bacterial abscess, or primary or metastatic cerebellar tumor. CT or MRI studies will reveal clinically significant processes of this type. Many of these lesions represent true neurologic emergencies, as sudden herniation, either rostrally through the tentorium or caudal herniation of cerebellar tonsils through the foramen magnum, can occur and is usually devastating. Acute surgical decompression may be required (Chap. 28). Lymphoma or progressive multifocal leukoencephalopathy (PML) in a patient with AIDS may present with an acute or subacute focal cerebellar syndrome. Chronic etiologies of progressive ataxia include multiple sclerosis (Chap. 39) and congenital lesions such as a Chiari malformation (Chap. 35) or a congenital cyst of the posterior fossa (Dandy-Walker syndrome).

THE INHERITED ATAXIAS

These may show autosomal dominant, autosomal recessive, or maternal (mitochondrial) modes of inheritance. A genomic classification (Table 31-2) has now largely superseded previous ones based on clinical expression alone.

Although the clinical manifestations and neuropathologic findings of cerebellar disease dominate the clinical picture, there may also be characteristic changes in the basal ganglia, brainstem, spinal cord, optic nerves, retina, and peripheral nerves. In large families with dominantly inherited ataxias, many gradations are observed from purely cerebellar manifestations to mixed cerebellar and brainstem disorders, cerebellar and basal ganglia syndromes, and spinal cord or peripheral nerve disease. Rarely, dementia is present as well. The clinical picture may be homogeneous within a family with dominantly inherited ataxia, but sometimes most affected family members show one characteristic syndrome, while one or several members have an entirely different phenotype.

AUTOSOMAL DOMINANT ATAXIAS

The autosomal spinocerebellar ataxias (SCAs) include SCA types 1 through 28, dentatorubropallidoluysian

TABLE 31-2

CLASSIFICATION OF THE SPINOCEREBELLAR ATAXIAS

NAME	LOCUS	PHENOTYPE
SCA1 (autosomal dominant type 1)	6p22-p23 with CAG repeats (exonic); leucine-rich acidic nuclear protein (LANP), region-specific interaction protein Ataxin-1	Ataxia with ophthalmoparesis, pyramidal and extrapyramidal findings; genetic testing is available; 6% of all autosomal dominant (AD) cerebellar ataxia
SCA2 (autosomal dominant type 2)	12q23-q24.1 with CAG repeats (exonic) Ataxin-2	Ataxia with slow saccades and minimal pyramidal and extrapyramidal findings; genetic testing available; 13% of all AD cerebellar ataxia
Machado-Joseph disease/SCA3 (autosomal dominant type 3)	14q24.3-q32 with CAG repeats (exonic); codes for ubiquitin protease (inactive with polyglutamine expansion); altered turnover of cellular proteins due to proteosome dysfunction MJD–ataxin-3	Ataxia with ophthalmoparesis and variable pyramidal, extrapyramidal, and amyotrophic signs; dementia (mild); 23% of all AD cerebellar ataxia; genetic testing available
SCA4 (autosomal dominant type 4)	16q22.1-ter; pleckstrin homology domain-containing protein, family G, member 4 (PLEKHG4; puratrophin-1: Purkinje cell atrophy associated protein-1, including spectrin repeat and the guanine-nucleotide exchange factor, GEF for Rho GTPases)	Ataxia with normal eye movements, sensory axonal neuropathy, and pyramidal signs; genetic testing available
SCA5 (autosomal dominant type 5)	11p12-q12; β-III spectrin mutations (SPTBN2); stabilizes glutamate transporter EAAT4; descendants of President Abraham Lincoln	Ataxia and dysarthria; genetic testing available
SCA6 (autosomal dominant type 6)	19p13.2 with CAG repeats in α_{1A}-voltage–dependent calcium channel gene (exonic); CACNA1A protein, P/Q type calcium channel subunit	Ataxia and dysarthria, nystagmus, mild proprioceptive sensory loss; genetic testing available
SCA7 (autosomal dominant type 7)	3p14.1-p21.1 with CAG repeats (exonic); ataxin-7; subunit of GCN5, histone acetyltransferase-containing complexes; ataxin-7 binding protein; Cbl-associated protein (CAP; SH3D5)	Ophthalmoparesis, visual loss, ataxia, dysarthria, extensor plantar response, pigmentary retinal degeneration; genetic testing available
SCA8 (autosomal dominant type 8)	13q21 with CTG repeats; noncoding; 3′ untranslated region of transcribed RNA; KLHL1AS	Gait ataxia, dysarthria, nystagmus, leg spasticity, and reduced vibratory sensation; genetic testing available
SCA10 (autosomal dominant type 10)	22q13; pentanucleotide repeat ATTCT repeat; noncoding, intron 9	Gait ataxia, dysarthria, nystagmus; partial complex and generalized motor seizures; polyneuropathy; genetic testing available
SCA11 (autosomal dominant type 11)	15q14-q21.3 by linkage	Slowly progressive gait and extremity ataxia, dysarthria, vertical nystagmus, hyperreflexia
SCA12 (autosomal dominant type 12)	5q31-q33 by linkage; CAG repeat; protein phosphatase 2A, regulatory subunit B (PPP2R2B); protein PP2A, serine/threonine phosphatase	Tremor, decreased movement, increased reflexes, dystonia, ataxia, dysautonomia, dementia, dysarthria; genetic testing available

(*continued*)

TABLE 31-2

CLASSIFICATION OF THE SPINOCEREBELLAR ATAXIAS (*CONTINUED*)

NAME	LOCUS	PHENOTYPE
SCA13 (autosomal dominant type 13)	19q13.3-q14.4	Ataxia, legs>arms; dysarthria, horizontal nystagmus; delayed motor development; mental developmental delay; tendon reflexes increased; MRI: cerebellar and pontine atrophy; genetic testing available
SCA14 (autosomal dominant type 14)	19q-13.4; protein kinase C_γ (PRKCG), missense mutations including in-frame deletion and a splice site mutation among others; serine/threonine kinase	Gait ataxia; leg>arm ataxia; dysarthria; pure ataxia with later onset; myoclonus; tremor of head and extremities; increased deep tendon reflexes at ankles; occasional dystonia and sensory neuropathy; genetic testing available
SCA15 (autosomal dominant type 15)	3p24.2-3pter	Gait and extremity ataxia, dysarthria; nystagmus; MRI: superior vermis atrophy; sparing of hemispheres and tonsils
SCA16 (autosomal dominant type 16)	8q22.1-24.1	Pure cerebellar ataxia and head tremor, gait ataxia, and dysarthria; horizontal gaze–evoked nystagmus; MR: cerebellar atrophy; no brainstem changes
SCA17 (autosomal dominant type 17)	6q27; CAG expansion in the TATA-binding protein (*TBP*) gene	Gait ataxia, dementia, parkinsonism, dystonia, chorea, seizures; hyperreflexia; dysarthria and dysphagia; MRI shows cerebral and cerebellar atrophy; genetic testing available
SCA18 (autosomal dominant type 18)	7q22-q32	Ataxia; motor/sensory neuropathy; head tremor; dysarthria; extensor plantar responses in some patients; sensory axonal neuropathy; EMG denervation; MRI: cerebellar atrophy
SCA19 (autosomal dominant type 19)	1p21-q21	Ataxia, tremor, cognitive impairment, myoclonus; MRI: atrophy of cerebellum
SCA20 (autosomal dominant)	11p13-q11	Dysarthria; gait ataxia; ocular gaze–evoked saccades; palatal tremor; dentate calcification on CT; MRI: cerebral atrophy
SCA21 (autosomal dominant)	7p21.3-p15.1	Ataxia, dysarthria, extrapyramidal features of akinesia, rigidity, tremor, cognitive defect; reduced deep tendon reflexes; MRI: cerebellar atrophy, normal basal ganglia and brainstem
SCA22 (autosomal dominant)	1p21-q23	Pure cerebellar ataxia; dysarthria; dysphagia; nystagmus; MRI: cerebellar atrophy
SCA23 (autosomal dominant)	20p13-12.3	Gait ataxia; dysarthria; extremity ataxia; ocular nystagmus, dysmetria; leg vibration loss; extensor plantar responses; MRI: cerebellar atrophy

(continued)

TABLE 31-2

CLASSIFICATION OF THE SPINOCEREBELLAR ATAXIAS (*CONTINUED*)

NAME	LOCUS	PHENOTYPE
SCA25 (autosomal dominant)	2p15-p21	Ataxia, nystagmus; vibratory loss in the feet; pain loss in some; abdominal pain; nausea and vomiting may be prominent; absent ankle reflexes; sensory nerve action potentials are absent; MRI: cerebellar atrophy, normal brainstem
SCA26 (autosomal dominant)	19p13.3	Gait ataxia; extremity ataxia; dysarthria; nystagmus; MRI: cerebellar atrophy
SCA27 (autosomal dominant)	13q34; fibroblast growth factor 14 protein; mutation F145S; produces reduced protein stability	Tremor extremities and head and orofacial dyskinesia; ataxia of arms>legs, gait ataxia; dysarthria; nystagmus; psychiatric symptoms; cognitive defect; MRI: cerebellar atrophy; genetic testing available
SCA28 (autosomal dominant)	18p11.22-q11.2	Extremity and gait ataxia; dysarthria; nystagmus; ophthalmoparesis; leg hyperreflexia and extensor plantar responses; MRI: cerebellar atrophy
SCA30 (autosomal dominant)	4q34.3-q35.1	Candidate gene *ODZ3*; gait ataxia, dysarthria, saccades; nystagmus, brisk tendon reflexes in legs; MRI: cerebellar atrophy
SCA31 (autosomal dominant)	16q22.1	Pentanucleotide $(TGGAA)_N$ repeat insertions; previously called SCA4; gait ataxia; limb dysmetria; MRI: cerebellar atrophy
Dentatorubropallidoluysian atrophy (autosomal dominant)	12p13.31 with CAG repeats (exonic) Atrophin 1	Ataxia, choreoathetosis, dystonia, seizures, myoclonus, dementia; genetic testing available
Friedreich's ataxia (autosomal recessive)	9q13-q21.1 with intronic GAA repeats, in intron at end of exon 1 Frataxin defective; abnormal regulation of mitochondrial iron metabolism; iron accumulates in mitochondria in yeast mutants	Ataxia, areflexia, extensor plantar responses, position sense deficits, cardiomyopathy, diabetes mellitus, scoliosis, foot deformities; optic atrophy; late-onset form, as late as 50 years with preserved deep tendon reflexes, slower progression, reduced skeletal deformities, associated with an intermediate number of GAA repeats and missense mutations in one allele of frataxin; genetic testing available
Friedreich's ataxia (autosomal recessive)	8q13.1-q13.3 (α-TTP deficiency)	Same as phenotype that maps to 9q but associated with vitamin E deficiency; genetic testing available
Sensory ataxic neuropathy and ophthalmoparesis (SANDO) with dysarthria (autosomal recessive)	15q25; mutations in DNA polymerase-gamma (POLG) gene that leads to mtDNA deletions	Young adult–onset ataxia, sensory neuropathy, ophthalmoparesis, hearing loss, gastric symptoms; a variant of progressive external ophthalmoplegia; MRI: cerebellar and thalamic abnormalities; mildly increased lactate and creatine kinase

(*continued*)

TABLE 31-2

CLASSIFICATION OF THE SPINOCEREBELLAR ATAXIAS (*CONTINUED*)

NAME	LOCUS	PHENOTYPE
Von Hippel-Lindau syndrome (autosomal dominant)	3p26-p25	Cerebellar hemangioblastoma; pheochromocytoma
Baltic myoclonus (Unverricht-Lundborg) (recessive)	21q22.3; cystatin B; extra repeats of 12–base pair tandem repeats	Myoclonus epilepsy; late-onset ataxia; responds to valproic acid, clonazepam; phenobarbital
Marinesco-Sjögren syndrome (recessive)	5q31; SIL 1 protein, nucleotide exchange factor for the heat-shock protein 70 (HSP70); chaperone HSPA5; homozygous 4-nucleotide duplication in exon 6; also compound heterozygote	Ataxia, dysarthria; nystagmus; retarded motor and mental maturation; rhabdomyolysis after viral illness; weakness; hypotonia; areflexia; cataracts in childhood; short stature; kyphoscoliosis; contractures; hypogonadism
Autosomal recessive spastic ataxia of Charlevoix-Saguenay (ARSACS)	Chromosome 13q12; SACS gene; loss of sacsin peptide activity	Childhood onset of ataxia, spasticity, dysarthria, distal muscle wasting, foot deformity, retinal striations, mitral valve prolapse
Kearns-Sayre syndrome (sporadic)	mtDNA deletion and duplication mutations	Ptosis, ophthalmoplegia, pigmentary retinal degeneration, cardiomyopathy, diabetes mellitus, deafness, heart block, increased CSF protein, ataxia
Myoclonic epilepsy and ragged red fiber syndrome (MERRF) (maternal inheritance)	Mutation in mtDNA of the $tRNA^{lys}$ at 8344; also mutation at 8356	Myoclonic epilepsy, ragged red fiber myopathy, ataxia
Mitochondrial encephalopathy, lactic acidosis, and stroke syndrome (MELAS) (maternal inheritance)	$tRNA^{leu}$ mutation at 3243; also at 3271 and 3252	Headache, stroke, lactic acidosis, ataxia
Neuropathy; ataxia; retinitis pigmentosa (NARP)	ATPase6 (Complex 5); mtDNA point mutation at 8993	Neuropathy; ataxia; retinitis pigmentosa; dementia; seizures
Episodic ataxia, type 1 (EA-1) (autosomal dominant)	12p13; potassium voltage-gated channel gene, *KCNA1*; Phe249Leu mutation; variable syndrome	Episodic ataxia for minutes; provoked by startle or exercise; with facial and hand myokymia; cerebellar signs are not progressive; choreoathetotic movements; responds to phenytoin; genetic testing available
Episodic ataxia, type 2 (EA-2) (autosomal dominant)	19p-13(*CACNA1A*) (allelic with SCA6) (α_{1A}-voltage–dependent calcium channel subunit); point mutations or small deletions; allelic with SCA6 and familial hemiplegic migraine	Episodic ataxia for days; provoked by stress, fatigue; with down-gaze nystagmus; vertigo; vomiting; headache; cerebellar atrophy results; progressive cerebellar signs; responds to acetazolamide; genetic testing available
Episodic ataxia, type 3 (autosomal dominant)	1q42	Episodic ataxia; 1 min to over 6 h; induced by movement; vertigo and tinnitus; headache; responds to acetazolamide
Episodic ataxia, type 4 (autosomal dominant)	Not mapped	Episodic ataxia; vertigo; diplopia; ocular slow pursuit defect; no response to acetazolamide
Episodic ataxia, type 5 (autosomal dominant)	2q22-q23; CACNB4β4 protein	Episodic ataxia; hours to weeks; seizures
Episodic ataxia, type 6	5p13; SLC1A3; glutamate transporter in astrocytes	Episodic ataxia; seizures; cognitive impairment; under 24 h

(*continued*)

TABLE 31-2

CLASSIFICATION OF THE SPINOCEREBELLAR ATAXIAS (*CONTINUED*)

NAME	LOCUS	PHENOTYPE
Episodic ataxia, type 7 (autosomal dominant)	19q13	Episodic ataxia; vertigo, weakness; less than 24 h
Episodic ataxia with seizures, migraine, and alternating hemiplegia (autosomal dominant)	SLC1A3; 5p13; EAAT1 protein; missense mutations; glial glutamate transporter (GLAST); 1047 C to G; proline to arginine	Ataxia, duration 2–4 days; episodic hypotonia; delayed motor milestones; seizures; migraine; alternating hemiplegia; mild truncal ataxia; coma; febrile illness as a trigger; MRI: cerebellar atrophy
Fragile X tremor/ataxia syndrome (FXTAS) X-linked dominant	Xq27.3; CGG premutation expansion in FMR1 gene; expansions of 55–200 repeats in 5′ UTR of the FMR-1 mRNA; presumed dominant toxic RNA effect	Late-onset ataxia with tremor, cognitive impairment, occasional parkinsonism; males typically affected, although affected females also reported; syndrome is of high concern if affected male has grandson with mental retardation (fragile X syndrome); MRI shows increased T2 signal in middle cerebellar peduncles, cerebellar atrophy, and occasional widespread brain atrophy; genetic testing available
Ataxia telangiectasia (autosomal recessive)	11q22-23; *ATM* gene for regulation of cell cycle; mitogenic signal transduction and meiotic recombination	Telangiectasia, ataxia, dysarthria, pulmonary infections, neoplasms of lymphatic system; IgA and IgG deficiencies; diabetes mellitus, breast cancer; genetic testing available
Early-onset cerebellar ataxia with retained deep tendon reflexes (autosomal recessive)	13q11-12	Ataxia; neuropathy; preserved deep tendon reflexes; impaired cognitive and visuospatial functions; MRI, cerebellar atrophy
Ataxia with oculomotor apraxia (AOA1) (autosomal recessive)	9p13; protein is member of histidine triad superfamily, role in DNA repair	Ataxia; dysarthria; limb dysmetria; dystonia; oculomotor apraxia; optic atrophy; motor neuropathy; late sensory loss (vibration); genetic testing available
Ataxia with oculomotor apraxia 2 (AOA2) (autosomal recessive)	9q34; senataxin protein, involved in RNA maturation and termination; helicase superfamily 1	Gait ataxia; choreoathetosis; dystonia; oculomotor apraxia; neuropathy, vibration loss, position sense loss, and mild light touch loss; absent leg deep tendon reflexes; extensor plantar response; genetic testing available
Cerebellar ataxia with muscle coenzyme Q10 deficiency (autosomal recessive)	9p13	Ataxia; hypotonia; seizures; mental retardation; increased deep tendon reflexes; extensor plantar responses; coenzyme Q10 levels reduced with about 25% of patients with a block in transfer of electrons to complex 3; may respond to coenzyme 10
Joubert syndrome (autosomal recessive)	9q34.3	Ataxia; ptosis; mental retardation; oculomotor apraxia; nystagmus; retinopathy; rhythmic tongue protrusion; episodic hyperpnea or apnea; dimples at wrists and elbows; telecanthus; micrognathia

(*continued*)

TABLE 31-2

CLASSIFICATION OF THE SPINOCEREBELLAR ATAXIAS (*CONTINUED*)

NAME	LOCUS	PHENOTYPE
Sideroblastic anemia and spinocerebellar ataxia (X-linked recessive)	Xq13; ATP-binding cassette 7 (ABCB7; ABC7) transporter; mitochondrial inner membrane; iron homeostasis; export from matrix to the intermembrane space	Ataxia; elevated free erythrocyte protoporphyrin levels; ring sideroblasts in bone marrow; heterozygous females may have mild anemia but not ataxia
Infantile-onset spinocerebellar ataxia of Nikali et al (autosomal recessive)	10q23.3-q24.1; twinkle protein (gene); homozygous for Tyr508Cys missense mutations	Infantile ataxia, sensory neuropathy; athetosis, hearing deficit, reduced deep tendon reflexes; ophthalmoplegia, optic atrophy; seizures; primary hypogonadism in females
Hypoceruloplasminemia with ataxia and dysarthria (autosomal recessive)	Ceruloplasmin gene; 3q23-q25 (trp 858 ter)	Gait ataxia and dysarthria; hyperreflexia; cerebellar atrophy by MRI; iron deposition in cerebellum, basal ganglia, thalamus, and liver; onset in the 4th decade
Spinocerebellar ataxia with neuropathy (SCAN1) (autosomal recessive)	Tyrosyl-DNA phosphodiesterase-1 (TDP-1) 14q31-q32	Onset in 2nd decade; gait ataxia, dysarthria, seizures, cerebellar vermis atrophy on MRI, dysmetria

Abbreviations: CSF, cerebrospinal fluid; EMG, electromyogram; MRI, magnetic resonance imaging.

atrophy (DRPLA), and episodic ataxia (EA) types 1 and 2 (Table 31-2). SCA1, SCA2, SCA3 (Machado-Joseph disease [MJD]), SCA6, SCA7, and SCA17 are caused by CAG triplet repeat expansions in different genes. SCA8 is due to an untranslated CTG repeat expansion, SCA12 is linked to an untranslated CAG repeat, and SCA10 is caused by an untranslated pentanucleotide repeat. The clinical phenotypes of these SCAs overlap. The genotype has become the gold standard for diagnosis and classification. CAG encodes glutamine, and these expanded CAG triplet repeat expansions result in expanded polyglutamine proteins, termed *ataxins*, that produce a toxic gain of function with autosomal dominant inheritance. Although the phenotype is variable for any given disease gene, a pattern of neuronal loss with gliosis is produced that is relatively unique for each ataxia. Immunohistochemical and biochemical studies have shown cytoplasmic (SCA2), neuronal (SCA1, MJD, SCA7), and nucleolar (SCA7) accumulation of the specific mutant polyglutamine-containing ataxin proteins. Expanded polyglutamine ataxins with more than ~40 glutamines are potentially toxic to neurons for a variety of reasons including the following: high levels of gene expression for the mutant polyglutamine ataxin in affected neurons; conformational change of the aggregated protein to a β-pleated structure; abnormal transport of the ataxin into the nucleus (SCA1, MJD, SCA7); binding to other polyglutamine proteins, including the TATA-binding transcription protein and the CREB-binding protein, impairing their functions; altering the efficiency of the ubiquitin-proteosome system of protein turnover; and inducing neuronal apoptosis. An earlier age of onset (anticipation) and more aggressive disease in subsequent generations are due to further expansion of the CAG triplet repeat and increased polyglutamine number in the mutant ataxin. The most common disorders are discussed later.

SCA1

SCA1 was previously referred to as *olivopontocerebellar atrophy*, but genomic data have shown that that entity represents several different genotypes with overlapping clinical features.

Symptoms and signs

SCA1 is characterized by the development in early or middle adult life of progressive cerebellar ataxia of the trunk and limbs, impairment of equilibrium and gait, slowness of voluntary movements, scanning speech, nystagmoid eye movements, and oscillatory tremor of the head and trunk. Dysarthria, dysphagia, and oculomotor and facial palsies may also occur. Extrapyramidal symptoms include rigidity, an immobile face, and parkinsonian tremor. The reflexes are usually normal, but knee and ankle jerks may be lost, and extensor plantar responses may occur. Dementia may be noted but is usually mild. Impairment of sphincter function is common, with urinary and sometimes fecal incontinence. Cerebellar and brainstem atrophy are evident on MRI (**Fig. 31-1**).

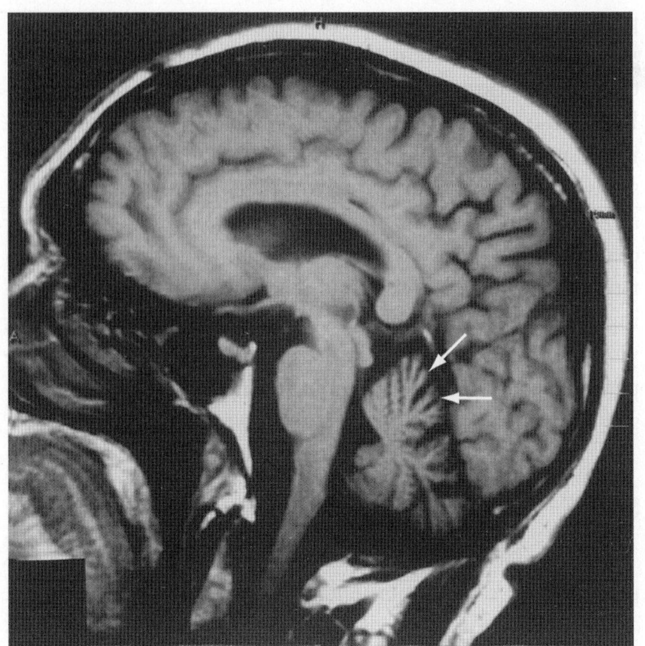

FIGURE 31-1
Sagittal MRI of the brain of a 60-year-old man with gait ataxia and dysarthria due to SCA1, illustrating cerebellar atrophy (*arrows*). MRI, magnetic resonance imaging; SCA1, spinocerebellar ataxia type 1.

Marked shrinkage of the ventral half of the pons, disappearance of the olivary eminence on the ventral surface of the medulla, and atrophy of the cerebellum are evident on gross postmortem inspection of the brain. Variable loss of Purkinje cells, reduced numbers of cells in the molecular and granular layer, demyelination of the middle cerebellar peduncle and the cerebellar hemispheres, and severe loss of cells in the pontine nuclei and olives are found on histologic examination. Degenerative changes in the striatum, especially the putamen, and loss of the pigmented cells of the substantia nigra may be found in cases with extrapyramidal features. More widespread degeneration in the central nervous system (CNS), including involvement of the posterior columns and the spinocerebellar fibers, is often present.

GENETIC CONSIDERATIONS

SCA1 encodes a gene product, called *ataxin-1*, which is a novel protein of unknown function. The mutant allele has 40 CAG repeats located within the coding region, whereas alleles from unaffected individuals have ≤36 repeats. A few patients with 38–40 CAG repeats have been described. There is a direct correlation between a larger number of repeats and a younger age of onset for SCA1. Juvenile patients have higher numbers of repeats, and anticipation is present in subsequent generations. Transgenic mice carrying SCA1 developed ataxia and Purkinje cell pathology. Nuclear localization, but not aggregation, of ataxin-1 appears to be required for cell death initiated by the mutant protein.

SCA2

Symptoms and signs

Another clinical phenotype, SCA2, has been described in patients from Cuba and India. Cuban patients probably are descendants of a common ancestor, and the population may be the largest homogeneous group of patients with ataxia yet described. The age of onset ranges from 2–65 years, and there is considerable clinical variability within families. Although neuropathologic and clinical findings are compatible with a diagnosis of SCA1, including slow saccadic eye movements, ataxia, dysarthria, parkinsonian rigidity, optic disc pallor, mild spasticity, and retinal degeneration, SCA2 is a unique form of cerebellar degenerative disease.

GENETIC CONSIDERATIONS

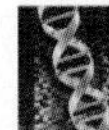

The gene in SCA2 families also contains CAG repeat expansions coding for a polyglutamine-containing protein, ataxin-2. Normal alleles contain 15–32 repeats; mutant alleles have 35–77 repeats.

MACHADO-JOSEPH DISEASE/SCA3

MJD was first described among the Portuguese and their descendants in New England and California. Subsequently, MJD has been found in families from Portugal, Australia, Brazil, Canada, China, England, France, India, Israel, Italy, Japan, Spain, Taiwan, and the United States. In most populations, it is the most common autosomal dominant ataxia.

Symptoms and signs

MJD has been classified into three clinical types. In type I MJD (amyotrophic lateral sclerosis–parkinsonism–dystonia type), neurologic deficits appear in the first two decades and involve weakness and spasticity of extremities, especially the legs, often with dystonia of the face, neck, trunk, and extremities. Patellar and ankle clonus are common, as are extensor plantar responses. The gait is slow and stiff, with a slightly broadened base and lurching from side to side; this gait results from spasticity, not true ataxia. There is no truncal titubation. Pharyngeal weakness and spasticity cause difficulty with speech and swallowing. Of note is the prominence of horizontal and vertical nystagmus, loss of fast saccadic eye movements, hypermetric and hypometric saccades, and impairment of upward vertical gaze. Facial fasciculations, facial myokymia, lingual fasciculations without atrophy, ophthalmoparesis, and ocular prominence are common early manifestations.

In type II MJD (ataxic type), true cerebellar deficits of dysarthria and gait and extremity ataxia begin in the second to fourth decades along with corticospinal and extrapyramidal deficits of spasticity, rigidity, and dystonia. Type II is the most common form of MJD. Ophthalmoparesis, upward vertical gaze deficits, and facial and lingual fasciculations are also present. Type II MJD can be distinguished from the clinically similar disorders SCA1 and SCA2.

Type III MJD (ataxic-amyotrophic type) presents in the fifth to the seventh decades with a pancerebellar disorder that includes dysarthria and gait and extremity ataxia. Distal sensory loss involving pain, touch, vibration, and position senses and distal atrophy are prominent, indicating the presence of peripheral neuropathy. The deep tendon reflexes are depressed to absent, and there are no corticospinal or extrapyramidal findings.

The mean age of onset of symptoms in MJD is 25 years. Neurologic deficits invariably progress and lead to death from debilitation within 15 years of onset, especially in patients with types I and II disease. Usually, patients retain full intellectual function.

The major pathologic findings are variable loss of neurons and glial replacement in the corpus striatum and severe loss of neurons in the pars compacta of the substantia nigra. A moderate loss of neurons occurs in the dentate nucleus of the cerebellum and in the red nucleus. Purkinje cell loss and granule cell loss occur in the cerebellar cortex. Cell loss also occurs in the dentate nucleus and in the cranial nerve motor nuclei. Sparing of the inferior olives distinguishes MJD from other dominantly inherited ataxias.

GENETIC CONSIDERATIONS

The gene for MJD maps to 14q24.3-q32. Unstable CAG repeat expansions are present in the MJD gene coding for a polyglutamine-containing protein named ataxin-3, or MJD-ataxin. An earlier age of onset is associated with longer repeats. Alleles from normal individuals have between 12 and 37 CAG repeats, while MJD alleles have 60–84 CAG repeats. Polyglutamine-containing aggregates of ataxin-3 (MJD-ataxin) have been described in neuronal nuclei undergoing degeneration. MJD-ataxin codes for a ubiquitin protease, which is inactive due to expanded polyglutamines. Proteosome function is impaired, resulting in altered clearance of proteins and cerebellar neuronal loss.

SCA6

Genomic screening for CAG repeats in other families with autosomal dominant ataxia and vibratory and proprioceptive sensory loss have yielded another locus. Of interest is that different mutations in the same gene for the α_{1A} voltage-dependent calcium channel subunit (CACNLIA4; also referred to as the *CACNA1A* gene) at 19p13 result in different clinical disorders. CAG repeat expansions (21–27 in patients; 4–16 triplets in normal individuals) result in late-onset progressive ataxia with cerebellar degeneration. Missense mutations in this gene result in familial hemiplegic migraine. Nonsense mutations resulting in termination of protein synthesis of the gene product yield hereditary paroxysmal cerebellar ataxia or EA. Some patients with familial hemiplegic migraine develop progressive ataxia and also have cerebellar atrophy.

SCA7

This disorder is distinguished from all other SCAs by the presence of retinal pigmentary degeneration. The visual abnormalities first appear as blue-yellow color blindness and proceed to frank visual loss with macular degeneration. In almost all other respects, SCA7 resembles several other SCAs in which ataxia is accompanied by various noncerebellar findings, including ophthalmoparesis and extensor plantar responses. The genetic defect is an expanded CAG repeat in the SCA7 gene at 3p14-p21.1. The expanded repeat size in SCA7 is highly variable. Consistent with this, the severity of clinical findings varies from essentially asymptomatic to mild late-onset symptoms to severe, aggressive disease in childhood with rapid progression. Marked anticipation has been recorded, especially with paternal transmission. The disease protein, ataxin-7, forms aggregates in nuclei of affected neurons, as has also been described for SCA1 and SCA3/MJD.

SCA8

This form of ataxia is caused by a CTG repeat expansion in an untranslated region of a gene on chromosome 13q21. There is marked maternal bias in transmission, perhaps reflecting contractions of the repeat during spermatogenesis. The mutation is not fully penetrant. Symptoms include slowly progressive dysarthria and gait ataxia beginning at ~40 years of age with a range between 20 and 65 years. Other features include nystagmus, leg spasticity, and reduced vibratory sensation. Severely affected individuals are nonambulatory by the fourth to sixth decades. MRI shows cerebellar atrophy. The mechanism of disease may involve a dominant "toxic" effect occurring at the RNA level, as occurs in myotonic dystrophy.

DENTATORUBROPALLIDOLUYSIAN ATROPHY

DRPLA has a variable presentation that may include progressive ataxia, choreoathetosis, dystonia, seizures, myoclonus, and dementia. DRPLA is due to unstable CAG triplet repeats in the open reading frame of a gene named *atrophin* located on chromosome 12p12-ter. Larger expansions are found in patients with earlier onset. The number of repeats is 49 in patients with DRPLA and ≤26 in normal individuals. Anticipation occurs in successive generations, with earlier onset of disease in association with an increasing CAG repeat number in children who inherit the disease from their father. One well-characterized family in North Carolina has a phenotypic variant known as the *Haw River syndrome*, now recognized to be due to the DRPLA mutation.

EPISODIC ATAXIA

EA types 1 and 2 are two rare dominantly inherited disorders that have been mapped to chromosomes 12p (a potassium channel gene) for type 1 and 19p for type 2. Patients with EA-1 have brief episodes of ataxia with myokymia and nystagmus that last only minutes. Startle, sudden change in posture, and exercise can induce episodes. Acetazolamide or anticonvulsants may be therapeutic. Patients with EA-2 have episodes of ataxia with nystagmus that can last for hours or days. Stress, exercise, or excessive fatigue may be precipitants. Acetazolamide may be therapeutic and can reverse the relative intracellular alkalosis detected by magnetic resonance spectroscopy. Stop codon, nonsense mutations causing EA-2 have been found in the *CACNA1A* gene, encoding the α_{1A} voltage-dependent calcium channel subunit (see "SCA6").

AUTOSOMAL RECESSIVE ATAXIAS

Friedreich's ataxia

This is the most common form of inherited ataxia, comprising one-half of all hereditary ataxias. It can occur in a classic form or in association with a genetically determined vitamin E deficiency syndrome; the two forms are clinically indistinguishable.

Symptoms and signs

Friedreich's ataxia presents before 25 years of age with progressive staggering gait, frequent falling, and titubation. The lower extremities are more severely involved than the upper ones. Dysarthria occasionally is the presenting symptom; rarely, progressive scoliosis, foot deformity, nystagmus, or cardiopathy is the initial sign.

The neurologic examination reveals nystagmus, loss of fast saccadic eye movements, truncal titubation, dysarthria, dysmetria, and ataxia of trunk and limb movements. Extensor plantar responses (with normal tone in trunk and extremities), absence of deep tendon reflexes, and weakness (greater distally than proximally) are usually found. Loss of vibratory and proprioceptive sensation occurs. The median age of death is 35 years. Women have a significantly better prognosis than men.

Cardiac involvement occurs in 90% of patients. Cardiomegaly, symmetric hypertrophy, murmurs, and conduction defects are reported. Moderate mental retardation or psychiatric syndromes are present in a small percentage of patients. A high incidence of diabetes mellitus (20%) is found and is associated with insulin resistance and pancreatic β-cell dysfunction. Musculoskeletal deformities are common and include pes cavus, pes equinovarus, and scoliosis. MRI of the spinal cord shows atrophy (Fig. 31-2).

The primary sites of pathology are the spinal cord, dorsal root ganglion cells, and the peripheral nerves. Slight atrophy of the cerebellum and cerebral gyri may occur. Sclerosis and degeneration occur predominantly in the spinocerebellar tracts, lateral corticospinal tracts, and posterior columns. Degeneration of the glossopharyngeal, vagus, hypoglossal, and deep cerebellar nuclei is described. The cerebral cortex is histologically normal except for loss of Betz cells in the precentral gyri. The peripheral nerves are extensively involved, with a loss of large myelinated fibers. Cardiac pathology consists of myocytic hypertrophy and fibrosis, focal vascular fibromuscular dysplasia with subintimal or medial deposition of periodic acid–Schiff (PAS)-positive material, myocytopathy with unusual pleomorphic nuclei, and focal degeneration of nerves and cardiac ganglia.

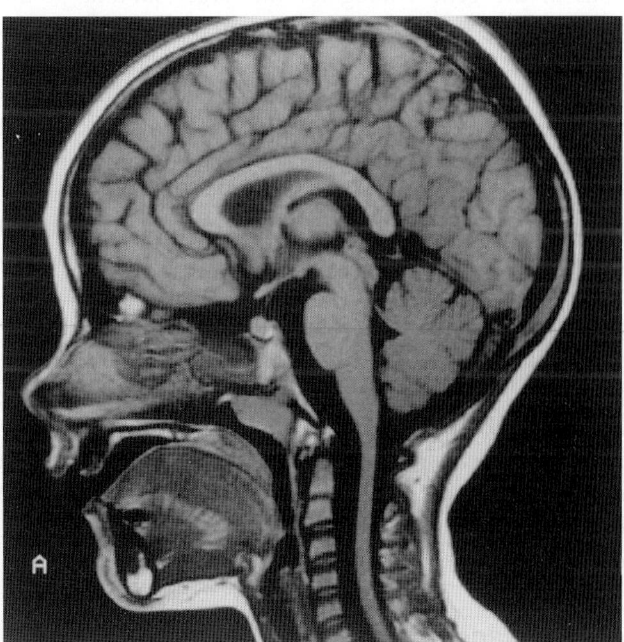

FIGURE 31-2
Sagittal MRI of the brain and spinal cord of a patient with Friedreich's ataxia, demonstrating spinal cord atrophy.

GENETIC CONSIDERATIONS

The classic form of Friedreich's ataxia has been mapped to 9q13-q21.1, and the mutant gene, *frataxin*, contains expanded GAA triplet repeats in the first intron. There is homozygosity for expanded GAA repeats in >95% of patients. Normal persons have 7–22 GAA repeats, and patients have 200–900 GAA repeats. A more varied clinical syndrome has been described in compound heterozygotes who have one copy of the GAA expansion and the other copy a point mutation in the *frataxin* gene. When the point mutation is located in the region of the gene that encodes the amino-terminal half of frataxin, the phenotype is milder, often consisting of a spastic gait, retained or exaggerated reflexes, no dysarthria, and mild or absent ataxia.

Patients with Friedreich's ataxia have undetectable or extremely low levels of *frataxin* mRNA, as compared with carriers and unrelated individuals; thus, disease appears to be caused by a loss of expression of the frataxin protein. Frataxin is a mitochondrial protein involved in iron homeostasis. Mitochondrial iron accumulation due to loss of the iron transporter coded by the mutant *frataxin* gene results in oxidized intramitochondrial iron. Excess oxidized iron results in turn in the oxidation of cellular components and irreversible cell injury.

Two forms of hereditary ataxia associated with abnormalities in the interactions of vitamin E (α-tocopherol) with very low density lipoprotein (VLDL) have been delineated. These are abetalipoproteinemia (Bassen-Kornzweig syndrome) and ataxia with vitamin E deficiency (AVED). Abetalipoproteinemia is caused by mutations in the gene coding for the larger subunit of the microsomal triglyceride transfer protein (MTP). Defects in MTP result in impairment of formation and secretion of VLDL in liver. This defect results in a deficiency of delivery of vitamin E to tissues, including the central and peripheral nervous system, as VLDL is the transport molecule for vitamin E and other fat-soluble substitutes. AVED is due to mutations in the gene for α-tocopherol transfer protein (α-TTP). These patients have an impaired ability to bind vitamin E into the VLDL produced and secreted by the liver, resulting in a deficiency of vitamin E in peripheral tissues. Hence, either absence of VLDL (abetalipoproteinemia) or impaired binding of vitamin E to VLDL (AVED) causes an ataxic syndrome. Once again, a genotype classification has proved to be essential in sorting out the various forms of the Friedreich's disease syndrome, which may be clinically indistinguishable.

Ataxia telangiectasia

Symptoms and signs

Patients with ataxia telangiectasia (AT) present in the first decade of life with progressive telangiectatic lesions associated with deficits in cerebellar function and nystagmus. The neurologic manifestations correspond to those in Friedreich's disease, which should be included in the differential diagnosis. Truncal and limb ataxia, dysarthria, extensor plantar responses, myoclonic jerks, areflexia, and distal sensory deficits may develop. There is a high incidence of recurrent pulmonary infections and neoplasms of the lymphatic and reticuloendothelial system in patients with AT. Thymic hypoplasia with cellular and humoral (IgA and IgG2) immunodeficiencies, premature aging, and endocrine disorders such as type 1 diabetes mellitus are described. There is an increased incidence of lymphomas, Hodgkin's disease, acute leukemias of the T cell type, and breast cancer.

The most striking neuropathologic changes include loss of Purkinje, granule, and basket cells in the cerebellar cortex as well as of neurons in the deep cerebellar nuclei. The inferior olives of the medulla may also have neuronal loss. There is a loss of anterior horn neurons in the spinal cord and of dorsal root ganglion cells associated with posterior column spinal cord demyelination. A poorly developed or absent thymus gland is the most consistent defect of the lymphoid system.

GENETIC CONSIDERATIONS

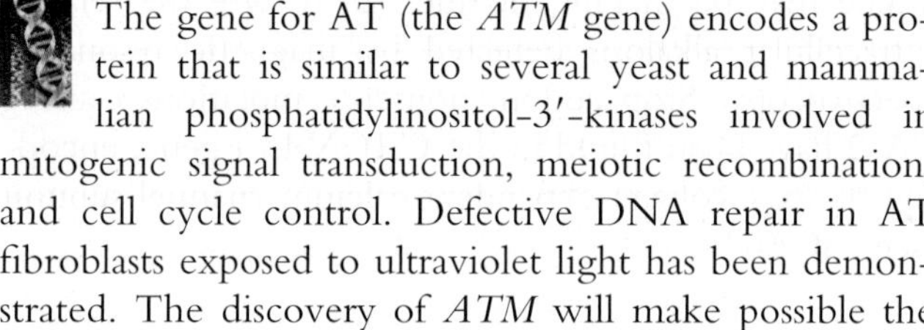

The gene for AT (the *ATM* gene) encodes a protein that is similar to several yeast and mammalian phosphatidylinositol-3′-kinases involved in mitogenic signal transduction, meiotic recombination, and cell cycle control. Defective DNA repair in AT fibroblasts exposed to ultraviolet light has been demonstrated. The discovery of *ATM* will make possible the identification of heterozygotes who are at risk for cancer (e.g., breast cancer) and permit early diagnosis.

MITOCHONDRIAL ATAXIAS

Spinocerebellar syndromes have been identified with mutations in mitochondrial DNA (mtDNA). Thirty pathogenic mtDNA point mutations and 60 different types of mtDNA deletions are known, several of which cause or are associated with ataxia (Chap. 48).

TREATMENT Ataxic Disorders

The most important goal in management of patients with ataxia is to identify treatable disease entities. Mass lesions must be recognized promptly and treated appropriately. Paraneoplastic disorders can often be identified by the clinical patterns of disease that they produce, measurement of specific autoantibodies, and uncovering the primary cancer; these disorders are often refractory to therapy, but some patients improve following removal of the tumor or immunotherapy (Chap. 44). Ataxia with anti-gliadin antibodies and gluten-sensitive enteropathy may improve with a gluten-free diet. Malabsorption syndromes leading to vitamin E deficiency may lead to ataxia. The vitamin E deficiency form of Friedreich's ataxia must be considered, and serum vitamin E levels measured. Vitamin E therapy is indicated for these rare patients. Vitamin B_1 and B_{12} levels in serum should be measured, and the vitamins administered to patients having deficient levels. Hypothyroidism is easily treated. The cerebrospinal fluid should be tested for a syphilitic infection in patients with progressive ataxia and other features of tabes dorsalis. Similarly, antibody titers for Lyme disease and *Legionella* should be measured and appropriate antibiotic therapy should be instituted in antibody-positive patients. Aminoacidopathies, leukodystrophies, urea-cycle abnormalities, and mitochondrial encephalomyopathies may produce ataxia, and some dietary or metabolic therapies are available for these disorders. The deleterious effects of phenytoin and alcohol on the cerebellum are well known, and these exposures should be avoided in patients with ataxia of any cause.

There is no proven therapy for any of the autosomal dominant ataxias (SCA1 to SCA28). There is preliminary evidence that idebenone, a free-radical scavenger, can improve myocardial hypertrophy in patients with classic Friedreich ataxia; there is no current evidence, however, that it improves neurologic function. A small preliminary study in a mixed population of patients with different inherited ataxias raised the possibility that the glutamate antagonist riluzole may offer modest benefit. Iron chelators and antioxidant drugs are potentially harmful in Friedreich's patients as they may increase heart muscle injury. Acetazolamide can reduce the duration of symptoms of episodic ataxia. At present, identification of an at-risk person's genotype, together with appropriate family and genetic counseling, can reduce the incidence of these cerebellar syndromes in future generations.

CHAPTER 32

AMYOTROPHIC LATERAL SCLEROSIS AND OTHER MOTOR NEURON DISEASES

Robert H. Brown, Jr.

AMYOTROPHIC LATERAL SCLEROSIS

Amyotrophic lateral sclerosis (ALS) is the most common form of progressive motor neuron disease. It is a prime example of a neurodegenerative disease and is arguably the most devastating of the neurodegenerative disorders.

PATHOLOGY

The pathologic hallmark of motor neuron degenerative disorders is death of lower motor neurons (consisting of anterior horn cells in the spinal cord and their brainstem homologues innervating bulbar muscles) and upper, or corticospinal, motor neurons (originating in layer five of the motor cortex and descending via the pyramidal tract to synapse with lower motor neurons, either directly or indirectly via interneurons) (Chap. 12). Although at its onset ALS may involve selective loss of function of only upper or lower motor neurons, it ultimately causes progressive loss of both categories of motor neurons. Indeed, in the absence of clear involvement of both motor neuron types, the diagnosis of ALS is questionable.

Other motor neuron diseases involve only particular subsets of motor neurons (Tables 32-1 and 32-2). Thus, in bulbar palsy and spinal muscular atrophy (SMA; also called *progressive muscular atrophy*), the lower motor neurons of brainstem and spinal cord, respectively, are most severely involved. By contrast, pseudobulbar palsy, primary lateral sclerosis (PLS), and familial spastic paraplegia (FSP) affect only upper motor neurons innervating the brainstem and spinal cord.

In each of these diseases, the affected motor neurons undergo shrinkage, often with accumulation of the pigmented lipid (lipofuscin) that normally develops in these cells with advancing age. In ALS, the motor neuron cytoskeleton is typically affected early in the illness. Focal enlargements are frequent in proximal motor axons; ultrastructurally, these "spheroids" are composed of accumulations of neurofilaments and other proteins. Also seen is proliferation of astroglia and microglia, the inevitable accompaniment of all degenerative processes in the central nervous system (CNS).

The death of the peripheral motor neurons in the brainstem and spinal cord leads to denervation and consequent atrophy of the corresponding muscle fibers. Histochemical and electrophysiologic evidence indicates that in the early phases of the illness denervated muscle can be reinnervated by sprouting of nearby distal motor nerve terminals, although reinnervation in this disease is considerably less extensive than in most other disorders affecting motor neurons (e.g., poliomyelitis, peripheral neuropathy). As denervation progresses, muscle atrophy is readily recognized in muscle biopsies and on clinical examination. This is the basis for the term *amyotrophy*. The loss of cortical motor neurons results in thinning of the corticospinal tracts that travel via the internal capsule (Fig. 32-1) and brainstem to the lateral and anterior white matter columns of the spinal cord. The loss of fibers in the lateral columns and resulting fibrillary gliosis impart a particular firmness (*lateral sclerosis*). A remarkable feature of the disease is the selectivity of neuronal cell death. By light microscopy, the entire sensory apparatus, the regulatory mechanisms for the control and coordination of movement, and the components of the brain that are needed for cognitive processes, remain intact. However, immunostaining indicates that neurons bearing ubiquitin, a marker for degeneration, are also detected in nonmotor systems. Moreover, studies of glucose metabolism in the illness also indicate that there is neuronal dysfunction outside of the motor system. Within the motor system, there is some selectivity of involvement. Thus, motor neurons required for ocular motility remain unaffected, as

TABLE 32-1

ETIOLOGY OF MOTOR NEURON DISORDERS

DIAGNOSTIC CATEGORY	INVESTIGATION
Structural lesions	MRI scan of head (including foramen magnum and cervical spine)
Parasagittal or foramen magnum tumors	
Cervical spondylosis	
Chiari malformation of syrinx	
Spinal cord arteriovenous malformation	
Infections	CSF exam, culture
Bacterial—tetanus, Lyme	Lyme titer
Viral—poliomyelitis, herpes zoster	Anti-viral antibody
Retroviral—myelopathy	HTLV-1 titers
Intoxications, physical agents	24-h urine for heavy metals
Toxins—lead, aluminum, others	Serum lead level
Drugs—strychnine, phenytoin	
Electric shock, x-irradiation	
Immunologic mechanisms	Complete blood count[a]
Plasma cell dyscrasias	Sedimentation rate[a]
Autoimmune polyradiculopathy	Total protein[a]
Motor neuropathy with conduction block	Anti-GM1 antibodies[a]
Paraneoplastic	Anti-Hu antibody
Paracarcinomatous	MRI scan, bone marrow biopsy
Metabolic	Fasting blood sugar[a]
Hypoglycemia	Routine chemistries including calcium[a]
Hyperparathyroidism	PTH
Hyperthyroidism	Thyroid function[a]
Deficiency of folate, vitamin B_{12}, vitamin E	Vitamin B_{12}, vitamin E, folate[a]
Deficiency of copper, zinc	Serum zinc, copper[a]
Malabsorption	24-h stool fat, carotene, prothrombin time
Mitochondrial dysfunction	Fasting lactate, pyruvate, ammonia
	Consider mtDNA
Hyperlipidemia	Lipid electrophoresis
Hyperglycinuria	Urine and serum amino acids
	CSF amino acids
Hereditary disorders	WBC DNA for mutational analysis
Superoxide dismutase	
TDP43	
FUS/TLS	
Androgen receptor defect (Kennedy's disease)	
Hexosaminidase deficiency	
Infantile α-glucosidase deficiency (Pompe's)	

[a]Denotes studies that should be obtained in all cases.

Abbreviations: CSF, cerebrospinal fluid; FUS/TLS, fused in sarcoma/translocated in liposarcoma; HTLV-1, human T cell lymphotropic virus; PTH, parathyroid; WBC, white blood cell.

do the parasympathetic neurons in the sacral spinal cord (the nucleus of Onufrowicz, or Onuf) that innervate the sphincters of the bowel and bladder.

CLINICAL MANIFESTATIONS

The manifestations of ALS are somewhat variable depending on whether corticospinal neurons or lower motor neurons in the brainstem and spinal cord are more prominently involved. With lower motor neuron dysfunction and early denervation, typically the first evidence of the disease is insidiously developing asymmetric weakness, usually first evident distally in one of the limbs. A detailed history often discloses recent development of cramping with volitional movements, typically in the early hours of the morning (e.g., while stretching in bed). Weakness caused by denervation is associated with progressive wasting and atrophy of muscles and, particularly early in the illness, spontaneous twitching of motor units, or fasciculations. In the hands, a preponderance of extensor over flexor weakness is common. When the initial denervation involves bulbar rather than limb

TABLE 32-2

SPORADIC MOTOR NEURON DISEASES

Chronic	Entity
Upper and lower motor neuron	Amyotrophic lateral sclerosis
Predominantly upper motor neuron	Primary lateral sclerosis
Predominantly lower motor neuron	Multifocal motor neuropathy with conduction block
	Motor neuropathy with paraproteinemia or cancer
	Motor predominant peripheral neuropathies
Other	
Associated with other neurodegenerative disorders	
Secondary motor neuron disorders (see Table 32-1)	
Acute	
Poliomyelitis	
Herpes zoster	
Coxsackie virus	

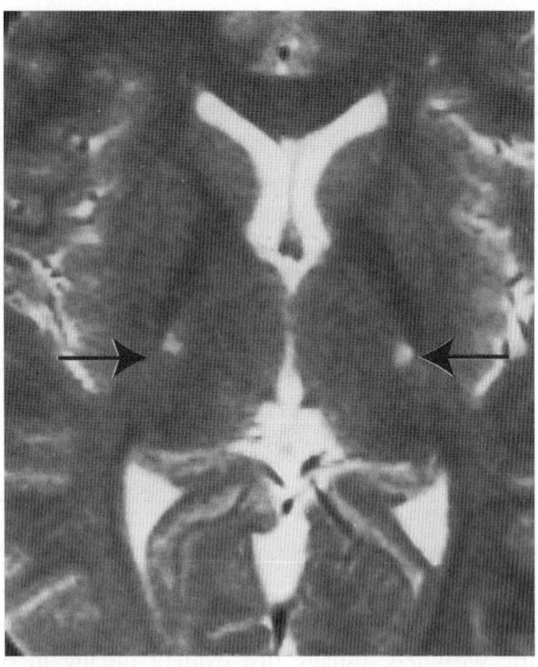

FIGURE 32-1

Amyotrophic lateral sclerosis. Axial T2-weighted MRI scan through the lateral ventricles of the brain reveals abnormal high signal intensity within the corticospinal tracts (*arrows*). This MRI feature represents an increase in water content in myelin tracts undergoing Wallerian degeneration secondary to cortical motor neuronal loss. This finding is commonly present in ALS, but can also be seen in AIDS-related encephalopathy, infarction, or other disease processes that produce corticospinal neuronal loss in a symmetric fashion.

muscles, the problem at onset is difficulty with chewing, swallowing, and movements of the face and tongue. Early involvement of the muscles of respiration may lead to death before the disease is far advanced elsewhere. With prominent corticospinal involvement, there is hyperactivity of the muscle-stretch reflexes (tendon jerks) and, often, spastic resistance to passive movements of the affected limbs. Patients with significant reflex hyperactivity complain of muscle stiffness often out of proportion to weakness. Degeneration of the corticobulbar projections innervating the brainstem results in dysarthria and exaggeration of the motor expressions of emotion. The latter leads to involuntary excess in weeping or laughing (pseudobulbar affect).

Virtually any muscle group may be the first to show signs of disease, but, as time passes, more and more muscles become involved until ultimately the disorder takes on a symmetric distribution in all regions. It is characteristic of ALS that, regardless of whether the initial disease involves upper or lower motor neurons, both will eventually be implicated. Even in the late stages of the illness, sensory, bowel and bladder, and cognitive functions are preserved. Even when there is severe brainstem disease, ocular motility is spared until the very late stages of the illness. Dementia is not a component of sporadic ALS. In some families, ALS is co-inherited with frontotemporal dementia, characterized by early behavioral abnormalities with prominent behavioral features indicative of frontal lobe dysfunction.

A committee of the World Federation of Neurology has established diagnostic guidelines for ALS. Essential for the diagnosis is simultaneous upper and lower motor neuron involvement with progressive weakness, and the exclusion of all alternative diagnoses. The disorder is ranked as "definite" ALS when three or four of the following are involved: bulbar, cervical, thoracic, and lumbosacral motor neurons. When two sites are involved, the diagnosis is "probable," and when only one site is implicated, the diagnosis is "possible." An exception is made for those who have progressive upper and lower motor neuron signs at only one site and a mutation in the gene encoding superoxide dismutase (SOD1; see later).

EPIDEMIOLOGY

The illness is relentlessly progressive, leading to death from respiratory paralysis; the median survival is from 3–5 years. There are very rare reports of stabilization or even regression of ALS. In most societies there is an incidence of 1–3 per 100,000 and a prevalence of 3–5 per 100,000. Several endemic foci of higher prevalence exist in the western Pacific (e.g., in specific regions of Guam or Papua New Guinea). In the United States and Europe, males are somewhat more frequently affected than females. Epidemiologic studies have incriminated risk factors for this disease including exposure to pesticides and insecticides, smoking, and, in one report, service in the military. While ALS is overwhelmingly a sporadic disorder, some 5–10% of cases are inherited as an autosomal dominant trait.

FAMILIAL ALS

Several forms of selective motor neuron disease are inheritable (Table 32-3). Familial ALS (FALS) involves both corticospinal and lower motor neurons. Apart from its inheritance as an autosomal dominant trait, it is clinically indistinguishable from sporadic ALS. Genetic studies have identified mutations in the genes encoding the cytosolic enzyme SOD1 (superoxide dismutase), and the RNA binding proteins TDP43 (encoded by the TAR DNA binding protein gene), and FUS/TLS (fused in sarcoma/translocated in liposarcoma), as the most common causes of FALS. Mutations in SOD1 account for about 20% of cases of FALS, while TDP43 and FUS/TLS each represent about 5% of familial cases.

Rare mutations in other genes are also clearly implicated in ALS-like diseases. Thus, a familial, dominantly inherited motor disorder that in some individuals closely mimics the ALS phenotype arises from mutations in a gene that encodes a vesicle-binding protein. A predominantly lower motor neuron disease with early hoarseness due to laryngeal dysfunction has been ascribed to mutations in the gene encoding the cellular accessory motor protein dynactin. Mutations in senataxin, a helicase, cause an early adult-onset, slowly evolving ALS variant. Kennedy's syndrome is an X-linked, adult-onset disorder that may mimic ALS, as described later.

Genetic analyses are also beginning to illuminate the pathogenesis of some childhood-onset motor neuron diseases. For example, a slowly disabling degenerative, predominantly upper motor neuron disease that starts in the first decade is caused by mutations in a gene that expresses a novel signaling molecule with properties of a guanine-exchange factor, termed *alsin*.

DIFFERENTIAL DIAGNOSIS

Because ALS is currently untreatable, it is imperative that potentially remediable causes of motor neuron dysfunction be excluded (Table 32-1). This is particularly true in cases that are atypical by virtue of (1) restriction to either upper or lower motor neurons, (2) involvement of neurons other than motor neurons, and (3) evidence of motor neuronal conduction block on electrophysiologic testing. Compression of the cervical spinal cord or cervicomedullary junction from tumors in the cervical regions or at the foramen magnum or from cervical spondylosis with osteophytes projecting into the vertebral canal can produce weakness, wasting, and fasciculations in the upper limbs and spasticity in the legs, closely resembling ALS. The absence of cranial nerve involvement may be helpful in differentiation, although some foramen magnum lesions may compress the twelfth cranial (hypoglossal) nerve, with resulting paralysis of the tongue. Absence of pain or of sensory changes, normal bowel and bladder function, normal roentgenographic studies of the spine, and normal cerebrospinal fluid (CSF) all favor ALS. Where doubt exists, MRI scans and contrast myelography should be performed to visualize the cervical spinal cord.

Another important entity in the differential diagnosis of ALS is *multifocal motor neuropathy with conduction block* (MMCB), discussed later. A diffuse, lower motor axonal neuropathy mimicking ALS sometimes evolves in association with hematopoietic disorders such as lymphoma or multiple myeloma. In this clinical setting, the presence of an M-component in serum should prompt consideration of a bone marrow biopsy. Lyme disease may also cause an axonal, lower motor neuropathy, although typically with intense proximal limb pain and a CSF pleocytosis.

Other treatable disorders that occasionally mimic ALS are chronic lead poisoning and thyrotoxicosis. These disorders may be suggested by the patient's social or occupational history or by unusual clinical features. When the family history is positive, disorders involving the genes encoding cytosolic SOD1, TDP43, FUS/TLS, as well as adult hexosaminidase A or α-glucosidase deficiency must be excluded. These are readily identified by appropriate laboratory tests. Benign fasciculations are occasionally a source of concern because on inspection they resemble the fascicular twitchings that accompany motor neuron degeneration. The absence of weakness, atrophy, or denervation phenomena on electrophysiologic examination usually excludes ALS or other serious neurologic disease. Patients who have recovered from poliomyelitis may experience a delayed deterioration of motor neurons that presents clinically with progressive weakness, atrophy, and fasciculations. Its cause is unknown, but it is thought to reflect sublethal prior injury to motor neurons by poliovirus.

Rarely, ALS develops concurrently with features indicative of more widespread neurodegeneration. Thus, one infrequently encounters otherwise typical ALS patients with a parkinsonian movement disorder or dementia. It remains unclear whether this reflects the unlikely simultaneous occurrence of two disorders or a primary defect triggering two forms of neurodegeneration. The latter is suggested by the observation that multisystem neurodegenerative diseases may be inherited. For example, prominent amyotrophy has been described as a dominantly inherited disorder

TABLE 32-3

GENETIC MOTOR NEURON DISEASES

DISEASE	LOCUS	GENE	INHERITANCE	ONSET	GENE FUNCTION	UNUSUAL FEATURES
I. Upper and Lower Motor Neurons (familial ALS)						
ALS1	21q	Superoxide dismutase	AD	Adult	Protein antioxidant	
ALS2	2q	Alsin	AR	Juvenile	GEF signalling	Severe corticobulbar, corticospinal features
ALS4	9q	Senataxin	AD	Late juvenile	DNA helicase	Late childhood onset
ALS6	16p	FUS/TLS	AD	Adult	DNA, RNA binding	
ALS8	20q	Vesicle-associated protein B	AD	Adult	Vesicular trafficking	
ALS9	14q	Angiogenin	AD	Adult	RNAse, angiogenesis	
ALS10	1q	TARDBP	AD	Adult	DNA, RNA binding	
ALS	2p	Dynactin	AD	Adult	Axonal transport	Vocal cord stridor in some families
ALS	17q	Paraoxonases 1-3	AD	Adult	Detoxify intoxicants	
ALS	mtDNA	Cytochrome c oxidase		Adult	ATP generation	
ALS	mtDNA	tRNA-isoleucine		Adult	ATP generation	
II. Lower Motor Neurons						
Spinal muscular atrophies	5q	Survival motor neuron	AR	Infancy	RNA metabolism	
GM2-gangliosidosis						
1. Sandhoff disease	5q	Hexosaminidase B	AR	Childhood	Ganglioside recycling	
2. AB variant	5q	GM2-activator protein	AR	Childhood	Ganglioside recycling	
3. Adult Tay-Sachs disease	15q	Hexosaminidase A	AR	Childhood	Ganglioside recycling	
X-linked spinobulbar muscular atrophy	Xq	Androgen receptor	XR	Adult	Nuclear signalling	
III. Upper Motor Neuron (Selected FSPs)						
SPG3A	14q	Atlastin	AD	Childhood	GTPase—vesicle recycling	Some peripheral neuropathy
SPG4	2p	Spastin	AD	Early adulthood	ATPase family—microtubule associate	± mental retardation, motor neuropathy

(continued)

TABLE 32-3

GENETIC MOTOR NEURON DISEASES (*CONTINUED*)

DISEASE	LOCUS	GENE	INHERITANCE	ONSET	GENE FUNCTION	UNUSUAL FEATURES
SPG6	15q	NIPA1	AD	Early adulthood	Membrane transporter or receptor	Deleted in Prader-Willi, Angelman
SPG8	8q	Strumpellin	AD	Early adulthood	Ubiquitous, spectrin-like	
SPG10	12q	Kinesin heavy chain KIF5A	AD	2nd–3rd decade	Motor-associated protein	± peripheral neuropathy, retardation
SPG13	2q	Heat shock protein 60	AD	Early adulthood	Chaperone protein	
SPG17	11q	Silver (BSCL2)	AD	Variable	Membrane protein in ER	Amyotrophy hands, feet
SPG31	2p	REEP1	AD	Early	Mitochondrial protein	Rarely, amyotrophy
SPG33	10q	ZFYVE27	AD	Adult	Interacts with spastin	Pes equinus
SPG42	3q	Acetyl-CoA-transporter	AD	Variable	Solute carrier	
SPG5	8q	Cytochrome P450	AR	Variable	Degrades endogenous substances	Sensory loss
SPG7	16q	Paraplegin	AR	Variable	Mitochondrial protein	Rarely, optic atrophy, ataxia, neuropathy
SPG11	15q	Spatacsin	AR	Childhood	Cytosolic, ? membrane-associated	Some sensory loss, thin corpus callosum
SPG15	14q	Spastizin	AR	Childhood	Zinc finger protein	Some amyotrophy, some CNS features including thin corpus callosum
SPG20	13q	Spartin	AR	Childhood	Endosomal-trafficking protein	Cerebellar, extrapyramidal signs, short stature, MR
SPG21	15q	Maspardin	AR	Childhood	Endosomal-trafficking protein	Cerebellar, extrapyramidal signs, short stature, MR
SPG35	16q	Fatty acid 2 hydrolase	AR	Childhood	Membrane protein	Multiple CNS features
SPG39	19p	Neuropathy target esterase	AR	Early childhood	Esterase	
SPG44	1q	Connexin 47	AR	Childhood	Gap junction protein	Possible mild CNS features
SPG2	Xq	Proteolipid protein	XR	Early childhood	Myelin protein	Sometimes multiple CNS features

(continued)

TABLE 32-3

GENETIC MOTOR NEURON DISEASES (*CONTINUED*)

DISEASE	LOCUS	GENE	INHERITANCE	ONSET	GENE FUNCTION	UNUSUAL FEATURES
SPG1	Xq	L1-CAM	XR	Infancy	Cell-adhesion molecule	
	Xq	Adrenoleukodystrophy	XR	Early adulthood	ATP-binding transporter protein	Possible adrenal insufficiency, CNS inflammation
IV. ALS-Plus Syndromes						
Amyotrophy with behavioral disorders	17q	Tau protein				
Parkinsonism						

Abbreviations: ALS, amyotrophic lateral sclerosis; BSCL2, Bernadelli-Seip congenital lipodystrophy 2B; FSP, familial spastic paraplegia; FUS/TLS, fused in sarcoma/translocated in liposarcoma; TDP43, Tar DNA binding protein 43 kd.

in individuals with bizarre behavior and a movement disorder suggestive of parkinsonism; many such cases have now been ascribed to mutations that alter the expression of tau protein in brain (Chap. 29). In other cases, ALS develops simultaneously with a striking frontotemporal dementia. These disorders may be dominantly co-inherited; in some families, this trait is linked to a locus on chromosome 9p, although the underlying genetic defect is not established. An ALS-like disorder has also been described in some individuals with chronic traumatic encephalopathy, associated with deposition of TDP43 and neurofibrillary tangles in motor neurons.

PATHOGENESIS

The cause of sporadic ALS is not well defined. Several mechanisms that impair motor neuron viability have been elucidated in mice and rats induced to develop motor neuron disease by SOD1 transgenes with ALS-associated mutations. It is evident that excitotoxic neurotransmitters such as glutamate participate in the death of motor neurons in ALS. This may be a consequence of diminished uptake of synaptic glutamate by an astroglial glutamate transporter, EAAT2. It is striking that one cellular defense against such excitotoxicity is the enzyme SOD1, which detoxifies the free radical superoxide anion. Precisely why SOD1 mutations are toxic to motor nerves is not established, although it is clear the effect is not simply loss of normal scavenging of the superoxide anion. The mutant protein is conformationally unstable and prone to aberrant catalytic reactions. In turn, these features lead to aggregation of SOD1 protein, impairment of axonal transport, reduced production of ATP and other perturbations of mitochondrial function, activation of neuroinflammatory cascades within the ALS spinal cord, and ultimately induction of cell death via pathways that are at least partially dependent on caspases.

It has recently been observed that mutations in the TDP43 and FUS/TLS genes also cause ALS. These multifunctional proteins bind RNA and DNA and shuttle between the nucleus and the cytoplasm, playing multiple roles in the control of cell proliferation, DNA repair and transcription, and gene translation, both in the cytoplasm and locally in dendritic spines in response to electrical activity. How mutations in FUS/TLS provoke motor neuron cell death is not clear, although this may represent loss of function of FUS/TLS in the nucleus or an acquired, toxic function of the mutant proteins in the cytosol.

Multiple recent studies have convincingly demonstrated that non-neuronal cells importantly influence the disease course, at least in ALS transgenic mice. A striking additional finding in neurodegenerative disorders is that miscreant proteins arising from gene defects in familial forms of these diseases are often implicated in sporadic forms of the same disorder. For example, germline mutations in the genes encoding beta-amyloid and alpha-synuclein cause familial forms of Alzheimer's and Parkinson's diseases (AD and PD), and posttranslational, noninherited abnormalities in these proteins are also central to sporadic AD and PD. Analogously, recent reports propose that nonheritable, posttranslational modifications in SOD1 are pathogenic in sporadic ALS.

TREATMENT Amyotrophic Lateral Sclerosis

No treatment arrests the underlying pathologic process in ALS. The drug riluzole (100 mg/d) was approved for ALS because it produces a modest lengthening of survival. In one trial, the survival rate at 18 months with riluzole was similar to placebo at 15 months. The mechanism of this effect is not known with certainty; riluzole may reduce excitotoxicity by diminishing glutamate release. Riluzole is generally well tolerated; nausea, dizziness, weight loss, and elevated liver enzymes occur occasionally. Pathophysiologic studies of mutant SOD1–related ALS in mice have disclosed diverse targets for therapy; consequently, multiple therapies are presently in clinical trials for ALS. These include studies of ceftriaxone, which may augment astroglial glutamate transport and thereby be anti-excitotoxic, and pramipexole and tamoxifen, which are neuroprotective. Interventions such as antisense oligonucleotides (ASO) that diminish expression of mutant SOD1 protein prolong survival in transgenic ALS mice and rats and are also now in trial for SOD1-mediated ALS.

In the absence of a primary therapy for ALS, a variety of rehabilitative aids may substantially assist ALS patients. Foot-drop splints facilitate ambulation by obviating the need for excessive hip flexion and by preventing tripping on a floppy foot. Finger extension splints can potentiate grip. Respiratory support may be life-sustaining. For patients electing against long-term ventilation by tracheostomy, positive-pressure ventilation by mouth or nose provides transient (several weeks) relief from hypercarbia and hypoxia. Also extremely beneficial for some patients is a respiratory device (Cough Assist Device) that produces an artificial cough. This is highly effective in clearing airways and preventing aspiration pneumonia. When bulbar disease prevents normal chewing and swallowing, gastrostomy is uniformly helpful, restoring normal nutrition and hydration. Fortunately, an increasing variety of speech synthesizers are now available to augment speech when there is advanced bulbar palsy. These facilitate oral communication and may be effective for telephone use.

In contrast to ALS, several of the disorders (Tables 32-1 and 32-3) that bear some clinical resemblance to ALS are treatable. For this reason, a careful search for causes of secondary motor neuron disease is warranted.

OTHER MOTOR NEURON DISEASES

SELECTED LOWER MOTOR NEURON DISORDERS

In these motor neuron diseases, the peripheral motor neurons are affected without evidence of involvement of the corticospinal motor system (Tables 32-1 to 32-3).

X-Linked spinobulbar muscular atrophy (Kennedy's disease)

This is an X-linked lower motor neuron disorder in which progressive weakness and wasting of limb and bulbar muscles begins in males in mid-adult life and is conjoined with androgen insensitivity manifested by gynecomastia and reduced fertility. In addition to gynecomastia, which may be subtle, two findings distinguishing this disorder from ALS are the absence of signs of pyramidal tract disease (spasticity) and the presence of a subtle sensory neuropathy in some patients. The underlying molecular defect is an expanded trinucleotide repeat (-CAG-) in the first exon of the androgen receptor gene on the X chromosome. DNA testing is available. An inverse correlation appears to exist between the number of -CAG- repeats and the age of onset of the disease.

Adult Tay-Sach's disease

Several reports have described adult-onset, predominantly lower motor neuropathies arising from deficiency of the enzyme β-hexosaminidase (hex A). These tend to be distinguishable from ALS because they are very slowly progressive; dysarthria and radiographically evident cerebellar atrophy may be prominent. In rare cases, spasticity may also be present, although it is generally absent.

Spinal muscular atrophy

The SMAs are a family of selective lower motor neuron diseases of early onset. Despite some phenotypic variability (largely in age of onset), the defect in the majority of families with SMA maps to a locus on chromosome 5 encoding a putative motor neuron survival protein (SMN, for survival motor neuron) that is important in the formation and trafficking of RNA complexes across the nuclear membrane. Neuropathologically these disorders are characterized by extensive loss of large motor neurons; muscle biopsy reveals evidence of denervation atrophy. Several clinical forms exist.

Infantile SMA (SMA I, Werdnig-Hoffmann disease) has the earliest onset and most rapidly fatal course. In some instances it is apparent even before birth, as indicated by decreased fetal movements late in the third trimester. Though alert, afflicted infants are weak and floppy (hypotonic) and lack muscle stretch reflexes. Death generally ensues within the first year of life. *Chronic childhood SMA* (SMA II) begins later in childhood and evolves with a more slowly progressive course. *Juvenile SMA* (SMA III, Kugelberg-Welander disease) manifests during late childhood and runs a slow, indolent course. Unlike most denervating diseases, in this chronic disorder weakness is greatest in the proximal muscles; indeed, the pattern of clinical weakness can suggest a primary myopathy such as limb-girdle dystrophy. Electrophysiologic and muscle biopsy evidence of denervation distinguish SMA III from the myopathic syndromes. There is no primary therapy for SMA, although remarkable recent experimental data indicate that it may be possible to deliver the missing SMN gene to motor neurons using intravenously delivered adeno-associated viruses (e.g., AAV9) immediately after birth.

Multifocal motor neuropathy with conduction block

In this disorder lower motor neuron function is regionally and chronically disrupted by remarkably focal blocks in conduction. Many cases have elevated serum titers of mono- and polyclonal antibodies to ganglioside GM1; it is hypothesized that the antibodies produce selective, focal, paranodal demyelination of motor neurons. MMCB is not typically associated with corticospinal signs. In contrast with ALS, MMCB may respond dramatically to therapy such as IV immunoglobulin or chemotherapy; it is thus imperative that MMCB be excluded when considering a diagnosis of ALS.

Other forms of lower motor neuron disease

In individual families, other syndromes characterized by selective lower motor neuron dysfunction in an SMA-like pattern have been described. There are rare X-linked and autosomal dominant forms of apparent SMA. There is an ALS variant of juvenile onset, the Fazio-Londe syndrome, that involves mainly the musculature innervated by the brainstem. A component of lower motor neuron dysfunction is also found in degenerative disorders such as Machado-Joseph disease and the related olivopontocerebellar degenerations (Chap. 31).

SELECTED DISORDERS OF THE UPPER MOTOR NEURON

Primary lateral sclerosis

This exceedingly rare disorder arises sporadically in adults in mid to late life. Clinically PLS is characterized by progressive spastic weakness of the limbs, preceded or followed by spastic dysarthria and dysphagia, indicating combined involvement of the corticospinal and corticobulbar tracts. Fasciculations, amyotrophy, and sensory changes are absent; neither electromyography nor muscle biopsy shows denervation. On neuropathologic examination there is selective loss of the large pyramidal cells in the precentral gyrus and degeneration of the corticospinal and corticobulbar projections. The peripheral motor neurons and other neuronal systems are spared. The course of PLS is variable; while long-term survival is documented, the course may be as aggressive as in ALS, with ~3-year survival from onset to death. Early in its course, PLS raises the question of multiple sclerosis or other demyelinating diseases such as adrenoleukodystrophy as diagnostic considerations (Chap. 39). A myelopathy suggestive of PLS is infrequently seen with infection with the retrovirus human T cell lymphotropic virus (HTLV-I) (Chap. 35). The clinical course and laboratory testing will distinguish these possibilities.

Familial spastic paraplegia

In its pure form, FSP is usually transmitted as an autosomal trait; most adult-onset cases are dominantly inherited. Symptoms usually begin in the third or fourth decade, presenting as progressive spastic weakness beginning in the distal lower extremities; however, there are variants with onset so early that the differential diagnosis includes cerebral palsy. FSP typically has a long survival, presumably because respiratory function is spared. Late in the illness there may be urinary urgency and incontinence and sometimes fecal incontinence; sexual function tends to be preserved.

In pure forms of FSP, the spastic leg weakness is often accompanied by posterior column (vibration and position) abnormalities and disturbance of bowel and bladder function. Some family members may have spasticity without clinical symptoms.

By contrast, particularly when recessively inherited, FSP may have complex or complicated forms in which altered corticospinal and dorsal column function is accompanied by significant involvement of other regions of the nervous system, including amyotrophy, mental retardation, optic atrophy, and sensory neuropathy.

Neuropathologically, in FSP there is degeneration of the corticospinal tracts, which appear nearly normal in the brainstem but show increasing atrophy at more caudal levels in the spinal cord; in effect, the pathologic picture is of a dying-back or distal axonopathy of long neuronal fibers within the CNS.

Defects at numerous loci underlie both dominantly and recessively inherited forms of FSP (Table 32-3). More than 20 FSP genes have now been identified. The gene most commonly implicated in dominantly inherited FSP is *spastin,* which encodes a microtubule interacting protein. The most common childhood-onset dominant form arises from mutations in the *atlastin* gene. A kinesin heavy-chain protein implicated in microtubule motor function was found to be defective in a family with dominantly inherited FSP of variable onset age.

An infantile-onset form of X-linked, recessive FSP arises from mutations in the gene for myelin proteolipid protein. This is an example of rather striking allelic variation, as most other mutations in the same gene cause not FSP but Pelizaeus-Merzbacher disease, a widespread disorder of CNS myelin. Another recessive variant is caused by defects in the *paraplegin* gene. Paraplegin has homology to metalloproteases that are important in mitochondrial function in yeast.

WEBSITES

Several websites provide valuable information on ALS including those offered by the Muscular Dystrophy Association (*www.mdausa.org*), the Amyotrophic Lateral Sclerosis Association (*www.alsa.org*), and the World Federation of Neurology and the Neuromuscular Unit at Washington University in St. Louis (*www.neuro.wustl.edu/neuromuscular*).

CHAPTER 33

DISORDERS OF THE AUTONOMIC NERVOUS SYSTEM

Phillip A. Low ■ John W. Engstrom

The autonomic nervous system (ANS) innervates the entire neuraxis and permeates all organ systems. It regulates blood pressure (BP), heart rate, sleep, and bladder and bowel function. It operates automatically; its full importance becomes recognized only when ANS function is compromised, resulting in dysautonomia. Hypothalamic disorders that cause disturbances in homeostasis are discussed in Chap. 38.

ANATOMIC ORGANIZATION

The activity of the ANS is regulated by central neurons responsive to diverse afferent inputs. After central integration of afferent information, autonomic outflow is adjusted to permit the functioning of the major organ systems in accordance with the needs of the organism as a whole. Connections between the cerebral cortex and the autonomic centers in the brainstem coordinate autonomic outflow with higher mental functions.

The preganglionic neurons of the parasympathetic nervous system leave the central nervous system (CNS) in the third, seventh, ninth, and tenth cranial nerves as well as the second and third sacral nerves, while the preganglionic neurons of the sympathetic nervous system exit the spinal cord between the first thoracic and the second lumbar segments (Fig. 33-1). These are thinly myelinated. The postganglionic neurons, located in ganglia outside the CNS, give rise to the postganglionic unmyelinated autonomic nerves that innervate organs and tissues throughout the body. Responses to sympathetic and parasympathetic stimulation are frequently antagonistic (Table 33-1), reflecting highly coordinated interactions within the CNS; the resultant changes in parasympathetic and sympathetic activity provide more precise control of autonomic responses than could be achieved by the modulation of a single system.

Acetylcholine (ACh) is the preganglionic neurotransmitter for both divisions of the ANS as well as the postganglionic neurotransmitter of the parasympathetic neurons; the preganglionic receptors are nicotinic, and the postganglionic are muscarinic in type. Norepinephrine (NE) is the neurotransmitter of the postganglionic sympathetic neurons, except for cholinergic neurons innervating the eccrine sweat glands.

CLINICAL EVALUATION

CLASSIFICATION

Disorders of the ANS may result from pathology of either the CNS or the peripheral nervous system (PNS) (Table 33-2). Signs and symptoms may result from interruption of the afferent limb, CNS processing centers, or efferent limb of reflex arcs controlling autonomic responses. For example, a lesion of the medulla produced by a posterior fossa tumor can impair BP responses to postural changes and result in orthostatic hypotension (OH). OH can also be caused by lesions of the spinal cord or peripheral vasomotor nerve fibers (e.g., diabetic autonomic neuropathy). Lesions of the efferent limb cause the most consistent and severe OH. The site of reflex interruption is usually established by the clinical context in which the dysautonomia arises, combined with judicious use of ANS testing and neuroimaging studies. The presence or absence of CNS signs, association with sensory or motor polyneuropathy, medical illnesses, medication use, and family history are often important considerations. Some syndromes do not fit easily into any classification scheme.

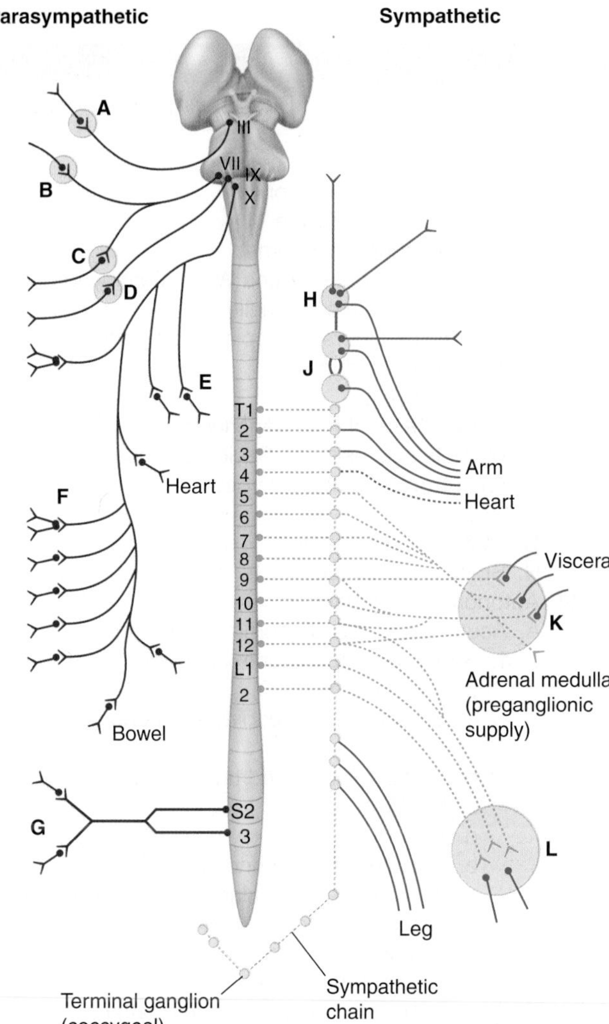

Parasympathetic system
from cranial nerves III, VII, IX, X
and from sacral nerves 2 and 3

- **A** Ciliary ganglion
- **B** Sphenopalatine (pterygopalatine) ganglion
- **C** Submandibular ganglion
- **D** Otic ganglion
- **E** Vagal ganglion cells in the heart wall
- **F** Vagal ganglion cells in bowel wall
- **G** Pelvic ganglia

Sympathetic system
from T1-L2
Preganglionic fibers ············
Postganglionic fibers ———

- **H** Superior cervical ganglion
- **J** Middle cervical ganglion and inferior cervical (stellate) ganglion including T1 ganglion
- **K** Coeliac and other abdominal ganglia
- **L** Lower abdominal sympathetic ganglia

FIGURE 33-1

Schematic representation of the autonomic nervous system. *(From M Moskowitz: Clin Endocrinol Metab 6:77, 1977.)*

SYMPTOMS OF AUTONOMIC DYSFUNCTION

Clinical manifestations can result from loss of function, overactivity, or dysregulation of autonomic circuits. Disorders of autonomic function should be considered in all patients with unexplained orthostatic hypotension, syncope, sleep dysfunction, altered sweating (hyperhidrosis or hypohidrosis), constipation, upper gastrointestinal symptoms (bloating, nausea, vomiting of old food), impotence, or bladder disorders (urinary frequency, hesitancy, or incontinence). Symptoms may be widespread or regional in distribution. An autonomic history focuses on systemic functions (BP, heart rate, sleep, fever, sweating) and involvement of individual organ systems (pupils, bowel, bladder, sexual function). The autonomic symptom profile is a self-report questionnaire that can be used for formal assessment. It is also important to recognize the modulating effects of age. For example, OH typically produces lightheadedness in the young, whereas cognitive slowing is more common in the elderly. Specific symptoms of orthostatic intolerance are diverse (Table 33-3). Autonomic symptoms may vary dramatically, reflecting the dynamic nature of autonomic control over homeostatic function. For example, OH might be manifest only in the early morning, following a meal, with exercise, or with raised ambient temperature, depending upon the regional vascular bed affected by dysautonomia.

Early symptoms may be overlooked. Impotence, although not specific for autonomic failure, often heralds autonomic failure in men and may precede other symptoms by years. A decrease in the frequency of spontaneous early morning erections may occur months before loss of nocturnal penile tumescence and development of total impotence. Bladder dysfunction may appear early in men and women, particularly in those with CNS involvement. Cold feet may indicate peripheral vasomotor constriction. Brain and spinal cord disease above the level of the lumbar spine results first in

TABLE 33-1

FUNCTIONAL CONSEQUENCES OF NORMAL ANS ACTIVATION

	SYMPATHETIC	PARASYMPATHETIC
Heart rate	Increased	Decreased
Blood pressure	Increased	Mildly decreased
Bladder	Increased sphincter tone	Voiding (decreased tone)
Bowel motility	Decreased motility	Increased
Lung	Bronchodilation	Bronchoconstriction
Sweat glands	Sweating	—
Pupils	Dilation	Constriction
Adrenal glands	Catecholamine release	—
Sexual function	Ejaculation, orgasm	Erection
Lacrimal glands	—	Tearing
Parotid glands	—	Salivation

TABLE 33-2

CLASSIFICATION OF CLINICAL AUTONOMIC DISORDERS

I. Autonomic disorders with brain involvement
  A. Associated with multisystem degeneration
    1. Multisystem degeneration: autonomic failure clinically prominent
      a. Multiple system atrophy (MSA)
      b. Parkinson's disease with autonomic failure
      c. Diffuse Lewy body disease (some cases)
    2. Multisystem degeneration: autonomic failure clinically not usually prominent
      a. Parkinson's disease
      b. Other extrapyramidal disorders (inherited spinocerebellar atrophies, progressive supranuclear palsy, corticobasal degeneration, Machado-Joseph disease, fragile X syndrome [FXTAS])
  B. Unassociated with multisystem degeneration (focal CNS disorders)
    1. Disorders mainly due to cerebral cortex involvement
      a. Frontal cortex lesions causing urinary/bowel incontinence
      b. Partial complex seizures (temporal lobe or anterior cingulate)
      c. Cerebral infarction of the insula
    2. Disorders of the limbic and paralimbic circuits
      a. Shapiro's syndrome (agenesis of corpus callosum, hyperhidrosis, hypothermia)
      b. Autonomic seizures
      c. Limbic encephalitis
    3. Disorders of the hypothalamus
      a. Wernicke-Korsakoff syndrome
      b. Diencephalic syndrome
      c. Neuroleptic malignant syndrome
      d. Serotonin syndrome
      e. Fatal familial insomnia
      f. Antidiuretic hormone syndromes (diabetes insipidus, inappropriate ADH secretion)
      g. Disturbances of temperature regulation (hyperthermia, hypothermia)
      h. Disturbances of sexual function
      i. Disturbances of appetite
      j. Disturbances of BP/HR and gastric function
      k. Horner's syndrome
    4. Disorders of the brainstem and cerebellum
      a. Posterior fossa tumors
      b. Syringobulbia and Arnold-Chiari malformation
      c. Disorders of BP control (hypertension, hypotension)
      d. Cardiac arrhythmias
      e. Central sleep apnea
      f. Baroreflex failure
      g. Horner's syndrome
      h. Vertebrobasilar and Wallenberg syndromes
      i. Brainstem encephalitis

II. Autonomic disorders with spinal cord involvement
  A. Traumatic quadriplegia
  B. Syringomyelia
  C. Subacute combined degeneration
  D. Multiple sclerosis and Devic's disease
  E. Amyotrophic lateral sclerosis
  F. Tetanus
  G. Stiff-man syndrome
  H. Spinal cord tumors

III. Autonomic neuropathies
  A. Acute/subacute autonomic neuropathies
    1. Subacute autoimmune autonomic ganglionopathy (AAG)
      a. Subacute paraneoplastic autonomic neuropathy
      b. Guillain-Barré syndrome
      c. Botulism
      d. Porphyria
      e. Drug-induced autonomic neuropathies-stimulants, drug withdrawal, vasoconstrictor, vasodilators, beta-receptor antagonists, beta-agonists
      f. Toxic autonomic neuropathies
      g. Subacute cholinergic neuropathy
  B. Chronic peripheral autonomic neuropathies
    1. Distal small fiber neuropathy
    2. Combined sympathetic and parasympathetic failure
      a. Amyloid
      b. Diabetic autonomic neuropathy
      c. Autoimmune autonomic ganglionopathy (paraneoplastic and idiopathic)
      d. Sensory neuronopathy with autonomic failure
      e. Familial dysautonomia (Riley-Day syndrome)
      f. Diabetic, uremic, or nutritional deficiency
      g. Dysautonomia of old age
    3. Disorders of reduced orthostatic intolerance-reflex syncope, POTS, associated with prolonged bed rest, associated with space flight, chronic fatigue

Abbreviations: BP, blood pressure; HR, heart rate; POTS, postural orthostatic tachycardia syndrome.

urinary frequency and small bladder volumes and eventually in incontinence (upper motor neuron or spastic bladder). By contrast, PNS disease of autonomic nerve fibers results in large bladder volumes, urinary frequency, and overflow incontinence (lower motor neuron flaccid bladder). Measurement of bladder volume (postvoid residual) is a useful bedside test for distinguishing between upper and lower motor neuron bladder dysfunction in the early stages of dysautonomia. Gastrointestinal autonomic dysfunction typically presents as severe constipation. Diarrhea occurs occasionally (as in diabetes mellitus) due to rapid transit of contents or uncoordinated small-bowel motor activity, or on an osmotic basis from bacterial overgrowth associated with small-bowel stasis. Impaired glandular secretory function may cause difficulty with food intake due to decreased salivation or eye irritation due to decreased lacrimation. Occasionally, temperature elevation and vasodilation

TABLE 33-3

SYMPTOMS OF ORTHOSTATIC INTOLERANCE	
Lightheadedness (dizziness)	88%
Weakness or tiredness	72%
Cognitive difficulty (thinking/concentrating)	47%
Blurred vision	47%
Tremulousness	38%
Vertigo	37%
Pallor	31%
Anxiety	29%
Palpitations	26%
Clammy feeling	19%
Nausea	18%

Source: From PA Low et al: Mayo Clin Proc 70:617, 1995.

can result from anhidrosis because sweating is normally important for heat dissipation. Lack of sweating after a hot bath, during exercise, or on a hot day can suggest sudomotor failure.

OH (also called *orthostatic or postural hypotension*) is perhaps the most disabling feature of autonomic dysfunction. The prevalence of OH is relatively high, especially when OH associated with aging and diabetes mellitus is included (Table 33-4). OH can cause a variety of symptoms, including dimming or loss of vision, lightheadedness, diaphoresis, diminished hearing, pallor, and weakness. Syncope results when the drop in BP impairs cerebral perfusion. Other manifestations of impaired baroreflexes are supine hypertension, a heart rate that is fixed regardless of posture, postprandial hypotension, and an excessively high nocturnal BP. Many patients with OH have a preceding diagnosis of hypertension or have concomitant supine hypertension, reflecting the great importance of baroreflexes in maintaining postural and supine normotension. The appearance of OH in patients receiving antihypertensive treatment may indicate overtreatment or the onset of an autonomic disorder. The most common causes of OH are not neurologic in origin; these must be distinguished from the neurogenic causes (Table 33-5). Neurocardiogenic and cardiac causes of syncope are considered in Chap. 10.

TABLE 33-4

PREVALENCE OF ORTHOSTATIC HYPOTENSION IN DIFFERENT DISORDERS

DISORDER	PREVALENCE
Aging	14–20%
Diabetic neuropathy	10%
Other autonomic neuropathies	10–50 per 100,000
Multiple system atrophy	5–15 per 100,000
Pure autonomic failure	10–30 per 100,000

APPROACH TO THE PATIENT: Orthostatic Hypotension and Other ANS Disorders

The first step in the evaluation of symptomatic OH is the exclusion of treatable causes. The history should include a review of medications that may affect the autonomic system (Table 33-6). The main classes of drugs that may cause OH are diuretics, antihypertensives, antidepressants, phenothiazines, ethanol, narcotics, insulin, dopamine agonists, barbiturates, and calcium channel-blocking agents. However, the precipitation of OH by medications may also be the first sign of an underlying autonomic disorder. The history may reveal an underlying cause for symptoms (e.g., diabetes, Parkinson's disease) or specific underlying mechanisms (e.g., cardiac pump failure, reduced intravascular volume). The relationship of symptoms to meals (splanchnic pooling), standing on awakening in the morning (intravascular volume depletion), ambient warming (vasodilatation), or exercise (muscle arteriolar vasodilatation) should be

TABLE 33-5

NONNEUROGENIC CAUSES OF ORTHOSTATIC HYPOTENSION

Cardiac pump failure
- Myocardial infarction
- Myocarditis
- Constrictive pericarditis
- Aortic stenosis
- Tachyarrhythmias
- Bradyarrhythmias
- Salt-losing nephropathy
- Adrenal insufficiency
- Diabetes insipidus
- Venous obstruction

Reduced intravascular volume
- Straining or heavy lifting, urination, defecation
- Dehydration
- Diarrhea, emesis
- Hemorrhage
- Burns

Metabolic
- Adrenocortical insufficiency
- Hypoaldosteronism
- Pheochromocytoma
- Severe potassium depletion

Venous pooling
- Alcohol
- Postprandial dilation of splanchnic vessel beds
- Vigorous exercise with dilation of skeletal vessel beds
- Heat: hot environment, hot showers and baths, fever
- Prolonged recumbency or standing
- Sepsis

Medications
- Antihypertensives
- Diuretics
- Vasodilators: nitrates, hydralazine
- Alpha- and beta-blocking agents
- CNS sedatives: barbiturates, opiates
- Tricyclic antidepressants
- Phenothiazines

TABLE 33-6

SOME DRUGS THAT AFFECT AUTONOMIC FUNCTION

SYMPTOM	DRUG CLASS	SPECIFIC EXAMPLES
Impotence	Opioids Anabolic steroids Some antiarrhythmics Some antihypertensives Some diuretics Some SSRIs	Tylenol #3 — Prazosin Clonidine Benazepril Venlafaxine
Urinary retention	Opioids Decongestants	Fentanyl Brompheniramine Diphenhydramine
Diaphoresis	Some antihypertensives Some SSRIs Opioids	Amlodipine Citalopram Morphine
Hypotension	Tricyclics Beta blockers Diuretics CCBs	Amitriptyline Propranolol HCTZ Verapamil

Abbreviations: CCBs, calcium channel blockers; HCTZ, hydrochlorothiazide; SSRIs, selective serotonin reuptake inhibitors.

sought. Standing time to first symptom and presyncope should be followed for management.

Physical examination includes measurement of supine and standing pulse and BP. OH is defined as a sustained drop in systolic (≥20 mmHg) or diastolic (≥10 mmHg) BP within 3 min of standing. In nonneurogenic causes of OH (such as hypovolemia), the BP drop is accompanied by a compensatory increase in heart rate of >15 beats/min. A clue that the patient has neurogenic OH is the aggravation or precipitation of OH by autonomic stressors (such as a meal, hot tub/hot bath, and exercise). Neurologic examination should include mental status (neurodegenerative disorders), cranial nerves (impaired downgaze with progressive supranuclear palsy; abnormal pupils with Horner's or Adie's syndrome), motor tone (Parkinson's disease and parkinsonian syndromes), and reflexes and sensation (polyneuropathies). In patients without a clear diagnosis initially, follow-up evaluations may reveal the underlying cause.

Disorders of autonomic function should be considered in patients with symptoms of altered sweating (hyperhidrosis or hypohidrosis), gastroparesis (bloating, nausea, vomiting of old food), constipation, impotence, or bladder dysfunction (urinary frequency, hesitancy, or incontinence).

AUTONOMIC TESTING Autonomic function tests are helpful when the history and examination findings are inconclusive; to detect subclinical involvement; or to follow the course of an autonomic disorder.

Heart Rate Variation with Deep Breathing This is a test of the parasympathetic component of cardiovascular reflexes, via the vagus nerve. Results are influenced by multiple factors including the subject's position (recumbent, sitting, or standing), rate and depth of respiration (6 breaths per minute and a forced vital capacity [FVC] >1.5 L are optimal), age, medications, weight, and degree of hypocapnia. Interpretation of results requires comparison of test data with results from age-matched controls collected under identical test conditions. For example, the lower limit of normal heart rate variation with deep breathing in persons <20 years is >15–20 beats/min, but for persons over age 60 it is 5–8 beats/min. Heart rate variation with deep breathing (respiratory sinus arrhythmia) is abolished by the muscarinic acetylcholine (ACh)-receptor antagonist atropine but is unaffected by sympathetic postganglionic blockade (e.g., propranolol).

Valsalva Response This response (Table 33-7) assesses integrity of the baroreflex control of heart rate (parasympathetic) and BP (adrenergic). Under normal conditions, increases in BP at the carotid bulb trigger a reduction in heart rate (increased vagal tone), and decreases in BP trigger an increase in heart rate (reduced vagal tone). The Valsalva response is tested in the supine position. The subject exhales against a closed glottis (or into a manometer maintaining a constant expiratory pressure of 40 mmHg) for 15 s while measuring changes in heart rate and beat-to-beat BP. There are four phases of BP and heart rate response to the Valsalva maneuver. Phases I and III are mechanical and related to changes in intrathoracic and intraabdominal pressure. In early phase II, reduced venous return results in a fall in stroke volume and BP, counteracted by a combination of reflex tachycardia and increased total peripheral resistance. Increased total peripheral resistance arrests the BP drop ~5–8 s after the onset of the maneuver. Late phase II begins with a progressive rise in BP toward or above baseline. Venous return and cardiac output return to normal in phase IV. Persistent peripheral arteriolar vasoconstriction and increased cardiac adrenergic tone result in a temporary BP overshoot and phase IV bradycardia (mediated by the baroreceptor reflex).

Autonomic function during the Valsalva maneuver can be measured using beat-to-beat blood pressure or heart rate changes. The *Valsalva ratio* is defined as the maximum phase II tachycardia divided by the minimum phase IV bradycardia (Table 33-8). The ratio reflects the integrity of the entire baroreceptor reflex arc and of sympathetic efferents to blood vessels.

Sudomotor Function Sweating is induced by release of ACh from sympathetic postganglionic fibers. The quantitative sudomotor axon reflex test (QSART) is a measure of regional autonomic function mediated by

TABLE 33-7

NORMAL BLOOD PRESSURE AND HEART RATE CHANGES DURING THE VALSALVA MANEUVER

PHASE	MANEUVER	BLOOD PRESSURE	HEART RATE	COMMENTS
I	Forced expiration against a partially closed glottis	Rises; aortic compression from raised intrathoracic pressure	Decreases	Mechanical
II *early*	Continued expiration	Falls; decreased venous return to the heart	Increases (reflex tachycardia)	Reduced vagal tone
II *late*	Continued expiration	Rises; reflex increase in peripheral vascular resistance	Increases at slower rate	Requires intact efferent sympathetic response
III	End of expiration	Falls; increased capacitance of pulmonary bed	Increases further	Mechanical
IV	Recovery	Rises; persistent vasoconstriction and increased cardiac output	Compensatory bradycardia	Requires intact efferent sympathetic response

ACh-induced sweating. A reduced or absent response indicates a lesion of the postganglionic sudomotor axon. For example, sweating may be reduced in the feet as a result of distal polyneuropathy (e.g., diabetes). The thermoregulatory sweat test (TST) is a qualitative measure of regional sweat production in response to an elevation of body temperature under controlled conditions. An indicator powder placed on the anterior surface of the body changes color with sweat production during temperature elevation. The pattern of color changes is a measure of regional sweat secretion. A postganglionic lesion is present if both QSART and TST show absent sweating. In a preganglionic lesion, QSART is normal but TST shows anhidrosis.

TABLE 33-8

NEURAL PATHWAYS UNDERLYING SOME STANDARDIZED AUTONOMIC TESTS

TEST EVALUATED	PROCEDURE	AUTONOMIC FUNCTION
HRDB	6 deep breaths/min	Cardiovagal function
Valsalva ratio	Expiratory pressure, 40 mmHg for 10–15 s	Cardiovagal function
QSART	Axon-reflex test 4 limb sites	Postganglionic sudomotor function
BP_{BB} to VM	BP_{BB} response to VM	Adrenergic function: baroreflex adrenergic control of vagal and vasomotor function
HUT	BP_{BB} and heart rate response to HUT	Adrenergic and cardiovagal responses to HUT

Abbreviations: BP_{BB}, beat-to-beat blood pressure; HRDB, heart rate response to deep breathing; HUT, head-up tilt; QSART, quantitative sudomotor axon-reflex test; VM, Valsalva maneuver.

Orthostatic BP Recordings Beat-to-beat BP measurements determined in supine, 70° tilt, and tilt-back positions are useful to quantitate orthostatic failure of BP control. Allow a 20-min period of rest in the supine position before assessing changes in BP during tilting. The BP change combined with heart rate monitoring is useful for the evaluation of patients with suspected OH or unexplained syncope.

Tilt Table Testing for Syncope The great majority of patients with syncope do not have autonomic failure. Tilt table testing can be used to make the diagnosis of vasovagal syncope with sensitivity, specificity, and reproducibility. A standardized protocol is used that specifies the tilt apparatus, angle and duration of tilt, and procedure for provocation of vasodilation (e.g., sublingual or spray nitroglycerin). A positive nitroglycerin-stimulated test predicts recurrence of syncope. Recommendations for the performance of tilt studies for syncope have been incorporated in consensus guidelines.

SPECIFIC SYNDROMES OF ANS DYSFUNCTION

MULTIPLE SYSTEM ATROPHY (CHAP. 30)

Multiple system atrophy (MSA) is an entity that comprises autonomic failure (OH or a neurogenic bladder) *and* either parkinsonism (MSA-p) or a cerebellar

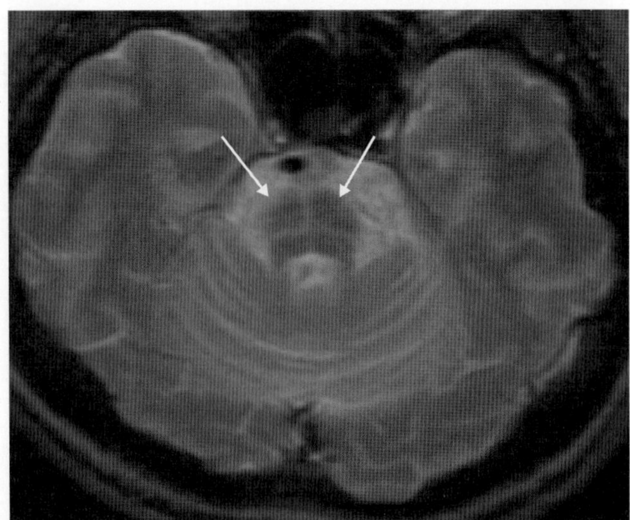

FIGURE 33-2
Multiple system atrophy, cerebellar type (MSA-c). Axial T2-weighted MRI at the level of the pons shows a characteristic hyperintense signal, the "hot cross buns" sign.

syndrome (MSA-c). MSA-p is the more common form; the parkinsonism is atypical in that it is usually unassociated with significant tremor or response to levodopa. Symptomatic OH within 1 year of onset of parkinsonism predicts eventual development of MSA-p in 75% of patients. Although autonomic abnormalities are common in advanced Parkinson's disease (Chap. 30), the severity and distribution of autonomic failure is more severe and more generalized in MSA. Brain MRI is a useful diagnostic adjunct; in MSA-p, iron deposition in the striatum may be evident as T2 hypointensity, and in MSA-c cerebellar atrophy is present with a characteristic T2 hyperintense signal ("hot cross buns sign") in the pons (Fig. 33-2). Cardiac postganglionic adrenergic innervation, measured by uptake of fluorodopamine on positron emission tomography, is markedly impaired in the dysautonomia of Parkinson's disease but is usually normal in MSA.

MSA generally progresses relentlessly to death 7–10 years after onset. Neuropathologic changes include neuronal loss and gliosis in many CNS regions, including the brainstem, cerebellum, striatum, and intermediolateral cell column of the thoracolumbar spinal cord. Management is symptomatic for neurogenic OH (see later in the chapter), gastrointestinal (GI), and urinary dysfunction. GI management includes frequent small meals, soft diet, stool softeners, and bulk agents. Gastroparesis is difficult to treat; metoclopramide stimulates gastric emptying but worsens parkinsonism by blocking central dopamine receptors. Domperidone has been used in other countries but is not available in the United States.

Autonomic dysfunction is also a common feature in dementia with Lewy bodies (Chap. 29); the severity is usually less than that found in MSA or Parkinson's disease. In multiple sclerosis (MS; Chap. 39), autonomic complications reflect the CNS location of MS involvement and generally worsen with disease duration and disability.

SPINAL CORD

Spinal cord lesions from any cause may result in focal autonomic deficits or autonomic hyperreflexia (e.g., spinal cord transection or hemisection) affecting bowel, bladder, sexual, temperature-regulation, or cardiovascular functions. Quadriparetic patients exhibit both supine hypertension and OH after upward tilting. *Autonomic dysreflexia* describes a dramatic increase in blood pressure in patients with traumatic spinal cord lesions above the C6 level, often in response to stimulation of the bladder, skin, or muscles. Suprapubic palpation of the bladder, a distended bladder, catheter insertion, catheter obstruction, or urinary infection are common triggers. Associated symptoms can include flushing, headache, or piloerection. Potential complications include intracranial vasospasm or hemorrhage, cardiac arrhythmia, and death. Awareness of the syndrome and monitoring of blood pressure during procedures in patients with acute or chronic spinal cord injury is essential. In patients with supine hypertension, BP can be lowered by tilting the head upward. Vasodilator drugs may be used to treat acute elevations in BP. Clonidine can be used prophylactically to reduce the hypertension resulting from bladder stimulation. Dangerous increases or decreases in body temperature may result from an inability to experience the sensory accompaniments of heat or cold exposure or the ability to control peripheral vasoconstriction or sweating below the level of the spinal cord injury.

PERIPHERAL NERVE AND NEUROMUSCULAR JUNCTION DISORDERS

Peripheral neuropathies (Chap. 45) are the most common cause of chronic autonomic insufficiency. Polyneuropathies that affect small myelinated and unmyelinated fibers of the sympathetic and parasympathetic nerves commonly occur in diabetes mellitus, amyloidosis, chronic alcoholism, porphyria, and Guillain-Barré syndrome. Neuromuscular junction disorders with autonomic involvement include botulism and Lambert-Eaton syndrome (Chap. 47).

Diabetes mellitus

Autonomic neuropathy typically begins ~10 years after the onset of diabetes and is slowly progressive.

Amyloidosis

Autonomic neuropathy occurs in both sporadic and familial forms of amyloidosis. The AL (immunoglobulin light chain) type is associated with primary amyloidosis or amyloidosis secondary to multiple myeloma. The ATTR type, with transthyretin as the primary protein component, is responsible for the most common form of inherited amyloidosis. Although patients usually present with a distal painful neuropathy accompanied by sensory loss, autonomic insufficiency can precede the development of the polyneuropathy or occur in isolation. Diagnosis can be made by protein electrophoresis of blood and urine, tissue biopsy (abdominal fat pad, rectal mucosa, or sural nerve) to search for amyloid deposits, and genetic testing for transthyretin mutations in familial cases. Treatment of familial cases with liver transplantation can be successful. The response of primary amyloidosis to melphalan and stem cell transplantation has been mixed. Death is usually due to cardiac or renal involvement. Postmortem studies reveal amyloid deposition in many organs, including two sites that contribute to autonomic failure: intraneural blood vessels and autonomic ganglia. Pathologic examination reveals a loss of unmyelinated and myelinated nerve fibers.

Alcoholic neuropathy

Abnormalities in parasympathetic vagal and efferent sympathetic function are usually mild in individuals with alcoholic polyneuropathy. Pathologic changes can be demonstrated in the parasympathetic (vagus) and sympathetic fibers, and in ganglia. OH is usually due to brainstem involvement. Impotence is a major problem, but concurrent gonadal hormone abnormalities may obscure the parasympathetic component. Clinical symptoms of autonomic failure generally appear when the polyneuropathy is severe, and there is usually coexisting Wernicke's encephalopathy (Chap. 28). Autonomic involvement may contribute to the high mortality rates associated with alcoholism (Chap. 56).

Porphyria

Although each of the porphyrias can cause autonomic dysfunction, the condition is most extensively documented in the acute intermittent type. Autonomic symptoms include tachycardia, sweating, urinary retention, hypertension, or (less commonly) hypotension. Other prominent symptoms include anxiety, abdominal pain, nausea, and vomiting. Abnormal autonomic function can occur both during acute attacks and during remissions. Elevated catecholamine levels during acute attacks correlate with the degree of tachycardia and hypertension that is present.

Guillain-Barré syndrome (Chap. 46)

BP fluctuations and arrhythmias can be severe. It is estimated that between 2 and 10% of patients with severe Guillain-Barré syndrome suffer fatal cardiovascular collapse. Gastrointestinal autonomic involvement, sphincter disturbances, abnormal sweating, and pupillary dysfunction also occur. Demyelination has been described in the vagus and glossopharyngeal nerves, the sympathetic chain, and the white rami communicantes. Interestingly, the degree of autonomic involvement appears to be independent of the severity of motor or sensory neuropathy.

Autoimmune autonomic neuropathy (AAN)

This disorder presents with the subacute development of autonomic disturbances with OH, enteric neuropathy (gastroparesis, ileus, constipation/diarrhea), and cholinergic failure; the latter consists of loss of sweating, sicca complex, and a tonic pupil. Autoantibodies against the ganglionic ACh receptor (A_3 AChR) are present in the serum of many patients and are now considered to be diagnostic of this syndrome. In general, the antibody titer correlates with the severity of autonomic failure. Symptoms of cholinergic failure are also associated with a high antibody titer. Onset of the neuropathy follows a viral infection in approximately half of cases. AAN is almost always monophasic; up to one-third of untreated patients experience significant functional improvement over time. There are isolated case reports of a beneficial response to plasmapheresis or intravenous immune globulin, but there are no clinical trials that systematically assess the effectiveness of immunomodulatory therapies. Symptomatic management of OH, gastroparesis, and sicca symptoms is essential. The spectrum of AAN is now broader than originally thought; some antibody-positive cases have an insidious onset and slow progression with a pure autonomic failure (see later) phenotype. A dramatic clinical response to repeated plasma exchange combined with immunosuppression was described in one patient with longstanding AAN.

AAN can have a paraneoplastic basis (Chap. 44). The clinical features of the autonomic neuropathy may be indistinguishable from a coexisting paraneoplastic syndrome, although quite often in the paraneoplastic cases, distinctive additional central features, such as cerebellar involvement or dementia, may be present (see Tables 44-1, 44-2, and 44-3). The neoplasm may be truly occult and possibly suppressed by the autoantibody.

Botulism

Botulinum toxin binds presynaptically to cholinergic nerve terminals and, after uptake into the cytosol, blocks ACh release. Manifestations consist of motor paralysis and autonomic disturbances that include blurred vision, dry mouth, nausea, unreactive or sluggishly reactive pupils, constipation, and urinary retention.

PURE AUTONOMIC FAILURE (PAF)

This sporadic syndrome consists of postural hypotension, impotence, bladder dysfunction, and defective sweating. The disorder begins in the middle decades and occurs in women more often than men. The symptoms can be disabling, but the disease does not shorten life span. The clinical and pharmacologic characteristics suggest primary involvement of postganglionic sympathetic neurons. There is a severe reduction in the density of neurons within sympathetic ganglia that results in low supine plasma NE levels and noradrenergic supersensitivity. Some studies have questioned the specificity of PAF as a distinct clinical entity. Some cases are ganglionic antibody–positive and thus represent a type of AAN. Between 10 and 15% of cases evolve into MSA.

POSTURAL ORTHOSTATIC TACHYCARDIA SYNDROME (POTS)

This syndrome is characterized by symptomatic orthostatic intolerance (not OH) and by either an increase in heart rate to >120 beats/min or an increase of 30 beats/min with standing that subsides on sitting or lying down. Women are affected approximately five times more often than men, and most develop the syndrome between the ages of 15 and 50. Approximately half of affected patients report an antecedent viral infection. Syncopal symptoms (lightheadedness, weakness, blurred vision) combined with symptoms of autonomic overactivity (palpitations, tremulousness, nausea) are common. Recurrent unexplained episodes of dysautonomia and fatigue also occur. The pathogenesis is unclear in most cases; hypovolemia, deconditioning, venous pooling, impaired brainstem regulation, or β-receptor supersensitivity may play a role. In one affected individual, a mutation in the NE transporter, which resulted in impaired NE clearance from synapses, was responsible. Some cases are due to an underlying limited autonomic neuropathy. Although ~80% of patients improve, only one-quarter eventually resume their usual daily activities (including exercise and sports). Expansion of fluid volume and postural training (see "Treatment: Autonomic Failure") are initial approaches to treatment. If these approaches are inadequate, then midodrine, fludrocortisone, phenobarbital, beta blockers, or clonidine may be used with some success. Reconditioning and a sustained exercise program are very important.

INHERITED DISORDERS

There are five known hereditary sensory and autonomic neuropathies (HSAN I–V). The most important ones are HSAN I and HSAN III (Riley-Day syndrome; familial dysautonomia). HSAN I is dominantly inherited and often presents as a distal small-fiber neuropathy (burning feet syndrome). The responsible gene, on chromosome 9q, is designated *SPTLC1*. SPTLC is an important enzyme in the regulation of ceramide. Cells from HSAN I patients affected by mutation of *SPTLC1* produce higher-than-normal levels of glucosyl ceramide, perhaps triggering apoptosis.

HSAN III, an autosomal recessive disorder of infants and children that occurs among Ashkenazi Jews, is much less prevalent than HSAN I. Decreased tearing, hyperhidrosis, reduced sensitivity to pain, areflexia, absent fungiform papillae on the tongue, and labile BP may be present. Episodic abdominal crises and fever are common. Pathologic examination of nerves reveals a loss of small myelinated and unmyelinated nerve fibers. The defective gene, named *IKBKAP*, is also located on the long arm of chromosome 9. Pathogenic mutations may prevent normal transcription of important molecules in neural development.

PRIMARY HYPERHIDROSIS

This syndrome presents with excess sweating of the palms of the hands and soles of the feet. The disorder affects 0.6–1.0% of the population; the etiology is unclear, but there may be a genetic component. While not dangerous, the condition can be socially embarrassing (e.g., shaking hands) or disabling (e.g., inability to write without soiling the paper). Onset of symptoms is usually in adolescence; the condition tends to improve with age. Topical antiperspirants are occasionally helpful. More useful are potent anticholinergic drugs such as glycopyrrolate (1–2 mg PO tid). T2 ganglionectomy or sympathectomy is successful in >90% of patients with palmar hyperhidrosis. The advent of endoscopic transaxillary T2 sympathectomy has lowered the complication rate of the procedure. The most common postoperative complication is compensatory hyperhidrosis, which improves spontaneously over months; other potential complications include recurrent hyperhidrosis (16%), Horner's syndrome (<2%), gustatory sweating, wound infection, hemothorax, and intercostal neuralgia. Local injection of botulinum toxin has also been used to block cholinergic, postganglionic sympathetic fibers to sweat glands in patients with palmar hyperhidrosis. This approach is limited by the need for repetitive injections (the effect usually lasts 4 months before waning), pain with injection, the high cost of botulinum toxin, and the possibility of temporary intrinsic hand muscle weakness.

ACUTE AUTONOMIC SYNDROMES

The physician may be confronted occasionally with an acute autonomic syndrome, either acute autonomic failure (acute AAN syndrome) or a state of sympathetic overactivity. An *autonomic storm* is an acute state of sustained sympathetic surge that results in variable combinations of alterations in blood pressure and heart rate, body temperature, respiration, and sweating. Causes of autonomic storm are brain and spinal cord injury, toxins and drugs, autonomic neuropathy, and chemodectomas (e.g., pheochromocytoma).

Brain injury is most commonly a cause of autonomic storm following severe head trauma and in postresuscitation encephalopathy following anoxic-ischemic brain injury. Autonomic storm can also occur with other acute intracranial lesions such as hemorrhage, cerebral infarction, rapidly expanding tumors, subarachnoid hemorrhage, hydrocephalus, or (less commonly) an acute spinal cord lesion. Lesions involving the diencephalon may be more prone to present with dysautonomia, but the most consistent setting is that of an acute intracranial catastrophe of sufficient size and rapidity to produce a massive catecholaminergic surge. The surge can cause seizures, neurogenic pulmonary edema, and myocardial injury. Manifestations include fever, tachycardia, hypertension, tachypnea, hyperhidrosis, pupillary dilatation, and flushing. Lesions of the afferent limb of the baroreflex can result in milder recurrent autonomic storms; many of these follow neck irradiation.

Drugs and toxins may also be responsible, including sympathomimetics such as phenylpropanolamine, cocaine, amphetamines, and tricyclic antidepressants; tetanus; and, less often, botulinum. Phenylpropanolamine, now off the market, was in the past a potent cause of this syndrome. Cocaine, including "crack," can cause a hypertensive state with CNS hyperstimulation. Tricyclic overdose, such as amitriptyline, can cause flushing, hypertension, tachycardia, fever, mydriasis, anhidrosis, and a toxic psychosis. *Neuroleptic malignant syndrome* refers to a syndrome of muscle rigidity, hyperthermia, and hypertension in psychotic patients treated with phenothiazines.

The hyperadrenergic state with Guillain-Barré syndrome can produce a moderate autonomic storm. Pheochromocytoma presents with a paroxysmal or sustained hyperadrenergic state, headache, hyperhidrosis, palpitations, anxiety, tremulousness, and hypertension.

Management of autonomic storm includes ruling out other causes of autonomic instability, including malignant hyperthermia, porphyria, and epilepsy. Sepsis and encephalitis need to be excluded with appropriate studies. An electroencephalogram (EEG) should be done to detect epileptiform activity; MRI of the brain and spine is often necessary. The patient should be managed in an intensive care unit. Management with morphine sulphate (10 mg every 4 h) and labetalol (100–200 mg twice daily) have worked relatively well. Treatment may need to be maintained for several weeks. For chronic and milder autonomic storm, propranolol and/or clonidine can be effective.

MISCELLANEOUS

Other conditions associated with autonomic failure include infections, poisoning (organophosphates), malignancy, and aging. Disorders of the hypothalamus can affect autonomic function and produce abnormalities in temperature control, satiety, sexual function, and circadian rhythms (Chap. 38).

REFLEX SYMPATHETIC DYSTROPHY AND CAUSALGIA

The failure to identify a primary role of the ANS in the pathogenesis of these disorders has resulted in a change of nomenclature. Complex regional pain syndrome (CRPS) types I and II are now used in place of reflex sympathetic dystrophy (RSD) and causalgia, respectively.

CRPS type I is a regional pain syndrome that usually develops after tissue trauma. Examples of associated trauma include myocardial infarction, minor shoulder or limb injury, and stroke. *Allodynia* (the perception of a nonpainful stimulus as painful), *hyperpathia* (an exaggerated pain response to a painful stimulus), and spontaneous pain occur. The symptoms are unrelated to the severity of the initial trauma and are not confined to the distribution of a single peripheral nerve. CRPS type II is a regional pain syndrome that develops after injury to a specific peripheral nerve, usually a major nerve trunk. Spontaneous pain initially develops within the territory of the affected nerve but eventually may spread outside the nerve distribution.

Pain is the primary clinical feature of CRPS. Vasomotor dysfunction, sudomotor abnormalities, or focal edema may occur alone or in combination but must be present for diagnosis. Limb pain syndromes that do not meet these criteria are best classified as "limb pain—not otherwise specified." In CRPS, localized sweating (increased resting sweat output) and changes in blood flow may produce temperature differences between affected and unaffected limbs.

CRPS type I (RSD) has classically been divided into three clinical phases but is now considered to be more variable. Phase I consists of pain and swelling in the distal extremity occurring within weeks to 3 months after the precipitating event. The pain is diffuse, spontaneous, and either burning, throbbing, or aching in quality. The involved extremity is warm and edematous, and the joints are tender. Increased sweating and hair growth develop. In phase II (3–6 months after onset), thin, shiny, cool skin appears. After an additional 3–6 months (phase III), atrophy of the skin and subcutaneous tissue plus flexion contractures complete the clinical picture.

The natural history of typical CRPS may be more benign than reflected in the literature. A variety of surgical and medical treatments have been developed, with conflicting reports of efficacy. Clinical trials suggest that early mobilization with physical therapy or a brief course of glucocorticoids may be helpful for CRPS type I. Other medical treatments include the use of adrenergic blockers, nonsteroidal anti-inflammatory drugs, calcium channel blockers, phenytoin, opioids, and calcitonin. Stellate ganglion blockade is a commonly used invasive technique that often provides temporary pain relief, but the efficacy of repetitive blocks is uncertain.

TREATMENT Autonomic Failure

Management of autonomic failure is aimed at specific treatment of the cause and alleviation of symptoms. Of particular importance is the removal of drugs or amelioration of underlying conditions that cause or aggravate the autonomic symptoms, especially in the elderly. For example, OH can be caused or aggravated by angiotensin-converting enzyme inhibitors, calcium channel-blocking agents, tricyclic antidepressants, levodopa, alcohol, or insulin. A summary of drugs that can cause OH by class, putative mechanism, and magnitude of the BP drop, is shown in Table 33-6.

PATIENT EDUCATION Only a minority of patients with OH require drug treatment. All patients should be taught the mechanisms of postural normotension (volume status, resistance and capacitance bed, autoregulation) and the nature of orthostatic stressors (time of day and the influence of meals, heat, standing, and exercise). Patients should learn to recognize orthostatic symptoms early (especially subtle cognitive symptoms, weakness, and fatigue) and to modify or avoid activities that provoke episodes. Other helpful measures may include keeping a BP log and dietary education (salt/fluids). Learning physical countermaneuvers that reduce standing OH and practicing postural and resistance training are helpful measures.

SYMPTOMATIC TREATMENT Nonpharmacologic approaches are summarized in Table 33-9. Adequate intake of salt and fluids to produce a voiding volume between 1.5 and 2.5 L of urine (containing >170 meq/L of Na^+) each 24 h is essential. Sleeping with the head of the bed elevated will minimize the effects of supine nocturnal hypertension. Prolonged recumbency should be avoided when possible. Patients are advised to sit with legs dangling over the edge of the bed for several minutes before attempting to stand in the morning; other postural stresses should be similarly approached in a gradual manner. One maneuver that can reduce OH is leg-crossing with maintained contraction of leg muscles for 30 s; this compresses leg veins and increases systemic resistance. Compressive garments, such as compression stockings and abdominal binders, are helpful on occasion but uncomfortable for some patients. Anemia should be corrected with erythropoietin, administered subcutaneously at doses of 25–75 U/kg three times per week. The hematocrit increases after 2–6 weeks. A weekly maintenance dose is usually necessary. The increased intravascular volume that accompanies the rise in hematocrit can exacerbate supine hypertension.

TABLE 33-9

INITIAL TREATMENT OF ORTHOSTATIC HYPOTENSION (OH)
Patient education: mechanisms and stressors of OH
High-salt diet (10–20 g/d)
High-fluid intake (2 L/D)
Elevate head of bed 10 cm (4 in.)
Maintain postural stimuli
Learn physical countermaneuvers
Compression garments
Correct anemia

If these measures are not sufficient, drug treatment may be necessary. Midodrine, a directly acting α_1-agonist that does not cross the blood-brain barrier, is effective. It has a duration of action of 2–4 h. The usual dose is 5–10 mg orally tid, but some patients respond best to a decremental dose (e.g., 15 mg on awakening, 10 mg at noon, and 5 mg in the afternoon). Midodrine should not be taken after 6 P.M. Side effects include pruritus, uncomfortable piloerection, and supine hypertension especially at higher doses. Pyridostigmine appears to improve OH without aggravating supine hypertension by enhancing ganglionic transmission (maximal when orthostatic, minimal supine). Fludrocortisone will reduce OH, but it aggravates supine hypertension. At doses between 0.1 mg/d and 0.3 mg bid orally, it enhances renal sodium conservation and increases the sensitivity of arterioles to NE. Susceptible patients may develop fluid overload, congestive heart failure, supine hypertension, or hypokalemia. Potassium supplements are often necessary with chronic administration of fludrocortisone. Sustained elevations of supine BP >180/110 mmHg should be avoided.

Postprandial OH may respond to several measures. Frequent, small, low-carbohydrate meals may diminish splanchnic shunting of blood after meals and reduce postprandial OH. Prostaglandin inhibitors (ibuprofen or indomethacin) taken with meals or midodrine (10 mg with the meal) can be helpful. The somatostatin analogue octreotide can be useful in the treatment of postprandial syncope by inhibiting the release of gastrointestinal peptides that have vasodilator and hypotensive effects. The subcutaneous dose ranges from 25 μg bid to 200 μg tid.

The patient should be taught to self-treat transient worsening of OH. Drinking two 250-mL (8-oz) glasses of water can raise standing BP 20–30 mmHg for about 2 h, beginning ~20 min after the fluid load. The patient can increase intake of salt and fluids (bouillon treatment), increase use of physical countermaneuvers, temporarily resort to a full-body stocking (compression pressure 30–40 mmHg), or increase the dose of midodrine. Supine hypertension (>180/110 mmHg) can be self-treated by avoiding the supine position and reducing fludrocortisone. A daily glass of wine, if requested by the patient, can be taken shortly before bedtime. If these simple measures are not adequate, drugs to be considered include oral hydralazine (25 mg qhs), oral Procardia (10 mg qhs), or a nitroglycerin patch.

CHAPTER 34

TRIGEMINAL NEURALGIA, BELL'S PALSY, AND OTHER CRANIAL NERVE DISORDERS

M. Flint Beal ■ Stephen L. Hauser

Symptoms and signs of cranial nerve pathology are common in internal medicine. They often develop in the context of a widespread neurologic disturbance, and in such situations cranial nerve involvement may represent the initial manifestation of the illness. In other disorders, involvement is largely restricted to one or several cranial nerves; these distinctive disorders are reviewed in this chapter. Disorders of ocular movement are discussed in Chap. 21, disorders of hearing in Chap. 24, and vertigo and disorders of vestibular function in Chap. 11.

FACIAL PAIN OR NUMBNESS

ANATOMIC CONSIDERATIONS

The trigeminal (fifth cranial) nerve supplies sensation to the skin of the face and anterior half of the head (Fig. 34-1). Its motor part innervates the masseter and pterygoid masticatory muscles.

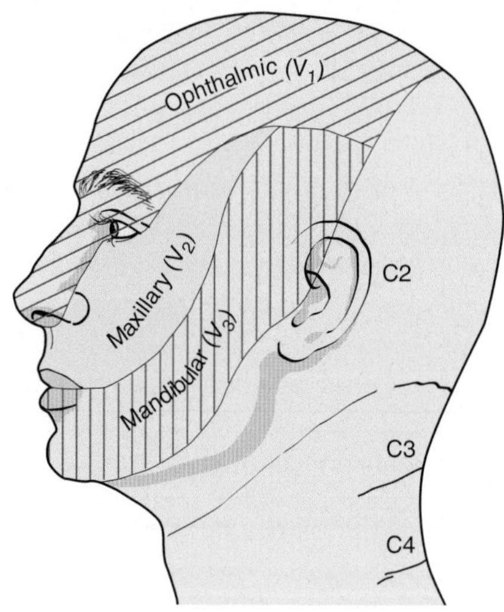

FIGURE 34-1
The three major sensory divisions of the trigeminal nerve consist of the ophthalmic, maxillary, and mandibular nerves.

TRIGEMINAL NEURALGIA (TIC DOULOUREUX)

Clinical manifestations

Trigeminal neuralgia is characterized by excruciating paroxysms of pain in the lips, gums, cheek, or chin and, very rarely, in the distribution of the ophthalmic division of the fifth nerve. The pain seldom lasts more than a few seconds or a minute or two but may be so intense that the patient winces, hence the term *tic*. The paroxysms, experienced as single jabs or clusters, tend to recur frequently, both day and night, for several weeks at a time. They may occur spontaneously or with movements of affected areas evoked by speaking, chewing, or smiling. Another characteristic feature is the presence of trigger zones, typically on the face, lips, or tongue, that provoke attacks; patients may report that tactile stimuli—e.g., washing the face, brushing the teeth, or exposure to a draft of air—generate excruciating pain. *An essential feature of trigeminal neuralgia is that objective signs of sensory loss cannot be demonstrated on examination.*

Trigeminal neuralgia is relatively common, with an estimated annual incidence of 4.5 per 100,000 individuals. Middle-aged and elderly persons are affected primarily, and ~60% of cases occur in women. Onset is typically sudden, and bouts tend to persist for weeks or months before remitting spontaneously. Remissions may be long-lasting, but in most patients the disorder ultimately recurs.

Pathophysiology

Symptoms result from ectopic generation of action potentials in pain-sensitive afferent fibers of the fifth cranial nerve root just before it enters the lateral surface of the pons. Compression or other pathology in the nerve leads to demyelination of large myelinated fibers that do not themselves carry pain sensation but become hyperexcitable and electrically coupled with smaller unmyelinated or poorly myelinated pain fibers in close proximity; this may explain why tactile stimuli, conveyed via the large myelinated fibers, can stimulate paroxysms of pain. Compression of the trigeminal nerve root by a blood vessel, most often the superior cerebellar artery or on occasion a tortuous vein, is the source of trigeminal neuralgia in a substantial proportion of patients. In cases of vascular compression, age-related brain sagging and increased vascular thickness and tortuosity may explain the prevalence of trigeminal neuralgia in later life.

Differential diagnosis

Trigeminal neuralgia must be distinguished from other causes of face and head pain (Chap. 8) and from pain arising from diseases of the jaw, teeth, or sinuses. Pain from migraine or cluster headache tends to be deep-seated and steady, unlike the superficial stabbing quality of trigeminal neuralgia; rarely, cluster headache is associated with trigeminal neuralgia, a syndrome known as *cluster-tic*. In temporal arteritis, superficial facial pain is present but is not typically shocklike, the patient frequently complains of myalgias and other systemic symptoms, and an elevated erythrocyte sedimentation rate (ESR) is usually present. When trigeminal neuralgia develops in a young adult or is bilateral, multiple sclerosis (MS) is a key consideration, and in such cases the cause is a demyelinating plaque at the root entry zone of the fifth nerve in the pons; often, evidence of facial sensory loss can be found on careful examination. Cases that are secondary to mass lesions—such as aneurysms, neurofibromas, acoustic schwannomas, or meningiomas—usually produce objective signs of sensory loss in the trigeminal nerve distribution (trigeminal neuropathy, see later in the chapter).

Laboratory evaluation

An ESR is indicated if temporal arteritis is suspected. In typical cases of trigeminal neuralgia, neuroimaging studies are usually unnecessary but may be valuable if MS is a consideration or in assessing overlying vascular lesions in order to plan for decompression surgery.

TREATMENT Trigeminal Neuralgia

Drug therapy with carbamazepine is effective in ~50–75% of patients. Carbamazepine should be started as a single daily dose of 100 mg taken with food and increased gradually (by 100 mg daily in divided doses every 1–2 days) until substantial (>50%) pain relief is achieved. Most patients require a maintenance dose of 200 mg qid. Doses >1200 mg daily provide no additional benefit. Dizziness, imbalance, sedation, and rare cases of agranulocytosis are the most important side effects of carbamazepine. If treatment is effective, it is usually continued for 1 month and then tapered as tolerated. Oxcarbazepine (300–1200 mg bid) is an alternative to carbamazepine, has less bone marrow toxicity, and probably is equally efficacious. If these agents are not well tolerated or are ineffective, lamotrigine 400 mg daily or phenytoin, 300–400 mg daily, are other options. Baclofen may also be administered, either alone or in combination with an anticonvulsant. The initial dose is 5–10 mg tid, gradually increasing as needed to 20 mg qid.

If drug treatment fails, surgical therapy should be offered. The most widely used method currently is microvascular decompression to relieve pressure on the trigeminal nerve as it exits the pons. This procedure requires a suboccipital craniotomy. Based on limited data, this procedure appears to have a >70% efficacy rate and a low rate of pain recurrence in responders; the response is better for classic tic-like symptoms than for nonlancinating facial pains. In a small number of cases, there is perioperative damage to the eighth or seventh cranial nerves or to the cerebellum, or a postoperative CSF leak syndrome. High-resolution magnetic resonance angiography is useful preoperatively to visualize the relationships between the fifth cranial nerve root and nearby blood vessels.

Gamma knife radiosurgery is also utilized for treatment and results in complete pain relief in more than two-thirds of patients and a low risk of persistent facial numbness; the response is sometimes long-lasting, but recurrent pain develops over 2–3 years in half of patients. Compared with surgical decompression, gamma knife surgery appears to be somewhat less effective but has few serious complications.

Another procedure, *radiofrequency thermal rhizotomy*, creates a heat lesion of the trigeminal (gasserian) ganglion or nerve. It is used less often now than in the past. Short-term relief is experienced by >95% of patients; however, long-term studies indicate that pain recurs in up to one-third of treated patients. Postoperatively, partial numbness of the face is common, masseter (jaw) weakness may occur especially following bilateral procedures, and corneal denervation with secondary keratitis can follow rhizotomy for first-division trigeminal neuralgia.

TRIGEMINAL NEUROPATHY

A variety of diseases may affect the trigeminal nerve (Table 34-1). Most present with sensory loss on the face or with weakness of the jaw muscles. Deviation of the jaw on opening indicates weakness of the pterygoids on the side to which the jaw deviates. Some cases are due to Sjögren's syndrome or a collagen-vascular disease such as systemic lupus erythematosus, scleroderma, or mixed connective tissue disease. Among infectious causes, herpes zoster and leprosy should be considered. Tumors of the middle cranial fossa (meningiomas), of the trigeminal nerve (schwannomas), or of the base of the skull (metastatic tumors) may cause a combination of motor and sensory signs. Lesions in the cavernous sinus can affect the first and second divisions of the trigeminal nerve, and lesions of the superior orbital fissure can affect the first (ophthalmic) division; the accompanying corneal anesthesia increases the risk of ulceration (neuro keratitis).

Loss of sensation over the chin (mental neuropathy) can be the only manifestation of systemic malignancy. Rarely, an idiopathic form of trigeminal neuropathy is observed. It is characterized by numbness and paresthesias, sometimes bilaterally, with loss of sensation in the territory of the trigeminal nerve but without weakness of the jaw. Gradual recovery is the rule. Tonic spasm of the masticatory muscles, known as *trismus*, is symptomatic of tetanus or may occur in patients treated with phenothiazine drugs.

TABLE 34-1

TRIGEMINAL NERVE DISORDERS

Nuclear (brainstem) lesions	**Peripheral nerve lesions**
Multiple sclerosis	Nasopharyngeal carcinoma
Stroke	Trauma
Syringobulbia	Guillain-Barré syndrome
Glioma	Sjögren's syndrome
Lymphoma	Collagen-vascular diseases
Preganglionic lesions	Sarcoidosis
Acoustic neuroma	Leprosy
Meningioma	Drugs (stilbamidine, trichloroethylene)
Metastasis	Idiopathic trigeminal neuropathy
Chronic meningitis	
Cavernous carotid aneurysm	
Gasserian ganglion lesions	
Trigeminal neuroma	
Herpes zoster	
Infection (spread from otitis media or mastoiditis)	

FACIAL WEAKNESS

ANATOMIC CONSIDERATIONS

(Fig. 34-2) The seventh cranial nerve supplies all the muscles concerned with facial expression. The sensory component is small (the nervus intermedius); it conveys taste sensation from the anterior two-thirds of the tongue and probably cutaneous impulses from the anterior wall of the external auditory canal. The motor nucleus of the seventh nerve lies anterior and lateral to the abducens nucleus. After leaving the pons, the seventh nerve enters the internal auditory meatus with the acoustic nerve. The nerve continues its course in its own bony channel, the facial canal, and exits from the skull via the stylomastoid foramen. It then passes through the parotid gland and subdivides to supply the facial muscles.

A complete interruption of the facial nerve at the stylomastoid foramen paralyzes all muscles of facial expression. The corner of the mouth droops, the creases and skinfolds are effaced, the forehead is unfurrowed, and the eyelids will not close. Upon attempted closure of the lids, the eye on the paralyzed side rolls upward (*Bell's phenomenon*). The lower lid sags and falls away from the conjunctiva, permitting tears to spill over the cheek. Food collects between the teeth and lips, and saliva may dribble from the corner of the mouth. The patient complains of a heaviness or numbness in the face, but sensory loss is rarely demonstrable and taste is intact.

If the lesion is in the middle-ear portion, taste is lost over the anterior two-thirds of the tongue on the same side. If the nerve to the stapedius is interrupted, there is hyperacusis (sensitivity to loud sounds). Lesions in the internal auditory meatus may affect the adjacent auditory and vestibular nerves, causing deafness, tinnitus, or dizziness. Intrapontine lesions that paralyze the face usually affect the abducens nucleus as well, and often the corticospinal and sensory tracts.

If the peripheral facial paralysis has existed for some time and recovery of motor function is incomplete, a continuous diffuse contraction of facial muscles may appear. The palpebral fissure becomes narrowed, and the nasolabial fold deepens. Attempts to move one group of facial muscles may result in contraction of all (associated movements, or *synkinesis*). Facial spasms, initiated by movements of the face, may develop (*hemifacial spasm*). Anomalous regeneration of seventh nerve fibers may result in other troublesome phenomena. If fibers originally connected with the orbicularis oculi come to innervate the orbicularis oris, closure of the lids may cause a retraction of the mouth, or if fibers originally connected with muscles of the face later innervate the lacrimal gland, anomalous tearing ("crocodile tears") may occur with any activity of the facial muscles, such

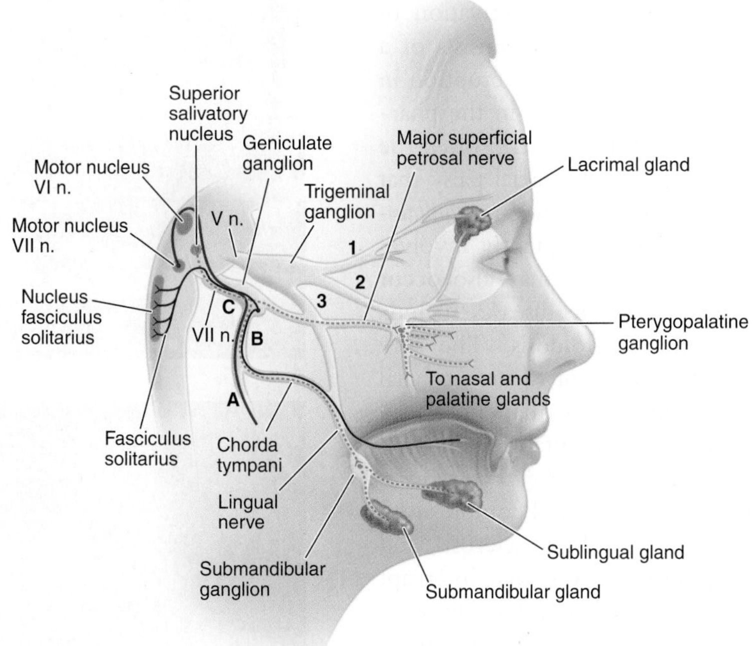

FIGURE 34-2

The facial nerve. A, B, and C denote lesions of the facial nerve at the stylomastoid foramen, distal and proximal to the geniculate ganglion, respectively. Green lines indicate the parasympathetic fibers, red line indicates motor fibers, and purple lines indicate visceral afferent fibers (taste). (*Adapted from MB Carpenter: Core Text of Neuroanatomy, 2nd ed. Baltimore, Williams & Wilkins, 1978.*)

as eating. Another facial synkinesia is triggered by jaw opening, causing closure of the eyelids on the side of the facial palsy (jaw-winking).

BELL'S PALSY

The most common form of facial paralysis is *Bell's palsy*. The annual incidence of this idiopathic disorder is ~25 per 100,000 annually, or about 1 in 60 persons in a lifetime.

Clinical manifestations

The onset of Bell's palsy is fairly abrupt, maximal weakness being attained by 48 h as a general rule. Pain behind the ear may precede the paralysis for a day or two. Taste sensation may be lost unilaterally, and hyperacusis may be present. In some cases there is mild cerebrospinal fluid lymphocytosis. MRI may reveal swelling and uniform enhancement of the geniculate ganglion and facial nerve and, in some cases, entrapment of the swollen nerve in the temporal bone. Approximately 80% of patients recover within a few weeks or months. Electromyography may be of some prognostic value; evidence of denervation after 10 days indicates there has been axonal degeneration, that there will be a long delay (3 months as a rule) before regeneration occurs, and that it may be incomplete. The presence of incomplete paralysis in the first week is the most favorable prognostic sign.

Pathophysiology

In acute Bell's palsy there is inflammation of the facial nerve with mononuclear cells, consistent with an infectious or immune cause. Herpes simplex virus (HSV) type 1 DNA was frequently detected in endoneurial fluid and posterior auricular muscle, suggesting that a reactivation of this virus in the geniculate ganglion may be responsible for most cases. Reactivation of varicella zoster virus is associated with Bell's palsy in up to one-third of cases, and may represent the second most frequent cause. A variety of other viruses have also been implicated less commonly. An increased incidence of Bell's palsy was also reported among recipients of inactivated intranasal influenza vaccine, and it was hypothesized that this could have resulted from the *Escherichia coli* enterotoxin used as adjuvant or to reactivation of latent virus.

Differential diagnosis

There are many other causes of acute facial palsy that must be considered in the differential diagnosis of Bell's palsy. Lyme disease can cause unilateral or bilateral facial palsies; in endemic areas, 10% or more of cases of facial palsy are likely due to infection with *Borrelia burgdorferi*. The *Ramsay Hunt syndrome*, caused by reactivation of herpes zoster in the geniculate ganglion, consists of a severe facial palsy associated with a vesicular eruption in the external auditory canal and sometimes in the pharynx and other parts of the cranial integument; often the eighth cranial nerve is affected as well. Facial palsy that is often bilateral occurs in sarcoidosis and in *Guillain-Barré syndrome* (Chap. 46). Leprosy frequently involves the facial nerve, and facial neuropathy may also occur in diabetes mellitus, connective tissue diseases including Sjögren's syndrome, and amyloidosis. The rare *Melkersson-Rosenthal syndrome* consists of recurrent facial paralysis; recurrent—and eventually permanent—facial (particularly labial) edema; and, less constantly, plication of the tongue. Its cause is unknown. *Acoustic neuromas* frequently involve the facial nerve by local compression. Infarcts, demyelinating lesions of multiple sclerosis, and tumors are the common pontine lesions that interrupt the facial nerve fibers; other signs of brainstem involvement are usually present. Tumors that invade the temporal bone (carotid body, cholesteatoma, dermoid) may produce a facial palsy, but the onset is insidious and the course progressive.

All these forms of nuclear or peripheral facial palsy must be distinguished from the supranuclear type. In the latter, the frontalis and orbicularis oculi muscles are involved less than those of the lower part of the face, since the upper facial muscles are innervated by corticobulbar pathways from both motor cortices, whereas the lower facial muscles are innervated only by the opposite hemisphere. In supranuclear lesions there may be a dissociation of emotional and voluntary facial movements and often some degree of paralysis of the arm and leg, or an aphasia (in dominant hemisphere lesions) is present.

Laboratory evaluation

The diagnosis of Bell's palsy can usually be made clinically in patients with (1) a typical presentation, (2) no risk factors or preexisting symptoms for other causes of facial paralysis, (3) absence of cutaneous lesions of herpes zoster in the external ear canal, and (4) a normal neurologic examination with the exception of the facial nerve. Particular attention to the eighth cranial nerve, which courses near to the facial nerve in the pontomedullary junction and in the temporal bone, and to other cranial nerves is essential. In atypical or uncertain cases, an ESR, testing for diabetes mellitus, a Lyme titer, angiotensin-converting enzyme and chest imaging studies for possible sarcoidosis, a lumbar puncture for possible Guillain-Barré syndrome, or MRI scanning may be indicated. MRI often shows swelling and enhancement of the facial nerve in idiopathic Bell's palsy **(Fig. 34-3)**.

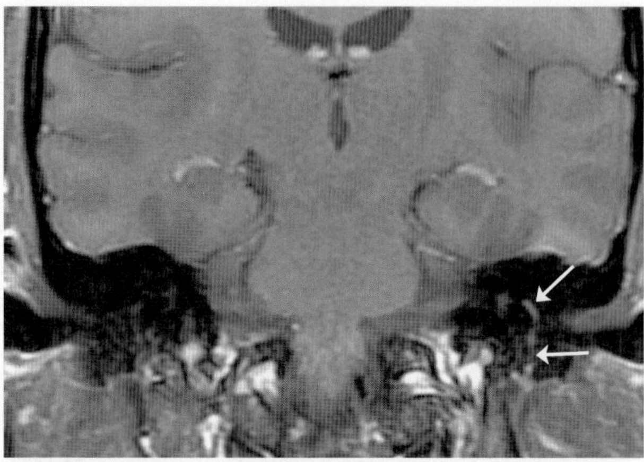

A

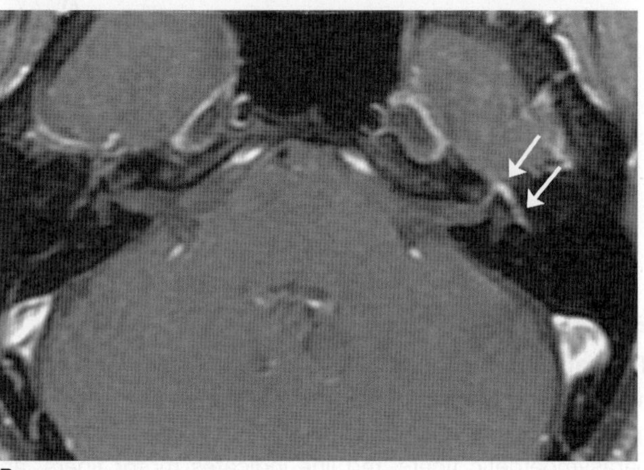

B

FIGURE 34-3

Axial and coronal T1-weighted images post-Gadolinium with fat suppression demonstrate diffuse smooth linear enhancement of the left facial nerve, involving the genu, tympanic, and mastoid segments within the temporal bone (*arrows*), without evidence of mass lesion. Although highly suggestive of Bell's palsy, similar findings may be seen with other etiologies such as Lyme disease, sarcoidosis, and perineural malignant spread.

TREATMENT **Bell's Palsy**

Symptomatic measures include (1) the use of paper tape to depress the upper eyelid during sleep and prevent corneal drying, and (2) massage of the weakened muscles. A course of glucocorticoids, given as prednisone 60–80 mg daily during the first 5 days and then tapered over the next 5 days, modestly shortens the recovery period and improves the functional outcome. Although two large recently published randomized trials found no added benefit of antiviral agents valacyclovir (1000 mg daily for 5–7 days) or acyclovir (400 mg five times daily for 10 days) compared to glucocorticoids alone, the overall weight of evidence suggests that the combination therapy with prednisone plus valacyclovir may be marginally better than prednisone alone, especially in patients with severe clinical presentations.

OTHER MOTOR DISORDERS OF THE FACE

Hemifacial spasm consists of painless irregular involuntary contractions on one side of the face. Most cases appear related to vascular compression of the exiting facial nerve in the pons. Other cases develop as a sequela to Bell's palsy or are secondary to compression and/or demyelination of the nerve by tumor, infection or multiple sclerosis. Mild cases can be treated with carbamazepine, gabapentin, or, if these drugs fail, with baclofen. Local injections of botulinum toxin into affected muscles can relieve spasms for 3–4 months, and the injections can be repeated. Refractory cases due to vascular compression usually respond to surgical decompression of the facial nerve. *Blepharospasm* is an involuntary recurrent spasm of both eyelids that usually occurs in elderly persons as an isolated phenomenon or with varying degrees of spasm of other facial muscles. Severe, persistent cases of blepharospasm can be treated by local injection of botulinum toxin into the orbicularis oculi. *Facial myokymia* refers to a fine rippling activity of the facial muscles; it may be caused by multiple sclerosis or follow Guillain-Barré syndrome (Chap. 46).

Facial hemiatrophy occurs mainly in women and is characterized by a disappearance of fat in the dermal and subcutaneous tissues on one side of the face. It usually begins in adolescence or early adult years and is slowly progressive. In its advanced form, the affected side of the face is gaunt, and the skin is thin, wrinkled, and brown. The facial hair may turn white and fall out, and the sebaceous glands become atrophic. Bilateral involvement may occur. A limited form of systemic sclerosis (scleroderma) may be the cause of some cases. Treatment is cosmetic, consisting of transplantation of skin and subcutaneous fat.

OTHER CRANIAL NERVE DISORDERS

GLOSSOPHARYNGEAL NEURALGIA

This form of neuralgia involves the ninth (glossopharyngeal) and sometimes portions of the tenth (vagus) cranial nerves. It resembles trigeminal neuralgia in many respects but is much less common. The pain is intense and paroxysmal; it originates on one side of the throat, approximately in the tonsillar fossa. In some cases the pain is localized in the ear or may radiate from the throat to the ear because of involvement of the tympanic branch of the glossopharyngeal nerve. Spasms of pain may be initiated by swallowing or coughing. There is no demonstrable motor or sensory deficit; the glossopharyngeal nerve supplies taste sensation to the posterior third of the tongue and, together with the vagus nerve, sensation to the posterior pharynx. Cardiac symptoms—bradycardia or asystole, hypotension, and fainting—have been reported. Medical therapy is similar to that for trigeminal neuralgia, and carbamazepine is generally the first choice. If drug therapy is unsuccessful, surgical procedures—including microvascular decompression if vascular compression is evident—or rhizotomy of glossopharyngeal and vagal fibers in the jugular bulb is frequently successful.

Very rarely, herpes zoster involves the glossopharyngeal nerve. Glossopharyngeal neuropathy in conjunction with vagus and accessory nerve palsies may also occur with a tumor or aneurysm in the posterior fossa or in the jugular foramen. Hoarseness due to vocal cord paralysis, some difficulty in swallowing, deviation of the soft palate to the intact side, anesthesia of the posterior wall of the pharynx, and weakness of the upper part of the trapezius and sternocleidomastoid muscles make up the jugular foramen syndrome (Table 34-2).

DYSPHAGIA AND DYSPHONIA

When the intracranial portion of one vagus (tenth cranial) nerve is interrupted, the soft palate droops ipsilaterally and does not rise in phonation. There is loss of the gag reflex on the affected side, as well as of the "curtain movement" of the lateral wall of the pharynx, whereby the faucial pillars move medially as the palate rises in saying "ah." The voice is hoarse and slightly nasal, and the vocal cord lies immobile midway between abduction and adduction. Loss of sensation at the external auditory meatus and the posterior pinna may also be present.

The pharyngeal branches of both vagal nerves may be affected in diphtheria; the voice has a nasal quality, and regurgitation of liquids through the nose occurs during the act of swallowing.

The vagus nerve may be involved at the meningeal level by neoplastic and infectious processes and within the medulla by tumors, vascular lesions (e.g., the lateral medullary syndrome), and motor neuron disease. This nerve may be involved by infection with varicella zoster virus. Polymyositis and dermatomyositis, which cause hoarseness and dysphagia by direct involvement of laryngeal and pharyngeal muscles, may be confused with diseases of the vagus nerves. Dysphagia is also a symptom in some patients with myotonic dystrophy.

The recurrent laryngeal nerves, especially the left, are most often damaged as a result of intrathoracic disease. Aneurysm of the aortic arch, an enlarged left atrium, and tumors of the mediastinum and bronchi are much more frequent causes of an isolated vocal cord palsy than are intracranial disorders. However, a substantial number of cases of recurrent laryngeal palsy remain idiopathic.

TABLE 34-2

CRANIAL NERVE SYNDROMES

SITE	CRANIAL NERVES	USUAL CAUSE
Sphenoid fissure (superior orbital)	III, IV, first division V, VI	Invasive tumors of sphenoid bone; aneurysms
Lateral wall of cavernous sinus	III, IV, first division V, VI, often with proptosis	Infection, thrombosis, aneurysm, or fistula of cavernous sinus; invasive tumors from sinuses and sella turcica; benign granuloma responsive to glucocorticoids
Retrosphenoid space	II, III, IV, V, VI	Large tumors of middle cranial fossa
Apex of petrous bone	V, VI	Petrositis; tumors of petrous bone
Internal auditory meatus	VII, VIII	Tumors of petrous bone (dermoids, etc.); infectious processes; acoustic neuroma
Pontocerebellar angle	V, VII, VIII, and sometimes IX	Acoustic neuroma; meningioma
Jugular foramen	IX, X, XI	Tumors and aneurysms
Posterior laterocondylar space	IX, X, XI, XII	Tumors of parotid gland and carotid body and metastatic tumors
Posterior retroparotid space	IX, X, XI, XII, and Horner syndrome	Tumors of parotid gland, carotid body, lymph nodes; metastatic tumor; tuberculous adenitis

When confronted with a case of laryngeal palsy, the physician must attempt to determine the site of the lesion. If it is intramedullary, there are usually other signs, such as ipsilateral cerebellar dysfunction, loss of pain and temperature sensation over the ipsilateral face and contralateral arm and leg, and an ipsilateral Horner syndrome. If the lesion is extramedullary, the glossopharyngeal and spinal accessory nerves are frequently involved (jugular foramen syndrome). If it is extracranial in the posterior laterocondylar or retroparotid space, there may be a combination of ninth, tenth, eleventh, and twelfth cranial nerve palsies and a Horner syndrome (Table 34-2). If there is no sensory loss over the palate and pharynx and no palatal weakness or dysphagia, the lesion is below the origin of the pharyngeal branches, which leave the vagus nerve high in the cervical region; the usual site of disease is then the mediastinum.

NECK WEAKNESS

Isolated involvement of the accessory (eleventh cranial) nerve can occur anywhere along its route, resulting in partial or complete paralysis of the sternocleidomastoid and trapezius muscles. More commonly, involvement occurs in combination with deficits of the ninth and tenth cranial nerves in the jugular foramen or after exit from the skull (Table 34-2). An idiopathic form of accessory neuropathy, akin to Bell's palsy, has been described, and it may be recurrent in some cases. Most but not all patients recover.

TONGUE PARALYSIS

The hypoglossal (twelfth cranial) nerve supplies the ipsilateral muscles of the tongue. The nucleus of the nerve or its fibers of exit may be involved by intramedullary lesions such as tumor, poliomyelitis, or most often motor neuron disease. Lesions of the basal meninges and the occipital bones (platybasia, invagination of occipital condyles, Paget's disease) may compress the nerve in its extramedullary course or in the hypoglossal canal. Isolated lesions of unknown cause can occur. Atrophy and fasciculation of the tongue develop weeks to months after interruption of the nerve.

MULTIPLE CRANIAL NERVE PALSIES

Several cranial nerves may be affected by the same disease process. In this situation, the main clinical problem is to determine whether the lesion lies within the brainstem or outside it. Lesions that lie on the surface of the brainstem are characterized by involvement of adjacent cranial nerves (often occurring in succession) and late and rather slight involvement of the long sensory and motor pathways and segmental structures lying within the brainstem. The opposite is true of primary lesions within the brainstem. The extramedullary lesion is more likely to cause bone erosion or enlargement of the foramens of exit of cranial nerves. The intramedullary lesion involving cranial nerves often produces a crossed sensory or motor paralysis (cranial nerve signs on one side of the body and tract signs on the opposite side).

Involvement of multiple cranial nerves outside the brainstem is frequently the result of trauma, localized infections including varicella zoster virus, infectious and noninfectious (especially carcinomatous) causes of meningitis (Chaps. 40 and 41), granulomatous diseases such as granulomatosis with polyangiitis (Wegener's), Behçet's disease, vascular disorders including those associated with diabetes, enlarging saccular aneurysms, or locally infiltrating tumors. Among the tumors, nasopharyngeal cancers, lymphomas, neurofibromas, meningiomas, chordomas, cholesteatomas, carcinomas, and sarcomas have all been observed to involve a succession of lower cranial nerves. Owing to their anatomic relationships, the multiple cranial nerve palsies form a number of distinctive syndromes, listed in Table 34-2. Sarcoidosis is the cause of some cases of multiple cranial neuropathy, and chronic glandular tuberculosis the cause of a few others. Platybasia, basilar invagination of the skull, and the Chiari malformation are additional causes. A purely motor disorder without atrophy always raises the question of myasthenia gravis (Chap. 47). As noted earlier, Guillain-Barré syndrome commonly affects the facial nerves bilaterally. In the Fisher variant of the Guillain-Barré syndrome, oculomotor paresis occurs with ataxia and areflexia in the limbs (Chap. 46). Wernicke encephalopathy can cause a severe ophthalmoplegia combined with other brainstem signs (Chap. 28).

The *cavernous sinus syndrome* (Fig. 34-4) is a distinctive and frequently life-threatening disorder. It often presents as orbital or facial pain; orbital swelling and chemosis due to occlusion of the ophthalmic veins; fever; oculomotor neuropathy affecting the third, fourth, and sixth cranial nerves; and trigeminal neuropathy affecting the ophthalmic (V_1) and occasionally the maxillary (V_2) divisions of the trigeminal nerve. Cavernous sinus thrombosis, often secondary to infection from orbital cellulitis (frequently *Staphylococcus aureus*), a cutaneous source on the face, or sinusitis (especially with mucormycosis in diabetic patients), is the most frequent cause; other etiologies include aneurysm of the carotid artery, a carotid-cavernous fistula (orbital bruit may be present), meningioma, nasopharyngeal carcinoma, other tumors, or an idiopathic granulomatous disorder (Tolosa-Hunt syndrome). The two cavernous sinuses directly communicate via intercavernous channels; thus, involvement on one side may extend to become bilateral. Early diagnosis is essential, especially when due to infection, and treatment depends on the underlying etiology.

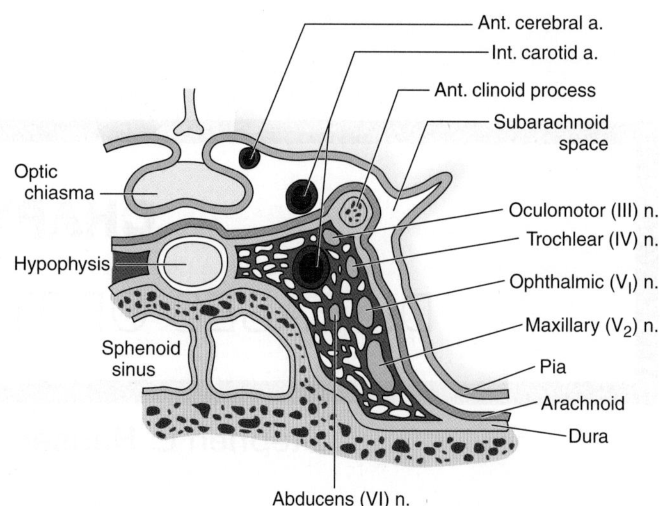

FIGURE 34-4
Anatomy of the cavernous sinus in coronal section, illustrating the location of the cranial nerves in relation to the vascular sinus, internal carotid artery (which loops anteriorly to the section), and surrounding structures.

In infectious cases, prompt administration of broad-spectrum antibiotics, drainage of any abscess cavities, and identification of the offending organism are essential. Anticoagulant therapy may benefit cases of primary thrombosis. Repair or occlusion of the carotid artery may be required for treatment of fistulas or aneurysms. The Tolosa-Hunt syndrome generally responds to glucocorticoids. A dramatic improvement in pain is usually evident within a few days; oral prednisone (60 mg daily) is usually continued for 2 weeks and then gradually tapered over a month, or longer if pain recurs.

An idiopathic form of multiple cranial nerve involvement on one or both sides of the face is occasionally seen. The syndrome consists of a subacute onset of boring facial pain, followed by paralysis of motor cranial nerves. The clinical features overlap those of the Tolosa-Hunt syndrome and appear to be due to idiopathic inflammation of the dura mater, which may be visualized by MRI. The syndrome is frequently responsive to glucocorticoids.

CHAPTER 35

DISEASES OF THE SPINAL CORD

Stephen L. Hauser ■ Allan H. Ropper

Diseases of the spinal cord are frequently devastating. They produce quadriplegia, paraplegia, and sensory deficits far beyond the damage they would inflict elsewhere in the nervous system because the spinal cord contains, in a small cross-sectional area, almost the entire motor output and sensory input of the trunk and limbs. Many spinal cord diseases are reversible if recognized and treated at an early stage (Table 35-1); thus, they are among the most critical of neurologic emergencies. The efficient use of diagnostic procedures, guided by knowledge of the anatomy and the clinical features of spinal cord diseases, is required for a successful outcome.

TABLE 35-1

TREATABLE SPINAL CORD DISORDERS

Compressive
- Epidural, intradural, or intramedullary neoplasm
- Epidural abscess
- Epidural hemorrhage
- Cervical spondylosis
- Herniated disk
- Posttraumatic compression by fractured or displaced vertebra or hemorrhage

Vascular
- Arteriovenous malformation
- Antiphospholipid syndrome and other hypercoagulable states

Inflammatory
- Multiple sclerosis
- Neuromyelitis optica
- Transverse myelitis
- Sarcoidosis
- Sjögren-related myelopathy
- Systemic lupus erythematosus
- Vasculitis

Infectious
- Viral: VZV, HSV-1 and -2, CMV, HIV, HTLV-I, others
- Bacterial and mycobacterial: *Borrelia*, *Listeria*, syphilis, others
- *Mycoplasma pneumoniae*
- Parasitic: schistosomiasis, toxoplasmosis

Developmental
- Syringomyelia
- Meningomyelocele
- Tethered cord syndrome

Metabolic
- Vitamin B_{12} deficiency (subacute combined degeneration)
- Copper deficiency

Abbreviations: CMV, cytomegalovirus; HSV, herpes simplex virus; HTLV, human T cell lymphotropic virus; VZV, varicella-zoster virus.

APPROACH TO THE PATIENT: Spinal Cord Disease

SPINAL CORD ANATOMY RELEVANT TO CLINICAL SIGNS The spinal cord is a thin, tubular extension of the central nervous system contained within the bony spinal canal. It originates at the medulla and continues caudally to the conus medullaris at the lumbar level; its fibrous extension, the filum terminale, terminates at the coccyx. The adult spinal cord is ~46 cm (18 in.) long, oval in shape, and enlarged in the cervical and lumbar regions, where neurons that innervate the upper and lower extremities, respectively, are located. The white matter tracts containing ascending sensory and descending motor pathways are located peripherally, whereas nerve cell bodies are clustered in an inner region shaped like a four-leaf clover that surrounds the central canal (anatomically an extension of the fourth ventricle). The membranes that cover the spinal cord—the pia, arachnoid, and dura—are continuous with those of the brain.

The spinal cord has 31 segments, each defined by a pair of exiting ventral motor roots and entering dorsal sensory roots. During embryologic development, growth of the cord lags behind that of the vertebral column, and the mature spinal cord ends at approximately the first lumbar vertebral body. The lower spinal nerves take an increasingly downward course to exit via intervertebral foramens. The first seven pairs of cervical spinal nerves exit above the same-numbered vertebral bodies, whereas all the subsequent nerves exit below the same-numbered vertebral bodies because of the presence of eight cervical spinal cord segments but only seven cervical vertebrae. The relationship between spinal cord segments and the corresponding vertebral bodies is shown in Table 35-2. These relationships assume particular importance for localization of lesions that cause spinal cord compression. Sensory loss below the circumferential level of the umbilicus, for example, corresponds to the T10 cord segment but indicates involvement of the cord adjacent to the seventh or eighth thoracic vertebral body (Figs. 15-2 and 15-3). In addition, at every level the main ascending and descending tracts are somatotopically organized with a laminated distribution that reflects the origin or destination of nerve fibers.

Determining the Level of the Lesion The presence of a horizontally defined level below which sensory, motor, and autonomic function is impaired is a hallmark of spinal cord disease. This *sensory level* is sought by asking the patient to identify a pinprick or cold stimulus applied to the proximal legs and lower trunk and successively moved up toward the neck on each side. Sensory loss below this level is the result of damage to the spinothalamic tract on the opposite side one to two segments higher in the case of a unilateral spinal cord lesion, and at the level of a bilateral lesion. The discrepancy in the level of a unilateral lesion is the result of the course of the second-order sensory fibers, which originate in the dorsal horn, and ascend for one or two levels as they cross anterior to the central canal to join the opposite spinothalamic tract. Lesions that transect the descending corticospinal and other motor tracts cause paraplegia or quadriplegia with heightened deep tendon reflexes, Babinski signs, and eventual spasticity (the upper motor neuron syndrome). Transverse damage to the cord also produces autonomic disturbances consisting of absent sweating below the implicated cord level and bladder, bowel, and sexual dysfunction.

The uppermost level of a spinal cord lesion can also be localized by attention to the *segmental signs* corresponding to disturbed motor or sensory innervation by an individual cord segment. A band of altered sensation (hyperalgesia or hyperpathia) at the upper end of the sensory disturbance, fasciculations or atrophy in muscles innervated by one or several segments, or a muted or absent deep tendon reflex may be noted at this level. These signs also can occur with focal root or peripheral nerve disorders; thus, they are most useful when they occur together with signs of long tract damage. With severe and acute transverse lesions, the limbs initially may be flaccid rather than spastic. This state of "spinal shock" lasts for several days, rarely for weeks, and should not be mistaken for extensive damage to the anterior horn cells over many segments of the cord or for an acute polyneuropathy.

The main features of transverse damage at each level of the spinal cord are summarized next.

Cervical Cord Upper cervical cord lesions produce quadriplegia and weakness of the diaphragm. Lesions at C4-C5 produce quadriplegia; at C5-C6, there is loss of power and reflexes in the biceps; at C7 weakness affects finger and wrist extensors and triceps; and at C8, finger and wrist flexion are impaired. Horner's syndrome (miosis, ptosis, and facial hypohidrosis) may accompany a cervical cord lesion at any level.

Thoracic Cord Lesions here are localized by the sensory level on the trunk and by the site of midline back pain that may accompany the syndrome. Useful markers for localization are the nipples (T4) and umbilicus (T10). Leg weakness and disturbances of bladder and bowel function accompany the paralysis. Lesions at T9-T10 paralyze the lower—but not the upper—abdominal muscles, resulting in upward movement of the umbilicus when the abdominal wall contracts (*Beevor's sign*).

Lumbar Cord Lesions at the L2-L4 spinal cord levels paralyze flexion and adduction of the thigh, weaken leg extension at the knee, and abolish the patellar reflex. Lesions at L5-S1 paralyze only movements of the foot and ankle, flexion at the knee, and extension of the thigh, and abolish the ankle jerks (S1).

Sacral Cord/Conus Medullaris The conus medullaris is the tapered caudal termination of the spinal cord, comprising the lower sacral and single coccygeal segments. The distinctive conus syndrome consists of

TABLE 35-2

SPINAL CORD LEVELS RELATIVE TO THE VERTEBRAL BODIES

SPINAL CORD LEVEL	CORRESPONDING VERTEBRAL BODY
Upper cervical	Same as cord level
Lower cervical	1 level higher
Upper thoracic	2 levels higher
Lower thoracic	2 to 3 levels higher
Lumbar	T10-T12
Sacral	T12-L1

bilateral saddle anesthesia (S3-S5), prominent bladder and bowel dysfunction (urinary retention and incontinence with lax anal tone), and impotence. The bulbocavernosus (S2-S4) and anal (S4-S5) reflexes are absent (Chap. 1). Muscle strength is largely preserved. By contrast, lesions of the cauda equina, the nerve roots derived from the lower cord, are characterized by low back and radicular pain, asymmetric leg weakness and sensory loss, variable areflexia in the lower extremities, and relative sparing of bowel and bladder function. Mass lesions in the lower spinal canal often produce a mixed clinical picture with elements of both cauda equina and conus medullaris syndromes. Cauda equina syndromes are also discussed in Chap. 9.

Special Patterns of Spinal Cord Disease

The locations of the major ascending and descending pathways of the spinal cord are shown in Fig. 35-1. Most fiber tracts—including the posterior columns and the spinocerebellar and pyramidal tracts—are situated on the side of the body they innervate. However, afferent fibers mediating pain and temperature sensation ascend in the spinothalamic tract contralateral to the side they supply. The anatomic configurations of these tracts produce characteristic syndromes that provide clues to the underlying disease process.

Brown-Sequard Hemicord Syndrome This consists of ipsilateral weakness (corticospinal tract) and loss of joint position and vibratory sense (posterior column), with contralateral loss of pain and temperature sense (spinothalamic tract) one or two levels below the lesion. Segmental signs, such as radicular pain, muscle atrophy, or loss of a deep tendon reflex, are unilateral. Partial forms are more common than the fully developed syndrome.

Central Cord Syndrome This syndrome results from selective damage to the gray matter nerve cells and crossing spinothalamic tracts surrounding the central canal. In the cervical cord, the central cord syndrome produces arm weakness out of proportion to leg weakness and a "dissociated" sensory loss, meaning loss of pain and temperature sensations over the shoulders, lower neck, and upper trunk (cape distribution), in contrast to preservation of light touch, joint position, and vibration sense in these regions. Spinal trauma, syringomyelia, and intrinsic cord tumors are the main causes.

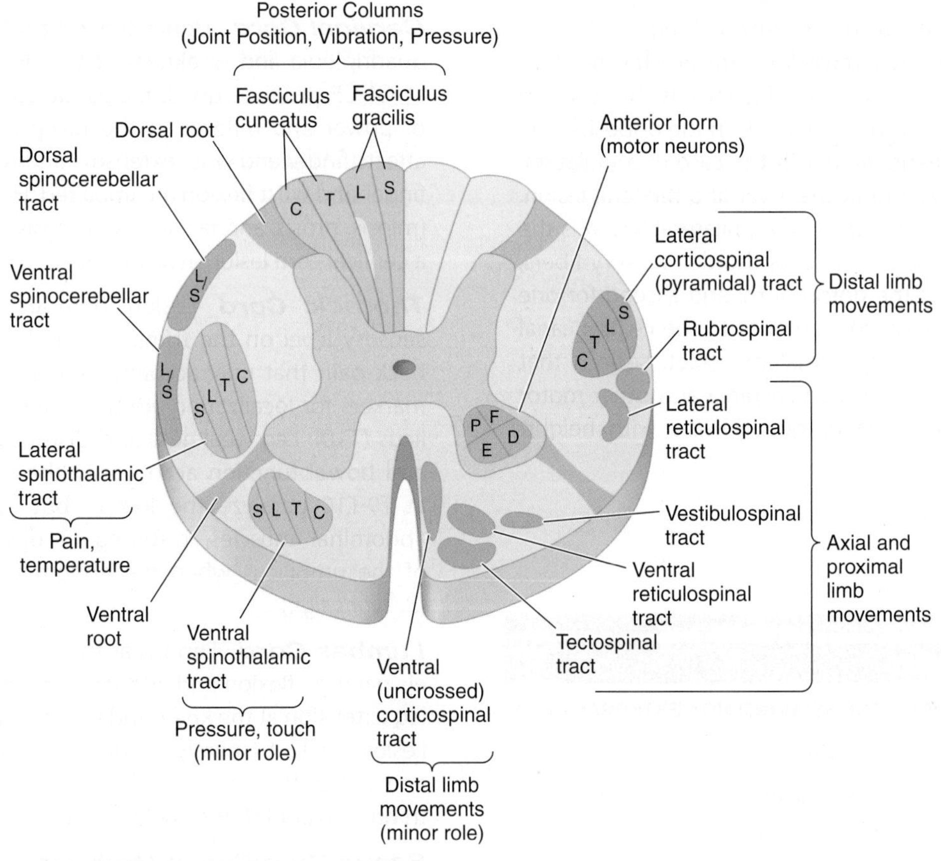

FIGURE 35-1

Transverse section through the spinal cord, composite representation, illustrating the principal ascending (*left*) and descending (*right*) pathways. The lateral and ventral spinothalamic tracts ascend contralateral to the side of the body that is innervated. C, cervical; D, distal; E, extensors; F, flexors; L, lumbar; P, proximal; S, sacral; T, thoracic.

Anterior Spinal Artery Syndrome Infarction of the cord is generally the result of occlusion or diminished flow in this artery. The result is extensive bilateral tissue destruction that spares the posterior columns. All spinal cord functions—motor, sensory, and autonomic—are lost below the level of the lesion, with the striking exception of retained vibration and position sensation.

Foramen Magnum Syndrome Lesions in this area interrupt decussating pyramidal tract fibers destined for the legs, which cross caudal to those of the arms, resulting in weakness of the legs (*crural paresis*). Compressive lesions near the foramen magnum may produce weakness of the ipsilateral shoulder and arm followed by weakness of the ipsilateral leg, then the contralateral leg, and finally the contralateral arm, an "around-the-clock" pattern that may begin in any of the four limbs. There is typically suboccipital pain spreading to the neck and shoulders.

Intramedullary and Extramedullary Syndromes It is useful to differentiate *intramedullary* processes, arising within the substance of the cord, from *extramedullary* ones that compress the spinal cord or its vascular supply. The differentiating features are only relative and serve as clinical guides. With extramedullary lesions, radicular pain is often prominent, and there is early sacral sensory loss (lateral spinothalamic tract) and spastic weakness in the legs (corticospinal tract) due to the superficial location of leg fibers in the corticospinal tract. Intramedullary lesions tend to produce poorly localized burning pain rather than radicular pain and to spare sensation in the perineal and sacral areas ("sacral sparing"), reflecting the laminated configuration of the spinothalamic tract with sacral fibers outermost; corticospinal tract signs appear later. Regarding extramedullary lesions, a further distinction is made between extradural and intradural masses, as the former are generally malignant and the latter benign (neurofibroma being a common cause). Consequently, a long duration of symptoms favors an intradural origin.

ACUTE AND SUBACUTE SPINAL CORD DISEASES

The initial symptoms of disease that evolve over days or weeks are focal neck or back pain, followed by various combinations of paresthesias, sensory loss, motor weakness, and sphincter disturbance evolving over hours to several days. There may be only mild sensory symptoms or a devastating functional transection of the cord. Partial lesions selectively involve the posterior columns or anterior spinothalamic tracts or are limited to one side of the cord. Paresthesias or numbness typically begins in the feet and ascends symmetrically or asymmetrically. These symptoms initially simulate Guillain-Barré syndrome, but involvement of the trunk with a sharply demarcated spinal cord level indicates the myelopathic nature of the process. In severe and abrupt cases, areflexia reflecting spinal shock may be present, but hyperreflexia supervenes over days or weeks; persistent areflexic paralysis with a sensory level indicates necrosis over multiple segments of the spinal cord.

APPROACH TO THE PATIENT: Compressive and Noncompressive Myelopathy

DISTINGUISHING COMPRESSIVE FROM NONCOMPRESSIVE MYELOPATHY The first priority is to exclude a treatable compression of the cord by a mass. The common causes are tumor, epidural abscess or hematoma, herniated disk, or vertebral pathology. Epidural compression due to malignancy or abscess often causes warning signs of neck or back pain, bladder disturbances, and sensory symptoms that precede the development of paralysis. Spinal subluxation, hemorrhage, and noncompressive etiologies such as infarction are more likely to produce myelopathy without antecedent symptoms. MRI with gadolinium infusion, centered on the clinically suspected level, is the initial diagnostic procedure; in some cases it is appropriate to image the entire spine (cervical through sacral regions) to search for additional clinically silent lesions. Once compressive lesions have been excluded, noncompressive causes of acute myelopathy that are intrinsic to the cord are considered, primarily vascular, inflammatory, and infectious etiologies.

COMPRESSIVE MYELOPATHIES

Neoplastic spinal cord compression

In adults, most neoplasms are epidural in origin, resulting from metastases to the adjacent spinal bones. The propensity of solid tumors to metastasize to the vertebral column probably reflects the high proportion of bone marrow located in the axial skeleton. Almost any malignant tumor can metastasize to the spinal column, with breast, lung, prostate, kidney, lymphoma, and plasma cell dyscrasia being particularly frequent. The thoracic spinal column is most commonly involved; exceptions are metastases from prostate and ovarian cancer, which occur disproportionately in the sacral and lumbar vertebrae, probably resulting from spread through Batson's plexus, a network of veins along the anterior epidural space. Retroperitoneal neoplasms (especially lymphomas or sarcomas) enter the spinal canal through the intervertebral foramens and produce radicular pain with signs of root weakness prior to cord compression.

Pain is usually the initial symptom of spinal metastasis; it may be aching and localized or sharp and radiating in quality and typically worsens with movement, coughing, or sneezing and characteristically awakens patients at night. A recent onset of persistent back pain, particularly if in the thoracic spine (which is uncommonly involved by spondylosis), should prompt consideration of vertebral metastasis. Rarely, pain is mild or absent. Plain radiographs of the spine and radionuclide bone scans have only a limited role in diagnosis because they do not identify 15–20% of metastatic vertebral lesions and fail to detect paravertebral masses that reach the epidural space through the intervertebral foramens. MRI provides excellent anatomic resolution of the extent of spinal tumors (Fig. 35-2) and is able to distinguish between malignant lesions and other masses—epidural abscess, tuberculoma, or epidural hemorrhage, among others—that present in a similar fashion. Vertebral metastases are usually hypointense relative to a normal bone marrow signal on T1-weighted MRI scans; after the administration of gadolinium, contrast enhancement may deceptively "normalize" the appearance of the tumor by increasing its intensity to that of normal bone marrow. Infections of the spinal column (osteomyelitis and related disorders) are distinctive in that, unlike tumor, they may cross the disk space to involve the adjacent vertebral body.

If spinal cord compression is suspected, imaging should be obtained promptly. If there are radicular symptoms but no evidence of myelopathy, it is usually safe to defer imaging for 24–48 h. Up to 40% of patients who present with cord compression at one level are found to have asymptomatic epidural metastases elsewhere; thus, the length of the spine should be imaged when epidural malignancy is in question.

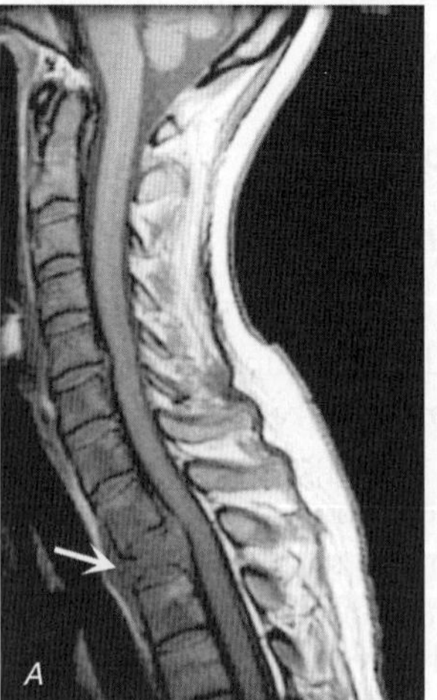

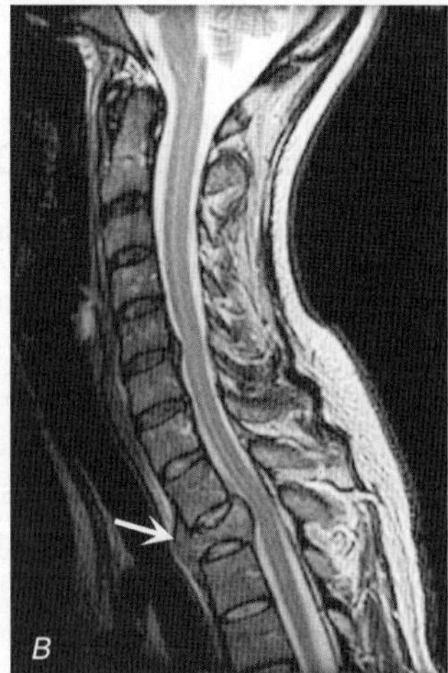

FIGURE 35-2

Epidural spinal cord compression due to breast carcinoma. Sagittal T1-weighted (*A*) and T2-weighted (*B*) MRI scans through the cervicothoracic junction reveal an infiltrated and collapsed second thoracic vertebral body with posterior displacement and compression of the upper thoracic spinal cord. The low-intensity bone marrow signal in *A* signifies replacement by tumor.

TREATMENT Neoplastic Spinal Cord Compression

Management of cord compression includes glucocorticoids to reduce cord edema, local radiotherapy (initiated as early as possible) to the symptomatic lesion, and specific therapy for the underlying tumor type. Glucocorticoids (dexamethasone, up to 40 mg daily) can be administered before the imaging study if the clinical suspicion is strong and continued at a lower dose until radiotherapy (generally 3000 cGy administered in 15 daily fractions) is completed. Radiotherapy appears to be effective even for most classically radioresistant metastases. A good response to radiotherapy can be expected in individuals who are ambulatory at presentation. Treatment usually prevents new weakness, and some recovery of motor function occurs in up to one-third of treated patients. Motor deficits (paraplegia or quadriplegia), once established for >12 h, do not usually improve, and beyond 48 h the prognosis for substantial motor recovery is poor. Although most patients do not experience recurrences in the months following radiotherapy, with survival beyond 2 years, recurrence becomes increasingly likely and can be managed with additional radiotherapy. New techniques, including intensity-modulated radiotherapy (IMRT), can deliver high doses of focused radiation with extreme precision, and preliminary data suggest that these methods produce similar rates of response compared to traditional radiotherapy. Biopsy of the epidural mass is unnecessary in patients with known primary cancer, but it is indicated if a history of underlying cancer is lacking. Surgery, either decompression by laminectomy or vertebral body resection, is usually considered when signs of cord compression worsen despite radiotherapy, when the maximum tolerated dose of radiotherapy has been delivered previously to the site, or when a vertebral compression fracture or spinal instability contributes to cord compression. The routine use of radiotherapy as first-line treatment for most cases of malignant spinal cord compression has recently been called into question by a randomized clinical trial indicating that surgery followed by radiotherapy is more effective than radiotherapy alone for patients with a single area of spinal cord compression by extradural tumor; patients with recurrent cord compression, brain metastases, radiosensitive tumors, or severe motor symptoms of >48 h duration were excluded from this study.

In contrast to tumors of the epidural space, most intradural mass lesions are slow-growing and benign.

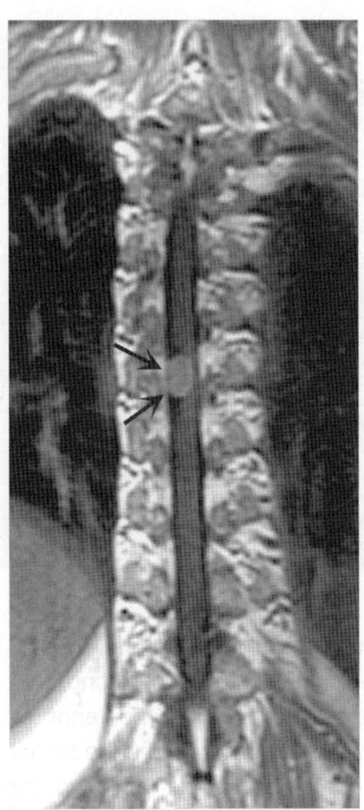

FIGURE 35-3
MRI of a thoracic meningioma. Coronal T1-weighted postcontrast image through the thoracic spinal cord demonstrates intense and uniform enhancement of a well-circumscribed extramedullary mass (*arrows*), which displaces the spinal cord to the left.

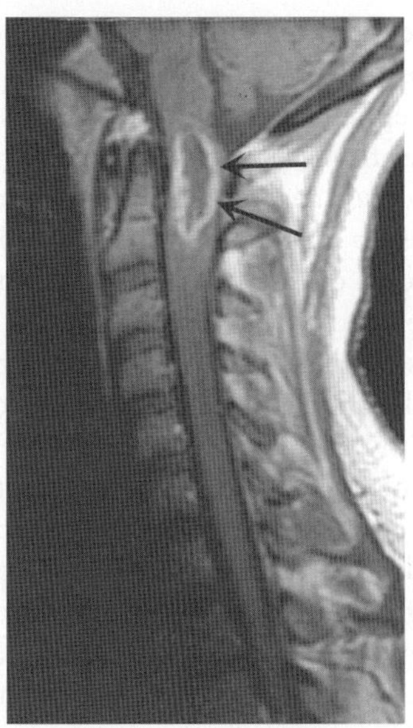

FIGURE 35-4
MRI of an intramedullary astrocytoma. Sagittal T1-weighted postcontrast image through the cervical spine demonstrates expansion of the upper cervical spine by a mass lesion emanating from within the spinal cord at the cervicomedullary junction. Irregular peripheral enhancement occurs within the mass (*arrows*).

Meningiomas and neurofibromas account for most of these, with occasional cases caused by chordoma, lipoma, dermoid, or sarcoma. Meningiomas (Fig. 35-3) are often located posterior to the thoracic cord or near the foramen magnum, although they can arise from the meninges anywhere along the spinal canal. Neurofibromas are benign tumors of the nerve sheath that typically arise near the posterior root; when multiple, neurofibromatosis is the likely etiology. Symptoms usually begin with radicular sensory symptoms followed by an asymmetric, progressive spinal cord syndrome. Therapy is by surgical resection.

Primary intramedullary tumors of the spinal cord are uncommon. They present as central cord or hemicord syndromes, often in the cervical region; there may be poorly localized burning pain in the extremities and sparing of sacral sensation. In adults, these lesions are ependymomas, hemangioblastomas, or low-grade astrocytomas (Fig. 35-4). Complete resection of an intramedullary ependymoma is often possible with microsurgical techniques. Debulking of an intramedullary astrocytoma can also be helpful, as these are often slowly growing lesions; the value of adjunctive radiotherapy and chemotherapy is uncertain. Secondary (metastatic) intramedullary tumors also occur, especially in patients with advanced metastatic disease (Chap. 37), although these are not nearly as frequent as brain metastases.

Spinal epidural abscess

Spinal epidural abscess presents as a clinical triad of midline dorsal pain, fever, and progressive limb weakness. Prompt recognition of this distinctive process will in most cases prevent permanent sequelae. Aching pain is almost always present, either over the spine or in a radicular pattern. The duration of pain prior to presentation is generally ≤2 weeks but may on occasion be several months or longer. Fever is usual, accompanied by elevated white blood cell count, sedimentation rate, and C-reactive protein. As the abscess expands, further spinal cord damage results from venous congestion and thrombosis. Once weakness and other signs of myelopathy appear, progression may be rapid. A more chronic sterile granulomatous form of abscess is also known, usually after treatment of an acute epidural infection.

Risk factors include an impaired immune status (diabetes mellitus, renal failure, alcoholism, malignancy), intravenous drug abuse, and infections of the skin or other tissues. Two-thirds of epidural infections result from hematogenous spread of bacteria from the skin (furunculosis), soft tissue (pharyngeal or dental abscesses), or deep viscera (bacterial endocarditis). The remainder arise from direct extension of a local infection to the subdural space; examples of local predisposing conditions are vertebral osteomyelitis, decubitus ulcers, lumbar puncture, epidural anesthesia, or spinal surgery. Most cases are due to *Staphylococcus aureus*; gram-negative bacilli, *Streptococcus*, anaerobes, and fungi can also cause epidural abscesses. Tuberculosis from an adjacent vertebral source (Pott's disease) remains an important cause in the underdeveloped world (Fig. 35-5).

MRI scans localize the abscess and exclude other causes of myelopathy. Lumbar puncture is only required if encephalopathy or other clinical signs raise the question of associated meningitis, a feature that is found in <25% of cases. The level of the puncture should be planned to minimize the risk of meningitis due to passage of the needle through infected tissue. A high cervical tap is sometimes the safest approach. CSF abnormalities in subdural abscess consist of pleocytosis with a preponderance of polymorphonuclear cells, an elevated protein level, and a reduced glucose level, but the responsible organism is not cultured unless there is associated meningitis. Blood cultures are positive in <25% of cases.

TREATMENT Spinal Epidural Abscess

Treatment is by decompressive laminectomy with debridement combined with long-term antibiotic treatment. Surgical evacuation prevents development of paralysis and may improve or reverse paralysis in evolution, but it is unlikely to improve deficits of more than several days duration. Broad-spectrum antibiotics should be started empirically before surgery and then modified on the basis of culture results; medication is continued for at least 4 weeks. If surgery is contraindicated or if there is a fixed paraplegia or quadriplegia that is unlikely to improve following surgery, long-term administration of systemic and oral antibiotics can be used; in such cases, the choice of antibiotics may be guided by results of blood cultures. However, paralysis may develop or progress during antibiotic therapy; thus, initial surgical management remains the treatment of choice unless the abscess is limited in size and causes few or no neurologic signs.

With prompt diagnosis and treatment of spinal epidural abscess, up to two-thirds of patients experience significant recovery.

Spinal epidural hematoma

Hemorrhage into the epidural (or subdural) space causes acute focal or radicular pain followed by variable signs of a spinal cord or conus medullaris disorder. Therapeutic anticoagulation, trauma, tumor, or blood dyscrasias are predisposing conditions. Rare cases complicate lumbar puncture or epidural anesthesia. MRI and CT confirm the clinical suspicion and can delineate the extent of the bleeding.

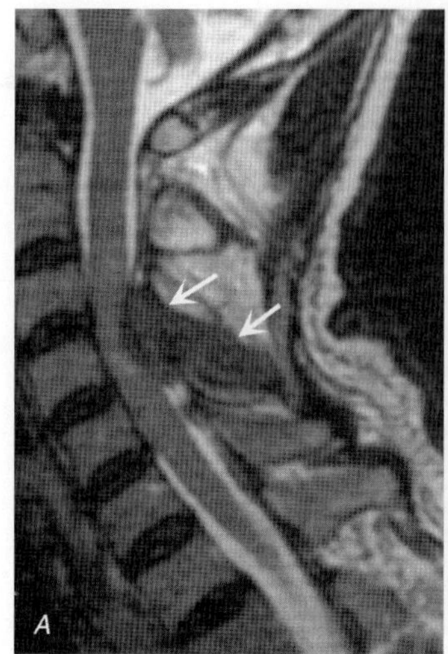

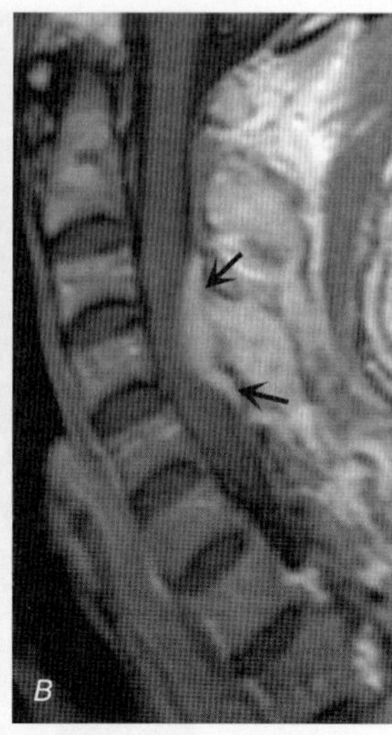

FIGURE 35-5

MRI of a spinal epidural abscess due to tuberculosis. ***A.*** Sagittal T2-weighted free spin-echo MR sequence. A hypointense mass replaces the posterior elements of C3 and extends epidurally to compress the spinal cord (*arrows*). ***B.*** Sagittal T1-weighted image after contrast administration reveals a diffuse enhancement of the epidural process (*arrows*) with extension into the epidural space.

Treatment consists of prompt reversal of any underlying clotting disorder and surgical decompression. Surgery may be followed by substantial recovery, especially in patients with some preservation of motor function preoperatively. Because of the risk of hemorrhage, lumbar puncture should be avoided whenever possible in patients with severe thrombocytopenia or other coagulopathies.

Hematomyelia

Hemorrhage into the substance of the spinal cord is a rare result of trauma, intraparenchymal vascular malformation (see later in the chapter), vasculitis due to polyarteritis nodosa or systemic lupus erythematosus (SLE), bleeding disorders, or a spinal cord neoplasm. Hematomyelia presents as an acute painful transverse myelopathy. With large lesions, extension into the subarachnoid space results in subarachnoid hemorrhage (Chap. 28). Diagnosis is by MRI or CT. Therapy is supportive, and surgical intervention is generally not useful. An exception is hematomyelia due to an underlying vascular malformation, for which selective spinal angiography may be indicated, followed by surgery to evacuate the clot and remove the underlying vascular lesion.

NONCOMPRESSIVE MYELOPATHIES

The most frequent causes of noncompressive acute transverse myelopathy (ATM) are spinal cord infarction; systemic inflammatory disorders, including SLE and

TABLE 35-3

EVALUATION OF ACUTE TRANSVERSE MYELOPATHY
1. MRI of spinal cord with and without contrast (exclude compressive causes).
2. CSF studies: Cell count, protein, glucose, IgG index/synthesis rate, oligoclonal bands, VDRL; Gram's stain, acid-fast bacilli, and India ink stains; PCR for VZV, HSV-2, HSV-1, EBV, CMV, HHV-6, enteroviruses, HIV; antibody for HTLV-I, *Borrelia burgdorferi, Mycoplasma pneumoniae,* and *Chlamydia pneumoniae;* viral, bacterial, mycobacterial, and fungal cultures.
3. Blood studies for infection: HIV; RPR; IgG and IgM enterovirus antibody; IgM mumps, measles, rubella, group B arbovirus, *Brucella melitensis, Chlamydia psittaci, Bartonella henselae,* schistosomal antibody; cultures for *B. melitensis.* Also consider nasal/pharyngeal/anal cultures for enteroviruses; stool O&P for *Schistosoma* ova.
4. Immune-mediated disorders: ESR; ANA; ENA; dsDNA; rheumatoid factor; anti-SSA; anti-SSB, complement levels; antiphospholipid and anticardiolipin antibodies; p-ANCA; antimicrosomal and antithyroglobulin antibodies; if Sjögren syndrome suspected, Schirmer test, salivary gland scintography, and salivary/lacrimal gland biopsy.
5. Sarcoidosis: Serum angiotensin-converting enzyme; serum Ca; 24-h urine Ca; chest x-ray; chest CT; total body gallium scan; lymph node biopsy.
6. Demyelinating disease: Brain MRI scan, evoked potentials, CSF oligoclonal bands, neuromyelitis optica antibody (anti-aquaporin-4 [NMO] antibody).
7. Vascular causes: CT myelogram; spinal angiogram.

Abbreviations: ANA, antinuclear antibodies; CMV, cytomegalovirus; EBV, Epstein-Barr virus; ENA, epithelial neutrophil-activating peptide; ESR, erythrocyte sedimentation rate; HHV, human herpes virus; HSV, herpes simplex virus; HTLV, human T cell leukemia/lymphoma virus; O&P, ova and parasites; p-ANCA, perinuclear antineutrophilic cytoplasmic antibodies; PCR, polymerase chain reaction; RPR, rapid plasma reagin (test); VDRL, Venereal Disease Research Laboratory; VZV, varicella-zoster virus.

sarcoidosis; demyelinating diseases, including multiple sclerosis (MS); neuromyelitis optica (NMO); postinfectious or idiopathic transverse myelitis, which is presumed to be an immune condition related to acute disseminated encephalomyelitis (Chap. 39); and infectious (primarily viral) causes. After spinal cord compression is excluded, the evaluation generally requires a lumbar puncture and a search for underlying systemic disease (Table 35-3).

Spinal cord infarction

The cord is supplied by three arteries that course vertically over its surface: a single anterior spinal artery and paired posterior spinal arteries. In addition to the vertebral arteries, the anterior spinal artery is fed by radicular vessels that arise at C6, at an upper thoracic level, and, most consistently, at T11-L2 (artery of Adamkiewicz). At each segment, paired penetrating vessels branch from the anterior spinal artery to supply the anterior two-thirds of the spinal cord; the posterior spinal arteries, which often become less distinct below the midthoracic level, supply the posterior columns.

Spinal cord ischemia can occur at any level; however, the presence of the artery of Adamkiewicz creates a watershed of marginal blood flow in the upper thoracic segments. With systemic hypotension or cross-clamping of the aorta, cord infarction occurs at the level of greatest ischemic risk, usually T3-T4, and also at boundary zones between the anterior and posterior spinal artery territories which may result in a rapidly progressive syndrome (over hours) of weakness and spasticity with little sensory change.

Acute infarction in the territory of the *anterior spinal artery* produces paraplegia or quadriplegia, dissociated sensory loss affecting pain and temperature sense but sparing vibration and position sense, and loss of sphincter control ("anterior cord syndrome"). Onset may be sudden and dramatic but more typically is progressive over minutes or a few hours, quite unlike stroke in the cerebral hemispheres. Sharp midline or radiating back pain localized to the area of ischemia is frequent. Areflexia due to spinal shock is often present initially; with time, hyperreflexia and spasticity appear. Less common is infarction in the territory of the *posterior spinal arteries,* resulting in loss of posterior column function.

Spinal cord infarction results from aortic atherosclerosis, dissecting aortic aneurysm (manifest as chest or back pain with diminished pulses in legs), vertebral artery occlusion or dissection in the neck, aortic surgery, or profound hypotension from any cause. Cardiogenic emboli and vasculitis related to collagen vascular disease (particularly SLE, Sjögren's syndrome, and the antiphospholipid antibody syndrome [see later]) are other causative conditions. Occasional cases develop from *embolism of nucleus pulposus* material into spinal vessels, usually from local spine trauma. In a substantial number of cases no cause can be found, and thromboembolism in arterial feeders is suspected. The MRI may fail to demonstrate limited infarctions of the cord, especially in the first day, but as often it becomes abnormal at the affected level.

In cord infarction due to presumed thromboembolism, acute anticoagulation is probably not indicated, with the exception of the unusual transient ischemic attack or incomplete infarction with a stuttering or progressive course. The antiphospholipid antibody syndrome is treated with anticoagulation. Drainage of spinal fluid has reportedly been successful in some cases of cord infarction but has not been studied systematically.

Inflammatory and immune myelopathies (myelitis)

This broad category includes the demyelinating conditions MS, NMO, and postinfectious myelitis, as well as sarcoidosis and connective tissue disease.

In approximately one-quarter of cases of myelitis, no underlying cause can be identified. Some will later manifest additional symptoms of an immune-mediated disease. *Recurrent episodes of myelitis* are usually due to one of the immune-mediated diseases or to infection with herpes simplex virus (HSV) type 2 (see later in the chapter).

Multiple sclerosis

MS (Chap. 39) may present with acute myelitis, particularly in individuals of Asian or African ancestry. In whites, MS rarely causes a complete transverse myelopathy (i.e., acute bilateral signs), but it is among the most common causes of a partial syndrome. MRI findings in MS-associated myelitis typically consist of mild swelling and edema of the cord and diffuse or multifocal areas of abnormal signal on T2-weighted sequences. Contrast enhancement, indicating disruption in the blood-brain barrier associated with inflammation, is present in many acute cases. A brain MRI is most helpful in gauging the likelihood that a case of myelitis represents an initial attack of MS. A normal scan indicates that the risk of evolution to MS is low, ~10–15% over 5 years; in contrast, the finding of multiple periventricular T2-bright lesions indicates a much higher risk, >50% over 5 years and >90% by 14 years. The CSF may be normal, but more often there is a mild mononuclear cell pleocytosis, with normal or mildly elevated CSF protein levels; oligoclonal bands are variable, but when bands are present, a diagnosis of MS is more likely.

There are no adequate trials of therapy for MS-associated transverse myelitis. Intravenous methylprednisolone (500 mg qd for 3 days) followed by oral prednisone (1 mg/kg per day for several weeks, then gradual taper) has been used as initial treatment. A course of plasma exchange is indicated for severe cases if glucocorticoids are ineffective.

Neuromyelitis optica

NMO is an immune-mediated demyelinating disorder consisting of a severe myelopathy that is typically longitudinally extensive, meaning that the lesion spans three or more vertebral segments. NMO is associated with optic neuritis that is often bilateral and may precede or follow myelitis by weeks or months, and also by brainstem and in some cases hypothalamic involvement. However, isolated recurrent myelitis without optic nerve involvemement can occur in NMO; affected individuals are usually female, and often of Asian ancestry. CSF studies reveal a variable mononuclear pleocytosis of up to several hundred cells per microliter; unlike MS, oligoclonal bands are generally absent. Diagnostic serum autoantibodies against the water channel protein aquaporin-4 are present in 60–70% of patients with NMO. NMO has also been associated with SLE and antiphospholipid antibodies (see later) as well as with other connective tissue diseases; rare cases are paraneoplastic in origin. Treatment is with glucocorticoids and, for refractory cases, plasma exchange (as for MS, discussed earlier). Preliminary data suggest that treatment with azathioprine, mycophenolate, or anti-CD20 (anti–B cell) monoclonal antibody may protect against subsequent relapses; treatment for 5 years or longer is generally recommended. NMO is discussed in Chap. 39.

Systemic immune-mediated disorders

Myelitis occurs in a small number of patients with SLE, many cases of which are associated with antiphospholipid antibodies. The CSF is usually normal or shows a mild lymphocytic pleocytosis; oligoclonal bands are a variable finding. Responses to glucocorticoids and/or cyclophosphamide have been reported, but there is no systematic evidence of their benefit. Other immune-mediated myelitides include cases associated with Sjögren's syndrome, mixed connective tissue disease, Behçet's syndrome, vasculitis with perinuclear antineutrophilic cytoplasmic antibodies (p-ANCA), and primary CNS vasculitis.

Another important consideration in this group is sarcoid mye-lopathy that may present as a slowly progressive or relapsing disorder. MRI reveals an edematous swelling of the spinal cord that may mimic tumor; there is almost always gadolinium enhancement of active lesions and in some cases of the adjacent surface of the cord; lesions may be single or multiple, and on axial images, enhancement of the central cord is usually present. The typical CSF profile consists of a variable lymphocytic pleocytosis and mildly elevated protein level; in a minority of cases reduced glucose and oligoclonal bands are found. The diagnosis is particularly difficult when systemic manifestations of sarcoid are minor or absent (nearly 50% of cases) or when other typical neurologic manifestations of the disease—such as cranial neuropathy, hypothalamic involvement, or meningeal enhancement visualized by MRI—are lacking. A slit-lamp examination of the eye to search for uveitis; chest x-ray and CT to assess pulmonary involvement; and mediastinal lymphadenopathy, serum or CSF angiotensin-converting enzyme (ACE; present in only a minority of cases), serum calcium, and a gallium scan may assist in the diagnosis. The usefulness of spinal fluid ACE is uncertain. Initial treatment is with oral glucocorticoids; immunosuppressant drugs are used for resistant cases.

Postinfectious myelitis

Many cases of myelitis, termed *postinfectious* or *postvaccinal,* follow an infection or vaccination. Numerous organisms have been implicated, including Epstein-Barr virus (EBV), cytomegalovirus (CMV), mycoplasma, influenza, measles, varicella, rubeola, and mumps. As in the related disorder acute disseminated encephalomyelitis (Chap. 39), postinfectious myelitis often begins as the patient appears to be recovering from an acute febrile infection, or in the subsequent days or weeks, but an infectious agent cannot be isolated from the nervous system or spinal fluid. The presumption is that the myelitis represents an autoimmune disorder triggered by infection and is not due to direct infection of the spinal cord. No randomized controlled trials of therapy exist; treatment is usually with glucocorticoids or, in fulminant cases, plasma exchange.

Acute infectious myelitis

Many viruses have been associated with an acute myelitis that is infectious in nature rather than postinfectious. Nonetheless, the two processes are often difficult to distinguish. Herpes zoster is the best characterized viral myelitis, but herpes simplex virus (HSV) types 1 and 2, EBV, CMV, and rabies virus are other well-described causes. HSV-2 (and less commonly HSV-1) produces a distinctive syndrome of recurrent sacral myelitis in association with outbreaks of genital herpes mimicking MS. Poliomyelitis is the prototypic viral myelitis, but it is more or less restricted to the gray matter of the cord. Chronic viral myelitic infections, such as that due to HIV, are discussed later.

Bacterial and mycobacterial myelitis (most are essentially abscesses) are far less common than viral causes and much less frequent than cerebral bacterial abscess. Almost any pathogenic species may be responsible, including *Listeria monocytogenes*, *Borrelia burgdorferi* (Lyme disease), and *Treponema pallidum* (syphilis). *Mycoplasma pneumoniae* may be a cause of myelitis, but its status is uncertain since many cases are more properly classified as postinfectious.

Schistosomiasis is an important cause of parasitic myelitis in endemic areas. The process is intensely inflammatory and granulomatous, caused by a local response to tissue-digesting enzymes from the ova of the parasite, typically *S. mansoni*. Toxoplasmosis can occasionally cause a focal myelopathy, and this diagnosis should be considered in patients with AIDS.

In cases of suspected viral myelitis, it may be appropriate to begin specific therapy pending laboratory confirmation. Herpes zoster, HSV, and EBV myelitis are treated with intravenous acyclovir (10 mg/kg q8h) or oral valacyclovir (2 g tid) for 10–14 days; CMV with ganciclovir (5 mg/kg IV bid) plus foscarnet (60 mg/kg IV tid), or cidofovir (5 mg/kg per week for 2 weeks).

CHRONIC MYELOPATHIES

SPONDYLITIC MYELOPATHY

Spondylitic myelopathy is one of the most common causes of chronic cord compression and of gait difficulty in the elderly. Neck and shoulder pain with stiffness are early symptoms; impingement of bone and soft tissue overgrowth on nerve roots results in radicular arm pain, most often in a C5 or C6 distribution. Compression of the cervical cord, which occurs in fewer than one-third of cases, produces a slowly progressive spastic paraparesis, at times asymmetric and often accompanied by paresthesias in the feet and hands. Vibratory sense is diminished in the legs, there is a Romberg sign, and occasionally there is a sensory level for vibration on the upper thorax. In some cases, coughing or straining produces leg weakness or radiating arm or shoulder pain. Dermatomal sensory loss in the arms, atrophy of intrinsic hand muscles, increased deep-tendon reflexes in the legs, and extensor plantar responses are common. Urinary urgency or incontinence occurs in advanced cases, but there are many alternative causes of these problems in older individuals. A tendon reflex in the arms is often diminished at some level, most often at the biceps (C5-C6). In individual cases, radicular, myelopathic, or combined signs may predominate. The diagnosis should be considered in cases of progressive cervical myelopathy, paresthesias of the feet and hands, or wasting of the hands.

Diagnosis is usually made by MRI and may be suspected from CT images; plain x-rays are less helpful. Extrinsic cord compression and deformation is appreciated on axial MRI views, and T2-weighted sequences may reveal areas of high signal intensity within the cord adjacent to the site of compression. A cervical collar may be helpful in milder cases, but definitive therapy consists of surgical decompression. Posterior laminectomy or an anterior approach with resection of the protruded disk and bony material may be required. Cervical spondylosis and related degenerative diseases of the spine are discussed in Chap. 9.

VASCULAR MALFORMATIONS OF THE CORD AND DURA

Vascular malformations of the cord and overlying dura are treatable causes of progressive myelopathy. Most common are fistulas located posteriorly along the surface of the cord or within the dura. Most dural arteriovenous (AV) fistulas are located at or below the midthoracic level, usually consisting of a direct connection between a radicular feeding artery in the nerve root sleeve with dural veins. The typical presentation is a middle-aged man with a progressive myelopathy that worsens slowly or intermittently and may have periods of remission resembling MS. Acute deterioration due to hemorrhage into the spinal cord or subarachnoid space may also occur but is rare. A saltatory progression is common and is the result of local ischemia and edema from venous congestion. Most patients have incomplete sensory, motor, and bladder disturbances. The motor disorder may predominate and produce a mixture of upper and restricted lower motor neuron signs, simulating amyotrophic lateral sclerosis (ALS). Pain over the dorsal spine, dysesthesias, or radicular pain may be present. Other symptoms suggestive of arteriovenous malformation (AVM) include intermittent claudication, symptoms that change with posture, exertion such as singing, menses, or fever. Less commonly, AVM disorders are intramedullary rather than dural. One classic syndrome presents as a progressive thoracic myelopathy with paraparesis developing over weeks or several months, characterized pathologically by abnormally thick, hyalinized vessels within the cord (Foix-Alajouanine syndrome).

Spinal bruits are infrequent but should be sought at rest and after exercise in suspected cases. A vascular nevus on the overlying skin may indicate an underlying vascular malformation (Klippel-Trénaunay-Weber syndrome). High-resolution MRI with contrast administration detects many but not all AVMs (Fig. 35-6). An uncertain proportion not detected by MRI may be visualized by CT myelography as enlarged vessels along the surface of the cord. Definitive diagnosis requires selective spinal angiography, which defines the feeding vessels and the extent of the malformation. Endovascular embolization of the major feeding vessels may stabilize a progressive neurologic deficit or allow for gradual recovery.

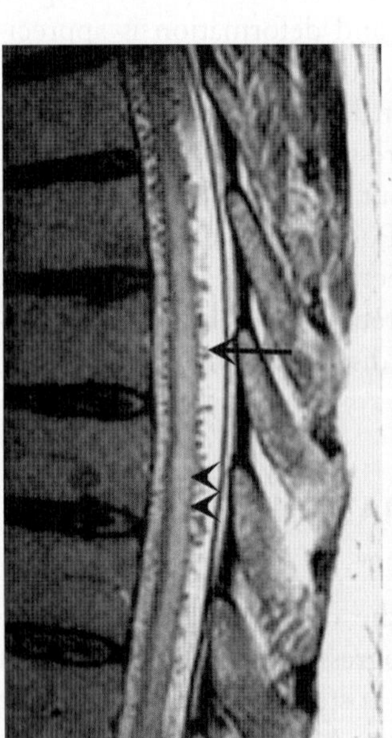

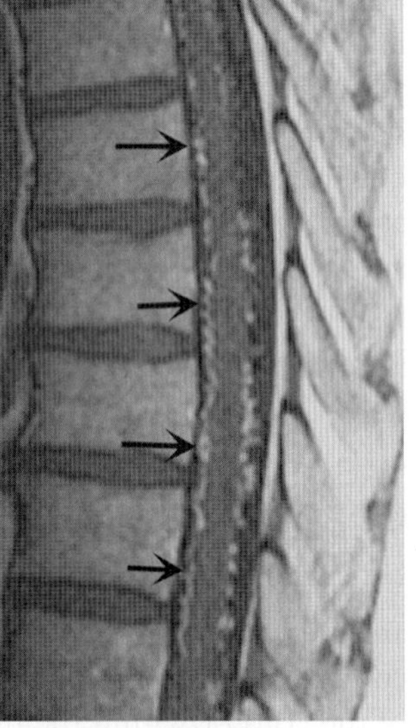

FIGURE 35-6

Arteriovenous malformation. Sagittal MR scans of the thoracic spinal cord: T2 fast spin-echo technique (***left***) and T1 postcontrast image (***right***). On the T2-weighted image (*left*), abnormally high signal intensity is noted in the central aspect of the spinal cord (*arrowheads*). Numerous punctate flow voids indent the dorsal and ventral spinal cord (*arrow*). These represent the abnormally dilated venous plexus supplied by a dural arteriovenous fistula. After contrast administration (*right*), multiple, serpentine, enhancing veins (*arrows*) on the ventral and dorsal aspect of the thoracic spinal cord are visualized, diagnostic of arteriovenous malformation. This patient was a 54-year-old man with a 4-year history of progressive paraparesis.

RETROVIRUS-ASSOCIATED MYELOPATHIES

The myelopathy associated with the human T cell lymphotropic virus type I (HTLV-I), formerly called *tropical spastic paraparesis*, is a slowly progressive spastic syndrome with variable sensory and bladder disturbance. Approximately half of patients have mild back or leg pain. The neurologic signs may be asymmetric, often lacking a well-defined sensory level; the only sign in the arms may be hyperreflexia after several years of illness. The onset is insidious, and the illness is slowly progressive at a variable rate; most patients are unable to walk within 10 years of onset. This presentation may resemble primary progressive MS or a thoracic AVM. Diagnosis is made by demonstration of HTLV-I–specific antibody in serum by enzyme-linked immunosorbent assay (ELISA), confirmed by radioimmunoprecipitation or Western blot analysis. There is no effective treatment, but symptomatic therapy for spasticity and bladder symptoms may be helpful.

A progressive myelopathy may also result from HIV infection (Chap. 42). It is characterized by vacuolar degeneration of the posterior and lateral tracts, resembling subacute combined degeneration (see later).

SYRINGOMYELIA

Syringomyelia is a developmental cavity of the cervical cord that is prone to enlarge and produce progressive myelopathy. Symptoms begin insidiously in adolescence or early adulthood, progress irregularly, and may undergo spontaneous arrest for several years. Many young patients acquire a cervical-thoracic scoliosis. More than half of all cases are associated with Chiari type 1 malformations in which the cerebellar tonsils protrude through the foramen magnum and into the cervical spinal canal. The pathophysiology of syrinx expansion is controversial, but some interference with the normal flow of CSF seems likely, perhaps by the Chiari malformation. Acquired cavitations of the cord in areas of necrosis are also termed *syrinx cavities*; these follow trauma, myelitis, necrotic spinal cord tumors, and chronic arachnoiditis due to tuberculosis and other etiologies.

The presentation is a central cord syndrome consisting of dissociated sensory loss (loss of pain and temperature sensation with sparing of touch and vibration) and areflexic weakness in the upper limbs. The sensory deficit has a distribution that is "suspended" over the nape of the neck, shoulders, and upper arms (cape distribution) or in the hands. Most cases begin asymmetrically with unilateral sensory loss in the hands that leads to injuries and burns that are not appreciated by the patient. Muscle wasting in the lower neck, shoulders, arms, and hands with asymmetric or absent reflexes in the arms reflects expansion of the cavity into the gray matter of the cord. As the cavity enlarges and further compresses the long tracts, spasticity and weakness of the legs, bladder and bowel dysfunction, and a Horner's syndrome appear. Some patients develop facial numbness and sensory loss from damage to the descending tract of the trigeminal nerve (C2 level or above). In cases with Chiari malformations, cough-induced headache and neck, arm, or facial pain are reported. Extension of the syrinx into the medulla, syringobulbia, causes palatal or vocal cord paralysis, dysarthria, horizontal or vertical nystagmus, episodic dizziness or vertigo, and tongue weakness with atrophy.

MRI scans accurately identify developmental and acquired syrinx cavities and their associated spinal cord enlargement (Fig. 35-7). MRI scans of the brain and the entire spinal cord should be obtained to delineate the full longitudinal extent of the syrinx, assess posterior fossa structures for the Chiari malformation, and determine whether hydrocephalus is present.

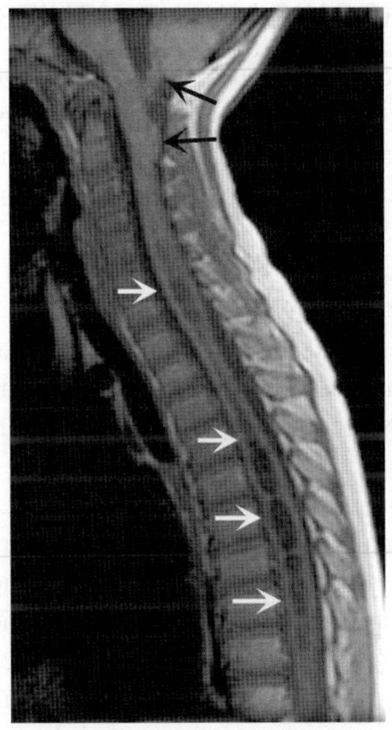

FIGURE 35-7
MRI of syringomyelia associated with a Chiari malformation. Sagittal T1-weighted image through the cervical and upper thoracic spine demonstrates descent of the cerebellar tonsils and vermis below the level of the foramen magnum (*black arrows*). Within the substance of the cervical and thoracic spinal cord, a CSF collection dilates the central canal (*white arrows*).

TREATMENT Syringomyelia

Treatment of syringomyelia is generally unsatisfactory. The Chiari tonsillar herniation is usually decompressed, generally by suboccipital craniectomy, upper cervical laminectomy, and placement of a dural graft. Obstruction of fourth ventricular outflow is reestablished by this procedure. If the syrinx cavity is large, some surgeons recommend direct decompression or drainage by one of a number of methods, but the added benefit of this procedure is uncertain, and morbidity is common. With Chiari malformations, shunting of hydrocephalus should generally precede any attempt to correct the syrinx. Surgery may stabilize the neurologic deficit, and some patients improve.

Syringomyelia secondary to trauma or infection is treated with a decompression and drainage procedure in which a small shunt is inserted between the syrinx cavity and the subarachnoid space; alternatively, the cavity can be fenestrated. Cases due to intramedullary spinal cord tumor are generally managed by resection of the tumor.

CHRONIC MYELOPATHY OF MULTIPLE SCLEROSIS

A chronic progressive myelopathy is the most frequent cause of disability in both primary progressive and secondary progressive forms of MS. Involvement is typically bilateral but asymmetric and produces motor, sensory, and bladder and bowel disturbances. Fixed motor disability appears to result from extensive loss of axons in the corticospinal tracts. Diagnosis is facilitated by identification of earlier attacks such as optic neuritis. MRI, CSF, and evoked-response testing are confirmatory. Therapy with interferon β, glatiramer acetate, or natalizumab is indicated for patients with progressive myelopathy, who also have coexisting MS relapses. These therapies are sometimes also offered to patients without relapses, despite the lack of evidence supporting their value in this setting. The value of anti-B cell therapy in primary progressive MS is under investigation. MS is discussed in Chap. 39.

SUBACUTE COMBINED DEGENERATION (VITAMIN B_{12} DEFICIENCY)

This treatable myelopathy presents with subacute paresthesias in the hands and feet, loss of vibration and position sensation, and a progressive spastic and ataxic weakness. Loss of reflexes due to an associated peripheral neuropathy in a patient who also has Babinski signs is an important diagnostic clue. Optic atrophy and irritability or other mental changes may be prominent in advanced cases but are rarely the presenting symptoms. The myelopathy of subacute combined degeneration tends to be diffuse rather than focal; signs are generally symmetric and reflect predominant involvement of the posterior and lateral tracts, including Romberg's sign. The diagnosis is confirmed by the finding of macrocytic red blood cells, a low serum B_{12} concentration, and elevated serum levels of homocysteine and methylmalonic acid. Treatment is by replacement therapy, beginning with 1000 μg of intramuscular vitamin B_{12} repeated at regular intervals or by subsequent oral treatment.

HYPOCUPRIC MYELOPATHY

This myelopathy is virtually identical to subacute combined degeneration (discussed earlier) and probably explains many cases previously described with normal serum levels of B_{12}. Low levels of serum copper are found and often there is also a low level of serum ceruloplasmin. Some cases follow gastrointestinal procedures that result in impaired copper absorption; others have been associated with excess zinc from health food supplements or, until recently, use of zinc-containing denture creams, which impair copper absorption via induction of metallothionein, a copper-binding protein. Many cases are idiopathic. Improvement or at least stabilization may be expected with reconstitution of copper stores by oral supplementation. The pathophysiology and pathology of the idiopathic form are not known.

TABES DORSALIS

The classic syndromes of tabes dorsalis and meningovascular syphilis of the spinal cord are now less frequent than in the past but must be considered in the differential diagnosis of spinal cord disorders. The characteristic symptoms of tabes are fleeting and repetitive lancinating pains, primarily in the legs or less often in the back, thorax, abdomen, arms, and face. Ataxia of the legs and gait due to loss of position sense occurs in half of patients. Paresthesias, bladder disturbances, and acute abdominal pain with vomiting (visceral crisis) occur in 15–30% of patients. The cardinal signs of tabes are loss of reflexes in the legs; impaired position and vibratory sense; Romberg's sign; and, in almost all cases, bilateral Argyll Robertson pupils, which fail to constrict to light but accommodate. Diabetic polyradiculopathy may simulate tabes.

FAMILIAL SPASTIC PARAPLEGIA

Many cases of slowly progressive myelopathy are genetic in origin (Chap. 32). More than 20 different causative loci have been identified, including autosomal dominant, autosomal recessive, and X-linked forms. Most patients present with almost imperceptibly progressive spasticity and weakness in the legs, usually but not always symmetric. Sensory symptoms and signs are absent or mild, but sphincter disturbances may be present. In some families additional neurologic signs are prominent, including nystagmus, ataxia, or optic atrophy. The onset may be as early as the first year of life or as late as middle adulthood. Only symptomatic therapies for the spasticity are currently available.

ADRENOMYELONEUROPATHY

This X-linked disorder is a variant of adrenoleukodystrophy. Affected males usually have a history of adrenal insufficiency beginning in childhood and then develop a progressive spastic (or ataxic) paraparesis beginning in early adulthood; some patients also have a mild peripheral neuropathy. Female heterozygotes may develop a slower, insidiously progressive spastic myelopathy beginning later in adulthood and without adrenal insufficiency. Diagnosis is usually made by demonstration of elevated levels of very long chain fatty acids in plasma and in cultured fibroblasts. The responsible gene encodes ADLP, a peroxisomal membrane transporter that is a member of the ATP-binding cassette (ABC) family. Steroid replacement is indicated if hypoadrenalism is present, and bone marrow transplantation and nutritional supplements have been attempted for this condition without clear evidence of efficacy.

OTHER CHRONIC MYELOPATHIES

Primary lateral sclerosis (Chap. 32) is a degenerative disorder characterized by progressive spasticity with weakness, eventually accompanied by dysarthria and dysphonia; bladder symptoms occur in approximately half of patients. Sensory function is spared. The disorder resembles ALS and is considered a variant of the motor neuron degenerations, but without the characteristic lower motor neuron disturbance. Some cases may represent familial spastic paraplegia, particularly autosomal recessive or X-linked varieties in which a family history may be absent.

Tethered cord syndrome is a developmental disorder of the lower spinal cord and nerve roots that rarely presents in adulthood as low back pain accompanied by a progressive lower spinal cord and/or nerve root syndrome. Some patients have a small leg or foot deformity indicating a long-standing process, and in others a dimple, patch of hair, or sinus tract on the skin overlying the lower back is the clue to a congenital lesion. Diagnosis is made by MRI, which demonstrates a low-lying conus medullaris and thickened filum terminale. The MRI may also reveal diastematomyelia (division of the lower spinal cord into two halves), lipomas, cysts, or other congenital abnormalities of the lower spine coexisting with the tethered cord. Treatment is with surgical release.

There are a number of rare toxic causes of spastic myelopathy, including lathyrism due to ingestion of chick peas containing the excitotoxin β-*N*-oxalylamino-L-alanine (BOAA), seen primarily in the developing world, and nitrous oxide inhalation producing a myelopathy identical to subacute combined degeneration. SLE, Sjögren's syndrome, and sarcoidosis may each cause a myelopathy without overt evidence of systemic disease. Cancer-related causes of chronic myelopathy, besides the common neoplastic compressive myelopathy discussed earlier, include radiation injury (Chap. 37) and rare paraneoplastic myelopathies. The latter are most often associated with lung or breast cancer and anti-Hu antibodies (Chap. 44); NMO can also be paraneoplastic in origin (Chap. 39). Metastases to the cord are probably more common than either of these in patients with cancer. Often, a cause of intrinsic myelopathy can be identified only through periodic reassessment.

REHABILITATION OF SPINAL CORD DISORDERS

The prospects for recovery from an acute destructive spinal cord lesion fade after ~6 months. There are currently no effective means to promote repair of injured spinal cord tissue; promising experimental approaches include the use of factors that influence reinnervation by axons of the corticospinal tract, nerve and neural sheath graft bridges, and the local introduction of stem cells. The disability associated with irreversible spinal cord damage is determined primarily by the level of the lesion and by whether the disturbance in function is complete or incomplete (Table 35-4). Even a complete high cervical cord lesion may be compatible with a productive life. The primary goals are development of a rehabilitation plan framed by realistic expectations and attention to the neurologic, medical, and psychological complications that commonly arise.

Many of the usual symptoms associated with medical illnesses, especially somatic and visceral pain, may be lacking because of the destruction of afferent pain pathways. Unexplained fever, worsening of spasticity, or deterioration in neurologic function should prompt a search for infection, thrombophlebitis, or an intraabdominal pathology. The loss of normal thermoregulation and inability to maintain normal body temperature can produce recurrent fever (*quadriplegic fever*), although most episodes of fever are due to infection of the urinary tract, lung, skin, or bone.

Bladder dysfunction generally results from loss of supraspinal innervation of the detrusor muscle of the bladder wall and the sphincter musculature. Detrusor spasticity is treated with anticholinergic drugs (oxybutynin, 2.5–5 mg qid) or tricyclic antidepressants that have anticholinergic properties (imipramine, 25–200 mg/d). Failure of the sphincter muscle to relax during bladder emptying (urinary dyssynergia) may be managed with the α-adrenergic blocking agent terazosin hydrochloride (1–2 mg tid or qid), with intermittent catheterization, or, if that is not feasible, by use of a condom catheter in men or a permanent indwelling catheter. Surgical options include the creation of an artificial bladder by isolating a segment of intestine that can be catheterized intermittently (enterocystoplasty) or can drain continuously to an external appliance (urinary conduit). Bladder areflexia due to acute spinal shock or conus lesions is best treated by catheterization. Bowel regimens and disimpaction are necessary in most patients to ensure at least biweekly evacuation and avoid colonic distention or obstruction.

Patients with acute cord injury are at risk for venous thrombosis and pulmonary embolism. During the first 2 weeks, use of calf-compression devices and anticoagulation with heparin (5000 U subcutaneously every 12 h) or warfarin (INR, 2–3) are recommended. In cases of persistent paralysis, anticoagulation should probably be continued for 3 months.

Prophylaxis against decubitus ulcers should involve frequent changes in position in a chair or bed, the use of special mattresses, and cushioning of areas where pressure sores often develop, such as the sacral prominence and heels. Early treatment of ulcers with careful cleansing, surgical or enzyme debridement of necrotic tissue, and appropriate dressing and drainage may prevent infection of adjacent soft tissue or bone.

TABLE 35-4

EXPECTED NEUROLOGIC FUNCTION FOLLOWING COMPLETE CORD LESIONS

LEVEL	SELF-CARE	TRANSFERS	MAXIMUM MOBILITY
High quadriplegia (C1-C4)	Dependent on others; requires respiratory support	Dependent on others	Motorized wheelchair
Low quadriplegia (C5-C8)	Partially independent with adaptive equipment	May be dependent or independent	May use manual wheelchair, drive an automobile with adaptive equipment
Paraplegia (below T1)	Independent	Independent	Ambulates short distances with aids

Source: Adapted from JF Ditunno, CS Formal: N Engl J Med 330:550, 1994; with permission.

Spasticity is aided by stretching exercises to maintain mobility of joints. Drug treatment is effective but may result in reduced function, as some patients depend upon spasticity as an aid to stand, transfer, or walk. Baclofen (15–240 mg/d in divided doses) is effective; it acts by facilitating γ-aminobutyric acid (GABA)-mediated inhibition of motor reflex arcs. Diazepam acts by a similar mechanism and is useful for leg spasms that interrupt sleep (2–4 mg at bedtime). Tizanidine (2–8 mg tid), an α_2-adrenergic agonist that increases presynaptic inhibition of motor neurons, is another option. For nonambulatory patients, the direct muscle inhibitor dantrolene (25–100 mg qid) may be used, but it is potentially hepatotoxic. In refractory cases, intrathecal baclofen administered via an implanted pump, botulinum toxin injections, or dorsal rhizotomy may be required to control spasticity.

Despite the loss of sensory function, many patients with spinal cord injury experience chronic pain sufficient to diminish their quality of life. Randomized controlled studies indicate that gabapentin or pregabalin is useful in this setting. Management of chronic pain is discussed in Chap. 7.

A paroxysmal autonomic hyperreflexia may occur following lesions above the major splanchnic sympathetic outflow at T6. Headache, flushing, and diaphoresis above the level of the lesion, as well as transient severe hypertension with bradycardia or tachycardia, are the major symptoms. The trigger is typically a noxious stimulus—for example, bladder or bowel distention, a urinary tract infection, or a decubitus ulcer. Treatment consists of removal of offending stimuli; ganglionic blocking agents (mecamylamine, 2.5–5 mg) or other short-acting antihypertensive drugs are useful in some patients.

Attention to these details allows longevity and a productive life for patients with complete transverse myelopathies.

CHAPTER 36

CONCUSSION AND OTHER HEAD INJURIES

Allan H. Ropper

Almost 10 million head injuries occur annually in the United States, about 20% of which are serious enough to cause brain damage. Among men <35 years, accidents, usually motor vehicle collisions, are the chief cause of death and >70% of these involve head injury. Furthermore, minor head injuries are so common that almost all physicians will be called upon to provide immediate care or to see patients who are suffering from various sequelae.

Medical personnel caring for head injury patients should be aware that (1) spinal injury often accompanies head injury, and care must be taken in handling the patient to prevent compression of the spinal cord due to instability of the spinal column; (2) intoxication is a common accompaniment of traumatic brain injury and, when appropriate, testing should be carried out for drugs and alcohol; and (3) additional injuries, including rupture of abdominal organs, may produce vascular collapse or respiratory distress that requires immediate attention.

TYPES OF HEAD INJURIES

CONCUSSION

This form of minor head injury refers to an immediate and transient loss of consciousness that is associated with a short period of amnesia. Many patients do not lose consciousness after a minor head injury but instead are dazed or confused, or feel stunned or "star struck." Severe concussion may precipitate a brief convulsion or autonomic signs such as facial pallor, bradycardia, faintness with mild hypotension, or sluggish pupillary reaction, but most patients are quickly neurologically normal.

The mechanics of a typical concussion involve sudden deceleration of the head when hitting a blunt object. This creates an anterior-posterior movement of the brain within the skull due to inertia and rotation of the cerebral hemispheres on the relatively fixed upper brainstem. Loss of consciousness in concussion is believed to result from a transient electrophysiologic dysfunction of the reticular activating system in the upper midbrain that is at the site of rotation (Chap. 17).

Gross and light-microscopic changes in the brain are usually absent following concussion but biochemical and ultrastructural changes, such as mitochondrial ATP depletion and local disruption of the blood-brain barrier, are transient abnormalities. CT and MRI scans are usually normal; however, a small number of patients will be found to have a skull fracture, an intracranial hemorrhage, or brain contusion.

A brief period of both retrograde and anterograde amnesia is characteristic of concussion and it recedes rapidly in alert patients. Memory loss spans the moments before impact but may encompass the previous days or weeks (rarely months). With severe injuries, the extent of retrograde amnesia roughly correlates with the severity of injury. Memory is regained from the most distant to more recent memories, with islands of amnesia occasionally remaining. The mechanism of amnesia is not known. Hysterical posttraumatic amnesia is not uncommon after head injury and should be suspected when inexplicable behavioral abnormalities occur, such as recounting events that cannot be recalled on later testing, a bizarre affect, forgetting one's own name, or a persistent anterograde deficit that is excessive in comparison with the degree of injury. Amnesia is discussed in Chap. 18.

A single, uncomplicated concussion only infrequently produces permanent neurobehavioral changes in patients who are free of preexisting psychiatric and neurologic problems. Nonetheless, residual problems in memory and concentration may have an anatomic correlate in microscopic cerebral lesions (later in the chapter).

CONTUSION, BRAIN HEMORRHAGE, AND AXONAL SHEARING LESIONS

A surface bruise of the brain, or *contusion*, consists of varying degrees of petechial hemorrhage, edema, and tissue destruction. Contusions and deeper hemorrhages result from mechanical forces that displace and compress the hemispheres forcefully and by deceleration of the brain against the inner skull, either under a point of impact (coup lesion) or, as the brain swings back, in the antipolar area (contrecoup lesion). Trauma sufficient to cause prolonged unconsciousness usually produces some degree of contusion. Blunt deceleration impact, as occurs against an automobile dashboard or from falling forward onto a hard surface, causes contusions on the orbital surfaces of the frontal lobes and the anterior and basal portions of the temporal lobes. With lateral forces, as from impact on an automobile door frame, contusions are situated on the lateral convexity of the hemisphere. The clinical signs of contusion are determined by the location and size of the lesion; often, there are no focal neurologic abnormalities, but these injured regions are later the sites of gliotic scars that may produce seizures. A hemiparesis or gaze preference is fairly typical of moderately sized contusions. Large bilateral contusions produce stupor with extensor posturing, while those limited to the frontal lobes cause a taciturn state. Contusions in the temporal lobe may cause delirium or an aggressive, combative syndrome.

Contusions are easily visible on CT and MRI scans, appearing as inhomogeneous hyperdensities on CT and as hyperintensities on MRI sequences that detect blood; there is usually localized brain edema (Fig. 36-1) and some subarachnoid bleeding. Blood in the cerebrospinal fluid (CSF) due to trauma may provoke a mild inflammatory reaction. Over a few days, contusions acquire a surrounding contrast enhancement and edema that may be mistaken for tumor or abscess. Glial and macrophage reactions result in chronic, scarred, hemosiderin-stained depressions on the cortex (*plaques jaunes*) that are the main source of posttraumatic epilepsy.

Torsional or shearing forces within the brain cause hemorrhages of the basal ganglia and other deep regions. Large hemorrhages after minor trauma suggest that there is a bleeding diathesis or cerebrovascular amyloidosis. For unexplained reasons, deep cerebral hemorrhages may not develop until several days after injury. Sudden neurologic deterioration in a comatose patient or a sudden rise in intracranial pressure (ICP) suggests this complication and should therefore prompt investigation with a CT scan.

A special type of deep white matter lesion consists of widespread mechanical disruption, or shearing, of axons at the time of impact. Most characteristic are small areas of tissue injury in the corpus callosum and dorsolateral pons. The presence of widespread axonal damage in both hemispheres, a state called *diffuse axonal injury* (DAI), has been proposed to explain persistent coma and the vegetative state after closed head injury (Chap. 17), but small ischemic-hemorrhagic lesions in the midbrain and thalamus are as often the cause. Only severe shearing lesions that contain blood are visualized by CT, usually in the corpus callosum and centrum semiovale (Fig. 36-2); however, selective imaging sequences of the MRI can demonstrate such lesions throughout the white matter.

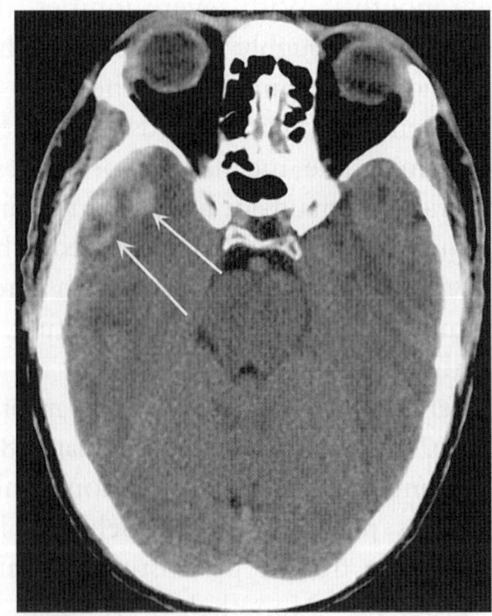

FIGURE 36-1
Traumatic cerebral contusion. Noncontrast CT scan demonstrating a hyperdense hemorrhagic region in the anterior temporal lobe.

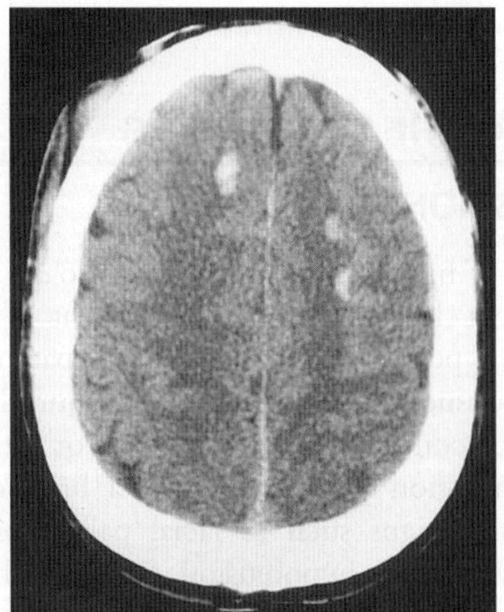

FIGURE 36-2
Multiple small areas of hemorrhage and tissue disruption in the white matter of the frontal lobes on noncontrast CT scan. These appear to reflect an extreme type of the diffuse axonal shearing lesions that occur with closed head injury.

SKULL FRACTURES

A blow to the skull that exceeds the elastic tolerance of the bone causes a fracture. Intracranial lesions accompany roughly two-thirds of skull fractures and the presence of a fracture increases many-fold the chances of an underlying subdural or epidural hematoma. Consequently, fractures are primarily markers of the site and severity of injury. They also provide potential pathways for entry of bacteria to the CSF with a risk of meningitis and for leakage of CSF outward through the dura. Severe orthostatic headache results from lowered pressure in the spinal fluid compartment.

Most fractures are linear and extend from the point of impact toward the base of the skull. Basilar skull fractures are often extensions of adjacent linear fractures over the convexity of the skull but may occur independently owing to stresses on the floor of the middle cranial fossa or occiput. Basilar fractures are usually parallel to the petrous bone or along the sphenoid bone and directed toward the sella turcica and ethmoidal groove. Although most basilar fractures are uncomplicated, they can cause CSF leakage, pneumocephalus, and cavernous-carotid fistulas. Hemotympanum (blood behind the tympanic membrane), delayed ecchymosis over the mastoid process (Battle sign), or periorbital ecchymosis ("raccoon sign") are associated with basilar fractures. Because routine x-ray examination may fail to disclose basilar fractures, they should be suspected if these clinical signs are present.

CSF may leak through the cribriform plate or the adjacent sinus and cause CSF rhinorrhea (a watery discharge from the nose). Persistent rhinorrhea and recurrent meningitis are indications for surgical repair of torn dura underlying the fracture. The site of the leak is often difficult to determine, but useful diagnostic tests include the instillation of water-soluble contrast into the CSF followed by CT with the patient in various positions, or injection of radionuclide compounds or fluorescein into the CSF and the insertion of absorptive nasal pledgets. The location of an intermittent leak is rarely delineated, and many resolve spontaneously.

Sellar fractures, even those associated with serious neuroendocrine dysfunction, may be radiologically occult or evident only by an air-fluid level in the sphenoid sinus. Fractures of the dorsum sella cause sixth or seventh nerve palsies or optic nerve damage.

Petrous bone fractures, especially those oriented along the long axis of the bone, may be associated with facial palsy, disruption of ear ossicles, and CSF otorrhea. Transverse petrous fractures are less common; they almost always damage the cochlea or labyrinths and often the facial nerve as well. External bleeding from the ear is usually from local abrasion of the external canal but can also result from petrous fracture.

Fractures of the frontal bone are usually depressed, involving the frontal and paranasal sinuses and the orbits. Depressed skull fractures are typically compound, but they are often asymptomatic because the impact energy is dissipated in breaking the bone; some have underlying brain contusions. Debridement and exploration of compound fractures are required in order to avoid infection; simple fractures do not require surgery.

CRANIAL NERVE INJURIES

The cranial nerves most often injured with head trauma are the olfactory, optic, oculomotor, and trochlear; the first and second branches of the trigeminal nerve; and the facial and auditory nerves. Anosmia and an apparent loss of taste (actually a loss of perception of aromatic flavors, with retained elementary taste perception) occur in ~10% of persons with serious head injuries, particularly from falls on the back of the head. This is the result of displacement of the brain and shearing of the fine olfactory nerve filaments that course through the cribriform bone. At least partial recovery of olfactory and gustatory function is expected, but if bilateral anosmia persists for several months, the prognosis is poor. Partial optic nerve injuries from closed trauma result in blurring of vision, central or paracentral scotomas, or sector defects. Direct orbital injury may cause short-lived blurred vision for close objects due to reversible iridoplegia. Diplopia limited to downward gaze and corrected when the head is tilted away from the side of the affected eye indicates trochlear (fourth nerve) nerve damage. It occurs frequently as an isolated problem after minor head injury or may develop for unknown reasons after a delay of several days. Facial nerve injury caused by a basilar fracture is present immediately in up to 3% of severe injuries; it may also be delayed 5-7 days. Fractures through the petrous bone, particularly the less common transverse type, are liable to produce facial palsy. Delayed palsy, the mechanism of which is unknown, has a good prognosis. Injury to the eighth cranial nerve from a fracture of the petrous bone causes loss of hearing, vertigo, and nystagmus immediately after injury. Deafness from eighth nerve injury is rare and must be distinguished from blood in the middle ear or disruption of the middle ear ossicles. Dizziness, tinnitus, and high-tone hearing loss occur from cochlear concussion.

SEIZURES

Convulsions are surprisingly uncommon immediately after a head injury, but a brief period of tonic extensor posturing or a few clonic movements of the limbs just after the moment of impact can occur. However, the cortical scars that evolve from contusions are highly epileptogenic and may later manifest as seizures, even after many months or years (Chap. 26). The severity of injury roughly determines the risk of future seizures. It has been estimated that 17% of individuals with brain contusion, subdural hematoma, or prolonged loss of consciousness will develop a seizure disorder and that this risk extends for an indefinite period of time, whereas the risk is ≤2% after mild injury. The majority of convulsions in the latter group occur within 5 years of injury but may be delayed for decades. Penetrating injuries have a much higher rate of subsequent epilepsy.

SUBDURAL AND EPIDURAL HEMATOMAS

Hemorrhages beneath the dura (subdural) or between the dura and skull (epidural) have characteristic clinical and radiologic features. They are associated with underlying contusions and other injuries, often making it difficult to determine the relative contribution of each component to the clinical state. The mass effect and raised ICP caused by these hematomas can be life threatening, making it imperative to identify them rapidly by CT or MRI scan and to remove them when appropriate.

Acute subdural hematoma (Fig. 36-3)

Direct cranial trauma may be minor and is not required for acute subdural hemorrhage to occur, especially in the elderly and those taking anticoagulant medications. Acceleration forces alone, as from whiplash, are sometimes sufficient to produce subdural hemorrhage. Up to one-third of patients have a lucid interval lasting minutes to hours before coma supervenes, but most are drowsy or comatose from the moment of injury. A unilateral headache and slightly enlarged pupil on the side of the hematoma are frequently, but not invariably, present. Stupor or coma, hemiparesis, and unilateral pupillary enlargement are signs of larger hematomas. In an acutely deteriorating patient, burr (drainage) holes or an emergency craniotomy are required. Small subdural hematomas may be asymptomatic and usually do not require evacuation if they do not expand.

A subacutely evolving syndrome due to subdural hematoma occurs days or weeks after injury with drowsiness, headache, confusion, or mild hemiparesis, usually in alcoholics and in the elderly and often after only minor trauma. On imaging studies subdural hematomas appear as crescentic collections over the convexity of one or both hemispheres, most commonly in the frontotemporal region, and less often in the inferior middle fossa or over the occipital poles (Fig. 36-3). Interhemispheric, posterior fossa, or bilateral convexity hematomas are less frequent and are difficult to diagnose clinically, although drowsiness and the neurologic signs expected from damage in each region can usually be detected. The bleeding that causes larger hematomas is primarily venous in origin, although additional arterial bleeding sites are sometimes found at operation, and a few large hematomas have a purely arterial origin.

Epidural hematoma (Fig. 36-4)

These evolve more rapidly than subdural hematomas and are correspondingly more treacherous. They occur in up to 10% of cases of severe head injury but are associated with underlying cortical damage less often than are subdural hematomas. Most patients are unconscious when first seen. A "lucid interval" of several minutes to hours before coma supervenes is most characteristic of epidural hemorrhage, but it is still uncommon, and epidural hemorrhage is not the only cause of this temporal

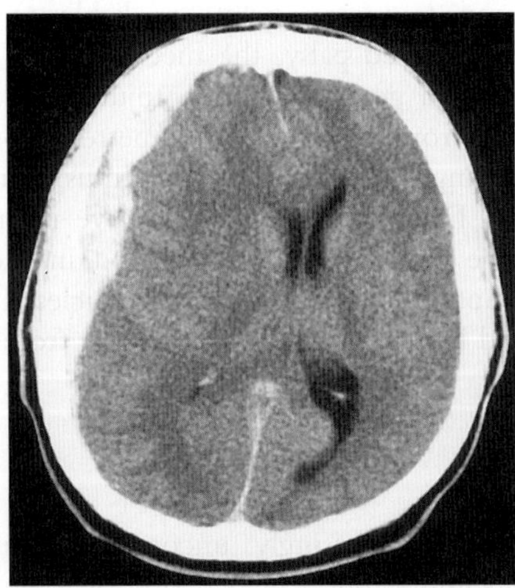

FIGURE 36-3
Acute subdural hematoma. Noncontrast CT scan reveals a hyperdense clot which has an irregular border with the brain and causes more horizontal displacement (mass effect) than might be expected from its thickness. The disproportionate mass effect is the result of the large rostral-caudal extent of these hematomas. Compare to Fig. 36-4.

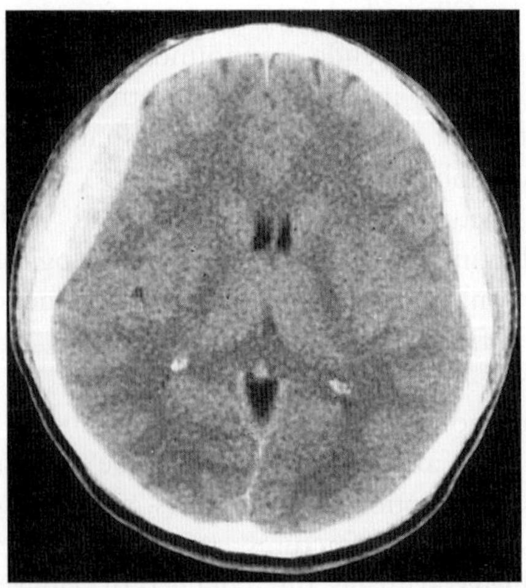

FIGURE 36-4
Acute epidural hematoma. The tightly attached dura is stripped from the inner table of the skull, producing a characteristic lenticular-shaped hemorrhage on noncontrast CT scan. Epidural hematomas are usually caused by tearing of the middle meningeal artery following fracture of the temporal bone.

sequence. Rapid surgical evacuation and ligation or cautery of the damaged vessel is indicated, usually the middle meningeal artery that has been lacerated by an overlying skull fracture.

Chronic subdural hematoma (Fig. 36-5)

A history of trauma may or may not be elicited in relation to chronic subdural hematoma; the injury may have been trivial and forgotten, particularly in the elderly and those with clotting disorders. Headache is common but not invariable. Additional features may include slowed thinking, vague change in personality, seizure, or a mild hemiparesis. The headache fluctuates in severity, sometimes with changes in head position. Bilateral chronic subdural hematomas produce perplexing clinical syndromes and the initial clinical impression may be of a stroke, brain tumor, drug intoxication, depression, or a dementing illness. Drowsiness, inattentiveness, and incoherence of thought are more generally prominent than focal signs such as hemiparesis. Rarely, chronic hematomas cause brief episodes of hemiparesis or aphasia that are indistinguishable from transient ischemic attacks. Patients with undetected bilateral subdural hematomas have a low tolerance for surgery, anesthesia, and drugs that depress the nervous system; drowsiness or confusion persist for long periods postoperatively.

CT without contrast initially shows a low-density mass over the convexity of the hemisphere (Fig. 36-5). Between 2 and 6 weeks after the initial bleeding the hemorrhage becomes isodense compared to adjacent brain and may be inapparent. Many subdural hematomas that are several weeks in age contain areas of blood and intermixed serous fluid. Bilateral chronic hematomas may fail to be detected because of the absence of lateral tissue shifts; this circumstance in an older patient is suggested by a "hypernormal" CT scan with fullness of the cortical sulci and small ventricles. Infusion of contrast material demonstrates enhancement of the vascular fibrous capsule surrounding the collection. MRI reliably identifies subacute and chronic hematomas.

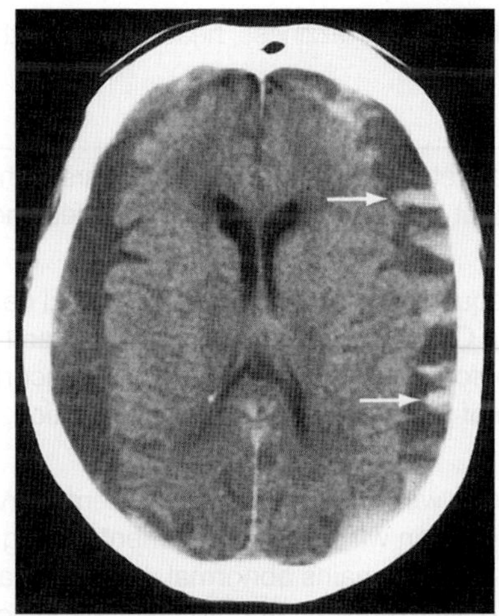

FIGURE 36-5
CT scan of chronic bilateral subdural hematomas of different ages. The collections began as acute hematomas and have become hypodense in comparison to the adjacent brain after a period during which they were isodense and difficult to appreciate. Some areas of resolving blood are contained on the more recently formed collection on the left (*arrows*).

Clinical observation coupled with serial imaging is a reasonable approach to patients with few symptoms, such as headache alone, and small chronic subdural collections. Treatment of minimally symptomatic chronic subdural hematoma with glucocorticoids is favored by some clinicians, but surgical evacuation is more often successful. The fibrous membranes that grow from the dura and encapsulate the collection require removal to prevent recurrent fluid accumulation. Small hematomas are resorbed, leaving only the organizing membranes. On imaging studies very chronic subdural hematomas are difficult to distinguish from hygromas, which are collections of CSF from a rent in the arachnoid membrane.

CLINICAL SYNDROMES AND TREATMENT OF HEAD INJURY

MINOR INJURY

The patient who has briefly lost consciousness or been stunned after a minor head injury usually becomes fully alert and attentive within minutes but may complain of headache, dizziness, faintness, nausea, a single episode of emesis, difficulty with concentration, a brief amnestic period, or slight blurring of vision. This typical concussion syndrome has a good prognosis with little risk of subsequent deterioration. Children are particularly prone to drowsiness, vomiting, and irritability, symptoms that are sometimes delayed for several hours after apparently minor injuries. Vasovagal syncope that follows injury may cause undue concern. Generalized or frontal headache is common in the following days. It may be migrainous (throbbing and hemicranial) in nature or aching and bilateral. After several hours of observation, patients with minor injury may be accompanied home and observed for a day by a family member or friend; written instructions to return if symptoms worsen should be provided.

Persistent severe headache and repeated vomiting in the context of normal alertness and no focal neurologic signs is usually benign, but CT should be obtained and a longer period of observation is appropriate. The decision to perform imaging tests also depends on clinical signs that indicate the impact was severe (e.g., prolonged concussion, periorbital or mastoid hematoma, repeated vomiting, palpable skull fracture), on the seriousness of other bodily injuries, and on the degree of surveillance that can be anticipated after discharge. Two studies have indicated that older age, two or more episodes of vomiting, >30 min of retrograde or persistent anterograde amnesia, seizure, and concurrent drug or alcohol intoxication are sensitive (but not specific) indicators of intracranial hemorrhage that justify CT scanning. It is appropriate to be more liberal in obtaining CT scans in children since a small number, even without loss of consciousness, will have intracranial lesions.

Concussion in sports

In the current absence of adequate data, a common sense approach to athletic concussion has been to avoid contact sports for at least several days after a mild injury, and for a longer period if there are more severe injuries or if there are protracted neurologic symptoms. The individual then undertakes a graduated program of activity until there are no further symptoms with exercise (Table 36-1). These guidelines are designed in part to avoid the extremely rare *second impact syndrome*, in which cerebral swelling follows a second minor head injury. There is some evidence that repeated concussions are associated with cumulative cognitive deficits, but this and the subsequent risk for dementia and Parkinson's disease are controversial.

INJURY OF INTERMEDIATE SEVERITY

Patients who are not fully alert or have persistent confusion, behavioral changes, extreme dizziness, or focal neurologic signs such as hemiparesis should be admitted to the hospital and have a CT scan. A cerebral contusion or hematoma is usually found. Common syndromes include: (1) delirium with a disinclination to be examined or moved, expletive speech, and resistance if disturbed (anterior temporal lobe contusions); (2) a quiet, disinterested, slowed mental state (abulia) alternating with irascibility (inferior frontal and frontopolar contusions); (3) a focal deficit such as aphasia or mild hemiparesis

TABLE 36-1

GUIDELINES FOR MANAGEMENT OF CONCUSSION IN SPORTS
Severity of Concussion
Grade 1: Transient confusion, no loss of consciousness (LOC), all symptoms resolve within 15 min. Grade 2: Transient confusion, no LOC, but concussive symptoms or mental status abnormalities persist longer than 15 min. Grade 3: Any LOC, either brief (seconds) or prolonged (minutes).
On-Site Evaluation
1. Mental status testing a. Orientation—time, place, person, circumstances of injury b. Concentration—digits backward, months of year in reverse order c. Memory—names of teams, details of contest, recent events, recall of three words and objects at 0 and 5 min 2. Finger-to-nose with eyes open and closed 3. Pupillary symmetry and reaction 4. Romberg and tandem gait 5. Provocative testing—40-yard sprint, 5 push ups, 5 sit ups, 5 knee bends (development of dizziness, headaches, or other symptoms is abnormal)
Management Guidelines
Grade 1: Remove from contest. Examine immediately and at 5-min intervals. May return to contest if exam clears within 15 min. A second grade 1 concussion eliminates player for 1 week, with return contingent upon normal neurologic assessment at rest and with exertion. Grade 2: Remove from contest, cannot return for at least 1 week. Examine at frequent intervals on sideline. Formal neurologic exam the next day. If headache or other symptoms persist for 1 week or longer, CT or MRI scan is indicated. After 1 full asymptomatic week, repeat neurologic assessment at rest and with exercise before cleared to resume play. A second grade 2 concussion eliminates player for at least 2 weeks following complete resolution of symptoms at rest or with exertion. If imaging shows abnormality, player is removed from play for the season. Grade 3: Transport by ambulance to emergency department if still unconscious or worrisome signs are present; cervical spine stabilization may be indicated. Neurologic exam and, when indicated, CT or MRI scan will guide subsequent management. Hospital admission indicated when signs of pathology are present or if mental status remains abnormal. If findings are normal at the time of the initial medical evaluation, the athlete may be sent home, but daily exams as an outpatient are indicated. A brief (LOC for seconds) grade 3 concussion eliminates player for 1 week, and a prolonged (LOC for minutes) grade 3 concussion for 2 weeks, following complete resolution of symptoms. A second grade 3 concussion should eliminate player from sports for at least 1 month following resolution of symptoms. Any abnormality on CT or MRI scans should result in termination of the season for the athlete, and return to play at any future time should be discouraged.

Source: Modified from Quality Standards Subcommittee of the American Academy of Neurology: *The American Academy of Neurology Practice Handbook*. The American Academy of Neurology, St. Paul, MN, 1997.

(due to subdural hematoma or convexity contusion, or, less often, carotid artery dissection); (4) confusion and inattention, poor performance on simple mental tasks, and fluctuating orientation (associated with several types of injuries, including those described earlier and with medial frontal contusions and interhemispheric subdural hematoma); (5) repetitive vomiting, nystagmus, drowsiness, and unsteadiness (labyrinthine concussion, but occasionally due to a posterior fossa subdural hematoma or vertebral artery dissection); and (6) diabetes insipidus (damage to the median eminence or pituitary stalk). *Injuries of this degree are often complicated by drug or alcohol intoxication, and clinically inapparent cervical spine injury may be present.*

After surgical removal of hematomas, most patients in this category improve over weeks. During the first week, the state of alertness, memory, and other cognitive functions often fluctuate, and agitation is common. Behavioral changes tend to be worse at night, as with many other encephalopathies, and may be treated with small doses of antipsychotic medications. Subtle abnormalities of attention, intellect, spontaneity, and memory return toward normal weeks or months after the injury, sometimes abruptly. Persistent cognitive problems are discussed later.

SEVERE INJURY

Patients who are comatose from the moment of injury require immediate neurologic attention and resuscitation. After intubation, with care taken to immobilize the cervical spine, the depth of coma, pupillary size and reactivity, limb movements, and Babinski responses are assessed. As soon as vital functions permit and cervical spine x-rays and a CT scan have been obtained, the patient should be transported to a critical care unit. Hypoxia should be reversed, and normal saline used as the resuscitation fluid in preference to albumin. The finding of an epidural or subdural hematoma or large intracerebral hemorrhage is an indication for prompt surgery and intracranial decompression in an otherwise salvageable patient. The use of prophylactic antiepileptic medications has been recommended but there is little supportive data. Management of raised ICP, a frequent feature of severe head injury, is discussed in Chap. 28.

GRADING AND PROGNOSIS

In severe head injury, the clinical features of eye opening, motor responses of the limbs, and verbal output have been found to be generally predictive of outcome. These three responses are assessed by the Glasgow Coma Scale; a score between 3 and 15 is assigned (Table 36-2). Over 85% of patients with aggregate scores of <5 die within 24 h. However, a number of patients with slightly higher scores, including a few without pupillary light responses, survive, suggesting that an initially aggressive approach is justified in most patients. Patients <20 years, particularly children, may make remarkable recoveries after having grave early neurologic signs. In one large study of severe head injury, 55% of children had a good outcome at 1 year, compared with 21% of adults. Older age, increased ICP, early hypoxia or hypotension, compression of the brainstem on CT or MRI, and a delay in the evacuation of large intracranial hemorrhages are indicators of a poor prognosis.

TABLE 36-2

GLASGOW COMA SCALE FOR HEAD INJURY

EYE OPENING (E)		VERBAL RESPONSE (V)	
Spontaneous	4	Oriented	5
To loud voice	3	Confused, disoriented	4
To pain	2	Inappropriate words	3
Nil	1	Incomprehensible sounds	2
		Nil	1

BEST MOTOR RESPONSE (M)	
Obeys	6
Localizes	5
Withdraws (flexion)	4
Abnormal flexion posturing	3
Extension posturing	2
Nil	1

Note: Coma score = E + M + V. Patients scoring 3 or 4 have an 85% chance of dying or remaining vegetative, while scores >11 indicate only a 5–10% likelihood of death or vegetative state and 85% chance of moderate disability or good recovery. Intermediate scores correlate with proportional chances of recovery.

POSTCONCUSSION SYNDROME

The *postconcussion syndrome* refers to a state following minor head injury consisting of fatigue, dizziness, headache, and difficulty in concentration. The syndrome simulates asthenia and anxious depression. Based on experimental models, it has been proposed that subtle axonal shearing lesions or as yet undefined biochemical alterations account for the cognitive symptoms. In moderate and severe trauma, neuropsychological changes such as difficulty with attention, memory and other cognitive deficits are undoubtedly present, sometimes severe, but many problems identified by formal testing do not affect daily functioning. Test scores tend to improve rapidly during the first 6 months after injury, then more slowly for years.

Management of the postconcussive syndrome requires the identification and treatment of depression, sleeplessness, anxiety, persistent headache, and dizziness. A clear explanation of the problems that may follow concussion has been shown to reduce subsequent complaints. Care is taken to avoid prolonged use of drugs that produce dependence. Headache may initially be treated with acetaminophen and small doses of amitryptiline. Vestibular exercises (Chap. 11) and small doses of vestibular suppressants such as promethazine (Phenergan) may be helpful when dizziness is the main problem. Patients who after minor or moderate injury have difficulty with memory or with complex cognitive tasks at work may be reassured that these problems usually improve over 6–12 months. It is sometimes helpful to obtain serial and quantified neuropsychological testing in order to adjust the work environment to the patient's abilities and to document improvement over time. Whether cognitive exercises are useful in contrast to rest and a reduction in mental challenges is uncertain. Previously energetic and resilient individuals usually have the best recoveries. In patients with persistent symptoms, the possibility exists of malingering or prolongation as a result of litigation.

CHAPTER 37

PRIMARY AND METASTATIC TUMORS OF THE NERVOUS SYSTEM

Lisa M. DeAngelis ■ Patrick Y. Wen

INTRODUCTION

Primary brain tumors are diagnosed in approximately 52,000 people each year in the United States. At least one-half of these tumors are malignant and associated with a high mortality rate. Glial tumors account for about 60% of all primary brain tumors, and 80% of those are malignant neoplasms. Meningiomas account for 25%, vestibular schwannomas 10%, and central nervous system (CNS) lymphomas about 2%. Brain metastases are three times more common than all primary brain tumors combined and are diagnosed in approximately 150,000 people each year. Metastases to the leptomeninges and epidural space of the spinal cord each occur in approximately 3–5% of patients with systemic cancer and are also a major cause of neurologic disability in this population.

APPROACH TO THE PATIENT: Primary and Metastatic Tumors of the Nervous System

CLINICAL FEATURES Brain tumors of any type can present with a variety of symptoms and signs that fall into two categories: general and focal; patients often have a combination of the two (Table 37-1). General or nonspecific symptoms include headache, cognitive difficulties, personality change, and gait disorder. Generalized symptoms arise when the enlarging tumor and its surrounding edema cause an increase in intracranial pressure or direct compression of cerebrospinal fluid (CSF) circulation leading to hydrocephalus. The classic headache associated with a brain tumor is most evident in the morning and improves during the day, but this particular pattern is actually seen in a minority of patients. Headache may be accompanied by nausea or vomiting when intracranial pressure is elevated. Headaches are often holocephalic but can be ipsilateral to the side of a tumor. Occasionally, headaches have features of a typical migraine with unilateral throbbing pain associated with visual scotoma. Personality changes may include apathy and withdrawal from social circumstances, mimicking depression. Focal or lateralizing findings include hemiparesis, aphasia, or visual field defect. Lateralizing symptoms such as hemiparesis are typically subacute and progressive. A visual field defect is often not noticed by the patient; its presence may only be revealed after it leads to an injury such as an automobile accident occurring in the blind visual field. Language difficulties may be mistaken for confusion. Seizures are a common presentation of brain tumors, occurring in about 25% of patients with brain metastases or malignant gliomas but can be the presenting symptom in up to 90% of patients with low-

TABLE 37-1

SYMPTOMS AND SIGNS AT PRESENTATION OF BRAIN TUMORS

	HIGH-GRADE GLIOMA (%)	LOW-GRADE GLIOMA (%)	MENINGIOMA (%)	METASTASES (%)
Generalized				
Impaired cognitive function	50	10	30	60
Hemiparesis	40	10	36	60
Headache	50	40	37	50
Lateralizing				
Seizures	20	70+	17	18
Aphasia	20	<5		18
Visual field deficit	—	—	—	7

grade gliomas. Most seizures have a focal signature that reflects their location in the brain and many proceed to secondary generalization. All generalized seizures that arise from a brain tumor will have a focal onset whether or not it is apparent clinically.

NEUROIMAGING Cranial MRI is the preferred diagnostic test for any patient suspected of having a brain tumor, and should be performed with gadolinium contrast administration. CT scan should be reserved for those patients unable to undergo MRI (e.g., pacemaker). Malignant brain tumors—whether primary or metastatic—typically enhance with gadolinium and may have central areas of necrosis; they are characteristically surrounded by edema of the neighboring white matter. Low-grade gliomas typically do not enhance with gadolinium and are best appreciated on fluid-attenuated inversion recovery (FLAIR) MR images. Meningiomas have a characteristic appearance on MRI as they are dural-based with a dural tail and compress but do not invade the brain. Dural metastases or a dural lymphoma can have a similar appearance. Imaging is characteristic for many primary and metastatic tumors, but occasionally there is diagnostic uncertainty based on imaging alone. In such patients a brain biopsy may be helpful in determining a definitive diagnosis. However, when a tumor is strongly suspected, the biopsy can be obtained as an intraoperative frozen section before a definitive resection is performed.

Functional MRI is useful in presurgical planning and defining eloquent sensory, motor, and language cortex. Positron emission tomography (PET) is useful in determining the metabolic activity of the lesions seen on MRI; MR perfusion and spectroscopy can provide information on blood flow or tissue composition. These techniques may help distinguish tumor progression from necrotic tissue as a consequence of treatment with radiation and chemotherapy or identify foci of high-grade tumor in an otherwise low-grade-appearing glioma.

Neuroimaging is the only test necessary to diagnose a brain tumor. Laboratory tests are rarely useful, although patients with metastatic disease may have elevation of a tumor marker in their serum that reflects the presence of brain metastases (e.g., human chorionic gonadotropin [βhCG] from testicular cancer). Additional testing such as cerebral angiogram, electroencephalogram (EEG), or lumbar puncture is rarely indicated or helpful.

TREATMENT Brain Tumors

Therapy of any intracranial malignancy requires both symptomatic and definitive treatments. Definitive treatment is based upon the specific tumor type and includes surgery, radiotherapy (RT), and chemotherapy. However, symptomatic treatments apply to brain tumors of any type. Most high-grade malignancies are accompanied by substantial surrounding edema, which contributes to neurologic disability and raised intracranial pressure. Glucocorticoids are highly effective at reducing perilesional edema and improving neurologic function, often within hours of administration. Dexamethasone has been the glucocorticoid of choice because of its relatively low mineralocorticoid activity. Initial doses are typically 12 mg to 16 mg a day in divided doses given orally or IV (both are equivalent). While glucocorticoids rapidly ameliorate symptoms and signs, their long-term use causes substantial toxicity including insomnia, weight gain, diabetes mellitus, steroid myopathy, and personality changes. Consequently, a taper is indicated as definitive treatment is administered and the patient improves.

Patients with brain tumors who present with seizures, require anticonvulsant drug therapy. There is no role for prophylactic anticonvulsant drugs in patients who have not had a seizure, thus their use should be restricted to those who have had a convincing ictal event. The agents of choice are those drugs that do not induce the hepatic microsomal enzyme system. These include levetiracetam, topiramate, lamotrigine, valproic acid, or lacosamide (Chap. 26). Other drugs such as phenytoin and carbamazepine are used less frequently because they are potent enzyme inducers that can interfere with both glucocorticoid metabolism and the metabolism of chemotherapeutic agents needed to treat the underlying systemic malignancy or the primary brain tumor.

Venous thromboembolic disease occurs in 20–30% of patients with high-grade gliomas and brain metastases. Therefore, anticoagulants should be used prophylactically during hospitalization and in patients who are nonambulatory. Those who have had either a deep vein thrombosis or pulmonary embolus can receive therapeutic doses of anticoagulation safely and without increasing the risk for hemorrhage into the tumor. Inferior vena cava filters are reserved for patients with absolute contraindications to anticoagulation such as recent craniotomy.

PRIMARY BRAIN TUMORS

PATHOGENESIS

No underlying cause has been identified for the majority of primary brain tumors. The only established risk factors are exposure to ionizing radiation (meningiomas, gliomas, and schwannomas) and immunosuppression (primary CNS lymphoma). Evidence for an association with exposure to electromagnetic fields including cellular telephones, head injury, foods containing *N*-nitroso compounds, or occupational risk factors, are unproven. A small minority of patients have a family history of brain tumors. Some of these familial cases are associated with genetic syndromes (Table 37-2).

As with other neoplasms, brain tumors arise as a result of a multistep process driven by the sequential acquisition of genetic alterations. These include loss of tumor suppressor genes (e.g., p53 and phosphatase and tensin homolog on chromosome 10 [PTEN]) and amplification and overexpression of protooncogenes such as the epidermal growth factor receptor (EGFR) and the platelet-derived growth factor receptors (PDGFR). The accumulation of these genetic abnormalities results in uncontrolled cell growth and tumor formation.

Important progress has been made in understanding the molecular pathogenesis of several types of brain tumors, including glioblastomas and medulloblastomas. Glioblastomas can be separated into two main subtypes based on genetic and biologic differences (Fig. 37-1). The majority are primary glioblastomas. These arise de

TABLE 37-2

GENETIC SYNDROMES ASSOCIATED WITH PRIMARY BRAIN TUMORS

SYNDROME	INHERITANCE	GENE/PROTEIN	ASSOCIATED TUMORS
Cowden's syndrome	AD	Mutations of PTEN (ch10p23)	Dysplastic cerebellar gangliocytoma (Lhermitte-Duclos disease), meningioma, astrocytoma Breast, endometrial, thyroid cancer, trichilemmomas
Familial schwannomatosis	Sporadic Hereditary	Mutations in INI1/SNF5 (ch22q11)	Schwannomas, gliomas
Gardner's syndrome	AD	Mutations in APC(ch5q21)	Medulloblastoma, glioblastoma, craniopharyngioma Familial polyposis, multiple osteomas, skin and soft tissue tumors
Gorlin syndrome (basal cell nevus syndrome)	AD	Mutations in Patched 1 gene (ch9q22.3)	Medulloblastomas Basal cell carcinoma
Li-Fraumeni syndrome	AD	Mutations in p53 (ch17p13.1)	Gliomas, medulloblastomas Sarcomas, breast cancer, leukemias, others
Multiple endocrine neoplasia 1 (Werner's syndrome)	AD	Mutations in Menin (ch11q13)	Pituitary adenoma, malignant schwannomas Parathyroid and pancreatic islet cell tumors
Neurofibromatosis type 1 (NF1)	AD	Mutations in NF1/ Neurofibromin (ch17q12-22)	Schwannomas, astrocytomas, optic nerve gliomas, meningiomas Neurofibromas, neurofibrosarcomas, others
Neurofibromatosis type 2 (NF2)	AD	Mutations in NF2/Merlin (ch22q12)	Bilateral vestibular schwannomas, astrocytomas, multiple meningiomas, ependymomas
Tuberous sclerosis (TSC) (Bourneville's disease)	AD	Mutations in TSC1/TSC2 (ch9q34/16)	Subependymal giant cell astrocytoma, ependymomas, glioma, ganglioneuroma, hamartoma
Turcot's syndrome	AD AR	Mutations in APC[a] (ch5) hMLH1 (ch3p21)	Gliomas, medulloblastomas Adenomatous colon polyps, adenocarcinoma
Von Hippel–Lindau (VHL)	AD	Mutations in VHL gene (ch3p25)	Hemangioblastomas Retinal angiomas, renal cell carcinoma, pheochromocytoma, pancreatic tumors and cysts, endolymphatic sac tumors of the middle ear

[a]Various DNA mismatch repair gene mutations may cause a similar clinical phenotype, also referred to as Turcot's syndrome, in which there is a predisposition to nonpolyposis colon cancer and brain tumors.

Abbreviations: AD, autosomal dominant; APC, adenomatous polyposis coli; AR, autosomal recessive; ch, chromosome; PTEN, phosphatase and tensin homologue; TSC, tuberous sclerosis complex.

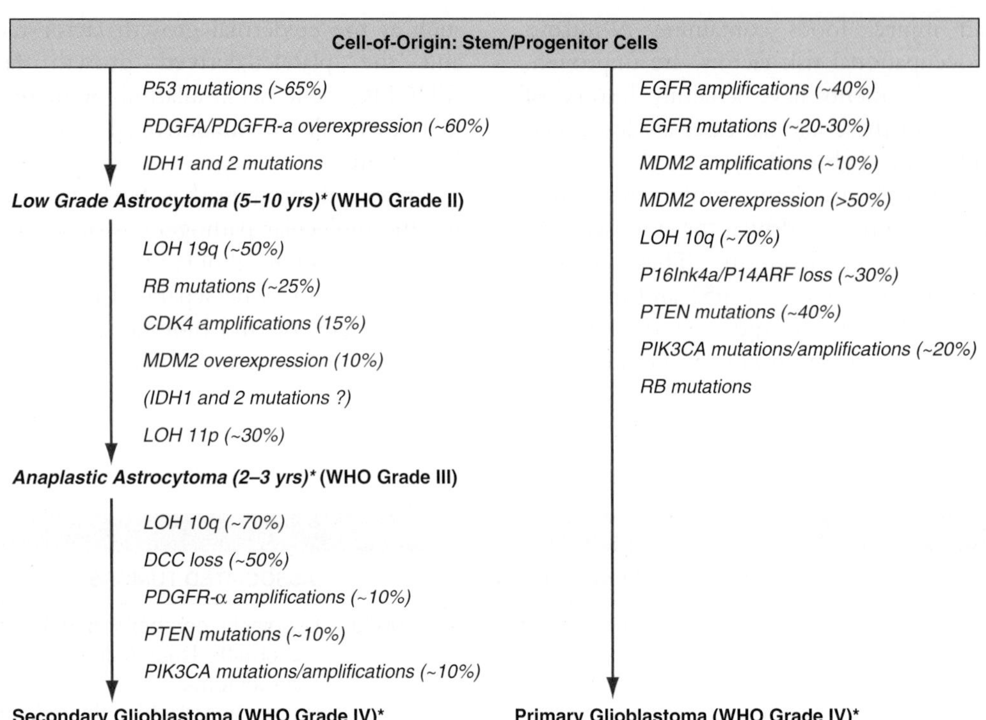

FIGURE 37-1

Genetic and chromosomal alterations involved in the development of primary and secondary glioblastomas. A *slash* indicates one or the other or both. *DCC*, deleted in colorectal carcinoma; *EGFR*, epidermal growth factor receptor; *IDH*, isocitrate dehydrogenase; *LOH*, loss of heterozygosity; *MDM2*, murine double minute 2; *PDGF*, platelet-derived growth factor; *PDGFR*, platelet-derived growth factor receptor; *PIK3CA*, phosphatidylinositol 3-kinase, catalytic; *PTEN*, phosphatase and tensin homologue; *RB*, retinoblastoma; WHO, World Health Organization.

novo and are characterized by EGFR amplification and mutations, and deletion or mutation of PTEN. Secondary glioblastomas arise in younger patients as lower-grade tumors and transform over a period of several years into glioblastomas. These tumors have inactivation of the p53 tumor suppressor gene, overexpression of PDGFR, and mutations of the isocitrate dehydrogenase 1 and 2 genes. Despite their genetic differences, primary and secondary glioblastomas are morphologically indistinguishable, although they are likely to respond differently to molecular therapies. The molecular subtypes of medulloblastomas are also being elucidated. Approximately 25% of medulloblastomas have activating mutations of the sonic hedgehog signaling pathway, raising the possibility that inhibitors of this pathway may have therapeutic potential.

The adult nervous system contains neural stem cells that are capable of self-renewal, proliferation, and differentiation into distinctive mature cell types. There is increasing evidence that neural stem cells, or related progenitor cells, can be transformed into tumor stem cells and give rise to primary brain tumors, including gliomas and medulloblastomas. These stem cells appear to be more resistant to standard therapies than the tumor cells themselves and contribute to the difficulty in eradicating these tumors. There is intense interest in developing therapeutic strategies that effectively target tumor stem cells.

INTRINSIC "MALIGNANT" TUMORS

ASTROCYTOMAS

These are infiltrative tumors with a presumptive glial cell of origin. The World Health Organization (WHO) classifies astrocytomas into four prognostic grades based on histologic features: grade I (pilocytic astrocytoma, subependymal giant cell astrocytoma); grade II (diffuse astrocytoma); grade III (anaplastic astrocytoma); and grade IV (glioblastoma). Grades I and II are considered low-grade, and grades III and IV high-grade, astrocytomas.

Low-grade astrocytoma

These tumors occur predominantly in children and young adults.

Grade I astrocytomas

Pilocytic astrocytomas (WHO grade I) are the most common tumor of childhood. They occur typically in the cerebellum but may also be found elsewhere in the neuraxis, including the optic nerves and brainstem. Frequently they appear as cystic lesions with an enhancing mural nodule. They are potentially curable if they can be completely resected. Giant cell subependymal astrocytomas are usually found in the ventricular wall of patients with tuberous sclerosis. They often do not require intervention but can be treated surgically or with inhibitors of the mammalian target of rapamycin (mTOR).

Grade II astrocytomas

These are infiltrative tumors that usually present with seizures in young adults. They appear as nonenhancing tumors with increased T2/FLAIR signal (Fig. 37-2). If feasible, patients should undergo maximal surgical resection, although complete resection is rarely possible because of the invasive nature of the tumor. Radiotherapy is helpful, but there is no difference in overall survival between radiotherapy administered postoperatively or delayed until the time of tumor progression. There is increasing evidence that chemotherapeutic agents such as temozolomide, an oral alkylating agent, can be helpful in some patients.

High-grade astrocytoma

Grade III (anaplastic) astrocytoma

These account for approximately 15–20% of high-grade astrocytomas. They generally present in the fourth and fifth decades of life as variably enhancing tumors. Treatment is the same as for glioblastoma, consisting of maximal safe surgical resection followed by radiotherapy with concurrent and adjuvant temozolomide, or with radiotherapy and adjuvant temozolomide alone.

Grade IV astrocytoma (glioblastoma)

Glioblastoma accounts for the majority of high-grade astrocytomas. They are the most common cause of malignant primary brain tumors, with over 10,000 cases diagnosed each year in the United States. Patients usually present in the sixth and seventh decades of life with headache, seizures, or focal neurologic deficits. The tumors appear as ring-enhancing masses with central necrosis and surrounding edema (Fig. 37-3). These are highly infiltrative tumors, and the areas of increased T2/FLAIR signal surrounding the main tumor mass contain invading tumor cells. Treatment involves maximal surgical resection followed by partial-field external beam radiotherapy (6000 cGy in thirty 200-cGy fractions) with concomitant temozolomide, followed by 6–12 months of adjuvant temozolomide. With this regimen, median survival is increased to 14.6 months compared to only 12 months with radiotherapy alone, and 2-year survival is increased to 27%, compared to 10% with radiotherapy alone. Patients whose tumor contains the DNA repair enzyme O^6-methylguanine-DNA methyltransferase (MGMT) are relatively resistant to temozolomide and have a worse prognosis compared to those whose tumors contain low levels of MGMT as a result of silencing of the MGMT gene by promoter hypermethylation. Implantation of biodegradable

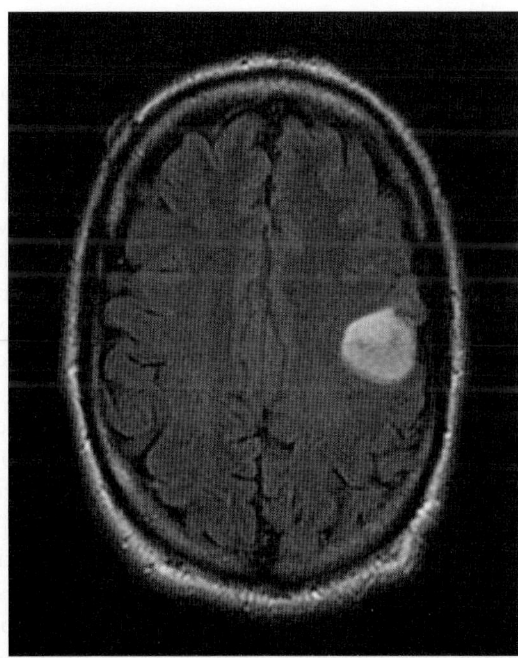

FIGURE 37-2
Fluid-attenuated inversion recovery (FLAIR) MRI of a left frontal low-grade astrocytoma. This lesion did not enhance.

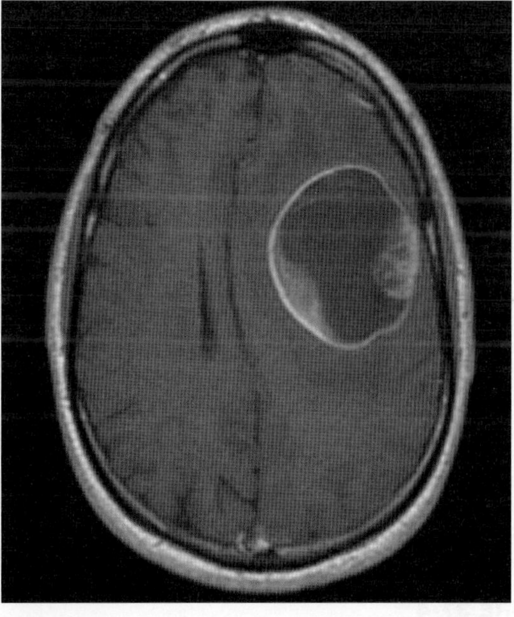

FIGURE 37-3
Postgadolinium T1 MRI of a large cystic left frontal glioblastoma.

polymers containing the chemotherapeutic agent carmustine into the tumor bed after resection of the tumor also produces a modest improvement in survival.

Despite optimal therapy, glioblastomas invariably recur. Treatment options for recurrent disease may include reoperation, carmustine wafers, and alternate chemotherapeutic regimens. Reirradiation is rarely helpful. Bevacizumab, a humanized vascular endothelial growth factor (VEGF) monoclonal antibody, has activity in recurrent glioblastoma, increasing progression-free survival and reducing peritumoral edema and glucocorticoid use (Fig. 37-4). Treatment decisions for patients with recurrent glioblastoma must be made on an individual basis, taking into consideration such factors as previous therapy, time to relapse, performance status, and quality of life. Whenever feasible, patients with recurrent disease should be enrolled in clinical trials. Novel therapies undergoing evaluation in patients with glioblastoma include targeted molecular agents directed at receptor tyrosine kinases and signal transduction pathways; antiangiogenic agents, especially those directed at the VEGF receptors; chemotherapeutic agents that cross the blood-brain barrier more effectively than currently available drugs; gene therapy; immunotherapy; and infusion of radiolabeled drugs and targeted toxins into the tumor and surrounding brain by means of convection-enhanced delivery.

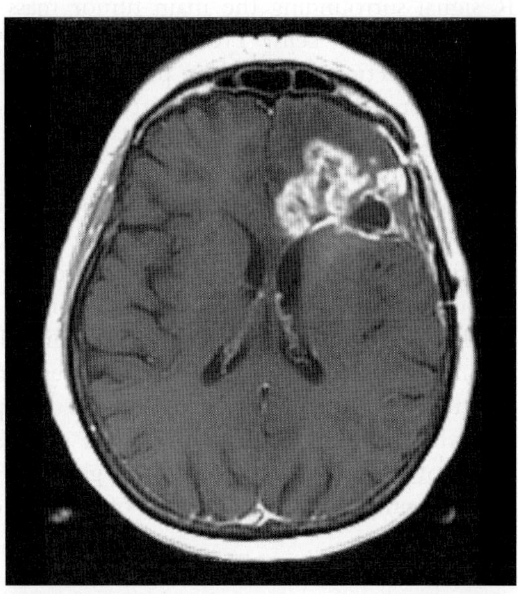

A

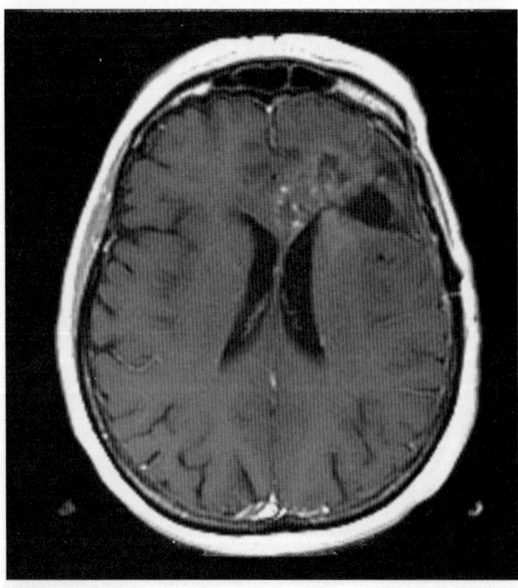

B

FIGURE 37-4
Postgadolinium T1 MRI of a recurrent glioblastoma before (***A***) and after (***B***) administration of bevacizumab. Note the decreased enhancement and mass effect.

The most important adverse prognostic factors in patients with high-grade astrocytomas are older age, histologic features of glioblastoma, poor Karnofsky performance status, and unresectable tumor. Patients with unmethylated MGMT promoter resulting in the presence of the repair enzyme in tumor cells and resistance to temozolomide also have a worse prognosis.

Gliomatosis cerebri

Rarely, patients may present with a highly infiltrating, nonenhancing tumor involving more than two lobes. These tumors do not qualify for the histologic diagnosis of glioblastoma but behave aggressively and have a similarly poor outcome. Treatment involves radiotherapy and temozolomide chemotherapy.

Oligodendroglioma

Oligodendrogliomas account for approximately 15–20% of gliomas. They are classified by the WHO into well-differentiated oligodendrogliomas (grade II) or anaplastic oligodendrogliomas (AOs) (grade III). Tumors with oligodendroglial components have distinctive features such as perinuclear clearing—giving rise to a "fried-egg" appearance—and a reticular pattern of blood vessel growth. Some tumors have both an oligodendroglial as well as an astrocytic component. These mixed tumors, or oligoastrocytomas (OAs), are also classified into well-differentiated OA (grade II) or anaplastic oligoastrocytomas (AOAs) (grade III).

Grade II oligodendrogliomas and OAs are generally more responsive to therapy and have a better prognosis than pure astrocytic tumors. These tumors present similarly to grade II astrocytomas in young adults. The tumors are nonenhancing and often partially calcified. They should be treated with surgery and, if necessary, radiotherapy and chemotherapy. Patients with oligodendrogliomas have a median survival in excess of 10 years.

Anaplastic oligodendrogliomas and AOAs present in the fourth and fifth decades as variably enhancing tumors. They are more responsive to therapy than grade III astrocytomas.

Co-deletion of chromosomes 1p and 19q, mediated by an unbalanced translocation of 19p to 1q, occurs in 61 to 89% of patients with AO and 14 to 20% of patients with AOA. Tumors with the 1p and 19q co-deletion are particularly sensitive to chemotherapy with procarbazine, lomustine (cyclohexylchloroethylnitrosourea [CCNU]), and vincristine (PCV) or temozolomide, as well as to radiotherapy. Median survival of patients with AO or AOA is approximately 3–6 years.

Ependymomas

Ependymomas are tumors derived from ependymal cells that line the ventricular surface. They account for approximately 5% of childhood tumors and frequently arise from the wall of the fourth ventricle in the posterior fossa. Although adults can have intracranial ependymomas, they occur more commonly in the spine, especially in the filum terminale of the spinal cord where they have a myxopapillary histology. Ependymomas that can be completely resected are potentially curable. Partially resected ependymomas will recur and require irradiation. The less common anaplastic ependymomas are more aggressive but can be treated in the same way as ependymomas. Subependymomas are slow-growing benign lesions arising in the wall of ventricles that often do not require treatment.

Other less common gliomas

Gangliogliomas and pleomorphic xanthoastrocytomas occur in young adults. They behave as more indolent forms of grade II gliomas and are treated in the same way. Brainstem gliomas usually occur in children or young adults. Despite treatment with radiotherapy and chemotherapy, the prognosis is poor with median survival of only 1 year. Gliosarcomas contain both an astrocytic as well as a sarcomatous component and are treated in the same way as glioblastomas.

PRIMARY CENTRAL NERVOUS SYSTEM LYMPHOMA

Primary central nervous system lymphoma (PCNSL) is a rare non-Hodgkin's lymphoma accounting for less than 3% of primary brain tumors. For unclear reasons, its incidence is increasing, particularly in immunocompetent individuals.

PCNSL in immunocompetent patients usually consists of diffuse large B-cell lymphomas. PCNSL may also occur in immunocompromised patients, usually those infected with the human immunodeficiency virus (HIV) or organ transplant recipients on immunosuppressive therapy. PCNSL in immunocompromised patients is typically large cell with immunoblastic and more aggressive features. These patients are usually severely immunocompromised with CD4 counts of less than 50/mL. The Epstein-Barr virus (EBV) frequently plays an important role in the pathogenesis of HIV-related PCNSL.

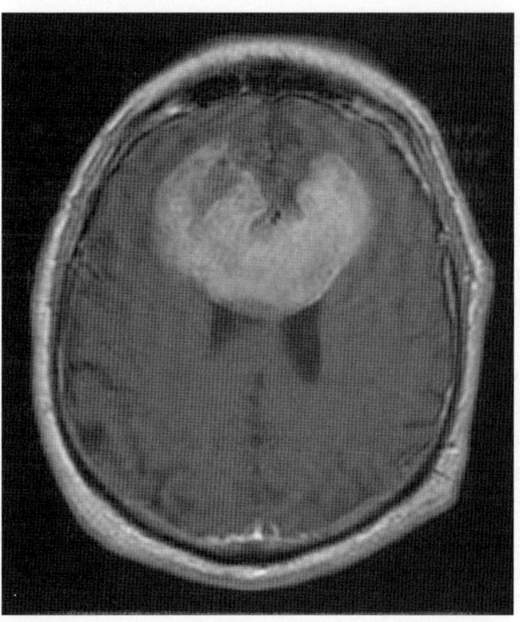

FIGURE 37-5
Postgadolinium T1 MRI demonstrating a large bifrontal primary central nervous system lymphoma (PCNSL). The periventricular location and diffuse enhancement pattern are characteristic of lymphoma.

Immunocompetent patients are older (median 60 years) compared to HIV-related PCNSL (median 31 years). PCNSL usually presents as a mass lesion, with neuropsychiatric symptoms, symptoms of increased intracranial pressure, lateralizing signs, or seizures.

On contrast-enhanced MRI, PCNSL usually appears as a densely enhancing tumor (Fig. 37-5). Immunocompetent patients have solitary lesions more often than immunosuppressed patients. Frequently there is involvement of the basal ganglia, corpus callosum, or periventricular region. Although the imaging features are often characteristic, PCNSL can sometimes be difficult to differentiate from high-grade gliomas, infections, or demyelination. Stereotactic biopsy is necessary to obtain a histologic diagnosis. Whenever possible, glucocorticoids should be withheld until after the biopsy has been obtained, since they have a cytolytic effect on lymphoma cells and may lead to nondiagnostic tissue. In addition, patients should be tested for HIV and the extent of disease assessed by performing positron emission tomography (PET) or computerized tomography (CT) of the body, MRI of the spine, CSF analysis, and slit-lamp examination of the eye. Bone marrow biopsy and testicular ultrasound are occasionally performed.

TREATMENT **Primary Central Nervous System Lymphoma**

Unlike other primary brain tumors, PCNSL is relatively sensitive to glucocorticoids, chemotherapy, and radiotherapy. Durable complete responses and long-term survival are possible with these treatments. High-dose methotrexate, a folate antagonist that interrupts DNA synthesis, produces response rates ranging from 35 to 80% and median survival up to 50 months. Combination of methotrexate with other chemotherapeutic agents such as cytarabine, as well as whole-brain radiotherapy, increases the response rate to 70–100%. However, radiotherapy is associated with delayed neurotoxicity, especially in patients over the age of 60 years. As a result radiotherapy is frequently omitted in older patients with PCNSL. There is emerging evidence that the anti-CD20 monoclonal antibody rituximab may have activity in PCNSL, although there remain concerns about its ability to pass through the blood-brain barrier as it becomes reconstituted with therapy. For some patients, high-dose chemotherapy with autologous stem cell rescue may offer the best chance of preventing relapse.

At least 50% of patients will eventually develop recurrent disease. Treatment options include radiotherapy for patients who have not had prior irradiation, re-treatment with methotrexate, as well as other agents such as temozolomide, rituximab, procarbazine, topotecan, and pemetrexed. High-dose chemotherapy with autologous stem cell rescue may have a role in selected patients with relapsed disease.

PCNSL IN IMMUNOCOMPROMISED PATIENTS PCNSL in immunocompromised patients often produces multiple-ring enhancing lesions that can be difficult to differentiate from metastases and infections such as toxoplasmosis. The diagnosis is usually established by examination of the cerebrospinal fluid for cytology and EBV DNA, toxoplasmosis serologic testing, brain PET imaging for hypermetabolism of the lesions consistent with tumor instead of infection, and, if necessary, brain biopsy. Since the advent of highly active antiretroviral drugs, the incidence of HIV-related PCNSL has declined. These patients may be treated with whole-brain radiotherapy, high-dose methotrexate, and initiation of highly active antiretroviral therapy. In organ transplant recipients, reduction of immunosuppression may improve outcome.

MEDULLOBLASTOMAS

Medulloblastomas are the most common malignant brain tumor of childhood, accounting for approximately 20% of all primary CNS tumors among children. They arise from granule cell progenitors or from multipotent progenitors from the ventricular zone. Approximately 5% of children have inherited disorders with germline mutations of genes that predispose to the development of medulloblastoma. The Gorlin syndrome, the most common of these inherited disorders, is due to mutations in the patched-1 (PTCH-1) gene, a key component in the sonic hedgehog pathway. Turcot's syndrome, caused by mutations in the adenomatous polyposis coli (APC) gene and familial adenomatous polyposis, has also been associated with an increased incidence of medulloblastoma. Histologically, medulloblastomas appear as highly cellular tumors with abundant dark staining, round nuclei, and rosette formation (Homer-Wright rosettes). They present with headache, ataxia, and signs of brainstem involvement. On MRI they appear as densely enhancing tumors in the posterior fossa, sometimes associated with hydrocephalus. Seeding of the CSF is common. Treatment involves maximal surgical resection, craniospinal irradiation, and chemotherapy with agents such as cisplatin, lomustine, cyclophosphamide, and vincristine. Approximately 70% of patients have long-term survival but usually at the cost of significant neurocognitive impairment. A major goal of current research is to improve survival while minimizing long-term complications.

PINEAL REGION TUMORS

A large number of tumors can arise in the region of the pineal gland. These typically present with headache, visual symptoms, and hydrocephalus. Patients may have Parinaud's syndrome characterized by impaired upgaze and accommodation. Some pineal tumors such as pineocytomas and benign teratomas can be treated simply by surgical resection. Germinomas respond to irradiation, while pineoblastomas and malignant germ cell tumors require craniospinal radiation and chemotherapy.

EXTRINSIC "BENIGN" TUMORS

MENINGIOMAS

Meningiomas are diagnosed with increasing frequency as more people undergo neuroimaging studies for various indications. They are now the most common primary brain tumor, accounting for approximately 32% of the total. Their incidence increases with age. They tend to be more common in women and in patients with neurofibromatosis type 2. They also occur more commonly in patients with a past history of cranial irradiation.

Meningiomas arise from the dura mater and are composed of neoplastic meningothelial (arachnoidal cap) cells. They are most commonly located over the cerebral convexities, especially adjacent to the sagittal sinus, but can also occur in the skull base and along the dorsum of the spinal cord. Meningiomas are classified by the WHO into three histologic grades of increasing aggressiveness: grade I (benign meningiomas), grade II (atypical meningiomas), and grade III (malignant meningiomas).

Many meningiomas are found incidentally following neuroimaging for unrelated reasons. They can also present with headaches, seizures, or focal neurologic deficits. On imaging studies they have a characteristic appearance usually consisting of a partially calcified, densely enhancing extraaxial tumor arising from the dura (Fig. 37-6). Occasionally they may have a dural tail, consisting of thickened, enhanced dura extending like a tail from the mass. The main differential diagnosis of meningioma is a dural metastasis.

If the meningioma is small and asymptomatic, no intervention is necessary and the lesion can be observed with serial MRI studies. Larger, symptomatic lesions should be resected surgically. If complete resection is achieved, the patient is cured. Incompletely resected tumors tend to recur, although the rate of recurrence can be very slow with grade I tumors. Tumors that cannot be resected, or can only be partially removed, may benefit from treatment with external beam radiotherapy or stereotactic radiosurgery (SRS). These treatments may also be helpful in patients whose tumor has recurred after surgery. Hormonal therapy and chemotherapy are currently unproven.

Rarer tumors that resemble meningiomas include hemangiopericytomas and solitary fibrous tumors. These are treated with surgery and radiotherapy but have a higher propensity to recur.

SCHWANNOMAS

These are generally benign tumors arising from the Schwann cells of cranial and spinal nerve roots. The most common schwannomas, termed *vestibular schwannomas* or *acoustic neuromas*, arise from the vestibular portion of the eighth cranial nerve and account for approximately 9% of primary brain tumors. Patients with neurofibromatosis type 2 have a high incidence of vestibular schwannomas that are frequently bilateral. Schwannomas arising from other cranial nerves, such as the trigeminal nerve (cranial nerve V), occur with much lower frequency. Neurofibromatosis type 1 is associated with an increased incidence of schwannomas of the spinal nerve roots.

Vestibular schwannomas may be found incidentally on neuroimaging or present with progressive unilateral hearing loss, dizziness, tinnitus, or less commonly, symptoms resulting from compression of the brainstem and cerebellum. On MRI they appear as densely enhancing lesions, enlarging the internal auditory canal and often extending into the cerebellopontine angle (Fig. 37-7). The differential diagnosis includes meningioma. Very small, asymptomatic lesions can be observed with serial MRIs. Larger lesions should be treated with surgery or stereotactic radiosurgery. The optimal treatment will depend on the size of the tumor,

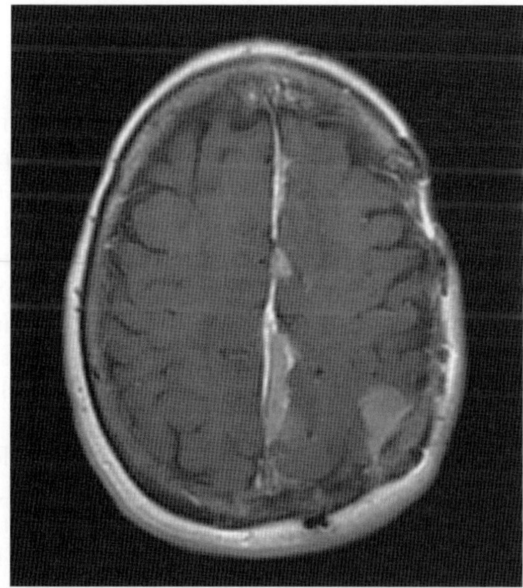

FIGURE 37-6
Postgadolinium T1 MRI demonstrating multiple meningiomas along the falx and left parietal cortex.

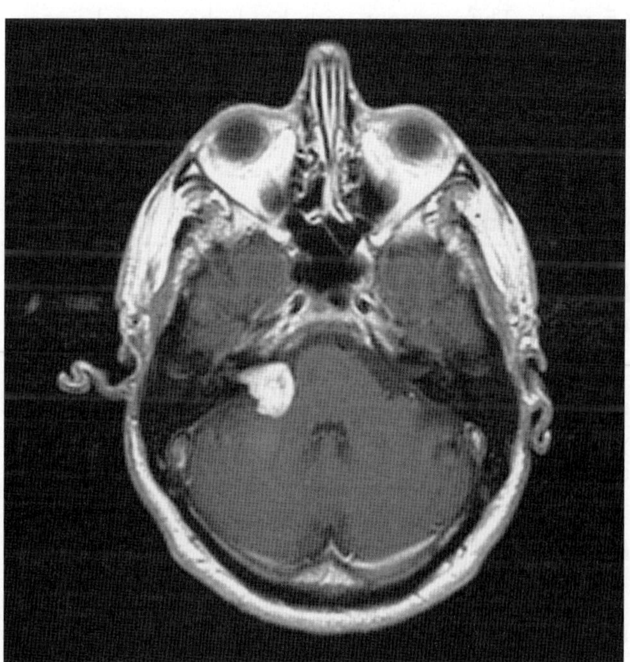

FIGURE 37-7
Postgadolinium MRI of a right vestibular schwannoma. The tumor can be seen to involve the internal auditory canal.

symptoms, and the patient's preference. In patients with small vestibular schwannomas and relatively intact hearing, early surgical intervention increases the chance of preserving hearing.

PITUITARY TUMORS (CHAP. 38)

These account for approximately 9% of primary brain tumors. They can be divided into functioning and nonfunctioning tumors. Functioning tumors are usually microadenomas (<1 cm in diameter) that secrete hormones and produce specific endocrine syndromes (e.g., acromegaly for growth hormone–secreting tumors, Cushing's syndrome for adrenocorticotropic hormone [ACTH]-secreting tumors, and galactorrhea, amenorrhea, and infertility for prolactin-secreting tumors]). Nonfunctioning pituitary tumors tend to be macroadenomas (>1 cm) that produce symptoms by mass effect, giving rise to headaches, visual impairment (such as bitemporal hemianopia), and hypopituitarism. Prolactin-secreting tumors respond well to dopamine agonists such as bromocriptine and cabergoline. Other pituitary tumors usually require treatment with surgery and sometimes radiotherapy or radiosurgery and hormonal therapy.

CRANIOPHARYNGIOMAS

Craniopharyngiomas are rare, usually suprasellar, partially calcified, solid, or mixed solid-cystic benign tumors that arise from remnants of Rathke's pouch. They have a bimodal distribution, occurring predominantly in children but also between the ages of 55 and 65 years. They present with headaches, visual impairment, and impaired growth in children and hypopituitarism in adults. Treatment involves surgery, radiotherapy, or the combination of the two.

OTHER BENIGN TUMORS

Dysembryoplastic neuroepithelial tumors (DNTs)

These are benign, supratentorial tumors, usually in the temporal lobes. They typically occur in children and young adults with a long-standing history of seizures. If the seizures are refractory, surgical resection is curative.

Epidermoid cysts

These consist of squamous epithelium surrounding a keratin-filled cyst. They are usually found in the cerebellopontine angle and the intrasellar and suprasellar regions. They may present with headaches, cranial nerve abnormalities, seizures, or hydrocephalus. Imaging studies demonstrate extraaxial lesions with characteristics that are similar to CSF but have restricted diffusion. Treatment involves surgical resection.

Dermoid cysts

Like epidermoid cysts, dermoid cysts arise from epithelial cells that are retained during closure of the neural tube. They contain both epidermal and dermal structures such as hair follicles, sweat glands, and sebaceous glands. Unlike epidermoid cysts, these tumors usually have a midline location. They occur most frequently in the posterior fossa, especially the vermis, fourth ventricle, and suprasellar cistern. Radiographically, dermoid cysts resemble lipomas, demonstrating T1 hyperintensity and variable signal on T2. Symptomatic dermoid cysts can be treated with surgery.

Colloid cysts

These usually arise in the anterior third ventricle and may present with headaches, hydrocephalus, and very rarely sudden death. Surgical resection is curative or a third ventriculostomy may relieve the obstructive hydrocephalus and be sufficient therapy.

NEUROCUTANEOUS SYNDROMES (PHAKOMATOSES)

A number of genetic disorders are characterized by cutaneous lesions and an increased risk of brain tumors. Most of these disorders have an autosomal dominance inheritance with variable penetrance.

NEUROFIBROMATOSIS TYPE 1 (NF1) (VON RECKLINGHAUSEN'S DISEASE)

NF1 is an autosomal dominant disorder with an incidence of approximately 1 in 2600–3000. Approximately half the cases are familial; the remainder are new mutations arising in patients with unaffected parents. The NF1 gene on chromosome 17q11.2 encodes a protein, *neurofibromin*, a guanosine triphosphatase (GTPase)-activating protein (GAP) that modulates signaling through the ras pathway. Mutations of the NF1 gene result in a large number of nervous system tumors including neurofibromas, plexiform neurofibromas, optic nerve gliomas, astrocytomas, and meningiomas. In addition to neurofibromas, which appear as multiple, soft, rubbery cutaneous tumors, other cutaneous manifestations of NF1 include café au lait spots and axillary freckling. NF1 is also associated with hamartomas of the iris termed Lisch nodules, pheochromocytomas, pseudoarthrosis of the tibia, scoliosis, epilepsy, and mental retardation.

NEUROFIBROMATOSIS TYPE 2 (NF2)

NF2 is less common than NF1, with an incidence of 1 in 25,000–40,000. It is an autosomal dominant disorder with full penetrance. As with NF1, approximately half the cases arise from new mutations. The NF2 gene on 22q encodes a cytoskeletal protein "merlin" (moesin, ezrin, radixin-like protein) that functions as a tumor suppressor. NF2 is characterized by bilateral vestibular schwannomas in over 90% of patients, multiple meningiomas, and spinal ependymomas and astrocytomas. Treatment of bilateral vestibular schwannomas can be challenging because the goal is to preserve hearing for as long as possible. These patients may also have posterior subcapsular lens opacities and retinal hamartomas.

TUBEROUS SCLEROSIS (BOURNEVILLE'S DISEASE)

This is an autosomal dominant disorder with an incidence of approximately 1 in 5000 to 10,000 live births. It is caused by mutations in either the TSC1 gene, which maps to chromosome 9q34, and encodes a protein termed *hamartin*, or mutations in the TSC2 gene, which maps to chromosome 16p13.3 and encodes the tuberin protein. Hamartin forms a complex with tuberin, which inhibits cellular signaling through the mammalian target of rapamycin (mTOR), and acts as a negative regulator of the cell cycle. Patients with tuberous sclerosis have seizures, mental retardation, adenoma sebaceum (facial angiofibromas), shagreen patch, hypomelanotic macules, periungual fibromas, renal angiomyolipomas, and cardiac rhabdomyomas. These patients have an increased incidence of subependymal nodules, cortical tubers, and subependymal giant cell astrocytomas (SEGA). Patients frequently require anticonvulsants for seizures. SEGAs often do not need treatment but occasionally require surgical resection. There is emerging evidence that mTOR inhibitors may have activity in SEGAs.

TUMORS METASTATIC TO THE BRAIN

Brain metastases arise from hematogenous spread and frequently arise from either a lung primary or are associated with pulmonary metastases. Most metastases develop at the gray matter–white matter junction in the watershed distribution of the brain where intravascular tumor cells lodge in terminal arterioles. The distribution of metastases in the brain approximates the proportion of blood flow such that about 85% of all metastases are supratentorial and 15% occur in the posterior fossa. The most common sources of brain metastases are lung and breast carcinomas; melanoma has the greatest propensity to metastasize to the brain, being found in 80% of patients at autopsy (Table 37-3). Other tumor types such as ovarian and esophageal carcinoma rarely metastasize to the brain. Prostate and breast cancer also have a propensity to metastasize to the dura and can mimic meningioma. Leptomeningeal metastases are common from hematologic malignancies and also breast and lung cancers. Spinal cord compression primarily arises in patients with prostate and breast cancer, tumors with a strong propensity to metastasize to the axial skeleton.

TABLE 37-3

FREQUENCY OF NERVOUS SYSTEM METASTASES BY COMMON PRIMARY TUMORS

	BRAIN %	LM %	ESCC %
Lung	41	17	15
Breast	19	57	22
Melanoma	10	12	4
Prostate	1	1	10
GIT	7	—	5
Renal	3	2	7
Lymphoma	<1	10	10
Sarcoma	7	1	9
Other	11	—	18

Abbreviations: ESCC, epidural spinal cord compression; GIT, gastrointestinal tract; LM, leptomeningeal metastases.

DIAGNOSIS OF METASTASES

Brain metastases are best visualized on MRI, where they usually appear as well-circumscribed lesions (Fig. 37-8). The amount of perilesional edema can be highly variable with large lesions causing minimal edema and sometimes very small lesions causing extensive edema. Enhancement may be in a ring pattern or diffuse. Occasionally, intracranial metastases will hemorrhage; although melanoma, thyroid, and kidney cancer have the greatest propensity to hemorrhage, the most common cause of a hemorrhagic metastasis is lung cancer because it accounts for the majority of brain metastases. The radiographic appearance of brain metastasis is nonspecific, and similar appearing lesions can occur with infection including brain abscesses and also with demyelinating lesions, sarcoidosis, radiation necrosis in a previously treated patient, or a primary brain tumor that may be a second malignancy in a patient with systemic cancer. However, biopsy is rarely necessary for diagnosis in most patients because imaging alone in the appropriate clinical situation usually suffices. This is straightforward for the majority

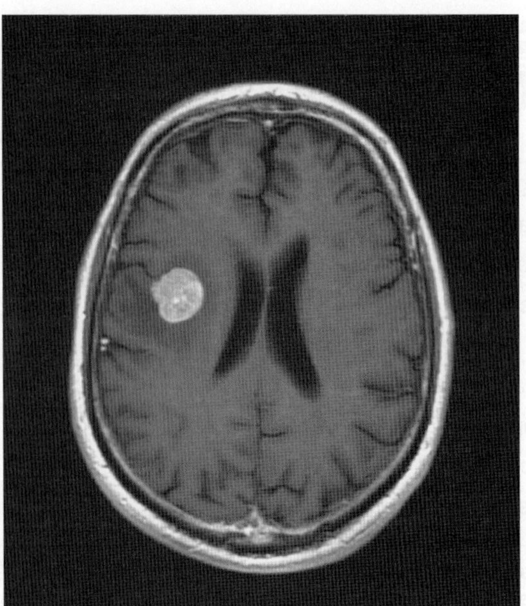

A

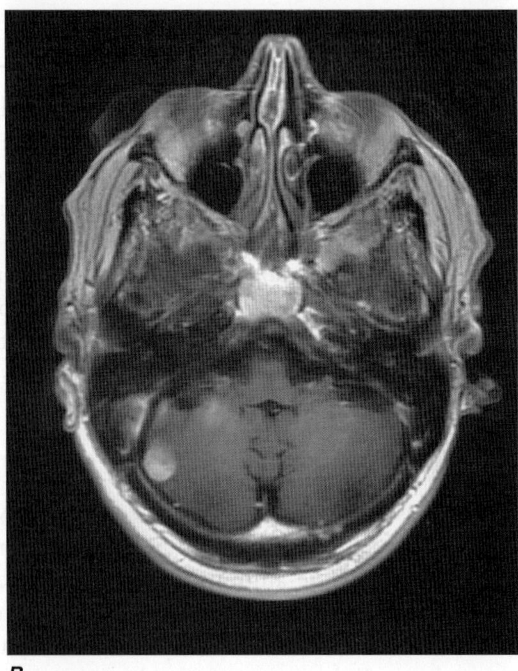

B

FIGURE 37-8

Postgadolinium T1 MRI of multiple brain metastases from non-small cell lung cancer involving the right frontal (***A***) and right cerebellar (***B***) hemispheres. Note the diffuse enhancement pattern and absence of central necrosis.

of patients with brain metastases because they have a known systemic cancer. However, in approximately 10% of patients a systemic cancer may present with a brain metastasis, and if there is not an easily accessible systemic site to biopsy, then a brain lesion must be removed for diagnostic purposes.

TREATMENT Tumors Metastatic to the Brain

DEFINITIVE TREATMENT The number and location of brain metastases often determine the therapeutic options. The patient's overall condition and the current or potential control of the systemic disease are also major determinants. Brain metastases are single in approximately one-half of patients and multiple in the other half.

RADIATION THERAPY The standard treatment for brain metastases has been whole-brain radiotherapy (WBRT) usually administered to a total dose of 3000 cGy in 10 fractions. This affords rapid palliation, and approximately 80% of patients improve with glucocorticoids and radiation therapy. However, it is not curative. Median survival is only 4–6 months. More recently, stereotactic radiosurgery (SRS) delivered through a variety of techniques including the gamma knife, linear accelerator, proton beam, and CyberKnife all can deliver highly focused doses of RT, usually in a single fraction. SRS can effectively sterilize the visible lesions and afford local disease control in 80–90% of patients. In addition, there are some patients who have clearly been cured of their brain metastases using SRS, whereas this is distinctly rare with WBRT. However, SRS can be used only for lesions 3 cm or less in diameter and should be confined to patients with only 1–3 metastases. The addition of WBRT to SRS improves disease control in the nervous system but does not prolong survival.

SURGERY Randomized controlled trials have demonstrated that surgical extirpation of a single brain metastasis followed by WBRT is superior to WBRT alone. Removal of two lesions or a single symptomatic mass, particularly if compressing the ventricular system, can also be useful. This is particularly useful in patients who have highly radioresistant lesions such as renal carcinoma. Surgical resection can afford rapid symptomatic improvement and prolonged survival. RT administered after complete resection of a brain metastasis improves disease control but does not prolong survival.

CHEMOTHERAPY Chemotherapy is rarely useful for brain metastases. Metastases from certain tumor types that are highly chemosensitive, such as germ cell tumors or small cell lung cancer, may respond to chemotherapeutic regimens chosen according to the underlying malignancy. Increasingly, there are data demonstrating responsiveness of brain metastases to chemotherapy including small molecule–targeted therapy when the lesion possesses the target. This has been best illustrated in patients with lung cancer harboring EGFR mutations that sensitize them to EGFR inhibitors. Antiangiogenic agents such as bevacizumab may also prove efficacious in the treatment of CNS metastases.

LEPTOMENINGEAL METASTASES

Leptomeningeal metastases are also identified as carcinomatous meningitis, meningeal carcinomatosis, or in the case of specific tumors, leukemic or lymphomatous meningitis. Among the hematologic malignancies, acute leukemia is the most common to metastasize to the subarachnoid space, and in lymphomas the aggressive diffuse lymphomas can metastasize to the subarachnoid space frequently as well. Among solid tumors, breast and lung carcinomas and melanoma most frequently spread in this fashion. Tumor cells reach the subarachnoid space via the arterial circulation or occasionally through retrograde flow in venous systems that drain metastases along the bony spine or cranium. In addition, leptomeningeal metastases may develop as a direct consequence of prior brain metastases and can develop in almost 40% of patients who have a metastasis resected from the cerebellum.

CLINICAL FEATURES

Leptomeningeal metastases are characterized clinically by multilevel symptoms and signs along the neuraxis. Combinations of lumbar and cervical radiculopathies, cranial neuropathies, seizures, confusion, and encephalopathy from hydrocephalus or raised intracranial pressure can be present. Focal deficits such as hemiparesis or aphasia are rarely due to leptomeningeal metastases unless there is direct brain infiltration and are more often associated with coexisting brain lesions. New onset limb pain in patients with breast, lung cancer, or melanoma should prompt consideration of leptomeningeal spread.

LABORATORY AND IMAGING DIAGNOSIS

Leptomeningeal metastases are particularly challenging to diagnose as identification of tumor cells in the subarachnoid compartment may be elusive. MR imaging can be definitive in patients when there are clear tumor nodules adherent to the cauda equina or spinal cord, enhancing cranial nerves, or subarachnoid enhancement on brain imaging (Fig. 37-9). Imaging is diagnostic in approximately 75% of patients and is more often positive in patients with solid tumors. Demonstration of tumor cells in the CSF is definitive and often considered the gold standard. However, CSF cytologic examination is positive in only 50% of patients on the first lumbar puncture and still misses 10% after three CSF samples. CSF cytologic examination is most useful in hematologic malignancies. Accompanying CSF abnormalities include an elevated protein concentration and an elevated white count. Hypoglycorrhachia is noted in less than 25% of patients

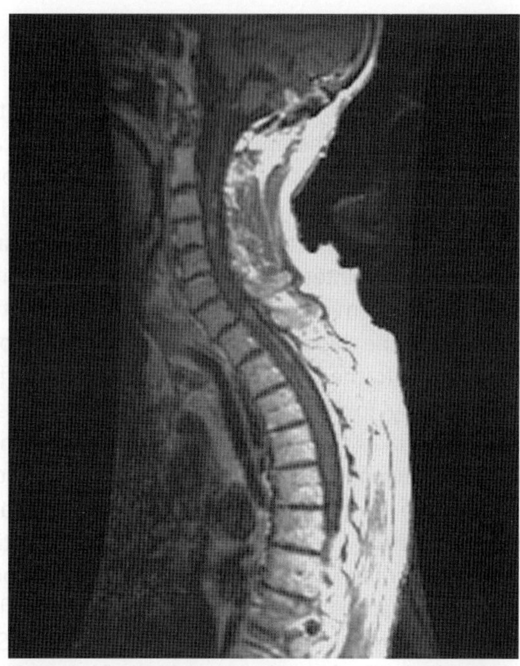

A

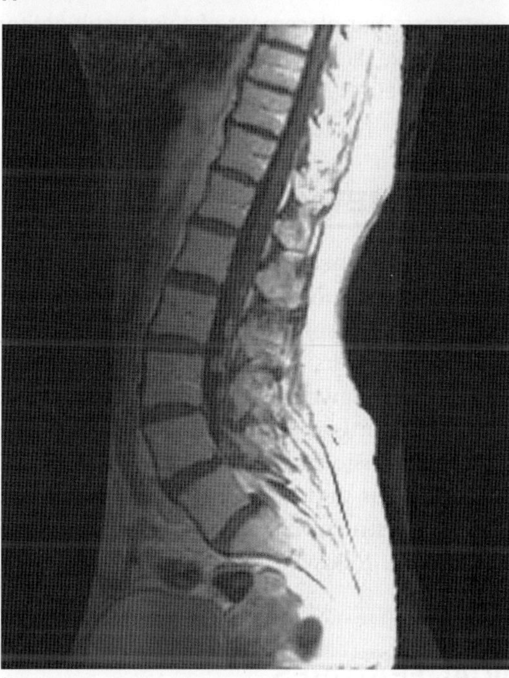

B

FIGURE 37-9
Postgadolinium MRI images of extensive leptomeningeal metastases from breast cancer. Nodules along the dorsal surface of the spinal cord (***A***) and cauda equina (***B***) are seen.

but is useful when present. Identification of tumor markers or molecular confirmation of clonal proliferation with techniques such as flow cytometry within the CSF can also be definitive when present. Tumor markers are usually specific to solid tumors, and chromosomal or molecular markers are most useful in patients with hematologic malignancies.

TREATMENT Leptomeningeal Metastases

The treatment of leptomeningeal metastasis is palliative as there is no curative therapy. RT to the symptomatically involved areas, such as skull base for cranial neuropathy, can relieve pain and sometimes improve function. Whole neuraxis RT has extensive toxicity with myelosuppression and gastrointestinal irritation as well as limited effectiveness. Systemic chemotherapy with agents that can penetrate the blood-CSF barrier may be helpful. Alternatively, intrathecal chemotherapy can be effective, particularly in hematologic malignancies. This is optimally delivered through an intraventricular cannula (Ommaya reservoir) rather than by lumbar puncture. Few drugs can be delivered safely into the subarachnoid space and they have a limited spectrum of antitumor activity, perhaps accounting for the relatively poor response to this approach. In addition, impaired CSF flow dynamics can compromise intrathecal drug delivery. Surgery has a limited role in the treatment of leptomeningeal metastasis, but placement of a ventriculoperitoneal shunt can relieve raised intracranial pressure. However, it compromises delivery of chemotherapy into the CSF.

EPIDURAL METASTASIS

Epidural metastasis occurs in 3–5% of patients with a systemic malignancy and causes neurologic compromise by compressing the spinal cord or cauda equina. The most common cancers that metastasize to the epidural space are those malignancies that spread to bone, such as breast and prostate. Lymphoma can cause bone involvement and compression but it can also invade the intervertebral foramens and cause spinal cord compression without bone destruction. The thoracic spine is affected most commonly, followed by the lumbar and then cervical spine.

CLINICAL FEATURES

Back pain is the presenting symptom of epidural metastasis in virtually all patients; the pain may precede neurologic findings by weeks or months. The pain is usually exacerbated by lying down; by contrast, arthritic pain is often relieved by recumbency. Leg weakness is seen in about 50% of patients as is sensory dysfunction. Sphincter problems are present in about 25% of patients at diagnosis.

DIAGNOSIS

Diagnosis is established by imaging, with MRI of the complete spine being the best test (Fig. 37-10). Contrast is not needed to identify spinal or epidural lesions.

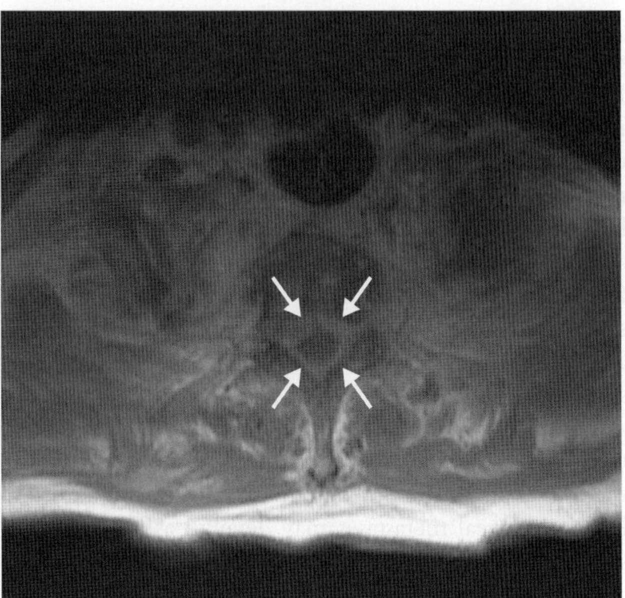

FIGURE 37-10
Postgadolinium T1 MRI showing circumferential epidural tumor around the thoracic spinal cord from esophageal cancer.

Any patient with cancer who has severe back pain should undergo an MRI. Plain films, bone scans, or even CT scans may show bone metastases, but only MRI can reliably delineate epidural tumor. For patients unable to have an MRI, CT myelography should be performed to outline the epidural space. The differential diagnosis of epidural tumor includes epidural abscess, acute or chronic hematomas, and rarely, extramedullary hematopoiesis.

TREATMENT Epidural Metastasis

Epidural metastasis requires immediate treatment. A randomized controlled trial demonstrated the superiority of surgical resection followed by RT compared to RT alone. However, patients must be able to tolerate surgery, and the surgical procedure of choice is a complete removal of the mass, which is typically anterior to the spinal canal, necessitating an extensive approach and resection. Otherwise, RT is the mainstay of treatment and can be used for patients with radiosensitive tumors, such as lymphoma, or for those unable to undergo surgery. Chemotherapy is rarely used for epidural metastasis unless the patient has minimal to no neurologic deficit and a highly chemosensitive tumor such as lymphoma or germinoma. Patients generally fare well if treated before there is severe neurologic deficit. Recovery after paraparesis is better after surgery than with RT alone, but survival is often short due to widespread metastatic tumor.

NEUROLOGIC TOXICITY OF THERAPY

TOXICITY FROM RADIOTHERAPY

Radiotherapy can cause a variety of toxicities in the CNS. These are usually described based on their relationship in time to the administration of RT, e.g., they can be acute (occurring within days of RT), early delayed (months), or late delayed (years). In general, the acute and early delayed syndromes resolve and do not result in persistent deficits, whereas the late delayed toxicities are usually permanent and sometimes progressive.

Acute toxicity

Acute cerebral toxicity usually occurs during RT to the brain. RT can cause a transient disruption of the blood-brain barrier, resulting in increased edema and elevated intracranial pressure. This is usually manifest as headache, lethargy, nausea and vomiting, and can be both prevented and treated with the administration of glucocorticoids. There is no acute RT toxicity that affects the spinal cord.

Early delayed toxicity

Early delayed toxicity is usually apparent weeks to months after completion of cranial irradiation and is likely due to focal demyelination. Clinically it may be asymptomatic or take the form of worsening or reappearance of a preexisting neurologic deficit. At times a contrast-enhancing lesion can be seen on MRI/CT that can mimic the tumor for which the patient received the RT. For patients with a malignant glioma, this has been described as "pseudoprogression" because it mimics tumor recurrence on MRI but actually represents inflammation and necrotic debris engendered by effective therapy. This is seen with increased frequency when chemotherapy, particularly temozolomide, is given concurrently with RT. Pseudoprogression can resolve on its own or, if very symptomatic, may require resection. A rare form of early delayed toxicity is the somnolence syndrome that occurs primarily in children and is characterized by marked sleepiness.

In the spinal cord, early delayed RT toxicity is manifest as a Lhermitte symptom with paresthesias of the limbs or along the spine when the patient flexes the neck. Although frightening, it is benign, resolves on its own, and does not portend more serious problems.

Late delayed toxicity

Late delayed toxicities are the most serious as they are often irreversible and cause severe neurologic deficits. In the brain, late toxicities can take several forms, the most common of which include radiation necrosis and leukoencephalopathy. Radiation necrosis is a focal mass of necrotic tissue that is contrast enhancing on CT/MRI and may be associated with significant edema. This may appear identical to pseudoprogression but is seen months to years after RT and is always symptomatic. Clinical symptoms and signs include seizure and lateralizing findings referable to the location of the necrotic mass. The necrosis is caused by the effect of RT on cerebral vasculature with resultant fibrinoid necrosis and occlusion of the blood vessels. It can mimic tumor radiographically, but unlike tumor it is typically hypometabolic on a PET scan and has reduced perfusion on perfusion MR sequences. It may require resection for diagnosis and treatment unless it can be managed with glucocorticoids. There are rare reports of improvement with hyperbaric oxygen or anticoagulation but the usefulness of these approaches is questionable.

Leukoencephalopathy is seen most commonly after WBRT as opposed to focal RT. On T2 or FLAIR MR sequences there is diffuse increased signal seen throughout the hemispheric white matter, often bilaterally and symmetrically. There tends to be a periventricular predominance that may be associated with atrophy and ventricular enlargement. Clinically, patients develop cognitive impairment, gait disorder, and later urinary incontinence, all of which can progress over time. These symptoms mimic those of normal pressure hydrocephalus, and placement of a ventriculoperitoneal shunt can improve function in some patients but does not reverse the deficits completely. Increased age is a risk factor for leukoencephalopathy but not for radiation necrosis. Necrosis appears to depend on an as yet unidentified predisposition.

Other late neurologic toxicities include endocrine dysfunction if the pituitary or hypothalamus was included in the RT port. A radiation-induced neoplasm can occur many years after therapeutic RT for either a prior CNS tumor or a head and neck cancer; accurate diagnosis requires surgical resection or biopsy. In addition, RT causes accelerated atherosclerosis, which can cause stroke either from intracranial vascular disease or carotid plaque from neck irradiation.

The peripheral nervous system is relatively resistant to RT toxicities. Peripheral nerves are rarely affected by RT, but the plexus is more vulnerable. Plexopathy develops more commonly in the brachial distribution than in the lumbosacral distribution. It must be differentiated from tumor progression in the plexus, which is usually accomplished with CT/MR imaging of the area or PET scan demonstrating tumor infiltrating the region. Clinically, tumor progression is usually painful whereas radiation-induced plexopathy is painless. Radiation plexopathy is also more commonly associated with lymphedema of the affected limb. Sensory loss and weakness are seen in both.

TOXICITY FROM CHEMOTHERAPY

Neurotoxicity is second to myelosuppression as the dose-limiting toxicity of chemotherapeutic agents (Table 37-4). Chemotherapy causes peripheral neuropathy from a number of commonly used agents, and the type of neuropathy can differ, depending upon the drug. Vincristine causes paresthesias but little sensory loss and is associated with motor dysfunction, autonomic impairment (frequently ileus), and rarely cranial nerve compromise. Cisplatin causes large fiber sensory loss resulting in sensory ataxia but little cutaneous sensory loss and no weakness. The taxanes also cause a predominately sensory neuropathy. Agents such as bortezomib and thalidomide also cause neuropathy.

Encephalopathy and seizures are common toxicities from chemotherapeutic drugs. Ifosfamide can cause a severe encephalopathy, which is reversible with discontinuation of the drug and the use of methylene blue for severely affected patients. Fludarabine also causes a severe global encephalopathy that may be permanent. Bevacizumab and other anti-VEGF agents can cause posterior reversible encephalopathy syndrome. Cisplatin can cause hearing loss and less frequently vestibular dysfunction.

TABLE 37-4

NEUROLOGIC SIGNS CAUSED BY AGENTS COMMONLY USED IN PATIENTS WITH CANCER

Acute encephalopathy (delirium)	Seizures
Methotrexate (high-dose IV, IT)	Methotrexate
Cisplatin	Etoposide (high-dose)
Vincristine	Cisplatin
Asparaginase	Vincristine
Procarbazine	Asparaginase
5-Flourouracil (± levamisole)	Nitrogen mustard
Cytarabine (high-dose)	Carmustine
Nitrosoureas (high-dose or arterial)	Dacarbazine (intraarterial or high-dose)
Ifosfamide	Busulfan (high-dose)
Etoposide (high-dose)	Myelopathy (intrathecal drugs)
Bevacizumab (PRES)	Methotrexate
Chronic encephalopathy (dementia)	Cytarabine
Methotrexate	Thiotepa
Carmustine	Peripheral neuropathy
Cytarabine	Vinca alkaloids
Fludarabine	Cisplatin
Visual loss	Procarbazine
Tamoxifen	Etoposide
Gallium nitrate	Teniposide
Cisplatin	Cytarabine
Fludarabine	Taxanes
Cerebellar dysfunction/ataxia	Suramin
5-Fluorouracil (± levamisole)	Bortezomib
Cytarabine	
Procarbazine	

Abbreviations: IT, intrathecal; IV, intravenous; PRES, posterior reversible encephalopathy syndrome.

CHAPTER 38

NEUROLOGIC DISORDERS OF THE PITUITARY AND HYPOTHALAMUS

Shlomo Melmed ■ J. Larry Jameson

The anterior pituitary often is referred to as the "master gland" because, together with the hypothalamus, it orchestrates the complex regulatory functions of many other endocrine glands. The anterior pituitary gland produces six major hormones: (1) prolactin (PRL), (2) growth hormone (GH), (3) adrenocorticotropic hormone (ACTH), (4) luteinizing hormone (LH), (5) follicle-stimulating hormone (FSH), and (6) thyroid-stimulating hormone (TSH) (**Table 38-1**). Pituitary hormones are secreted in a pulsatile manner, reflecting stimulation by

TABLE 38-1

ANTERIOR PITUITARY HORMONE EXPRESSION AND REGULATION

CELL	CORTICOTROPE	SOMATOTROPE	LACTOTROPE	THYROTROPE	GONADOTROPE
Tissue-specific transcription factor	T-Pit	Prop-1, Pit-1	Prop-1, Pit-1	Prop-1, Pit-1, TEF	SF-1, DAX-1
Fetal appearance	6 weeks	8 weeks	12 weeks	12 weeks	12 weeks
Hormone	POMC	GH	PRL	TSH	FSH LH
Protein	Polypeptide	Polypeptide	Polypeptide	Glycoprotein α, β subunits	Glycoprotein α, β subunits
Amino acids	266 (ACTH 1–39)	191	199	211	210 204
Stimulators	CRH, AVP, gp-130 cytokines	GHRH, ghrelin	Estrogen, TRH, VIP	TRH	GnRH, activins, estrogen
Inhibitors	Glucocorticoids	Somatostatin, IGF-I	Dopamine	T_3, T_4, dopamine, somatostatin, glucocorticoids	Sex steroids, inhibin
Target gland	Adrenal	Liver, other tissues	Breast, other tissues	Thyroid	Ovary, testis
Trophic effect	Steroid production	IGF-I production, growth induction, insulin antagonism	Milk production	T_4 synthesis and secretion	Sex steroid production, follicle growth, germ cell maturation
Normal range	ACTH, 4–22 pg/L	<0.5 μg/L[a]	M <15; F <20 μg/L	0.1–5 mU/L	M, 5–20 IU/L, F (basal), 5–20 IU/L

[a]Hormone secretion integrated over 24 h.

Abbreviations: M, male; F, female. For other abbreviations, see text.

Source: Adapted from I Shimon, S Melmed, in S Melmed, P Conn (eds): *Endocrinology: Basic and Clinical Principles*. Totowa, NJ, Humana, 2005.

an array of specific hypothalamic releasing factors. Each of these pituitary hormones elicits specific responses in peripheral target tissues. The hormonal products of those peripheral glands, in turn, exert feedback control at the level of the hypothalamus and pituitary to modulate pituitary function (Fig. 38-1). Pituitary tumors cause characteristic hormone-excess syndromes. Hormone deficiency may be inherited or acquired. Fortunately, there are efficacious treatments for the various pituitary hormone-excess and -deficiency syndromes. Nonetheless, these diagnoses are often elusive; this emphasizes the importance of recognizing subtle clinical manifestations and performing the correct laboratory diagnostic tests.

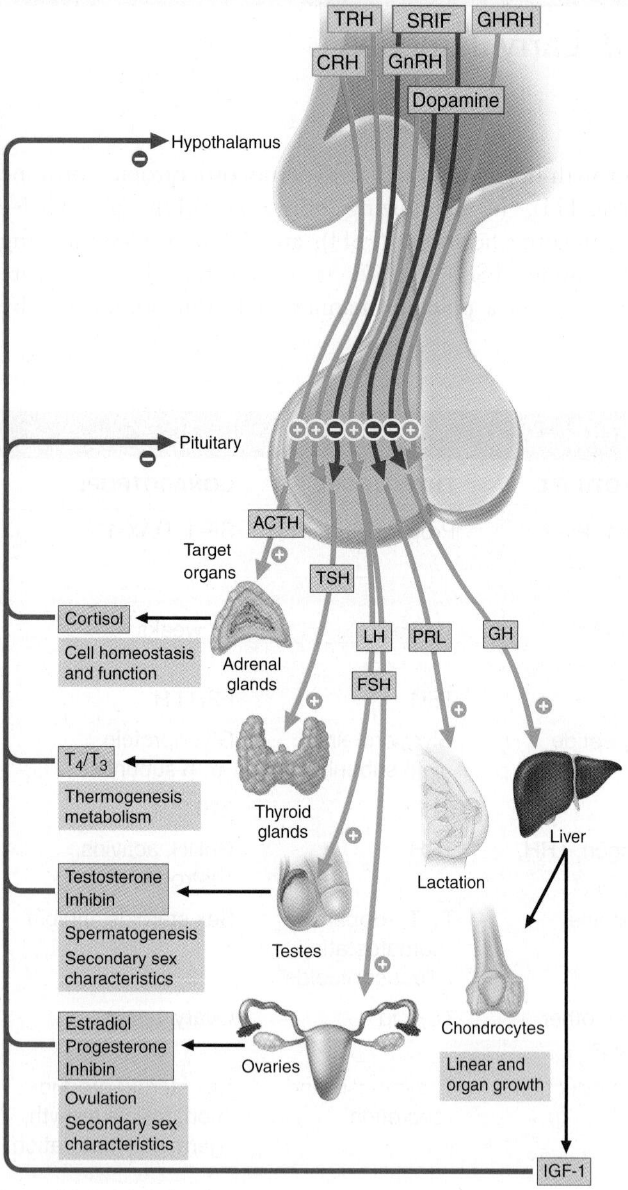

FIGURE 38-1
Diagram of pituitary axes. Hypothalamic hormones regulate anterior pituitary trophic hormones that in turn determine target gland secretion. Peripheral hormones feed back to regulate hypothalamic and pituitary hormones. For abbreviations, see text.

ANATOMY AND DEVELOPMENT

ANATOMY

The pituitary gland weighs ~600 mg and is located within the sella turcica ventral to the diaphragma sella; it consists of anatomically and functionally distinct anterior and posterior lobes. The bony sella is contiguous to vascular and neurologic structures, including the cavernous sinuses, cranial nerves, and optic chiasm. Thus, expanding intrasellar pathologic processes may have significant central mass effects in addition to their endocrinologic impact.

Hypothalamic neural cells synthesize specific releasing and inhibiting hormones that are secreted directly into the portal vessels of the pituitary stalk. Blood supply of the pituitary gland comes from the superior and inferior hypophyseal arteries (Fig. 38-2). The hypothalamic-pituitary portal plexus provides the major blood source for the anterior pituitary, allowing reliable transmission of hypothalamic peptide pulses without significant

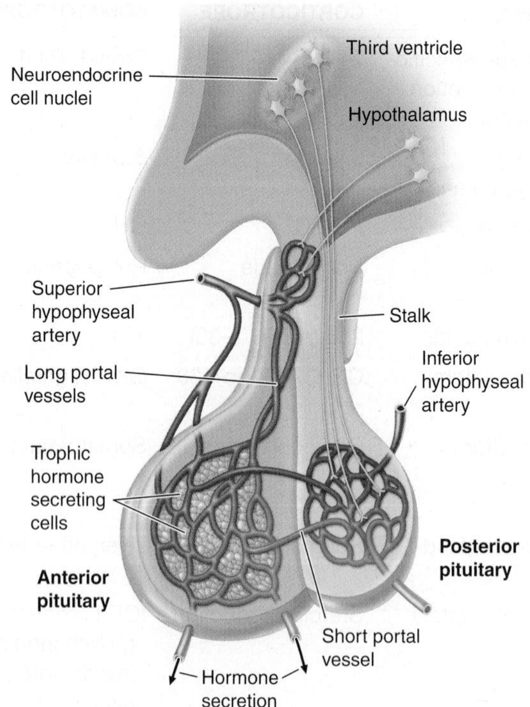

FIGURE 38-2
Diagram of hypothalamic-pituitary vasculature. The hypothalamic nuclei produce hormones that traverse the portal system and impinge on anterior pituitary cells to regulate pituitary hormone secretion. Posterior pituitary hormones are derived from direct neural extensions.

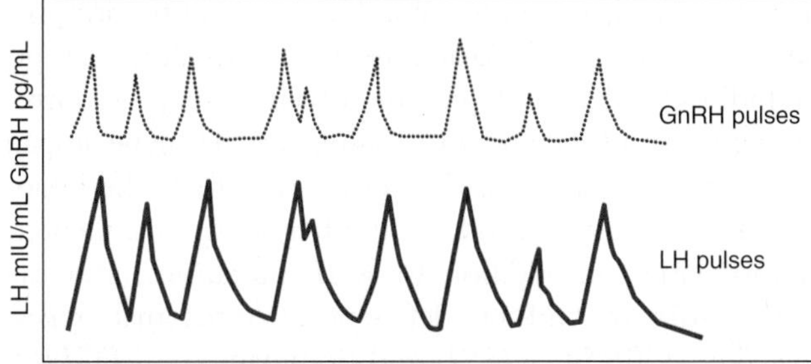

FIGURE 38-3
Hypothalamic gonadotropin-releasing hormone (GnRH) pulses induce secretory pulses of luteinizing hormone (LH).

systemic dilution; consequently, pituitary cells are exposed to releasing or inhibiting factors and in turn release their hormones as discrete pulses (Fig. 38-3).

The posterior pituitary is supplied by the inferior hypophyseal arteries. In contrast to the anterior pituitary, the posterior lobe is directly innervated by hypothalamic neurons (supraopticohypophyseal and tuberohypophyseal nerve tracts) via the pituitary stalk. Thus, posterior pituitary production of vasopressin (antidiuretic hormone [ADH]) and oxytocin is particularly sensitive to neuronal damage by lesions that affect the pituitary stalk or hypothalamus.

PITUITARY DEVELOPMENT

The embryonic differentiation and maturation of anterior pituitary cells have been elucidated in considerable detail. Pituitary development from Rathke's pouch involves a complex interplay of lineage-specific transcription factors expressed in pluripotent precursor cells and gradients of locally produced growth factors (Table 38-1). The transcription factor Prop-1 induces pituitary development of Pit-1-specific lineages as well as gonadotropes. The transcription factor Pit-1 determines cell-specific expression of GH, PRL, and TSH in somatotropes, lactotropes, and thyrotropes. Expression of high levels of estrogen receptors in cells that contain Pit-1 favors PRL expression, whereas thyrotrope embryonic factor (TEF) induces TSH expression. Pit-1 binds to GH, PRL, and TSH gene regulatory elements as well as to recognition sites on its own promoter, providing a mechanism for maintaining specific pituitary phenotypic stability. Gonadotrope cell development is further defined by the cell-specific expression of the nuclear receptors steroidogenic factor (SF-1) and *d*osage-sensitive sex reversal, *a*drenal hypoplasia critical region, on chromosome *X*, gene *1* (DAX-1). Development of corticotrope cells, which express the proopiomelanocortin (POMC) gene, requires the T-Pit transcription factor. Abnormalities of pituitary development caused by mutations of Pit-1, Prop-1, SF-1, DAX-1, and T-Pit result in a series of rare, selective or combined pituitary hormone deficits.

HYPOTHALAMIC AND ANTERIOR PITUITARY INSUFFICIENCY

Hypopituitarism results from impaired production of one or more of the anterior pituitary trophic hormones. Reduced pituitary function can result from inherited disorders; more commonly, hypopituitarism is acquired and reflects the compressive mass effects of tumors or the consequences of inflammation or vascular damage. These processes also may impair synthesis or secretion of hypothalamic hormones, with resultant pituitary failure (Table 38-2).

TABLE 38-2

ETIOLOGY OF HYPOPITUITARISM[a]
Development/structural
Transcription factor defect
Pituitary dysplasia/aplasia
Congenital CNS mass, encephalocele
Primary empty sella
Congenital hypothalamic disorders (septo-optic dysplasia, Prader-Willi syndrome, Laurence-Moon-Biedl syndrome, Kallmann syndrome)
Traumatic
Surgical resection
Radiation damage
Head injuries
Neoplastic
Pituitary adenoma
Parasellar mass (germinoma, ependymoma, glioma)
Rathke's cyst
Craniopharyngioma
Hypothalamic hamartoma, gangliocytoma
Pituitary metastases (breast, lung, colon carcinoma)
Lymphoma and leukemia
Meningioma
Infiltrative/inflammatory
Lymphocytic hypophysitis
Hemochromatosis
Sarcoidosis
Histiocytosis X
Granulomatous hypophysitis
Vascular
Pituitary apoplexy
Pregnancy-related (infarction with diabetes; postpartum necrosis)
Sickle cell disease
Arteritis
Infections
Fungal (histoplasmosis)
Parasitic (toxoplasmosis)
Tuberculosis
Pneumocystis carinii

[a]Trophic hormone failure associated with pituitary compression or destruction usually occurs sequentially: GH > FSH > LH > TSH > ACTH. During childhood, growth retardation is often the presenting feature, and in adults, hypogonadism is the earliest symptom.

DEVELOPMENTAL AND GENETIC CAUSES OF HYPOPITUITARISM

Pituitary dysplasia

Pituitary dysplasia may result in aplastic, hypoplastic, or ectopic pituitary gland development. Because pituitary development follows midline cell migration from the nasopharyngeal Rathke's pouch, midline craniofacial disorders may be associated with pituitary dysplasia. Acquired pituitary failure in the newborn also can be caused by birth trauma, including cranial hemorrhage, asphyxia, and breech delivery.

Septo-optic dysplasia

Hypothalamic dysfunction and hypopituitarism may result from dysgenesis of the septum pellucidum or corpus callosum. Affected children have mutations in the *HESX1* gene, which is involved in early development of the ventral prosencephalon. These children exhibit variable combinations of cleft palate, syndactyly, ear deformities, hypertelorism, optic atrophy, micropenis, and anosmia. Pituitary dysfunction leads to diabetes insipidus, GH deficiency and short stature, and, occasionally, TSH deficiency.

Tissue-specific factor mutations

Several pituitary cell–specific transcription factors, such as Pit-1 and Prop-1, are critical for determining the development and committed function of differentiated anterior pituitary cell lineages. Autosomal dominant or recessive Pit-1 mutations cause combined GH, PRL, and TSH deficiencies. These patients usually present with growth failure and varying degrees of hypothyroidism. The pituitary may appear hypoplastic on MRI.

Prop-1 is expressed early in pituitary development and appears to be required for Pit-1 function. Familial and sporadic *PROP1* mutations result in combined GH, PRL, TSH, and gonadotropin deficiency. Over 80% of these patients have growth retardation; by adulthood, all are deficient in TSH and gonadotropins, and a small minority later develop ACTH deficiency. Because of gonadotropin deficiency, these individuals do not enter puberty spontaneously. In some cases, the pituitary gland is enlarged. *TPIT* mutations result in ACTH deficiency associated with hypocortisolism.

Developmental hypothalamic dysfunction

Kallmann syndrome

Kallmann syndrome results from defective hypothalamic gonadotropin-releasing hormone (GnRH) synthesis and is associated with anosmia or hyposmia due to olfactory bulb agenesis or hypoplasia. The syndrome also may be associated with color blindness, optic atrophy, nerve deafness, cleft palate, renal abnormalities, cryptorchidism, and neurologic abnormalities such as mirror movements. Defects in the X-linked *KAL* gene impair embryonic migration of GnRH neurons from the hypothalamic olfactory placode to the hypothalamus. Genetic abnormalities, in addition to *KAL* mutations, also can cause isolated GnRH deficiency. Autosomal recessive (i.e., *GPR54, KISS1*) and dominant (i.e., *FGFR1*) modes of transmission have been described, and there is a growing list of genes associated with GnRH deficiency (*GNRH1, PROK2, PROKR2, CH7, PCSK1, FGF8, TAC3, TACR3*). GnRH deficiency prevents progression through puberty. Males present with delayed puberty and pronounced hypogonadal features, including micropenis, probably the result of low testosterone levels during infancy. Females present with primary amenorrhea and failure of secondary sexual development.

Kallmann syndrome and other causes of congenital GnRH deficiency are characterized by low LH and FSH levels and low concentrations of sex steroids (testosterone or estradiol). In sporadic cases of isolated gonadotropin deficiency, the diagnosis is often one of exclusion after other causes of hypothalamic-pituitary dysfunction have been eliminated. Repetitive GnRH administration restores normal pituitary gonadotropin responses, pointing to a hypothalamic defect.

Long-term treatment of men with human chorionic gonadotropin (hCG) or testosterone restores pubertal development and secondary sex characteristics; women can be treated with cyclic estrogen and progestin. Fertility also may be restored by the administration of gonadotropins or by using a portable infusion pump to deliver subcutaneous, pulsatile GnRH.

Bardet-Biedl syndrome

This is a rare genetically heterogeneous disorder characterized by mental retardation, renal abnormalities, obesity, and hexadactyly, brachydactyly, or syndactyly. Central diabetes insipidus may or may not be associated. GnRH deficiency occurs in 75% of males and half of affected females. Retinal degeneration begins in early childhood, and most patients are blind by age 30. Numerous subtypes of Bardet-Biedl syndrome (BBS) have been identified, with genetic linkage to at least nine different loci. Several of the loci encode genes involved in basal body cilia function, and this may account for the diverse clinical manifestations.

Leptin and leptin receptor mutations

Deficiencies of leptin or its receptor cause a broad spectrum of hypothalamic abnormalities, including hyperphagia, obesity, and central hypogonadism. Decreased GnRH production in these patients results in attenuated pituitary FSH and LH synthesis and release.

Prader-Willi syndrome

This is a contiguous gene syndrome that results from deletion of the paternal copies of the imprinted *SNRPN* gene, the *NECDIN* gene, and possibly other genes on chromosome 15q. Prader-Willi syndrome is associated with hypogonadotropic hypogonadism, hyperphagia-obesity, chronic muscle hypotonia, mental retardation, and adult-onset diabetes mellitus. Multiple somatic defects also involve the skull, eyes, ears, hands, and feet. Diminished hypothalamic oxytocin- and vasopressin-producing nuclei have been reported. Deficient GnRH synthesis is suggested by the observation that chronic GnRH treatment restores pituitary LH and FSH release.

ACQUIRED HYPOPITUITARISM

Hypopituitarism may be caused by accidental or neurosurgical trauma; vascular events such as apoplexy; pituitary or hypothalamic neoplasms, craniopharyngioma, lymphoma, or metastatic tumors; inflammatory disease such as lymphocytic hypophysitis; infiltrative disorders such as sarcoidosis, hemochromatosis, and tuberculosis; or irradiation.

Increasing evidence suggests that patients with brain injury, including sports trauma, subarachnoid hemorrhage, and irradiation, have transient hypopituitarism and require intermittent long-term endocrine follow-up, as permanent hypothalamic or pituitary dysfunction will develop in 25–40% of these patients.

Hypothalamic infiltration disorders

These disorders—including sarcoidosis, histiocytosis X, amyloidosis, and hemochromatosis—frequently involve both hypothalamic and pituitary neuronal and neurochemical tracts. Consequently, diabetes insipidus occurs in half of patients with these disorders. Growth retardation is seen if attenuated GH secretion occurs before pubertal epiphyseal closure. Hypogonadotropic hypogonadism and hyperprolactinemia are also common.

Inflammatory lesions

Pituitary damage and subsequent dysfunction can be seen with chronic infections such as tuberculosis, with opportunistic fungal infections associated with AIDS, and in tertiary syphilis. Other inflammatory processes, such as granulomas and sarcoidosis, may mimic the features of a pituitary adenoma. These lesions may cause extensive hypothalamic and pituitary damage, leading to trophic hormone deficiencies.

Cranial irradiation

Cranial irradiation may result in long-term hypothalamic and pituitary dysfunction, especially in children and adolescents, as they are more susceptible to damage after whole-brain or head and neck therapeutic irradiation. The development of hormonal abnormalities correlates strongly with irradiation dosage and the time interval after completion of radiotherapy. Up to two-thirds of patients ultimately develop hormone insufficiency after a median dose of 50 Gy (5000 rad) directed at the skull base. The development of hypopituitarism occurs over 5–15 years and usually reflects hypothalamic damage rather than primary destruction of pituitary cells. Although the pattern of hormone loss is variable, GH deficiency is most common, followed by gonadotropin and ACTH deficiency. When deficiency of one or more hormones is documented, the possibility of diminished reserve of other hormones is likely. Accordingly, anterior pituitary function should be continually evaluated over the long term in previously irradiated patients, and replacement therapy instituted when appropriate (discussed later).

Lymphocytic hypophysitis

This occurs most often in postpartum women; it usually presents with hyperprolactinemia and MRI evidence of a prominent pituitary mass that often resembles an adenoma, with mildly elevated PRL levels. Pituitary failure caused by diffuse lymphocytic infiltration may be transient or permanent but requires immediate evaluation and treatment. Rarely, isolated pituitary hormone deficiencies have been described, suggesting a selective autoimmune process targeted to specific cell types. Most patients manifest symptoms of progressive mass effects with headache and visual disturbance. The erythrocyte sedimentation rate often is elevated. As the MRI image may be indistinguishable from that of a pituitary adenoma, hypophysitis should be considered in a postpartum woman with a newly diagnosed pituitary mass before an unnecessary surgical intervention is undertaken. The inflammatory process often resolves after several months of glucocorticoid treatment, and pituitary function may be restored, depending on the extent of damage.

Pituitary apoplexy

Acute intrapituitary hemorrhagic vascular events can cause substantial damage to the pituitary and surrounding sellar structures. Pituitary apoplexy may occur spontaneously in a preexisting adenoma; postpartum (Sheehan's syndrome); or in association with diabetes, hypertension, sickle cell anemia, or acute shock. The hyperplastic enlargement of the pituitary, which occurs normally during pregnancy, increases the risk for hemorrhage and infarction. Apoplexy is an endocrine emergency that may result in severe hypoglycemia, hypotension and shock, central nervous system (CNS) hemorrhage, and death. Acute symptoms may include severe headache with signs of meningeal irritation, bilateral visual changes, ophthalmoplegia, and, in severe cases, cardiovascular collapse and loss of consciousness. Pituitary CT or MRI may reveal signs of intratumoral or sellar hemorrhage, with deviation of the pituitary stalk and compression of pituitary tissue.

Patients with no evident visual loss or impaired consciousness can be observed and managed conservatively with high-dose glucocorticoids. Those with significant or progressive visual loss or loss of consciousness require urgent surgical decompression. Visual recovery after sellar surgery is inversely correlated with the length of time after the acute event. Therefore, severe ophthalmoplegia or visual deficits are indications for early surgery. Hypopituitarism is very common after apoplexy.

Empty sella

A partial or apparently totally empty sella is often an incidental MRI finding. These patients usually have normal pituitary function, implying that the surrounding rim of pituitary tissue is fully functional. Hypopituitarism, however, may develop insidiously. Pituitary masses also may undergo clinically silent infarction and involution with development of a partial or totally empty sella by cerebrospinal fluid (CSF) filling the dural herniation. Rarely, small but functional pituitary adenomas may arise within the rim of pituitary tissue, and they are not always visible on MRI.

PRESENTATION AND DIAGNOSIS

The clinical manifestations of hypopituitarism depend on which hormones are lost and the extent of the hormone deficiency. GH deficiency causes growth disorders in children and leads to abnormal body composition in adults (discussed later). Gonadotropin deficiency causes menstrual disorders and infertility in women and decreased sexual function, infertility, and loss of secondary sexual characteristics in men. TSH and ACTH deficiency usually develop later in the course of pituitary failure. TSH deficiency causes growth retardation in children and features of hypothyroidism in children and adults. The secondary form of adrenal insufficiency caused by ACTH deficiency leads to hypocortisolism with relative preservation of mineralocorticoid production. PRL deficiency causes failure of lactation. When lesions involve the posterior pituitary, polyuria and polydipsia reflect loss of vasopressin secretion. Epidemiologic studies have documented an increased mortality rate in patients with long-standing pituitary damage, primarily from increased cardiovascular and cerebrovascular disease. Previous head or neck irradiation is also a determinant of increased mortality rates in patients with hypopituitarism.

LABORATORY INVESTIGATION

Biochemical diagnosis of pituitary insufficiency is made by demonstrating low levels of trophic hormones in the setting of low levels of target hormones. For example, low free thyroxine in the setting of a low or inappropriately normal TSH level suggests secondary hypothyroidism. Similarly, a low testosterone level without elevation of gonadotropins suggests hypogonadotropic hypogonadism. Provocative tests may be required to assess pituitary reserve (Table 38-3). GH responses to insulin-induced hypoglycemia, arginine, L-dopa, growth hormone–releasing hormone (GHRH), or growth hormone–releasing peptides (GHRPs) can be used to assess GH reserve. Corticotropin-releasing hormone (CRH) administration induces ACTH release, and administration of synthetic ACTH (cosyntropin) evokes adrenal cortisol release as an indirect indicator of pituitary ACTH reserve. ACTH reserve is most reliably assessed by measuring ACTH and cortisol levels during insulin-induced hypoglycemia. However, this test should be performed cautiously in patients with suspected adrenal insufficiency because of enhanced susceptibility to hypoglycemia and hypotension. Administering insulin to induce hypoglycemia is contraindicated in patients with active coronary artery disease or seizure disorders.

TREATMENT Hypopituitarism

Hormone replacement therapy, including glucocorticoids, thyroid hormone, sex steroids, growth hormone, and vasopressin, is usually safe and free of complications. Treatment regimens that mimic physiologic hormone production allow for maintenance of satisfactory clinical homeostasis. Effective dosage schedules are outlined in Table 38-4. Patients in need of glucocorticoid replacement require careful dose adjustments during stressful events such as acute illness, dental procedures, trauma, and acute hospitalization.

HYPOTHALAMIC, PITUITARY, AND OTHER SELLAR MASSES

PITUITARY TUMORS

Pituitary adenomas are the most common cause of pituitary hormone hypersecretion and hyposecretion syndromes in adults. They account for ~15% of all intracranial neoplasms and have been identified with a population prevalence of ~80/100,000. At autopsy, up to one-quarter of all pituitary glands harbor an unsuspected microadenoma (<10 mm diameter). Similarly, pituitary imaging detects small clinically inapparent pituitary lesions in at least 10% of individuals.

TABLE 38-3

TESTS OF PITUITARY SUFFICIENCY

HORMONE	TEST	BLOOD SAMPLES	INTERPRETATION
Growth hormone	Insulin tolerance test: regular insulin (0.05–0.15 U/kg IV)	–30, 0, 30, 60, 120 min for glucose and GH	Glucose <40 mg/dL; GH should be >3 μg/L
	GHRH test: 1 μg/kg IV	0, 15, 30, 45, 60, 120 min for GH	Normal response is GH >3 μg/L
	L-Arginine test: 30 g IV over 30 min	0, 30, 60, 120 min for GH	Normal response is GH >3 μg/L
	L-Dopa test: 500 mg PO	0, 30, 60, 120 min for GH	Normal response is GH >3 μg/L
Prolactin	TRH test: 200–500 μg IV	0, 20, and 60 min for TSH and PRL	Normal prolactin is >2 μg/L and increase >200% of baseline
ACTH	Insulin tolerance test: regular insulin (0.05–0.15 U/kg IV)	–30, 0, 30, 60, 90 min for glucose and cortisol	Glucose <40 mg/dL Cortisol should increase by >7 μg/dL or to >20 μg/dL
	CRH test: 1 μg/kg ovine CRH IV at 8 A.M.	0, 15, 30, 60, 90, 120 min for ACTH and cortisol	Basal ACTH increases 2- to 4-fold and peaks at 20–100 pg/mL Cortisol levels >20–25 μg/dL
	Metyrapone test: metyrapone (30 mg/kg) at midnight	Plasma 11-deoxycortisol and cortisol at 8 A.M.; ACTH can also be measured	Plasma cortisol should be <4 μg/dL to assure an adequate response Normal response is 11-deoxycortisol >7.5 μg/dL or ACTH >75 pg/mL
	Standard ACTH stimulation test: ACTH 1-24 (cosyntropin), 0.25 mg IM or IV	0, 30, 60 min for cortisol and aldosterone	Normal response is cortisol >21 μg/dL and aldosterone response of >4 ng/dL above baseline
	Low-dose ACTH test: ACTH 1-24 (cosyntropin), 1 μg IV	0, 30, 60 min for cortisol	Cortisol should be >21 μg/dL
	3-day ACTH stimulation test consists of 0.25 mg ACTH 1-24 given IV over 8 h each day		Cortisol >21 μg/dL
TSH	Basal thyroid function tests: T_4, T_3, TSH	Basal measurements	Low free thyroid hormone levels in the setting of TSH levels that are not appropriately increased indicate pituitary insufficiency
	TRH test: 200–500 μg IV	0, 20, 60 min for TSH and PRL[a]	TSH should increase by >5 mU/L unless thyroid hormone levels are increased
LH, FSH	LH, FSH, testosterone, estrogen	Basal measurements	Basal LH and FSH should be increased in postmenopausal women Low testosterone levels in the setting of low LH and FSH indicate pituitary insufficiency
	GnRH test: GnRH (100 μg) IV	0, 30, 60 min for LH and FSH	In most adults, LH should increase by 10 IU/L and FSH by 2 IU/L Normal responses are variable
Multiple hormones	Combined anterior pituitary test: GHRH (1 μg/kg), CRH (1 μg/kg), GnRH (100 μg), TRH (200 μg) are given IV	–30, 0, 15, 30, 60, 90, 120 min for GH, ACTH, cortisol, LH, FSH, and TSH	Combined or individual releasing hormone responses must be elevated in the context of basal target gland hormone values and may not be uniformly diagnostic (see text)

[a]Evoked PRL response indicates lactotrope integrity.

Note: For abbreviations, see text.

TABLE 38-4

HORMONE REPLACEMENT THERAPY FOR ADULT HYPOPITUITARISM[a]

TROPHIC HORMONE DEFICIT	HORMONE REPLACEMENT
ACTH	Hydrocortisone (10–20 mg A.M.; 5–10 mg P.M.) Cortisone acetate (25 mg A.M.; 12.5 mg P.M.) Prednisone (5 mg A.M.)
TSH	L-Thyroxine (0.075–0.15 mg daily)
FSH/LH	Males Testosterone enanthate (200 mg IM every 2 weeks) Testosterone skin patch (5 mg/d) Females Conjugated estrogen (0.65–1.25 mg qd for 25 days) Progesterone (5–10 mg qd) on days 16–25 Estradiol skin patch (0.5 mg, every other day) For fertility: Menopausal gonadotropins, human chorionic gonadotropins
GH	Adults: Somatotropin (0.1–1.25 mg SC qd) Children: Somatotropin (0.02–0.05 [mg/kg per day])
Vasopressin	Intranasal desmopressin (5–20 μg twice daily) Oral 300–600 μg qd

[a]All doses shown should be individualized for specific patients and should be reassessed during stress, surgery, or pregnancy.
Note: For abbreviations, see text.

TABLE 38-5

CLASSIFICATION OF PITUITARY ADENOMAS[a]

ADENOMA CELL ORIGIN	HORMONE PRODUCT	CLINICAL SYNDROME
Lactotrope	PRL	Hypogonadism, galactorrhea
Gonadotrope	FSH, LH, subunits	Silent or hypogonadism
Somatotrope	GH	Acromegaly/ gigantism
Corticotrope	ACTH	Cushing's disease
Mixed growth hormone and prolactin cell	GH, PRL	Acromegaly, hypogonadism, galactorrhea
Other plurihormonal cell	Any	Mixed
Acidophil stem cell	PRL, GH	Hypogonadism, galactorrhea, acromegaly
Mammosomatotrope	PRL, GH	Hypogonadism, galactorrhea, acromegaly
Thyrotrope	TSH	Thyrotoxicosis
Null cell	None	Pituitary failure
Oncocytoma	None	Pituitary failure

[a]Hormone-secreting tumors are listed in decreasing order of frequency. All tumors may cause local pressure effects, including visual disturbances, cranial nerve palsy, and headache.
Note: For abbreviations, see text.
Source: Adapted from S Melmed, in JL Jameson (ed): *Principles of Molecular Medicine,* Totowa, NJ, Humana Press, 1998.

Pathogenesis

Pituitary adenomas are benign neoplasms that arise from one of the five anterior pituitary cell types. The clinical and biochemical phenotypes of pituitary adenomas depend on the cell type from which they are derived. Thus, tumors arising from lactotrope (PRL), somatotrope (GH), corticotrope (ACTH), thyrotrope (TSH), or gonadotrope (LH, FSH) cells hypersecrete their respective hormones (Table 38-5). Plurihormonal tumors that express combinations of GH, PRL, TSH, ACTH, and the glycoprotein hormone α or β subunit may be diagnosed by careful immunocytochemistry or may manifest as clinical syndromes that combine features of these hormonal hypersecretory syndromes. Morphologically, these tumors may arise from a single polysecreting cell type or include cells with mixed function within the same tumor.

Hormonally active tumors are characterized by autonomous hormone secretion with diminished feedback responsiveness to physiologic inhibitory pathways. Hormone production does not always correlate with tumor size. Small hormone-secreting adenomas may cause significant clinical perturbations, whereas larger adenomas that produce less hormone may be clinically silent and remain undiagnosed (if no central compressive effects occur). About one-third of all adenomas are clinically nonfunctioning and produce no distinct clinical hypersecretory syndrome. Most of them arise from gonadotrope cells and may secrete small amounts of α- and β-glycoprotein hormone subunits or, very rarely, intact circulating gonadotropins. True pituitary carcinomas with documented extracranial metastases are exceedingly rare.

Almost all pituitary adenomas are monoclonal in origin, implying the acquisition of one or more somatic mutations that confer a selective growth advantage. Consistent with their clonal origin, complete surgical resection of small pituitary adenomas usually cures hormone hypersecretion. Nevertheless, hypothalamic hormones such as GHRH and CRH also enhance mitotic activity of their respective pituitary target cells in addition to their role in pituitary hormone regulation. Thus, patients who harbor rare abdominal or chest tumors that elaborate ectopic GHRH or CRH may present with somatotrope or corticotrope hyperplasia with GH or ACTH hypersecretion.

Several etiologic genetic events have been implicated in the development of pituitary tumors. The pathogenesis of sporadic forms of acromegaly has been particularly informative as a model of tumorigenesis. GHRH, after binding to its G protein–coupled somatotrope receptor, utilizes cyclic AMP (adenosine monophosphate) as a second messenger to stimulate GH secretion and somatotrope proliferation. A subset (~35%) of GH-secreting pituitary tumors contain sporadic mutations in Gsα (Arg 201 → Cys or His; Gln 227 → Arg). These mutations attenuate intrinsic GTPase activity, resulting in constitutive elevation of cyclic AMP, Pit-1 induction, and activation of cyclic AMP response element binding protein (CREB), thereby promoting somatotrope cell proliferation and GH secretion.

Characteristic loss of heterozygosity (LOH) in various chromosomes has been documented in large or invasive macroadenomas, suggesting the presence of putative tumor suppressor genes at these loci. LOH of chromosome regions on 11q13, 13, and 9 is present in up to 20% of sporadic pituitary tumors, including GH-, PRL-, and ACTH-producing adenomas and some nonfunctioning tumors.

Compelling evidence also favors growth factor promotion of pituitary tumor proliferation. Basic fibroblast growth factor (bFGF) is abundant in the pituitary and has been shown to stimulate pituitary cell mitogenesis. Other factors involved in initiation and promotion of pituitary tumors include loss of negative-feedback inhibition (as seen with primary hypothyroidism or hypogonadism) and estrogen-mediated or paracrine angiogenesis. Growth characteristics and neoplastic behavior also may be influenced by several activated oncogenes, including *RAS* and pituitary tumor transforming gene (*PTTG*), or inactivation of growth suppressor genes, including *MEG3*.

Genetic syndromes associated with pituitary tumors

Several familial syndromes are associated with pituitary tumors, and the genetic mechanisms for some of them have been unraveled (Table 38-6).

Multiple endocrine neoplasia (MEN) 1 is an autosomal dominant syndrome characterized primarily by a genetic predisposition to parathyroid, pancreatic islet, and pituitary adenomas. MEN1 is caused by inactivating germline mutations in *MENIN*, a constitutively expressed tumor-suppressor gene located on chromosome 11q13. Loss of heterozygosity, or a somatic mutation of the remaining normal *MENIN* allele, leads to tumorigenesis. About half of affected patients develop prolactinomas; acromegaly and Cushing's syndrome are less commonly encountered.

TABLE 38-6

FAMILIAL PITUITARY TUMOR SYNDROMES

	GENE MUTATED	CLINICAL FEATURES
Multiple endocrine neoplasia 1 (MEN1)	*MEN1* (11q13)	Hyperparathyroidism Pancreatic neuroendocrine tumors Foregut carcinoids Adrenal adenomas Skin lesions Pituitary adenomas (40%)
Multiple endocrine neoplasia 4 (MEN4)	*CDKNIB (12p13)*	Hyperparathyroidsm Pituitary adenomas Other tumors
Carney complex	*PRKAR1A 17q23-24*	Pituitary hyperplasia and adenomas (10%) Atrial myxomas Schwannomas Adrenal hyperplasia Lentigines
Familial pituitary adenomas	*AIP (11q13.3)*	Acromegaly/gigantism (15%)

Carney syndrome is characterized by spotty skin pigmentation, myxomas, and endocrine tumors, including testicular, adrenal, and pituitary adenomas. Acromegaly occurs in about 20% of these patients. A subset of patients have mutations in the R1α regulatory subunit of protein kinase A (*PRKAR1A*).

McCune-Albright syndrome consists of polyostotic fibrous dysplasia, pigmented skin patches, and a variety of endocrine disorders, including acromegaly, adrenal adenomas, and autonomous ovarian function. Hormonal hypersecretion results from constitutive cyclic AMP production caused by inactivation of the GTPase activity of Gsα. The Gsα mutations occur postzygotically, leading to a mosaic pattern of mutant expression.

Familial acromegaly is a rare disorder in which family members may manifest either acromegaly or gigantism. The disorder is associated with LOH at a chromosome 11q13 locus distinct from that of *MENIN*. A subset of families with a predisposition for familial pituitary tumors, especially acromegaly, have been found to harbor inactivating mutations in the *AIP* gene, which encodes the aryl hydrocarbon receptor interacting protein.

OTHER SELLAR MASSES

Craniopharyngiomas are benign, suprasellar cystic masses that present with headaches, visual field deficits, and variable degrees of hypopituitarism. They are derived from Rathke's pouch and arise near the pituitary stalk, commonly extending into the suprasellar cistern. Craniopharyngiomas are often large, cystic, and locally invasive. Many are partially calcified, exhibiting a characteristic appearance on skull x-ray and CT images. More than half of all patients present before age 20, usually with signs of increased intracranial pressure, including headache, vomiting, papilledema, and hydrocephalus. Associated symptoms include visual field abnormalities, personality changes and cognitive deterioration, cranial nerve damage, sleep difficulties, and weight gain. Hypopituitarism can be documented in about 90%, and diabetes insipidus occurs in about 10% of patients. About half of affected children present with growth retardation. MRI is generally superior to CT for evaluating cystic structure and tissue components of craniopharyngiomas. CT is useful to define calcifications and evaluate invasion into surrounding bony structures and sinuses.

Treatment usually involves transcranial or transsphenoidal surgical resection followed by postoperative radiation of residual tumor. Surgery alone is curative in less than half of patients because of recurrences due to adherence to vital structures or because of small tumor deposits in the hypothalamus or brain parenchyma. The goal of surgery is to remove as much tumor as possible without risking complications associated with efforts to remove firmly adherent or inaccessible tissue. In the absence of radiotherapy, about 75% of craniopharyngiomas recur, and 10-year survival is less than 50%. In patients with incomplete resection, radiotherapy improves 10-year survival to 70–90% but is associated with increased risk of secondary malignancies. Most patients require lifelong pituitary hormone replacement.

Developmental failure of Rathke's pouch obliteration may lead to *Rathke's cysts*, which are small (<5 mm) cysts entrapped by squamous epithelium and are found in about 20% of individuals at autopsy. Although Rathke's cleft cysts do not usually grow and are often diagnosed incidentally, about a third present in adulthood with compressive symptoms, diabetes insipidus, and hyperprolactinemia due to stalk compression. Rarely, hydrocephalus develops. The diagnosis is suggested preoperatively by visualizing the cyst wall on MRI, which distinguishes these lesions from craniopharyngiomas. Cyst contents range from CSF-like fluid to mucoid material. *Arachnoid cysts* are rare and generate an MRI image that is isointense with cerebrospinal fluid.

Sella chordomas usually present with bony clival erosion, local invasiveness, and, on occasion, calcification. Normal pituitary tissue may be visible on MRI, distinguishing chordomas from aggressive pituitary adenomas. Mucinous material may be obtained by fine-needle aspiration.

Meningiomas arising in the sellar region may be difficult to distinguish from nonfunctioning pituitary adenomas. Meningiomas typically enhance on MRI and may show evidence of calcification or bony erosion. Meningiomas may cause compressive symptoms.

Histiocytosis X includes a variety of syndromes associated with foci of eosinophilic granulomas. Diabetes insipidus, exophthalmos, and punched-out lytic bone lesions (*Hand-Schüller-Christian disease*) are associated with granulomatous lesions visible on MRI, as well as a characteristic axillary skin rash. Rarely, the pituitary stalk may be involved.

Pituitary metastases occur in ~3% of cancer patients. Bloodborne metastatic deposits are found almost exclusively in the posterior pituitary. Accordingly, diabetes insipidus can be a presenting feature of lung, gastrointestinal, breast, and other pituitary metastases. About half of pituitary metastases originate from breast cancer; about 25% of patients with metastatic breast cancer have such deposits. Rarely, pituitary stalk involvement results in anterior pituitary insufficiency. The MRI diagnosis of a metastatic lesion may be difficult to distinguish from an aggressive pituitary adenoma; the diagnosis may require histologic examination of excised tumor tissue. Primary or metastatic lymphoma, leukemias, and plasmacytomas also occur within the sella.

Hypothalamic hamartomas and *gangliocytomas* may arise from astrocytes, oligodendrocytes, and neurons with varying degrees of differentiation. These tumors may overexpress hypothalamic neuropeptides, including GnRH, GHRH, and CRH. With GnRH-producing tumors, children present with precocious puberty, psychomotor delay, and laughing-associated seizures. Medical treatment of GnRH-producing hamartomas with long-acting GnRH analogues effectively suppresses gonadotropin secretion and controls premature pubertal development. Rarely, hamartomas also are associated with craniofacial abnormalities; imperforate anus; cardiac, renal, and lung disorders; and pituitary failure as features of *Pallister-Hall syndrome*, which is caused by mutations in the carboxy terminus of the *GLI3* gene. Hypothalamic hamartomas are often contiguous with the pituitary, and preoperative MRI diagnosis may not be possible. Histologic evidence of hypothalamic neurons in tissue resected at transsphenoidal surgery may be the first indication of a primary hypothalamic lesion.

Hypothalamic gliomas and *optic gliomas* occur mainly in childhood and usually present with visual loss. Adults have more aggressive tumors; about a third are associated with neurofibromatosis.

Brain germ cell tumors may arise within the sellar region. They include *dysgerminomas*, which frequently are associated with diabetes insipidus and visual loss. They rarely metastasize. *Germinomas, embryonal carcinomas, teratomas*, and *choriocarcinomas* may arise in the parasellar region and produce hCG. These germ cell tumors present with precocious puberty, diabetes insipidus, visual field defects, and thirst disorders. Many patients are GH-deficient with short stature.

METABOLIC EFFECTS OF HYPOTHALAMIC LESIONS

Lesions involving the anterior and preoptic hypothalamic regions cause paradoxical vasoconstriction, tachycardia, and hyperthermia. Acute hyperthermia usually is due to a hemorrhagic insult, but poikilothermia may also occur. Central disorders of thermoregulation result from posterior hypothalamic damage. The *periodic hypothermia syndrome* is characterized by episodic attacks of rectal temperatures <30°C (86°F), sweating, vasodilation, vomiting, and bradycardia. Damage to the ventromedial hypothalamic nuclei by craniopharyngiomas, hypothalamic trauma, or inflammatory disorders may be associated with *hyperphagia* and *obesity*. This region appears to contain an energy-satiety center where melanocortin receptors are influenced by leptin, insulin, POMC products, and gastrointestinal peptides. Polydipsia and hypodipsia are associated with damage to central osmoreceptors located in preoptic nuclei. Slow-growing hypothalamic lesions can cause increased somnolence and disturbed sleep cycles as well as obesity, hypothermia, and emotional outbursts. Lesions of the central hypothalamus may stimulate sympathetic neurons, leading to elevated serum catecholamine and cortisol levels. These patients are predisposed to cardiac arrhythmias, hypertension, and gastric erosions.

TABLE 38-7

FEATURES OF SELLAR MASS LESIONS[a]

IMPACTED STRUCTURE	CLINICAL IMPACT
Pituitary	Hypogonadism Hypothyroidism Growth failure and adult hyposomatotropism Hypoadrenalism
Optic chiasm	Loss of red perception Bitemporal hemianopia Superior or bitemporal field defect Scotoma Blindness
Hypothalamus	Temperature dysregulation Appetite and thirst disorders Obesity Diabetes insipidus Sleep disorders Behavioral dysfunction Autonomic dysfunction
Cavernous sinus	Opthalmoplegia with or without ptosis or diplopia Facial numbness
Frontal lobe	Personality disorder Anosmia
Brain	Headache Hydrocephalus Psychosis Dementia Laughing seizures

[a]As the intrasellar mass expands, it first compresses intrasellar pituitary tissue, then usually invades dorsally through the dura to lift the optic chiasm or laterally to the cavernous sinuses. Bony erosion is rare, as is direct brain compression. Microadenomas may present with headache.

EVALUATION

Local mass effects

Clinical manifestations of sellar lesions vary, depending on the anatomic location of the mass and the direction of its extension (Table 38-7). The dorsal sellar diaphragm presents the least resistance to soft tissue expansion from the sella; consequently, pituitary adenomas frequently extend in a suprasellar direction. Bony invasion may occur as well.

Headaches are common features of small intrasellar tumors, even with no demonstrable suprasellar extension. Because of the confined nature of the pituitary, small changes in intrasellar pressure stretch the dural plate; however, headache severity correlates poorly with adenoma size or extension.

Suprasellar extension can lead to visual loss by several mechanisms, the most common being compression of the optic chiasm, but rarely, direct invasion of the optic nerves or obstruction of CSF flow leading to secondary visual disturbances also occurs. Pituitary stalk compression by a hormonally active or inactive intrasellar mass may compress the portal vessels, disrupting pituitary access to hypothalamic hormones and dopamine; this results in early hyperprolactinemia and later concurrent loss of other pituitary hormones. This "stalk section" phenomenon may also be caused by trauma, whiplash injury with posterior clinoid stalk compression, or skull base fractures. Lateral mass invasion may impinge on the cavernous sinus and compress its neural contents, leading to cranial nerve III, IV, and VI palsies as well as effects on the ophthalmic and maxillary branches of the fifth cranial nerve (Chap. 34). Patients may present with diplopia, ptosis, ophthalmoplegia, and decreased facial sensation, depending on the extent of neural damage. Extension into the sphenoid sinus indicates that the pituitary mass has eroded through the sellar floor. Aggressive tumors rarely invade the palate roof and cause nasopharyngeal obstruction, infection, and

CSF leakage. Temporal and frontal lobe involvement may rarely lead to uncinate seizures, personality disorders, and anosmia. Direct hypothalamic encroachment by an invasive pituitary mass may cause important metabolic sequelae, including precocious puberty or hypogonadism, diabetes insipidus, sleep disturbances, dysthermia, and appetite disorders.

MRI

Sagittal and coronal T1-weighted MRI imaging before and after administration of gadolinium allows precise visualization of the pituitary gland with clear delineation of the hypothalamus, pituitary stalk, pituitary tissue and surrounding suprasellar cisterns, cavernous sinuses, sphenoid sinus, and optic chiasm. Pituitary gland height ranges from 6 mm in children to 8 mm in adults; during pregnancy and puberty, the height may reach 10–12 mm. The upper aspect of the adult pituitary is flat or slightly concave, but in adolescent and pregnant individuals, this surface may be convex, reflecting physiologic pituitary enlargement. The stalk should be midline and vertical. CT scan is reserved to define the extent of bony erosion or the presence of calcification.

Anterior pituitary gland soft tissue consistency is slightly heterogeneous on MRI, and signal intensity resembles that of brain matter on T1-weighted imaging (Fig. 38-4). Adenoma density is usually lower than that of surrounding normal tissue on T1-weighted imaging, and the signal intensity increases with T2-weighted images. The high phospholipid content of the posterior pituitary results in a "pituitary bright spot."

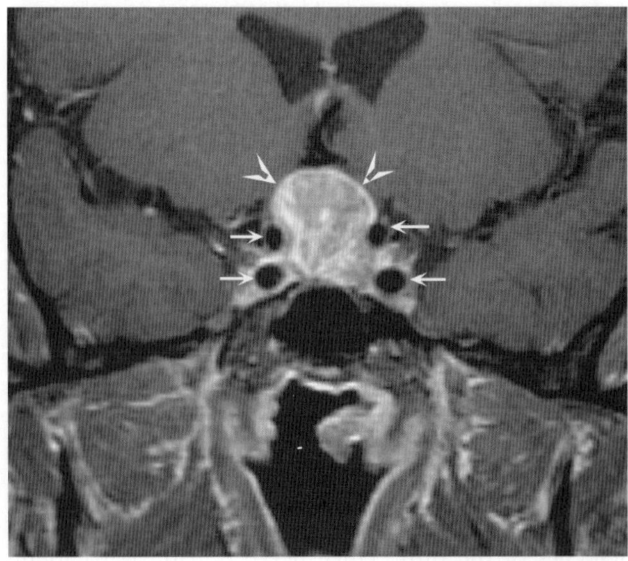

FIGURE 38-4

Pituitary adenoma. Coronal T1-weighted postcontrast MR image shows a homogeneously enhancing mass (*arrowheads*) in the sella turcica and suprasellar region compatible with a pituitary adenoma; the small arrows outline the carotid arteries.

Sellar masses are encountered commonly as incidental findings on MRI, and most of them are pituitary adenomas (incidentalomas). In the absence of hormone hypersecretion, these small intrasellar lesions can be monitored safely with MRI, which is performed annually and then less often if there is no evidence of further growth. Resection should be considered for incidentally discovered macroadenomas, as about one-third become invasive or cause local pressure effects. If hormone hypersecretion is evident, specific therapies are indicated. When larger masses (>1 cm) are encountered, they should also be distinguished from nonadenomatous lesions. Meningiomas often are associated with bony hyperostosis; craniopharyngiomas may be calcified and are usually hypodense, whereas gliomas are hyperdense on T2-weighted images.

Ophthalmologic evaluation

Because optic tracts may be contiguous to an expanding pituitary mass, reproducible visual field assessment using perimetry techniques should be performed on all patients with sellar mass lesions that abut the optic chiasm (Chap. 21). Bitemporal hemianopia or superior bitemporal defects are classically observed, reflecting the location of these tracts within the inferior and posterior part of the chiasm. Homonymous cuts reflect postchiasmal lesions, and monocular field cuts prechiasmal lesions. Loss of red perception is an early sign of optic tract pressure. Early diagnosis reduces the risk of blindness, scotomas, or other visual disturbances.

Laboratory investigation

The presenting clinical features of functional pituitary adenomas (e.g., acromegaly, prolactinomas, or Cushing's syndrome) should guide the laboratory studies (Table 38-8). However, for a sellar mass with no obvious clinical features of hormone excess, laboratory studies are geared toward determining the nature of the tumor and assessing the possible presence of hypopituitarism. When a pituitary adenoma is suspected based on MRI, initial hormonal evaluation usually includes (1) basal PRL; (2) insulin-like growth factor (IGF) I; (3) 24-h urinary free cortisol (UFC) and/or overnight oral dexamethasone (1 mg) suppression test; (4) α subunit, FSH, and LH; and (5) thyroid function tests. Additional hormonal evaluation may be indicated based on the results of these tests. Pending more detailed assessment of hypopituitarism, a menstrual history, measurement of testosterone and 8 A.M. cortisol levels, and thyroid function tests usually identify patients with pituitary hormone deficiencies that require hormone replacement before further testing or surgery.

TABLE 38-8

SCREENING TESTS FOR FUNCTIONAL PITUITARY ADENOMAS

	TEST	COMMENTS
Acromegaly	Serum IGF-I	Interpret IGF-I relative to age- and sex-matched controls
	Oral glucose tolerance test with GH obtained at 0, 30, and 60 min	Normal subjects should suppress growth hormone to <1 μg/L
Prolactinoma	Serum PRL	Exclude medications
		MRI of the sella should be ordered if prolactin is elevated
Cushing's disease	24-h urinary free cortisol	Ensure urine collection is total and accurate
	Dexamethasone (1 mg) at 11 P.M. and fasting plasma cortisol measured at 8 A.M.	Normal subjects suppress to <5 μg/dL
	ACTH assay	Distinguishes adrenal adenoma (ACTH suppressed) from ectopic ACTH or Cushing's disease (ACTH normal or elevated)

Note: For abbreviations, see text.

Histologic evaluation

Immunohistochemical staining of pituitary tumor specimens obtained at transsphenoidal surgery confirms clinical and laboratory studies and provides a histologic diagnosis when hormone studies are equivocal and in cases of clinically nonfunctioning tumors. Occasionally, ultrastructural assessment by electron microscopy is required for diagnosis.

TREATMENT Hypothalamic, Pituitary, and Other Sellar Masses

OVERVIEW Successful management of sellar masses requires accurate diagnosis as well as selection of optimal therapeutic modalities. Most pituitary tumors are benign and slow-growing. Clinical features result from local mass effects and hormonal hypo- or hypersecretion syndromes caused directly by the adenoma or occurring as a consequence of treatment. Thus, lifelong management and follow-up are necessary for these patients.

MRI with gadolinium enhancement for pituitary visualization, new advances in transsphenoidal surgery and in stereotactic radiotherapy (including gamma-knife radiotherapy), and novel therapeutic agents have improved pituitary tumor management. The goals of pituitary tumor treatment include normalization of excess pituitary secretion, amelioration of symptoms and signs of hormonal hypersecretion syndromes, and shrinkage or ablation of large tumor masses with relief of adjacent structure compression. Residual anterior pituitary function should be preserved during treatment and sometimes can be restored by removing the tumor mass. Ideally, adenoma recurrence should be prevented.

TRANSSPHENOIDAL SURGERY Transsphenoidal rather than transfrontal resection is the desired surgical approach for pituitary tumors, except for the rare invasive suprasellar mass surrounding the frontal or middle fossa or the optic nerves or invading posteriorly behind the clivus. Intraoperative microscopy facilitates visual distinction between adenomatous and normal pituitary tissue as well as microdissection of small tumors that may not be visible by MRI (Fig. 38-5). Transsphenoidal surgery also avoids the cranial invasion and manipulation of brain tissue required by subfrontal surgical approaches. Endoscopic techniques with three-dimensional intraoperative localization have also improved visualization and access to tumor tissue.

In addition to correction of hormonal hypersecretion, pituitary surgery is indicated for mass lesions that impinge on surrounding structures. Surgical decompression and resection are required for an expanding pituitary mass accompanied by persistent headache, progressive visual field defects, cranial nerve palsies, hydrocephalus, and, occasionally, intrapituitary hemorrhage and apoplexy. Transsphenoidal surgery sometimes is used for pituitary tissue biopsy to establish a histologic diagnosis.

Whenever possible, the pituitary mass lesion should be selectively excised; normal pituitary tissue should be manipulated or resected only when critical for effective mass dissection. Nonselective hemihypophysectomy or total hypophysectomy may be indicated if no hypersecreting mass lesion is clearly discernible, multifocal lesions are present, or the remaining nontumorous pituitary tissue is obviously necrotic. This strategy, however, increases the likelihood of hypopituitarism and the need for lifelong hormone replacement.

Preoperative mass effects, including visual field defects and compromised pituitary function, may be reversed by surgery, particularly when the deficits are not long-standing. For large and invasive tumors, it is

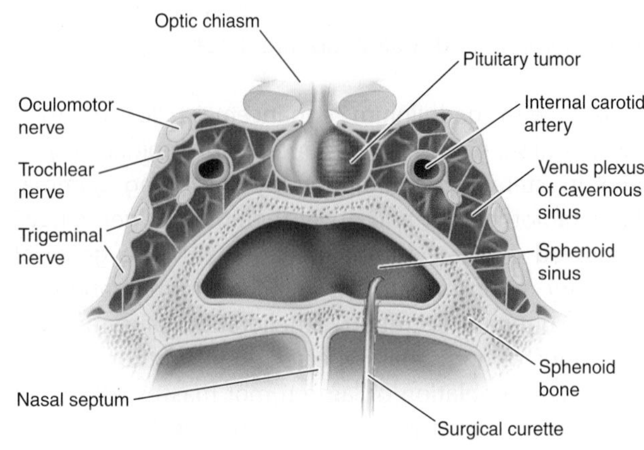

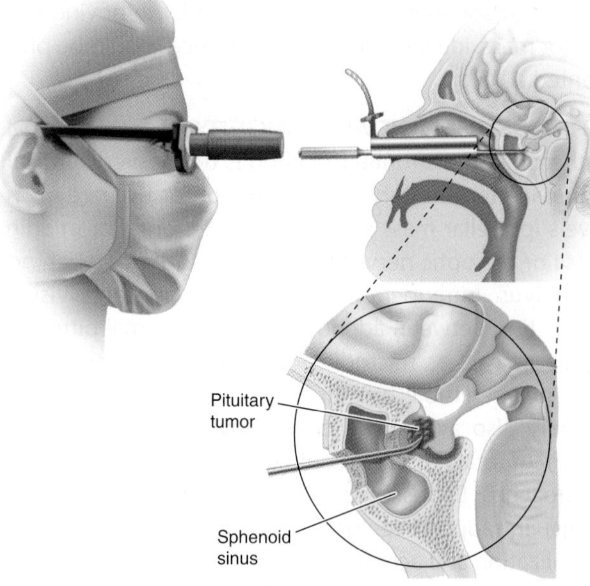

FIGURE 38-5

Transsphenoidal resection of pituitary mass via the endonasal approach. (*Adapted from R Fahlbusch: Endocrinol Metab Clin 21:669, 1992.*)

necessary to determine the optimal balance between maximal tumor resection and preservation of anterior pituitary function, especially for preserving growth and reproductive function in younger patients. Similarly, tumor invasion outside the sella is rarely amenable to surgical cure; the surgeon must judge the risk-versus-benefit ratio of extensive tumor resection.

Side Effects Tumor size, the degree of invasiveness, and experience of the surgeon largely determine the incidence of surgical complications. Operative mortality rate is about 1%. Transient diabetes insipidus and hypopituitarism occur in up to 20% of patients. Permanent diabetes insipidus, cranial nerve damage, nasal septal perforation, or visual disturbances may be encountered in up to 10% of patients. CSF leaks occur in 4% of patients. Less common complications include carotid artery injury, loss of vision, hypothalamic damage, and meningitis. Permanent side effects are rare after surgery for microadenomas.

RADIATION Radiation is used either as a primary therapy for pituitary or parasellar masses or, more commonly, as an adjunct to surgery or medical therapy. Focused megavoltage irradiation is achieved by precise MRI localization, using a high-voltage linear accelerator and accurate isocentric rotational arcing. A major determinant of accurate irradiation is reproduction of the patient's head position during multiple visits and maintenance of absolute head immobility. A total of <50 Gy (5000 rad) is given as 180-cGy (180-rad) fractions divided over about 6 weeks. Stereotactic radiosurgery delivers a large single high-energy dose from a cobalt 60 source (gamma knife), linear accelerator, or cyclotron. Long-term effects of gamma-knife surgery are unclear but appear to be similar to those encountered with conventional radiation.

The role of radiation therapy in pituitary tumor management depends on multiple factors, including the nature of the tumor, the age of the patient, and the availability of surgical and radiation expertise. Because of its relatively slow onset of action, radiation therapy is usually reserved for postsurgical management. As an adjuvant to surgery, radiation is used to treat residual tumor and in an attempt to prevent regrowth. Irradiation offers the only means for potentially ablating significant postoperative residual nonfunctioning tumor tissue. In contrast, PRL- and GH-secreting tumor tissues are amenable to medical therapy.

Side Effects In the short term, radiation may cause transient nausea and weakness. Alopecia and loss of taste and smell may be more long-lasting. Failure of pituitary hormone synthesis is common in patients who have undergone head and neck or pituitary-directed irradiation. More than 50% of patients develop loss of GH, ACTH, TSH, and/or gonadotropin secretion within 10 years, usually due to hypothalamic damage. Lifelong follow-up with testing of anterior pituitary hormone reserve is therefore required after radiation treatment. Optic nerve damage with impaired vision due to optic neuritis is reported in about 2% of patients who undergo pituitary irradiation. Cranial nerve damage is uncommon now that radiation doses are ≤2 Gy (200 rad) at any one treatment session and the maximum dose is <50 Gy (5000 rad). The use of stereotactic radiotherapy may reduce damage to adjacent structures. Radiotherapy for pituitary tumors has been associated with adverse mortality rates, mainly from cerebrovascular disease. The cumulative risk of developing a secondary tumor after conventional radiation is 1.3% after 10 years and 1.9% after 20 years.

Medical Medical therapy for pituitary tumors is highly specific and depends on tumor type. For prolactinomas, dopamine agonists are the treatment of choice. For acromegaly, somatostatin analogues and GH receptor antagonists are indicated. For TSH-secreting tumors, somatostatin analogues and occasionally dopamine agonists are indicated. ACTH-secreting tumors and nonfunctioning tumors are generally not responsive to medications and require surgery and/or irradiation.

PROLACTIN

SYNTHESIS

PRL consists of 198 amino acids and has a molecular mass of 21,500 kDa; it is weakly homologous to GH and human placental lactogen (hPL), reflecting the duplication and divergence of a common GH-PRL-hPL precursor gene. PRL is synthesized in lactotropes, which constitute about 20% of anterior pituitary cells. Lactotropes and somatotropes are derived from a common precursor cell that may give rise to a tumor that secretes both PRL and GH. Marked lactotrope cell hyperplasia develops during pregnancy and the first few months of lactation. These transient functional changes in the lactotrope population are induced by estrogen.

SECRETION

Normal adult serum PRL levels are about 10–25 μg/L in women and 10–20 μg/L in men. PRL secretion is pulsatile, with the highest secretory peaks occurring during rapid eye movement sleep. Peak serum PRL levels (up to 30 μg/L) occur between 4:00 and 6:00 A.M. The circulating half-life of PRL is about 50 min.

PRL is unique among the pituitary hormones in that the predominant central control mechanism is inhibitory, reflecting dopamine-mediated suppression of PRL release. This regulatory pathway accounts for the spontaneous PRL hypersecretion that occurs with pituitary stalk section, often a consequence of compressive mass lesions at the skull base. Pituitary dopamine type 2 (D_2) receptors mediate inhibition of PRL synthesis and secretion. Targeted disruption (gene knockout) of the murine D_2 receptor in mice results in hyperprolactinemia and lactotrope proliferation. As discussed later, dopamine agonists play a central role in the management of hyperprolactinemic disorders.

Thyrotropin-releasing hormone (TRH) (pyro Glu-His-Pro-NH_2) is a hypothalamic tripeptide that elicits prolactin release within 15–30 min after intravenous injection. The physiologic relevance of TRH for PRL regulation is unclear, and it appears primarily to regulate TSH. *Vasoactive intestinal peptide* (VIP) also induces PRL release, whereas glucocorticoids and thyroid hormone weakly suppress PRL secretion.

Serum PRL levels rise transiently after exercise, meals, sexual intercourse, minor surgical procedures, general anesthesia, chest wall injury, acute myocardial infarction, and other forms of acute stress. PRL levels increase markedly (about tenfold) during pregnancy and decline rapidly within 2 weeks of parturition. If breast-feeding is initiated, basal PRL levels remain elevated; suckling stimulates reflex increases in PRL levels that last for about 30–45 min. Breast suckling activates neural afferent pathways in the hypothalamus that induce PRL release. With time, suckling-induced responses diminish and interfeeding PRL levels return to normal.

ACTION

The PRL receptor is a member of the type I cytokine receptor family that also includes GH and interleukin (IL) 6 receptors. Ligand binding induces receptor dimerization and intracellular signaling by Janus kinase (JAK), which stimulates translocation of the signal transduction and activators of transcription (STAT) family to activate target genes. In the breast, the lobuloalveolar epithelium proliferates in response to PRL, placental lactogens, estrogen, progesterone, and local paracrine growth factors, including IGF-I.

PRL acts to induce and maintain lactation, decrease reproductive function, and suppress sexual drive. These functions are geared toward ensuring that maternal lactation is sustained and not interrupted by pregnancy. PRL inhibits reproductive function by suppressing hypothalamic GnRH and pituitary gonadotropin secretion and by impairing gonadal steroidogenesis in both women and men. In the ovary, PRL blocks folliculogenesis and inhibits granulosa cell aromatase activity, leading to hypoestrogenism and anovulation. PRL also has a luteolytic effect, generating a shortened, or inadequate, luteal phase of the menstrual cycle. In men, attenuated LH secretion leads to low testosterone levels and decreased spermatogenesis. These hormonal changes decrease libido and reduce fertility in patients with hyperprolactinemia.

HYPERPROLACTINEMIA

Etiology

Hyperprolactinemia is the most common pituitary hormone hypersecretion syndrome in both men and women. PRL-secreting pituitary adenomas (prolactinomas) are the most common cause of PRL levels >200 μg/L (discussed later). Less pronounced PRL elevation can also be seen with microprolactinomas but is more commonly caused by drugs, pituitary stalk compression, hypothyroidism, or renal failure (Table 38-9).

Pregnancy and lactation are the important physiologic causes of hyperprolactinemia. Sleep-associated hyperprolactinemia reverts to normal within an hour of awakening. Nipple stimulation and sexual orgasm also may increase PRL. Chest wall stimulation or trauma (including chest surgery and herpes zoster) invoke the reflex suckling arc with resultant hyperprolactinemia. Chronic renal failure elevates PRL by decreasing peripheral clearance. Primary hypothyroidism is associated with mild hyperprolactinemia, probably because of compensatory TRH secretion.

Lesions of the hypothalamic-pituitary region that disrupt hypothalamic dopamine synthesis, portal vessel delivery, or lactotrope responses are associated with hyperprolactinemia. Thus, hypothalamic tumors, cysts, infiltrative disorders, and radiation-induced damage cause elevated PRL levels, usually in the range of 30–100 μg/L. Plurihormonal adenomas (including GH and ACTH tumors) may hypersecrete PRL directly. Pituitary masses, including clinically nonfunctioning pituitary tumors, may compress the pituitary stalk to cause hyperprolactinemia.

Drug-induced inhibition or disruption of dopaminergic receptor function is a common cause of hyperprolactinemia (Table 38-9). Thus, antipsychotics and antidepressants are a relatively common cause of mild hyperprolactinemia. Most patients receiving risperidone have elevated prolactin levels, sometimes exceeding 200 μg/L. Methyldopa inhibits dopamine synthesis and verapamil blocks dopamine release, also leading to hyperprolactinemia. Hormonal agents that induce PRL include estrogens and TRH.

Presentation and diagnosis

Amenorrhea, galactorrhea, and infertility are the hallmarks of hyperprolactinemia in women. If hyperprolactinemia develops before menarche, primary amenorrhea results. More commonly, hyperprolactinemia develops later in life and leads to oligomenorrhea and ultimately to amenorrhea. If hyperprolactinemia is sustained, vertebral bone mineral density can be reduced compared with age-matched controls, particularly when it is associated with pronounced hypoestrogenemia. Galactorrhea is present in up to 80% of hyperprolactinemic women. Although usually bilateral and spontaneous, it may be unilateral or expressed only manually. Patients also may complain of decreased libido, weight gain, and mild hirsutism.

In men with hyperprolactinemia, diminished libido, infertility, and visual loss (from optic nerve compression) are the usual presenting symptoms. Gonadotropin suppression leads to reduced testosterone, impotence,

TABLE 38-9

ETIOLOGY OF HYPERPROLACTINEMIA

I. Physiologic hypersecretion
- Pregnancy
- Lactation
- Chest wall stimulation
- Sleep
- Stress

II. Hypothalamic–pituitary stalk damage
- Tumors
  - Craniopharyngioma
  - Suprasellar pituitary mass
  - Meningioma
  - Dysgerminoma
  - Metastases
- Empty sella
- Lymphocytic hypophysitis
- Adenoma with stalk compression
- Granulomas
- Rathke's cyst
- Irradiation
- Trauma
  - Pituitary stalk section
  - Suprasellar surgery

III. Pituitary hypersecretion
- Prolactinoma
- Acromegaly

IV. Systemic disorders
- Chronic renal failure
- Hypothyroidism
- Cirrhosis
- Pseudocyesis
- Epileptic seizures

V. Drug-induced hypersecretion
- Dopamine receptor blockers
  - Atypical antipsychotics: risperidone
  - Phenothiazines: chlorpromazine, perphenazine
  - Butyrophenones: haloperidol
  - Thioxanthenes
  - Metoclopramide
- Dopamine synthesis inhibitors
  - α-Methyldopa
- Catecholamine depletors
  - Reserpine
- Opiates
- H_2 antagonists
  - Cimetidine, ranitidine
- Imipramines
  - Amitriptyline, amoxapine
- Serotonin reuptake inhibitors
  - Fluoxetine
- Calcium channel blockers
  - Verapamil
  - Estrogens
  - TRH

Note: Hyperprolactinemia >200 μg/L almost invariably is indicative of a prolactin-secreting pituitary adenoma. Physiologic causes, hypothyroidism, and drug-induced hyperprolactinemia should be excluded before extensive evaluation.

and oligospermia. True galactorrhea is uncommon in men with hyperprolactinemia. If the disorder is longstanding, secondary effects of hypogonadism are evident, including osteopenia, reduced muscle mass, and decreased beard growth.

The diagnosis of idiopathic hyperprolactinemia is made by exclusion of known causes of hyperprolactinemia in the setting of a normal pituitary MRI. Some of these patients may harbor small microadenomas below visible MRI sensitivity (~2 mm).

GALACTORRHEA

Galactorrhea, the inappropriate discharge of milk-containing fluid from the breast, is considered abnormal if it persists longer than 6 months after childbirth or discontinuation of breast-feeding. Postpartum galactorrhea associated with amenorrhea is a self-limiting disorder usually associated with moderately elevated PRL levels. Galactorrhea may occur spontaneously, or it may be elicited by nipple pressure. In both men and women, galactorrhea may vary in color and consistency (transparent, milky, or bloody) and arise either unilaterally or bilaterally. Mammography or ultrasound is indicated for bloody discharges (particularly from a single nipple), which may be caused by breast cancer. Galactorrhea is commonly associated with hyperprolactinemia caused by any of the conditions listed in Table 38-9. Acromegaly is associated with galactorrhea in about one-third of patients. Treatment of galactorrhea usually involves managing the underlying disorder (e.g., replacing T_4 for hypothyroidism, discontinuing a medication, treating prolactinoma).

Laboratory investigation

Basal, fasting morning PRL levels (normally <20 μg/L) should be measured to assess hypersecretion. Both false-positive and false-negative results may be encountered. In patients with markedly elevated PRL levels (>1000 μg/L), reported results may be falsely lowered because of assay artifacts; sample dilution is required to measure these high values accurately. Falsely elevated values may be caused by aggregated forms of circulating PRL, which are usually biologically inactive (macroprolactinemia). Hypothyroidism should be excluded by measuring TSH and T_4 levels.

TREATMENT **Hyperprolactinemia**

Treatment of hyperprolactinemia depends on the cause of elevated PRL levels. Regardless of the etiology, however, treatment should be aimed at normalizing PRL levels to alleviate suppressive effects on gonadal function, halt galactorrhea, and preserve bone mineral density. Dopamine agonists are effective for most causes of hyperprolactinemia (see the treatment section for prolactinoma later in this chapter) regardless of the underlying cause.

If the patient is taking a medication known to cause hyperprolactinemia, the drug should be withdrawn, if possible. For psychiatric patients who require neuroleptic agents, supervised dose titration or the addition of a dopamine agonist can help restore normoprolactinemia and alleviate reproductive symptoms. However, dopamine agonists sometimes worsen the underlying psychiatric condition, especially at high doses. Hyperprolactinemia usually resolves after adequate thyroid hormone replacement in hypothyroid patients or after renal transplantation in patients undergoing dialysis. Resection of hypothalamic or sellar mass lesions can reverse hyperprolactinemia caused by stalk compression and reduced dopamine tone. Granulomatous infiltrates occasionally respond to glucocorticoid administration. In patients with irreversible hypothalamic damage, no treatment may be warranted. In up to 30% of patients with hyperprolactinemia—usually without a visible pituitary microadenoma—the condition may resolve spontaneously.

PROLACTINOMA

Etiology and prevalence

Tumors arising from lactotrope cells account for about half of all functioning pituitary tumors, with a population prevalence of ~10/100,000 in men and ~30/100,000 in women. Mixed tumors that secrete combinations of GH and PRL, ACTH and PRL, and rarely TSH and PRL are also seen. These plurihormonal tumors are usually recognized by immunohistochemistry, sometimes without apparent clinical manifestations from the production of additional hormones. Microadenomas are classified as <1 cm in diameter and usually do not invade the parasellar region. Macroadenomas are >1 cm in diameter and may be locally invasive and impinge on adjacent structures. The female:male ratio for microprolactinomas is 20:1, whereas the sex ratio is near 1:1 for macroadenomas. Tumor size generally correlates directly with PRL concentrations; values >250 μg/L usually are associated with macroadenomas. Men tend to present with larger tumors than women, possibly because the features of male hypogonadism are less readily evident. PRL levels remain stable in most patients, reflecting the slow growth of these tumors. About 5% of microadenomas progress in the long term to macroadenomas.

Presentation and diagnosis

Women usually present with amenorrhea, infertility, and galactorrhea. If the tumor extends outside the sella, visual field defects or other mass effects may be seen. Men often present with impotence, loss of libido, infertility, or signs of central CNS compression, including headaches and visual defects. Assuming that physiologic and medication-induced causes of hyperprolactinemia are excluded (Table 38-9), the diagnosis of prolactinoma is likely with a PRL level >200 μg/L. PRL levels <100 μg/L may be caused by microadenomas, other sellar lesions that decrease dopamine inhibition, or non-neoplastic causes of hyperprolactinemia. For this reason, an MRI should be performed in all patients with hyperprolactinemia. It is important to remember that hyperprolactinemia caused secondarily by the mass effects of nonlactotrope lesions is also corrected by treatment with dopamine agonists despite failure to shrink the underlying mass. Consequently, PRL suppression by dopamine agonists does not necessarily indicate that the underlying lesion is a prolactinoma.

TREATMENT Prolactinoma

As microadenomas rarely progress to become macroadenomas, no treatment may be needed if fertility is not desired. Estrogen replacement is indicated to prevent bone loss and other consequences of hypoestrogenemia and does not appear to increase the risk of tumor enlargement; these patients should be monitored by regular serial PRL and MRI measurements.

For symptomatic microadenomas, therapeutic goals include control of hyperprolactinemia, reduction of tumor size, restoration of menses and fertility, and resolution of galactorrhea. Dopamine agonist doses should be titrated to achieve maximal PRL suppression and restoration of reproductive function (Fig. 38-6). A normalized PRL level does not ensure reduced tumor size. However, tumor shrinkage usually is not seen in those who do not respond with lowered PRL levels. For macroadenomas, formal visual field testing should be performed before initiating dopamine agonists. MRI and visual fields should be assessed at 6- to 12-month intervals until the mass shrinks and annually thereafter until maximum size reduction has occurred.

MEDICAL Oral dopamine agonists (cabergoline and bromocriptine) are the mainstay of therapy for patients with micro- or macroprolactinomas. Dopamine agonists suppress PRL secretion and synthesis as well as lactotrope cell proliferation. In patients with microadenomas who have achieved normoprolactinemia and significant reduction of tumor mass, the dopamine agonist may be withdrawn after 2 years. These patients should be monitored carefully for evidence of prolactinoma recurrence. About 20% of patients (especially males) are resistant to dopaminergic treatment; these adenomas may exhibit

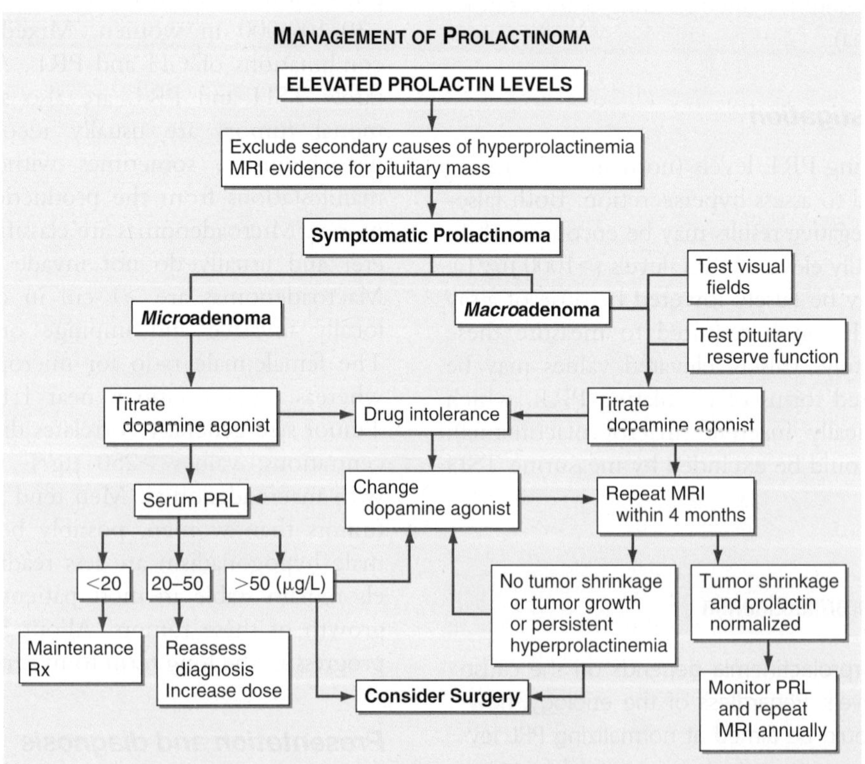

FIGURE 38-6
Management of prolactinoma. MRI, magnetic resonance imaging; PRL, prolactin.

decreased D_2 dopamine receptor numbers or a postreceptor defect. D_2 receptor gene mutations in the pituitary have not been reported.

Cabergoline An ergoline derivative, cabergoline is a long-acting dopamine agonist with high D_2 receptor affinity. The drug effectively suppresses PRL for >14 days after a single oral dose and induces prolactinoma shrinkage in most patients. Cabergoline (0.5 to 1.0 mg twice weekly) achieves normoprolactinemia and resumption of normal gonadal function in ~80% of patients with microadenomas; galactorrhea improves or resolves in 90% of patients. Cabergoline normalizes PRL and shrinks ~70% of macroprolactinomas. Mass effect symptoms, including headaches and visual disorders, usually improve dramatically within days after cabergoline initiation; improvement of sexual function requires several weeks of treatment but may occur before complete normalization of prolactin levels. After initial control of PRL levels has been achieved, cabergoline should be reduced to the lowest effective maintenance dose. In ~5% of treated patients harboring a microadenoma, hyperprolactinemia may resolve and not recur when dopamine agonists are discontinued after long-term treatment. Cabergoline also may be effective in patients resistant to bromocriptine. Adverse effects and drug intolerance are encountered less commonly than with bromocriptine.

Bromocriptine The ergot alkaloid bromocriptine mesylate is a dopamine receptor agonist that suppresses prolactin secretion. Because it is short-acting, the drug is preferred when pregnancy is desired. In microadenomas bromocriptine rapidly lowers serum prolactin levels to normal in up to 70% of patients, decreases tumor size, and restores gonadal function. In patients with macroadenomas, prolactin levels are also normalized in 70% of patients and tumor mass shrinkage (≥50%) is achieved in most patients.

Therapy is initiated by administering a low bromocriptine dose (0.625–1.25 mg) at bedtime with a snack, followed by gradually increasing the dose. Most patients are controlled with a daily dose of ≤7.5 mg (2.5 mg tid).

Side Effects Side effects of dopamine agonists include constipation, nasal stuffiness, dry mouth, nightmares, insomnia, and vertigo; decreasing the dose usually alleviates these problems. Nausea, vomiting, and postural hypotension with faintness may occur in ~25% of patients after the initial dose. These symptoms may persist in some patients. In general, fewer side effects are reported with cabergoline. For the approximately 15% of patients who are intolerant of oral bromocriptine, cabergoline may be better tolerated. Intravaginal administration of bromocriptine is often efficacious in patients with intractable gastrointestinal side effects. Auditory hallucinations, delusions, and mood swings have been reported in up to 5% of patients and may be due to the dopamine agonist properties or to the lysergic acid derivative of the compounds. Rare reports of leukopenia, thrombocytopenia, pleural fibrosis, cardiac arrhythmias, and hepatitis have been described. Patients with Parkinson's disease who receive at least 3 mg of cabergoline daily have been reported to be at risk for development of cardiac valve regurgitation. Studies analyzing over 500 prolactinoma patients receiving recommended doses of cabergoline (up to 2 mg weekly) have shown no evidence for an increased incidence of valvular disorders. Nevertheless, as no controlled prospective studies are available, it is prudent to perform echocardiograms before initiating standard-dose cabergoline therapy.

Surgery Indications for surgical adenoma debulking include dopamine resistance or intolerance and the presence of an invasive macroadenoma with compromised vision that fails to improve after drug treatment. Initial PRL normalization is achieved in about 70% of microprolactinomas after surgical resection, but only 30% of macroadenomas can be resected successfully. Follow-up studies have shown that hyperprolactinemia recurs in up to 20% of patients within the first year after surgery; long-term recurrence rates exceed 50% for macroadenomas. Radiotherapy for prolactinomas is reserved for patients with aggressive tumors that do not respond to maximally tolerated dopamine agonists and/or surgery.

PREGNANCY The pituitary increases in size during pregnancy, reflecting the stimulatory effects of estrogen and perhaps other growth factors on pituitary vascularity and lactotrope cell hyperplasia. About 5% of microadenomas significantly increase in size, but 15–30% of macroadenomas grow during pregnancy. Bromocriptine has been used for more than 30 years to restore fertility in women with hyperprolactinemia, without evidence of teratogenic effects. Nonetheless, most authorities recommend strategies to minimize fetal exposure to the drug. For women taking bromocriptine who desire pregnancy, mechanical contraception should be used through three regular menstrual cycles to allow for conception timing. When pregnancy is confirmed, bromocriptine should be discontinued and PRL levels followed serially, especially if headaches or visual symptoms occur. For women harboring macroadenomas, regular visual field testing is recommended, and the drug should be reinstituted if tumor growth is apparent. Although pituitary MRI may be safe during pregnancy, this procedure should be reserved for symptomatic patients with severe headache and/or visual field defects. Surgical decompression may be indicated if vision is threatened. Although comprehensive data support the efficacy and relative safety of bromocriptine-facilitated fertility, patients should be advised of potential unknown deleterious effects and the risk of tumor growth during pregnancy. As cabergoline is long-acting with a high D_2-receptor affinity, it is not recommended for use in women when fertility is desired.

GROWTH HORMONE

SYNTHESIS

GH is the most abundant anterior pituitary hormone, and GH-secreting somatotrope cells constitute up to 50% of the total anterior pituitary cell population. Mammosomatotrope cells, which coexpress PRL with GH, can be identified by using double immunostaining techniques. Somatotrope development and GH transcription are determined by expression of the cell-specific Pit-1 nuclear transcription factor. Five distinct genes encode GH and related proteins. The pituitary GH gene (*hGH-N*) produces two alternatively spliced products that give rise to 22-kDa GH (191 amino acids) and a less abundant 20-kDa GH molecule with similar biologic activity. Placental syncytiotrophoblast cells express a GH variant (*hGH-V*) gene; the related hormone human chorionic somatotropin (HCS) is expressed by distinct members of the gene cluster.

SECRETION

GH secretion is controlled by complex hypothalamic and peripheral factors. *GHRH* is a 44-amino-acid hypothalamic peptide that stimulates GH synthesis and release. Ghrelin, an octanoylated gastric-derived peptide, and synthetic agonists of the *GHS-R* induce GHRH and also directly stimulate GH release. *Somatostatin* (somatotropin-release inhibiting factor [SRIF]) is synthesized in the medial preoptic area of the hypothalamus and inhibits GH secretion. GHRH is secreted in discrete spikes that elicit GH pulses, whereas SRIF sets basal GH secretory tone. SRIF also is expressed in many extrahypothalamic tissues, including the CNS, gastrointestinal tract, and pancreas, where it also acts to inhibit islet hormone secretion. *IGF-I*, the peripheral target hormone for GH, feeds back to inhibit GH; estrogen induces GH, whereas chronic glucocorticoid excess suppresses GH release.

Surface receptors on the somatotrope regulate GH synthesis and secretion. The GHRH receptor is a G protein–coupled receptor (GPCR) that signals through the intracellular cyclic AMP pathway to stimulate somatotrope cell proliferation as well as GH production. Inactivating mutations of the GHRH receptor cause profound dwarfism (discussed later). A distinct surface receptor for ghrelin, the gastric-derived GH secretagogue, is expressed in the hypothalamus and pituitary. Somatostatin binds to five distinct receptor subtypes (SSTR1 to SSTR5); SSTR2 and SSTR5 subtypes preferentially suppress GH (and TSH) secretion.

GH secretion is pulsatile, with highest peak levels occurring at night, generally correlating with sleep onset. GH secretory rates decline markedly with age so that hormone levels in middle age are about 15% of pubertal levels. These changes are paralleled by an age-related decline in lean muscle mass. GH secretion is also reduced in obese individuals, though IGF-I levels may not be suppressed, suggesting a change in the setpoint for feedback control. Elevated GH levels occur within an hour of deep sleep onset as well as after exercise, physical stress, and trauma and during sepsis. Integrated 24-h GH secretion is higher in women and is also enhanced by estrogen replacement. Using standard assays, random GH measurements are undetectable in ~50% of daytime samples obtained from healthy subjects and are also undetectable in most obese and elderly subjects. Thus, single random GH measurements do not distinguish patients with adult GH deficiency from normal persons.

GH secretion is profoundly influenced by nutritional factors. Using newer ultrasensitive GH assays with a sensitivity of 0.002 μg/L, a glucose load suppresses GH to <0.7 μg/L in women and to <0.07 μg/L in men. Increased GH pulse frequency and peak amplitudes occur with chronic malnutrition or prolonged fasting. GH is stimulated by intravenous L-arginine, dopamine, and apomorphine (a dopamine receptor agonist), as well as by α-adrenergic pathways. β-Adrenergic blockage induces basal GH and enhances GHRH- and insulin-evoked GH release.

ACTION

The pattern of GH secretion may affect tissue responses. The higher GH pulsatility observed in men compared with the relatively continuous GH secretion in women may be an important biologic determinant of linear growth patterns and liver enzyme induction.

The 70-kDa peripheral GH receptor protein has structural homology with the cytokine/hematopoietic superfamily. A fragment of the receptor extracellular domain generates a soluble GH binding protein (GHBP) that interacts with GH in the circulation. The liver and cartilage contain the greatest number of GH receptors. GH binding to preformed receptor dimers is followed by internal rotation and subsequent signaling through the JAK/STAT pathway. Activated STAT proteins translocate to the nucleus, where they modulate expression of GH-regulated target genes. GH analogues that bind to the receptor but are incapable of mediating receptor signaling are potent antagonists of GH action. A GH receptor antagonist (pegvisomant) is approved for treatment of acromegaly.

GH induces protein synthesis and nitrogen retention and impairs glucose tolerance by antagonizing insulin action. GH also stimulates lipolysis, leading to increased circulating fatty acid levels, reduced omental fat mass, and enhanced lean body mass. GH promotes sodium, potassium, and water retention and elevates serum levels of inorganic phosphate. Linear bone growth occurs as a result of complex hormonal and growth factor actions, including those of IGF-I. GH stimulates epiphyseal prechondrocyte differentiation. These precursor cells produce IGF-I locally, and their proliferation is also responsive to the growth factor.

INSULIN-LIKE GROWTH FACTORS

Although GH exerts direct effects in target tissues, many of its physiologic effects are mediated indirectly through IGF-I, a potent growth and differentiation factor. The liver is the major source of circulating IGF-I. In peripheral tissues, IGF-I exerts local paracrine actions that appear to be both dependent on and independent of GH. Thus, GH administration induces circulating IGF-I as well as stimulating local IGF-I production in multiple tissues.

Both IGF-I and IGF-II are bound to high-affinity circulating IGF-binding proteins (IGFBPs) that regulate IGF bioactivity. Levels of IGFBP3 are GH-dependent, and it serves as the major carrier protein for circulating IGF-I. GH deficiency and malnutrition usually are associated with low IGFBP3 levels. IGFBP1 and IGFBP2 regulate local tissue IGF action but do not bind appreciable amounts of circulating IGF-I.

Serum IGF-I concentrations are profoundly affected by physiologic factors. Levels increase during puberty, peak at 16 years, and subsequently decline by >80% during the aging process. IGF-I concentrations are higher in women than in men. Because GH is the major determinant of hepatic IGF-I synthesis, abnormalities of GH synthesis or action (e.g., pituitary failure, GHRH receptor defect, GH receptor defect) reduce IGF-I levels. Hypocaloric states are associated with GH resistance; IGF-I levels are therefore low with cachexia, malnutrition, and sepsis. In acromegaly, IGF-I levels are invariably high and reflect a log-linear relationship with GH concentrations.

IGF-I physiology

IGF-I has been approved for use in patients with GH-resistance syndromes. Injected IGF-I (100 μg/kg) induces hypoglycemia, and lower doses improve insulin sensitivity in patients with severe insulin resistance and diabetes. In cachectic subjects, IGF-I infusion (12 μg/kg per hour) enhances nitrogen retention and lowers cholesterol levels. Longer-term subcutaneous IGF-I injections enhance protein synthesis and are anabolic. Although bone formation markers are induced, bone turnover also may be stimulated by IGF-I.

IGF-I side effects are dose-dependent, and overdose may result in hypoglycemia, hypotension, fluid retention, temporomandibular jaw pain, and increased intracranial pressure, all of which are reversible. Avascular femoral head necrosis has been reported. Chronic excess IGF-I administration presumably would result in features of acromegaly.

DISORDERS OF GROWTH AND DEVELOPMENT

Skeletal maturation and somatic growth

The growth plate is dependent on a variety of hormonal stimuli, including GH, IGF-I, sex steroids, thyroid hormones, paracrine growth factors, and cytokines. The growth-promoting process also requires caloric energy, amino acids, vitamins, and trace metals and consumes about 10% of normal energy production. Malnutrition impairs chondrocyte activity and reduces circulating IGF-I and IGFBP3 levels.

Linear bone growth rates are very high in infancy and are pituitary-dependent. Mean growth velocity is ~6 cm/year in later childhood and usually is maintained within a given range on a standardized percentile chart. Peak growth rates occur during midpuberty when bone age is 12 (girls) or 13 (boys). Secondary sexual development is associated with elevated sex steroids that cause progressive epiphyseal growth plate closure. *Bone age* is delayed in patients with all forms of true GH deficiency or GH receptor defects that result in attenuated GH action.

Short stature may occur as a result of constitutive intrinsic growth defects or because of acquired extrinsic factors that impair growth. In general, delayed bone age in a child with short stature is suggestive of a hormonal or systemic disorder, whereas normal bone age in a short child is more likely to be caused by a genetic cartilage dysplasia or growth plate disorder.

GH deficiency in children

GH deficiency

Isolated GH deficiency is characterized by short stature, micropenis, increased fat, high-pitched voice, and a propensity to hypoglycemia due to relatively unopposed insulin action. Familial modes of inheritance are seen in one-third of these individuals and may be autosomal dominant, recessive, or X-linked. About 10% of children with GH deficiency have mutations in the *GH-N* gene, including gene deletions and a wide range of point mutations. Mutations in transcription factors Pit-1 and Prop-1, which control somatotrope development result in GH deficiency in combination with other pituitary hormone deficiencies, which may become manifest only in adulthood. The diagnosis of *idiopathic GH deficiency* (IGHD) should be made only after known molecular defects have been rigorously excluded.

GHRH receptor mutations

Recessive mutations of the GHRH receptor gene in subjects with severe proportionate dwarfism are associated with low basal GH levels that cannot be stimulated by exogenous GHRH, GHRP, or insulin-induced hypoglycemia, as well as anterior pituitary hypoplasia. The syndrome exemplifies the importance of the GHRH receptor for somatotrope cell proliferation and hormonal responsiveness.

Growth hormone insensitivity

This is caused by defects of GH receptor structure or signaling. Homozygous or heterozygous mutations of the GH receptor are associated with partial or complete GH insensitivity and growth failure (*Laron syndrome*). The diagnosis is based on normal or high GH levels, with decreased circulating GHBP, and low IGF-I levels. Very rarely, defective IGF-I, IGF-I receptor, or IGF-I signaling defects are also encountered. *STAT5B* mutations result in immunodeficiency with abrogated GH signaling, leading to short stature with normal or elevated GH levels and low IGF-I levels.

Nutritional short stature

Caloric deprivation and malnutrition, uncontrolled diabetes, and chronic renal failure represent secondary causes of abrogated GH receptor function. These conditions also stimulate production of proinflammatory cytokines, which act to exacerbate the block of GH-mediated signal transduction. Children with these conditions typically exhibit features of acquired short stature with normal or elevated GH, and low IGF-I levels. Circulating GH receptor antibodies may rarely cause peripheral GH insensitivity.

Psychosocial short stature

Emotional and social deprivation lead to growth retardation accompanied by delayed speech, discordant hyperphagia, and an attenuated response to administered GH. A nurturing environment restores growth rates.

Presentation and diagnosis

Short stature is commonly encountered in clinical practice, and the decision to evaluate these children requires clinical judgment in association with auxologic data and family history. Short stature should be evaluated comprehensively if a patient's height is >3 standard deviations (SD) below the mean for age or if the growth rate has decelerated. Skeletal maturation is best evaluated by measuring a radiologic bone age, which is based mainly on the degree of wrist bone growth plate fusion. Final height can be predicted using standardized scales (Bayley-Pinneau or Tanner-Whitehouse) or estimated by adding 6.5 cm (boys) or subtracting 6.5 cm (girls) from the midparental height.

Laboratory investigation

Because GH secretion is pulsatile, GH deficiency is best assessed by examining the response to provocative stimuli, including exercise, insulin-induced hypoglycemia, and other pharmacologic tests that normally increase GH to >7 μg/L in children. Random GH measurements do not distinguish normal children from those with true GH deficiency. Adequate adrenal and thyroid hormone replacement should be assured before testing. Age- and sex-matched IGF-I levels are not sufficiently sensitive or specific to make the diagnosis but can be useful to confirm GH deficiency. Pituitary MRI may reveal pituitary mass lesions or structural defects. Molecular analyses for known mutations should be undertaken when the cause of short stature remains cryptic, or when additional clinical features suggest a gentic cause.

TREATMENT Disorders of Growth and Development

Replacement therapy with recombinant GH (0.02–0.05 mg/kg per day subcutaneously) restores growth velocity in GH-deficient children to ~10 cm/year. If pituitary insufficiency is documented, other associated hormone deficits should be corrected—especially adrenal steroids. GH treatment is also moderately effective for accelerating growth rates in children with Turner's syndrome and chronic renal failure.

In patients with GH insensitivity and growth retardation due to mutations of the GH receptor, treatment with IGF-I bypasses the dysfunctional GH receptor.

ADULT GH DEFICIENCY (AGHD)

This disorder usually is caused by hypothalamic or pituitary somatotrope damage. Acquired pituitary hormone deficiency follows a typical pattern in which loss of adequate GH reserve foreshadows subsequent hormone deficits. The sequential order of hormone loss is usually GH → FSH/LH → TSH → ACTH.

Presentation and diagnosis

The clinical features of AGHD include changes in body composition, lipid metabolism, and quality of life and

TABLE 38-10

FEATURES OF ADULT GROWTH HORMONE DEFICIENCY
Clinical
Impaired quality of life
Decreased energy and drive
Poor concentration
Low self-esteem
Social isolation
Body composition changes
Increased body fat mass
Central fat deposition
Increased waist-hip ratio
Decreased lean body mass
Reduced exercise capacity
Reduced maximum O_2 uptake
Impaired cardiac function
Reduced muscle mass
Cardiovascular risk factors
Impaired cardiac structure and function
Abnormal lipid profile
Decreased fibrinolytic activity
Atherosclerosis
Omental obesity
Imaging
Pituitary: mass or structural damage
Bone: reduced bone mineral density
Abdomen: excess omental adiposity
Laboratory
Evoked GH <3 ng/mL
IGF-I and IGFBP3 low or normal
Increased LDL cholesterol
Concomitant gonadotropin, TSH, and/or ACTH reserve deficits may be present

Abbreviation: LDL, low-density lipoprotein. For other abbreviations, see text.

cardiovascular dysfunction (Table 38-10). Body composition changes are common and include reduced lean body mass, increased fat mass with selective deposition of intraabdominal visceral fat, and increased waist-to-hip ratio. Hyperlipidemia, left ventricular dysfunction, hypertension, and increased plasma fibrinogen levels also may be present. Bone mineral content is reduced, with resultant increased fracture rates. Patients may experience social isolation, depression, and difficulty maintaining gainful employment. Adult hypopituitarism is associated with a threefold increase in cardiovascular mortality rates in comparison to age- and sex-matched controls, and this may be due to GH deficiency, as patients in these studies were replaced with other deficient pituitary hormones.

Laboratory investigation

AGHD is rare, and in light of the nonspecific nature of associated clinical symptoms, patients appropriate for testing should be selected carefully on the basis of well-defined criteria. With few exceptions, testing should be restricted to patients with the following predisposing factors: (1) pituitary surgery, (2) pituitary or hypothalamic tumor or granulomas, (3) history of cranial irradiation, (4) radiologic evidence of a pituitary lesion, (5) childhood requirement for GH replacement therapy, and rarely (6) unexplained low age- and sex-matched IGF-I levels. The transition of a GH-deficient adolescent to adulthood requires retesting to document subsequent adult GH deficiency. Up to 20% of patients previously treated for childhood-onset GH deficiency are found to be GH-sufficient on repeat testing as adults.

A significant proportion (~25%) of truly GH-deficient adults have low-normal IGF-I levels. Thus, as in the evaluation of GH deficiency in children, valid age- and sex-matched IGF-I measurements provide a useful index of therapeutic responses but are not sufficiently sensitive for diagnostic purposes. The most validated test to distinguish pituitary-sufficient patients from those with AGHD is insulin-induced (0.05–0.1 U/kg) hypoglycemia. After glucose reduction to ~40 mg/dL, most individuals experience neuroglycopenic symptoms, and peak GH release occurs at 60 min and remains elevated for up to 2 h. About 90% of healthy adults exhibit GH responses >5 μg/L; AGHD is defined by a peak GH response to hypoglycemia of <3 μg/L. Although insulin-induced hypoglycemia is safe when performed under appropriate supervision, it is contraindicated in patients with diabetes, ischemic heart disease, cerebrovascular disease, or epilepsy and in elderly patients. Alternative stimulatory tests include intravenous arginine (30 g), GHRH (1 μg/kg), GHRP-6 (90 μg), and glucagon (1 mg). Combinations of these tests may evoke GH secretion in subjects who are not responsive to a single test.

TREATMENT Adult GH Deficiency

Once the diagnosis of AGHD is unequivocally established, replacement of GH may be indicated. Contraindications to therapy include the presence of an active neoplasm, intracranial hypertension, and uncontrolled diabetes and retinopathy. The starting dose of 0.1–0.2 mg/d should be titrated (up to a maximum of 1.25 mg/d) to maintain IGF-I levels in the mid-normal range for age- and sex-matched controls (Fig. 38-7). Women require higher doses than men, and elderly patients require less GH. Long-term GH maintenance sustains normal IGF-I levels and is associated with persistent body composition changes (e.g., enhanced lean body mass and lower body fat). High-density lipoprotein cholesterol increases, but total cholesterol and insulin levels

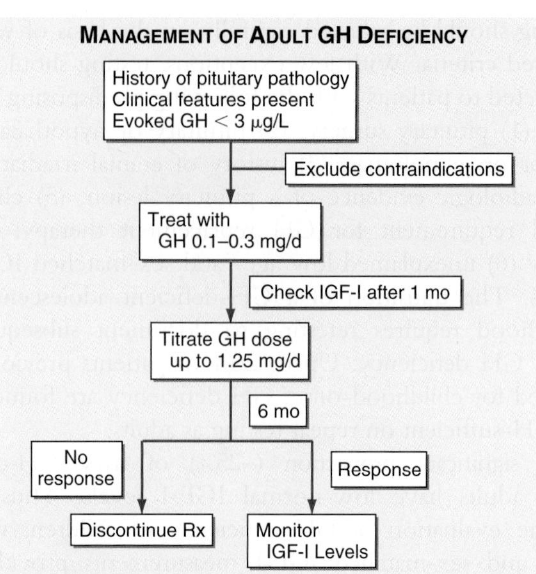

FIGURE 38-7

Management of adult growth hormone (GH) deficiency. IGF, insulin-like growth factor.

do not change significantly. Lumbar spine bone mineral density increases, but this response is gradual (>1 year). Many patients note significant improvement in quality of life when evaluated by standardized questionnaires. The effect of GH replacement on mortality rates in GH-deficient patients is currently the subject of long-term prospective investigation.

About 30% of patients exhibit reversible dose-related fluid retention, joint pain, and carpal tunnel syndrome, and up to 40% exhibit myalgias and paresthesia. Patients receiving insulin require careful monitoring for dosing adjustments, as GH is a potent counterregulatory hormone for insulin action. Patients with type 2 diabetes mellitus initially develop further insulin resistance. However, glycemic control improves with the sustained loss of abdominal fat associated with long-term GH replacement. Headache, increased intracranial pressure, hypertension, and tinnitus occur rarely. Pituitary tumor regrowth and progression of skin lesions or other tumors are being assessed in long-term surveillance programs. To date, development of these potential side effects does not appear significant.

ACROMEGALY

Etiology

GH hypersecretion is usually the result of a somatotrope adenoma but may rarely be caused by extrapituitary lesions (Table 38-11). In addition to more common GH-secreting somatotrope adenomas, mixed mammosomatotrope tumors and acidophilic stem-cell adenomas secrete both GH and PRL. In patients with acidophilic stem-cell adenomas, features of hyperprolactinemia (hypogonadism and galactorrhea) predominate over the less clinically evident signs of acromegaly. Occasionally, mixed plurihormonal tumors are encountered that also secrete ACTH, the glycoprotein hormone α subunit, or TSH in addition to GH. Patients with partially empty sellas may present with GH hypersecretion due to a small GH-secreting adenoma within the compressed rim of pituitary tissue; some of these may reflect the spontaneous necrosis of tumors that were previously larger. GH-secreting tumors rarely arise from ectopic pituitary tissue remnants in the nasopharynx or midline sinuses.

There are case reports of ectopic GH secretion by tumors of pancreatic, ovarian, lung, or hematopoietic origin. Rarely, excess GHRH production may cause acromegaly because of chronic stimulation of somatotropes. These patients present with classic features of acromegaly, elevated GH levels, pituitary enlargement

TABLE 38-11

CAUSES OF ACROMEGALY

	PREVALENCE, %
Excess Growth Hormone Secretion	
Pituitary	98
Densely or sparsely granulated GH cell adenoma	60
Mixed GH cell and PRL cell adenoma	25
Mammosomatrope cell adenoma	10
Plurihormonal adenoma	
GH cell carcinoma or metastases	
Multiple endocrine neoplasia 1 (GH cell adenoma)	
McCune-Albright syndrome	
Ectopic sphenoid or parapharyngeal sinus pituitary adenoma	
Extrapituitary tumor	
Pancreatic islet cell tumor	<1
Lymphoma	
Excess Growth Hormone–Releasing Hormone Secretion	
Central	<1
Hypothalamic hamartoma, choristoma, ganglioneuroma	<1
Peripheral	<1
Bronchial carcinoid, pancreatic islet cell tumor, small cell lung cancer, adrenal adenoma, medullary thyroid carcinoma, pheochromocytoma	

Source: Adapted from S Melmed: N Engl J Med 322:966, 1990.
Abbreviations: GH, growth hormone; PRL, prolactin.

on MRI, and pathologic characteristics of pituitary hyperplasia. The most common cause of GHRH-mediated acromegaly is a chest or abdominal carcinoid tumor. Although these tumors usually express positive GHRH immunoreactivity, clinical features of acromegaly are evident in only a minority of patients with carcinoid disease. Excessive GHRH also may be elaborated by hypothalamic tumors, usually choristomas or neuromas.

Presentation and diagnosis

Protean manifestations of GH and IGF-I hypersecretion are indolent and often are not clinically diagnosed for 10 years or more. Acral bony overgrowth results in frontal bossing, increased hand and foot size, mandibular enlargement with prognathism, and widened space between the lower incisor teeth. In children and adolescents, initiation of GH hypersecretion before epiphyseal long bone closure is associated with development of pituitary gigantism (Fig. 38-8). Soft tissue swelling results in increased heel pad thickness, increased shoe or glove size, ring tightening, characteristic coarse facial features, and a large fleshy nose. Other commonly encountered clinical features include hyperhidrosis, a deep and hollow-sounding voice, oily skin, arthropathy, kyphosis, carpal tunnel syndrome, proximal muscle weakness and fatigue, acanthosis nigricans, and skin tags. Generalized visceromegaly occurs, including cardiomegaly, macroglossia, and thyroid gland enlargement.

The most significant clinical impact of GH excess occurs with respect to the cardiovascular system. Coronary heart disease, cardiomyopathy with arrhythmias, left ventricular hypertrophy, decreased diastolic function, and hypertension ultimately occur in most patients if untreated. Upper airway obstruction with sleep apnea occurs in more than 60% of patients and is associated with both soft tissue laryngeal airway obstruction and central sleep dysfunction. Diabetes mellitus develops in 25% of patients with acromegaly, and most patients are intolerant of a glucose load (as GH counteracts the action of insulin). Acromegaly is associated with an increased risk of colon polyps and mortality from colonic malignancy; polyps are diagnosed in up to one-third of patients. Overall mortality is increased about threefold and is due primarily to cardiovascular and cerebrovascular disorders and respiratory disease. Unless GH levels are controlled, survival is reduced by an average of 10 years compared with an age-matched control population.

Laboratory investigation

Age- and sex-matched serum IGF-I levels are elevated in acromegaly. Consequently, an IGF-I level provides a useful laboratory screening measure when clinical

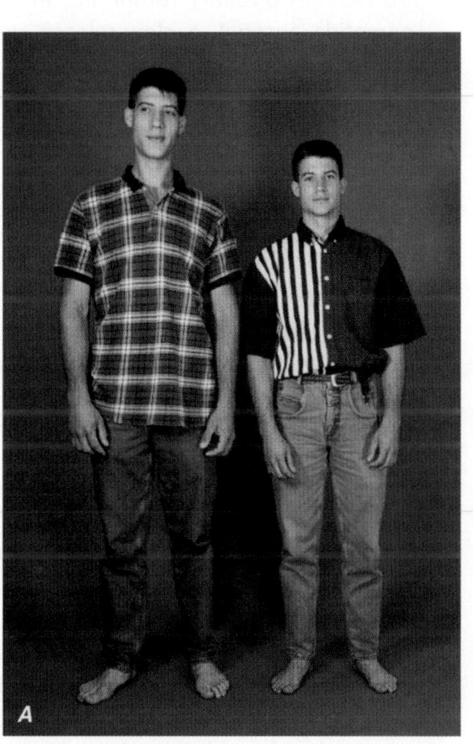

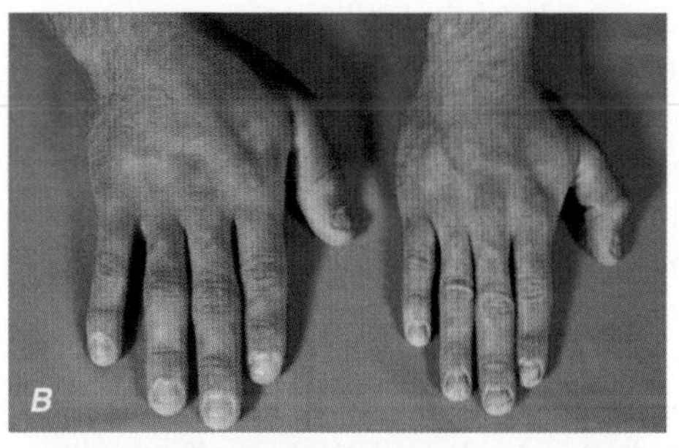

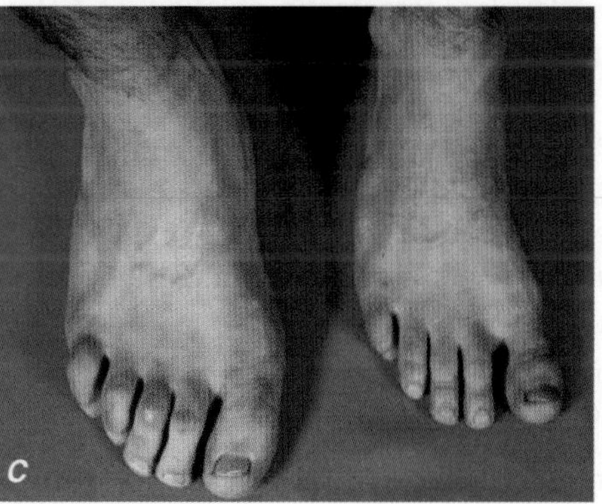

FIGURE 38-8

Features of acromegaly/gigantism. A 22-year-old man with gigantism due to excess growth hormone is shown to the left of his identical twin. The increased height and prognathism (***A***) and enlarged hand (***B***) and foot (***C***) of the affected twin are apparent. Their clinical features began to diverge at the age of approximately 13 years. (*Reproduced from R Gagel, IE McCutcheon: N Engl J Med 340:524, 1999; with permission.*)

features raise the possibility of acromegaly. Due to the pulsatility of GH secretion, measurement of a single random GH level is not useful for the diagnosis or exclusion of acromegaly and does not correlate with disease severity. The diagnosis of acromegaly is confirmed by demonstrating the failure of GH suppression to <0.4 μg/L within 1–2 h of an oral glucose load (75 g). When newer ultrasensitive GH assays are used, normal nadir GH levels are even lower (<0.05 μg/L). About 20% of patients exhibit a paradoxical GH rise after glucose. PRL should be measured, as it is elevated in ~25% of patients with acromegaly. Thyroid function, gonadotropins, and sex steroids may be attenuated because of tumor mass effects. Because most patients will undergo surgery with glucocorticoid coverage, tests of ACTH reserve in asymptomatic patients are more efficiently deferred until after surgery.

TREATMENT Acromegaly

The goal of treatment is to control GH and IGF-I hypersecretion, ablate or arrest tumor growth, ameliorate comorbidities, restore mortality rates to normal, and preserve pituitary function.

Surgical resection of GH-secreting adenomas is the initial treatment for most patients (Fig. 38-9). Somatostatin analogues are used as adjuvant treatment for preoperative shrinkage of large invasive macroadenomas, immediate relief of debilitating symptoms, and reduction of GH hypersecretion; in frail patients experiencing morbidity; and in patients who decline surgery or, when surgery fails, to achieve biochemical control. Irradiation or repeat surgery may be required for patients who cannot tolerate or do not respond to adjunctive medical therapy. The high rate of late hypopituitarism and the slow rate (5–15 years) of biochemical response are the main disadvantages of radiotherapy. Irradiation is also relatively ineffective in normalizing IGF-I levels. Stereotactic ablation of GH-secreting adenomas by gamma-knife radiotherapy is promising, but initial reports suggest that long-term results and side effects are similar to those observed with conventional radiation. Somatostatin analogues may be required while awaiting the full benefits of radiotherapy. Systemic sequelae of acromegaly, including cardiovascular disease, diabetes, and arthritis, should be managed aggressively. Mandibular surgical repair may be indicated.

SURGERY Transsphenoidal surgical resection by an experienced surgeon is the preferred primary treatment for both microadenomas (cure rate ~70%) and macroadenomas (<50% cured). Soft tissue swelling improves immediately after tumor resection. GH levels return to normal within an hour, and IGF-I levels are normalized within 3–4 days. In ~10% of patients, acromegaly may recur several years after apparently successful surgery; hypopituitarism develops in up to 15% of patients after surgery.

SOMATOSTATIN ANALOGUES Somatostatin analogues exert their therapeutic effects through SSTR2 and SSTR5 receptors, both of which invariably are expressed by GH-secreting tumors. Octreotide acetate is an eight-amino-acid synthetic somatostatin analogue. In contrast to native somatostatin, the analogue is relatively resistant to plasma degradation. It has a 2-h serum half-life and possesses 40-fold greater potency than native somatostatin to suppress GH. Octreotide is administered by subcutaneous injection, beginning with 50 μg tid; the dose can be increased gradually up to 1500 μg/d. Fewer than 10% of patients do not respond to the analogue. Octreotide suppresses integrated GH levels and normalizes IGF-I levels in ~75% of treated patients.

The long-acting somatostatin depot formulations, octreotide and lanreotide, are the preferred medical treatment for patients with acromegaly. *Sandostatin-LAR* is a sustained-release, long-acting formulation of octreotide incorporated into microspheres that sustain drug levels for several weeks after intramuscular injection. GH suppression occurs for as long as 6 weeks after a 30-mg intramuscular injection; long-term monthly treatment sustains GH and IGF-I suppression and also reduces pituitary tumor size in ~50% of patients. *Lanreotide* autogel, a slow-release depot somatostatin preparation, is a cyclic somatostatin octapeptide analogue that suppresses GH and IGF-I hypersecretion after a 60-mg subcutaneous injection. Long-term monthly administration controls GH hypersecretion in two-thirds of treated patients and improves patient compliance because of the long interval required between drug injections. Rapid relief of headache and soft tissue swelling occurs in ~75% of patients within days to weeks of somatostatin analogue initiation. Most patients report symptomatic improvement, including amelioration of headache, perspiration, obstructive apnea, and cardiac failure.

Side Effects Somatostatin analogues are well tolerated in most patients. Adverse effects are short-lived and mostly relate to drug-induced suppression of gastrointestinal motility and secretion. Nausea, abdominal discomfort, fat malabsorption, diarrhea, and flatulence occur in one-third of patients, and these symptoms usually remit within 2 weeks. Octreotide suppresses postprandial gallbladder contractility and delays gallbladder emptying; up to 30% of patients develop long-term echogenic sludge or asymptomatic cholesterol gallstones. Other side effects include mild glucose intolerance due to transient insulin suppression, asymptomatic bradycardia, hypothyroxinemia, and local injection site discomfort.

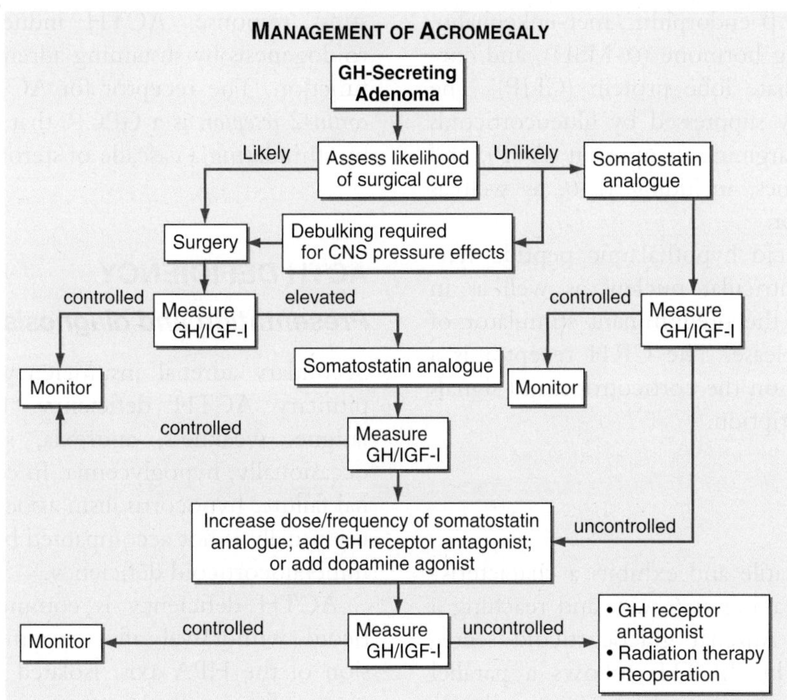

FIGURE 38-9

Management of acromegaly. GH, growth hormone; CNS, central nervous system; IGF, insulin-like growth factor. (*Adapted from S Melmed et al: J Clin Endocrinol Metab 94:1509–1517, 2009; © The Endocrine Society.*)

GH RECEPTOR ANTAGONIST Pegvisomant antagonizes endogenous GH action by blocking peripheral GH binding to its receptor. Consequently, serum IGF-I levels are suppressed, reducing the deleterious effects of excess endogenous GH. Pegvisomant is administered by daily subcutaneous injection (10–20 mg) and normalizes IGF-I in >90% of patients. GH levels, however, remain elevated as the drug does not have antitumor actions. Side effects include reversible liver enzyme elevation, lipodystrophy, and injection site pain. Tumor size should be monitored by MRI.

Combined treatment with monthly somatostatin analogues and weekly or biweekly pegvisomant injections has been used effectively in resistant patients.

DOPAMINE AGONISTS Bromocriptine and cabergoline may modestly suppress GH secretion in some patients. High doses of bromocriptine (≥20 mg/d) or cabergoline (0.5 mg/d) are usually required to achieve modest GH therapeutic efficacy. Combined treatment with octreotide and cabergoline may induce additive biochemical control compared with either drug alone.

RADIATION External radiation therapy or high-energy stereotactic techniques are used as adjuvant therapy for acromegaly. An advantage of radiation is that patient compliance with long-term treatment is not required. Tumor mass is reduced, and GH levels are attenuated over time. However, 50% of patients require at least 8 years for GH levels to be suppressed to <5 μg/L; this level of GH reduction is achieved in about 90% of patients after 18 years but represents suboptimal GH suppression. Patients may require interim medical therapy for several years before attaining maximal radiation benefits. Most patients also experience hypothalamic-pituitary damage, leading to gonadotropin, ACTH, and/or TSH deficiency within 10 years of therapy.

In summary, surgery is the preferred primary treatment for GH-secreting microadenomas (Fig. 38-9). The high frequency of GH hypersecretion after macroadenoma resection usually necessitates adjuvant or primary medical therapy for these larger tumors. Patients unable to receive or respond to unimodal medical treatment may benefit from combined treatments or can be offered radiation.

ADRENOCORTICOTROPIC HORMONE

SYNTHESIS

ACTH-secreting corticotrope cells constitute about 20% of the pituitary cell population. ACTH (39 amino acids) is derived from the POMC precursor protein (266 amino acids) that also generates several other peptides, including β-lipotropin, β-endorphin, met-enkephalin, α-melanocyte-stimulating hormone (α-MSH), and corticotropin-like intermediate lobe protein (CLIP). The POMC gene is potently suppressed by glucocorticoids and induced by CRH, arginine vasopressin (AVP), and proinflammatory cytokines, including IL-6, as well as leukemia inhibitory factor.

CRH, a 41-amino-acid hypothalamic peptide synthesized in the paraventricular nucleus as well as in higher brain centers, is the predominant stimulator of ACTH synthesis and release. The CRH receptor is a GPCR that is expressed on the corticotrope and signals to induce POMC transcription.

SECRETION

ACTH secretion is pulsatile and exhibits a characteristic circadian rhythm, peaking at 6 A.M. and reaching a nadir about midnight. Adrenal glucocorticoid secretion, which is driven by ACTH, follows a parallel diurnal pattern. ACTH circadian rhythmicity is determined by variations in secretory pulse amplitude rather than changes in pulse frequency. Superimposed on this endogenous rhythm, ACTH levels are increased by physical and psychological stress, exercise, acute illness, and insulin-induced hypoglycemia.

Loss of cortisol feedback inhibition, as occurs in primary adrenal failure, results in extremely high ACTH levels. Glucocorticoid-mediated negative regulation of the hypothalamic-pituitary-adrenal (HPA) axis occurs as a consequence of both hypothalamic CRH suppression and direct attenuation of pituitary POMC gene expression and ACTH release.

Acute inflammatory or septic insults activate the HPA axis through the integrated actions of proinflammatory cytokines, bacterial toxins, and neural signals. The overlapping cascade of ACTH-inducing cytokines (tumor necrosis factor [TNF]; IL-1, -2, and -6; and leukemia inhibitory factor) activates hypothalamic CRH and AVP secretion, pituitary POMC gene expression, and local pituitary paracrine cytokine networks. The resulting cortisol elevation restrains the inflammatory response and enables host protection. Concomitantly, cytokine-mediated central glucocorticoid receptor resistance impairs glucocorticoid suppression of the HPA. Thus, the neuroendocrine stress response reflects the net result of highly integrated hypothalamic, intrapituitary, and peripheral hormone and cytokine signals.

ACTION

The major function of the HPA axis is to maintain metabolic homeostasis and mediate the neuroendocrine stress response. ACTH induces adrenocortical steroidogenesis by sustaining adrenal cell proliferation and function. The receptor for ACTH, designated *melanocortin-2 receptor*, is a GPCR that induces steroidogenesis by stimulating a cascade of steroidogenic enzymes.

ACTH DEFICIENCY

Presentation and diagnosis

Secondary adrenal insufficiency occurs as a result of pituitary ACTH deficiency. It is characterized by fatigue, weakness, anorexia, nausea, vomiting, and, occasionally, hypoglycemia. In contrast to primary adrenal failure, hypocortisolism associated with pituitary failure usually is not accompanied by hyperpigmentation or mineralocorticoid deficiency.

ACTH deficiency is commonly due to glucocorticoid withdrawal after treatment-associated suppression of the HPA axis. Isolated ACTH deficiency may occur after surgical resection of an ACTH-secreting pituitary adenoma that has suppressed the HPA axis; this phenomenon is suggestive of a surgical cure. The mass effects of other pituitary adenomas or sellar lesions may lead to ACTH deficiency, but usually in combination with other pituitary hormone deficiencies. Partial ACTH deficiency may be unmasked in the presence of an acute medical or surgical illness, when clinically significant hypocortisolism reflects diminished ACTH reserve. Rarely, *TPIT* or *POMC* mutations result in primary ACTH deficiency.

Laboratory diagnosis

Inappropriately low ACTH levels in the setting of low cortisol levels are characteristic of diminished ACTH reserve. Low basal serum cortisol levels are associated with blunted cortisol responses to ACTH stimulation and impaired cortisol response to insulin-induced hypoglycemia, or testing with metyrapone or CRH.

TREATMENT ACTH Deficiency

Glucocorticoid replacement therapy improves most features of ACTH deficiency. The total daily dose of hydrocortisone replacement preferably should not exceed 25 mg daily, divided into two or three doses. Prednisone (5 mg each morning) is longer-acting and has fewer mineralocorticoid effects than hydrocortisone. Some authorities advocate lower maintenance doses in an effort to avoid cushingoid side effects. Doses should be increased severalfold during periods of acute illness or stress.

CUSHING'S SYNDROME (ACTH-PRODUCING ADENOMA)

Etiology and prevalence

Pituitary corticotrope adenomas account for 70% of patients with endogenous causes of Cushing's syndrome. However, it should be emphasized that iatrogenic hypercortisolism is the most common cause of cushingoid features. Ectopic tumor ACTH production, cortisol-producing adrenal adenomas, adrenal carcinoma, and adrenal hyperplasia account for the other causes; rarely, ectopic tumor CRH production is encountered.

ACTH-producing adenomas account for about 10–15% of all pituitary tumors. Because the clinical features of Cushing's syndrome often lead to early diagnosis, most ACTH-producing pituitary tumors are relatively small microadenomas. However, macroadenomas also are seen while some ACTH-expressing adenomas are clinically silent. Cushing's disease is 5–10 times more common in women than in men. These pituitary adenomas exhibit unrestrained ACTH secretion, with resultant hypercortisolemia. However, they retain partial suppressibility in the presence of high doses of administered glucocorticoids, providing the basis for dynamic testing to distinguish pituitary from nonpituitary causes of Cushing's syndrome.

Presentation and diagnosis

The diagnosis of Cushing's syndrome presents two great challenges: (1) to distinguish patients with pathologic cortisol excess from those with physiologic or other disturbances of cortisol production and (2) to determine the etiology of cortisol excess.

Typical features of chronic cortisol excess include thin skin, central obesity, hypertension, plethoric moon facies, purple striae and easy bruisability, glucose intolerance or diabetes mellitus, gonadal dysfunction, osteoporosis, proximal muscle weakness, signs of hyperandrogenism (acne, hirsutism), and psychological disturbances (depression, mania, and psychoses) (Table 38-12). Hematopoietic features of hypercortisolism include leukocytosis, lymphopenia, and eosinopenia. Immune suppression includes delayed hypersensitivity. These protean yet commonly encountered manifestations of hypercortisolism make it challenging to decide which patients mandate formal laboratory evaluation. Certain features make pathologic causes of hypercortisolism more likely; they include characteristic central redistribution of fat, thin skin with striae and bruising, and proximal muscle weakness. In children and in young females, early osteoporosis may be particularly prominent. The primary cause of death is cardiovascular disease, but infections and risk of suicide are also increased.

TABLE 38-12

CLINICAL FEATURES OF CUSHING'S SYNDROME (ALL AGES)

SYMPTOMS/SIGNS	FREQUENCY, %
Obesity or weight gain (>115% ideal body weight)	80
Thin skin	80
Moon facies	75
Hypertension	75
Purple skin striae	65
Hirsutism	65
Menstrual disorders (usually amenorrhea)	60
Plethora	60
Abnormal glucose tolerance	55
Impotence	55
Proximal muscle weakness	50
Truncal obesity	50
Acne	45
Bruising	45
Mental changes	45
Osteoporosis	40
Edema of lower extremities	30
Hyperpigmentation	20
Hypokalemic alkalosis	15
Diabetes mellitus	15

Source: Adapted from MA Magiokou et al, in ME Wierman (ed): *Diseases of the Pituitary.* Totowa, NJ, Humana, 1997.

Rapid development of features of hypercortisolism associated with skin hyperpigmentation and severe myopathy suggests an ectopic source of ACTH. Hypertension, hypokalemic alkalosis, glucose intolerance, and edema are also more pronounced in these patients. Serum potassium levels <3.3 mmol/L are evident in ~70% of patients with ectopic ACTH secretion but are seen in <10% of patients with pituitary-dependent Cushing's syndrome.

Laboratory investigation

The diagnosis of Cushing's syndrome is based on laboratory documentation of endogenous hypercortisolism. Measurement of 24-h urine free cortisol (UFC) is a precise and cost-effective screening test. Alternatively, the failure to suppress plasma cortisol after an overnight 1-mg dexamethasone suppression test can be used to identify patients with hypercortisolism. As nadir levels of cortisol occur at night, elevated midnight samples of cortisol are suggestive of Cushing's syndrome. Basal plasma ACTH levels often distinguish patients with ACTH-independent (adrenal or exogenous glucocorticoid) from those with ACTH-dependent (pituitary, ectopic ACTH) Cushing's syndrome. Mean basal ACTH levels are about eightfold higher in patients with ectopic ACTH secretion than in those with pituitary ACTH-secreting adenomas. However, extensive overlap of ACTH levels in these two disorders precludes using ACTH measurements to make the distinction. Instead, dynamic testing based on differential sensitivity to glucocorticoid feedback or ACTH stimulation in response to CRH or cortisol reduction is used to distinguish ectopic from pituitary sources of excess ACTH (Table 38-13). Very rarely, circulating CRH levels are elevated, reflecting ectopic tumor-derived secretion of CRH and often ACTH.

Most ACTH-secreting pituitary tumors are <5 mm in diameter, and about half are undetectable by sensitive MRI. The high prevalence of incidental pituitary microadenomas diminishes the ability to distinguish ACTH-secreting pituitary tumors accurately from nonsecreting incidentalomas.

Inferior petrosal venous sampling

Because pituitary MRI with gadolinium enhancement is insufficiently sensitive to detect small (<2 mm) pituitary ACTH-secreting adenomas, bilateral inferior petrosal sinus ACTH sampling before and after CRH administration may be required to distinguish these lesions from ectopic ACTH-secreting tumors that may have similar clinical and biochemical characteristics. Simultaneous assessment of ACTH in each inferior petrosal vein and in the peripheral circulation provides a strategy for confirming and localizing pituitary ACTH production. Sampling is performed at baseline and 2, 5, and 10 min after intravenous bovine CRH (1 μg/kg) injection. An increased ratio (>2) of inferior petrosal:peripheral vein ACTH confirms pituitary Cushing's syndrome. After CRH injection, peak petrosal:peripheral ACTH ratios ≥3 confirm the presence of a pituitary ACTH-secreting tumor. The sensitivity of this test is >95%, with very rare false-positive results. False-negative results may be encountered in patients with aberrant venous drainage. Petrosal sinus catheterizations are technically difficult, and about 0.05% of patients develop neurovascular complications. The procedure should not be performed

TABLE 38-13

DIFFERENTIAL DIAGNOSIS OF ACTH-DEPENDENT CUSHING'S SYNDROME[a]

	ACTH-SECRETING PITUITARY TUMOR	ECTOPIC ACTH SECRETION
Etiology	Pituitary corticotrope adenoma Plurihormonal adenoma	Bronchial, abdominal carcinoid Small cell lung cancer Thymoma
Sex	F > M	M > F
Clinical features	Slow onset	Rapid onset Pigmentation Severe myopathy
Serum potassium <3.3 μg/L	<10%	75%
24-h urinary free cortisol (UFC)	High	High
Basal ACTH level	Inappropriately high	Very high
Dexamethasone suppression		
1 mg overnight		
Low dose (0.5 mg q6h)	Cortisol >5 μg/dL	Cortisol >5 μg/dL
High dose (2 mg q6h)	Cortisol <5 μg/dL	Cortisol >5 μg/dL
UFC >80% suppressed	Microadenomas: 90% Macroadenomas: 50%	10%
Inferior petrosal sinus sampling (IPSS)		
Basal		
IPSS: peripheral	>2	<2
CRH-induced		
IPSS: peripheral	>3	<3

[a]ACTH-independent causes of Cushing's syndrome are diagnosed by suppressed ACTH levels and an adrenal mass in the setting of hypercortisolism. Iatrogenic Cushing's syndrome is excluded by history.

Abbreviations: ACTH, adrenocorticotropic hormone; CRH, corticotropin-releasing hormone; F, female; M, male.

in patients with hypertension or in the presence of a well-visualized pituitary adenoma on MRI.

TREATMENT Cushing's Syndrome

Selective transsphenoidal resection is the treatment of choice for Cushing's disease (Fig. 38-10). The remission rate for this procedure is ~80% for microadenomas but <50% for macroadenomas. After successful tumor resection, most patients experience a postoperative period of symptomatic ACTH deficiency that may last up to 12 months. This usually requires low-dose cortisol replacement, as patients experience both steroid withdrawal symptoms and have a suppressed HPA axis. Biochemical recurrence occurs in approximately 5% of patients in whom surgery was initially successful.

When initial surgery is unsuccessful, repeat surgery is sometimes indicated, particularly when a pituitary source for ACTH is well documented. In older patients, in whom issues of growth and fertility are less important, hemi- or total hypophysectomy may be necessary if a discrete pituitary adenoma is not recognized. Pituitary irradiation may be used after unsuccessful surgery, but it cures only about 15% of patients. Because the effects of radiation are slow and only partially effective in adults, steroidogenic inhibitors are used in combination with pituitary irradiation to block adrenal effects of persistently high ACTH levels.

Ketoconazole, an imidazole derivative antimycotic agent, inhibits several P450 enzymes and effectively lowers cortisol in most patients with Cushing's disease when administered twice daily (600–1200 mg/d). Elevated hepatic transaminases, gynecomastia, impotence, gastrointestinal upset, and edema are common side effects. *Metyrapone* (2–4 g/d) inhibits 11β-hydroxylase activity and normalizes plasma cortisol in up to 75% of patients. Side effects include nausea and vomiting, rash, and exacerbation of acne or hirsutism. *Mitotane* (*o,p′*-DDD; 3–6 g/d orally in four divided doses) suppresses cortisol hypersecretion by inhibiting 11β-hydroxylase and cholesterol side-chain cleavage enzymes and by destroying adrenocortical cells. Side effects of mitotane include gastrointestinal symptoms, dizziness, gynecomastia, hyperlipidemia, skin rash, and hepatic enzyme elevation. It also may lead to hypoaldosteronism. Other agents include *aminoglutethimide* (250 mg tid), trilostane (200–1000 mg/d), *cyproheptadine* (24 mg/d), and IV etomidate (0.3 mg/kg per hour). Glucocorticoid insufficiency is a potential side effect of agents used to block steroidogenesis.

The use of steroidogenic inhibitors has decreased the need for bilateral adrenalectomy. Removal of both adrenal glands corrects hypercortisolism but may be associated with significant morbidity rates and necessitates permanent glucocorticoid and mineralocorticoid replacement. Adrenalectomy in the setting of residual corticotrope adenoma tissue predisposes to the development of *Nelson's syndrome*, a disorder characterized by rapid pituitary tumor enlargement and increased pigmentation secondary to high ACTH levels. Radiation therapy may be indicated to prevent the development of Nelson's syndrome after adrenalectomy.

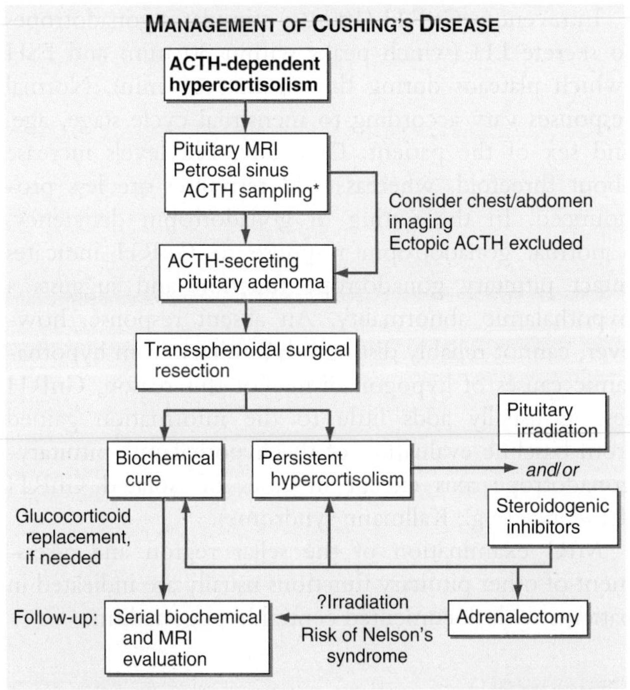

FIGURE 38-10

Management of Cushing's syndrome. ACTH, adrenocorticotropin hormone; MRI, magnetic resonance imaging. *Not usually required.

GONADOTROPINS: FSH AND LH

SYNTHESIS AND SECRETION

Gonadotrope cells constitute about 10% of anterior pituitary cells and produce two gonadotropins—LH and FSH. Like TSH and hCG, LH and FSH are glycoprotein hormones that consist of α and β subunits. The α subunit is common to these glycoprotein hormones; specificity is conferred by the β subunits, which are expressed by separate genes.

Gonadotropin synthesis and release are dynamically regulated. This is particularly true in women, in whom rapidly fluctuating gonadal steroid levels vary throughout the menstrual cycle. Hypothalamic GnRH, a 10-amino-acid peptide, regulates the synthesis and secretion of both LH and FSH. GnRH is secreted in discrete pulses every 60–120 min, and the pulses in turn elicit LH and FSH pulses (Fig. 38-3). The pulsatile mode of GnRH input is essential to its action; pulses prime gonadotrope responsiveness, whereas continuous GnRH exposure induces desensitization. Based on this phenomenon, long-acting GnRH agonists are used to suppress gonadotropin levels in children with precocious puberty and in men with prostate cancer and are used in some ovulation-induction protocols to reduce levels of endogenous gonadotropins. Estrogens act at both the hypothalamus and the pituitary to modulate gonadotropin secretion. Chronic estrogen exposure is inhibitory, whereas rising estrogen levels, as occur during the preovulatory surge, exert positive feedback to increase gonadotropin pulse frequency and amplitude. Progesterone slows GnRH pulse frequency but enhances gonadotropin responses to GnRH. Testosterone feedback in men also occurs at the hypothalamic and pituitary levels and is mediated in part by its conversion to estrogens.

Although GnRH is the main regulator of LH and FSH secretion, FSH synthesis is also under separate control by the gonadal peptides inhibin and activin, which are members of the transforming growth factor β (TGF-β) family. Inhibin selectively suppresses FSH, whereas activin stimulates FSH synthesis.

ACTION

The gonadotropin hormones interact with their respective GPCRs expressed in the ovary and testis, evoking germ cell development and maturation and steroid hormone biosynthesis. In women, FSH regulates ovarian follicle development and stimulates ovarian estrogen production. LH mediates ovulation and maintenance of the corpus luteum. In men, LH induces Leydig cell testosterone synthesis and secretion and FSH stimulates seminiferous tubule development and regulates spermatogenesis.

GONADOTROPIN DEFICIENCY

Hypogonadism is the most common presenting feature of adult hypopituitarism even when other pituitary hormones are also deficient. It is often a harbinger of hypothalamic or pituitary lesions that impair GnRH production or delivery through the pituitary stalk. As noted earlier, hypogonadotropic hypogonadism is a common presenting feature of hyperprolactinemia.

A variety of inherited and acquired disorders are associated with *isolated hypogonadotropic hypogonadism* (IHH). Hypothalamic defects associated with GnRH deficiency include two X-linked disorders, Kallmann syndrome (discussed earlier) and mutations in the *DAX1* gene, as well as dominant mutations in *FGFR1*. Mutations in *GPR54*, kisspeptin, the GnRH receptor, and the LH β or FSH β subunit genes are additional causes of selective gonadotropin deficiency. Acquired forms of GnRH deficiency leading to hypogonadotropism are seen in association with anorexia nervosa, stress, starvation, and extreme exercise but also may be idiopathic. Hypogonadotropic hypogonadism in these disorders is reversed by removal of the stressful stimulus or by caloric replenishment.

Presentation and diagnosis

In premenopausal women, hypogonadotropic hypogonadism presents as diminished ovarian function leading to oligomenorrhea or amenorrhea, infertility, decreased vaginal secretions, decreased libido, and breast atrophy. In hypogonadal adult men, secondary testicular failure is associated with decreased libido and potency, infertility, decreased muscle mass with weakness, reduced beard and body hair growth, soft testes, and characteristic fine facial wrinkles. Osteoporosis occurs in both untreated hypogonadal women and men.

Laboratory investigation

Central hypogonadism is associated with low or inappropriately normal serum gonadotropin levels in the setting of low sex hormone concentrations (testosterone in men, estradiol in women). Because gonadotropin secretion is pulsatile, valid assessments may require repeated measurements or the use of pooled serum samples. Men have reduced sperm counts.

Intravenous GnRH (100 μg) stimulates gonadotropes to secrete LH (which peaks within 30 min) and FSH (which plateaus during the ensuing 60 min). Normal responses vary according to menstrual cycle stage, age, and sex of the patient. Generally, LH levels increase about threefold, whereas FSH responses are less pronounced. In the setting of gonadotropin deficiency, a normal gonadotropin response to GnRH indicates intact pituitary gonadotrope function and suggests a hypothalamic abnormality. An absent response, however, cannot reliably distinguish pituitary from hypothalamic causes of hypogonadism. For this reason, GnRH testing usually adds little to the information gained from baseline evaluation of the hypothalamic-pituitary-gonadotrope axis except in cases of isolated GnRH deficiency (e.g., Kallmann syndrome).

MRI examination of the sellar region and assessment of other pituitary functions usually are indicated in patients with documented central hypogonadism.

TREATMENT Gonadotropin Deficiency

In males, testosterone replacement is necessary to achieve and maintain normal growth and development of the external genitalia, secondary sex characteristics, male sexual behavior, and androgenic anabolic effects, including maintenance of muscle function and bone mass. Testosterone may be administered by intramuscular injections every 1–4 weeks or by using skin patches that are replaced daily. Testosterone gels are also available. Gonadotropin injections (hCG or human menopausal gonadotropin [hMG]) over 12–18 months are used to restore fertility. Pulsatile GnRH therapy (25–150 ng/kg every 2 h), administered by a subcutaneous infusion pump, is also effective for treatment of hypothalamic hypogonadism when fertility is desired.

In premenopausal women, cyclical replacement of estrogen and progesterone maintains secondary sexual characteristics and integrity of genitourinary tract mucosa and prevents premature osteoporosis. Gonadotropin therapy is used for ovulation induction. Follicular growth and maturation are initiated using hMG or recombinant FSH; hCG or human luteinizing hormone (hLH) is subsequently injected to induce ovulation. As in men, pulsatile GnRH therapy can be used to treat hypothalamic causes of gonadotropin deficiency.

NONFUNCTIONING AND GONADOTROPIN-PRODUCING PITUITARY ADENOMAS

Etiology and prevalence

Nonfunctioning pituitary adenomas include those that secrete little or no pituitary hormones as well as tumors that produce too little hormone to result in recognizable clinical features. They are the most common type of pituitary adenoma and are usually macroadenomas at the time of diagnosis because clinical features are not apparent until tumor mass effects occur. Based on immunohistochemistry, most clinically nonfunctioning adenomas can be shown to originate from gonadotrope cells. These tumors typically produce small amounts of intact gonadotropins (usually FSH) as well as uncombined α, LH β, and FSH β subunits. Tumor secretion may lead to elevated α and FSH β subunits and, rarely, to increased LH β subunit levels. Some adenomas express α subunits without FSH or LH. TRH administration often induces an atypical increase of tumor-derived gonadotropins or subunits.

Presentation and diagnosis

Clinically nonfunctioning tumors often present with optic chiasm pressure and other symptoms of local expansion or may be incidentally discovered on an MRI performed for another indication (incidentaloma). Rarely, menstrual disturbances or ovarian hyperstimulation occur in women with large tumors that produce FSH and LH. More commonly, adenoma compression of the pituitary stalk or surrounding pituitary tissue leads to attenuated LH and features of hypogonadism. PRL levels are usually slightly increased, also because of stalk compression. It is important to distinguish this circumstance from true prolactinomas, as nonfunctioning tumors do not shrink in response to treatment with dopamine agonists.

Laboratory investigation

The goal of laboratory testing in clinically nonfunctioning tumors is to classify the type of the tumor, identify hormonal markers of tumor activity, and detect possible hypopituitarism. Free α subunit levels may be elevated in 10–15% of patients with nonfunctioning tumors. In female patients, peri- or postmenopausal basal FSH concentrations are difficult to distinguish from tumor-derived FSH elevation. Premenopausal women have cycling FSH levels, also preventing clear-cut diagnostic distinction from tumor-derived FSH. In men, gonadotropin-secreting tumors may be diagnosed because of slightly increased gonadotropins (FSH > LH) in the setting of a pituitary mass. Testosterone levels are usually low despite the normal or increased LH level, perhaps reflecting reduced LH bioactivity or the loss of normal LH pulsatility. Because this pattern of hormone test results is also seen in primary gonadal failure and, to some extent, with aging, the finding of increased gonadotropins alone is insufficient for the diagnosis of a gonadotropin-secreting tumor. In the majority of patients with gonadotrope adenomas, TRH administration stimulates LH β subunit secretion; this response is not seen in normal individuals. GnRH testing, however, is not helpful for making the diagnosis. For nonfunctioning and gonadotropin-secreting tumors, the diagnosis usually rests on immunohistochemical analyses of surgically resected tumor tissue, as the mass effects of these tumors usually necessitate resection.

Although acromegaly or Cushing's syndrome usually presents with unique clinical features, clinically inapparent (silent) somatotrope or corticotrope adenomas may only be diagnosed by immunostaining of resected tumor tissue. If PRL levels are <100 μg/L in a patient harboring a pituitary mass, a nonfunctioning adenoma causing pituitary stalk compression should be considered.

TREATMENT **Nonfunctioning and Gonadotropin-Producing Pituitary Adenomas**

Asymptomatic small nonfunctioning microadenomas adenomas with no threat to vision may be followed with regular MRI and visual field testing without immediate intervention. However, for macroadenomas, transsphenoidal surgery is indicated to reduce tumor size and relieve mass

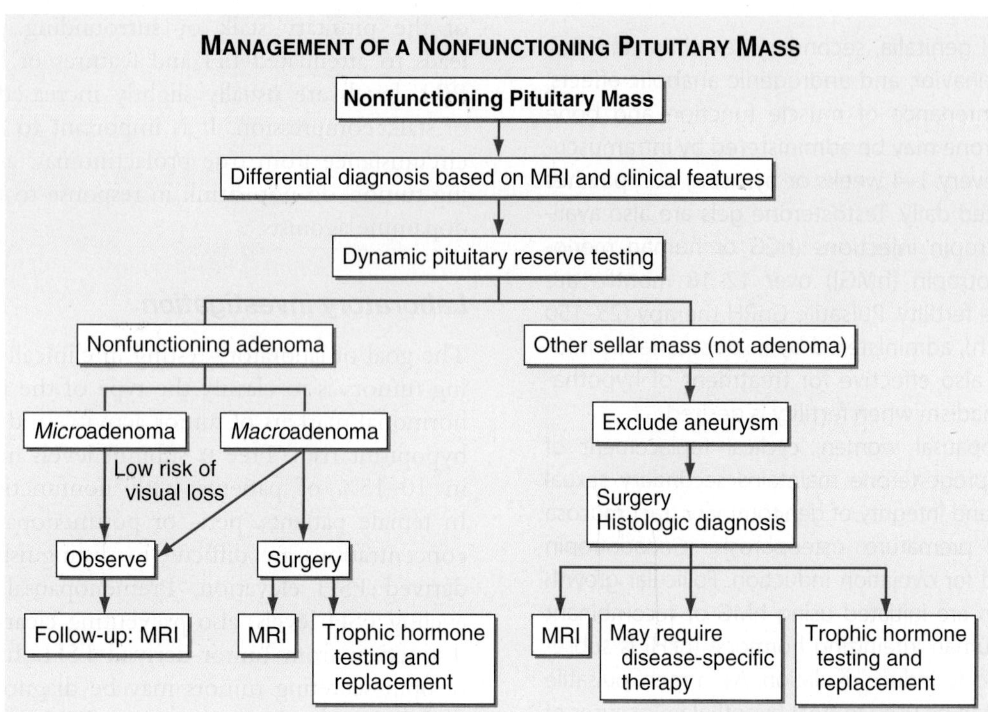

FIGURE 38-11
Management of a nonfunctioning pituitary mass.

effects (Fig. 38-11). Although it is not usually possible to remove all adenoma tissue surgically, vision improves in 70% of patients with preoperative visual field defects. Preexisting hypopituitarism that results from tumor mass effects may improve or resolve completely. Beginning about 6 months postoperatively, MRI scans should be performed yearly to detect tumor regrowth. Within 5–6 years after successful surgical resection, ~15% of nonfunctioning tumors recur. When substantial tumor remains after transsphenoidal surgery, adjuvant radiotherapy may be indicated to prevent tumor regrowth. Radiotherapy may be deferred if no postoperative residual mass is evident.

Nonfunctioning pituitary tumors respond poorly to dopamine agonist treatment and somatostatin analogues are largely ineffective for shrinking these tumors. The selective GnRH antagonist Nal-Glu GnRH suppresses FSH hypersecretion but has no effect on adenoma size.

THYROID-STIMULATING HORMONE

SYNTHESIS AND SECRETION

TSH-secreting thyrotrope cells constitute 5% of the anterior pituitary cell population. TSH is structurally related to LH and FSH. It shares a common α subunit with these hormones but contains a specific TSH β subunit. TRH is a hypothalamic tripeptide (pyroglutamyl histidylprolinamide) that acts through a GPCR to stimulate TSH synthesis and secretion; it also stimulates the lactotrope cell to secrete PRL. TSH secretion is stimulated by TRH, whereas thyroid hormones, dopamine, somatostatin, and glucocorticoids suppress TSH by overriding TRH induction.

Thyrotrope growth and TSH secretion are both induced when negative feedback inhibition by thyroid hormones is removed. Thus, thyroid damage (including surgical thyroidectomy), radiation-induced hypothyroidism, chronic thyroiditis, and prolonged goitrogen exposure are associated with increased TSH. Long-standing untreated hypothyroidism can lead to thyrotrope hyperplasia and pituitary enlargement, which may be evident on MRI.

ACTION

TSH is secreted in pulses, though the excursions are modest in comparison to other pituitary hormones because of the low amplitude of the pulses and the relatively long half-life of TSH. Consequently, single determinations of TSH suffice to assess its circulating levels. TSH binds to a GPCR on thyroid follicular cells to stimulate thyroid hormone synthesis and release.

TSH DEFICIENCY

Features of central hypothyroidism due to TSH deficiency mimic those seen with primary hypothyroidism but are generally less severe. Pituitary hypothyroidism is characterized by low basal TSH levels in the setting of low free thyroid hormone. In contrast, patients with hypothyroidism of hypothalamic origin (presumably due to a lack of endogenous TRH) may exhibit normal or even slightly elevated TSH levels. The TSH produced in this circumstance appears to have reduced biologic activity because of altered glycosylation.

TRH (200 μg) injected intravenously causes a two- to threefold increase in TSH (and PRL) levels within 30 min. Although TRH testing can be used to assess TSH reserve, abnormalities of the thyroid axis usually can be detected based on basal free T_4 and TSH levels, and TRH testing is rarely indicated.

Thyroid-replacement therapy should be initiated after adequate adrenal function has been established. Dose adjustment is based on thyroid hormone levels and clinical parameters rather than the TSH level.

TSH-SECRETING ADENOMAS

TSH-producing macroadenomas are rare but are often large and locally invasive when they occur. Patients usually present with thyroid goiter and hyperthyroidism, reflecting overproduction of TSH. Diagnosis is based on demonstrating elevated serum free T_4 levels, inappropriately normal or high TSH secretion, and MRI evidence of a pituitary adenoma.

It is important to exclude other causes of inappropriate TSH secretion, such as resistance to thyroid hormone, an autosomal dominant disorder caused by mutations in the thyroid hormone β receptor. The presence of a pituitary mass and elevated α subunit levels are suggestive of a TSH-secreting tumor. Dysalbuminemic hyperthyroxinemia syndromes, caused by mutations in serum thyroid hormone binding proteins, are also characterized by elevated thyroid hormone levels, but with normal rather than suppressed TSH levels. Moreover, free thyroid hormone levels are normal in these disorders, most of which are familial.

TREATMENT TSH-Secreting Adenomas

The initial therapeutic approach is to remove or debulk the tumor mass surgically, usually using a transsphenoidal approach. Total resection is not often achieved as most of these adenomas are large and locally invasive. Normal circulating thyroid hormone levels are achieved in about two-thirds of patients after surgery. Thyroid ablation or antithyroid drugs (methimazole and propylthiouracil) can be used to reduce thyroid hormone levels. Somatostatin analogue treatment effectively normalizes TSH and α subunit hypersecretion, shrinks the tumor mass in 50% of patients, and improves visual fields in 75% of patients; euthyroidism is restored in most patients. Because somatostatin analogues markedly suppress TSH, biochemical hypothyroidism often requires concomitant thyroid hormone replacement, which may also further control tumor growth.

CHAPTER 39

MULTIPLE SCLEROSIS AND OTHER DEMYELINATING DISEASES

Stephen L. Hauser ■ Douglas S. Goodin

Demyelinating disorders are immune-mediated conditions characterized by preferential destruction of central nervous system (CNS) myelin. The peripheral nervous system (PNS) is spared, and most patients have no evidence of an associated systemic illness. Multiple sclerosis (MS), the most common disease in this category, is second only to trauma as a cause of neurologic disability beginning in early to middle adulthood.

MULTIPLE SCLEROSIS

Multiple sclerosis (MS) is a chronic disease characterized by inflammation, demyelination, gliosis (scarring), and neuronal loss; the course can be relapsing-remitting or progressive. Lesions of MS typically occur at different times and in different CNS locations (i.e., disseminated in time and space). MS affects ~350,000 individuals in the United States and 2.5 million individuals worldwide. Manifestations of MS vary from a benign illness to a rapidly evolving and incapacitating disease requiring profound lifestyle adjustments.

PATHOGENESIS

Anatomy

New MS lesions begin with perivenular cuffing by inflammatory mononuclear cells, predominantly T cells and macrophages, which also infiltrate the surrounding white matter. At sites of inflammation, the blood-brain barrier (BBB) is disrupted, but unlike vasculitis, the vessel wall is preserved. Involvement of the humoral immune system is also evident; small numbers of B lymphocytes also infiltrate the nervous system, and myelin-specific autoantibodies are present on degenerating myelin sheaths. As lesions evolve, there is prominent astrocytic proliferation (gliosis). Surviving oligodendrocytes or those that differentiate from precursor cells can partially remyelinate the surviving naked axons, producing so-called shadow plaques. In many lesions, oligodendrocyte precursor cells are present in large numbers but fail to differentiate and remyelinate. Over time, ectopic lymphocyte follicles appear in perivascular and perimeningeal regions, consisting of aggregates of T and B cells and resembling secondary lymphoid structures. Although relative sparing of axons is typical of MS, partial or total axonal destruction can also occur, especially within highly inflammatory lesions. Thus, MS is not solely a disease of myelin, and neuronal pathology is increasingly recognized as a major contributor to irreversible neurologic disability. Inflammation and plaque formation are present in the cerebral cortex, and significant axon loss indicating death of neurons is widespread, specially in advanced cases (see "Neurodegeneration," later in this chapter).

Physiology

Nerve conduction in myelinated axons occurs in a saltatory manner, with the nerve impulse jumping from one node of Ranvier to the next without depolarization of the axonal membrane underlying the myelin sheath between nodes (Fig. 39-1). This produces considerably faster conduction velocities (~70 m/s) than the slow velocities (~1 m/s) produced by continuous propagation in unmyelinated nerves. Conduction block occurs when the nerve impulse is unable to traverse the demyelinated segment. This can happen when the resting axon membrane becomes hyperpolarized due to the exposure of voltage-dependent potassium channels that are normally buried underneath the myelin sheath. A temporary conduction block often follows a demyelinating event before sodium channels (originally

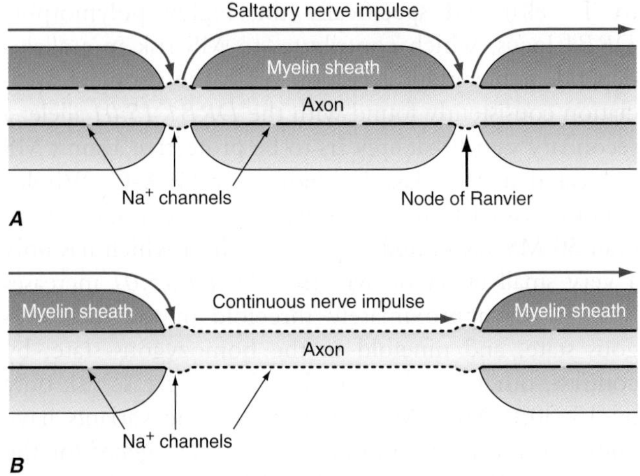

FIGURE 39-1
Nerve conduction in myelinated and demyelinated axons. ***A.*** Saltatory nerve conduction in myelinated axons occurs with the nerve impulse jumping from one node of Ranvier to the next. Sodium channels (shown as breaks in the solid black line) are concentrated at the nodes where axonal depolarization occurs. ***B.*** Following demyelination, additional sodium channels are redistributed along the axon itself, thereby allowing continuous propagation of the nerve action potential despite the absence of myelin.

concentrated at the nodes) redistribute along the naked axon (Fig. 39-1). This redistribution ultimately allows continuous propagation of nerve action potentials through the demyelinated segment. Conduction block may be incomplete, affecting high- but not low-frequency volleys of impulses. Variable conduction block can occur with raised body temperature or metabolic alterations and may explain clinical fluctuations that vary from hour to hour or appear with fever or exercise. Conduction slowing occurs when the demyelinated segments of the axonal membrane is reorganized to support continuous (slow) nerve impulse propagation.

Epidemiology

MS is approximately threefold more common in women than men. The age of onset is typically between 20 and 40 years (slightly later in men than in women), but the disease can present across the life span. In ~10% of cases it begins before age 18 years, and in a small percentage, it begins before the age of 10 years.

Geographic gradients have been repeatedly observed in MS, with the highest known prevalence for MS (250 per 100,000) in the Orkney Islands, located north of Scotland. In other temperate zone areas (e.g., northern North America, northern Europe, southern Australia, and south New Zealand), the prevalence of MS is 0.1–0.2%. By contrast, in the tropics (e.g., Asia, equatorial Africa, and the Middle East), the prevalence is often ten- to twentyfold less.

One proposed explanation for the latitude effect on MS is that there is a protective effect of sun exposure. Exposure of the skin to ultraviolet-B (UVB) radiation from the sun is essential for the biosynthesis of vitamin D, and this endogenous production is the most important source of vitamin D in most individuals. At high latitudes, the amount of UVB radiation reaching the earth's surface is often insufficient, particularly during winter months, and, consequently, low serum levels of vitamin D are common in temperate zones. Prospective studies have confirmed that vitamin D deficiency is associated with an increase in MS risk and preliminary data also suggest that ongoing deficiency may increase the relapse rate in established MS. Immunoregulatory effects of vitamin D could explain this apparent relationship.

At least three sequential (population-wide) environmental events are implicated in the causal pathway leading to MS. The first factor seems to occur either in utero or in the early postnatal period and is supported, in part, by the almost twofold increase in MS risk for dizygotic twins of MS probands (5.4%) compared to siblings (2.9%). It is also supported by the month-of-birth effect (in the northern hemisphere), in which May babies are significantly more likely, and November babies less likely, to develop MS compared to babies born in other months. Importantly, a recently published population-based study in the southern hemisphere (Australia) found a similar (but inverted) month-of-birth effect with the zenith in risk occurring for November/December babies and the nadir occurring for May/June babies. This month-of-birth effect provides evidence for an early environmental event, involved in MS pathogenesis, that is both coupled to the solar cycle and time-locked to birth.

A second factor seems to occur during adolescence. Thus, several studies suggest that when individuals move (prior to their adolescent years) from an area of high MS prevalence to an area of low prevalence (or vice versa), their MS risk becomes similar to that of the region to which they moved. By contrast, when they make the same move after adolescence, their MS risk remains similar to that of the region from which they moved.

Because both of these first two factors occur well before the onset of clinically evident MS, presumably other factors are also necessary. In addition, the identification of possible point epidemics suggests a possible role for infectious agents, although the only (partially) convincing example of this occurred in the Faeroe Islands north of Denmark after the British occupation during World War II.

The prevalence of MS has increased steadily (and dramatically) in several regions around the world over the past half-century, presumably reflecting the impact of some environmental shift. Moreover, the fact that this increase has occurred primarily (or exclusively) in women indicates that women are more responsive to whatever this environmental change has been. Interestingly, recent epidemiologic data suggest that the latitude effect on MS currently may be decreasing. The reason for these changes are not known but, potentially, could be related to the increased use of sun block, which (at SPF-15) blocks 94% of the incoming UVB radiation, and which would be expected to exacerbate any population-wide vitamin D deficiency and might also mitigate the impact of differences in UVB exposure.

MS risk also correlates with high socioeconomic status, which may reflect improved sanitation and delayed initial exposures to infectious agents. By analogy, some viral infections (e.g., poliomyelitis and measles viruses) produce neurologic sequelae more frequently when the age of initial infection is delayed. Evidence of a remote Epstein-Barr virus (EBV) infection playing some role in MS is supported by a number of epidemiologic and laboratory studies. A higher risk of infectious mononucleosis (associated with relatively late EBV infection) and higher antibody titers to latency-associated EBV nuclear antigen are associated with MS. At this time, however, a causal role for EBV is not definitively established.

GENETIC CONSIDERATIONS

Whites are inherently at higher risk for MS than Africans or Asians, even when residing in a similar environment. MS also aggregates within some families, and adoption, half-sibling, twin, and spousal studies indicate that familial aggregation is due to genetic, and not environmental, factors (Table 39-1).

Whites to MS is polygenic, with each gene contributing a relatively small amount to the overall risk. Despite this, the influence of genetics on MS pathogenesis is substantial. The major histocompatibility complex (MHC) on chromosome 6 is by far the strongest MS susceptibility region in the genome. Fine mapping studies implicate primarily the class II region (encoding HLA molecules involved in presenting peptide antigens to T cells) and specifically the highly polymorphic *DRB1* locus, which contributes to MS risk in a allele-dependent hierarchical fashion, with the strongest association consistently found with the *DRB1*15:01* allele; a secondary signal that appears to be protective against MS is located in the class 1 region near HLA-C. Whole-genome association studies have now identified more than 50 MS susceptibility genes, each of which has only a very small effect on MS risk. *DRB1*15:01* increases MS risk by approximately threefold in the heterozygous state, and ninefold in the homozygous state; by contrast, other MS-associated variants increase risk only by 15–30%. Most MS-associated genetic variants have known roles in the immune system (i.e., genes for the interleukin [IL]-7 receptor [CD127], the IL-2 receptor [CD25], and the T cell co-stimulatory molecule LFA-3 [CD58]); some variants also influence susceptibility to other autoimmune diseases in addition to MS. The variants identified thus far all lack specificity and sensitivity for MS; thus they are not useful for diagnosis or to predict the future course of the disease.

TABLE 39-1

RISK OF DEVELOPING MS	
1 in 3	If an identical twin has MS
1 in 15	If a fraternal twin has MS
1 in 25	If a sibling has MS
1 in 50	If a parent or half-sibling has MS
1 in 100	If a first cousin has MS
1 in 1000	If a spouse has MS
1 in 1000	If no one in the family has MS

Immunology

Autoreactive T lymphocytes

Myelin basic protein (MBP) is an important T cell antigen in experimental allergic encephalomyelitis (EAE), a laboratory model, and probably also in human MS. Activated MBP-reactive T cells have been identified in the blood, in cerebrospinal fluid (CSF), and within MS lesions. Moreover, *DRB1*15:01* may influence the autoimmune response because it binds with high affinity to a fragment of MBP (spanning amino acids 89–96), stimulating T cell responses to this self-protein. Two different populations of proinflammatory T cells are likely to mediate autoimmunity in MS. T-helper type 1 (T_H1) cells producing interferon γ (IFN-γ) are one key effector population, and more recently a role for highly proinflammatory T_H17 T cells has been established. T_H17 cells are induced by transforming growth factor β (TGF-β) and IL-6, and are amplified by IL-21 and IL-23. T_H17 cells, and levels of their corresponding cytokine IL-17, are increased in MS lesions and also in the circulation of people with active MS. High circulating levels of IL-17 may also be a marker of a more severe course of MS. T_H1 cytokines including interleukin (IL) 2, tumor necrosis factor (TNF) α, and interferon (IFN) γ also play key roles in activating and maintaining autoimmune responses, and TNF-α and IFN-γ may directly injure oligodendrocytes or the myelin membrane.

Humoral autoimmunity

B cell activation and antibody responses also appear to be necessary for the full development of demyelinating lesions to occur, both in experimental models and in human MS. Increased numbers of clonally expanded B cells with properties of postgerminal center memory or antibody-producing lymphocytes are present in MS lesions and in CSF. Myelin-specific autoantibodies, some directed against myelin oligodendrocyte glycoprotein (MOG), have been detected bound to vesiculated myelin debris in MS plaques. In the CSF, elevated levels of locally synthesized immunoglobulins and oligoclonal antibodies derived from expansion of clonally restricted plasma cells are also characteristic of MS. The pattern of oligoclonal banding is unique to each individual, and attempts to identify the targets of these antibodies have been largely unsuccessful.

Triggers

Serial MRI studies in early relapsing-remitting MS reveal that bursts of focal inflammatory disease activity occur far more frequently than would have been predicted by the frequency of relapses. Thus, early in MS most disease activity is clinically silent. The triggers causing these bursts are unknown, although the fact that patients may experience relapses after nonspecific upper respiratory infections suggests that either molecular mimicry between viruses and myelin antigens or viral super-antigens activating pathogenic T cells may be responsible.

Neurodegeneration

Axonal damage occurs in every newly formed MS lesion, and cumulative axonal loss is considered to be the major cause of progressive and irreversible neurologic disability in MS. As many as 70% of axons are lost from the lateral corticospinal (e.g., motor) tracts in patients with advanced paraparesis from MS, and longitudinal MRI studies suggest there is progressive axonal loss over time within established, inactive lesions. Knowledge of the mechanisms responsible for axonal injury is incomplete and, despite the fact that axonal transactions are most conspicuous in acute inflammatory lesions, it is still unclear whether demyelination is a prerequisite for axonal injury in MS. Demyelination can result in reduced trophic support for axons, redistribution of ion channels, and destabilization of action potential membrane potentials. Axons can adapt initially to these injuries; with time distal and retrograde degeneration often occurs. Therefore, promotion of remyelination and preservation of oligodendrocytes early in the disease course remain important therapeutic goals in MS. Some evidence suggests that axonal damage is mediated directly by resident and invading inflammatory cells and their toxic products, in particular by microglia, macrophages, and CD8 T lymphocytes. Activated microglia are particularly likely to cause axonal injury through the release of NO and oxygen radicals and via glutamate, which is toxic to oligodendrocytes and neurons. Interestingly, NMDA (glutamate) receptors are expressed on naked axon membranes that have undergone demyelination, perhaps providing a mechanism for glutamate-mediated calcium entry and cell death.

CLINICAL MANIFESTATIONS

The onset of MS may be abrupt or insidious. Symptoms may be severe or seem so trivial that a patient may not seek medical attention for months or years. Indeed, at autopsy, approximately 0.1% of individuals who were asymptomatic during life will be found, unexpectedly, to have pathologic evidence of MS. Similarly, in the modern era, an MRI scan obtained for an unrelated reason may show evidence of asymptomatic MS. Symptoms of MS are extremely varied and depend on the location and severity of lesions within the CNS (Table 39-2). Examination often reveals evidence of neurologic dysfunction, often in asymptomatic locations. For example, a patient may present with symptoms in one leg but signs in both.

Weakness of the limbs may manifest as loss of strength, speed, or dexterity, as fatigue, or a disturbance of gait. Exercise-induced weakness is a characteristic symptom of MS. The weakness is of the upper motor neuron type (Chap. 12) and is usually accompanied by other pyramidal signs such as spasticity, hyperreflexia, and Babinski's signs. Occasionally a tendon reflex may be lost (simulating a lower motor neuron lesion) if an MS lesion disrupts the afferent reflex fibers in the spinal cord (Fig. 12-2).

TABLE 39-2
INITIAL SYMPTOMS OF MS

SYMPTOM	PERCENT OF CASES	SYMPTOM	PERCENT OF CASES
Sensory loss	37	Lhermitte's	3
Optic neuritis	36	Pain	3
Weakness	35	Dementia	2
Paresthesias	24	Visual loss	2
Diplopia	15	Facial palsy	1
Ataxia	11	Impotence	1
Vertigo	6	Myokymia	1
Paroxysmal attacks	4	Epilepsy	1
Bladder	4	Falling	1

Source: After WB Matthews et al: *McAlpine's Multiple Sclerosis*, New York, Churchill Livingstone, 1991.

Spasticity (Chap. 12) is commonly associated with spontaneous and movement-induced muscle spasms. More than 30% of MS patients have moderate to severe spasticity, especially in the legs. This is often accompanied by painful spasms interfering with ambulation, work, or self-care. Occasionally spasticity provides support for the body weight during ambulation, and in these cases treatment of spasticity may actually do more harm than good.

Optic neuritis (ON) presents as diminished visual acuity, dimness, or decreased color perception (desaturation) in the central field of vision. These symptoms can be mild or may progress to severe visual loss. Rarely, there is complete loss of light perception. Visual symptoms are generally monocular but may be bilateral. Periorbital pain (aggravated by eye movement) often precedes or accompanies the visual loss. An afferent pupillary defect (Chap. 21) is usually present. Funduscopic examination may be normal or reveal optic disc swelling (papillitis). Pallor of the optic disc (optic atrophy) commonly follows ON. Uveitis is uncommon and should raise the possibility of alternative diagnoses such as sarcoid or lymphoma.

Visual blurring in MS may result from ON or diplopia (double vision); if the symptom resolves when either eye is covered, the cause is diplopia.

Diplopia may result from internuclear ophthalmoplegia (INO) or from palsy of the sixth cranial nerve (rarely the third or fourth). An INO consists of impaired adduction of one eye due to a lesion in the ipsilateral medial longitudinal fasciculus (Chap. 21). Prominent nystagmus is often observed in the abducting eye, along with a small skew deviation. A bilateral INO is particularly suggestive of MS. Other common gaze disturbances in MS include (1) a horizontal gaze palsy, (2) a "one and a half" syndrome (horizontal gaze palsy plus an INO), and (3) acquired pendular nystagmus.

Sensory symptoms are varied and include both paresthesias (e.g., tingling, prickling sensations, formications, "pins and needles," or painful burning) and hypesthesia (e.g., reduced sensation, numbness, or a "dead" feeling). Unpleasant sensations (e.g., feelings that body parts are swollen, wet, raw, or tightly wrapped) are also common. Sensory impairment of the trunk and legs below a horizontal line on the torso (a sensory level) indicates that the spinal cord is the origin of the sensory disturbance. It is often accompanied by a bandlike sensation of tightness around the torso. Pain is a common symptom of MS, experienced by >50% of patients. Pain can occur anywhere on the body and can change locations over time.

Ataxia usually manifests as cerebellar tremors (Chap. 31). Ataxia may also involve the head and trunk or the voice, producing a characteristic cerebellar dysarthria (scanning speech).

Bladder dysfunction is present in >90% of MS patients, and in a third of patients, dysfunction results in weekly or more frequent episodes of incontinence. During normal reflex voiding, relaxation of the bladder sphincter (α-adrenergic innervation) is coordinated with contraction of the detrusor muscle in the bladder wall (muscarinic cholinergic innervation). *Detrusor hyperreflexia*, due to impairment of suprasegmental inhibition, causes urinary frequency, urgency, nocturia, and uncontrolled bladder emptying. *Detrusor sphincter dyssynergia*, due to loss of synchronization between detrusor and sphincter muscles, causes difficulty in initiating and/or stopping the urinary stream, producing hesitancy, urinary retention, overflow incontinence, and recurrent infection.

Constipation occurs in >30% of patients. Fecal urgency or *bowel incontinence* is less common (15%) but can be socially debilitating.

Cognitive dysfunction can include memory loss, impaired attention, difficulties in executive functioning, memory, problem solving, slowed information processing, and problems shifting between cognitive tasks. Euphoria (elevated mood) was once thought to be characteristic of MS but is actually uncommon, occurring in <20% of patients. Cognitive dysfunction sufficient to impair activities of daily living is rare.

Depression, experienced by approximately half of patients, can be reactive, endogenous, or part of the illness itself, and can contribute to fatigue. *Fatigue* is experienced by 90% of patients; this symptom is the most common reason for work-related disability in MS. Fatigue can be exacerbated by elevated temperatures, by depression, by expending exceptional effort to accomplish basic activities of daily living, or by sleep disturbances (e.g., from frequent nocturnal awakenings to urinate).

Sexual dysfunction may manifest as decreased libido, impaired genital sensation, impotence in men, and diminished vaginal lubrication or adductor spasms in women.

Facial weakness due to a lesion in the pons may resemble idiopathic Bell's palsy (Chap. 34). Unlike Bell's palsy, facial weakness in MS is usually not associated with ipsilateral loss of taste sensation or retroauricular pain.

Vertigo may appear suddenly from a brainstem lesion, superficially resembling acute labyrinthitis (Chap. 11). *Hearing loss* may also occur in MS but is uncommon.

Ancillary symptoms

Heat sensitivity refers to neurologic symptoms produced by an elevation of the body's core temperature. For example, unilateral visual blurring may occur during a hot shower or with physical exercise (*Uhthoff's symptom*). It is also common for MS symptoms to worsen transiently, sometimes dramatically, during febrile illnesses (see "Acute Attacks or Initial Demyelinating Episodes," later). Such heat-related symptoms probably result from transient conduction block (discussed earlier).

Lhermitte's symptom is an electric shock–like sensation (typically induced by flexion or other movements of the neck) that radiates down the back into the legs. Rarely, it radiates into the arms. It is generally self-limited but may persist for years. Lhermitte's symptom can also occur with other disorders of the cervical spinal cord (e.g., cervical spondylosis).

Paroxysmal symptoms are distinguished by their brief duration (10 s to 2 min), high frequency (5–40 episodes per day), lack of any alteration of consciousness or change in background electroencephalogram during episodes, and a self-limited course (generally lasting weeks to months). They may be precipitated by hyperventilation or movement. These syndromes may include Lhermitte's symptom; tonic contractions of a limb, face, or trunk (tonic seizures); paroxysmal dysarthria and ataxia; paroxysmal sensory disturbances; and several other less well characterized syndromes. Paroxysmal symptoms probably result from spontaneous discharges, arising at the edges of demyelinated plaques and spreading to adjacent white matter tracts.

Trigeminal neuralgia, hemifacial spasm, and *glossopharyngeal neuralgia* (Chap. 34) can occur when the demyelinating lesion involves the root entry (or exit) zone of the fifth, seventh, and ninth cranial nerve, respectively. Trigeminal neuralgia (tic douloureux) is a very brief lancinating facial pain often triggered by an afferent input from the face or teeth. Most cases of trigeminal neuralgia are not MS related; however, atypical features such as onset before age 50 years, bilateral symptoms, objective sensory loss, or nonparoxysmal pain should raise concerns that MS could be responsible.

Facial myokymia consists of either persistent rapid flickering contractions of the facial musculature (especially the lower portion of the orbicularis oculi) or a contraction that slowly spreads across the face. It results from lesions of the corticobulbar tracts or brainstem course of the facial nerve.

DISEASE COURSE

Four clinical types of MS have been described (Fig. 39-2):

1. *Relapsing/remitting MS* (RRMS) accounts for 85% of MS cases at onset and is characterized by discrete attacks that generally evolve over days to weeks (rarely over hours). There is often complete recovery over the ensuing weeks to months (Fig. 39-2*A*). However, when ambulation is severely impaired during an attack, approximately half will fail to improve. Between attacks, patients are neurologically stable.

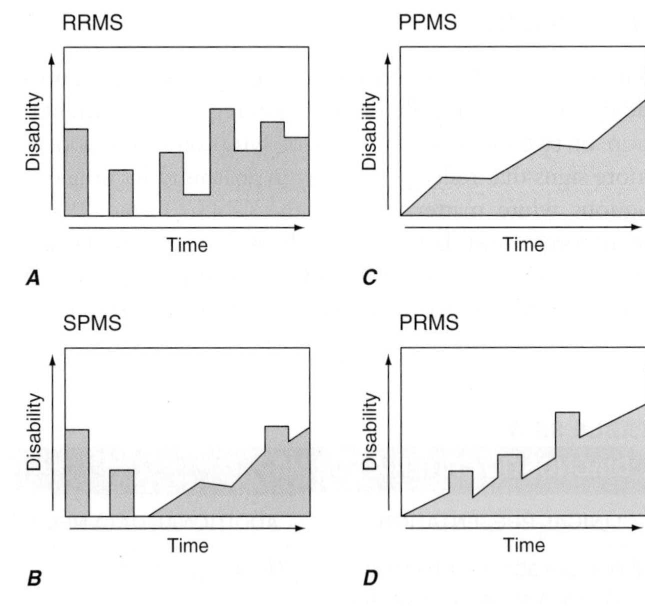

FIGURE 39-2

Clinical course of multiple sclerosis (MS). ***A.*** Relapsing/remitting MS. ***B.*** Secondary progressive MS. ***C.*** Primary progressive MS. ***D.*** Progressive/relapsing MS.

1. *Secondary progressive MS* (SPMS) always begins as RRMS (Fig. 39-2*B*). At some point, however, the clinical course changes so that the patient experiences a steady deterioration in function unassociated with acute attacks (which may continue or cease during the progressive phase). SPMS produces a greater amount of fixed neurologic disability than RRMS. For a patient with RRMS, the risk of developing SPMS is ~2% each year, meaning that the great majority of RRMS ultimately evolves into SPMS. SPMS appears to represent a late stage of the same underlying illness as RRMS.

1. *Primary progressive MS* (PPMS) accounts for ~15% of cases. These patients do not experience attacks but only a steady functional decline from disease onset (Fig. 39-2*C*). Compared to RRMS, the sex distribution is more even, the disease begins later in life (mean age ~40 years), and disability develops faster (at least relative to the onset of the first clinical symptom). Despite these differences, PPMS appears to represent the same underlying illness as RRMS.
2. *Progressive/relapsing MS* (PRMS) overlaps PPMS and SPMS and accounts for ~5% of MS patients. Like patients with PPMS, these patients experience a steady deterioration in their condition from disease onset. However, like SPMS patients, they experience occasional attacks superimposed upon their progressive course (Fig. 39-2*D*).

DIAGNOSIS

There is no definitive diagnostic test for MS. Diagnostic criteria for clinically definite MS require documentation of two or more episodes of symptoms and two or more signs that reflect pathology in anatomically noncontiguous white matter tracts of the CNS (Table 39-3). Symptoms must last for >24 h and occur as distinct episodes that are separated by a month or more. At least one of the two required signs must be present on neurologic examination. The second may be documented by abnormal paraclinical tests such as MRI or evoked potentials (EPs). Similarly, in the most recent diagnostic scheme, the second clinical event (in time) may be supported solely by paraclinical information, usually the development of new focal white matter lesions on MRI. In patients who experience gradual progression of disability for ≥6 months without superimposed relapses, documentation of intrathecal IgG synthesis may be used to support the diagnosis.

TABLE 39-3

DIAGNOSTIC CRITERIA FOR MS

CLINICAL PRESENTATION	ADDITIONAL DATA NEEDED FOR MS DIAGNOSIS
2 or more attacks; objective clinical evidence of 2 or more lesions or objective clinical evidence of 1 lesion with reasonable historical evidence of a prior attack	None
2 or more attacks; objective clinical evidence of 1 lesion	Dissemination in space, demonstrated by • ≥1 T2 lesion on MRI in at least two out of four MS-typical regions of the CNS (periventricular, juxtacortical, infratentorial, or spinal cord) OR • Await a further clinical attack implicating a different CNS site
1 attack; objective clinical evidence of 2 or more lesions	Dissemination in time, demonstrated by • Simultaneous presence of asymptomatic gadolinium-enhancing and nonenhancing lesions at any time OR • A new T2 and/or gadolinium-enhancing lesion(s) on follow-up MRI, irrespective of its timing with reference to a baseline scan OR • Await a second clinical attack
1 attack; objective clinical evidence of 1 lesion (clinically isolated syndrome)	Dissemination in space and time, demonstrated by: For dissemination in space • ≥1 T2 lesion in at least two out of four MS-typical regions of the CNS (periventricular, juxtacortical, infratentorial, or spinal cord) OR • Await a second clinical attack implicating a different CNS site **AND** For dissemination in time • Simultaneous presence of asymptomatic gadolinium-enhancing and nonenhancing lesions at any time OR • A new T2 and/or gadolinium-enhancing lesion(s) on follow-up MRI, irrespective of its timing with reference to a baseline scan **OR** • Await a second clinical attack
Insidious neurologic progression suggestive of MS (PPMS)	One year of disease progression (retrospectively or prospectively determined) **PLUS** Two out of the three following criteria Evidence for dissemination in space in the brain based on ≥1 T2⁺ lesions in the MS-characteristic periventricular, juxtacortical, or infratentorial regions Evidence for dissemination in space in the spinal cord based on ≥2 T2⁺ lesions in the cord Positive CSF (isoelectric focusing evidence of oligoclonal bands and/or elevated IgG index)

Source: From CH Polman et al: Ann Neurol 69:292, 2011.

DIAGNOSTIC TESTS

Magnetic resonance imaging

MRI has revolutionized the diagnosis and management of MS (Fig. 39-3); characteristic abnormalities are found in >95% of patients, although more than 90% of the lesions visualized by MRI are asymptomatic. An increase in vascular permeability from a breakdown of the BBB is detected by leakage of intravenous gadolinium (Gd) into the parenchyma. Such leakage occurs early in the development of an MS lesion and serves as a useful marker of inflammation. Gd enhancement persists for approximately 1 month, and the residual MS plaque remains visible indefinitely as a focal area of hyperintensity (a lesion) on spin-echo (T2-weighted) and proton-density images. Lesions are frequently oriented perpendicular to the ventricular surface, corresponding to the pathologic pattern of perivenous demyelination (Dawson's fingers). Lesions are multifocal within the brain, brainstem, and spinal cord. Lesions larger than 6 mm

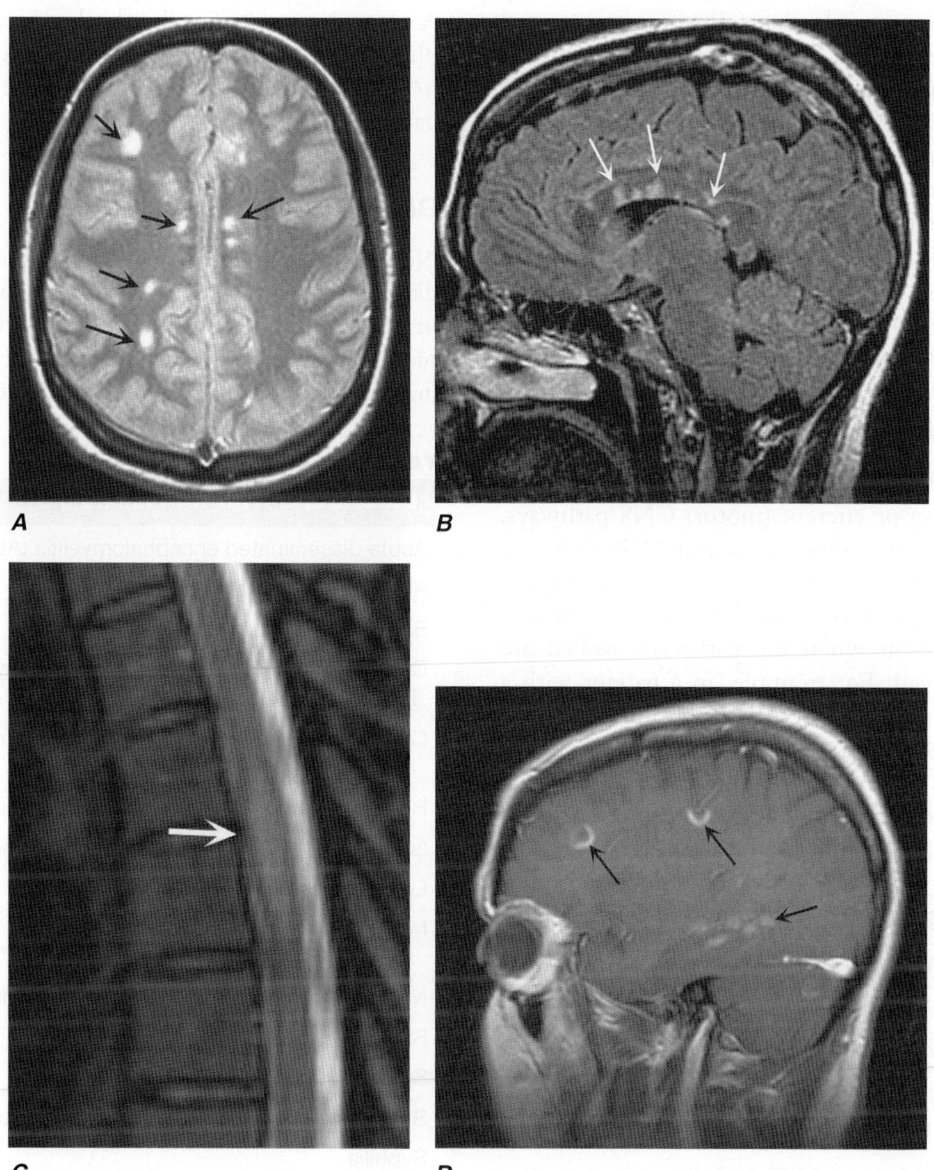

FIGURE 39-3

MRI findings in MS. ***A.*** Axial first-echo image from T2-weighted sequence demonstrates multiple bright signal abnormalities in white matter, typical for MS. ***B.*** Sagittal T2-weighted FLAIR (fluid attenuated inversion recovery) image in which the high signal of CSF has been suppressed. CSF appears dark, while areas of brain edema or demyelination appear high in signal as shown here in the corpus callosum (*arrows*). Lesions in the anterior corpus callosum are frequent in MS and rare in vascular disease. ***C.*** Sagittal T2-weighted fast spin echo image of the thoracic spine demonstrates a fusiform high-signal-intensity lesion in the mid-thoracic spinal cord. ***D.*** Sagittal T1-weighted image obtained after the intravenous administration of gadolinium DTPA reveals focal areas of blood-brain barrier disruption, identified as high-signal-intensity regions (*arrows*).

located in the corpus callosum, periventricular white matter, brainstem, cerebellum, or spinal cord are particularly helpful diagnostically. Different criteria for the use of MRI in the diagnosis of MS have been proposed (Table 39-3).

The total volume of T2-weighted signal abnormality (the "burden of disease") shows a significant (albeit weak) correlation with clinical disability, as do measures of brain atrophy. Approximately one-third of T2-weighted lesions appear as hypointense lesions (black holes) on T1-weighted imaging. Black holes may be a marker of irreversible demyelination and axonal loss, although even this measure depends on the timing of the image acquisition (e.g., most acute Gd-enhancing T2 lesions are T1 dark).

Newer MRI measures such as magnetization transfer ratio (MTR) imaging, and proton magnetic resonance spectroscopic imaging (MRSI) may ultimately serve as surrogate markers of clinical disability. MRSI can quantitate molecules such as *N*-acetyl aspartate, which is a marker of axonal integrity, and MTR may be able to distinguish demyelination from edema.

Evoked potentials

EP testing assesses function in afferent (visual, auditory, and somatosensory) or efferent (motor) CNS pathways. EPs use computer averaging to measure CNS electric potentials evoked by repetitive stimulation of selected peripheral nerves or of the brain. These tests provide the most information when the pathways studied are clinically uninvolved. For example, in a patient with a remitting and relapsing spinal cord syndrome with sensory deficits in the legs, an abnormal somatosensory EP following posterior tibial nerve stimulation provides little new information. By contrast, an abnormal visual EP in this circumstance would permit a diagnosis of clinically definite MS (Table 39-3). Abnormalities on one or more EP modalities occur in 80–90% of MS patients. EP abnormalities are not specific to MS, although a marked delay in the latency of a specific EP component (as opposed to a reduced amplitude or distorted wave-shape) is suggestive of demyelination.

Cerebrospinal fluid

CSF abnormalities found in MS include a mononuclear cell pleocytosis and an increased level of intrathecally synthesized IgG. The total CSF protein is usually normal or slightly elevated. Various formulas distinguish intrathecally synthesized IgG from IgG that may have entered the CNS passively from the serum. One formula, the CSF IgG index, expresses the ratio of IgG to albumin in the CSF divided by the same ratio in the serum. The IgG synthesis rate uses serum and CSF IgG and albumin measurements to calculate the rate of CNS IgG synthesis.

The measurement of oligoclonal banding (OCB) in the CSF also assesses intrathecal production of IgG. OCBs are detected by agarose gel electrophoresis. Two or more OCBs are found in 75–90% of patients with MS. OCBs may be absent at the onset of MS, and in individual patients the number of bands may increase with time. It is important that paired serum samples be studied to exclude a peripheral (i.e., non-CNS) origin of any OCBs detected in the CSF.

A mild CSF pleocytosis (>5 cells/μL) is present in ~25% of cases, usually in young patients with RRMS. A pleocytosis of >75 cells/μL, the presence of polymorphonuclear leukocytes, or a protein concentration >1 g/L (>100 mg/dL) in CSF should raise concern that the patient may not have MS.

DIFFERENTIAL DIAGNOSIS

No single clinical sign or test is diagnostic of MS. The diagnosis is readily made in a young adult with relapsing and remitting symptoms involving different areas of CNS white matter. The possibility of an alternative diagnosis should always be considered (Table 39-4),

TABLE 39-4

DISORDERS THAT CAN MIMIC MS
Acute disseminated encephalomyelitis (ADEM)
Antiphospholipid antibody syndrome
Behçet's disease
Cerebral autosomal dominant arteriopathy, subcortical infarcts, and leukoencephalopathy (CADASIL)
Congenital leukodystrophies (e.g., adrenoleukodystrophy, metachromatic leukodystrophy)
Human immunodeficiency virus (HIV) infection
Ischemic optic neuropathy (arteritic and nonarteritic)
Lyme disease
Mitochondrial encephalopathy with lactic acidosis and stroke (MELAS)
Neoplasms (e.g., lymphoma, glioma, meningioma)
Sarcoid
Sjögren's syndrome
Stroke and ischemic cerebrovascular disease
Syphilis
Systemic lupus erythematosus and related collagen vascular disorders
Tropical spastic paraparesis (HTLV I/II infection)
Vascular malformations (especially spinal dural AV fistulas)
Vasculitis (primary CNS or other)
Vitamin B_{12} deficiency

Abbreviations: AV, arteriovenous; CNS, central nervous system; HTLV, human T cell lymphotropic virus.

particularly when (1) symptoms are localized exclusively to the posterior fossa, craniocervical junction, or spinal cord; (2) the patient is aged <15 or >60 years; (3) the clinical course is progressive from onset; (4) the patient has never experienced visual, sensory, or bladder symptoms; or (5) laboratory findings (e.g., MRI, CSF, or EPs) are atypical. Similarly, uncommon or rare symptoms in MS (e.g., aphasia, parkinsonism, chorea, isolated dementia, severe muscular atrophy, peripheral neuropathy, episodic loss of consciousness, fever, headache, seizures, or coma) should increase concern about an alternative diagnosis. Diagnosis is also difficult in patients with a rapid or explosive (stroke-like) onset or with mild symptoms and a normal neurologic examination. Rarely, intense inflammation and swelling may produce a mass lesion that mimics a primary or metastatic tumor. The specific tests required to exclude alternative diagnoses will vary with each clinical situation; however, an erythrocyte sedimentation rate, serum B_{12} level, ANA, and treponemal antibody should probably be obtained in all patients with suspected MS.

PROGNOSIS

Most patients with clinically evident MS ultimately experience progressive neurologic disability. In older studies, 15 years after onset, only 20% of patients had no functional limitation, and between one-third and one-half progressed to SPMS and required assistance with ambulation; furthermore, 25 years after onset, ~80% of MS patients reached this level of disability. For unclear reasons, the long-term prognosis for untreated MS appears to have improved in recent years. In addition, the development of disease-modifying therapies for MS also appears to have favorably improved the long-term outlook. Although the prognosis in an individual is difficult to establish, certain clinical features suggest a more favorable prognosis. These include ON or sensory symptoms at onset, fewer than two relapses in the first year of illness, and minimal impairment after 5 years. By contrast, patients with truncal ataxia, action tremor, pyramidal symptoms, or a progressive disease course are more likely to become disabled. Patients with a long-term favorable course are likely to have developed fewer MRI lesions during the early years of disease, and vice versa. Importantly, some MS patients have a benign variant of MS and never develop neurologic disability. The likelihood of having benign MS is thought to be <20%. Patients with benign MS 15 years after onset who have entirely normal neurologic examinations are likely to maintain their benign course.

In patients with their first demyelinating event (i.e., a clinically isolated syndrome), the brain MRI provides prognostic information. With three or more typical T2-weighted lesions, the risk of developing MS after 20 years is ~80%. Conversely, with a normal brain MRI, the likelihood of developing MS is <20%. Similarly, two or more Gd-enhancing lesions at baseline is highly predictive of future MS, as is the appearance of either new T2-weighted lesions or new Gd enhancement ≥3 months after the initial episode.

Mortality as a direct consequence of MS is uncommon, although it has been estimated that the 25-year survival is only 85% of expected. Death can occur during an acute MS attack, although this is distinctly rare. More commonly, death occurs as a complication of MS (e.g., pneumonia in a debilitated individual). Death can also result from suicide.

Effect of pregnancy

Pregnant MS patients experience fewer attacks than expected during gestation (especially in the last trimester), but more attacks than expected in the first 3 months postpartum. When considering the pregnancy year as a whole (i.e., 9 months pregnancy plus 3 months postpartum), the overall disease course is unaffected. Decisions about childbearing should thus be made based on (1) the mother's physical state, (2) her ability to care for the child, and (3) the availability of social support. Disease-modifying therapy is generally discontinued during pregnancy, although the actual risk from the interferons and glatiramer acetate (discussed later) appears to be low.

TREATMENT Multiple Sclerosis

Therapy for MS can be divided into several categories: (1) treatment of acute attacks, (2) treatment with disease-modifying agents that reduce the biological activity of MS, and (3) symptomatic therapy. Treatments that promote remyelination or neural repair do not currently exist but would be highly desirable.

The Expanded Disability Status Score (EDSS) is a useful measure of neurologic impairment in MS (Table 39-5). Most patients with EDSS scores <3.5 have RRMS, walk normally, and are generally not disabled; by contrast, patients with EDSS scores >5.5 have progressive MS (SPMS or PPMS), are gait-impaired, and, typically, are occupationally disabled.

ACUTE ATTACKS OR INITIAL DEMYELINATING EPISODES When patients experience acute deterioration, it is important to consider whether this change reflects new disease activity or a "pseudoexacerbation" resulting from an increase in ambient temperature, fever, or an infection. When the clinical change is thought to reflect a pseudoexacerbation, glucocorticoid treatment is inappropriate. Glucocorticoids are used to manage either first attacks or acute exacerbations.

TABLE 39-5

SCORING SYSTEMS FOR MS

Kurtzke Expanded Disability Status Score (EDSS)

0.0 = Normal neurologic exam (all grade 0 in functional status [FS])
1.0 = No disability, minimal signs in one FS (i.e., grade 1)
1.5 = No disability, minimal signs in more than one FS (more than one grade 1)
2.0 = Minimal disability in one FS (one FS grade 2, others 0 or 1)
2.5 = Minimal disability in two FS (two FS grade 2, others 0 or 1)
3.0 = Moderate disability in one FS (one FS grade 3, others 0 or 1) or mild disability in three or four FS (three/four FS grade 2, others 0 or 1) though fully ambulatory
3.5 = Fully ambulatory but with moderate disability in one FS (one grade 3) and one or two FS grade 2; or two FS grade 3; or five FS grade 2 (others 0 or 1)
4.0 = Ambulatory without aid or rest for ~500 m
4.5 = Ambulatory without aid or rest for ~300 m
5.0 = Ambulatory without aid or rest for ~200 m
5.5 = Ambulatory without aid or rest for ~100 m
6.0 = Unilateral assistance required to walk about 100 m with or without resting
6.5 = Constant bilateral assistance required to walk about 20 m without resting
7.0 = Unable to walk beyond about 5 m even with aid; essentially restricted to wheelchair; wheels self and transfers alone
7.5 = Unable to take more than a few steps; restricted to wheelchair; may need aid to transfer
8.0 = Essentially restricted to bed or chair or perambulated in wheelchair, but out of bed most of day; retains many self-care functions; generally has effective use of arms
8.5 = Essentially restricted to bed much of the day; has some effective use of arm(s); retains some self-care functions
9.0 = Helpless bed patient; can communicate and eat
9.5 = Totally helpless bed patient; unable to communicate or eat
10.0 = Death due to MS

Functional Status (FS) Score

A. Pyramidal functions
0 = Normal
1 = Abnormal signs without disability
2 = Minimal disability
3 = Mild or moderate paraparesis or hemiparesis, or severe monoparesis
4 = Marked paraparesis or hemiparesis, moderate quadriparesis, or monoplegia
5 = Paraplegia, hemiplegia, or marked quadriparesis
6 = Quadriplegia

B. Cerebellar functions
0 = Normal
1 = Abnormal signs without disability
2 = Mild ataxia
3 = Moderate truncal or limb ataxia
4 = Severe ataxia all limbs
5 = Unable to perform coordinated movements due to ataxia

C. Brainstem functions
0 = Normal
1 = Signs only
2 = Moderate nystagmus or other mild disability
3 = Severe nystagmus, marked extraocular weakness, or moderate disability of other cranial nerves
4 = Marked dysarthria or other marked disability
5 = Inability to swallow or speak

D. Sensory functions
0 = Normal
1 = Vibration or figure-writing decrease only, in 1 or 2 limbs
2 = Mild decrease in touch or pain or position sense, and/or moderate decrease in vibration in 1 or 2 limbs, or vibratory decrease alone in 3 or 4 limbs
3 = Moderate decrease in touch or pain or position sense, and/or essentially lost vibration in 1 or 2 limbs, or mild decrease in touch or pain, and/or moderate decrease in all proprioceptive tests in 3 or 4 limbs
4 = Marked decrease in touch or pain or loss of proprioception, alone or combined, in 1 or 2 limbs or moderate decrease in touch or pain and/or severe proprioceptive decrease in more than 2 limbs
5 = Loss (essentially) of sensation in 1 or 2 limbs or moderate decrease in touch or pain and/or loss of proprioception for most of the body below the head
6 = Sensation essentially lost below the head

E. Bowel and bladder functions
0 = Normal
1 = Mild urinary hesitancy, urgency, or retention
2 = Moderate hesitancy, urgency, retention of bowel or bladder, or rare urinary incontinence
3 = Frequent urinary incontinence
4 = In need of almost constant catheterization
5 = Loss of bladder function
6 = Loss of bowel and bladder function

F. Visual (or optic) functions
0 = Normal
1 = Scotoma with visual acuity (corrected) better than 20/30
2 = Worse eye with scotoma with maximal visual acuity (corrected) of 20/30 to 20/59
3 = Worse eye with large scotoma, or moderate decrease in fields, but with maximal visual acuity (corrected) of 20/60 to 20/99
4 = Worse eye with marked decrease of fields and maximal acuity (corrected) of 20/100 to 20/200; grade 3 plus maximal acuity of better eye of 20/60 or less
5 = Worse eye with maximal visual acuity (corrected) less than 20/200; grade 4 plus maximal acuity of better eye of 20/60 or less
6 = Grade 5 plus maximal visual acuity of better eye of 20/60 or less

G. Cerebral (or mental) functions
0 = Normal
1 = Mood alteration only (does not affect EDSS score)
2 = Mild decrease in mentation
3 = Moderate decrease in mentation
4 = Marked decrease in mentation
5 = Chronic brain syndrome—severe or incompetent

Source: After JF Kurtzke: Neurology 33:1444, 1983.

They provide short-term clinical benefit by reducing the severity and shortening the duration of attacks. Whether treatment provides any long-term benefit on the course of the illness is less clear. Therefore, mild attacks are often not treated. Physical and occupational therapy can help with mobility and manual dexterity.

Glucocorticoid treatment is usually administered as intravenous methylprednisolone, 500–1000 mg/d for 3–5 days, either without a taper or followed by a course of oral prednisone beginning at a dose of 60–80 mg/d and gradually tapered over 2 weeks. Orally administered methylprednisolone or dexamethasone (in equivalent dosages) can be substituted for the intravenous portion of the therapy, although GI complications are more common by this route. Outpatient treatment is almost always possible.

Side effects of short-term glucocorticoid therapy include fluid retention, potassium loss, weight gain, gastric disturbances, acne, and emotional lability. Concurrent use of a low-salt, potassium-rich diet and avoidance of potassium-wasting diuretics is advisable. Lithium carbonate (300 mg orally bid) may help to manage emotional lability and insomnia associated with glucocorticoid therapy. Patients with a history of peptic ulcer disease may require cimetidine (400 mg bid) or ranitidine (150 mg bid). Proton pump inhibitors such as pantoprazole (40 mg orally bid) may reduce the likelihood of gastritis, especially when large doses are administered orally. Plasma exchange (5–7 exchanges: 40–60 mL/kg per exchange, every other day for 14 days) may benefit patients with fulminant attacks of demyelination (from MS and other fulminant causes) that are unresponsive to glucocorticoids. However, the cost is high, and conclusive evidence of efficacy is lacking.

DISEASE-MODIFYING THERAPIES FOR RELAPSING FORMS OF MS (RRMS, SPMS WITH EXACERBATIONS) Seven such agents are approved by the U.S. Food and Drug Administration (FDA): (1) IFN-β-1a (Avonex), (2) IFN-β-1a (Rebif), (3) IFN-β-1b (Betaseron), (4) glatiramer acetate (Copaxone), (5) natalizumab (Tysabri), (6) fingolimod (Gilenya), and (7) mitoxantrone (Novantrone). An eighth, cladribine (Leustatin), is currently awaiting an FDA decision on its approval. Each of these treatments is also used in SPMS patients who continue to experience attacks, because SPMS can be difficult to distinguish from RRMS, and because the available clinical trials suggest that such patients also derive therapeutic benefit. In Phase III clinical trials, recipients of IFN-β-1b, IFN-β-1a, glatiramer acetate, natalizumab, and fingolimod experienced fewer clinical exacerbations and fewer new MRI lesions compared to placebo recipients (Table 39-6). Mitoxantrone (Novantrone), an immune suppressant, has also been approved in the United States, although because of its potential toxicity it is generally reserved for patients with progressive disability who have failed other treatments. When considering the data in Table 39-6, however, it is important to note that the relative efficacy of the different agents cannot be determined by cross-trial comparisons. Relative efficacy can only be determined from a non-biased head-to-head clinical trial.

Interferon-β IFN-β is a class I interferon originally identified by its antiviral properties. Efficacy in MS probably results from immunomodulatory properties, including (1) downregulating expression of MHC molecules on antigen-presenting cells, (2) inhibiting proinflammatory and increasing regulatory cytokine levels, (3) inhibition of T cell proliferation, and (4) limiting the trafficking of inflammatory cells in the CNS. IFN-β reduces the attack rate and improves disease severity measures such as EDSS progression and MRI-documented disease burden. IFN-β should be considered in patients with either RRMS or SPMS with superimposed relapses. In patients with SPMS but without relapses, efficacy has not been established. Head-to-head trials suggest that higher IFN-β doses have slightly greater efficacy but are also more likely to induce neutralizing antibodies, which may reduce the clinical benefit (discussed later). IFN-β-1a (Avonex), 30 μg, is administered by intramuscular injection once every week. IFN-β-1a (Rebif), 44 μg, is administered by subcutaneous injection three times per week. IFN-β-1b (Betaseron), 250 μg, is administered by subcutaneous injection every other day.

Common side effects of IFN-β therapy include flulike symptoms (e.g., fevers, chills, and myalgias) and mild abnormalities on routine laboratory evaluation (e.g., elevated liver function tests or lymphopenia). Rarely, more severe hepatotoxicity may occur. Subcutaneous IFN-β also causes reactions at the injection site (e.g., pain, redness, induration, or, rarely, skin necrosis). Side effects can usually be managed with concomitant nonsteroidal anti-inflammatory medications and with the use of an autoinjector. Depression, increased spasticity, and cognitive changes have been reported, although these symptoms can also be due to the underlying disease. In any event, side effects to IFN-β therapy usually subside with time.

Approximately 2–10% of IFN-β-1a (Avonex) recipients, 15–25% of IFN-β-1a (Rebif) recipients, and 30–40% of IFN-β-1b (Betaseron) recipients develop neutralizing antibodies to IFN-β, which may disappear over time. Two very large randomized trials (one with more than 2000 patients) provide unequivocal evidence that neutralizing antibodies reduce efficacy as determined by several MRI outcomes. Paradoxically, however, these same trials, despite abundant statistical power, failed to demonstrate any concomitant impact on the clinical

TABLE 39-6

TWO-YEAR OUTCOMES FOR FDA-APPROVED THERAPIES FOR MULTIPLE SCLEROSIS[a]

	CLINICAL OUTCOMES[b]		MRI OUTCOMES[c]	
DOSE, ROUTE, AND SCHEDULE	**ATTACK RATE, MEAN**	**CHANGE IN DISEASE SEVERITY**	**NEW T2 LESIONS[d]**	**TOTAL BURDEN OF DISEASE**
IFN-β-1b, 250 μg SC qod	–34%[e]	–29% (ns)	–83%[f]	–17%[e]
IFN-β-1a, 30 μg IM qw	–18%[g]	–37%[g]	–36%[f]	–4% (ns)
IFN-β-1a, 44 μg SC tiw	–32%[e]	–30%[g]	–78%[e]	–15%[e]
GA, 20 mg SC qd	–29%[f]	–12% (ns)	–38%[f]	–8%[f]
MTX, 12 mg/m² IV q3mo	–66%[e]	–75%[g]	–79%[g]	nr
NTZ, 300 mg IV qmo	–68%[e]	–42%[e]	–83%[e]	–18%[e]
FGM, 0.5 mg PO qd	–55%[e]	–27%[f]	–74%[e]	–23%[e]
CLD[h], 3.5 mg/kg PO qyr	–58%[e]	–33%[g]	–73%[e]	nr

[a]Percentage reductions (or increases) have been calculated by dividing the reported rates in the treated group by the comparable rates in the placebo group, except for MRI disease burden, which was calculated as the difference in the median percentage change between the treated and placebo groups.

[b]Severity = 1 point EDSS progression, sustained for 3 months (in the IFN-β-1a 30 μg qw trial, this change was sustained for 6 months; in the IFN-β-1b trial, this was over 3 years).

[c]Different studies measured these MRI measures differently, making comparisons difficult (numbers for new T2 represent the best case scenario for each trial).

[d]New lesions seen on T2-weighted MRI.

[e]$p = .001$.

[f]$p = .01$.

[g]$p = .05$.

[h]Not FDA-approved at time of publication.

Abbreviations: IFN-β, interferon β; GA, glatiramer acetate; MTX, mitoxantrone; NTZ, natalizumab; FGM, fingolimod; CLD, cladribine; IM, intramuscular; SC, subcutaneous; IV, intravenous; PO, oral; qod, every other day; qw, once per week; tiw, three times per week; qd, daily; q3mo, once every 3 months; qmo, once per month; qyr, once per year; ns, not significant; nr, not reported.

outcomes of disability and relapse rate. The reason for this clinical-radiologic dissociation is unresolved. Fortunately, however, there are few situations where measurement of antibodies is necessary. Thus, for a patient doing well on therapy, the presence of antibodies should not affect treatment. Conversely, for a patient doing poorly on therapy, alternative treatment should be considered, even if there are no detectable antibodies.

Glatiramer Acetate Glatiramer acetate is a synthetic, random polypeptide composed of four amino acids (L-glutamic acid, L-lysine, L-alanine, and L-tyrosine). Its mechanism of action may include (1) induction of antigen-specific suppressor T cells; (2) binding to MHC molecules, thereby displacing bound MBP; or (3) altering the balance between proinflammatory and regulatory cytokines. Glatiramer acetate reduces the attack rate (whether measured clinically or by MRI) in RRMS. Glatiramer acetate may also benefit disease severity measures, although this is less well established than for the relapse rate. Therefore, glatiramer acetate should be considered in RRMS patients. Its usefulness in progressive disease is entirely unknown. Head-to-head clinical trials suggest that glatiramer acetate has about equal efficacy to high IFN-β doses. Glatiramer acetate, 20 mg, is administered by subcutaneous injection every day. Injection-site reactions also occur with glatiramer acetate. Initially, these were thought to be less severe than with IFN-β-1b, although two recent head-to-head comparisons of high-dose IFN-β to glatiramer acetate did not bear out this impression. In addition, approximately 15% of patients experience one or more episodes of flushing, chest tightness, dyspnea, palpitations, and anxiety after injection. This systemic reaction is unpredictable, brief (duration <1 h), and tends not to recur. Finally, some patients experience lipoatrophy, which, on occasion, can be disfiguring and require cessation of treatment.

Natalizumab Natalizumab (Tysabri) is a humanized monoclonal antibody directed against the α_4 subunit of $\alpha_4\beta_1$ integrin, a cellular adhesion molecule expressed on the surface of lymphocytes. It prevents lymphocytes from binding to endothelial cells, thereby preventing lymphocytes from penetrating the BBB and entering the CNS. Natalizumab greatly reduces the attack rate and significantly improves all measures of disease severity in MS. Moreover, it is well tolerated and the dosing schedule of monthly intravenous infusions make it very convenient for patients.

However, because of the development of progressive multifocal leukoencephalopathy (PML) in approximately 0.2% of patients treated with natalizumab for more than 2 years, natalizumab is currently recommended only for patients who have failed other therapies or who have particularly aggressive disease presentations. Its usefulness in the treatment of progressive disease has not been studied. Head-to-head data for natalizumab against low-dose (weekly) IFN-β showed a clear superiority of natalizumab in RRMS; the trial design, however, was biased against IFN-β (i.e., patients recruited could already be considered IFN-β treatment failures). Natalizumab, 300 μg, is administered by IV infusion each month. Treatment with natalizumab is, in general, well tolerated. A small percentage (<10%) of patients experience hypersensitivity reactions (including anaphylaxis) and ~6% develop neutralizing antibodies to the molecule.

The major concern with long-term treatment is the risk of PML. Because the risk is extremely low during the first year of treatment with natalizumab, we currently recommend treatment for periods of 12–18 months only for most patients; after this time, a change to another disease-modifying therapy should be considered. Recently, a blood test to detect antibodies against the PML (JC) virus has shown promise in identifying individuals who are at risk for this complication. In preliminary studies, approximately half of the adult population are antibody-positive, indicating that they experienced an asymptomatic infection with the virus at some time in the past, and to date all cases of natalizumab-associated PML have occurred in seropositive individuals.

Fingolimod Fingolimod (Gilenya) is a sphingosine-1-phosphate (S1P) inhibitor and it prevents the egress of lymphocytes from the secondary lymphoid organs such as the lymph nodes and spleen. Its mechanism of action is probably due, in part, to the trapping of lymphocytes in the periphery and the prevention, thereby, of lymphocytes reaching the brain. However, because S1P receptors are widely expressed in the CNS tissue and because fingolimod is able to cross the BBB, it may also have central effects. Fingolimod reduces the attack rate and significantly improves all measures of disease severity in MS. It is well tolerated, and the oral dosing schedule makes it very convenient for patients. Moreover, from the clinical trial data presented thus far, it seems to be a reasonably safe therapy and it is approved for first-line use by the FDA. However, as with any new therapy, long-term safety remains to be established. A large head-to-head phase III randomized study demonstrated the clear superiority of fingolimod over low dose (weekly) IFN-β. Fingolimod, 0.5 mg, is administered orally each day. Treatment with fingolimod is also, in general, well tolerated. Mild abnormalities on routine laboratory evaluation (e.g., elevated liver function tests or lymphopenia) are more common than in controls. Although rarely severe, sometimes discontinuation of the medication is necessary. First-degree heart block and bradycardia can also occur, the latter necessitating the prolonged (6-h) observation of patients receiving their first dose.

Teriflunomide Teriflunomide (Aubagio) is an oral inhibitor of the enzyme dihydroorotate dehydrogenase involved in pyramiding synthesis. Clinical trials using once daily dosages of 7 or 14 mg revealed modest effects on relapse rate (approximately 30% compared to placebo), and an effect on disability at the higher dose. Possible side effects include hepatic toxicity, nausea, and hair thinning. Teriflunomide can remain in the blood for many months following administration and is considered teratogenic.

Mitoxantrone Hydrochloride Mitoxantrone (Novantrone), an anthracenedione, exerts its antineoplastic action by (1) intercalating into DNA and producing both strand breaks and interstrand cross-links, (2) interfering with RNA synthesis, and (3) inhibiting topoisomerase II (involved in DNA repair). The FDA approved mitoxantrone on the basis of a single (relatively small) phase III clinical trial in Europe, in addition to an even smaller phase II study completed earlier. Mitoxantrone received (from the FDA) the broadest indication of any current treatment for MS. Thus, mitoxantrone is indicated for use in SPMS, in PRMS, and in patients with worsening RRMS (defined as patients whose neurologic status remains significantly abnormal between MS attacks). Despite this broad indication, however, the data supporting its efficacy are weaker than for other approved therapies.

Mitoxantrone can be cardiotoxic (e.g., cardiomyopathy, reduced left ventricular ejection fraction, and irreversible congestive heart failure). As a result, a cumulative dose >140 mg/m^2 is not recommended. At currently approved doses (12 mg/m^2 every 3 months), the maximum duration of therapy can be only 2–3 years. Furthermore, >40% of women will experience amenorrhea, which may be permanent. Finally, there is risk of acute leukemia, and this complication has already been reported in several mitoxantrone-treated MS patients.

Given these risks, mitoxantrone should not be used as a first-line agent in either RRMS or relapsing SPMS. It is reasonable to consider mitoxantrone in selected patients with a progressive course who have failed other approved therapies.

Cladribine Cladribine (Leustatin) is a purine analog that inhibits DNA synthesis and repair, and acts as a general immunosuppressant. Cladribine reduces the attack rate and significantly improves several measures of disease severity in MS. It seems to be well tolerated and the easy oral dosing schedule of only taking the drug for 2 weeks/year make it very convenient for patients. Again, however, the principal concern is long-term safety, a concern that is heightened by the long-term immunosuppression that occurs in some patients and, also, by the fact that, in the pivotal RCT, 10 neoplasms and all 20 herpes zoster cases occurred in Leustatin-treated patients.

Initiating and Changing Treatment Currently, most patients with relapsing forms of MS receive IFN-β or glatiramer acetate as first-line therapy. Although approved for first-line use, the role of fingolimod in this situation has yet to be defined. Regardless of which agent is chosen first, treatment should probably be changed in patients who continue to have frequent attacks or progressive disability (Fig. 39-4). The value of combination therapy is unknown.

The long-term efficacy of these treatments remains uncertain, although several recent studies suggest that these agents can improve the long-term outcome of MS, especially when administered early in the RRMS stage of the illness. Beneficial effects seen in early MS include a reduction in the relapse rate, a reduction in CNS inflammation as measured by MRI, and a prolongation in the time to reach certain disability outcomes such as SPMS and requiring assistance to ambulate. Unfortunately, however, already established progressive symptoms do not respond well to treatment with these disease-modifying therapies. Because progressive symptoms are likely to result from delayed effects of earlier focal demyelinating episodes, many experts now believe that very early treatment with a disease-modifying drug is appropriate for most MS patients. It is reasonable to delay initiating treatment in patients with (1) normal neurologic exams, (2) a single attack or a low attack frequency, and (3) a low burden of disease as assessed by brain MRI. Untreated patients, however, should be followed closely with periodic brain MRI scans; the need for therapy is reassessed if scans reveal evidence of ongoing, subclinical disease.

DISEASE-MODIFYING THERAPIES FOR PROGRESSIVE MS

SPMS High-dose IFN-β probably has a beneficial effect in patients with SPMS who are still experiencing acute relapses. IFN-β is probably ineffective in patients with SPMS who are not having acute attacks. Glatiramer acetate and natalizumab have not been studied in this

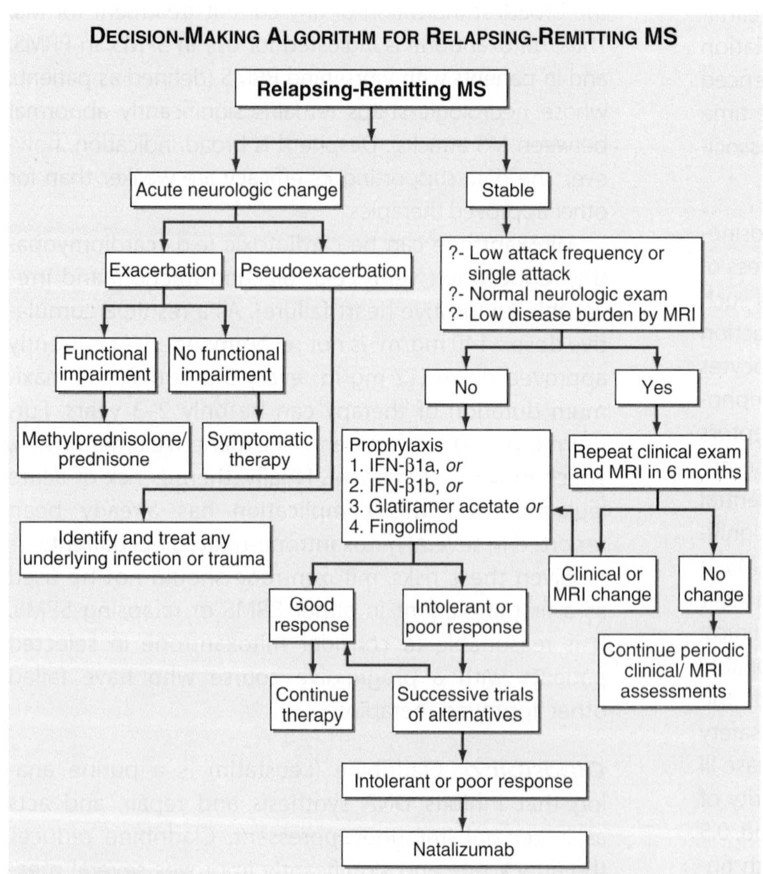

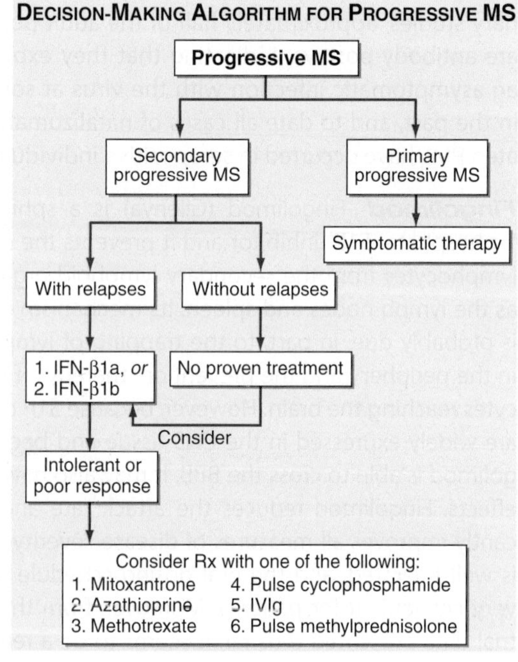

FIGURE 39-4
Therapeutic decision-making for MS.

patient population. Although mitoxantrone has been approved for patients with progressive MS, this is not the population studied in the pivotal trial. Therefore, no evidence-based recommendation can be made with regard to its use in this setting.

PPMS No therapies have been convincingly shown to modify the course of PPMS. A phase III clinical trial of glatiramer acetate in PPMS was stopped because of lack of efficacy. A phase II/III trial of rituximab in PPMS was also negative, but in a preplanned secondary analysis treatment appeared to slow disability progression in patients with gadolinium-enhancing lesions at entry; a follow-up trial with the humanized anti-CD20 therapy ocrelizumab will soon begin. A trial of mitoxantrone in PPMS is ongoing.

OFF-LABEL TREATMENT OPTIONS FOR RRMS AND SPMS *Azathioprine* (2–3 mg/kg per day) has been used primarily in SPMS. Meta-analysis of published trials suggests that azathioprine is marginally effective at lowering relapse rates, although a benefit on disability progression has not been demonstrated.

Methotrexate (7.5–20 mg/week) was shown in one study to slow the progression of upper-extremity dysfunction in SPMS. Because of the possibility of developing irreversible liver damage, some experts recommend a blind liver biopsy after 2 years of therapy.

Cyclophosphamide (700 mg/m^2, every other month) may be helpful for treatment-refractory patients who are (1) otherwise in good health, (2) ambulatory, and (3) <40 years of age. Because cyclophosphamide can be used for periods in excess of 3 years, it may be preferable to mitoxantrone in these circumstances.

Intravenous immunoglobulin (IVIg), administered in monthly pulses (up to 1 g/kg) for up to 2 years, appears to reduce annual exacerbation rates. However, its use is limited because of its high cost, questions about optimal dose, and uncertainty about its effect on long-term disability outcome.

Methylprednisolone administered in one study as monthly high-dose intravenous pulses reduced disability progression (discussed earlier).

OTHER THERAPEUTIC CLAIMS Many purported treatments for MS have never been subjected to scientific scrutiny. These include dietary therapies (e.g., the Swank diet in addition to others), megadose vitamins, calcium orotate, bee stings, cow colostrum, hyperbaric oxygen, Procarin (a combination of histamine and caffeine), chelation, acupuncture, acupressure, various Chinese herbal remedies, and removal of mercury-amalgam tooth fillings, among many others. Patients should avoid costly or potentially hazardous unproven treatments. Many such treatments lack biologic plausibility. For example, no reliable case of mercury poisoning resembling typical MS has ever been described.

Although potential roles for EBV, HHV-6, or chlamydia have been suggested for MS, these reports are unconfirmed, and treatment with antiviral agents or antibiotics is not currently appropriate.

Most recently, chronic cerebrospinal insufficiency (CCSVI) has been proposed as a cause of multiple sclerosis and vascular-surgical intervention recommended. However, the failure of independent investigators to even approximate the initial claims of 100% sensitivity and 100% specificity for the diagnostic procedure raised considerable doubt that CCSVI is a real entity. Certainly, any potentially dangerous surgery should be avoided until more rigorous science is available.

SYMPTOMATIC THERAPY For all patients, it is useful to encourage attention to a healthy lifestyle, including maintaining an optimistic outlook, a healthy diet, and regular exercise as tolerated (swimming is often well tolerated because of the cooling effect of cold water). It is reasonable also to correct vitamin D deficiency with oral vitamin D, and to recommend dietary supplementation with long-chain (omega-3) unsaturated fatty acids (present in oily fish such as salmon) because of their immunomodulatory properties. *Ataxia/tremor* is often intractable. Clonazepam, 1.5–20 mg/d; Mysoline, 50–250 mg/d; propranolol, 40–200 mg/d; or ondansetron, 8–16 mg/d, may help. Wrist weights occasionally reduce tremor in the arm or hand. Thalamotomy or deep-brain stimulation has been tried with mixed success.

Spasticity and *spasms* may improve with physical therapy, regular exercise, and stretching. Avoidance of triggers (e.g., infections, fecal impactions, bed sores) is extremely important. Effective medications include baclofen (Lioresal) (20–120 mg/d), diazepam (2–40 mg/d), tizanidine (8–32 mg/d), dantrolene (25–400 mg/d), and cyclobenzaprine hydrochloride (10–60 mg/d). For severe spasticity, a baclofen pump (delivering medication directly into the CSF) can provide substantial relief.

Weakness can sometimes be improved with the use of potassium channel blockers such as 4-amino pyridine (10–40 mg/d) and 3,4-di-aminopyridine (40–80 mg/d), particularly in the setting where lower extremity weakness interferes with the patient's ability to ambulate. The FDA has approved 4-amino pyridine (at 20 mg/d), and this can be obtained either as dalfampridine (Ampyra) or, more cheaply, through a compounding pharmacy. The principal concern with the use of these agents is the possibility of inducing seizures at high doses.

Pain is treated with anticonvulsants (carbamazepine, 100–1000 mg/d; phenytoin, 300–600 mg/d; gabapentin,

300–3600 mg/d; or pregabalin, 50–300 mg/d), antidepressants (amitriptyline, 25–150 mg/d; nortriptyline, 25–150 mg/d; desipramine, 100–300 mg/d; or venlafaxine, 75–225 mg/d), or antiarrhythmics (mexiletine, 300–900 mg/d). If these approaches fail, patients should be referred to a comprehensive pain management program.

Bladder dysfunction management is best guided by urodynamic testing. Evening fluid restriction or frequent voluntary voiding may help *detrusor hyperreflexia*. If these methods fail, propantheline bromide (10–15 mg/d), oxybutynin (5–15 mg/d), hyoscyamine sulfate (0.5–0.75 mg/d), tolterodine tartrate (2–4 mg/d), or solifenacin (5–10 mg/d) may help. Coadministration of pseudoephedrine (30–60 mg) is sometimes beneficial.

Detrusor/sphincter dyssynergia may respond to phenoxybenzamine (10–20 mg/d) or terazosin hydrochloride (1–20 mg/d). Loss of reflex bladder wall contraction may respond to bethanechol (30–150 mg/d). However, both conditions often require catheterization.

Urinary tract infections should be treated promptly. Patients with large postvoid residual urine volumes are predisposed to infections. Prevention by urine acidification (with cranberry juice or vitamin C) inhibits some bacteria. Prophylactic administration of antibiotics is sometimes necessary but may lead to colonization by resistant organisms. Intermittent catheterization may help to prevent recurrent infections.

Treatment of *constipation* includes high-fiber diets and fluids. Natural or other laxatives may help. *Fecal incontinence* may respond to a reduction in dietary fiber.

Depression should be treated. Useful drugs include the selective serotonin reuptake inhibitors (fluoxetine, 20–80 mg/d; or sertraline, 50–200 mg/d), the tricyclic antidepressants (amitriptyline, 25–150 mg/d; nortriptyline, 25–150 mg/d; or desipramine, 100–300 mg/d), and the non-tricyclic antidepressants (venlafaxine, 75–225 mg/d).

Fatigue may improve with assistive devices, help in the home, or successful management of spasticity. Patients with frequent nocturia may benefit from anticholinergic medication at bedtime. Primary MS fatigue may respond to amantadine (200 mg/d), methylphenidate (5–25 mg/d), or modafinil (100–400 mg/d).

Cognitive problems may respond to the cholinesterase inhibitor donepezil hydrochloride (10 mg/d).

Paroxysmal symptoms respond dramatically to low-dose anticonvulsants (acetazolamide, 200–600 mg/d; carbamazepine, 50–400 mg/d; phenytoin, 50–300 mg/d; or gabapentin, 600–1800 mg/d).

Heat sensitivity may respond to heat avoidance, air-conditioning, or cooling garments.

Sexual dysfunction may be helped by lubricants to aid in genital stimulation and sexual arousal. Management of pain, spasticity, fatigue, and bladder/bowel dysfunction may also help. Sildenafil (50–100 mg), tadalafil (5–20 mg), or vardenafil (5–20 mg) taken 1–2 h before sex are now the standard treatments for maintaining erections.

PROMISING EXPERIMENTAL THERAPIES

Numerous clinical trials are currently underway. These include (1) dimethyl fumarate (BG-12), an oral immunomodulator that reduced relapses and disability accumulation in phase 3 trials; (2) monoclonal antibodies against CD20 to deplete B cells, against the IL-2 receptor, or against CD52 to induce global lymphocyte depletion; and (3) novel oral sphingosine-1-phosphate receptor antagonists to sequester lymphocytes in the secondary lymphoid organs.

CLINICAL VARIANTS OF MS

Neuromyelitis optica (NMO), or Devic's syndrome, is an aggressive inflammatory disorder consisting most typically of attacks of acute ON and myelitis. Attacks of ON can be bilateral (rare in MS) or unilateral; myelitis can be severe and transverse (rare in MS) and is typically longitudinally extensive, involving three or more contiguous vertebral segments. Attacks of ON may be precede or follow an attack of myelitis by days, months, or years, or vice versa. In contrast to MS, progressive symptoms do not occur in NMO. The brain MRI was classically thought to be normal at the onset of NMO, but recent studies now indicate that asymptomatic lesions sometimes resembling typical MS are common. Lesions involving the hypothalamus, periaqueductal region of the brainstem, or "cloud-like" white matter lesions in the cerebral hemispheres are suggestive of NMO. Brainstem disease can present with nausea and vertigo, and large hemispheral lesions can present as encephalopathy or seizures. Spinal cord MRI typically reveals a focal enhancing region of swelling and cavitation, extending over three or more spinal cord segments and often located in central gray matter structures. Histopathology of these lesions may reveal thickening of blood-vessel walls, demyelination, deposition of antibody and complement, a characteristic loss of astrocytes, and aquaporin-4 staining not seen in MS.

NMO, which is uncommon in whites compared with Asians and Africans, is best understood as a syndrome with diverse causes. Up to 40% of patients have a systemic autoimmune disorder, often systemic lupus erythematosus, Sjögren's syndrome, p-ANCA (perinuclear antineutrophil cytoplasmic antibody)–associated vasculitis, myasthenia gravis, Hashimoto's thyroiditis, or mixed connective tissue disease. In others, onset may be associated with acute infection with varicella-zoster virus, EBV, HIV, or tuberculosis. Rare cases appear to be paraneoplastic and associated with breast, lung, or other cancers. NMO is often idiopathic, however. NMO is usually disabling over time; in one series, respiratory failure from cervical myelitis was present in one-third of patients, and 8 years after onset 60% of patients were blind and more than half had permanent paralysis of one or more limbs.

A highly specific autoantibody directed against the water channel protein aquaporin-4 is present in the sera of 60–70% of patients who have a clinical diagnosis of NMO. Seropositive patients have a very high risk for future relapses. Aquaporin-4 is localized to the foot processes of astrocytes in close apposition to endothelial surfaces. It is likely that aquaporin-4 antibodies are directly pathogenic in NMO, as passive transfer of antibodies from NMO patients into laboratory animals reproduced histologic features of the disease.

When MS affects individuals of African or Asian ancestry, there is a propensity for demyelinating lesions to involve predominantly the optic nerve and spinal cord, an MS subtype termed "opticospinal MS." Interestingly, some individuals with opticospinal MS are seropositive for aquaporin-4 antibodies, suggesting that such cases represent an NMO spectrum disorder.

Acute MS (Marburg's variant) is a fulminant demyelinating process that in some cases progresses inexorably to death within 1–2 years. Typically, there are no remissions. When acute MS presents as a solitary, usually cavitary, lesion, a brain tumor is often suspected. In such cases, a brain biopsy is usually required to establish the diagnosis. An antibody-mediated process appears to be responsible for most cases. Marburg's variant does not seem to follow infection or vaccination, and it is unclear whether this syndrome represents an extreme form of MS or another disease altogether. No controlled trials of therapy exist; high-dose glucocorticoids, plasma exchange, and cyclophosphamide have been tried, with uncertain benefit.

TREATMENT Neuromyelitis Optica

Disease-modifying therapies have not been rigorously studied in NMO. Acute attacks of NMO are usually treated with high-dose glucocorticoids (Solu-Medrol 1–2 g/d for 5–10 days followed by a prednisone taper). Because of the likelihood that NMO is antibody-mediated, plasma exchange (typically 7 qod exchanges of 1.5 plasma volumes) has also been used empirically for acute episodes that fail to respond to glucocorticoids. Prophylaxis against relapses can be achieved in some patients with one of the following regimens: mycophenolate mofetil (250 mg bid gradually increasing to 1000 mg bid); B cell depletion with anti-CD20 monoclonal antibody (Rituxan); or a combination of glucocorticoids (500 mg IV methylprednisolone daily for 5 days; then oral prednisone 1 mg/kg per day × 2 months, followed by slow taper) plus azathioprine (2 mg/kg per day started on week 3). By contrast, available evidence suggests that use of IFN-β is ineffective and paradoxically may increase the risk of NMO relapses.

ACUTE DISSEMINATED ENCEPHALOMYELITIS (ADEM)

ADEM has a monophasic course and is most frequently associated with an antecedent infection (postinfectious encephalomyelitis); approximately 5% of ADEM cases follow immunization (postvaccinal encephalomyelitis). ADEM is more common in children than adults. The hallmark of ADEM is the presence of widely scattered small foci of perivenular inflammation and demyelination in contrast to larger confluent demyelinating lesions typical of MS. In the most explosive form of ADEM, acute hemorrhagic leukoencephalitis, the lesions are vasculitic and hemorrhagic, and the clinical course is devastating.

Postinfectious encephalomyelitis is most frequently associated with the viral exanthems of childhood. Infection with measles virus is the most common antecedent (1 in 1000 cases). Worldwide, measles encephalomyelitis is still common, although use of the live measles vaccine has dramatically reduced its incidence in developed countries. An ADEM-like illness rarely follows vaccination with live measles vaccine (1–2 in 10^6 immunizations). ADEM is now most frequently associated with varicella (chickenpox) infections (1 in 4000–10,000 cases). It may also follow infection with rubella, mumps, influenza, parainfluenza, Epstein-Barr, HIV, and other viruses, and *Mycoplasma*. Some patients may have a nonspecific upper respiratory tract infection or no known antecedent illness. In addition to measles, postvaccinal encephalomyelitis may also follow the administration of smallpox (5 cases per million), the Semple rabies, and Japanese encephalitis vaccines. Modern vaccines that do not require viral culture in CNS tissue have reduced the ADEM risk.

All forms of ADEM presumably result from a cross-reactive immune response to the infectious agent or vaccine that then triggers an inflammatory demyelinating response. Autoantibodies to MBP and to other myelin antigens have been detected in the CSF from many patients with ADEM. Attempts to demonstrate direct viral invasion of the CNS have been unsuccessful.

CLINICAL MANIFESTATIONS

In severe cases, onset is abrupt and progression rapid (hours to days). In postinfectious ADEM, the neurologic syndrome generally begins late in the course of the viral illness as the exanthem is fading. Fever reappears, and headache, meningismus, and lethargy progressing to coma may develop. Seizures are common. Signs of disseminated neurologic disease are consistently present (e.g., hemiparesis or quadriparesis, extensor plantar responses, lost or hyperactive tendon reflexes, sensory loss, and brainstem involvement). In ADEM due to chickenpox, cerebellar involvement is often conspicuous. CSF protein is modestly elevated (0.5–1.5 g/L [50–150 mg/dL]). Lymphocytic pleocytosis, generally 200 cells/μL, occurs in 80% of patients. Occasional patients have higher counts or a mixed polymorphonuclear-lymphocytic pattern during the initial days of the illness. Transient CSF oligoclonal banding has been reported. MRI usually reveals extensive changes in the brain and spinal cord, consisting of white matter hyperintensities on T2 and FLAIR sequences with gadolinium enhancement on T1-weighted sequences.

DIAGNOSIS

The diagnosis is easily established when there is a history of recent vaccination or viral exanthematous illness. In severe cases with predominantly cerebral involvement, acute encephalitis due to infection with herpes simplex or other viruses including HIV may be difficult to exclude (Chap. 40); other considerations include hypercoagulable states including the antiphospholipid antibody syndrome, vasculitis, neurosarcoid, or metastatic cancer. An explosive presentation of MS can mimic ADEM, and especially in adults, it may not be possible to distinguish these conditions at onset. The simultaneous onset of disseminated symptoms and signs is common in ADEM and rare in MS. Similarly, meningismus, drowsiness, coma, or seizures suggest ADEM rather than MS. Unlike MS, in ADEM optic nerve involvement is generally bilateral and transverse myelopathy complete. MRI findings that favor ADEM include extensive and relatively symmetric white matter abnormalities, basal ganglia or cortical gray matter lesions, and Gd enhancement of all abnormal areas. By contrast, oligoclonal bands in the CSF are more common in MS. In one study of adult patients initially thought to have ADEM, 30% experienced additional relapses over a follow-up period of 3 years and they were now classified as having MS. Occasional patients with "recurrent ADEM" have also been reported especially in children; however, it is not possible to distinguish this entity from atypical MS.

TREATMENT Acute Disseminated Encephalomyelitis

Initial treatment is with high-dose glucocorticoids as for exacerbations of NMO (discussed earlier); depending on the response, treatment may need to be continued for 4–8 weeks. Patients who fail to respond within a few days may benefit from a course of plasma exchange or intravenous immunoglobulin. The prognosis reflects the severity of the underlying acute illness. Measles encephalomyelitis is associated with a mortality rate of 5–20%, and most survivors have permanent neurologic sequelae. Children who recover may have persistent seizures and behavioral and learning disorders.

CHAPTER 40

MENINGITIS, ENCEPHALITIS, BRAIN ABSCESS, AND EMPYEMA

Karen L. Roos ■ Kenneth L. Tyler

Acute infections of the nervous system are among the most important problems in medicine because early recognition, efficient decision-making, and rapid institution of therapy can be lifesaving. These distinct clinical syndromes include acute bacterial meningitis, viral meningitis, encephalitis, focal infections such as brain abscess and subdural empyema, and infectious thrombophlebitis. Each may present with a nonspecific prodrome of fever and headache, which in a previously healthy individual may initially be thought to be benign, until (with the exception of viral meningitis) altered consciousness, focal neurologic signs, or seizures appear. Key goals of early management are to emergently distinguish between these conditions, identify the responsible pathogen, and initiate appropriate antimicrobial therapy.

APPROACH TO THE PATIENT: Meningitis, Encephalitis, Brain Abscess, and Empyema

(Fig. 40-1) The first task is to identify whether an infection predominantly involves the subarachnoid space (*meningitis*) or whether there is evidence of either generalized or focal involvement of brain tissue in the cerebral hemispheres, cerebellum, or brainstem. When brain tissue is directly injured by a viral infection, the disease is referred to as *encephalitis*, whereas focal infections involving brain tissue are classified as either *cerebritis* or *abscess*, depending on the presence or absence of a capsule.

Nuchal rigidity ("stiff neck") is the pathognomonic sign of meningeal irritation and is present when the neck resists passive flexion. Kernig's and Brudzinski's signs are also classic signs of meningeal irritation. *Kernig's sign* is elicited with the patient in the supine position. The thigh is flexed on the abdomen, with the knee flexed; attempts to passively extend the knee elicit pain when meningeal irritation is present. *Brudzinski's sign* is elicited with the patient in the supine position and is positive when passive flexion of the neck results in spontaneous flexion of the hips and knees. Although commonly tested on physical examinations, the sensitivity and specificity of Kernig's and Brudzinski's signs are uncertain. Both may be absent or reduced in very young or elderly patients, immunocompromised individuals, or patients with a severely depressed mental status. The high prevalence of cervical spine disease in older individuals may result in false-positive tests for nuchal rigidity.

Initial management can be guided by several considerations: (1) Empirical therapy should be initiated promptly whenever bacterial meningitis is a significant diagnostic consideration. (2) All patients who have had recent head trauma, are immunocompromised, have known malignant lesions or central nervous system (CNS) neoplasms, or have focal neurologic findings, papilledema, or a depressed level of consciousness should undergo CT or MRI of the brain prior to lumbar puncture (LP). In these cases empirical antibiotic therapy should not be delayed pending test results but should be administered prior to neuroimaging and LP. (3) A significantly depressed level of consciousness (e.g., somnolence, coma), seizures, or focal neurologic deficits do not occur in viral meningitis; patients with these symptoms should be hospitalized for further evaluation and treated empirically for bacterial and viral meningoencephalitis. (4) Immunocompetent patients with a normal level of consciousness, no prior antimicrobial treatment, and a cerebrospinal fluid (CSF) profile consistent with viral meningitis (lymphocytic pleocytosis and a normal glucose concentration) can often be treated

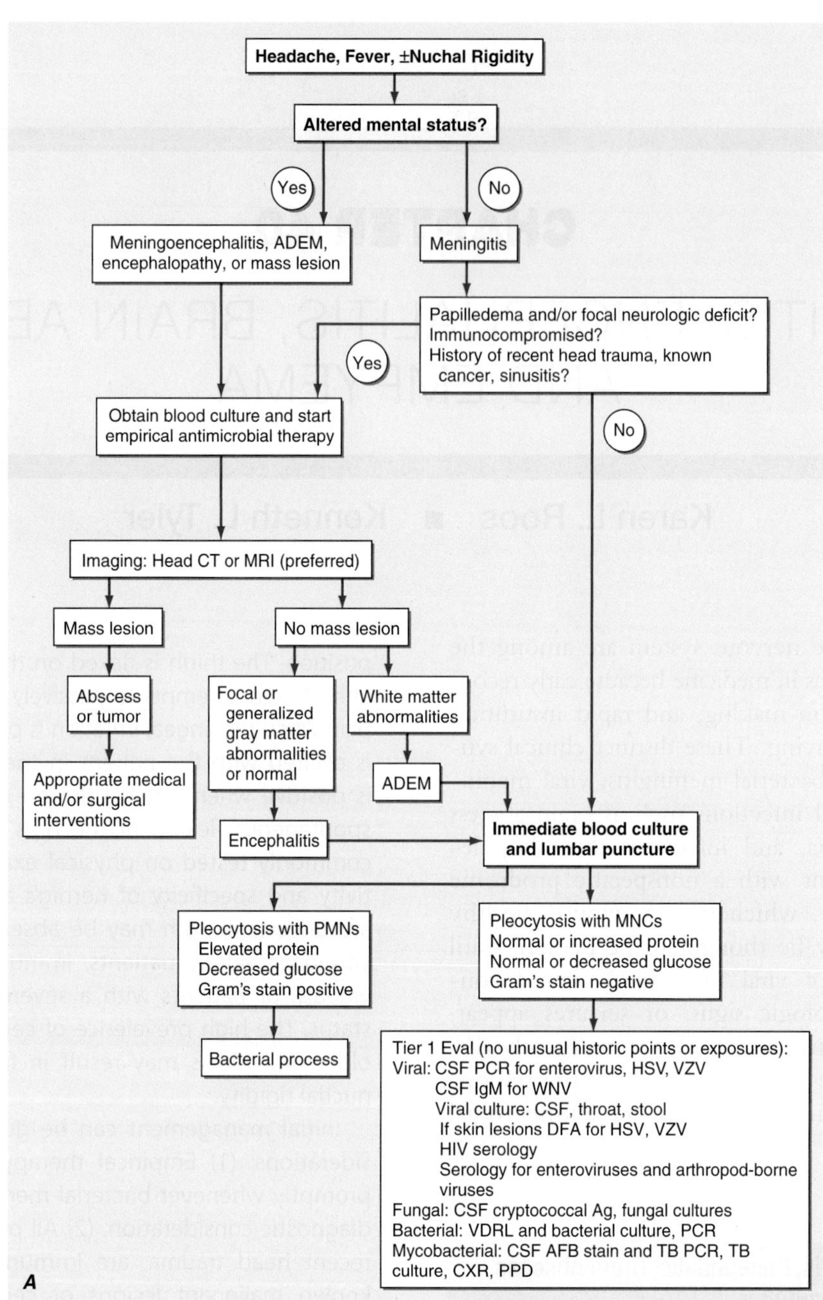

FIGURE 40-1

The management of patients with suspected CNS infection. ADEM, acute disseminated encephalomyelitis; AFB, acid-fast bacillus; Ag, antigen; CSF, cerebrospinal fluid; CT, computed tomography; CTFV, Colorado tick fever virus; CXR, chest x-ray; DFA, direct fluorescent antibody; EBV, Epstein-Barr virus; HHV, human herpesvirus; HSV, herpes simplex virus; LCMV, lymphocytic choriomeningitis virus; MNCs, mononuclear cells; MRI, magnetic resonance imaging; PCR, polymerase chain reaction; PMNs, polymorphonuclear leukocytes; PPD, purified protein derivative; TB, tuberculosis; VDRL, Venereal Disease Research Laboratory; VZV, varicella-zoster virus; WNV, West Nile virus.

as outpatients if appropriate contact and monitoring can be ensured. Failure of a patient with suspected viral meningitis to improve within 48 h should prompt a reevaluation including follow-up neurologic and general medical examination and repeat imaging and laboratory studies, often including a second LP.

ACUTE BACTERIAL MENINGITIS

DEFINITION

Bacterial meningitis is an acute purulent infection within the subarachnoid space. It is associated with a CNS inflammatory reaction that may result in decreased

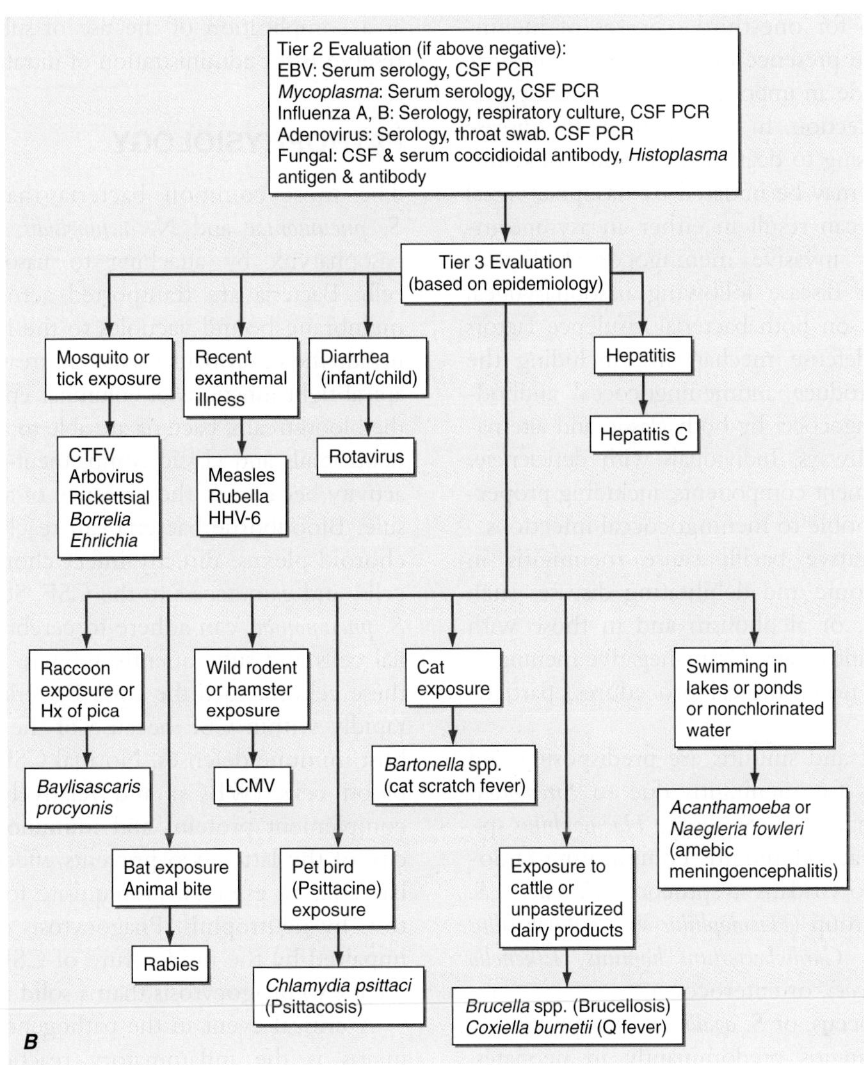

FIGURE 40-1 *(continued)*

consciousness, seizures, raised intracranial pressure (ICP), and stroke. The meninges, the subarachnoid space, and the brain parenchyma are all frequently involved in the inflammatory reaction (*meningoencephalitis*).

EPIDEMIOLOGY

Bacterial meningitis is the most common form of suppurative CNS infection, with an annual incidence in the United States of >2.5 cases/100,000 population. The organisms most often responsible for community-acquired bacterial meningitis are *Streptococcus pneumoniae* (~50%), *Neisseria meningitidis* (~25%), group B streptococci (~15%), and *Listeria monocytogenes* (~10%). *Haemophilus influenzae* type b accounts for <10% of cases of bacterial meningitis in most series. *N. meningitidis* is the causative organism of recurring epidemics of meningitis every 8 to 12 years.

ETIOLOGY

S. pneumoniae is the most common cause of meningitis in adults >20 years of age, accounting for nearly half the reported cases (1.1 per 100,000 persons per year). There are a number of predisposing conditions that increase the risk of pneumococcal meningitis, the most important of which is pneumococcal pneumonia. Additional risk factors include coexisting acute or chronic pneumococcal sinusitis or otitis media, alcoholism, diabetes, splenectomy, hypogammaglobulinemia, complement deficiency, and head trauma with basilar skull fracture and CSF rhinorrhea. The mortality rate remains ~20% despite antibiotic therapy.

The incidence of meningitis due to *N. meningitidis* has decreased with the routine immunization of 11- to 18-year-olds with the tetravalent (serogroups A, C, W-135, and Y) meningococcal glycoconjugate vaccine. The vaccine does not contain serogroup B, which is responsible for one-third of cases of meningococcal disease. The presence of petechial or purpuric skin lesions can provide an important clue to the diagnosis of meningococcal infection. In some patients the disease is fulminant, progressing to death within hours of symptom onset. Infection may be initiated by nasopharyngeal colonization, which can result in either an asymptomatic carrier state or invasive meningococcal disease. The risk of invasive disease following nasopharyngeal colonization depends on both bacterial virulence factors and host immune defense mechanisms, including the host's capacity to produce antimeningococcal antibodies and to lyse meningococci by both classic and alternative complement pathways. Individuals with deficiencies of any of the complement components, including properdin, are highly susceptible to meningococcal infections.

Enteric gram-negative bacilli cause meningitis in individuals with chronic and debilitating diseases such as diabetes, cirrhosis, or alcoholism and in those with chronic urinary tract infections. Gram-negative meningitis can also complicate neurosurgical procedures, particularly craniotomy.

Otitis, mastoiditis, and sinusitis are predisposing and associated conditions for meningitis due to *Streptococci* sp., gram-negative anaerobes, *S. aureus, Haemophilus* sp., and Enterobacteriaceae. Meningitis complicating endocarditis may be due to viridans streptococci, *S. aureus, S. bovis,* the HACEK group (*Haemophilus* sp., *Actinobacillus actinomycetemcomitans, Cardiobacterium hominis, Eikenella corrodens, Kingella kingae*), or enterococci.

Group B streptococcus, or *S. agalactiae*, was previously responsible for meningitis predominantly in neonates, but it has been reported with increasing frequency in individuals >50 years of age, particularly those with underlying diseases.

L. monocytogenes is an increasingly important cause of meningitis in neonates (<1 month of age), pregnant women, individuals >60 years, and immunocompromised individuals of all ages. Infection is acquired by ingesting foods contaminated by *Listeria*. Foodborne human listerial infection has been reported from contaminated coleslaw, milk, soft cheeses, and several types of "ready-to-eat" foods, including delicatessen meat and uncooked hotdogs.

The frequency of *H. influenzae* type b meningitis in children has declined dramatically since the introduction of the Hib conjugate vaccine, although rare cases of Hib meningitis in vaccinated children have been reported. More frequently, *H. influenzae* causes meningitis in unvaccinated children and older adults, and non-b *H. influenzae* is an emerging pathogen.

Staphylococcus aureus and coagulase-negative staphylococci are important causes of meningitis that occurs following invasive neurosurgical procedures, particularly shunting procedures for hydrocephalus, or as a complication of the use of subcutaneous Ommaya reservoirs for administration of intrathecal chemotherapy.

PATHOPHYSIOLOGY

The most common bacteria that cause meningitis, *S. pneumoniae* and *N. meningitidis*, initially colonize the nasopharynx by attaching to nasopharyngeal epithelial cells. Bacteria are transported across epithelial cells in membrane-bound vacuoles to the intravascular space or invade the intravascular space by creating separations in the apical tight junctions of columnar epithelial cells. Once in the bloodstream, bacteria are able to avoid phagocytosis by neutrophils and classic complement-mediated bactericidal activity because of the presence of a polysaccharide capsule. Bloodborne bacteria can reach the intraventricular choroid plexus, directly infect choroid plexus epithelial cells, and gain access to the CSF. Some bacteria, such as *S. pneumoniae*, can adhere to cerebral capillary endothelial cells and subsequently migrate through or between these cells to reach the CSF. Bacteria are able to multiply rapidly within CSF because of the absence of effective host immune defenses. Normal CSF contains few white blood cells (WBCs) and relatively small amounts of complement proteins and immunoglobulins. The paucity of the latter two prevents effective opsonization of bacteria, an essential prerequisite for bacterial phagocytosis by neutrophils. Phagocytosis of bacteria is further impaired by the fluid nature of CSF, which is less conducive to phagocytosis than a solid tissue substrate.

A critical event in the pathogenesis of bacterial meningitis is the inflammatory reaction induced by the invading bacteria. Many of the neurologic manifestations and complications of bacterial meningitis result from the immune response to the invading pathogen rather than from direct bacteria-induced tissue injury. As a result, neurologic injury can progress even after the CSF has been sterilized by antibiotic therapy.

The lysis of bacteria with the subsequent release of cell-wall components into the subarachnoid space is the initial step in the induction of the inflammatory response and the formation of a purulent exudate in the subarachnoid space (Fig. 40-2). Bacterial cell-wall components, such as the lipopolysaccharide (LPS) molecules of gram-negative bacteria and teichoic acid and peptidoglycans of *S. pneumoniae*, induce meningeal inflammation by stimulating the production of inflammatory cytokines and chemokines by microglia, astrocytes, monocytes, microvascular endothelial cells, and CSF leukocytes. In experimental models of meningitis, cytokines including tumor necrosis factor alpha (TNF-α) and interleukin 1 β (IL-1β) are present in CSF within 1–2 h of intracisternal inoculation of LPS. This cytokine response is quickly followed by an increase in CSF protein concentration and leukocytosis.

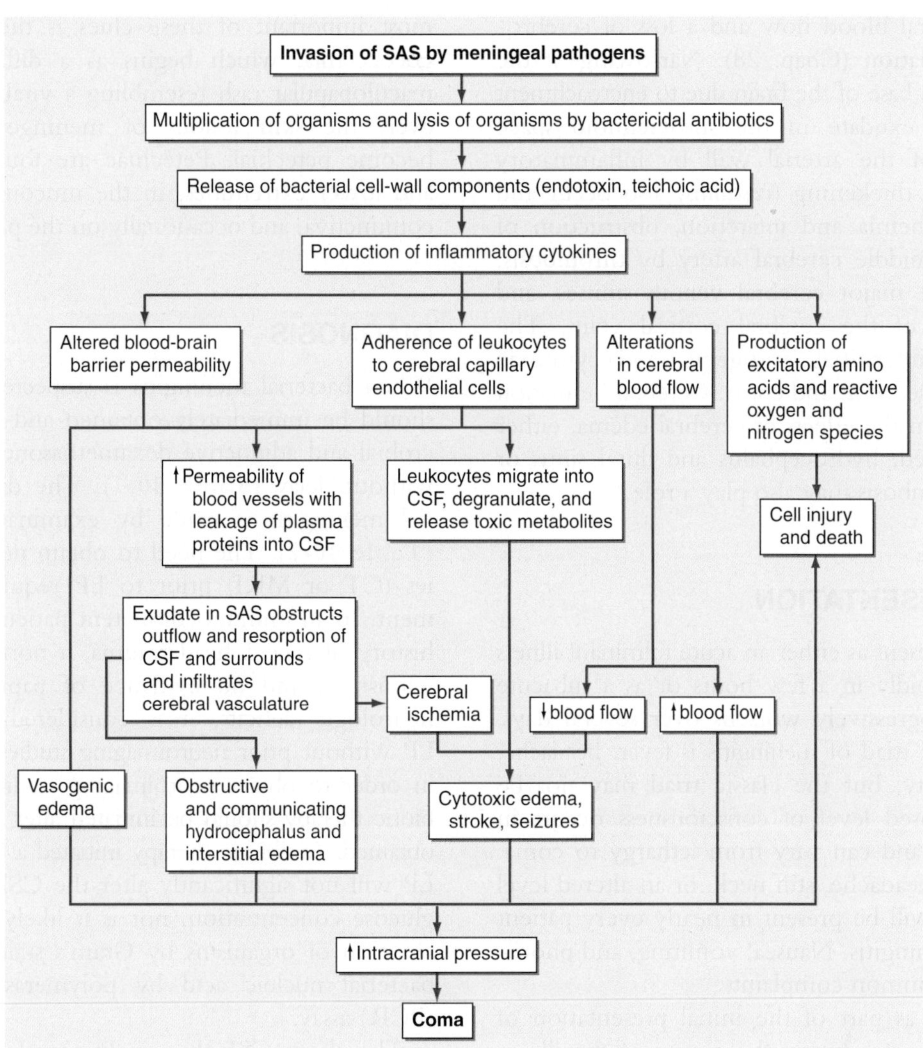

FIGURE 40-2

The pathophysiology of the neurologic complications of bacterial meningitis. CSF, cerebrospinal fluid; SAS, subarachnoid space.

Chemokines (cytokines that induce chemotactic migration in leukocytes) and a variety of other proinflammatory cytokines are also produced and secreted by leukocytes and tissue cells that are stimulated by IL-1β and TNF-α. In addition, bacteremia and the inflammatory cytokines induce the production of excitatory amino acids, reactive oxygen and nitrogen species (free oxygen radicals, nitric oxide, and peroxynitrite), and other mediators that can induce death of brain cells, especially in the dentate gyrus of the hippocampus.

Much of the pathophysiology of bacterial meningitis is a direct consequence of elevated levels of CSF cytokines and chemokines. TNF-α and IL-1β act synergistically to increase the permeability of the blood-brain barrier, resulting in induction of vasogenic edema and the leakage of serum proteins into the subarachnoid space (Fig. 40-2). The subarachnoid exudate of proteinaceous material and leukocytes obstructs the flow of CSF through the ventricular system and diminishes the resorptive capacity of the arachnoid granulations in the dural sinuses, leading to obstructive and communicating hydrocephalus and concomitant interstitial edema.

Inflammatory cytokines upregulate the expression of selectins on cerebral capillary endothelial cells and leukocytes, promoting leukocyte adherence to vascular endothelial cells and subsequent migration into the CSF. The adherence of leukocytes to capillary endothelial cells increases the permeability of blood vessels, allowing for the leakage of plasma proteins into the CSF, which adds to the inflammatory exudate. Neutrophil degranulation results in the release of toxic metabolites that contribute to cytotoxic edema, cell injury, and death. Contrary to previous beliefs, CSF leukocytes probably do little to contribute to the clearance of CSF bacterial infection.

During the very early stages of meningitis, there is an increase in cerebral blood flow, soon followed by a decrease in cerebral blood flow and a loss of cerebrovascular autoregulation (Chap. 28). Narrowing of the large arteries at the base of the brain due to encroachment by the purulent exudate in the subarachnoid space and infiltration of the arterial wall by inflammatory cells with intimal thickening (*vasculitis*) also occur and may result in ischemia and infarction, obstruction of branches of the middle cerebral artery by thrombosis, thrombosis of the major cerebral venous sinuses, and thrombophlebitis of the cerebral cortical veins. The combination of interstitial, vasogenic, and cytotoxic edema leads to raised ICP and coma. Cerebral herniation usually results from the effects of cerebral edema, either focal or generalized; hydrocephalus and dural sinus or cortical vein thrombosis may also play a role.

CLINICAL PRESENTATION

Meningitis can present as either an acute fulminant illness that progresses rapidly in a few hours or as a subacute infection that progressively worsens over several days. The classic clinical triad of meningitis is fever, headache, and nuchal rigidity, but the classic triad may not be present. A decreased level of consciousness occurs in >75% of patients and can vary from lethargy to coma. Fever and either headache, stiff neck, or an altered level of consciousness will be present in nearly every patient with bacterial meningitis. Nausea, vomiting, and photophobia are also common complaints.

Seizures occur as part of the initial presentation of bacterial meningitis or during the course of the illness in 20–40% of patients. Focal seizures are usually due to focal arterial ischemia or infarction, cortical venous thrombosis with hemorrhage, or focal edema. Generalized seizure activity and status epilepticus may be due to hyponatremia, cerebral anoxia, or, less commonly, the toxic effects of antimicrobial agents such as high-dose penicillin.

Raised ICP is an expected complication of bacterial meningitis and the major cause of obtundation and coma in this disease. More than 90% of patients will have a CSF opening pressure >180 mmH_2O, and 20% have opening pressures >400 mmH_2O. Signs of increased ICP include a deteriorating or reduced level of consciousness, papilledema, dilated poorly reactive pupils, sixth nerve palsies, decerebrate posturing, and the Cushing reflex (bradycardia, hypertension, and irregular respirations). The most disastrous complication of increased ICP is cerebral herniation. The incidence of herniation in patients with bacterial meningitis has been reported to occur in as few as 1% to as many as 8% of cases.

Attention to clinical features that are hallmarks of infection with certain pathogens may provide invaluable clues to the diagnosis of individual organisms. The most important of these clues is the rash of meningococcemia, which begins as a diffuse erythematous maculopapular rash resembling a viral exanthem; however, the skin lesions of meningococcemia rapidly become petechial. Petechiae are found on the trunk and lower extremities, in the mucous membranes and conjunctiva, and occasionally on the palms and soles.

DIAGNOSIS

When bacterial meningitis is suspected, blood cultures should be immediately obtained and empirical antimicrobial and adjunctive dexamethasone therapy initiated without delay (Table 40-1). The diagnosis of bacterial meningitis is made by examination of the CSF (Table 40-2). The need to obtain neuroimaging studies (CT or MRI) prior to LP requires clinical judgment. In an immunocompetent patient with no known history of recent head trauma, a normal level of consciousness, and no evidence of papilledema or focal neurologic deficits, it is considered safe to perform LP without prior neuroimaging studies. If LP is delayed in order to obtain neuroimaging studies, empirical antibiotic therapy should be initiated after blood cultures are obtained. Antibiotic therapy initiated a few hours prior to LP will not significantly alter the CSF WBC count or glucose concentration, nor is it likely to prevent visualization of organisms by Gram's stain or detection of bacterial nucleic acid by polymerase chain reaction (PCR) assay.

The classic CSF abnormalities in bacterial meningitis (Table 40-2) are (1) polymorphonuclear (PMN) leukocytosis (>100 cells/μL in 90%), (2) decreased glucose concentration (<2.2 mmol/L [<40 mg/dL] and/or CSF/serum glucose ratio of <0.4 in ~60%), (3) increased protein concentration (>0.45 g/L [>45 mg/dL] in 90%), and (4) increased opening pressure (>180 mmH_2O in 90%). CSF bacterial cultures are positive in >80% of patients, and CSF Gram's stain demonstrates organisms in >60%.

CSF glucose concentrations <2.2 mmol/L (<40 mg/dL) are abnormal, and a CSF glucose concentration of zero can be seen in bacterial meningitis. Use of the CSF/serum glucose ratio corrects for hyperglycemia that may mask a relative decrease in the CSF glucose concentration. The CSF glucose concentration is low when the CSF/serum glucose ratio is <0.6. A CSF/serum glucose ratio <0.4 is highly suggestive of bacterial meningitis but may also be seen in other conditions, including fungal, tuberculous, and carcinomatous meningitis. It takes from 30 min to several hours for the concentration of CSF glucose to reach equilibrium with blood glucose levels; therefore, administration of 50 mL of 50% glucose (D50) prior to LP, as commonly occurs in emergency room settings, is unlikely to alter CSF glucose

TABLE 40-1

ANTIBIOTICS USED IN EMPIRICAL THERAPY OF BACTERIAL MENINGITIS AND FOCAL CNS INFECTIONS[a]

INDICATION	ANTIBIOTIC
Preterm infants to infants <1 mon	Ampicillin + cefotaxime
Infants 1–3 mo	Ampicillin + cefotaxime or ceftriaxone
Immunocompetent children >3 mo and adults <55	Cefotaxime, ceftriaxone or cefepime + vancomycin
Adults >55 and adults of any age with alcoholism or other debilitating illnesses	Ampicillin + cefotaxime, ceftriaxone or cefepime + vancomycin
Hospital-acquired meningitis, posttraumatic or postneurosurgery meningitis, neutropenic patients, or patients with impaired cell-mediated immunity	Ampicillin + ceftazidime or meropenem + vancomycin

ANTIMICROBIAL AGENT	TOTAL DAILY DOSE AND DOSING INTERVAL: CHILD (>1 MONTH)	ADULT
Ampicillin	200 (mg/kg)/d, q4h	12 g/d, q4h
Cefepime	150 (mg/kg)/d, q8h	6 g/d, q8h
Cefotaxime	200 (mg/kg)/d, q6h	12 g/d, q4h
Ceftriaxone	100 (mg/kg)/d, q12h	4 g/d, q12h
Ceftazidime	150 (mg/kg)/d, q8h	6 g/d, q8h
Gentamicin	7.5 (mg/kg)/d, q8h[b]	7.5 (mg/kg)/d, q8h
Meropenem	120 (mg/kg)/d, q8h	3 g/d, q8h
Metronidazole	30 (mg/kg)/d, q6h	1500–2000 mg/d, q6h
Nafcillin	100–200 (mg/kg)/d, q6h	9–12 g/d, q4h
Penicillin G	400,000 (U/kg)/d, q4h	20–24 million U/d, q4h
Vancomycin	60 (mg/kg)/d, q6h	2 g/d, q12h[b]

[a]All antibiotics are administered intravenously; doses indicated assume normal renal and hepatic function.

[b]Doses should be adjusted based on serum peak and trough levels: gentamicin therapeutic level: peak: 5–8 μg/mL; trough: <2 μg/mL; vancomycin therapeutic level: peak: 25–40 μg/mL; trough: 5–15 μg/mL.

concentration significantly unless more than a few hours have elapsed between glucose administration and LP.

A 16S rRNA conserved sequence broad-based bacterial PCR can detect small numbers of viable and nonviable organisms in CSF and is expected to be useful for

TABLE 40-2

CEREBROSPINAL FLUID (CSF) ABNORMALITIES IN BACTERIAL MENINGITIS

Opening pressure	>180 mmH_2O
White blood cells	10/μL to 10,000/μL; neutrophils predominate
Red blood cells	Absent in nontraumatic tap
Glucose	<2.2 mmol/L (<40 mg/dL)
CSF/serum glucose	<0.4
Protein	>0.45 g/L (>45 mg/dL)
Gram's stain	Positive in >60%
Culture	Positive in >80%
Latex agglutination	May be positive in patients with meningitis due to *S. pneumoniae*, *N. meningitidis*, *H. influenzae* type b, *E. coli*, group B streptococci
Limulus lysate	Positive in cases of gram-negative meningitis
PCR	Detects bacterial DNA

Abbreviation: PCR, polymerase chain reaction.

making a diagnosis of bacterial meningitis in patients who have been pretreated with oral or parenteral antibiotics and in whom Gram's stain and CSF culture are negative. When the broad-range PCR is positive, a PCR that uses specific bacterial primers to detect the nucleic acid of *S. pneumoniae, N. meningitidis, Escherichia coli, L. monocytogenes, H. influenzae*, and *S. agalactiae* can be obtained based on the clinical suspicion of the meningeal pathogen. The latex agglutination (LA) test for the detection of bacterial antigens of *S. pneumoniae, N. meningitidis, H. influenzae* type b, group B streptococcus, and *E. coli* K1 strains in the CSF has been useful for making a diagnosis of bacterial meningitis but is being replaced by the CSF bacterial PCR assay. The CSF LA test has a *specificity* of 95–100% for *S. pneumoniae* and *N. meningitidis*, so a positive test is virtually diagnostic of bacterial meningitis caused by these organisms. However, the *sensitivity* of the CSF LA test is only 70–100% for detection of *S. pneumoniae* and 33–70% for detection of *N. meningitidis* antigens, so a negative test does not exclude infection by these organisms. The Limulus amebocyte lysate assay is a rapid diagnostic test for the detection of gram-negative endotoxin in CSF and thus for making a diagnosis of gram-negative bacterial meningitis. The test has a specificity of 85–100% and a sensitivity approaching 100%. Thus, a positive Limulus amebocyte lysate assay occurs in virtually all patients with gram-negative bacterial meningitis, but false positives may occur.

Almost all patients with bacterial meningitis will have neuroimaging studies performed during the course of their illness. MRI is preferred over CT because of its superiority in demonstrating areas of cerebral edema and ischemia. In patients with bacterial meningitis, diffuse meningeal enhancement is often seen after the administration of gadolinium. Meningeal enhancement is not diagnostic of meningitis but occurs in any CNS disease associated with increased blood-brain barrier permeability.

Petechial skin lesions, if present, should be biopsied. The rash of meningococcemia results from the dermal seeding of organisms with vascular endothelial damage, and biopsy may reveal the organism on Gram's stain.

DIFFERENTIAL DIAGNOSIS

Viral meningoencephalitis, and particularly herpes simplex virus (HSV) encephalitis, can mimic the clinical presentation of bacterial meningitis (see "Viral Encephalitis," later in the chapter). HSV encephalitis typically presents with headache, fever, altered consciousness, focal neurologic deficits (e.g., dysphasia, hemiparesis), and focal or generalized seizures. The findings on CSF studies, neuroimaging, and electroencephalogram (EEG) distinguish HSV encephalitis from bacterial meningitis. The typical CSF profile with viral CNS infections is a lymphocytic pleocytosis with a normal glucose concentration, in contrast to PMN pleocytosis and hypoglycorrhachia characteristic of bacterial meningitis. MRI abnormalities (other than meningeal enhancement) are not seen in uncomplicated bacterial meningitis. By contrast, in HSV encephalitis, on T2-weighted and fluid-attenuated inversion recovery (FLAIR) MRI images, high signal intensity lesions are seen in the orbitofrontal, anterior, and medial temporal lobes in the majority of patients within 48 h of symptom onset. Some patients with HSV encephalitis have a distinctive periodic pattern on EEG (discussed later).

Rickettsial disease can resemble bacterial meningitis. Rocky Mountain spotted fever (RMSF) is transmitted by a tick bite and caused by the bacteria *Rickettsia rickettsii*. The disease may present acutely with high fever, prostration, myalgia, headache, nausea, and vomiting. Most patients develop a characteristic rash within 96 h of the onset of symptoms. The rash is initially a diffuse erythematous maculopapular rash that may be difficult to distinguish from that of meningococcemia. It progresses to a petechial rash, then to a purpuric rash and, if untreated, to skin necrosis or gangrene. The color of the lesions changes from bright red to very dark red, then yellowish-green to black. The rash typically begins in the wrist and ankles and then spreads distally and proximally within a matter of a few hours, involving the palms and soles. Diagnosis is made by immunofluorescent staining of skin biopsy specimens. Ehrlichioses are also transmitted by a tick bite. These are small gram-negative coccobacilli of which two species cause human disease. *Anaplasma phagocytophilum* causes human granulocytic ehrlichiosis (anaplasmosis), and *Ehrlichia chaffeensis* causes human monocytic ehrlichiosis. The clinical and laboratory manifestations of the infections are similar. Patients present with fever, headache, nausea, and vomiting. Twenty percent of patients have a maculopapular or petechial rash. There is laboratory evidence of leukopenia, thrombocytopenia, and anemia, and mild to moderate elevations in alanine aminotransferases, alkaline phosphatase, and lactate dehydrogenase. Patients with RMSF and those with ehrlichial infections may have an altered level of consciousness ranging from mild lethargy to coma, confusion, focal neurologic signs, cranial nerve palsies, hyperreflexia, and seizures.

Focal suppurative CNS infections (discussed later), including subdural and epidural empyema and brain abscess, should also be considered, especially when focal neurologic findings are present. MRI should be performed promptly in all patients with suspected meningitis who have focal features, both to detect the intracranial infection and to search for associated areas of infection in the sinuses or mastoid bones.

A number of noninfectious CNS disorders can mimic bacterial meningitis. Subarachnoid hemorrhage (SAH; Chap. 28) is generally the major consideration. Other possibilities include chemical meningitis due to rupture of tumor contents into the CSF (e.g., from a cystic glioma or craniopharyngioma epidermoid or dermoid cyst); drug-induced hypersensitivity meningitis; carcinomatous or lymphomatous meningitis; meningitis associated with inflammatory disorders such as sarcoid, systemic lupus erythematosus (SLE), and Behçet's syndrome; pituitary apoplexy; and uveomeningitic syndromes (Vogt-Koyanagi-Harada syndrome).

On occasion, subacutely evolving meningitis (Chap. 41) may be considered in the differential diagnosis of acute meningitis. The principal causes include *Mycobacterium tuberculosis*, *Cryptococcus neoformans*, *Histoplasma capsulatum*, *Coccidioides immitis*, and *Treponema pallidum*.

TREATMENT Acute Bacterial Meningitis

EMPIRICAL ANTIMICROBIAL THERAPY

(Table 40-1) Bacterial meningitis is a medical emergency. The goal is to begin antibiotic therapy within 60 min of a patient's arrival in the emergency room. Empirical antimicrobial therapy is initiated in patients with suspected bacterial meningitis before the results of CSF Gram's stain and culture are known. *S. pneumoniae* and *N. meningitidis* are the most common etiologic organisms of community-acquired bacterial meningitis. Due to the emergence of penicillin- and cephalosporin-resistant *S. pneumoniae*, empirical therapy of community-acquired suspected bacterial meningitis in children and adults should include a combination of dexamethasone, a third- or fourth-generation cephalosporin (e.g., ceftriaxone, cefotaxime, or cefepime), and vancomycin, plus acyclovir, as HSV encephalitis is the leading disease in the differential diagnosis, and doxycycline during tick season to treat tick-borne bacterial infections. Ceftriaxone or cefotaxime provide good coverage for susceptible *S. pneumoniae*, group B streptococci, and *H. influenzae* and adequate coverage for *N. meningitidis*. Cefepime is a broad-spectrum fourth-generation cephalosporin with in vitro activity similar to that of cefotaxime or ceftriaxone against *S. pneumoniae* and *N. meningitidis* and greater activity against *Enterobacter* species and *Pseudomonas aeruginosa*. In clinical trials, cefepime has been demonstrated to be equivalent to cefotaxime in the treatment of penicillin-sensitive pneumococcal and meningococcal meningitis, and it has been used successfully in some patients with meningitis due to *Enterobacter* species and *P. aeruginosa*. Ampicillin should be added to the empirical regimen for coverage of *L. monocytogenes* in individuals <3 months of age, those >55, or those with suspected impaired cell-mediated immunity because of chronic illness, organ transplantation, pregnancy, malignancy, or immunosuppressive therapy. Metronidazole is added to the empirical regimen to cover gram-negative anaerobes in patients with otitis, sinusitis, or mastoiditis. In hospital-acquired meningitis, and particularly meningitis following neurosurgical procedures, staphylococci and gram-negative organisms including *P. aeruginosa* are the most common etiologic organisms. In these patients, empirical therapy should include a combination of vancomycin and ceftazidime, cefepime, or meropenem. Ceftazidime, cefepime, or meropenem should be substituted for ceftriaxone or cefotaxime in neurosurgical patients and in neutropenic patients, as ceftriaxone and cefotaxime do not provide adequate activity against CNS infection with *P. aeruginosa*. Meropenem is a carbapenem antibiotic that is highly active in vitro against *L. monocytogenes*, has been demonstrated to be effective in cases of meningitis caused by *P. aeruginosa*, and shows good activity against penicillin-resistant pneumococci. In experimental pneumococcal meningitis, meropenem was comparable to ceftriaxone and inferior to vancomycin in sterilizing CSF cultures. The number of patients with bacterial meningitis enrolled in clinical trials of meropenem has not been sufficient to definitively assess the efficacy of this antibiotic.

SPECIFIC ANTIMICROBIAL THERAPY

Meningococcal Meningitis (Table 40-3) Although ceftriaxone and cefotaxime provide adequate empirical coverage for *N. meningitidis*, penicillin G remains the antibiotic of choice for meningococcal meningitis caused by susceptible strains. Isolates of *N. meningitidis* with moderate resistance to penicillin have been identified, but patients infected with these strains have still been successfully treated with penicillin. CSF isolates of *N. meningitidis* should be tested for penicillin and ampicillin susceptibility, and if resistance is found, cefotaxime or ceftriaxone should be substituted for penicillin. A 7-day course of intravenous antibiotic therapy is adequate for uncomplicated meningococcal meningitis. The index case and all close contacts should receive chemoprophylaxis with a 2-day regimen of rifampin (600 mg every 12 h for 2 days in adults and 10 mg/kg every 12 h for 2 days in children >1 year). Rifampin is not recommended in pregnant women. Alternatively, adults can be treated with one dose of azithromycin (500 mg), or one intramuscular dose of ceftriaxone (250 mg). Close contacts are defined as those individuals who have had contact with oropharyngeal secretions, either through kissing or by sharing toys, beverages, or cigarettes.

TABLE 40-3

ANTIMICROBIAL THERAPY OF CNS BACTERIAL INFECTIONS BASED ON PATHOGEN[a]

ORGANISM	ANTIBIOTIC
Neisseria meningitides	
Penicillin-sensitive	Penicillin G or ampicillin
Penicillin-resistant	Ceftriaxone or cefotaxime
Streptococcus pneumoniae	
Penicillin-sensitive	Penicillin G
Penicillin-intermediate	Ceftriaxone or cefotaxime or cefepime
Penicillin-resistant	(Ceftriaxone or cefotaxime or cefepime) + vancomycin
Gram-negative bacilli (except *Pseudomonas* spp.)	Ceftriaxone or cefotaxime
Pseudomonas aeruginosa	Ceftazidime or cefepime or meropenem
Staphylococci spp.	
Methicillin-sensitive	Nafcillin
Methicillin-resistant	Vancomycin
Listeria monocytogenes	Ampicillin + gentamicin
Haemophilus influenzae	Ceftriaxone or cefotaxime or cefepime
Streptococcus agalactiae	Penicillin G or ampicillin
Bacteroides fragilis	Metronidazole
Fusobacterium spp.	Metronidazole

[a]Doses are as indicated in Table 40-1.

Pneumococcal Meningitis Antimicrobial therapy of pneumococcal meningitis is initiated with a cephalosporin (ceftriaxone, cefotaxime, or cefepime) and vancomycin. All CSF isolates of *S. pneumoniae* should be tested for sensitivity to penicillin and the cephalosporins. Once the results of antimicrobial susceptibility tests are known, therapy can be modified accordingly (Table 40-3). For *S. pneumoniae* meningitis, an isolate of *S. pneumoniae* is considered to be susceptible to penicillin with a minimal inhibitory concentration (MIC) <0.06 μg/mL, to have intermediate resistance when the MIC is 0.1–1.0 μg/mL, and to be highly resistant when the MIC >1.0 μg/mL. Isolates of *S. pneumoniae* that have cephalosporin MICs ≤0.5 μg/mL are considered sensitive to the cephalosporins (cefotaxime, ceftriaxone, cefepime). Those with MICs of 1 μg/mL are considered to have intermediate resistance, and those with MICs ≥2 μg/mL are considered resistant. For meningitis due to pneumococci, with cefotaxime or ceftriaxone MICs ≤0.5 μg/mL, treatment with cefotaxime or ceftriaxone is usually adequate. For MIC >1 μg/mL, vancomycin is the antibiotic of choice. Rifampin can be added to vancomycin for its synergistic effect but is inadequate as monotherapy because resistance develops rapidly when it is used alone.

A 2-week course of intravenous antimicrobial therapy is recommended for pneumococcal meningitis.

Patients with *S. pneumoniae* meningitis should have a repeat LP performed 24–36 h after the initiation of antimicrobial therapy to document sterilization of the CSF. Failure to sterilize the CSF after 24–36 h of antibiotic therapy should be considered presumptive evidence of antibiotic resistance. Patients with penicillin- and cephalosporin-resistant strains of *S. pneumoniae* who do not respond to intravenous vancomycin alone may benefit from the addition of intraventricular vancomycin. The intraventricular route of administration is preferred over the intrathecal route because adequate concentrations of vancomycin in the cerebral ventricles are not always achieved with intrathecal administration.

***Listeria* Meningitis** Meningitis due to *L. monocytogenes* is treated with ampicillin for at least 3 weeks (Table 40-3). Gentamicin is added in critically ill patients (2 mg/kg loading dose, then 7.5 mg/kg per day given every 8 h and adjusted for serum levels and renal function). The combination of trimethoprim (10–20 mg/kg per day) and sulfamethoxazole (50–100 mg/kg per day) given every 6 h may provide an alternative in penicillin-allergic patients.

Staphylococcal Meningitis Meningitis due to susceptible strains of *S. aureus* or coagulase-negative staphylococci is treated with nafcillin (Table 40-3). Vancomycin is the drug of choice for methicillin-resistant staphylococci and for patients allergic to penicillin. In these patients, the CSF should be monitored during therapy. If the CSF is not sterilized after 48 h of intravenous vancomycin therapy, then either intraventricular or intrathecal vancomycin, 20 mg once daily, can be added.

Gram-Negative Bacillary Meningitis The third-generation cephalosporins—cefotaxime, ceftriaxone, and ceftazidime—are equally efficacious for the treatment of gram-negative bacillary meningitis, with the exception of meningitis due to *P. aeruginosa*, which should be treated with ceftazidime, cefepime, or meropenem (Table 40-3). A 3-week course of intravenous antibiotic therapy is recommended for meningitis due to gram-negative bacilli.

ADJUNCTIVE THERAPY The release of bacterial cell-wall components by bactericidal antibiotics leads to the production of the inflammatory cytokines IL-1β and TNF-α in the subarachnoid space. Dexamethasone exerts its beneficial effect by inhibiting the synthesis of IL-1β and TNF-α at the level of mRNA, decreasing CSF outflow resistance, and stabilizing the blood-brain barrier. The rationale for giving dexamethasone 20 min before antibiotic therapy is that dexamethasone inhibits the production of TNF-α by macrophages and microglia only if it is administered before these cells are activated by endotoxin. Dexamethasone does not alter TNF-α production once it has been induced. The results of clinical trials of dexamethasone therapy in children, predominantly with meningitis due to *H. influenzae* and *S. pneumoniae*, have demonstrated its efficacy in decreasing meningeal inflammation and neurologic sequelae such as the incidence of sensorineural hearing loss.

A prospective European trial of adjunctive therapy for acute bacterial meningitis in 301 adults found that dexamethasone reduced the number of unfavorable outcomes (15 vs. 25%, $p = .03$) including death (7 vs. 15%, $p = .04$). The benefits were most striking in patients with pneumococcal meningitis. Dexamethasone (10 mg intravenously) was administered 15–20 min before the first dose of an antimicrobial agent, and the same dose was repeated every 6 h for 4 days. These results were confirmed in a second trial of dexamethasone in adults with pneumococcal meningitis. Therapy with dexamethasone should ideally be started 20 min before, or not later than concurrent with, the first dose of antibiotics. It is unlikely to be of significant benefit if started >6 h after antimicrobial therapy has been initiated. Dexamethasone may decrease the penetration of vancomycin into CSF, and it delays the sterilization of CSF in experimental models of *S. pneumoniae* meningitis. As a result, its potential benefit should be carefully weighed when vancomycin is the antibiotic of choice. Alternatively, vancomycin can be administered by the intraventricular route.

One of the concerns for using dexamethasone in adults with bacterial meningitis is that in experimental models of meningitis, dexamethasone therapy increased hippocampal cell injury and reduced learning capacity. This has not been the case in clinical series. The efficacy of dexamethasone therapy in preventing neurologic sequelae is different between high- and low-income countries. Three large randomized trials in low-income countries (sub-Saharan Africa, Southeast Asia) failed to show benefit in subgroups of patients. The lack of efficacy of dexamethasone in these trials has been attributed to late presentation to the hospital with more advanced disease, antibiotic pretreatment, malnutrition, infection with HIV, and treatment of patients with probable, but not microbiologically proven, bacterial meningitis. The results of these clinical trials suggest that patients in sub-Saharan Africa and those in low-income countries with negative CSF Gram's stain and culture should not be treated with dexamethasone.

INCREASED INTRACRANIAL PRESSURE Emergency treatment of increased ICP includes elevation of the patient's head to 30–45°, intubation and hyperventilation (Pa_{CO2} 25–30 mmHg), and mannitol. Patients with increased ICP should be managed in an intensive care unit; accurate ICP measurements are best obtained with an ICP monitoring device.

Treatment of increased intracranial pressure is discussed in detail in Chap. 28.

PROGNOSIS

Mortality rate is 3–7% for meningitis caused by *H. influenzae*, *N. meningitidis*, or group B streptococci; 15% for that due to *L. monocytogenes*; and 20% for *S. pneumoniae*. In general, the risk of death from bacterial meningitis increases with (1) decreased level of consciousness on admission, (2) onset of seizures within 24 h of admission, (3) signs of increased ICP, (4) young age (infancy) and age >50, (5) the presence of comorbid conditions including shock and/or the need for mechanical ventilation, and (6) delay in the initiation of treatment. Decreased CSF glucose concentratio (<2.2 mmol/L [<40 mg/dL]) and markedly increased CSF protein concentration (>3 g/L [>300 mg/dL]) have been predictive of increased mortality and poorer outcomes in some series. Moderate or severe sequelae occur in ~25% of survivors, although the exact incidence varies with the infecting organism. Common sequelae include decreased intellectual function, memory impairment, seizures, hearing loss and dizziness, and gait disturbances.

ACUTE VIRAL MENINGITIS

CLINICAL MANIFESTATIONS

Immunocompetent adult patients with viral meningitis usually present with headache, fever, and signs of meningeal irritation coupled with an inflammatory CSF profile (discussed later). Headache is almost invariably present and often characterized as frontal or retroorbital and frequently associated with photophobia and pain on moving the eyes. Nuchal rigidity is present in most cases but may be mild and present only near the limit of neck anteflexion. Constitutional signs can include malaise, myalgia, anorexia, nausea and vomiting, abdominal pain, and/or diarrhea. Patients often have mild lethargy or drowsiness; however, profound alterations in consciousness, such as stupor, coma, or marked confusion do not occur in viral meningitis and suggest the presence of encephalitis or other alternative diagnoses. Similarly, seizures or focal neurologic signs or symptoms or neuroimaging abnormalities indicative of brain parenchymal involvement are not typical of viral meningitis and suggest the presence of encephalitis or another CNS infectious or inflammatory process.

ETIOLOGY

Using a variety of diagnostic techniques, including CSF PCR, culture, and serology, a specific viral cause can be found in 75–90% of cases of viral meningitis. The most important agents are enteroviruses (including echoviruses and coxsackieviruses in addition to numbered enteroviruses), HSV type 2 (HSV-2), HIV, and arboviruses (Table 40-4). CSF cultures are positive in 30–70% of patients, the frequency of isolation depending on the specific viral agent. Approximately two-thirds of culture-negative cases of "aseptic" meningitis have a specific viral etiology identified by CSF PCR testing (discussed later).

TABLE 40-4

VIRUSES CAUSING ACUTE MENINGITIS AND ENCEPHALITIS IN NORTH AMERICA

ACUTE MENINGITIS

Common	Less Common
Enteroviruses (coxsackieviruses, echoviruses, and human enteroviruses 68–71)	Varicella-zoster virus Epstein-Barr virus
Herpes simplex virus 2	Lymphocytic choriomeningitis virus
Arthropod-borne viruses	
HIV	

ACUTE ENCEPHALITIS

Common	Less Common
Herpesviruses	Rabies
Herpes simplex virus 1	Eastern equine encephalitis virus
Varicella-zoster virus	Western equine encephalitis virus
Epstein-Barr virus	Powassan virus
Arthropod-borne viruses	Cytomegalovirus[a]
La Crosse virus	Enteroviruses[a]
West Nile virus	Colorado tick fever
St. Louis encephalitis virus	Mumps

[a]Immunocompromised host.

EPIDEMIOLOGY

Viral meningitis is not a nationally reportable disease; however, it has been estimated that the incidence is ~75,000 cases per year. In temperate climates, there is a substantial increase in cases during the summer and early fall months, reflecting the seasonal predominance of enterovirus and arthropod-borne virus (arbovirus) infections, with a peak monthly incidence of about 1 reported case per 100,000 population.

LABORATORY DIAGNOSIS

CSF examination

The most important laboratory test in the diagnosis of viral meningitis is examination of the CSF. The typical profile is a lymphocytic pleocytosis (25–500 cells/μL), a normal or slightly elevated protein concentration (0.2–0.8 g/L [20–80 mg/dL]), a normal glucose concentration, and a normal or mildly elevated opening pressure (100–350 mmH_2O). Organisms are *not* seen on Gram's stain of CSF. Rarely, PMNs may predominate in the first 48 h of illness, especially with infections due to echovirus 9, West Nile virus, eastern equine encephalitis (EEE) virus, or mumps. A pleocytosis of polymorphonuclear neutrophils occurs in 45% of patients with West Nile virus (WNV) meningitis and can persist for a week or longer before shifting to a lymphocytic pleocytosis. Despite these exceptions, the presence of a CSF PMN pleocytosis in a patient with suspected viral meningitis in whom a specific diagnosis has not been established should prompt consideration of alternative diagnoses, including bacterial meningitis or parameningeal infections. The total CSF cell count in viral meningitis is typically 25–500/μL, although cell counts of several thousand/μL are occasionally seen, especially with infections due to lymphocytic choriomeningitis virus (LCMV) and mumps virus. The CSF glucose concentration is typically normal in viral infections, although it may be decreased in 10–30% of cases due to mumps or LCMV. Rare instances of decreased CSF glucose concentration occur in cases of meningitis due to echoviruses and other enteroviruses, HSV-2, and varicella-zoster virus (VZV). As a rule, a lymphocytic pleocytosis with a low glucose concentration should suggest fungal or tuberculous meningitis, *Listeria* meningoencephalitis, or noninfectious disorders (e.g., sarcoid, neoplastic meningitis).

A number of tests measuring levels of various CSF proteins, enzymes, and mediators—including C-reactive protein, lactic acid, lactate dehydrogenase, neopterin, quinolinate, IL-1β, IL-6, soluble IL-2 receptor, β_2-microglobulin, and TNF—have been proposed as potential discriminators between viral and bacterial meningitis or as markers of specific types of viral infection (e.g., infection with HIV), but they remain of uncertain sensitivity and specificity and are not widely used for diagnostic purposes.

Polymerase chain reaction amplification of viral nucleic acid

Amplification of viral-specific DNA or RNA from CSF using PCR amplification has become the single most important method for diagnosing CNS viral infections. In both enteroviral and HSV infections of the CNS, PCR has become the diagnostic procedure of choice and is substantially more sensitive than viral cultures. HSV PCR is also an important diagnostic test in patients with recurrent episodes of "aseptic" meningitis, many of whom have amplifiable HSV DNA in CSF despite negative viral cultures. CSF PCR is also used routinely to diagnose CNS viral infections caused by cytomegalovirus (CMV), Epstein-Barr virus (EBV), VZV, and human herpesvirus 6 (HHV-6). CSF PCR tests are available for WNV but are not as sensitive as detection of WNV-specific CSF IgM. PCR is also useful in the diagnosis of CNS infection caused by *Mycoplasma pneumoniae,* which can mimic viral meningitis and encephalitis.

Viral culture

The sensitivity of CSF cultures for the diagnosis of viral meningitis and encephalitis, in contrast to its utility in bacterial infections, is generally poor. In addition to CSF, specific viruses may also be isolated from throat swabs, stool, blood, and urine. Enteroviruses and adenoviruses may be found in feces; arboviruses, some enteroviruses, and LCMV in blood; mumps and CMV in urine; and enteroviruses, mumps, and adenoviruses in throat washings. During enteroviral infections, viral shedding in stool may persist for several weeks. The presence of enterovirus in stool is not diagnostic and may result from residual shedding from a previous enteroviral infection; it also occurs in some asymptomatic individuals during enteroviral epidemics.

Serologic studies

For some viruses, including many arboviruses such as WNV, serologic studies remain a crucial diagnostic tool. Serum antibody determination is less useful for viruses with high seroprevalence rates in the general population such as HSV, VZV, CMV, and EBV. For viruses with low seroprevalence rates, diagnosis of acute viral infection can be made by documenting seroconversion between acute-phase and convalescent sera (typically obtained after 2–4 weeks) or by demonstrating the presence of virus-specific IgM antibodies. Documentation of synthesis of virus-specific antibodies in CSF, as shown by an increased IgG index or the presence of CSF IgM antibodies, is more useful than serum serology alone and can provide presumptive evidence of CNS infection. Although serum and CSF IgM antibodies generally persist for only a few months after acute infection, there are exceptions to this rule. For example, WNV IgM has been shown to persist in some patients for >1 year following acute infection. Unfortunately, the delay between onset of infection and the host's generation of a virus-specific antibody response often means that serologic data are useful mainly for the retrospective establishment of a specific diagnosis, rather than in aiding acute diagnosis or management.

CSF oligoclonal gamma globulin bands occur in association with a number of viral infections. The associated antibodies are often directed against viral proteins. Oligoclonal bands also occur commonly in certain noninfectious neurologic diseases (e.g., multiple sclerosis) and may be found in nonviral infections (e.g., neurosyphilis, Lyme neuroborreliosis).

Other laboratory studies

All patients with suspected viral meningitis should have a complete blood count and differential, liver and renal function tests, erythrocyte sedimentation rate (ESR), and C-reactive protein, electrolytes, glucose, creatine kinase, aldolase, amylase, and lipase. Neuroimaging studies (MRI, CT) are not necessary in patients with uncomplicated viral meningitis but should be performed in patients with altered consciousness, seizures, focal neurologic signs or symptoms, or atypical CSF profiles.

DIFFERENTIAL DIAGNOSIS

The most important issue in the differential diagnosis of viral meningitis is to consider diseases that can mimic viral meningitis, including (1) untreated or partially treated bacterial meningitis; (2) early stages of meningitis caused by fungi, mycobacteria, or *Treponema pallidum* (neurosyphilis), in which a lymphocytic pleocytosis is common, cultures may be slow growing or negative, and hypoglycorrhachia may not be present early; (3) meningitis caused by agents such as *Mycoplasma*, *Listeria* spp., *Brucella* spp., *Coxiella* spp., *Leptospira* spp., and *Rickettsia* spp.; (4) parameningeal infections; (5) neoplastic meningitis; and (6) meningitis secondary to noninfectious inflammatory diseases, including hypersensitivity meningitis, SLE and other rheumatologic diseases, sarcoidosis, Behçet's syndrome, and the uveomeningitic syndromes. Studies in children >28 days of age suggest that the presence of CSF protein >0.5 g/L (sensitivity 89%, specificity 78%), and elevated serum procalcitonin levels >0.5 ng/mL (sensitivity 89%, specificity 89%) were clues to the presence of bacterial as opposed to "aseptic" meningitis. A variety of clinical algorithms for differentiating bacterial from aseptic meningitis have been promulgated, although none have been widely validated. One such prospectively validated system, the *bacterial meningitis score*, suggests that the probability of bacterial meningitis is 0.1% or less (negative predictive value 99.9%, 95% CI 99.6–100%) in children with CSF pleocytosis who have: (1) a negative CSF Gram's stain, (2) CSF neutrophil count <1000 cells/μL, (3) CSF protein <80 mg/dL, (4) peripheral absolute neutrophil count of <10,000 cells/μL, and (5) no prior history or current presence of seizures.

SPECIFIC VIRAL ETIOLOGIES

Enteroviruses (EV) are the most common cause of viral meningitis, accounting for >85% of cases in which a specific etiology can be identified. Cases may either be sporadic or occur in clusters. Recent outbreaks of EV meningitis in the United States have been associated with coxsackievirus B5 and echovirus strains 6, 9, and 30. Coxsackievirus strains A9, B3, and B4 are more commonly associated with individual cases. EV71 has produced large epidemics of neurologic disease outside the United States, especially in Southeast Asia, but most recently reported cases in the United States have been sporadic. Enteroviruses are the most likely cause of viral meningitis in the summer and fall months, especially in children (<15 years), although cases occur at reduced frequency year round. Although the incidence of enteroviral meningitis declines with increasing age, some outbreaks have preferentially affected older children and adults. Meningitis outside the neonatal period is usually benign. Patients present with sudden onset of fever; headache; nuchal rigidity; and often constitutional signs, including vomiting, anorexia, diarrhea, cough, pharyngitis, and myalgias. The physical examination should include a careful search for stigmata of enterovirus infection, including exanthems, hand-foot-mouth disease, herpangina, pleurodynia, myopericarditis, and hemorrhagic conjunctivitis. The CSF profile is typically a lymphocytic pleocytosis (100–1000 cells/μL) with normal glucose and normal or mildly elevated protein concentration. However, up to 15% of patients, most commonly young infants rather than older children or adults, have a normal CSF leukocyte count. In rare cases, PMNs may predominate during the first 48 h of illness. CSF reverse transcriptase PCR (RT-PCR) is the diagnostic procedure of choice and is both sensitive (>95%) and specific (>100%). CSF PCR has the highest sensitivity if performed within 48 h of symptom onset, with sensitivity declining rapidly after day 5 of symptoms. Treatment is supportive, and patients usually recover without sequelae. Chronic and severe infections can occur in neonates and in individuals with hypo- or agammaglobulinemia.

Arbovirus infections occur predominantly in the summer and early fall. Arboviral meningitis should be considered when clusters of meningitis and encephalitis cases occur in a restricted geographic region during the summer or early fall. In the United States the most important causes of arboviral meningitis and encephalitis are West Nile virus, St. Louis encephalitis virus, and the California encephalitis group of viruses. In WNV epidemics, avian deaths may serve as sentinel infections for subsequent human disease. A history of tick exposure or travel or residence in the appropriate geographic area should suggest the possibility of Colorado tick fever virus or Powassan virus infection, although nonviral tick-borne diseases, including RMSF and Lyme neuroborreliosis, may present similarly. Arbovirus meningoencephalitis is typically associated with a CSF lymphocytic pleocytosis, normal glucose concentration, and normal or mildly elevated protein concentration. However, 40–45% of patients with WNV meningoencephalitis have CSF neutrophilia, which can persist for a week or more. The rarity of hypoglycorrhachia in WNV infection as well as the absence of positive Gram's stains and the negative cultures helps distinguish these patients from those with bacterial meningitis. The presence of increased numbers of plasmacytoid cells or Mollaret-like large mononuclear cells in the CSF may be a clue to the diagnosis of WNV infection. Definitive diagnosis of arboviral meningoencephalitis is based on demonstration of viral-specific IgM in CSF or seroconversion. CSF PCR tests are available for some viruses in selected diagnostic laboratories and at the Centers for Disease Control and Prevention (CDC), but in the case of WNV, sensitivity (~70%) of CSF PCR is less than that of CSF serology.

HSV-2 meningitis has been increasingly recognized as a major cause of viral meningitis in adults, and overall it is probably second in importance to enteroviruses as a cause of viral meningitis, accounting for 5% of total cases overall and undoubtedly a higher frequency of those cases occurring in adults and/or outside of the summer-fall period when enterovirus infections are increasingly common. HSV meningitis occurs in ~25-35% of women and ~10-15% of men at the time of an initial (primary) episode of genital herpes. Of these patients, 20% go on to have recurrent attacks of meningitis. Diagnosis of HSV meningitis is usually by HSV CSF PCR as cultures may be negative, especially in patients with recurrent meningitis. Demonstration of intrathecal synthesis of HSV-specific antibody may also be useful in diagnosis, although antibody tests are less sensitive and less specific than PCR and may not become positive until after the first week of infection. In contrast to HSV encephalitis in adults in which >90% of cases are due to HSV-1, the overwhelming majority of HSV meningitis is due to HSV-2. Although a history of or the presence of HSV genital lesions is an important diagnostic clue, many patients with HSV meningitis give no history and have no evidence of active genital herpes at the time of presentation. Most cases of recurrent viral or "aseptic" meningitis, including cases previously diagnosed as Mollaret's meningitis, are likely due to HSV.

VZV meningitis should be suspected in the presence of concurrent chickenpox or shingles. However, it is important to recognize that in some series, up to 40% of VZV meningitis cases have been reported to occur in the absence of rash. The frequency of VZV as a cause of meningitis is extremely variable, ranging from as low as 3% to as high as 20% in different series. Diagnosis is usually based on CSF PCR, although the sensitivity of this test may not be as high as for the other herpesviruses. In patients with negative CSF PCR results, the diagnosis of VZV CNS infection can be made by the demonstration of VZV-specific intrathecal antibody synthesis and/or the presence of VZV CSF IgM antibodies, or by positive CSF cultures.

EBV infections may also produce aseptic meningitis, with or without associated infectious mononucleosis. The presence of atypical lymphocytes in the CSF or peripheral blood is suggestive of EBV infection but may occasionally be seen with other viral infections. EBV is almost never cultured from CSF. Serum and CSF serology can help establish the presence of acute infection, which is characterized by IgM viral capsid antibodies (VCAs), antibodies to early antigens (EAs), and the absence of antibodies to EBV-associated nuclear antigen (EBNA). CSF PCR is another important diagnostic test, although positive results may reflect viral reactivation associated with other infectious or inflammatory processes.

HIV meningitis should be suspected in any patient presenting with a viral meningitis with known or suspected risk factors for HIV infection. Meningitis may occur following primary infection with HIV in 5–10% of cases and less commonly at later stages of illness. Cranial nerve palsies, most commonly involving cranial nerves V, VII, or VIII, are more common in HIV meningitis than in other viral infections. Diagnosis can be confirmed by detection of HIV genome in blood or CSF. Seroconversion may be delayed, and patients with negative HIV serologies who are suspected of having HIV meningitis should be monitored for delayed seroconversion. For further discussion of HIV infection, see Chap. 42.

Mumps should be considered when meningitis occurs in the late winter or early spring, especially in males (male/female ratio 3:1). With the widespread use of the live attenuated mumps vaccine in the United States since 1967, the incidence of mumps meningitis has fallen by >95%; however, mumps remains a potential source of infection in nonimmunized individuals and populations. Rare cases (10–100:100,000 vaccinated individuals) of vaccine-associated mumps meningitis have been described, with onset typically 2–4 weeks after vaccination. The presence of parotitis, orchitis, oophoritis, pancreatitis, or elevations in serum lipase and amylase is suggestive of mumps meningitis; however, their absence does not exclude the diagnosis. Clinical meningitis was previously estimated to occur in 10–30% of patients with mumps parotitis; however, in a recent U.S. outbreak of nearly 2600 cases of mumps, only 11 cases of meningitis were identified, suggesting the incidence may be lower than previously suspected. Mumps infection confers lifelong immunity, so a documented history of previous infection excludes this diagnosis. Patients with meningitis have a CSF pleocytosis that can exceed 1000 cells/μL in 25%. Lymphocytes predominate in 75%, although CSF neutrophilia occurs in 25%. Hypoglycorrhachia occurs in 10–30% of patients and may be a clue to the diagnosis when present. Diagnosis is typically made by culture of virus from CSF or by detecting IgM antibodies or seroconversion. CSF PCR is available in some diagnostic and research laboratories.

LCMV infection should be considered when aseptic meningitis occurs in the late fall or winter and in individuals with a history of exposure to house mice (*Mus musculus*), pet or laboratory rodents (e.g., hamsters, rats, mice), or their excreta. Some patients have an associated rash, pulmonary infiltrates, alopecia, parotitis, orchitis, or myopericarditis. Laboratory clues to the diagnosis of LCMV, in addition to the clinical findings noted earlier, may include the presence of leukopenia, thrombocytopenia, or abnormal liver function tests. Some cases present with a marked CSF pleocytosis (>1000 cells/μL) and hypoglycorrhachia (<30%). Diagnosis is based on serology and/or culture of virus from CSF.

TREATMENT Acute Viral Meningitis

Treatment of almost all cases of viral meningitis is primarily symptomatic and includes use of analgesics, antipyretics, and antiemetics. Fluid and electrolyte status should be monitored. Patients with suspected bacterial meningitis should receive appropriate empirical therapy pending culture results (discussed earlier). Hospitalization may not be required in immunocompetent patients with presumed viral meningitis and no focal signs or symptoms, no significant alteration in consciousness, and a classic CSF profile (lymphocytic pleocytosis, normal glucose, negative Gram's stain) if adequate provision for monitoring at home and medical follow-up can be ensured. Immunocompromised patients; patients with significant alteration in consciousness, seizures, or the presence of focal signs and symptoms suggesting the possibility of encephalitis or parenchymal brain involvement; and those patients who have an atypical CSF profile should be hospitalized. Oral or intravenous acyclovir may be of benefit in patients with meningitis caused by HSV-1 or -2 and in cases of severe EBV or VZV infection. Data concerning treatment of HSV, EBV, and VZV meningitis are extremely limited. Seriously ill patients should probably receive intravenous acyclovir (15–30 mg/kg per day in three divided doses), which can be followed by an oral drug such as acyclovir (800 mg, five times daily), famciclovir (500 mg tid), or valacyclovir (1000 mg tid) for a total course of 7–14 days. Patients who are less ill can be treated with oral drugs alone. Patients with HIV meningitis should receive highly active antiretroviral therapy (Chap. 42).

Patients with viral meningitis who are known to have deficient humoral immunity (e.g., X-linked agammaglobulinemia) and who are not already receiving either intramuscular gamma globulin or intravenous immunoglobulin (IVIg) should be treated with these agents. Intraventricular administration of immunoglobulin through an Ommaya reservoir has been tried in some patients with chronic enteroviral meningitis who have not responded to intramuscular or intravenous immunoglobulin.

An investigational drug, pleconaril, has shown efficacy against a variety of enteroviral infections and has good oral bioavailability and excellent CNS penetration. Clinical trials in patients with enteroviral meningitis indicated that pleconaril decreased the duration of symptoms compared to placebo; however, the drug is not likely to be marketed and is not generally available, due to its modest benefit in trials of non-CNS EV infections.

Vaccination is an effective method of preventing the development of meningitis and other neurologic complications associated with poliovirus, mumps, and measles infection. A live attenuated VZV vaccine (Varivax) is available in the United States. Clinical studies indicate an effectiveness rate of 70–90% for this vaccine, but a booster may be required to maintain immunity. An inactivated varicella vaccine is available for transplant recipients.

PROGNOSIS

In adults, the prognosis for full recovery from viral meningitis is excellent. Rare patients complain of persisting headache, mild mental impairment, incoordination, or generalized asthenia for weeks to months. The outcome in infants and neonates (<1 year) is less certain; intellectual impairment, learning disabilities, hearing loss, and other lasting sequelae have been reported in some studies.

VIRAL ENCEPHALITIS

DEFINITION

In contrast to viral meningitis, where the infectious process and associated inflammatory response are limited largely to the meninges, in encephalitis the brain parenchyma is also involved. Many patients with encephalitis also have evidence of associated meningitis (meningoencephalitis) and, in some cases, involvement of the spinal cord or nerve roots (encephalomyelitis, encephalomyeloradiculitis).

CLINICAL MANIFESTATIONS

In addition to the acute febrile illness with evidence of meningeal involvement characteristic of meningitis, the patient with encephalitis commonly has an altered level of consciousness (confusion, behavioral abnormalities), or a depressed level of consciousness ranging from mild lethargy to coma, and evidence of either focal or diffuse neurologic signs and symptoms. Patients with encephalitis may have hallucinations, agitation, personality change, behavioral disorders, and, at times, a frankly psychotic state. Focal or generalized seizures occur in many patients with encephalitis. Virtually every possible type of focal neurologic disturbance has been reported in viral encephalitis; the signs and symptoms reflect the sites of infection and inflammation. The most commonly encountered focal findings are aphasia, ataxia, upper or lower motor neuron patterns of weakness, involuntary movements (e.g., myoclonic jerks, tremor), and cranial nerve deficits (e.g., ocular palsies, facial weakness). Involvement of the hypothalamic-pituitary axis may result in temperature dysregulation, diabetes insipidus, or the development of the syndrome of inappropriate secretion of antidiuretic hormone (SIADH). Even though neurotropic viruses typically cause pathologic injury in distinct regions of the CNS, variations in clinical presentations make it impossible to reliably establish the etiology of a specific case of encephalitis on clinical grounds alone (see "Differential Diagnosis," later in the chapter).

ETIOLOGY

In the United States, there are ~20,000 reported cases of encephalitis per year, although the actual number of cases is likely to be significantly larger. Despite comprehensive diagnostic efforts, the majority of cases of acute encephalitis of suspected viral etiology remain of unknown cause. Hundreds of viruses are capable of causing encephalitis, although only a limited subset is responsible for most cases in which a specific cause is identified (Table 40-4). The most commonly identified viruses causing sporadic cases of acute encephalitis in immunocompetent adults are herpesviruses (HSV, VZV, EBV). Epidemics of encephalitis are caused by arboviruses, which belong to several different viral taxonomic groups including *Alphaviruses* (e.g., EEE virus, western equine encephalitis virus), *Flaviviruses* (e.g., WNV, St. Louis encephalitis virus, Japanese encephalitis virus, Powassan virus), and *Bunyaviruses* (e.g., California encephalitis virus serogroup, LaCrosse virus). Historically, the largest number of cases of arbovirus encephalitis in the United States has been due to St. Louis encephalitis virus and the California encephalitis virus serogroup. However, since 2002, WNV has been responsible for the majority of arbovirus meningitis and encephalitis cases in the United States. The 2003 epidemic was the largest epidemic of arboviral neuroinvasive disease (encephalitis + meningitis) ever recorded in the United States, with 2866 cases and 264 deaths. In 2004–2007, WNV has accounted for between 1142 and 1459 confirmed cases of neuroinvasive disease per year in the United States and 100–177 deaths. In 2008 and 2009 there was an unexpected and dramatic decline in both the number of WNV neuroinvasive cases (2008 = 687, 2009 = 335) and the number of deaths (2008 = 44, 2009 = 30). New causes of viral CNS infections are constantly appearing, as evidenced by the recent outbreak of cases of encephalitis in Southeast Asia caused by Nipah virus, a newly identified member of the Paramyxoviridae family; of meningitis in Europe caused by Toscana virus, an arbovirus belonging to the Bunyavirus family; and of neurologic disorders associated with major epidemics of Chikungunya virus, a togavirus, in Africa, India, and Southeast Asia.

LABORATORY DIAGNOSIS

CSF examination

CSF examination should be performed in all patients with suspected viral encephalitis unless contraindicated by the presence of severely increased ICP. The characteristic CSF profile is indistinguishable from that of viral meningitis and typically consists of a lymphocytic pleocytosis, a mildly elevated protein concentration, and a normal glucose concentration. A CSF pleocytosis (>5 cells/μL) occurs in >95% of immunocompetent patients with documented viral encephalitis. In rare cases, a pleocytosis may be absent on the initial LP but present on subsequent LPs. Patients who are severely immunocompromised by HIV infection, glucocorticoid or other immunosuppressant drugs, chemotherapy, or lymphoreticular malignancies may fail to mount a CSF inflammatory response. CSF cell counts exceed 500/μL in only about 10% of patients with encephalitis. Infections with certain arboviruses (e.g., EEE virus or California encephalitis virus), mumps, and LCMV may occasionally result in cell counts >1000/μL, but this degree of pleocytosis should suggest the possibility of nonviral infections or other inflammatory processes. Atypical lymphocytes in the CSF may be seen in EBV infection and less commonly with other viruses, including CMV, HSV, and enteroviruses. Increased numbers of plasmacytoid or Mollaret-like large mononuclear cells have been reported in WNV encephalitis. Polymorphonuclear pleocytosis occurs in ~45% of patients with WNV encephalitis and is also a common feature in CMV myeloradiculitis in immunocompromised patients. Large numbers of CSF PMNs may be present in patients with encephalitis due to EEE virus, echovirus 9, and, more rarely, other enteroviruses. However, persisting CSF neutrophilia should prompt consideration of bacterial infection, leptospirosis, amebic infection, and noninfectious processes such as acute hemorrhagic leukoencephalitis. About 20% of patients with encephalitis will have a significant number of red blood cells (>500/μL) in the CSF in a nontraumatic tap. The pathologic correlate of this finding may be a hemorrhagic encephalitis of the type seen with HSV; however, CSF red blood cells occur with similar frequency and in similar numbers in patients with nonherpetic focal encephalitides. A decreased CSF glucose concentration is distinctly unusual in viral encephalitis and should suggest the possibility of bacterial, fungal, tuberculous, parasitic, leptospiral, syphilitic, sarcoid, or neoplastic meningitis. Rare patients with mumps, LCMV, or advanced HSV encephalitis and many patients with CMV myeloradiculitis have low CSF glucose concentrations.

CSF PCR

CSF PCR has become the primary diagnostic test for CNS infections caused by CMV, EBV, HHV-6, and enteroviruses (see "Viral Meningitis," earlier in the chapter). In the case of VZV CNS infection, CSF PCR and detection of virus-specific IgM or intrathecal antibody synthesis both provide important aids to diagnosis. The sensitivity and specificity of CSF PCRs varies with the virus being tested. The sensitivity (~96%) and specificity (~99%) of HSV CSF PCR is equivalent to or exceeds that of brain biopsy. It is important to recognize that HSV CSF PCR results need to be interpreted after considering the likelihood of disease in the patient being tested, the timing of the test in relationship to onset of symptoms, and the prior use of antiviral therapy. A negative HSV CSF PCR test performed by a qualified laboratory at the appropriate time during illness in a patient with a high likelihood of HSV encephalitis based on clinical and laboratory abnormalities significantly reduces the likelihood of HSV encephalitis but does not exclude it. For example, in a patient with a pretest probability of 35% of having HSV encephalitis, a negative HSV CSF PCR reduces the posttest probability to ~2%, and for a patient with a pretest probability of 60%, a negative test reduces the posttest probability to ~6%. In both situations a positive test makes the diagnosis almost certain (98–99%). There have been several recent reports of initially negative HSV CSF PCR tests that were obtained early (≤72 h) following symptom onset and that became positive when repeated 1–3 days later. The frequency of positive HSV CSF PCRs in patients with herpes encephalitis also decreases as a function of the duration of illness, with only ~20% of cases remaining positive after ≥14 days. PCR results are generally not affected by ≤1 week of antiviral therapy. In one study, 98% of CSF specimens remained PCR-positive during the first week of initiation of antiviral therapy, but the numbers fell to ~50% by 8–14 days and to ~21% by >15 days after initiation of antiviral therapy.

The sensitivity and specificity of CSF PCR tests for viruses other than herpes simplex have not been definitively characterized. Enteroviral CSF PCR appears to have a sensitivity and specificity of >95%. The specificity of EBV CSF PCR has not been established. Positive EBV CSF PCRs associated with positive tests for other pathogens have been reported and may reflect reactivation of EBV latent in lymphocytes that enter the CNS as a result of an unrelated infectious or inflammatory process. In patients with CNS infection due to VZV, CSF antibody and PCR studies should be considered complementary, as patients may have evidence of intrathecal synthesis of VZV-specific antibodies and negative CSF PCRs. In the case of WNV infection, CSF PCR appears to be less sensitive (~70% sensitivity) than detection of WNV-specific CSF IgM, although PCR testing remains useful in immunocompromised patients who may not mount an effective anti-WNV antibody response.

CSF culture

CSF culture is generally of limited utility in the diagnosis of acute viral encephalitis. Culture may be insensitive (e.g., >95% of patients with HSV encephalitis have negative CSF cultures as do virtually all patients with EBV-associated CNS disease) and often takes too long to significantly affect immediate therapy.

Serologic studies and antigen detection

The basic approach to the serodiagnosis of viral encephalitis is identical to that discussed earlier for viral meningitis. Demonstration of WNV IgM antibodies is diagnostic of WNV encephalitis as IgM antibodies do not cross the blood-brain barrier, and their presence in CSF is therefore indicative of intrathecal synthesis. Timing of antibody collection may be important as the rate of CSF WNV IgM seropositivity increases by ~10% per day during the first week after illness onset, reaching 80% or higher on day 7 after symptom onset. In patients with HSV encephalitis, both antibodies to HSV-1 glycoproteins and glycoprotein antigens have been detected in the CSF. Optimal detection of both HSV antibodies and antigen typically occurs after the first week of illness, limiting the utility of these tests in acute diagnosis. Nonetheless, HSV CSF antibody testing is of value in selected patients whose illness is >1 week in duration and who are CSF PCR–negative for HSV. In the case of VZV infection, CSF antibody tests may be positive when PCR fails to detect viral DNA, and both tests should be considered complementary rather than mutually exclusive.

MRI, CT, EEG

Patients with suspected encephalitis almost invariably undergo neuroimaging studies and often EEG. These tests help identify or exclude alternative diagnoses and assist in the differentiation between a focal, as opposed to a diffuse, encephalitic process. Focal findings in a patient with encephalitis should always raise the possibility of HSV encephalitis. Examples of focal findings include: (1) areas of increased signal intensity in the frontotemporal, cingulate, or insular regions of the brain on T2-weighted, FLAIR, or diffusion-weighted MRI (Fig. 40-3); (2) focal areas of low absorption, mass effect, and contrast enhancement on CT; or (3) periodic focal temporal lobe spikes on a background of slow or low-amplitude ("flattened") activity on EEG. Approximately 10% of patients with PCR-documented HSV encephalitis will have a normal MRI, although nearly 80% will have abnormalities in the temporal lobe, and an additional 10% in extratemporal regions. The lesions are typically hyperintense on T2-weighted images. The addition of FLAIR and diffusion-weighted images to the standard MRI sequences enhances sensitivity. Children with HSV encephalitis may have atypical patterns of MRI lesions and often show involvement of brain regions outside the frontotemporal areas. CT is less sensitive than MRI and is normal in up to 20–35% of patients. EEG abnormalities occur in >75% of PCR-documented cases of HSV encephalitis; they typically involve the temporal lobes but are often nonspecific. Some patients with HSV encephalitis have a distinctive EEG pattern consisting of periodic, stereotyped, sharp-and-slow complexes originating in one or both temporal lobes and repeating at regular intervals of 2–3 s. The periodic complexes are typically noted between days 2 and 15 of the illness and are present in two-thirds of pathologically proven cases of HSV encephalitis.

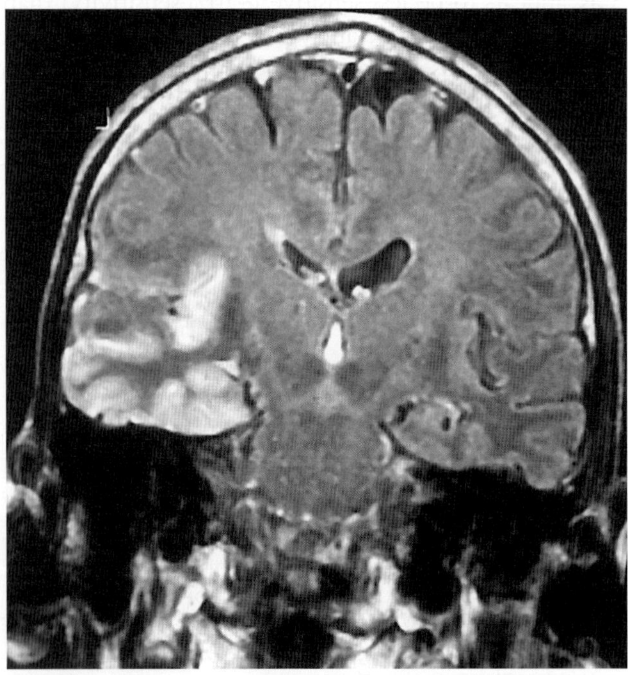

FIGURE 40-3
Coronal FLAIR magnetic resonance image from a patient with herpes simplex encephalitis. Note the area of increased signal in the right temporal lobe (*left side of image*) confined predominantly to the gray matter. This patient had predominantly unilateral disease; bilateral lesions are more common but may be quite asymmetric in their intensity.

Significant MRI abnormalities are found in only ~two-thirds of patients with WNV encephalitis, a frequency less than that with HSV encephalitis. When present, abnormalities often involve deep brain structures, including the thalamus, basal ganglia, and brainstem, rather than the cortex and may only be apparent on FLAIR images. EEGs in patients with WNV encephalitis typically show generalized slowing that may be more anteriorly prominent rather than the temporally predominant pattern of sharp or periodic discharges more characteristic of HSV encephalitis. Patients with VZV encephalitis may show multifocal areas of hemorrhagic and ischemic infarction, reflecting the tendency of this virus to produce a CNS vasculopathy rather than a true encephalitis. Immunocompromised adult patients with CMV often have enlarged ventricles with areas of increased T2 signal on MRI outlining the ventricles and subependymal enhancement on T1-weighted post-contrast images. Table 40-5 highlights specific diagnostic test results in encephalitis that can be useful in clinical decision-making.

Brain biopsy

Brain biopsy is now generally reserved for patients in whom CSF PCR studies fail to lead to a specific diagnosis, who have focal abnormalities on MRI, and who continue to show progressive clinical deterioration despite treatment with acyclovir and supportive therapy.

DIFFERENTIAL DIAGNOSIS

Infection by a variety of other organisms can mimic viral encephalitis. In studies of biopsy-proven HSV

TABLE 40-5

USE OF DIAGNOSTIC TESTS IN ENCEPHALITIS

The best test for WNV encephalitis is the *CSF IgM antibody test*. The prevalence of positive CSF IgM tests increases by about 10% per day after illness onset and reaches 70–80% by the end of the first week. Serum WNV IgM can provide evidence for recent WNV infection, but in the absence of other findings does not establish the diagnosis of neuroinvasive disease (meningitis, encephalitis, acute flaccid paralysis).

Approximately 80% of patients with proven HSV encephalitis have *MRI* abnormalities involving the temporal lobes. This percentage likely increases to >90% when FLAIR and DWI MR sequences are also utilized. The absence of temporal lobe lesions on MR reduces the likelihood of HSV encephalitis and should prompt consideration of other diagnostic possibilities.

The *CSF HSV PCR* test may be negative in the first 72 h of symptoms of HSV encephalitis. A repeat study should be considered in patients with an initial early negative PCR in whom diagnostic suspicion of HSV encephalitis remains high and no alternative diagnosis has yet been established.

Detection of *intrathecal synthesis* (increased CSF/serum HSV antibody ratio corrected for breakdown of the blood-brain barrier) of *HSV-specific antibody* may be useful in diagnosis of HSV encephalitis in patients in whom only late (>1 week post-onset) CSF specimens are available and PCR studies are negative. Serum serology alone is of no value in diagnosis of HSV encephalitis due to the high seroprevalence rate in the general population.

Negative *CSF viral cultures* are of no value in excluding the diagnosis of HSV or EBV encephalitis.

VZV CSF IgM antibodies may be present in patients with a negative VZV CSF PCR. Both tests should be performed in patients with suspected VZV CNS disease.

The specificity of *EBV CSF PCR* for diagnosis of CNS infection is unknown. Positive tests may occur in patients with a CSF pleocytosis due to other causes. Detection of EBV CSF IgM or intrathecal synthesis of antibody to VCA supports the diagnosis of EBV encephalitis. Serological studies consistent with acute EBV infection (e.g., IgM VCA, presence of antibodies against EA but not against EBNA) can help support the diagnosis.

Abbreviations: CNS, central nervous system; CSF, cerebrospinal fluid; DWI, diffusion-weighted imaging; EA, early antigen; EBNA, EBV-associated nuclear antigen; EBV, Epstein-Barr virus; FLAIR, fluid-attenuated inversion recovery; HSV, herpes simplex virus; IgM, immunoglobulin M; MRI, magnetic resonance imaging; PCR, polymerase chain reaction; VCA, viral capsid antibody; VZV, varicella-zoster virus; WNV, West Nile virus.

encephalitis, common infectious mimics of focal viral encephalitis included mycobacteria, fungi, rickettsia, *Listeria, Mycoplasma,* and other bacteria (including *Bartonella* sp.).

Infection caused by the ameba *Naegleria fowleri* can also cause acute meningoencephalitis (primary amebic meningoencephalitis), whereas that caused by *Acanthamoeba* and *Balamuthia* more typically produces subacute or chronic granulomatous amebic meningoencephalitis. *Naegleria* thrive in warm, iron-rich pools of water, including those found in drains, canals, and both natural and human-made outdoor pools. Infection has typically occurred in immunocompetent children with a history of swimming in potentially infected water. The CSF, in contrast to the typical profile seen in viral encephalitis, often resembles that of bacterial meningitis with a neutrophilic pleocytosis and hypoglycorrhachia. Motile trophozoites can be seen in a wet mount of warm, fresh CSF. There have been an increasing number of cases of *Balamuthia mandrillaris* amebic encephalitis mimicking acute viral encephalitis in children and immunocompetent adults. This organism has also been associated with encephalitis in recipients of transplanted organs from a donor with unrecognized infection. No effective treatment has been identified, and mortality approaches 100%.

Encephalitis can be caused by the raccoon pinworm *Baylisascaris procyonis*. Clues to the diagnosis include a history of raccoon exposure, especially of playing in or eating dirt potentially contaminated with raccoon feces. Most patients are children, and many have an associated eosinophilia.

Once nonviral causes of encephalitis have been excluded, the major diagnostic challenge is to distinguish HSV from other viruses that cause encephalitis. This distinction is particularly important because in virtually every other instance the therapy is supportive, whereas specific and effective antiviral therapy is available for HSV, and its efficacy is enhanced when it is instituted early in the course of infection. HSV encephalitis should be considered when clinical features suggesting involvement of the inferomedial frontotemporal regions of the brain are present, including prominent olfactory or gustatory hallucinations, anosmia, unusual or bizarre behavior or personality alterations, or memory disturbance. HSV encephalitis should always be suspected in patients with signs and symptoms consistent with acute encephalitis with focal findings on clinical examination, neuroimaging studies, or EEG. The diagnostic procedure of choice in these patients is CSF PCR analysis for HSV. A positive CSF PCR establishes the diagnosis, and a negative test dramatically reduces the likelihood of HSV encephalitis (discussed earlier).

The anatomic distribution of lesions may provide an additional clue to diagnosis. Patients with rapidly progressive encephalitis and prominent brainstem signs, symptoms, or neuroimaging abnormalities may be infected by flaviviruses (WNV, St. Louis encephalitis virus, Japanese encephalitis virus), HSV, rabies, or *L. monocytogenes*. Significant involvement of deep gray matter structures, including the basal ganglia and thalamus, should also suggest possible flavivirus infection. These patients may present clinically with prominent movement disorders (tremor, myoclonus) or parkinsonian features. Patients with WNV infection can also present with a poliomyelitis-like acute flaccid paralysis, as can patients infected with enterovirus 71 and, less commonly, other enteroviruses. Acute flaccid paralysis is characterized by the acute onset of a lower motor neuron type of weakness with flaccid tone, reduced or absent reflexes, and relatively preserved sensation. Despite an aggressive World Health Organization poliovirus eradication initiative, 1733 cases of wild-type poliovirus-induced poliomyelitis were reported worldwide in 2009, with 73% occurring in India and Nigeria. There have been recent small outbreaks of poliomyelitis associated with vaccine strains of virus that have reverted to virulence through mutation or recombination with circulating wild-type enteroviruses in Hispaniola, China, the Philippines, Indonesia, Nigeria, and Madagascar.

Epidemiologic factors may provide important clues to the diagnosis of viral meningitis or encephalitis. Particular attention should be paid to the season of the year; the geographic location and travel history; and possible exposure to animal bites or scratches, rodents, and ticks. Although transmission from the bite of an infected dog remains the most common cause of rabies worldwide, in the United States very few cases of dog rabies occur, and the most common risk factor is exposure to bats—although a clear history of a bite or scratch is often lacking. The classic clinical presentation of encephalitic (furious) rabies is of fever, fluctuating consciousness, and autonomic hyperactivity. Phobic spasms of the larynx, pharynx, neck muscles, and diaphragm can be triggered by attempts to swallow water (*hydrophobia*) or by inspiration (*aerophobia*). Patients may also present with paralytic (dumb) rabies characterized by acute ascending paralysis. Rabies due to the bite of a bat has a different clinical presentation than classic rabies due to a dog or wolf bite. Patients present with focal neurologic deficits, myoclonus, seizures, and hallucinations; phobic spasms are not a typical feature. Patients with rabies have a CSF lymphocytic pleocytosis and may show areas of increased T2 signal abnormality in the brainstem, hippocampus, and hypothalamus. Diagnosis can be made by finding rabies virus antigen in brain tissue or in the neural innervation of hair follicles at the nape of the neck. PCR amplification of viral nucleic acid from CSF and saliva or tears may also enable diagnosis. Serology is frequently negative in both serum and CSF in the first week after onset of infection, which limits its acute diagnostic utility. No specific therapy is available, and cases are almost invariably fatal, with isolated survivors having devastating neurologic sequelae.

State public health authorities provide a valuable resource concerning isolation of particular agents in individual regions. Regular updates concerning the number, type, and distribution of cases of arboviral encephalitis can be found on the CDC and U.S. Geological Survey (USGS) websites (*http://www.cdc.gov* and *http://diseasemaps.usgs.gov*).

The major noninfectious etiologies that should be included in the differential diagnosis of acute encephalitis are nonvasculitic autoimmune inflammatory meningoencephalitis, which is frequently associated with serum antithyroid microsomal and antithyroglobulin antibodies (Hashimoto's encephalopathy); paraneoplastic and non-paraneoplastic encephalitis associated with antineuronal antibodies (Chap. 44); acute disseminated encephalomyelitis and related fulminant demyelinating disorders (Chap. 39); and lymphoma. Finally, Creutzfeldt-Jakob disease (Chap. 43) can rarely present in an explosive fashion mimicking viral encephalitis.

TREATMENT Viral Encephalitis

Specific antiviral therapy should be initiated when appropriate. Vital functions, including respiration and blood pressure, should be monitored continuously and supported as required. In the initial stages of encephalitis, many patients will require care in an intensive care unit. Basic management and supportive therapy should include careful monitoring of ICP, fluid restriction, avoidance of hypotonic intravenous solutions, and suppression of fever. Seizures should be treated with standard anticonvulsant regimens, and prophylactic therapy should be considered in view of the high frequency of seizures in severe cases of encephalitis. As with all seriously ill, immobilized patients with altered levels of consciousness, encephalitis patients are at risk for aspiration pneumonia, stasis ulcers and decubiti, contractures, deep venous thrombosis and its complications, and infections of indwelling lines and catheters.

Acyclovir is of benefit in the treatment of HSV and should be started empirically in patients with suspected viral encephalitis, especially if focal features are present, while awaiting viral diagnostic studies. Treatment should be discontinued in patients found not to have HSV encephalitis, with the possible exception of patients with severe encephalitis due to VZV or EBV. HSV, VZV, and EBV all encode an enzyme, deoxypyrimidine (thymidine) kinase, that phosphorylates acyclovir to produce acyclovir-5′-monophosphate. Host cell enzymes then phosphorylate this compound to form a triphosphate derivative. It is the triphosphate that acts as an antiviral agent by inhibiting viral DNA polymerase and by causing premature termination of nascent viral DNA chains. The specificity of action depends on the fact that uninfected cells do not phosphorylate significant amounts of acyclovir to acyclovir-5′-monophosphate. A second level of specificity is provided by the fact that the acyclovir triphosphate is a more potent inhibitor of viral DNA polymerase than of the analogous host cell enzymes.

Adults should receive a dose of 10 mg/kg of acyclovir intravenously every 8 h (30 mg/kg per day total dose) for 14–21 days. CSF PCR can be repeated at the completion of this course, with PCR-positive patients receiving additional treatment, followed by a repeat CSF PCR test. Neonatal HSV CNS infection is less responsive to acyclovir therapy than HSV encephalitis in adults; it is recommended that neonates with HSV encephalitis receive 20 mg/kg of acyclovir every 8 h (60 mg/kg per day total dose) for a minimum of 21 days.

Prior to intravenous administration, acyclovir should be diluted to a concentration ≤7 mg/mL. (A 70-kg person would receive a dose of 700 mg, which would be diluted in a volume of 100 mL.) Each dose should be infused slowly over 1 h, rather than by rapid or bolus infusion, to minimize the risk of renal dysfunction. Care should be taken to avoid extravasation or intramuscular or subcutaneous administration. The alkaline pH of acyclovir can cause local inflammation and phlebitis (9%). Dose adjustment is required in patients with impaired renal glomerular filtration. Penetration into CSF is excellent, with average drug levels ~50% of serum levels. Complications of therapy include elevations in blood urea nitrogen and creatinine levels (5%), thrombocytopenia (6%), gastrointestinal toxicity (nausea, vomiting, diarrhea) (7%), and neurotoxicity (lethargy or obtundation, disorientation, confusion, agitation, hallucinations, tremors, seizures) (1%). Acyclovir resistance may be mediated by changes in either the viral deoxypyrimidine kinase or DNA polymerase. To date, acyclovir-resistant isolates have not been a significant clinical problem in immunocompetent individuals. However, there have been reports of clinically virulent acyclovir-resistant HSV isolates from sites outside the CNS in immunocompromised individuals, including those with AIDS.

Oral antiviral drugs with efficacy against HSV, VZV, and EBV, including acyclovir, famciclovir, and valacyclovir, have not been evaluated in the treatment of encephalitis either as primary therapy or as supplemental therapy following completion of a course of parenteral acyclovir. A National Institute of Allergy and Infectious Disease (NIAID)/National Institute of Neurological Disorders and Stroke–sponsored phase III trial of supplemental oral valacyclovir therapy (2 g tid for 3 months) following the initial 14- to 21-day course of therapy with parenteral acyclovir is ongoing in patients with HSV encephalitis (*www.clinicaltrials.gov*, identifier NCT00031486); this may help clarify the role of extended oral antiviral therapy.

Ganciclovir and foscarnet, either alone or in combination, are often utilized in the treatment of CMV-related CNS infections, although their efficacy remains unproven. Cidofovir (see later) may provide an alternative in patients who fail to respond to ganciclovir and foscarnet, although data concerning its use in CMV CNS infections are extremely limited.

Ganciclovir is a synthetic nucleoside analogue of 2′-deoxyguanosine. The drug is preferentially phosphorylated by virus-induced cellular kinases. Ganciclovir triphosphate acts as a competitive inhibitor of the CMV DNA polymerase, and its incorporation into nascent viral DNA results in premature chain termination. Following intravenous administration, CSF concentrations of ganciclovir are 25–70% of coincident plasma levels. The usual dose for treatment of severe neurologic illnesses is 5 mg/kg every 12 h given intravenously at a constant rate over 1 h. Induction therapy is followed by maintenance therapy of 5 mg/kg every day for an indefinite period. Induction therapy should be continued until patients show a decline in CSF pleocytosis and a reduction in CSF CMV DNA copy number on quantitative PCR testing (where available). Doses should be adjusted in patients with renal insufficiency. Treatment is often limited by the development of granulocytopenia and thrombocytopenia (20–25%), which may require reduction in or discontinuation of therapy. Gastrointestinal side effects, including nausea, vomiting, diarrhea, and abdominal pain, occur in ~20% of patients. Some patients treated with ganciclovir for CMV retinitis have developed retinal detachment, but the causal relationship to ganciclovir treatment is unclear. Valganciclovir is an orally bioavailable prodrug that can generate high serum levels of ganciclovir, although studies of its efficacy in treating CMV CNS infections are limited.

Foscarnet is a pyrophosphate analogue that inhibits viral DNA polymerases by binding to the pyrophosphate-binding site. Following intravenous infusion, CSF concentrations range from 15 to 100% of coincident plasma levels. The usual dose for serious CMV-related neurologic illness is 60 mg/kg every 8 h administered by constant infusion over 1 h. Induction therapy for 14–21 days is followed by maintenance therapy (60–120 mg/kg per day). Induction therapy may need to be extended in patients who fail to show a decline in CSF pleocytosis and a reduction in CSF CMV DNA copy number on quantitative PCR tests (where available). Approximately one-third of patients develop renal impairment during treatment, which is reversible following discontinuation of therapy in most, but not all, cases. This is often associated with elevations in serum creatinine and proteinuria and is less frequent in patients who are adequately hydrated. Many patients experience fatigue and nausea. Reduction in serum calcium, magnesium, and potassium occur in ~15% of patients and may be associated with tetany, cardiac rhythm disturbances, or seizures.

Cidofovir is a nucleotide analogue that is effective in treating CMV retinitis and equivalent to or better than ganciclovir in some experimental models of murine CMV encephalitis, although data concerning its efficacy in human CMV CNS disease are limited. The usual dose is 5 mg/kg intravenously once weekly for 2 weeks, then biweekly for two or more additional doses, depending on clinical response. Patients must be prehydrated with normal saline (e.g., 1 L over 1–2 h) prior to each dose and treated with probenecid (e.g., 1 g 3 h before cidofovir and 1 g 2 and 8 h after cidofovir). Nephrotoxicity is common; the dose should be reduced if renal function deteriorates.

Intravenous ribavirin (15–25 mg/kg per day in divided doses given every 8 h) has been reported to be of benefit in isolated cases of severe encephalitis due to California encephalitis (LaCrosse) virus. Ribavirin might be of benefit for the rare patients, typically infants or young children, with severe adenovirus or rotavirus encephalitis and in patients with encephalitis due to LCMV or other arenaviruses. However, clinical trials are lacking. Hemolysis, with resulting anemia, has been the major side effect limiting therapy.

No specific antiviral therapy of proven efficacy is currently available for treatment of WNV encephalitis. Patients have been treated with α-interferon, ribavirin, WNV-specific antisense oligonucleotides (*ClinicalTrials.gov*, identifier NCT0091845), an Israeli IVIg preparation that contains high-titer anti-WNV antibody (Omr-IgG-am) (*ClinicalTrials.gov*, identifier NCT00069316 and 0068055), and humanized monoclonal antibodies directed against the viral envelope glycoprotein (*ClinicalTrials.gov*, identifier NCT00927953 and 00515385). WNV chimeric vaccines, in which WNV envelope and premembrane proteins are inserted into the background of another flavivirus, are already undergoing human clinical testing for safety and immunogenicity (*ClinicalTrials.gov*, identifier NCT00746798 and 00442169). Both chimeric and killed inactivated WNV vaccines have been found to be safe and effective in preventing equine WNV infection, and several effective flavivirus vaccines are already in human use, creating optimism that a safe and effective human WNV vaccine can also be developed.

SEQUELAE

There is considerable variation in the incidence and severity of sequelae in patients surviving viral encephalitis. In the case of EEE virus infection, nearly 80% of survivors have severe neurologic sequelae. At the other extreme are infections due to EBV, California encephalitis virus, and Venezuelan equine encephalitis virus, where severe sequelae are unusual. For example, approximately 5–15% of children infected with LaCrosse virus have a residual seizure disorder, and 1% have persistent hemiparesis. Detailed information about sequelae in patients with HSV encephalitis treated with acyclovir is available from the NIAID-Collaborative Antiviral Study Group (CASG) trials. Of 32 acyclovir-treated patients, 26 survived (81%). Of the 26 survivors, 12 (46%) had no or only minor sequelae, 3 (12%) were moderately impaired (gainfully employed but not functioning at their previous level), and 11 (42%) were severely impaired (requiring continuous supportive care). The incidence and severity of sequelae were directly related to the age of the patient and the level of consciousness at the time of initiation of therapy. Patients with severe neurologic impairment (Glasgow coma score 6) at initiation of therapy either died or survived with severe sequelae. Young patients (<30 years) with good neurologic function at initiation of therapy did substantially better (100% survival, 62% with no or mild sequelae) compared with their older counterparts (>30 years; 64% survival, 57% no or mild sequelae). Some recent studies using quantitative HSV CSF PCR tests indicate that clinical outcome following treatment also correlates with the amount of HSV DNA present in CSF at the time of presentation. Many patients with WNV infection have sequelae, including cognitive impairment; weakness; and hyper- or hypokinetic movement disorders, including tremor, myoclonus, and parkinsonism. In a large longitudinal study of prognosis in 156 patients with WNV infection, the mean time to achieve recovery (defined as 95% of maximal predicted score on specific validated tests) was 112–148 days for fatigue, 121–175 days for physical function, 131–139 days for mood, and 302–455 days for mental function (the longer interval in each case representing patients with neuroinvasive disease).

SUBACUTE MENINGITIS

CLINICAL MANIFESTATIONS

Patients with subacute meningitis typically have an unrelenting headache, stiff neck, low-grade fever, and lethargy for days to several weeks before they present for evaluation. Cranial nerve abnormalities and night sweats may be present. This syndrome overlaps that of chronic meningitis, discussed in detail in Chap. 41.

ETIOLOGY

Common causative organisms include *M. tuberculosis*, *C. neoformans*, *H. capsulatum*, *C. immitis*, and *T. pallidum*. Initial infection with *M. tuberculosis* is acquired by inhalation of aerosolized droplet nuclei. Tuberculous meningitis in adults does not develop acutely from hematogenous spread of tubercle bacilli to the meninges.

Rather, millet seed–sized (miliary) tubercles form in the parenchyma of the brain during hematogenous dissemination of tubercle bacilli in the course of primary infection. These tubercles enlarge and are usually caseating. The propensity for a caseous lesion to produce meningitis is determined by its proximity to the subarachnoid space (SAS) and the rate at which fibrous encapsulation develops. Subependymal caseous foci cause meningitis via discharge of bacilli and tuberculous antigens into the SAS. Mycobacterial antigens produce an intense inflammatory reaction that leads to the production of a thick exudate that fills the basilar cisterns and surrounds the cranial nerves and major blood vessels at the base of the brain.

Fungal infections are typically acquired by the inhalation of airborne fungal spores. The initial pulmonary infection may be asymptomatic or present with fever, cough, sputum production, and chest pain. The pulmonary infection is often self-limited. A localized pulmonary fungal infection can then remain dormant in the lungs until there is an abnormality in cell-mediated immunity that allows the fungus to reactivate and disseminate to the CNS. The most common pathogen causing fungal meningitis is *C. neoformans*. This fungus is found worldwide in soil and bird excreta. *H. capsulatum* is endemic to the Ohio and Mississippi River valleys of the central United States and to parts of Central and South America. *C. immitis* is endemic to the desert areas of the southwest United States, northern Mexico, and Argentina.

Syphilis is a sexually transmitted disease that is manifest by the appearance of a painless chancre at the site of inoculation. *T. pallidum* invades the CNS early in the course of syphilis. Cranial nerves VII and VIII are most frequently involved.

LABORATORY DIAGNOSIS

The classic CSF abnormalities in tuberculous meningitis are as follows: (1) elevated opening pressure, (2) lymphocytic pleocytosis (10–500 cells/μL), (3) elevated protein concentration in the range of 1–5 g/L, and (4) decreased glucose concentration in the range of 1.1–2.2 mmol/L (20–40 mg/dL). *The combination of unrelenting headache, stiff neck, fatigue, night sweats, and fever with a CSF lymphocytic pleocytosis and a mildly decreased glucose concentration is highly suspicious for tuberculous meningitis.* The last tube of fluid collected at LP is the best tube to send for a smear for acid-fast bacilli (AFB). If there is a pellicle in the CSF or a cobweb-like clot on the surface of the fluid, AFB can best be demonstrated in a smear of the clot or pellicle. Positive smears are typically reported in only 10–40% of cases of tuberculous meningitis in adults. Cultures of CSF take 4–8 weeks to identify the organism and are positive in ~50% of adults. Culture remains the gold standard to make the diagnosis of tuberculous meningitis. PCR for the detection of *M. tuberculosis* DNA should be sent on CSF if available, but the sensitivity and specificity on CSF have not been defined. The Centers for Disease Control and Prevention recommend the use of nucleic acid amplification tests for the diagnosis of pulmonary tuberculosis.

The characteristic CSF abnormalities in fungal meningitis are a mononuclear or lymphocytic pleocytosis, an increased protein concentration, and a decreased glucose concentration. There may be eosinophils in the CSF in *C. immitis* meningitis. Large volumes of CSF are often required to demonstrate the organism on india ink smear or grow the organism in culture. If spinal fluid examined by LP on two separate occasions fails to yield an organism, CSF should be obtained by high-cervical or cisternal puncture.

The cryptococcal polysaccharide antigen test is a highly sensitive and specific test for cryptococcal meningitis. A reactive CSF cryptococcal antigen test establishes the diagnosis. The detection of the histoplasma polysaccharide antigen in CSF establishes the diagnosis of a fungal meningitis but is not specific for meningitis due to *H. capsulatum*. It may be falsely positive in coccidioidal meningitis. The CSF complement fixation antibody test is reported to have a specificity of 100% and a sensitivity of 75% for coccidioidal meningitis.

The diagnosis of syphilitic meningitis is made when a reactive serum treponemal test (fluorescent treponemal antibody absorption test [FTA-ABS] or microhemagglutination assay–*T. pallidum* [MHA-TP]) is associated with a CSF lymphocytic or mononuclear pleocytosis and an elevated protein concentration, or when the CSF Venereal Disease Research Laboratory (VDRL) is positive. A reactive CSF FTA-ABS is not definitive evidence of neurosyphilis. The CSF FTA-ABS can be falsely positive from blood contamination. A negative CSF VDRL does not rule out neurosyphilis. A negative CSF FTA-ABS or MHA-TP rules out neurosyphilis.

TREATMENT Subacute Meningitis

Empirical therapy of tuberculous meningitis is often initiated on the basis of a high index of suspicion without adequate laboratory support. Initial therapy is a combination of isoniazid (300 mg/d), rifampin (10 mg/kg per day), pyrazinamide (30 mg/kg per day in divided doses), ethambutol (15–25 mg/kg per day in divided doses), and pyridoxine (50 mg/d). When the antimicrobial sensitivity of the *M. tuberculosis* isolate is known, ethambutol can be discontinued. If the clinical response is good, pyrazinamide can be discontinued after 8 weeks and isoniazid and rifampin continued alone for the next 6–12 months. A 6-month course of therapy is acceptable, but therapy should be prolonged for 9–12 months in patients who have an inadequate resolution of symptoms of meningitis or who have positive mycobacterial cultures of CSF during the course of therapy. Dexamethasone therapy is recommended for HIV-negative patients with tuberculous meningitis. The dose is 12–16 mg per day for 3 weeks, then tapered over 3 weeks.

Meningitis due to *C. neoformans* in non-HIV, non-transplant patients is treated with induction therapy with amphotericin B (AmB) (0.7 mg/kg IV per day) plus flucytosine (100 mg/kg per day in four divided doses) for at least 4 weeks if CSF culture results are negative after 2 weeks of treatment. Therapy should be extended for a total of 6 weeks in the patient with neurologic complications. Induction therapy is followed by consolidation therapy with fluconazole 400 mg per day for 8 weeks. Organ transplant recipients are treated with liposomal AmB (3–4 mg/kg per day) or AmB lipid complex (ABLC) 5 mg/kg per day plus flucytosine (100 mg/kg per day in four divided doses) for at least 2 weeks or until CSF culture is sterile. Follow CSF yeast cultures for sterilization rather than the cryptococcal antigen titer. This treatment is followed by an 8- to 10-week course of fluconazole (400–800 mg/d [6–12 mg/kg] PO). If the CSF culture is sterile after 10 weeks of acute therapy, the dose of fluconazole is decreased to 200 mg/d for 6 months to a year. Patients with HIV infection are treated with AmB or a lipid formulation plus flucytosine for at least 2 weeks, followed by fluconazole for a minimum of 8 weeks. HIV-infected patients may require indefinite maintenance therapy with fluconazole 200 mg/d. Meningitis due to *H. capsulatum* is treated with AmB (0.7–1.0 mg/kg per day) for 4–12 weeks. A total dose of 30 mg/kg is recommended. Therapy with AmB is not discontinued until fungal cultures are sterile. After completing a course of AmB, maintenance therapy with itraconazole 200 mg twice daily is initiated and continued for at least 6 months to a year. *C. immitis* meningitis is treated with either high-dose fluconazole (1000 mg daily) as monotherapy or intravenous AmB (0.5–0.7 mg/kg per day) for >4 weeks. Intrathecal AmB (0.25–0.75 mg/d three times weekly) may be required to eradicate the infection. Lifelong therapy with fluconazole (200–400 mg daily) is recommended to prevent relapse. AmBisome (5 mg/kg per day) or AmB lipid complex (5 mg/kg per day) can be substituted for AmB in patients who have or who develop significant renal dysfunction. The most common complication of fungal meningitis is hydrocephalus. Patients who develop hydrocephalus should receive a CSF diversion device. A ventriculostomy can be used until CSF fungal cultures are sterile, at which time the ventriculostomy is replaced by a ventriculoperitoneal shunt.

Syphilitic meningitis is treated with aqueous penicillin G in a dose of 3–4 million units intravenously every 4 h for 10–14 days. An alternative regimen is 2.4 million units of procaine penicillin G intramuscularly daily with 500 mg of oral probenecid four times daily for 10–14 days. Either regimen is followed with 2.4 million units of benzathine penicillin G intramuscularly once a week for 3 weeks. The standard criterion for treatment success is reexamination of the CSF. The CSF should be reexamined at 6-month intervals for 2 years. The cell count is expected to normalize within 12 months, and the VDRL titer to decrease by two dilutions or revert to nonreactive within 2 years of completion of therapy. Failure of the CSF pleocytosis to resolve or an increase in the CSF VDRL titer by two or more dilutions requires retreatment.

CHRONIC ENCEPHALITIS

PROGRESSIVE MULTIFOCAL LEUKOENCEPHALOPATHY

Clinical features and pathology

Progressive multifocal leukoencephalopathy (PML) is characterized pathologically by multifocal areas of demyelination of varying size distributed throughout the brain but sparing the spinal cord and optic nerves. In addition to demyelination, there are characteristic cytologic alterations in both astrocytes and oligodendrocytes. Astrocytes are enlarged and contain hyperchromatic, deformed, and bizarre nuclei and frequent mitotic figures. Oligodendrocytes have enlarged, densely staining nuclei that contain viral inclusions formed by crystalline arrays of JC virus (JCV) particles. Patients often present with visual deficits (45%), typically a homonymous hemianopia; mental impairment (38%) (dementia, confusion, personality change); weakness, including hemi- or monoparesis; and ataxia. Seizures occur in ~20% of patients, predominantly in those with lesions abutting the cortex.

Almost all patients have an underlying immunosuppressive disorder. In recent series, the most common associated conditions were AIDS (80%), hematologic malignancies (13%), transplant recipients (5%), and chronic inflammatory diseases (2%). It has been estimated that up to 5% of AIDS patients will develop PML. There have been more than 30 reported cases of PML occurring in patients being treated for multiple sclerosis and inflammatory bowel disease with natalizumab, a humanized monoclonal antibody that inhibits lymphocyte trafficking into CNS and bowel mucosa by binding to α_4 integrins. Risk in these patients has been estimated at 1 PML case per 1000 treated patients after a mean of 18 months of therapy. Additional cases have been reported in patients receiving other humanized monoclonal antibodies with immunomodulatory activity including efalizumab and rituximab.

The basic clinical and diagnostic features appear to be similar to those seen in PML related to HIV and other forms of immunosuppression.

Diagnostic studies

The diagnosis of PML is frequently suggested by MRI. MRI reveals multifocal asymmetric, coalescing white matter lesions located periventricularly, in the centrum semiovale, in the parietal-occipital region, and in the cerebellum. These lesions have increased signal on T2 and FLAIR images and decreased signal on T1-weighted images. PML lesions are classically nonenhancing (90%) but may rarely show ring enhancement, especially in more immunocompetent patients. PML lesions are not typically associated with edema or mass effect. CT scans, which are less sensitive than MRI for the diagnosis of PML, often show hypodense nonenhancing white matter lesions.

The CSF is typically normal, although mild elevation in protein and/or IgG may be found. Pleocytosis occurs in <25% of cases, is predominantly mononuclear, and rarely exceeds 25 cells/μL. PCR amplification of JCV DNA from CSF has become an important diagnostic tool. The presence of a positive CSF PCR for JCV DNA in association with typical MRI lesions in the appropriate clinical setting is diagnostic of PML, reflecting the assay's relatively high specificity (92–100%); however, sensitivity is variable and a negative CSF PCR does not exclude the diagnosis. In HIV-negative patients and HIV-positive patients not receiving highly active antiviral therapy (HAART), sensitivity is likely 70–90%. In HAART-treated patients, sensitivity may be closer to 60%, reflecting the lower JCV CSF viral load in this relatively more immunocompetent group. Studies with quantitative JCV CSF PCR indicate that patients with low JCV loads (<100 copies/μL) have a generally better prognosis than those with higher viral loads. Patients with negative CSF PCR studies may require brain biopsy for definitive diagnosis. In biopsy or necropsy specimens of brain, JCV antigen and nucleic acid can be detected by immunocytochemistry, in situ hybridization, or PCR amplification. Detection of JCV antigen or genomic material should only be considered diagnostic of PML if accompanied by characteristic pathologic changes, since both antigen and genomic material have been found in the brains of normal patients.

Serologic studies are of no utility in diagnosis due to high basal seroprevalence level (>80%).

TREATMENT Progressive Multifocal Leukoencephalopathy

No effective therapy for PML is available. There are case reports of potential beneficial effects of the 5-HT2a receptor antagonist mirtazapine, which may inhibit binding of JCV to its receptor on oligodendrocytes. Retrospective noncontrolled studies have also suggested a possible beneficial effect of treatment with interferon-alpha. Neither of these agents has been tested in randomized controlled clinical trials. A clinical trial to evaluate the efficacy of the antimalarial drug mefloquine, which inhibits JCV replication in cell culture, is underway (*www.clinicaltrials.gov*, identifier NCT00746941). Intravenous and/or intrathecal cytarabine were not shown to be of benefit in a randomized controlled trial in HIV-associated PML, although some experts suggest that cytarabine may have therapeutic efficacy in situations where breakdown of the blood-brain barrier allows sufficient CSF penetration. A randomized controlled trial of cidofovir in HIV-associated PML also failed to show significant benefit. Since PML almost invariably occurs in immunocompromised individuals, any therapeutic interventions designed to enhance or restore immunocompetence should be considered. Perhaps the most dramatic demonstration of this is disease stabilization and, in rare cases, improvement associated with the improvement in the immune status of HIV-positive patients with AIDS following institution of HAART. In HIV-positive PML patients treated with HAART, 1-year survival is ~50%, although up to 80% of survivors may have significant neurologic sequelae. HIV-positive PML patients with higher CD4 counts (>300/μL^3) and low or nondetectable HIV viral loads have a better prognosis than those with lower CD4 counts and higher viral loads. Although institution of HAART enhances survival in HIV + PML patients, the associated immune reconstitution in patients with an underlying opportunistic infection such as PML may also result in a severe CNS inflammatory syndrome (immune reconstitution inflammatory syndrome [IRIS]) associated with clinical worsening, CSF pleocytosis, and the appearance of new enhancing MRI lesions. Patients receiving natalizumab or other immunomodulatory antibodies, who are suspected of having PML, should have therapy halted and circulating antibodies removed by plasma exchange.

SUBACUTE SCLEROSING PANENCEPHALITIS (SSPE)

SSPE is a rare chronic, progressive demyelinating disease of the CNS associated with a chronic nonpermissive infection of brain tissue with measles virus. The frequency has been estimated at 1 in 100,000–500,000 measles cases. An average of five cases per year are reported in the United States. The incidence has declined dramatically since the introduction of a measles vaccine. Most patients give a history of primary measles infection at an early age (2 years), which is followed after a latent interval of 6–8 years by the development of a progressive neurologic disorder. Some 85% of patients are between

5 and 15 years old at diagnosis. Initial manifestations include poor school performance and mood and personality changes. Typical signs of a CNS viral infection, including fever and headache, do not occur. As the disease progresses, patients develop progressive intellectual deterioration, focal and/or generalized seizures, myoclonus, ataxia, and visual disturbances. In the late stage of the illness, patients are unresponsive, quadriparetic, and spastic, with hyperactive tendon reflexes and extensor plantar responses.

Diagnostic studies

MRI is often normal early, although areas of increased T2 signal develop in the white matter of the brain and brainstem as disease progresses. The EEG may initially show only nonspecific slowing, but with disease progression, patients develop a characteristic periodic pattern with bursts of high-voltage, sharp, slow waves every 3–8 s, followed by periods of attenuated ("flat") background. The CSF is acellular with a normal or mildly elevated protein concentration and a markedly elevated gamma globulin level (>20% of total CSF protein). CSF antimeasles antibody levels are invariably elevated, and oligoclonal antimeasles antibodies are often present. Measles virus can be cultured from brain tissue using special cocultivation techniques. Viral antigen can be identified immunocytochemically, and viral genome can be detected by in situ hybridization or PCR amplification.

TREATMENT Subacute Sclerosing Panencephalitis

No definitive therapy for SSPE is available. Treatment with isoprinosine (Inosiplex, 100 mg/kg per day), alone or in combination with intrathecal or intraventricular alpha interferon, has been reported to prolong survival and produce clinical improvement in some patients but has never been subjected to a controlled clinical trial.

PROGRESSIVE RUBELLA PANENCEPHALITIS

This is an extremely rare disorder that primarily affects males with congenital rubella syndrome, although isolated cases have been reported following childhood rubella. After a latent period of 8–19 years, patients develop progressive neurologic deterioration. The manifestations are similar to those seen in SSPE. CSF shows a mild lymphocytic pleocytosis, slightly elevated protein concentration, markedly increased gamma globulin, and rubella virus–specific oligoclonal bands. No therapy is available. Universal prevention of both congenital and childhood rubella through the use of the available live attenuated rubella vaccine would be expected to eliminate the disease.

BRAIN ABSCESS

DEFINITION

A brain abscess is a focal, suppurative infection within the brain parenchyma, typically surrounded by a vascularized capsule. The term *cerebritis* is often employed to describe a nonencapsulated brain abscess.

EPIDEMIOLOGY

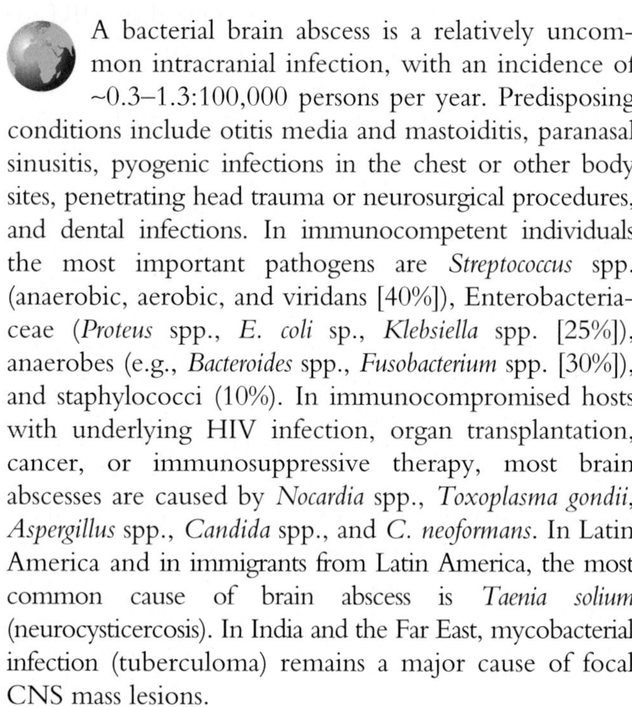

A bacterial brain abscess is a relatively uncommon intracranial infection, with an incidence of ~0.3–1.3:100,000 persons per year. Predisposing conditions include otitis media and mastoiditis, paranasal sinusitis, pyogenic infections in the chest or other body sites, penetrating head trauma or neurosurgical procedures, and dental infections. In immunocompetent individuals the most important pathogens are *Streptococcus* spp. (anaerobic, aerobic, and viridans [40%]), Enterobacteriaceae (*Proteus* spp., *E. coli* sp., *Klebsiella* spp. [25%]), anaerobes (e.g., *Bacteroides* spp., *Fusobacterium* spp. [30%]), and staphylococci (10%). In immunocompromised hosts with underlying HIV infection, organ transplantation, cancer, or immunosuppressive therapy, most brain abscesses are caused by *Nocardia* spp., *Toxoplasma gondii*, *Aspergillus* spp., *Candida* spp., and *C. neoformans*. In Latin America and in immigrants from Latin America, the most common cause of brain abscess is *Taenia solium* (neurocysticercosis). In India and the Far East, mycobacterial infection (tuberculoma) remains a major cause of focal CNS mass lesions.

ETIOLOGY

A brain abscess may develop (1) by direct spread from a contiguous cranial site of infection, such as paranasal sinusitis, otitis media, mastoiditis, or dental infection; (2) following head trauma or a neurosurgical procedure; or (3) as a result of hematogenous spread from a remote site of infection. In up to 25% of cases, no obvious primary source of infection is apparent (cryptogenic brain abscess).

Approximately one-third of brain abscesses are associated with otitis media and mastoiditis, often with an associated cholesteatoma. Otogenic abscesses occur predominantly in the temporal lobe (55–75%) and cerebellum (20–30%). In some series, up to 90% of cerebellar abscesses are otogenic. Common organisms include streptococci, *Bacteroides* spp., *Pseudomonas* spp., *Haemophilus* spp., and Enterobacteriaceae. Abscesses that develop as a result of direct spread of infection from the frontal, ethmoidal, or sphenoidal sinuses and those that occur due to dental infections are usually located in the frontal lobes. Approximately 10% of brain abscesses are associated with paranasal sinusitis, and this association is particularly strong in young males in their second and third decades of life. The most common pathogens in brain abscesses associated with paranasal sinusitis are streptococci (especially *S. milleri*), *Haemophilus* spp., *Bacteroides* spp., *Pseudomonas* spp., and *S. aureus*. Dental infections are associated with ~2% of brain abscesses, although it is often suggested that many "cryptogenic" abscesses are in fact due to dental infections. The most common pathogens in this setting are streptococci, staphylococci, *Bacteroides* spp., and *Fusobacterium* spp.

Hematogenous abscesses account for ~25% of brain abscesses. Hematogenous abscesses are often multiple, and multiple abscesses often (50%) have a hematogenous origin. These abscesses show a predilection for the territory of the middle cerebral artery (i.e., posterior frontal or parietal lobes). Hematogenous abscesses are often located at the junction of the gray and white matter and are often poorly encapsulated. The microbiology of hematogenous abscesses is dependent on the primary source of infection. For example, brain abscesses that develop as a complication of infective endocarditis are often due to viridans streptococci or *S. aureus*. Abscesses associated with pyogenic lung infections such as lung abscess or bronchiectasis are often due to streptococci, staphylococci, *Bacteroides* spp., *Fusobacterium* spp., or Enterobacteriaceae. Abscesses that follow penetrating head trauma or neurosurgical procedures are frequently due to methicillin-resistant *S. aureus* (MRSA), *S. epidermidis*, Enterobacteriaceae, *Pseudomonas* spp., and *Clostridium* spp. Enterobacteriaceae and *P. aeruginosa* are important causes of abscesses associated with urinary sepsis. Congenital cardiac malformations that produce a right-to-left shunt, such as tetralogy of Fallot, patent ductus arteriosus, and atrial and ventricular septal defects, allow bloodborne bacteria to bypass the pulmonary capillary bed and reach the brain. Similar phenomena can occur with pulmonary arteriovenous malformations. The decreased arterial oxygenation and saturation from the right-to-left shunt and polycythemia may cause focal areas of cerebral ischemia, thus providing a nidus for microorganisms that bypassed the pulmonary circulation to multiply and form an abscess. Streptococci are the most common pathogens in this setting.

PATHOGENESIS AND HISTOPATHOLOGY

Results of experimental models of brain abscess formation suggest that for bacterial invasion of brain parenchyma to occur, there must be preexisting or concomitant areas of ischemia, necrosis, or hypoxemia in brain tissue. The intact brain parenchyma is relatively resistant to infection. Once bacteria have established infection, brain abscess frequently evolves through a series of stages, influenced by the nature of the infecting organism and by the immunocompetence of the host. The early cerebritis stage (days 1–3) is characterized by a perivascular infiltration of inflammatory cells, which surround a central core of coagulative necrosis. Marked edema surrounds the lesion at this stage. In the late cerebritis stage (days 4–9), pus formation leads to enlargement of the necrotic center, which is surrounded at its border by an inflammatory infiltrate of macrophages and fibroblasts. A thin capsule of fibroblasts and reticular fibers gradually develops, and the surrounding area of cerebral edema becomes more distinct than in the previous stage. The third stage, early capsule formation (days 10–13), is characterized by the formation of a capsule that is better developed on the cortical than on the ventricular side of the lesion. This stage correlates with the appearance of a ring-enhancing capsule on neuroimaging studies. The final stage, late capsule formation (day 14 and beyond), is defined by a well-formed necrotic center surrounded by a dense collagenous capsule. The surrounding area of cerebral edema has regressed, but marked gliosis with large numbers of reactive astrocytes has developed outside the capsule. This gliotic process may contribute to the development of seizures as a sequelae of brain abscess.

CLINICAL PRESENTATION

A brain abscess typically presents as an expanding intracranial mass lesion rather than as an infectious process. Although the evolution of signs and symptoms is extremely variable, ranging from hours to weeks or even months, most patients present to the hospital 11–12 days following onset of symptoms. The classic clinical triad of headache, fever, and a focal neurologic deficit is present in <50% of cases. The most common symptom in patients with a brain abscess is headache, occurring in >75% of patients. The headache is often characterized as a constant, dull, aching sensation, either hemicranial or generalized, and it becomes progressively more severe and refractory to therapy. Fever is present in only 50% of patients at the time of diagnosis, and its absence should not exclude the diagnosis. The new onset of focal or generalized seizure activity is a presenting sign in 15–35% of patients. Focal neurologic deficits including hemiparesis, aphasia, or visual field defects are part of the initial presentation in >60% of patients.

The clinical presentation of a brain abscess depends on its location, the nature of the primary infection if present, and the level of the ICP. Hemiparesis is the most common localizing sign of a frontal lobe abscess. A temporal lobe abscess may present with a disturbance of language (dysphasia) or an upper homonymous quadrantanopia. Nystagmus and ataxia are signs of a cerebellar abscess. Signs of raised ICP—papilledema, nausea and vomiting, and drowsiness or confusion—can be the dominant presentation of some abscesses, particularly those in the cerebellum. Meningismus is not present unless the abscess has ruptured into the ventricle or the infection has spread to the subarachnoid space.

DIAGNOSIS

Diagnosis is made by neuroimaging studies. MRI (Fig. 40-4) is better than CT for demonstrating abscesses in the early (cerebritis) stages and is superior to CT for identifying abscesses in the posterior fossa. Cerebritis appears on MRI as an area of low-signal intensity on T1-weighted images with irregular postgadolinium enhancement and as an area of increased signal intensity on T2-weighted images. Cerebritis is often not visualized by CT scan but, when present, appears as an area of hypodensity. On a contrast-enhanced CT scan, a mature brain abscess appears as a focal area of hypodensity surrounded by ring enhancement with surrounding edema (hypodensity). On contrast-enhanced T1-weighted MRI, a mature brain abscess has a capsule that enhances surrounding a hypodense center and surrounded by a hypodense area of edema. On T2-weighted MRI, there is a hyperintense central area of pus surrounded by a well-defined hypointense capsule and a hyperintense surrounding area of edema. It is important to recognize that the CT and MR appearance, particularly of the capsule, may be altered by treatment with glucocorticoids. The distinction between a brain abscess and other focal CNS lesions such as primary or metastatic tumors may be facilitated by the use of diffusion-weighted imaging sequences on which brain abscesses typically show increased signal due to restricted diffusion.

Microbiologic diagnosis of the etiologic agent is most accurately determined by Gram's stain and culture of abscess material obtained by CT-guided stereotactic needle aspiration. Aerobic and anaerobic bacterial cultures and mycobacterial and fungal cultures should be obtained. Up to 10% of patients will also have positive blood cultures. LP should not be performed in patients with known or suspected focal intracranial infections such as abscess or empyema; CSF analysis contributes nothing to diagnosis or therapy, and LP increases the risk of herniation.

Additional laboratory studies may provide clues to the diagnosis of brain abscess in patients with a CNS mass lesion. About 50% of patients have a peripheral leukocytosis, 60% an elevated ESR, and 80% an elevated C-reactive protein. Blood cultures are positive in ~10% of cases overall but may be positive in >85% of patients with abscesses due to *Listeria*.

DIFFERENTIAL DIAGNOSIS

Conditions that can cause headache, fever, focal neurologic signs, and seizure activity include brain abscess, subdural empyema, bacterial meningitis, viral meningoencephalitis, superior sagittal sinus thrombosis, and acute disseminated encephalomyelitis. When fever is absent, primary and metastatic brain tumors become the major differential diagnosis. Less commonly, cerebral infarction or hematoma can have an MRI or CT appearance resembling brain abscess.

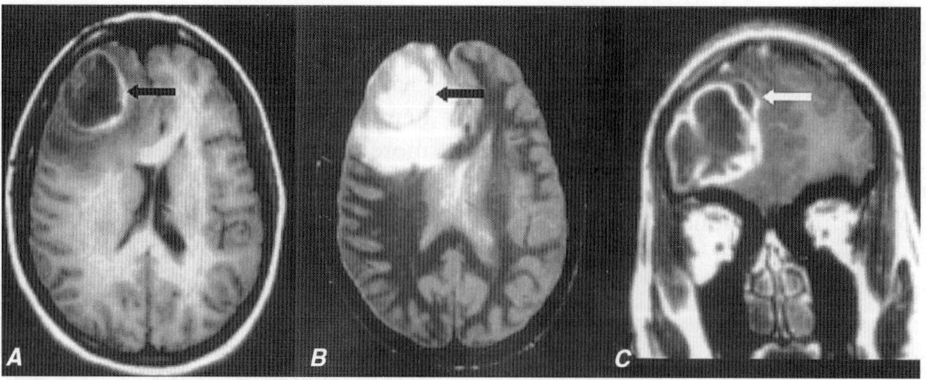

FIGURE 40-4

Pneumococcal brain abscess. Note that the abscess wall has hyperintense signal on the axial T1-weighted MRI (***A***, *black arrow*), hypointense signal on the axial proton density images (***B***, *black arrow*), and enhances prominently after gadolinium administration on the coronal T1-weighted image (**C**). The abscess is surrounded by a large amount of vasogenic edema and has a small "daughter" abscess (***C***, *white arrow*). (*Courtesy of Joseph Lurito, MD; with permission.*)

TREATMENT **Brain Abscess**

Optimal therapy of brain abscesses involves a combination of high-dose parenteral antibiotics and neurosurgical drainage. Empirical therapy of community-acquired brain abscess in an immunocompetent patient typically includes a third- or fourth-generation cephalosporin (e.g., cefotaxime, ceftriaxone, or cefepime) and metronidazole (see Table 40-1 for antibiotic dosages). In patients with penetrating head trauma or recent neurosurgical procedures, treatment should include ceftazidime as the third-generation cephalosporin to enhance coverage of *Pseudomonas* spp. and vancomycin for coverage of staphylococci. Meropenem plus vancomycin also provides good coverage in this setting.

Aspiration and drainage of the abscess under stereotactic guidance are beneficial for both diagnosis and therapy. Empirical antibiotic coverage should be modified based on the results of Gram's stain and culture of the abscess contents. Complete excision of a bacterial abscess via craniotomy or craniectomy is generally reserved for multiloculated abscesses or those in which stereotactic aspiration is unsuccessful.

Medical therapy alone is not optimal for treatment of brain abscess and should be reserved for patients whose abscesses are neurosurgically inaccessible, for patients with small (<2–3 cm) or nonencapsulated abscesses (cerebritis), and patients whose condition is too tenuous to allow performance of a neurosurgical procedure. All patients should receive a minimum of 6–8 weeks of parenteral antibiotic therapy. The role, if any, of supplemental oral antibiotic therapy following completion of a standard course of parenteral therapy has never been adequately studied.

In addition to surgical drainage and antibiotic therapy, patients should receive prophylactic anticonvulsant therapy because of the high risk (~35%) of focal or generalized seizures. Anticonvulsant therapy is continued for at least 3 months after resolution of the abscess, and decisions regarding withdrawal are then based on the EEG. If the EEG is abnormal, anticonvulsant therapy should be continued. If the EEG is normal, anticonvulsant therapy can be slowly withdrawn, with close follow-up and repeat EEG after the medication has been discontinued.

Glucocorticoids should not be given routinely to patients with brain abscesses. Intravenous dexamethasone therapy (10 mg every 6 h) is usually reserved for patients with substantial periabscess edema and associated mass effect and increased ICP. Dexamethasone should be tapered as rapidly as possible to avoid delaying the natural process of encapsulation of the abscess.

Serial MRI or CT scans should be obtained on a monthly or twice-monthly basis to document resolution of the abscess. More frequent studies (e.g., weekly) are probably warranted in the subset of patients who are receiving antibiotic therapy alone. A small amount of enhancement may remain for months after the abscess has been successfully treated.

PROGNOSIS

The mortality rate of brain abscess has declined in parallel with the development of enhanced neuroimaging techniques, improved neurosurgical procedures for stereotactic aspiration, and improved antibiotics. In modern series, the mortality rate is typically <15%. Significant sequelae, including seizures, persisting weakness, aphasia, or mental impairment, occur in ≥20% of survivors.

NONBACTERIAL CAUSES OF INFECTIOUS FOCAL CNS LESIONS

ETIOLOGY

Neurocysticercosis is the most common parasitic disease of the CNS worldwide. Humans acquire cysticercosis by the ingestion of food contaminated with the eggs of the parasite *T. solium*. Toxoplasmosis is a parasitic disease caused by *T. gondii* and acquired from the ingestion of undercooked meat and from handling cat feces.

CLINICAL PRESENTATION

The most common manifestation of neurocysticercosis is new-onset partial seizures with or without secondary generalization. Cysticerci may develop in the brain parenchyma and cause seizures or focal neurologic deficits. When present in the subarachnoid or ventricular spaces, cysticerci can produce increased ICP by interference with CSF flow. Spinal cysticerci can mimic the presentation of intraspinal tumors. When the cysticerci first lodge in the brain, they frequently cause little in the way of an inflammatory response. As the cysticercal cyst degenerates, it elicits an inflammatory response that may present clinically as a seizure. Eventually the cyst dies, a process that may take several years and is typically associated with resolution of the inflammatory response and, often, abatement of seizures.

Primary *Toxoplasma* infection is often asymptomatic. However, during this phase parasites may spread to the CNS, where they become latent. Reactivation of CNS infection is almost exclusively associated with immunocompromised hosts, particularly those with HIV infection. During this phase patients present with headache, fever, seizures, and focal neurologic deficits.

DIAGNOSIS

The lesions of neurocysticercosis are readily visualized by MRI or CT scans. Lesions with viable parasites appear as cystic lesions. The scolex can often be visualized on MRI. Lesions may appear as contrast-enhancing lesions surrounded by edema. A very early sign of cyst death is hypointensity of the vesicular fluid on T2-weighted images when compared with CSF. Parenchymal brain calcifications are the most common finding and evidence that the parasite is no longer viable. MRI findings of toxoplasmosis consist of multiple lesions in the deep white matter, the thalamus, and basal ganglia and at the gray-white junction in the cerebral hemispheres. With contrast administration, the majority of the lesions enhance in a ringed, nodular, or homogeneous pattern and are surrounded by edema. In the presence of the characteristic neuroimaging abnormalities of *T. gondii* infection, serum IgG antibody to *T. gondii* should be obtained and, when positive, the patient should be treated.

TREATMENT Infectious Focal CNS Lesions

Anticonvulsant therapy is initiated when the patient with neurocysticercosis presents with a seizure. There is controversy about whether or not anthelmintic therapy should be given to all patients, and recommendations are based on the stage of the lesion. Cysticerci appearing as cystic lesions in the brain parenchyma with or without pericystic edema or in the subarachnoid space at the convexity of the cerebral hemispheres should be treated with anticysticidal therapy. Cysticidal drugs accelerate the destruction of the parasites, resulting in a faster resolution of the infection. Albendazole and praziquantel are used in the treatment of neurocysticercosis. Approximately 85% of parenchymal cysts are destroyed by a single course of albendazole, and ~75% are destroyed by a single course of praziquantel. The dose of albendazole is 15 mg/kg per day in two doses for 8 days. The dose of praziquantel is 50 mg/kg per day for 15 days, although a number of other dosage regimens are also frequently cited. Prednisone or dexamethasone is given with anticysticidal therapy to reduce the host inflammatory response to degenerating parasites. Many, but not all, experts recommend anticysticidal therapy for lesions that are surrounded by a contrast-enhancing ring. There is universal agreement that calcified lesions do not need to be treated with anticysticidal therapy. Antiepileptic therapy can be stopped once the follow-up CT scan shows resolution of the lesion. Long-term antiepileptic therapy is recommended when seizures occur after resolution of edema and resorption or calcification of the degenerating cyst.

CNS toxoplasmosis is treated with a combination of sulfadiazine, 1.5–2.0 g orally qid, plus pyrimethamine, 100 mg orally to load, then 75–100 mg orally qd, plus folinic acid, 10–15 mg orally qd. Folinic acid is added to the regimen to prevent megaloblastic anemia. Therapy is continued until there is no evidence of active disease on neuroimaging studies, which typically takes at least 6 weeks, and then the dose of sulfadiazine is reduced to 2–4 g/d and pyrimethamine to 50 mg/d. Clindamycin plus pyrimethamine is an alternative therapy for patients who cannot tolerate sulfadiazine, but the combination of pyrimethamine and sulfadiazine is more effective.

SUBDURAL EMPYEMA

A subdural empyema (SDE) is a collection of pus between the dura and arachnoid membranes (Fig. 40-5).

EPIDEMIOLOGY

SDE is a rare disorder that accounts for 15–25% of focal suppurative CNS infections. Sinusitis is the most common predisposing condition and typically involves the frontal sinuses, either alone or in combination with the ethmoid and maxillary sinuses. Sinusitis-associated empyema has a striking predilection for young males, possibly reflecting sex-related differences in sinus anatomy and development. It has been suggested that SDE may complicate 1–2% of cases of frontal sinusitis severe enough to require hospitalization. As a consequence of this epidemiology, SDE shows an ~3:1 male/female predominance, with 70% of cases occurring in the second and third decades of life. SDE may also develop as a complication of head trauma or neurosurgery. Secondary infection of a subdural effusion may also result in empyema, although secondary infection of hematomas, in the absence of a prior neurosurgical procedure, is rare.

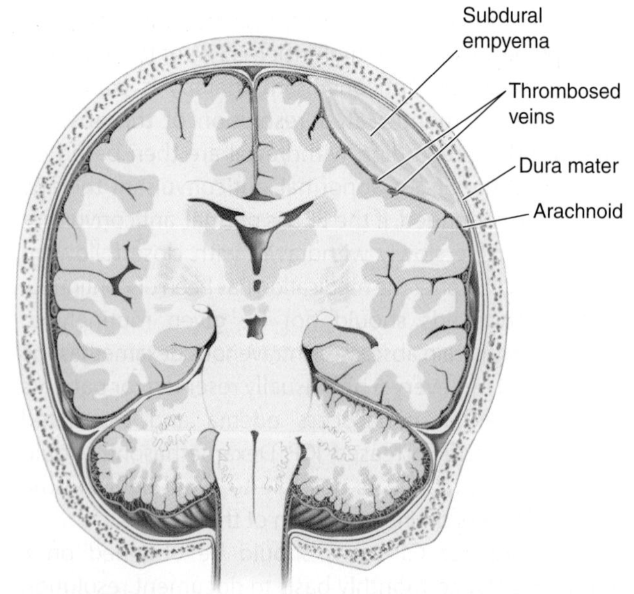

FIGURE 40-5
Subdural empyema.

ETIOLOGY

Aerobic and anaerobic streptococci, staphylococci, Enterobacteriaceae, and anaerobic bacteria are the most common causative organisms of sinusitis-associated SDE. Staphylococci and gram-negative bacilli are often the etiologic organisms when SDE follows neurosurgical procedures or head trauma. Up to one-third of cases are culture-negative, possibly reflecting difficulty in obtaining adequate anaerobic cultures.

PATHOPHYSIOLOGY

Sinusitis-associated SDE develops as a result of either retrograde spread of infection from septic thrombophlebitis of the mucosal veins draining the sinuses or contiguous spread of infection to the brain from osteomyelitis in the posterior wall of the frontal or other sinuses. SDE may also develop from direct introduction of bacteria into the subdural space as a complication of a neurosurgical procedure. The evolution of SDE can be extremely rapid because the subdural space is a large compartment that offers few mechanical barriers to the spread of infection. In patients with sinusitis-associated SDE, suppuration typically begins in the upper and anterior portions of one cerebral hemisphere and then extends posteriorly. SDE is often associated with other intracranial infections, including epidural empyema (40%), cortical thrombophlebitis (35%), and intracranial abscess or cerebritis (>25%). Cortical venous infarction produces necrosis of underlying cerebral cortex and subcortical white matter, with focal neurologic deficits and seizures (discussed later).

CLINICAL PRESENTATION

A patient with SDE typically presents with fever and a progressively worsening headache. The diagnosis of SDE should always be suspected in a patient with known sinusitis who presents with new CNS signs or symptoms. Patients with underlying sinusitis frequently have symptoms related to this infection. As the infection progresses, focal neurologic deficits, seizures, nuchal rigidity, and signs of increased ICP commonly occur. Headache is the most common complaint at the time of presentation; initially it is localized to the side of the subdural infection, but then it becomes more severe and generalized. Contralateral hemiparesis or hemiplegia is the most common focal neurologic deficit and can occur from the direct effects of the SDE on the cortex or as a consequence of venous infarction. Seizures begin as partial motor seizures that then become secondarily generalized. Seizures may be due to the direct irritative effect of the SDE on the underlying cortex or result from cortical venous infarction (discussed earlier). In untreated SDE, the increasing mass effect and increase in ICP cause progressive deterioration in consciousness, leading ultimately to coma.

DIAGNOSIS

MRI (Fig. 40-6) is superior to CT in identifying SDE and any associated intracranial infections. The administration of gadolinium greatly improves diagnosis by enhancing the rim of the empyema and allowing the empyema to be clearly delineated from the underlying brain parenchyma. Cranial MRI is also extremely valuable in identifying sinusitis, other focal CNS infections, cortical venous infarction, cerebral edema, and cerebritis. CT may show a crescent-shaped hypodense lesion over one or both hemispheres or in the interhemispheric fissure. Frequently the degree of mass effect, exemplified by midline shift, ventricular compression, and sulcal effacement, is far out of proportion to the mass of the SDE.

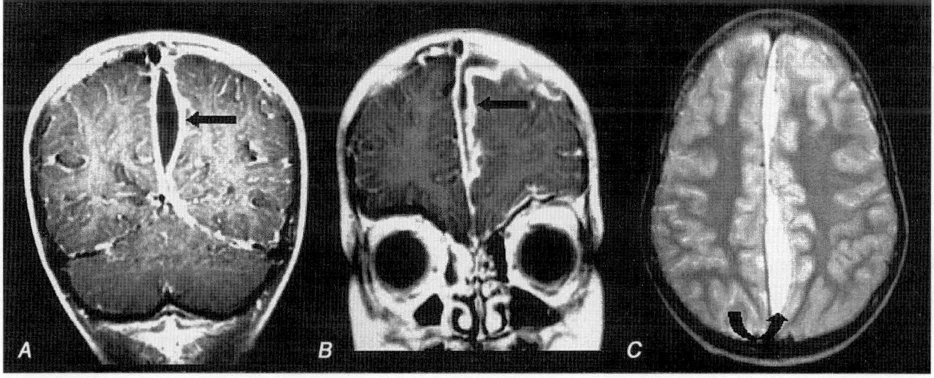

FIGURE 40-6
Subdural empyema. There is marked enhancement of the dura and leptomeninges (***A***, ***B***, *straight arrows*) along the left medial hemisphere. The pus is hypointense on T1-weighted images (***A***, ***B***) but markedly hyperintense on the proton density–weighted (***C***, *curved arrow*) image. (*Courtesy of Joseph Lurito, MD; with permission.*)

CSF examination should be avoided in patients with known or suspected SDE as it adds no useful information and is associated with the risk of cerebral herniation.

DIFFERENTIAL DIAGNOSIS

The differential diagnosis of the combination of headache, fever, focal neurologic signs, and seizure activity that progresses rapidly to an altered level of consciousness includes subdural hematoma, bacterial meningitis, viral encephalitis, brain abscess, superior sagittal sinus thrombosis, and acute disseminated encephalomyelitis. The presence of nuchal rigidity is unusual with brain abscess or epidural empyema and should suggest the possibility of SDE when associated with significant focal neurologic signs and fever. Patients with bacterial meningitis also have nuchal rigidity but do not typically have focal deficits of the severity seen with SDE.

TREATMENT Subdural Empyema

SDE is a medical emergency. Emergent neurosurgical evacuation of the empyema, either through craniotomy, craniectomy, or burr-hole drainage, is the definitive step in the management of this infection. Empirical antimicrobial therapy for community-acquired SDE should include a combination of a third-generation cephalosporin (e.g., cefotaxime or ceftriaxone), vancomycin, and metronidazole (see Table 40-1 for dosages). Patients with hospital-acquired SDE may have infections due to *Pseudomonas* spp. or MRSA and should receive coverage with a carbapenem (e.g., meropenem) and vancomycin. Metronidazole is not necessary for anti-anaerobic therapy when meropenem is being used. Parenteral antibiotic therapy should be continued for a minimum of 3–4 weeks after SDE drainage. Patients with associated cranial osteomyelitis may require longer therapy. Specific diagnosis of the etiologic organisms is made based on Gram's stain and culture of fluid obtained via either burr holes or craniotomy; the initial empirical antibiotic coverage can be modified accordingly.

PROGNOSIS

Prognosis is influenced by the level of consciousness of the patient at the time of hospital presentation, the size of the empyema, and the speed with which therapy is instituted. Long-term neurologic sequelae, which include seizures and hemiparesis, occur in up to 50% of cases.

CRANIAL EPIDURAL ABSCESS

Cranial epidural abscess is a suppurative infection occurring in the potential space between the inner skull table and dura (Fig. 40-7).

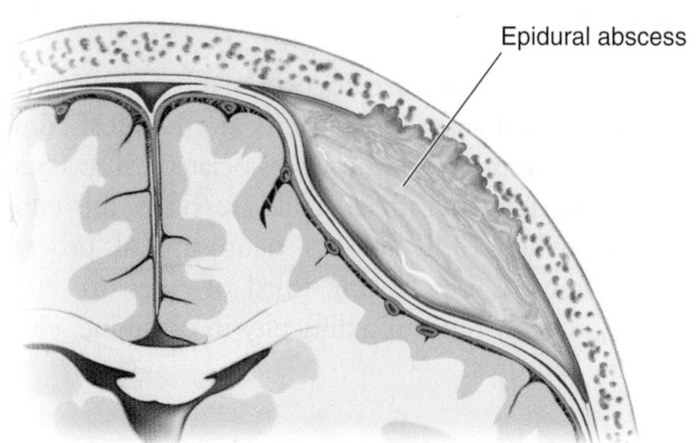

FIGURE 40-7
Cranial epidural abscess is a collection of pus between the dura and the inner table of the skull.

ETIOLOGY AND PATHOPHYSIOLOGY

Cranial epidural abscess is less common than either brain abscess or SDE and accounts for <2% of focal suppurative CNS infections. A cranial epidural abscess develops as a complication of a craniotomy or compound skull fracture or as a result of spread of infection from the frontal sinuses, middle ear, mastoid, or orbit. An epidural abscess may develop contiguous to an area of osteomyelitis, when craniotomy is complicated by infection of the wound or bone flap, or as a result of direct infection of the epidural space. Infection in the frontal sinus, middle ear, mastoid, or orbit can reach the epidural space through retrograde spread of infection from septic thrombophlebitis in the emissary veins that drain these areas or by way of direct spread of infection through areas of osteomyelitis. Unlike the subdural space, the epidural space is really a potential rather than an actual compartment. The dura is normally tightly adherent to the inner skull table, and infection must dissect the dura away from the skull table as it spreads. As a result, epidural abscesses are often smaller than SDEs. Cranial epidural abscesses, unlike brain abscesses, only rarely result from hematogenous spread of infection from extracranial primary sites. The bacteriology of a cranial epidural abscess is similar to that of SDE (discussed earlier). The etiologic organisms of an epidural abscess that arises from frontal sinusitis, middle-ear infections, or mastoiditis are usually streptococci or anaerobic organisms. Staphylococci or gram-negative organisms are the usual cause of an epidural abscess that develops as a complication of craniotomy or compound skull fracture.

CLINICAL PRESENTATION

Patients present with fever (60%), headache (40%), nuchal rigidity (35%), seizures (10%), and focal deficits (5%). Development of symptoms may be insidious, as the empyema usually enlarges slowly in the confined anatomic space between the dura and the inner table of the skull. Periorbital edema and Potts puffy tumor, reflecting underlying associated frontal bone osteomyelitis, are present in ~40%. In patients with a recent neurosurgical procedure, wound infection is invariably present, but other symptoms may be subtle and can include altered mental status (45%), fever (35%), and headache (20%). The diagnosis should be considered when fever and headache follow recent head trauma or occur in the setting of frontal sinusitis, mastoiditis, or otitis media.

DIAGNOSIS

Cranial MRI with gadolinium enhancement is the procedure of choice to demonstrate a cranial epidural abscess. The sensitivity of CT is limited by the presence of signal artifacts arising from the bone of the inner skull table. The CT appearance of an epidural empyema is that of a lens or crescent-shaped hypodense extraaxial lesion. On MRI, an epidural empyema appears as a lentiform or crescent-shaped fluid collection that is hyperintense compared to CSF on T2-weighted images. On T1-weighted images, the fluid collection may be either isointense or hypointense compared to brain. Following the administration of gadolinium, there is linear enhancement of the dura on T1-weighted images. In distinction to subdural empyema, signs of mass effect or other parenchymal abnormalities are uncommon.

TREATMENT Epidural Abscess

Immediate neurosurgical drainage is indicated. Empirical antimicrobial therapy, pending the results of Gram's stain and culture of the purulent material obtained at surgery, should include a combination of a third-generation cephalosporin, vancomycin, and metronidazole (Table 40-1). Ceftazidime or meropenem should be substituted for ceftriaxone or cefotaxime in neurosurgical patients. Metronidazole is not necessary for anti-anaerobic coverage in patients receiving meropenem. When the organism has been identified, antimicrobial therapy can be modified accordingly. Antibiotics should be continued for 3–6 weeks after surgical drainage. Patients with associated osteomyelitis may require additional therapy.

PROGNOSIS

The mortality rate is <5% in modern series, and full recovery is the rule in most survivors.

SUPPURATIVE THROMBOPHLEBITIS

DEFINITION

Suppurative intracranial thrombophlebitis is septic venous thrombosis of cortical veins and sinuses. This may occur as a complication of bacterial meningitis; SDE; epidural abscess; or infection in the skin of the face, paranasal sinuses, middle ear, or mastoid.

ANATOMY AND PATHOPHYSIOLOGY

The cerebral veins and venous sinuses have no valves; therefore, blood within them can flow in either direction. The superior sagittal sinus is the largest of the venous sinuses (Fig. 40-8). It receives blood from the frontal, parietal, and occipital superior cerebral veins and the diploic veins, which communicate with the meningeal veins. Bacterial meningitis is a common predisposing condition for septic thrombosis of the superior sagittal sinus. The diploic veins, which drain into the superior sagittal sinus, provide a route for the spread of infection from the meninges, especially in cases where there is purulent exudate near areas of the superior sagittal sinus. Infection can also spread to the superior sagittal sinus from nearby SDE or epidural abscess. Dehydration from vomiting, hypercoagulable states, and immunologic abnormalities, including the presence of circulating antiphospholipid antibodies, also contribute to cerebral venous sinus thrombosis. Thrombosis may extend from one sinus to another, and at autopsy thrombi of different histologic ages can often be detected in several sinuses. Thrombosis of the superior sagittal sinus is often associated with thrombosis of superior cortical veins and small parenchymal hemorrhages.

The superior sagittal sinus drains into the transverse sinuses (Fig. 40-8). The transverse sinuses also receive venous drainage from small veins from both the middle ear and mastoid cells. The transverse sinus becomes the sigmoid sinus before draining into the internal jugular vein. Septic transverse/sigmoid sinus thrombosis can be a complication of acute and chronic otitis media or mastoiditis. Infection spreads from the mastoid air

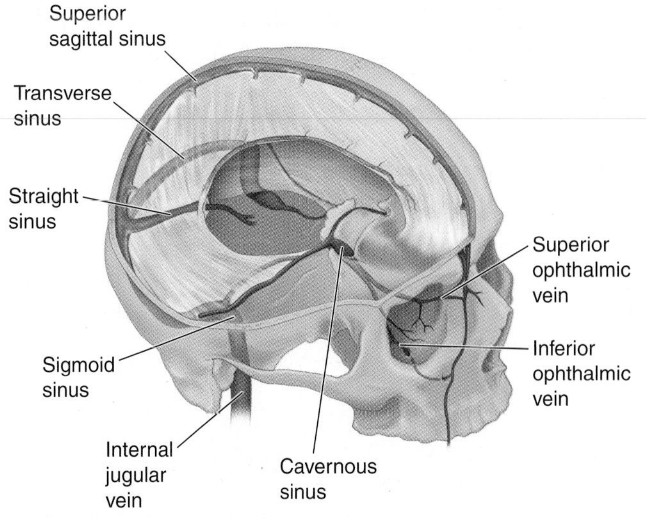

FIGURE 40-8
Anatomy of the cerebral venous sinuses.

cells to the transverse sinus via the emissary veins or by direct invasion. The cavernous sinuses are inferior to the superior sagittal sinus at the base of the skull. The cavernous sinuses receive blood from the facial veins via the superior and inferior ophthalmic veins. Bacteria in the facial veins enter the cavernous sinus via these veins. Bacteria in the sphenoid and ethmoid sinuses can spread to the cavernous sinuses via the small emissary veins. The sphenoid and ethmoid sinuses are the most common sites of primary infection resulting in septic cavernous sinus thrombosis.

CLINICAL MANIFESTATIONS

Septic thrombosis of the superior sagittal sinus presents with headache, fever, nausea and vomiting, confusion, and focal or generalized seizures. There may be a rapid development of stupor and coma. Weakness of the lower extremities with bilateral Babinski's signs or hemiparesis is often present. When superior sagittal sinus thrombosis occurs as a complication of bacterial meningitis, nuchal rigidity and Kernig's and Brudzinski's signs may be present.

The oculomotor nerve, the trochlear nerve, the abducens nerve, the ophthalmic and maxillary branches of the trigeminal nerve, and the internal carotid artery all pass through the cavernous sinus (see Fig. 34-4). The symptoms of *septic cavernous sinus thrombosis* are fever, headache, frontal and retroorbital pain, and diplopia. The classic signs are ptosis, proptosis, chemosis, and extraocular dysmotility due to deficits of cranial nerves III, IV, and VI; hyperesthesia of the ophthalmic and maxillary divisions of the fifth cranial nerve and a decreased corneal reflex may be detected. There may be evidence of dilated, tortuous retinal veins and papilledema.

Headache and earache are the most frequent symptoms of *transverse sinus thrombosis*. A transverse sinus thrombosis may also present with otitis media, sixth nerve palsy, and retroorbital or facial pain (*Gradenigo's syndrome*). Sigmoid sinus and internal jugular vein thrombosis may present with neck pain.

DIAGNOSIS

The diagnosis of septic venous sinus thrombosis is suggested by an absent flow void within the affected venous sinus on MRI and confirmed by magnetic resonance venography, CT angiogram, or the venous phase of cerebral angiography. The diagnosis of thrombophlebitis of intracerebral and meningeal veins is suggested by the presence of intracerebral hemorrhage but requires cerebral angiography for definitive diagnosis.

TREATMENT Suppurative Thrombophlebitis

Septic venous sinus thrombosis is treated with antibiotics, hydration, and removal of infected tissue and thrombus in septic lateral or cavernous sinus thrombosis. The choice of antimicrobial therapy is based on the bacteria responsible for the predisposing or associated condition. Optimal duration of therapy is unknown, but antibiotics are usually continued for 6 weeks or until there is radiographic evidence of resolution of thrombosis. Anticoagulation with dose-adjusted intravenous heparin is recommended for aseptic venous sinus thrombosis and in the treatment of septic venous sinus thrombosis complicating bacterial meningitis in patients who have progressive neurologic deterioration despite antimicrobial therapy and intravenous fluids. The presence of a small intracerebral hemorrhage from septic thrombophlebitis is not an absolute contraindication to heparin therapy. Successful management of aseptic venous sinus thrombosis has been reported with surgical thrombectomy, catheter-directed urokinase therapy, and with a combination of intrathrombus recombinant tissue plasminogen activator (rtPA) and intravenous heparin, but there is not enough data to recommend these therapies in septic venous sinus thrombosis.

CHAPTER 41

CHRONIC AND RECURRENT MENINGITIS

Walter J. Koroshetz ■ Morton N. Swartz

Chronic inflammation of the meninges (pia, arachnoid, and dura) can produce profound neurologic disability and may be fatal if not successfully treated. The condition is most commonly diagnosed when a characteristic neurologic syndrome exists for >4 weeks and is associated with a persistent inflammatory response in the cerebrospinal fluid (CSF) (white blood cell count >5/μL). The causes are varied, and appropriate treatment depends on identification of the etiology. Five categories of disease account for most cases of chronic meningitis: (1) meningeal infections, (2) malignancy, (3) noninfectious inflammatory disorders, (4) chemical meningitis, and (5) parameningeal infections.

CLINICAL PATHOPHYSIOLOGY

Neurologic manifestations of chronic meningitis (Table 41-1) are determined by the anatomic location of the inflammation and its consequences. Persistent headache with or without stiff neck, hydrocephalus, cranial neuropathies, radiculopathies, and cognitive or personality changes are the cardinal features. These can occur alone or in combination. When they appear in combination, widespread dissemination of the inflammatory process along CSF pathways has occurred. In some cases, the presence of an underlying systemic illness points to a specific agent or class of agents as the probable cause. The diagnosis of chronic meningitis is usually made when the clinical presentation prompts the astute physician to examine the CSF for signs of inflammation. CSF is produced by the choroid plexus of the cerebral ventricles, exits through narrow foramina into the subarachnoid space surrounding the brain and spinal cord, circulates around the base of the brain and over the cerebral hemispheres, and is resorbed by arachnoid villi projecting into the superior sagittal sinus. CSF flow provides a pathway for rapid spread of infectious and other infiltrative processes over the brain, spinal cord, and cranial and spinal nerve roots. Spread from the subarachnoid space into brain parenchyma may occur via the arachnoid cuffs that surround blood vessels that penetrate brain tissue (Virchow-Robin spaces).

TABLE 41-1

SYMPTOMS AND SIGNS OF CHRONIC MENINGITIS

SYMPTOM	SIGN
Chronic headache	+/− Papilledema
Neck or back pain	Brudzinski's or Kernig's sign of meningeal irritation
Change in personality	Altered mental status—drowsiness, inattention, disorientation, memory loss, frontal release signs (grasp, suck, snout), perseveration
Facial weakness	Peripheral seventh CN palsy
Double vision	Palsy of CNs III, IV, VI
Visual loss	Papilledema, optic atrophy
Hearing loss	Eighth CN palsy
Arm or leg weakness	Myelopathy or radiculopathy
Numbness in arms or legs	Myelopathy or radiculopathy
Sphincter dysfunction	Myelopathy or radiculopathy Frontal lobe dysfunction (hydrocephalus)
Clumsiness	Ataxia

Abbreviation: CN, cranial nerve.

Intracranial meningitis

Nociceptive fibers of the meninges are stimulated by the inflammatory process, resulting in headache or neck or back pain. Obstruction of CSF pathways at the foramina or arachnoid villi may produce *hydrocephalus* and symptoms of raised intracranial pressure (ICP), including headache, vomiting, apathy or drowsiness, gait instability, papilledema, visual loss, impaired upgaze, or palsy of the sixth cranial nerve (CN) (Chap. 34). Cognitive and behavioral changes during the course of chronic meningitis may also result from vascular damage, which may similarly produce seizures, stroke, or myelopathy. Inflammatory deposits seeded via the CSF circulation are often prominent around the brainstem and cranial nerves and along the undersurface of the frontal and temporal lobes. Such cases, termed *basal meningitis*, often present as multiple cranial neuropathies, with visual loss (CN II), facial weakness (CN VII), hearing loss (CN VIII), diplopia (CNs III, IV, and VI), sensory or motor abnormalities of the oropharynx (CNs IX, X, and XII), decreased olfaction (CN I), or facial sensory loss and masseter weakness (CN V).

Spinal meningitis

Injury may occur to motor and sensory roots as they traverse the subarachnoid space and penetrate the meninges. These cases present as multiple radiculopathies with combinations of radicular pain, sensory loss, motor weakness, and sphincter dysfunction. Meningeal inflammation can encircle the cord, resulting in myelopathy. Patients with slowly progressive involvement of multiple cranial nerves and/or spinal nerve roots are likely to have chronic meningitis. Electrophysiologic testing (electromyography, nerve conduction studies, and evoked response testing) may be helpful in determining whether there is involvement of cranial and spinal nerve roots.

Systemic manifestations

In some patients, evidence of systemic disease provides clues to the underlying cause of chronic meningitis. A careful history and physical examination are essential before embarking on a diagnostic workup, which may be costly, prolonged, and associated with risk from invasive procedures. A complete history of travel, sexual practice, and exposure to infectious agents should be sought. Infectious causes are often associated with fever, malaise, anorexia, and signs of localized or disseminated infection outside the nervous system. Infectious causes are of major concern in the immunosuppressed patient, especially in patients with AIDS, in whom chronic meningitis may present without headache or fever. Noninfectious inflammatory disorders often produce systemic manifestations, but meningitis may be the initial manifestation. Carcinomatous meningitis may or may not be accompanied by clinical evidence of the primary neoplasm.

APPROACH TO THE PATIENT Chronic Meningitis

The occurrence of chronic headache, hydrocephalus, cranial neuropathy, radiculopathy, and/or cognitive decline in a patient should prompt consideration of a lumbar puncture for evidence of meningeal inflammation. On occasion, the diagnosis is made when an imaging study (CT or MRI) shows contrast enhancement of the meninges, which is always abnormal with the exception of dural enhancement after lumbar puncture, neurosurgical procedures, or spontaneous CSF leakage. Once chronic meningitis is confirmed by CSF examination, effort is focused on identifying the cause (Tables 41-2 and 41-3) by (1) further analysis of the CSF, (2) diagnosis of an underlying systemic infection or noninfectious inflammatory condition, or (3) pathologic examination of meningeal biopsy specimens.

Two clinical forms of chronic meningitis exist. In the first, the symptoms are chronic and persistent, whereas in the second there are recurrent, discrete episodes of illness. In the latter group, all symptoms, signs, and CSF parameters of meningeal inflammation resolve completely between episodes without specific therapy. In such patients, the likely etiologies include herpes simplex virus (HSV) type 2; chemical meningitis due to leakage into CSF of contents from an epidermoid tumor, craniopharyngioma, or cholesteatoma; primary inflammatory conditions, including Vogt-Koyanagi-Harada syndrome, Behçet's syndrome, and systemic lupus erythematosus; and drug hypersensitivity with repeated administration of the offending agent.

The epidemiologic history is of considerable importance and may provide direction for selection of laboratory studies. Pertinent features include a history of tuberculosis or exposure to a likely case; past travel to areas endemic for fungal infections (the San Joaquin Valley in California and southwestern states for coccidioidomycosis, midwestern states for histoplasmosis, southeastern states for blastomycosis); travel to the Mediterranean region or ingestion of imported unpasteurized dairy products (*Brucella*); time spent in wooded areas endemic for Lyme disease; exposure to sexually transmitted disease (syphilis); exposure of an immunocompromised host to pigeons and their droppings (*Cryptococcus*); gardening (*Sporothrix schenkii*); ingestion of poorly cooked meat or contact with a household cat (*Toxoplasma gondii*); residence in Thailand or Japan (*Gnathostoma spinigerum*), Latin America (*Paracoccidioides brasiliiensis*), or the South Pacific (*Angiostrongylus cantonensis*); rural residence and raccoon exposure (*Baylisascaris procyonis*); and residence in Latin America, the Philippines, or Southeast Asia when eosinophilic meningitis is present (*Taenia solium*).

The presence of focal cerebral signs in a patient with chronic meningitis suggests the possibility of a brain abscess or other parameningeal infection; identification of a potential source of infection (chronic draining ear, sinusitis, right-to-left cardiac or pulmonary shunt, chronic pleuropulmonary infection) supports this diagnosis.

TABLE 41-2

INFECTIOUS CAUSES OF CHRONIC MENINGITIS

CAUSATIVE AGENT	CSF FORMULA	HELPFUL DIAGNOSTIC TESTS	RISK FACTORS AND SYSTEMIC MANIFESTATIONS
Common Bacterial Causes			
Partially treated suppurative meningitis	Mononuclear or mixed mononuclear-polymorphonuclear cells	CSF culture and Gram's stain	History consistent with acute bacterial meningitis and incomplete treatment
Parameningeal infection	Mononuclear or mixed polymorphonuclear-mononuclear cells	Contrast-enhanced CT or MRI to detect parenchymal, subdural, epidural, or sinus infection	Otitis media, pleuropulmonary infection, right-to-left cardiopulmonary shunt for brain abscess; focal neurologic signs; neck, back, ear, or sinus tenderness
Mycobacterium tuberculosis	Mononuclear cells except polymorphonuclear cells in early infection (commonly <500 WBC/μL); low CSF glucose, high protein	Tuberculin skin test may be negative; AFB culture of CSF (sputum, urine, gastric contents if indicated); tuberculostearic acid detection in CSF; identify tubercle bacillus on acid-fast stain of CSF or protein pellicle; PCR	Exposure history; previous tuberculous illness; immunosuppressed or AIDS; young children; fever, meningismus, night sweats, miliary TB on x-ray or liver biopsy; stroke due to arteritis
Lyme disease (Bannwarth's syndrome) *Borrelia burgdorferi*	Mononuclear cells; elevated protein	Serum Lyme antibody titer; Western blot confirmation; (patients with syphilis may have false-positive Lyme titer)	History of tick bite or appropriate exposure history; erythema chronicum migrans skin rash; arthritis, radiculopathy, Bell's palsy, meningoencephalitis–multiple sclerosis-like syndrome
Syphilis (secondary, tertiary) *Treponema pallidum*	Mononuclear cells; elevated protein	CSF VDRL; serum VDRL (or RPR); fluorescent treponemal antibody-absorbed (FTA) or MHA-TP; serum VDRL may be negative in tertiary syphilis	Appropriate exposure history; HIV-seropositive individuals at increased risk of aggressive infection; "dementia"; cerebral infarction due to endarteritis
Uncommon Bacterial Causes			
Actinomyces	Polymorphonuclear cells	Anaerobic culture	Parameningeal abscess or sinus tract (oral or dental focus); pneumonitis
Nocardia	Polymorphonuclear; occasionally mononuclear cells; often low glucose	Isolation may require weeks; weakly acid fast	Associated brain abscess may be present
Brucella	Mononuclear cells (rarely polymorphonuclear); elevated protein; often low glucose	CSF antibody detection; serum antibody detection	Intake of unpasteurized dairy products; exposure to goats, sheep, cows; fever, arthralgia, myalgia, vertebral osteomyelitis
Whipple's disease *Tropheryma whippelii*	Mononuclear cells	Biopsy of small bowel or lymph node; CSF PCR for *T. whippelii*; brain and meningeal biopsy (with PAS stain and EM examination)	Diarrhea, weight loss, arthralgias, fever; dementia, ataxia, paresis, ophthalmoplegia, oculomasticatory myoclonus
Rare Bacterial Causes			
Leptospirosis (occasionally if left untreated may last 3–4 weeks)			

(continued)

TABLE 41-2

INFECTIOUS CAUSES OF CHRONIC MENINGITIS (*CONTINUED*)

CAUSATIVE AGENT	CSF FORMULA	HELPFUL DIAGNOSTIC TESTS	RISK FACTORS AND SYSTEMIC MANIFESTATIONS
Fungal Causes			
Cryptococcus neoformans	Mononuclear cells; count not elevated in some patients with AIDS	India ink or fungal wet mount of CSF (budding yeast); blood and urine cultures; antigen detection in CSF	AIDS and immune suppression; pigeon exposure; skin and other organ involvement due to disseminated infection
Coccidioides immitis	Mononuclear cells (sometimes 10–20% eosinophils); often low glucose	Antibody detection in CSF and serum	Exposure history—southwestern US; increased virulence in dark-skinned races
Candida sp.	Polymorphonuclear or mononuclear	Fungal stain and culture of CSF	IV drug abuse; post surgery; prolonged intravenous therapy; disseminated candidiasis
Histoplasma capsulatum	Mononuclear cells; low glucose	Fungal stain and culture of large volumes of CSF; antigen detection in CSF, serum, and urine; antibody detection in serum, CSF	Exposure history—Ohio and central Mississippi River Valley; AIDS; mucosal lesions
Blastomyces dermatitidis	Mononuclear cells	Fungal stain and culture of CSF; biopsy and culture of skin, lung lesions; antibody detection in serum	Midwestern and southeastern US; usually systemic infection; abscesses, draining sinus, ulcers
Aspergillus sp.	Mononuclear or polymorphonuclear	CSF culture	Sinusitis; granulocytopenia or immunosuppression
Sporothrix schenckii	Mononuclear cells	Antibody detection in CSF and serum; CSF culture	Traumatic inoculation; IV drug use; ulcerated skin lesion
Rare Fungal Causes			
Xylohypha (formerly *Cladosporium*) *trichoides* and other dark-walled (demateaceous) fungi such as *Curvularia*, *Drechslera*, *Mucor*, and, after water aspiration, *Pseudoallescheria boydii*			
Protozoal Causes			
Toxoplasma gondii	Mononuclear cells	Biopsy or response to empirical therapy in clinically appropriate context (including presence of antibody in serum)	Usually with intracerebral abscesses; common in HIV-seropositive patients
Trypanosomiasis Trypanosoma *gambiense*, *T. rhodesiense*	Mononuclear cells, elevated protein	Elevated CSF IgM; identification of trypanosomes in CSF and blood smear	Endemic in Africa; chancre, lymphadenopathy; prominent sleep disorder
Rare Protozoal Causes			
Acanthamoeba sp. causing granulomatous amebic encephalitis and meningoencephalitis in immunocompromised and debilitated individuals. *Balamuthia mandrillaris* causing chronic meningoencephalitis in immunocompetent hosts.			
Helminthic Causes			
Cysticercosis (infection with cysts of *Taenia solium*)	Mononuclear cells; may have eosinophils; glucose level may be low	Indirect hemagglutination assay in CSF; ELISA immunoblotting in serum	Usually with multiple cysts in basal meninges and hydrocephalus; cerebral cysts, muscle calcification
Gnathostoma spinigerum	Eosinophils, mononuclear cells	Peripheral eosinophilia	History of eating raw fish; common in Thailand and Japan; subarachnoid hemorrhage; painful radiculopathy
Angiostrongylus cantonensis	Eosinophils, mononuclear cells	Recovery of worms from CSF	History of eating raw shellfish; common in tropical Pacific regions; often benign

TABLE 41-2

INFECTIOUS CAUSES OF CHRONIC MENINGITIS (*CONTINUED*)

CAUSATIVE AGENT	CSF FORMULA	HELPFUL DIAGNOSTIC TESTS	RISK FACTORS AND SYSTEMIC MANIFESTATIONS
Baylisascaris procyonis (raccoon ascarid)	Eosinophils, mononuclear cells		Infection follows accidental ingestion of *B. procyonis* eggs from raccoon feces; fatal meningoencephalitis
Rare Helminthic Causes			
Trichinella spiralis (trichinosis); *Fasciola hepatica* (liver fluke), *Echinococcus* cysts; *Schistosoma* sp. The former may produce a lymphocytic pleocytosis, whereas the latter two may produce an eosinophilic response in CSF associated with cerebral cysts (*Echinococcus*) or granulomatous lesions of brain or spinal cord			
Viral Causes			
Mumps	Mononuclear cells	Antibody in serum	No prior mumps or immunization; may produce meningoencephalitis; may persist for 3–4 weeks
Lymphocytic choriomeningitis	Mononuclear cells	Antibody in serum	Contact with rodents or their excreta; may persist for 3–4 weeks
Echovirus	Mononuclear cells; may have low glucose	Virus isolation from CSF	Congenital hypogammaglobulinemia; history of recurrent meningitis
HIV (acute retroviral syndrome)	Mononuclear cells	p24 antigen in serum and CSF; high level of HIV viremia	HIV risk factors; rash, fever, lymphadenopathy; lymphopenia in peripheral blood; syndrome may persist long enough to be considered as "chronic meningitis"; or chronic meningitis may develop in later stages (AIDS) due to HIV
Herpes simplex (HSV)	Mononuclear cells	PCR for HSV, CMV DNA; CSF antibody for HSV, EBV	Recurrent meningitis due to HSV-2 (rarely HSV-1) often associated with genital recurrences; EBV associated with myeloradiculopathy, CMV with polyradiculopathy

Abbreviations: AFB, acid-fast bacillus; CMV, cytomegalovirus; CSF, cerebrospinal fluid; CT, computed tomography; EBV, Epstein-Barr virus; ELISA, enzyme-linked immunosorbent assay; EM, electron microscopy; FTA, fluorescent treponemal antibody absorption test; HSV, herpes simplex virus; MHA-TP, microhemagglutination assay–*T. pallidum*; MRI, magnetic resonance imaging; PAS, periodic acid–Schiff; PCR, polymerase chain reaction; RPR, rapid plasma reagin test; TB, tuberculosis; VDRL, Venereal Disease Research Laboratory test.

In some cases, diagnosis may be established by recognition and biopsy of unusual skin lesions (Behçet's syndrome, cryptococcosis, blastomycosis, SLE, Lyme disease, IV drug use, sporotrichosis, trypanosomiasis) or enlarged lymph nodes (lymphoma, tuberculosis, sarcoid, infection with HIV, secondary syphilis, or Whipple's disease). A careful ophthalmologic examination may reveal uveitis [Vogt-Koyanagi-Harada syndrome, sarcoid, or central nervous system (CNS) lymphoma], keratoconjunctivitis sicca (Sjögren's syndrome), or iridocyclitis (Behçet's syndrome) and is essential to assess visual loss from papilledema. Aphthous oral lesions, genital ulcers, and hypopyon suggest Behçet's syndrome. Hepatosplenomegaly suggests lymphoma, sarcoid, tuberculosis, or brucellosis. Herpetic lesions in the genital area or on the thighs suggest HSV-2 infection. A breast nodule, a suspicious pigmented skin lesion, focal bone pain, or an abdominal mass directs attention to possible carcinomatous meningitis.

TABLE 41-3

NONINFECTIOUS CAUSES OF CHRONIC MENINGITIS

CAUSATIVE AGENTS	CSF FORMULA	HELPFUL DIAGNOSTIC TESTS	RISK FACTORS AND SYSTEMIC MANIFESTATIONS
Malignancy	Mononuclear cells, elevated protein, low glucose	Repeated cytologic examination of large volumes of CSF; CSF exam by polarizing microscopy; clonal lymphocyte markers; deposits on nerve roots or meninges seen on myelogram or contrast-enhanced MRI; meningeal biopsy	Metastatic cancer of breast, lung, stomach, or pancreas; melanoma, lymphoma, leukemia; meningeal gliomatosis; meningeal sarcoma; cerebral dysgerminoma; meningeal melanoma or B cell lymphoma
Chemical compounds (may cause recurrent meningitis)	Mononuclear or PMNs, low glucose, elevated protein; xanthochromia from subarachnoid hemorrhage in week prior to presentation with "meningitis"	Contrast-enhanced CT scan or MRI Cerebral angiogram to detect aneurysm	History of recent injection into the subarachnoid space; history of sudden onset of headache; recent resection of acoustic neuroma or craniopharyngioma; epidermoid tumor of brain or spine, sometimes with dermoid sinus tract; pituitary apoplexy
Primary Inflammation			
CNS sarcoidosis	Mononuclear cells; elevated protein; often low glucose	Serum and CSF angiotensin-converting enzyme levels; biopsy of extraneural affected tissues or brain lesion/meningeal biopsy	CN palsy, especially of CN VII; hypothalamic dysfunction, especially diabetes insipidus; abnormal chest radiograph; peripheral neuropathy or myopathy
Vogt-Koyanagi-Harada syndrome (recurrent meningitis)	Mononuclear cells		Recurrent meningoencephalitis with uveitis, retinal detachment, alopecia, lightening of eyebrows and lashes, dysacousia, cataracts, glaucoma
Isolated granulomatous angiitis of the nervous system	Mononuclear cells, elevated protein	Angiography or meningeal biopsy	Subacute dementia; multiple cerebral infarctions; recent zoster ophthalmicus
Systemic lupus erythematosus	Mononuclear or PMNs	Anti-DNA antibody, antinuclear antibodies	Encephalopathy; seizures; stroke; transverse myelopathy; rash; arthritis
Behçet's syndrome (recurrent meningitis)	Mononuclear or PMNs, elevated protein		Oral and genital aphthous ulcers; iridocyclitis; retinal hemorrhages; pathergic lesions at site of skin puncture
Chronic benign lymphocytic meningitis	Mononuclear cells		Recovery in 2–6 months, diagnosis by exclusion
Mollaret's meningitis (recurrent meningitis)	Large endothelial cells and PMNs in first hours, followed by mononuclear cells	PCR for herpes; MRI/CT to rule out epidermoid tumor or dural cyst	Recurrent meningitis; exclude HSV-2; rare cases due to HSV-1; occasional case associated with dural cyst
Drug hypersensitivity	PMNs; occasionally mononuclear cells or eosinophils	Complete blood count (eosinophilia)	Exposure to nonsteroidal anti-inflammatory agents, sulfonamides, isoniazid, tolmetin, ciprofloxacin, penicillin, carbamazaepine, lamotrigine, IV immunoglobulin, OKT3 antibodies, phenazopyridine; improvement after discontinuation of drug; recurrence with repeat exposure

TABLE 41-3

NONINFECTIOUS CAUSES OF CHRONIC MENINGITIS (*CONTINUED*)

CAUSATIVE AGENTS	CSF FORMULA	HELPFUL DIAGNOSTIC TESTS	RISK FACTORS AND SYSTEMIC MANIFESTATIONS
Granulomatosis with polyangiitis (Wegener's)	Mononuclear cells	Chest and sinus radiographs; urinalysis; ANCA antibodies in serum	Associated sinus, pulmonary, or renal lesions; CN palsies; skin lesions; peripheral neuropathy
Other: multiple sclerosis, Sjögren's syndrome, neonatal-onset multisystemic inflammatory disease (NOMID), and rarer forms of vasculitis (e.g., Cogan's syndrome)			

Abbreviations: ANCA, anti-neutrophil cytoplasmic antibodies; CN, cranial nerve; CSF, cerebrospinal fluid; CT, computed tomography; HSV, herpes simplex virus; MRI, magnetic resonance imaging; PCR, polymerase chain reaction; PMNs, polymorphonuclear cells.

IMAGING Once the clinical syndrome is recognized as a potential manifestation of chronic meningitis, proper analysis of the CSF is essential. However, if the possibility of raised ICP exists, a brain imaging study should be performed before lumbar puncture. If ICP is elevated because of a mass lesion, brain swelling, or a block in ventricular CSF outflow (obstructive hydrocephalus), then lumbar puncture carries the potential risk of brain herniation. Obstructive hydrocephalus usually requires direct ventricular drainage of CSF. In patients with open CSF flow pathways, elevated ICP can still occur due to impaired resorption of CSF by arachnoid villi. In such patients, lumbar puncture is usually safe, but repetitive or continuous lumbar drainage may be necessary to prevent abrupt deterioration and death from raised ICP. In some patients, especially with cryptococcal meningitis, fatal levels of raised ICP can occur without enlarged ventricles.

Contrast-enhanced MRI or CT studies of the brain and spinal cord can identify meningeal enhancement, parameningeal infections (including brain abscess), encasement of the spinal cord (malignancy or inflammation and infection), or nodular deposits on the meninges or nerve roots (malignancy or sarcoidosis) (**Fig. 41-1**). Imaging studies are also useful to localize areas of meningeal disease prior to meningeal biopsy.

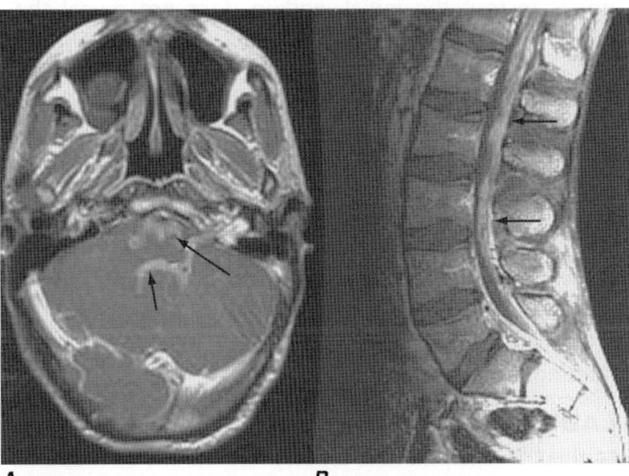

FIGURE 41-1
Primary central nervous system lymphoma. A 24-year-old man, immunosuppressed due to intestinal lymphangiectasia, developed multiple cranial neuropathies. CSF findings consisted of 100 lymphocytes/μL and a protein of 2.5 g/L (250 mg/dL); cytology and cultures were negative. Gadolinium-enhanced T1 MRI revealed diffuse, multifocal meningeal enhancement surrounding the brainstem (***A***), spinal cord, and cauda equina (***B***).

Cerebral angiography may be indicated in patients with chronic meningitis and stroke to identify cerebral arteritis (granulomatous angiitis, other inflammatory arteritides, or infectious arteritis).

CEREBROSPINAL FLUID ANALYSIS The CSF pressure should be measured and samples sent for bacterial, fungal, and tuberculous culture; Venereal Disease Research Laboratory (VDRL) test; cell count and differential; Gram's stain; and measurement of glucose and protein. Wet mount for fungus and parasites, India ink preparation and culture, culture for fastidious bacteria and fungi, assays for cryptococcal antigen and oligoclonal immunoglobulin bands, and cytology should be performed. Other specific CSF tests (Tables 41-2 and 41-3) or blood tests and cultures should be ordered as indicated on the basis of the history, physical examination, or preliminary CSF results (i.e., eosinophilic, mononuclear, or polymorphonuclear meningitis). Rapid diagnosis may be facilitated by serologic tests and polymerase chain reaction (PCR) testing to identify DNA sequences in the CSF that are specific for the suspected pathogen.

In most categories of chronic (not recurrent) meningitis, mononuclear cells predominate in the CSF. When neutrophils predominate after 3 weeks of illness, the principal etiologic considerations are *Nocardia asteroides*, *Actinomyces israelii*, *Brucella*, *Mycobacterium tuberculosis* (5–10% of early cases only), various fungi (*Blastomyces dermatitidis*, *Candida albicans*, *Histoplasma capsulatum*,

Aspergillus spp., *Pseudallescheria boydii, Cladophialophora bantiana*), and noninfectious causes (SLE, exogenous chemical meningitis). When eosinophils predominate or are present in limited numbers in a primarily mononuclear cell response in the CSF, the differential diagnosis includes parasitic diseases (*A. cantonensis, G. spinigerum, B. procyonis*, or *Toxocara canis* infection, cysticercosis, schistosomiasis, echinococcal disease, *T. gondii* infection), fungal infections (6–20% eosinophils along with a predominantly lymphocyte pleocytosis, particularly with coccidioidal meningitis), neoplastic disease (lymphoma, leukemia, metastatic carcinoma), or other inflammatory processes (sarcoidosis, hypereosinophilic syndrome).

It is often necessary to broaden the number of diagnostic tests if the initial workup does not reveal the cause. In addition, repeated samples of large volumes of CSF may be required to diagnose certain infectious and malignant causes of chronic meningitis. For instance, lymphomatous or carcinomatous meningitis may be diagnosed by examination of sections cut from a cell block formed by spinning down the sediment from a large volume of CSF. The diagnosis of fungal meningitis may require large volumes of CSF for culture of sediment. If standard lumbar puncture is unrewarding, a cervical cisternal tap to sample CSF near to the basal meninges may be fruitful.

LABORATORY INVESTIGATION In addition to the CSF examination, an attempt should be made to uncover pertinent underlying illnesses. Tuberculin skin test, chest radiograph, urine analysis and culture, blood count and differential, renal and liver function tests, alkaline phosphatase, sedimentation rate, antinuclear antibody, anti-Ro, anti-La antibody, and serum angiotensin-converting enzyme level are often indicated. Liver or bone marrow biopsy may be diagnostic in some cases of miliary tuberculosis, disseminated fungal infection, sarcoidosis, or metastatic malignancy. Abnormalities discovered on chest radiograph or chest CT can be pursued by bronchoscopy or transthoracic needle biopsy.

MENINGEAL BIOPSY A meningeal biopsy should be strongly considered in patients who are severely disabled, who need chronic ventricular decompression, or whose illness is progressing rapidly. The activities of the surgeon, pathologist, microbiologist, and cytologist should be coordinated so that a large enough sample is obtained and the appropriate cultures and histologic and molecular studies, including electron-microscopic and PCR studies, are performed. The diagnostic yield of meningeal biopsy can be increased by targeting regions that enhance with contrast on MRI or CT. With current microsurgical techniques, most areas of the basal meninges can be accessed for biopsy via a limited craniotomy. In a series from the Mayo Clinic reported by Cheng et al., MRI demonstrated meningeal enhancement in 47% of patients undergoing meningeal biopsy. Biopsy of an enhancing region was diagnostic in 80% of cases; biopsy of nonenhancing regions was diagnostic in only 9%; sarcoid (31%) and metastatic adenocarcinoma (25%) were the most common conditions identified. Tuberculosis is the most common condition identified in many reports from outside the United States.

APPROACH TO THE ENIGMATIC CASE In approximately one-third of cases, the diagnosis is not known despite careful evaluation of CSF and potential extraneural sites of disease. A number of the organisms that cause chronic meningitis may take weeks to be identified by cultures. In enigmatic cases, several options are available, determined by the extent of the clinical deficits and rate of progression. It is prudent to wait until cultures are finalized if the patient is asymptomatic or symptoms are mild and not progressive. Unfortunately, in many cases progressive neurologic deterioration occurs, and rapid treatment is required. Ventricular-peritoneal shunts may be placed to relieve hydrocephalus, but the risk of disseminating the undiagnosed inflammatory process into the abdomen must be considered.

Empirical Treatment Diagnosis of the causative agent is essential because effective therapies exist for many etiologies of chronic meningitis, but if the condition is left untreated, progressive damage to the CNS and cranial nerves and roots is likely to occur. Occasionally, empirical therapy must be initiated when all attempts at diagnosis fail. In general, empirical therapy in the United States consists of antimycobacterial agents, amphotericin for fungal infection, or glucocorticoids for noninfectious inflammatory causes. It is important to direct empirical therapy of lymphocytic meningitis at tuberculosis, particularly if the condition is associated with hypoglycorrhachia and sixth and other CN palsies, since untreated disease is fatal in 4–8 weeks. In the Mayo Clinic series, the most useful empirical therapy was administration of glucocorticoids rather than antituberculous therapy. Carcinomatous or lymphomatous meningitis may be difficult to diagnose initially, but the diagnosis becomes evident with time.

THE IMMUNOSUPPRESSED PATIENT

Chronic meningitis is not uncommon in the course of HIV infection. Pleocytosis and mild meningeal signs often occur at the onset of HIV infection, and occasionally low-grade meningitis persists. Toxoplasmosis commonly presents as intracranial abscesses and may also be associated with meningitis. Other important causes of chronic meningitis in AIDS include infection with *Cryptococcus*, *Nocardia*, *Candida*, or other fungi; syphilis; and lymphoma (Fig. 41-1). Toxoplasmosis, cryptococcosis, nocardiosis, and other fungal infections are important etiologic considerations in individuals with immunodeficiency states other than AIDS, including those due to immunosuppressive medications. Because of the increased risk of chronic meningitis and the attenuation of clinical signs of meningeal irritation in immunosuppressed individuals, CSF examination should be performed for any persistent headache or unexplained change in mental state.

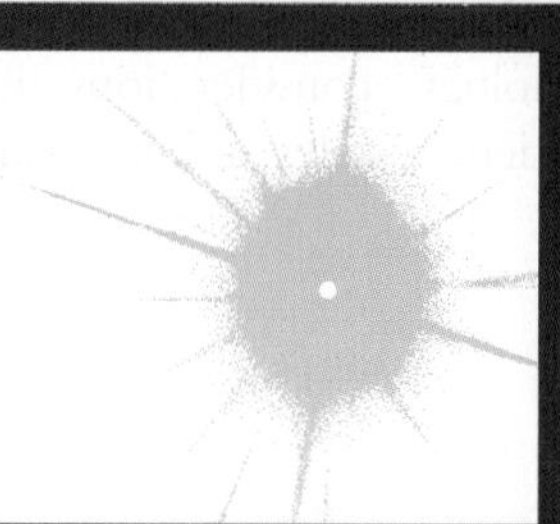

CHAPTER 42

HIV NEUROLOGY

Anthony S. Fauci ■ H. Clifford Lane

Clinical disease of the nervous system accounts for a significant degree of morbidity in a high percentage of patients with HIV infection. Neurologic problems occur throughout the course of infection and may be inflammatory, demyelinating, or degenerative in nature. These problems fall into four basic categories: neurologic disease caused by HIV itself, HIV-related neoplasms, opportunistic infections of the nervous system, and adverse effects of medical therapy (Table 42-1).

TABLE 42-1

NEUROLOGIC DISEASES IN PATIENTS WITH HIV INFECTION
Opportunistic infections
Toxoplasmosis
Cryptococcosis
Progressive multifocal leukoencephalopathy
Cytomegalovirus
Syphilis
Mycobacterium tuberculosis
HTLV-I infection
Amebiasis
Neoplasms
Primary CNS lymphoma
Kaposi's sarcoma
Result of HIV-1 infection
Aseptic meningitis
HIV-associated neurocognitive disorders, including HIV encephalopathy/AIDS dementia complex
Result of HIV-1 infection (con't)
Myelopathy
Vacuolar myelopathy
Pure sensory ataxia
Paresthesia/dysesthesia
Peripheral neuropathy
Acute inflammatory demyelinating polyneuropathy (Guillain-Barré syndrome)
Chronic inflammatory demyelinating polyneuropathy (CIDP)
Mononeuritis multiplex
Distal symmetric polyneuropathy
Myopathy

AIDS CLASSIFICATION

The current CDC classification system for HIV-infected adolescents and adults categorizes persons on the basis of clinical conditions associated with HIV infection and CD4+ T lymphocyte counts. The system is based on three ranges of CD4+ T lymphocyte counts and three clinical categories and is represented by a matrix of nine mutually exclusive categories (Tables 42-2 and 42-3). Using this system, any HIV-infected individual with a CD4+ T cell count of <200/μL has AIDS by definition, regardless of the presence of symptoms or opportunistic diseases (Table 42-2). Once individuals have had a clinical condition in category B, their disease classification cannot be reverted back to category A, even if the condition resolves; the same holds true for category C in relation to category B.

The definition of AIDS is indeed complex and comprehensive and was established not for the practical care of patients, but for surveillance purposes. Thus, the clinician should not focus on whether or not the patient fulfills the strict definition of AIDS, but should view HIV disease as a spectrum ranging from primary infection, with or without the acute syndrome, to the asymptomatic stage, to advanced disease.

ETIOLOGIC AGENT

HIV is the etiologic agent of AIDS; it belongs to the family of human retroviruses (Retroviridae) and the subfamily of lentiviruses. Nononcogenic lentiviruses cause disease in other animal species, including sheep, horses, goats, cattle, cats, and monkeys. The four recognized human retroviruses belong to two distinct groups: the human T lymphotropic viruses (HTLV)-I and HTLV-II, which are transforming retroviruses; and the human immunodeficiency viruses, HIV-1 and HIV-2, which

TABLE 42-2

1993 REVISED CLASSIFICATION SYSTEM FOR HIV INFECTION AND EXPANDED AIDS SURVEILLANCE CASE DEFINITION FOR ADOLESCENTS AND ADULTS

	CLINICAL CATEGORIES		
CD4+ T CELL CATEGORIES	**A ASYMPTOMATIC, ACUTE (PRIMARY) HIV OR PGL**	**B SYMPTOMATIC, NOT A OR C CONDITIONS**	**C AIDS-INDICATOR CONDITIONS**
>500/μL	A1	B1	C1
200–499/μL	A2	B2	C2
<200/μL	A3	B3	C3

Abbreviation: PGL, progressive generalized lymphadenopathy.
Source: MMWR 42(No. RR-17), December 18, 1992.

TABLE 42-3

CLINICAL CATEGORIES OF HIV INFECTION

Category A: Consists of one or more of the conditions listed below in an adolescent or adult (>13 years) with documented HIV infection. Conditions listed in categories B and C must not have occurred.

- Asymptomatic HIV infection
- Persistent generalized lymphadenopathy
- Acute (primary) HIV infection with accompanying illness or history of acute HIV infection

Category B: Consists of symptomatic conditions in an HIV-infected adolescent or adult that are not included among conditions listed in clinical category C and that meet at least one of the following criteria: (1) The conditions are attributed to HIV infection or are indicative of a defect in cell-mediated immunity; or (2) the conditions are considered by physicians to have a clinical course or to require management that is complicated by HIV infection. Examples include, but are not limited to, the following:

- Bacillary angiomatosis
- Candidiasis, oropharyngeal (thrush)
- Candidiasis, vulvovaginal; persistent, frequent, or poorly responsive to therapy
- Cervical dysplasia (moderate or severe)/cervical carcinoma in situ
- Constitutional symptoms, such as fever (38.5°C) or diarrhea lasting >1 month
- Hairy leukoplakia, oral
- Herpes zoster (shingles), involving at least two distinct episodes or more than one dermatome
- Idiopathic thrombocytopenic purpura
- Listeriosis
- Pelvic inflammatory disease, particularly if complicated by tuboovarian abscess
- Peripheral neuropathy

Category C: Conditions listed in the AIDS surveillance case definition.

- Candidiasis of bronchi, trachea, or lungs
- Candidiasis, esophageal
- Cervical cancer, invasive[a]
- Coccidioidomycosis, disseminated or extrapulmonary
- Cryptococcosis, extrapulmonary
- Cryptosporidiosis, chronic intestinal (>1 month's duration)
- Cytomegalovirus disease (other than liver, spleen, or nodes)
- Cytomegalovirus retinitis (with loss of vision)
- Encephalopathy, HIV-related
- Herpes simplex: chronic ulcer(s) (>1 month's duration); or bronchitis, pneumonia, or esophagitis
- Histoplasmosis, disseminated or extrapulmonary
- Isosporiasis, chronic intestinal (>1 month's duration)
- Kaposi's sarcoma
- Lymphoma, Burkitt's (or equivalent term)
- Lymphoma, primary, of brain
- *Mycobacterium avium* complex or *M. kansasii*, disseminated or extrapulmonary
- *Mycobacterium tuberculosis*, any site (pulmonary[a] or extrapulmonary)
- *Mycobacterium*, other species or unidentified species, disseminated or extrapulmonary
- *Pneumocystis jiroveci* pneumonia
- Pneumonia, recurrent[a]
- Progressive multifocal leukoencephalopathy
- *Salmonella* septicemia, recurrent
- Toxoplasmosis of brain
- Wasting syndrome due to HIV

[a]Added in the 1993 expansion of the AIDS surveillance case definition.
Source: MMWR 42(No. RR-17), December 18, 1992.

cause cytopathic effects either directly or indirectly. The most common cause of HIV disease throughout the world, and certainly in the United States, is HIV-1, which comprises several subtypes with different geographic distributions. HIV-2 was first identified in 1986 in West African patients and was originally confined to West Africa. However, a number of cases that can be traced to West Africa or to sexual contacts with West Africans have been identified throughout the world.

MORPHOLOGY OF HIV

Electron microscopy shows that the HIV virion is an icosahedral structure (Fig. 42-1*A*) containing numerous external spikes formed by the two major envelope proteins, the external gp120 and the transmembrane gp41. The virion buds from the surface of the infected cell and incorporates a variety of host proteins, including major histocompatibility complex (MHC) class I and II antigens, into its lipid bilayer. The structure of HIV-1 is schematically diagrammed in Fig. 42-1*B*.

REPLICATION CYCLE OF HIV

HIV is an RNA virus whose hallmark is the reverse transcription of its genomic RNA to DNA by the enzyme *reverse transcriptase*. The replication cycle of HIV begins with the high-affinity binding of the gp120 protein via a portion of its V1 region near the N terminus to its receptor on the host cell surface, the CD4 molecule (Fig. 42-2). The CD4 molecule is a 55-kDa protein found predominantly on a subset of T lymphocytes that are responsible for helper function in the immune system. It is also expressed on the surface of monocytes/macrophages and dendritic/Langerhans cells. Once gp120 binds to CD4, the gp120 undergoes a conformational change that facilitates binding to one of a group of co-receptors. The two major co-receptors for HIV-1 are CCR5 and CXCR4. Both receptors belong to the family of seven-transmembrane-domain G protein–coupled cellular receptors, and the use of one or the other or both receptors by the virus for entry into the cell is an important determinant of the cellular tropism of the virus. Certain dendritic cells express a diversity of C-type lectin receptors on their surface, one of which is called *DC-SIGN*, that also bind with high affinity to the HIV gp120 envelope protein, allowing the dendritic cell to facilitate the binding of virus to the CD4+ T cell upon engagement of dendritic cells with CD4+ T cells. Following binding of the envelope protein to the CD4 molecule associated with the previously -mentioned conformational change in the viral envelope gp120, fusion with the host cell membrane occurs via the newly exposed gp41 molecule penetrating the plasma membrane of the target cell and then coiling

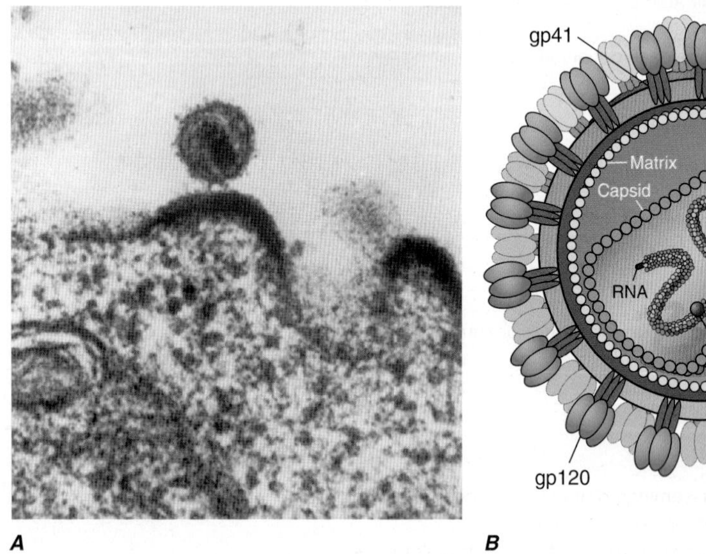

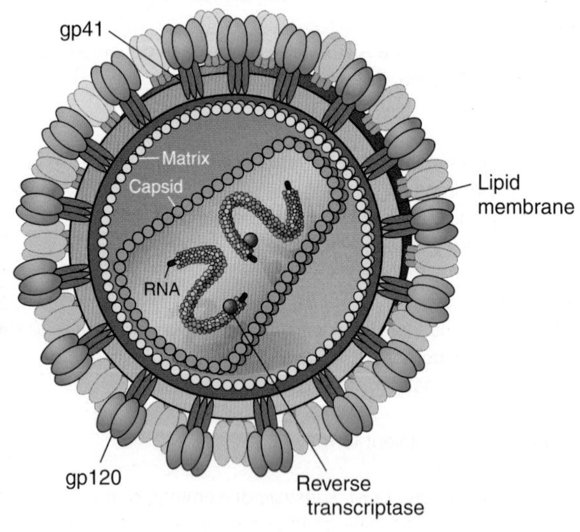

FIGURE 42-1
A.* Electron micrograph of HIV.** Figure illustrates a typical virion following budding from the surface of a CD4+ T lymphocyte, together with two additional incomplete virions in the process of budding from the cell membrane. ***B. Structure of HIV-1, including the gp120 outer membrane, gp41 transmembrane components of the envelope, genomic RNA, enzyme reverse transcriptase, p18(17) inner membrane (matrix), and p24 core protein (capsid). (*Copyright by George V. Kelvin. Adapted from RC Gallo: Sci Am 256:46, 1987.*)

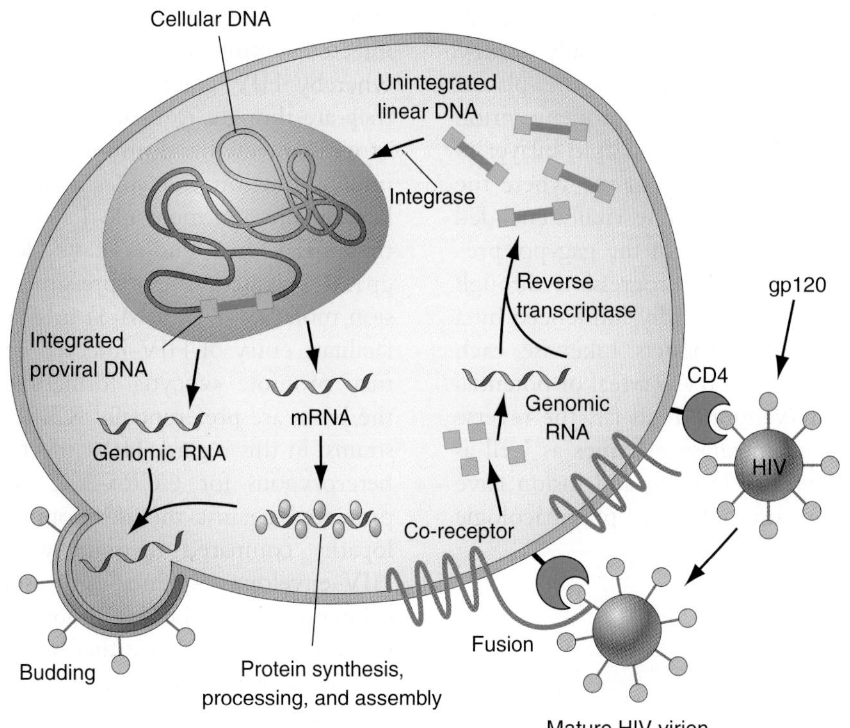

FIGURE 42-2
The replication cycle of HIV. See text for description. (*Adapted from AS Fauci: Nature 384:529, 1996.*)

upon itself to bring the virion and target cell together. Following fusion, the preintegration complex, composed of viral RNA and viral enzymes and surrounded by a capsid protein coat, is released into the cytoplasm of the target cell. As the preintegration complex traverses the cytoplasm to reach the nucleus, the viral reverse transcriptase enzyme catalyzes the reverse transcription of the genomic RNA into DNA, and the protein coat opens to release the resulting double-stranded HIV-DNA. At this point in the replication cycle, the viral genome is vulnerable to cellular factors that can block the progression of infection. In particular, the cytoplasmic TRIM5-α protein in rhesus macaque cells blocks SIV replication at a point shortly after the virus fuses with the host cell. Although the exact mechanisms of action of TRIM5-α remain unclear, the human form is inhibited by cyclophilin A and is not effective in restricting HIV replication in human cells. The recently described APOBEC family of cellular proteins also inhibits progression of virus infection after virus has entered the cell. APOBEC proteins bind to nascent reverse transcripts and deaminate viral cytidine, causing hypermutation of HIV genomes. It is still not clear whether (1) viral replication is inhibited by the binding of APOBEC to the virus genome with subsequent accumulation of reverse transcripts, or (2) by the hypermutations caused by the enzymatic deaminase activity of APOBEC proteins. HIV has evolved a powerful strategy to protect itself from APOBEC. The viral protein Vif targets APOBEC for proteasomal degradation.

With activation of the cell, the viral DNA accesses the nuclear pore and is exported from the cytoplasm to the nucleus, where it is integrated into the host cell chromosomes through the action of another virally encoded enzyme, *integrase*. HIV provirus (DNA) selectively integrates into the nuclear DNA preferentially within introns of active genes and regional hotspots. This provirus may remain transcriptionally inactive (latent) or it may manifest varying levels of gene expression, up to active production of virus.

Cellular activation plays an important role in the replication cycle of HIV and is critical to the pathogenesis of HIV disease. Following initial binding and internalization of virions into the target cell, incompletely reverse-transcribed DNA intermediates are labile in quiescent cells and do not integrate efficiently into the host cell genome unless cellular activation occurs shortly after infection. Furthermore, some degree of activation of the host cell is required for the initiation of transcription of the integrated proviral DNA into either genomic RNA or mRNA. This latter process may not necessarily be associated with the detectable expression of the classic cell surface markers of activation. In this regard, activation of HIV expression from the latent state depends on the interaction of a number of cellular and viral factors. Following transcription, HIV mRNA is translated into proteins that undergo modification through glycosylation, myristylation, phosphorylation, and cleavage. The viral particle is formed by the assembly of HIV proteins, enzymes, and genomic RNA at the plasma membrane of the cells. Budding of the progeny virion occurs through specialized regions in the lipid bilayer of the host cell membrane known as *lipid rafts*, where the core acquires its external envelope. The virally encoded protease then catalyzes the cleavage of the gag-pol precursor to yield the mature virion. Progression through the virus replication cycle is profoundly influenced by a variety of viral regulatory gene products. Likewise, each point in the replication cycle of HIV is a real or potential target for therapeutic intervention. Thus far, the reverse transcriptase, protease, and integrase enzymes as well as the process of virus–target cell binding and fusion have proven clinically to be susceptible to pharmacologic disruption.

PATHOPHYSIOLOGY AND PATHOGENESIS

The hallmark of HIV disease is a profound immunodeficiency resulting primarily from a progressive quantitative and qualitative deficiency of the subset of T lymphocytes referred to as *helper T cells* occurring in a setting of polyclonal immune activation. The *helper* subset of T cells is defined phenotypically by the presence on its surface of the CD4 molecule, which serves as the primary cellular receptor for HIV. When the number of CD4+ T cells declines below a certain level, the patient is at high risk for developing a variety of opportunistic diseases, particularly the infections and neoplasms that are AIDS-defining illnesses. Some features of AIDS, such as Kaposi sarcoma and certain neurologic abnormalities, cannot be explained completely by the immunosuppressive effects of HIV, since these complications may occur prior to the development of severe immunologic impairment.

NEUROPATHOGENESIS

While there has been a remarkable decrease in the incidence of HIV encephalopathy among those with access to treatment in the era of effective ARV therapy, HIV-infected individuals can still experience a variety of neurologic abnormalities due either to opportunistic infections and neoplasms or to direct effects of HIV or its products. With regard to the latter, HIV has been demonstrated in the brain and CSF of infected individuals with and without neuropsychiatric abnormalities. The main cell types that are infected in the brain in vivo are the perivascular macrophages and the microglial cells; monocytes that have already been infected in the blood can migrate into the brain, where they then reside as macrophages, or macrophages can be directly infected within the brain. The precise mechanisms whereby HIV enters the brain are unclear; however, they are thought to relate, at least in part, to the ability of virus-infected and immune-activated macrophages to induce adhesion molecules such as E-selectin and vascular cell adhesion molecule-1 (VCAM-1) on brain endothelium. Other studies have demonstrated that HIV gp120 enhances the expression of intercellular adhesion molecule-1 (ICAM-1) in glial cells; this effect may facilitate entry of HIV-infected cells into the CNS and may promote syncytia formation. Virus isolates from the brain are preferentially R5 strains as opposed to X4 strains; in this regard, HIV-infected individuals who are heterozygous for *CCR5-Δ32* appear to be relatively protected against the development of HIV encephalopathy compared to wild-type individuals. Distinct HIV envelope sequences are associated with the clinical expression of the AIDS dementia complex. There is no convincing evidence that brain cells other than those of monocyte/macrophage lineage can be productively infected in vivo.

HIV-infected individuals may manifest white matter lesions as well as neuronal loss. Given the absence of evidence of HIV infection of neurons either in vivo or in vitro, it is highly unlikely that direct infection of these cells accounts for their loss. Rather, the HIV-mediated effects on neurons and oligodendrocytes are thought to involve indirect pathways whereby viral proteins, particularly gp120 and Tat, trigger the release of endogenous neurotoxins from macrophages and to a lesser extent from astrocytes. In addition, it has been demonstrated that both HIV-1 Nef and Tat can induce chemotaxis of leukocytes, including monocytes, into the CNS. Neurotoxins can be released from monocytes as a consequence of infection and/or immune activation. Monocyte-derived neurotoxic factors have been reported to kill neurons via the *N*-methyl-D-aspartate (NMDA) receptor. In addition, HIV gp120 shed by virus-infected monocytes could cause neurotoxicity by antagonizing the function of vasoactive intestinal peptide (VIP), by elevating intracellular calcium levels, and by decreasing nerve growth factor levels in the cerebral cortex. A variety of monocyte-derived cytokines can contribute directly or indirectly to the neurotoxic effects in HIV infection; these include TNF-α, IL-1, IL-6, TGF-β, IFN-γ, platelet-activating factor, and endothelin. Furthermore, among the CC-chemokines, elevated levels of monocyte chemotactic protein (MCP) 1 in the brain and CSF have been shown to correlate best with the presence and degree of HIV encephalopathy. In addition, infection and/or activation of monocyte-lineage cells can result in increased production of eicosanoids, quinolinic acid, nitric oxide, excitatory amino acids such as L-cysteine and glutamate, arachidonic acid, platelet activating factor, free radicals, TNF-α, and TGF-β, which may contribute to neurotoxicity. Astrocytes may play diverse roles in HIV neuropathogenesis. Reactive gliosis or astrocytosis has been demonstrated in the brains of HIV-infected individuals, and TNF-α and IL-6 have been shown to induce astrocyte proliferation. In addition, astrocyte-derived IL-6 can induce HIV expression in infected cells in vitro. Furthermore, it has been suggested that astrocytes may downregulate macrophage-produced neurotoxins. It has been reported that HIV-infected individuals with the E4 allele for apolipoprotein E (apo E) are at increased risk for AIDS encephalopathy and peripheral neuropathy. The likelihood that HIV or its products are involved in neuropathogenesis is supported by the observation that neuropsychiatric abnormalities may undergo remarkable and rapid improvement upon the initiation of combination antiretroviral therapy (cART).

It has also been suggested that the CNS may serve as a relatively sequestered site for a reservoir of latently infected cells that might be a barrier for the eradication of the virus by cART.

CLINICAL MANIFESTATIONS

Clinical disease of the nervous systems accounts for a significant degree of morbidity in a high percentage of patients with HIV infection (Table 42-1). The neurologic problems that occur in HIV-infected individuals may be either primary to the pathogenic processes of HIV infection or secondary to opportunistic infections or neoplasms. Among the more frequent opportunistic diseases that involve the CNS are toxoplasmosis, cryptococcosis, progressive multifocal leukoencephalopathy, and primary CNS lymphoma. Other less common problems include mycobacterial infections; syphilis; and infection with CMV, HTLV-I, *T. cruzi*, or *Acanthamoeba*. Overall, secondary diseases of the CNS occur in approximately one-third of patients with AIDS. These data antedate the widespread use of cART, and this frequency is considerably less in patients receiving effective antiretroviral drugs. Primary processes related to HIV infection of the nervous system are reminiscent of those seen with other lentiviruses, such as the Visna-Maedi virus of sheep.

NEUROLOGIC DISEASES CAUSED BY HIV

HIV-associated cognitive impairment

The term *HIV-associated neurocognitive disorders* (HAND) is used to describe a spectrum of disorders that range from asymptomatic neurocognitive impairment (ANI) to minor neurocognitive disorder (MND) to clinically severe dementia. The most severe form, *HIV-associated dementia (HAD), also referred to as the AIDS dementia complex, or HIV encephalopathy*, is considered an AIDS-defining illness. Most HIV-infected patients have some neurologic problem during the course of their disease. Even in the setting of suppressive cART, approximately 50% of HIV-infected individuals can be shown to have mild to moderate neurocognitive impairment using sensitive neuropsychiatric testing. Virtually all patients with HIV infection have some degree of nervous system involvement with the virus. This is evidenced by the fact that CSF findings are abnormal in ~90% of patients, even during the asymptomatic phase of HIV infection. CSF abnormalities include pleocytosis (50–65% of patients), detection of viral RNA (~75%), elevated CSF protein (35%), and evidence of intrathecal synthesis of anti-HIV antibodies (90%). It is important to point out that evidence of infection of the CNS with HIV does not imply impairment of cognitive function. The neurologic function of an HIV-infected individual should be considered normal unless clinical signs and symptoms suggest otherwise.

HIV-associated dementia (also known as HIV encephalopathy) consists of a constellation of signs and symptoms of CNS disease. While this is generally a late complication of HIV infection that progresses slowly over months, it can be seen in patients with CD4+ T cell counts >350 cells/μL. A major feature of this entity is the development of dementia, defined as a decline in cognitive ability from a previous level. It may present as impaired ability to concentrate, increased forgetfulness, difficulty reading, or increased difficulty performing complex tasks. Initially these symptoms may be indistinguishable from findings of situational depression or fatigue. In contrast to "cortical" dementia (such as Alzheimer's disease), aphasia, apraxia, and agnosia are uncommon, leading some investigators to classify HIV-associated dementia as a "subcortical dementia" characterized by defects in short-term memory and executive function. In addition to dementia, patients with HIV-associated dementia may also have motor and behavioral abnormalities. Among the motor problems are unsteady gait, poor balance, tremor, and difficulty with rapid alternating movements. Increased tone and deep tendon reflexes may be found in patients with spinal cord involvement. Late stages may be complicated by bowel and/or bladder incontinence. Behavioral problems include apathy and lack of initiative, with progression to a vegetative state in some instances. Some patients develop a state of agitation or mild mania. These changes usually occur without significant changes in level of alertness. This is in contrast to the finding of somnolence in patients with dementia due to toxic/metabolic encephalopathies.

HIV-associated dementia is the initial AIDS-defining illness in ~3% of patients with HIV infection and thus only rarely precedes clinical evidence of immunodeficiency. Clinically significant encephalopathy eventually

TABLE 42-4

CLINICAL STAGING OF HIV ENCEPHALOPATHY (AIDS DEMENTIA COMPLEX)

STAGE	DEFINITION
0 (Normal)	Normal mental and motor function.
0.5 (Equivocal/subclinical)	Absent, minimal, or equivocal symptoms without impairment of work or capacity to perform activities of daily living. Mild signs (snout response, slowed ocular or extremity movements) may be present. Gait and strength are normal.
1 (Mild)	Able to perform all but the more demanding aspects of work or activities of daily living but with unequivocal evidence (signs or symptoms that may include performance on neuropsychological testing) of functional, intellectual, or motor impairment. Can walk without assistance.
2 (Moderate)	Able to perform basic activities of self-care but cannot work or maintain the more demanding aspects of daily life. Ambulatory, but may require a single prop.
3 (Severe)	Major intellectual incapacity (cannot follow news or personal events, cannot sustain complex conversation, considerable slowing of all output) or motor disability (cannot walk unassisted, usually with slowing and clumsiness of arms as well).
4 (End-stage)	Nearly vegetative. Intellectual and social comprehension and output are at a rudimentary level. Nearly or absolutely mute. Paraparetic or paraplegic with urinary and fecal incontinence.

Source: Adapted from JJ Sidtis, RW Price: Neurology 40:197, 1990.

develops in ~25% of untreated patients with AIDS. As immunologic function declines, the risk and severity of HIV encephalopathy increase. Autopsy series suggest that 80–90% of patients with HIV infection have histologic evidence of CNS involvement. Several classification schemes have been developed for grading HIV-associated dementia; a commonly used clinical staging system is outlined in Table 42-4.

The precise cause of HIV-associated dementia remains unclear, although the condition is thought to be a result of a combination of direct effects of HIV on the CNS and associated immune activation. HIV has been found in the brains of patients with HIV-associated dementia by Southern blot, in situ hybridization, PCR, and electron microscopy. Multinucleated giant cells, macrophages, and microglial cells appear to be the main cell types harboring virus in the CNS. Histologically, the major changes are seen in the subcortical areas of the brain and include pallor and gliosis, multinucleated giant cell encephalitis, and vacuolar myelopathy. Less commonly, diffuse or focal spongiform changes occur in the white matter. Areas of the brain involved in motor, language, and judgment are most severely affected.

There are no specific criteria for a diagnosis of HIV-associated dementia, and this syndrome must be differentiated from a number of other diseases that affect the CNS of HIV-infected patients. The diagnosis of dementia depends upon demonstrating a decline in cognitive function. This can be accomplished objectively with the use of a Mini-Mental Status Examination (MMSE) in patients for whom prior scores are available. For this reason, it is advisable for all patients with a diagnosis of HIV infection to have a baseline MMSE. However, changes in MMSE scores may be absent in patients with mild HIV-associated dementia. Imaging studies of the CNS, by either MRI or CT, often demonstrate evidence of cerebral atrophy (Fig. 42-3). MRI may also reveal small areas of increased density on T2-weighted images. Lumbar puncture is an important element of the evaluation of patients with HIV infection and neurologic abnormalities. It is generally most helpful in ruling out or

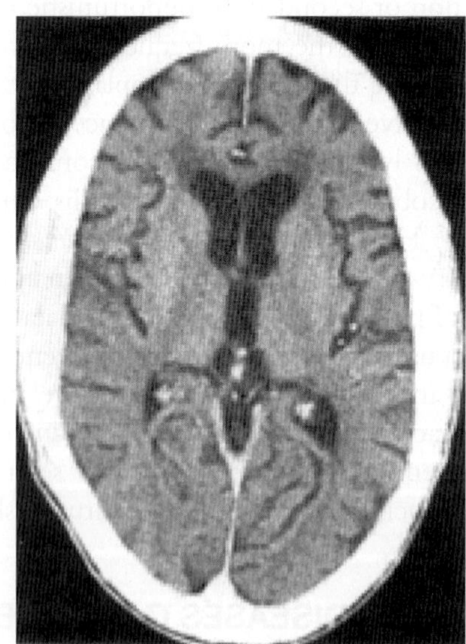

FIGURE 42-3

AIDS dementia complex. Postcontrast CT scan through the lateral ventricles of a 47-year-old man with AIDS, altered mental status, and dementia. The lateral and third ventricles and the cerebral sulci are abnormally prominent. Mild white matter hypodensity is also seen adjacent to the frontal horns of the lateral ventricles.

making a diagnosis of opportunistic infections. In HIV-associated dementia, patients may have the nonspecific findings of an increase in CSF cells and protein level. While HIV RNA can often be detected in the spinal fluid and HIV can be cultured from the CSF, this finding is not specific for HIV-associated dementia. There appears to be no correlation between the presence of HIV in the CSF and the presence of HIV-associated dementia. Elevated levels of macrophage chemoattractant protein (MCP-1), β_2-microglobulin, neopterin, and quinolinic acid (a metabolite of tryptophan reported to cause CNS injury) have been noted in the CSF of patients with HIV-associated dementia. These findings suggest that these factors as well as inflammatory cytokines may be involved in the pathogenesis of this syndrome.

Combination antiretroviral therapy is of benefit in patients with HIV-associated dementia. Improvement in neuropsychiatric test scores has been noted for both adult and pediatric patients treated with antiretrovirals. The rapid improvement in cognitive function noted with the initiation of cART suggests that at least some component of this problem is quickly reversible, again supporting at least a partial role of soluble mediators in the pathogenesis. It should also be noted that these patients have an increased sensitivity to the side effects of neuroleptic drugs. The use of these drugs for symptomatic treatment is associated with an increased risk of extrapyramidal side effects; therefore, patients with HIV-associated dementia who receive these agents must be monitored carefully. It is felt by many physicians that the decrease in the prevalence of severe cases of HIV-associated dementia brought about by cART has resulted in an increase in the prevalence of milder forms of this disorder.

Aseptic meningitis

Aseptic meningitis may be seen in any but the very late stages of HIV infection. In the setting of acute primary infection patients may experience a syndrome of headache, photophobia, and meningismus. Rarely, an acute encephalopathy due to encephalitis may occur. Cranial nerve involvement may be seen, predominantly cranial nerve VII but occasionally V and/or VIII. CSF findings include a lymphocytic pleocytosis, elevated protein level, and normal glucose level. This syndrome, which cannot be clinically differentiated from other viral meningitides (Chap. 41), usually resolves spontaneously within 2–4 weeks; however, in some patients, signs and symptoms may become chronic. Aseptic meningitis may occur any time in the course of HIV infection; however, it is rare following the development of AIDS. This fact suggests that clinical aseptic meningitis in the context of HIV infection is an immune-mediated disease.

HIV myelopathy

Spinal cord disease, or myelopathy, is present in ~20% of patients with AIDS, often as part of HIV-associated neurocognitive disorder. In fact, 90% of the patients with HIV-associated myelopathy have some evidence of dementia, suggesting that similar pathologic processes may be responsible for both conditions. Three main types of spinal cord disease are seen in patients with AIDS. The first of these is a vacuolar myelopathy. This condition is pathologically similar to subacute combined degeneration of the cord such as occurs with pernicious anemia. Although vitamin B_{12} deficiency can be seen in patients with AIDS as a primary complication of HIV infection, it does not appear to be responsible for the myelopathy seen in the majority of patients. Vacuolar myelopathy is characterized by a subacute onset and often presents with gait disturbances, predominantly ataxia and spasticity; it may progress to include bladder and bowel dysfunction. Physical findings include evidence of increased deep tendon reflexes and extensor plantar responses. The second form of spinal cord disease involves the dorsal columns and presents as a pure sensory ataxia. The third form is also sensory in nature and presents with paresthesias and dysesthesias of the lower extremities. In contrast to the cognitive problems, these spinal cord syndromes do not respond well to antiretroviral drugs, and therapy is mainly supportive.

One important disease of the spinal cord that also involves the peripheral nerves is a *myelopathy* and *polyradiculopathy* seen in association with CMV infection. This entity is generally seen late in the course of HIV infection and is fulminant in onset, with lower extremity and sacral paresthesias, difficulty in walking, areflexia, ascending sensory loss, and urinary retention. The clinical course is rapidly progressive over a period of weeks. CSF examination reveals a predominantly neutrophilic pleocytosis, and CMV DNA can be detected by CSF PCR. Therapy with ganciclovir or foscarnet can lead to rapid improvement, and prompt initiation of foscarnet or ganciclovir therapy is important in minimizing the degree of permanent neurologic damage. Combination therapy with both drugs should be considered in patients who have been previously treated for CMV disease. Other diseases involving the spinal cord in patients with HIV infection include HTLV-I-associated myelopathy (HAM), neurosyphilis, infection with herpes simplex or varicella-zoster, TB, and lymphoma.

HIV neuropathy

Peripheral neuropathies are common in patients with HIV infection. They occur at all stages of illness and take a variety of forms. Early in the course of HIV infection, an acute inflammatory demyelinating polyneuropathy resembling Guillain-Barré syndrome may occur (Chap. 46). In other patients, a progressive or relapsing-remitting inflammatory neuropathy resembling chronic inflammatory demyelinating polyneuropathy (CIDP) has been noted. Patients commonly present with progressive weakness, areflexia, and minimal sensory changes. CSF examination often reveals a mononuclear pleocytosis, and peripheral nerve biopsy demonstrates a perivascular infiltrate suggesting an autoimmune etiology. Plasma exchange or IVIg has been tried with variable success. Because of the immunosuppressive effects of glucocorticoids, they should be reserved for severe cases of CIDP refractory to other measures. Another autoimmune peripheral neuropathy seen in patients with AIDS is mononeuritis multiplex (due to a necrotizing arteritis of peripheral nerves). The most common peripheral neuropathy in patients with HIV infection is a *distal sensory polyneuropathy*, also referred to as painful sensory neuropathy, predominantly sensory neuropathy, or distal symmetric peripheral neuropathy. This condition may be a direct consequence of HIV infection or a side effect of dideoxynucleoside therapy. It is more common in taller individuals, older individuals, and those with lower CD4 counts. Two-thirds of patients with AIDS may be shown by electrophysiologic studies to have some evidence of peripheral nerve disease. Presenting symptoms are usually painful burning sensations in the feet and lower extremities. Findings on examination include a stocking-type sensory loss to pinprick, temperature, and touch sensation and a loss of ankle reflexes. Motor changes are mild and are usually limited to weakness of the intrinsic foot muscles. Response of this condition to antiretrovirals has been variable, perhaps because antiretrovirals are responsible for the problem in some instances. When due to dideoxynucleoside therapy, patients with lower extremity peripheral neuropathy may complain of a sensation that they are walking on ice. Other entities in the differential diagnosis of peripheral neuropathy include diabetes mellitus, vitamin B_{12} deficiency, and side effects from metronidazole or dapsone. For distal symmetric polyneuropathy that fails to resolve following the discontinuation of dideoxynucleosides, therapy is symptomatic; gabapentin, carbamazepine, tricyclics, or analgesics may be effective for dysesthesias. Treatment-naive patients may respond to cART.

HIV myopathy

Myopathy may complicate the course of HIV infection; causes include HIV infection itself, zidovudine, and the generalized wasting syndrome. HIV-associated myopathy may range in severity from an asymptomatic elevation in creatine kinase levels to a subacute syndrome characterized by proximal muscle weakness and myalgias. Quite pronounced elevations in creatine kinase may occur in asymptomatic patients, particularly after exercise. The clinical significance of this as an isolated laboratory finding is unclear. A variety of both inflammatory and noninflammatory pathologic processes have been noted in patients with more severe myopathy, including myofiber necrosis with inflammatory cells, nemaline rod bodies, cytoplasmic bodies, and mitochondrial abnormalities. Profound muscle wasting, often with muscle pain, may be seen after prolonged zidovudine therapy. This toxic side effect of the drug is dose-dependent and is related to its ability to interfere with the function of mitochondrial polymerases. It is reversible following discontinuation of the drug. Red ragged fibers are a histologic hallmark of zidovudine-induced myopathy.

HIV-related neoplasms

Systemic lymphoma

Lymphomas occur with an increased frequency in patients with congenital or acquired T cell immunodeficiencies. AIDS is no exception; at least 6% of all patients with AIDS develop lymphoma at some time during the course of their illness. This is a 120-fold increase in incidence compared to the general population. In contrast to the situation with Kaposi's sarcoma, primary CNS lymphoma, and most opportunistic infections, the incidence of AIDS-associated systemic lymphomas has not experienced as dramatic a decrease as a consequence of the widespread use of effective cART. Lymphoma occurs in all risk groups, with the highest incidence in patients with hemophilia and the lowest incidence in patients from the Caribbean or Africa with heterosexually acquired infection. Lymphoma is a late manifestation of HIV infection, generally occurring in patients with CD4+ T cell counts <200/μL. As HIV disease progresses, the risk of lymphoma increases. The attack rate for lymphoma increases exponentially with increasing duration of HIV infection and decreasing level of immunologic function. At 3 years following a diagnosis of HIV infection, the risk of lymphoma is 0.8% per year; by 8 years after infection, it is 2.6% per year. As individuals with HIV infection live longer as a consequence of improved cART and better treatment and prophylaxis of opportunistic infections, it is anticipated that the incidence of lymphomas may increase.

The clinical presentation of lymphoma in patients with HIV infection is quite varied, ranging from focal seizures to rapidly growing mass lesions in the oral mucosa to persistent unexplained fever. At least 80% of patients present with extranodal disease, and a similar percentage have B-type symptoms of fever, night sweats, or weight loss. Virtually any site in the body may be involved. The most common extranodal site is the CNS, which is involved in approximately one-third of all patients with lymphoma. Approximately 60% of these cases are primary CNS lymphoma.

CNS lymphoma

Primary CNS lymphoma accounts for ~20% of the cases of lymphoma in patients with HIV infection. In contrast to HIV-associated Burkitt's lymphoma, primary CNS lymphomas are usually positive for EBV. In one study, the incidence of Epstein-Barr positivity was 100%. This malignancy does not have a predilection for any particular age group. The median CD4+ T cell count at the time of diagnosis is ~50/μL. Thus, CNS lymphoma generally presents at a later stage of HIV infection than systemic lymphoma. This fact may at least in part explain the poorer prognosis for this subset of patients.

Primary CNS lymphoma generally presents with focal neurologic deficits, including cranial nerve findings, headaches, and/or seizures. MRI or CT generally reveals a limited number (one to three) of 3- to 5-cm lesions (Fig. 42-4). The lesions often show ring enhancement on contrast administration and may occur in any location. Locations that are most commonly involved with CNS lymphoma are deep in the white matter. Contrast enhancement is usually less pronounced than that seen with toxoplasmosis. The main diseases in the differential diagnosis are cerebral toxoplasmosis and cerebral Chagas' disease. In addition to the 20% of lymphomas in HIV-infected individuals that are primary CNS lymphomas, CNS disease is also seen in HIV-infected patients with systemic lymphoma. Approximately 20% of patients with systemic lymphoma have CNS disease in the form of leptomeningeal involvement. This fact underscores the importance of lumbar puncture in the staging evaluation of patients with systemic lymphoma.

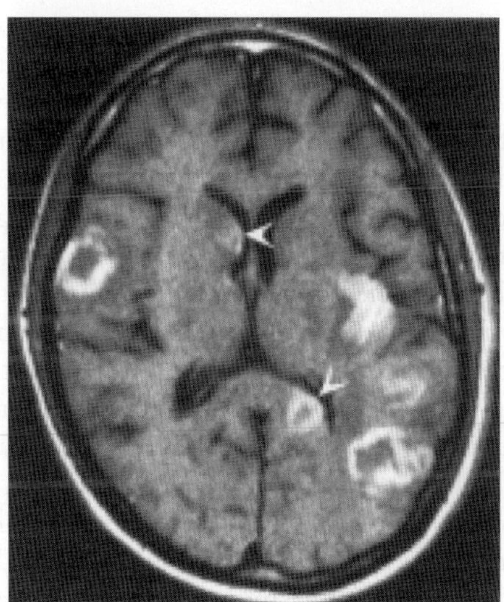

FIGURE 42-4
Central nervous system lymphoma. Postcontrast T1-weighted MR scan in a patient with AIDS, an altered mental status, and hemiparesis. Multiple enhancing lesions, some ring-enhancing, are present. The left Sylvian lesion shows gyral and subcortical enhancement, and the lesions in the caudate and splenium (*arrowheads*) show enhancement of adjacent ependymal surfaces.

Both conventional and unconventional approaches have been employed in an attempt to treat HIV-related lymphomas. Systemic lymphoma is generally treated by the oncologist with combination chemotherapy. Earlier disappointing figures are being replaced with more optimistic results for the treatment of systemic lymphoma following the availability of more effective cART and the use of rituximab in CD20+ tumors. While there is controversy regarding the use of antiretrovirals during chemotherapy, there is no question that their use overall in patients with HIV lymphoma has improved survival. As in most situations in patients with HIV disease, those with the higher CD4+ T cell counts tend to do better. Response rates as high as 72% with a median survival of 33 months and disease-free intervals up to 9 years have been reported. Treatment of primary CNS lymphoma remains a significant challenge. Treatment is complicated by the fact that this illness usually occurs in patients with advanced HIV disease. Palliative measures such as radiation therapy provide some relief. The prognosis remains poor in this group, with a 2-year survival of 29%.

HIV-related opportunistic infections

The most common HIV-related neurologic opportunistic infections are toxoplasmosis, cryptococcal infections, and progressive multifocal leukoencephalopathy. The risk of many such infections correlates well with the CD4+ T cell count (Fig. 42-5). A selected group of common and important opportunistic infections of the nervous system in patients with HIV is discussed next.

Cryptococcosis

C. neoformans is the leading infectious cause of meningitis in patients with AIDS. It is the initial AIDS-defining illness in ~2% of patients and generally occurs in patients with CD4+ T cell counts <100/μL. Cryptococcal meningitis is particularly common in patients with AIDS in Africa, occurring in ~5% of patients. Most patients present with a picture of subacute meningoencephalitis with fever, nausea, vomiting, altered mental status, headache, and meningeal signs. The incidence of seizures and focal neurologic deficits is low. The CSF profile may be normal or may show only modest elevations in WBC or protein levels and decreases in glucose. In addition to meningitis, patients may develop cryptococcomas and cranial nerve involvement. Approximately one-third of patients also have pulmonary disease. Uncommon manifestations of cryptococcal infection

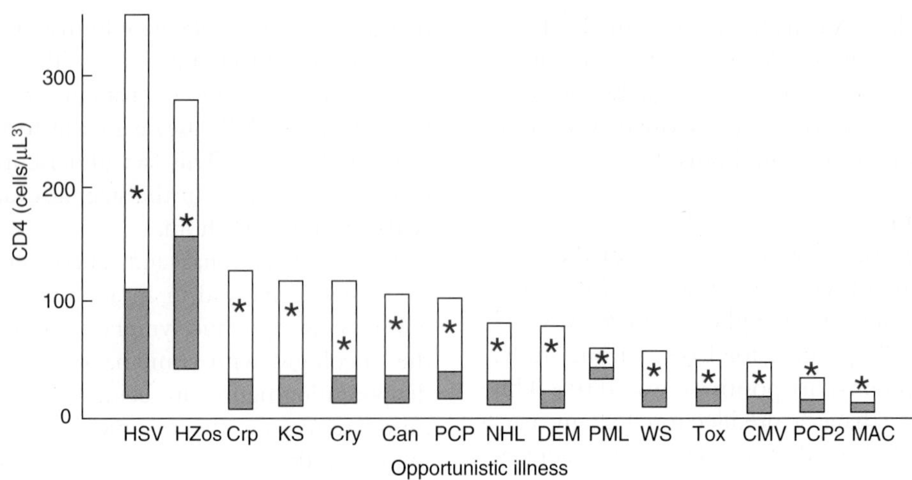

FIGURE 42-5

Relationship between CD4+ T cell counts and the development of opportunistic diseases. Boxplot of the median (line inside the box), first quartile (bottom of the box), third quartile (top of the box), and mean (asterisk) CD4+ lymphocyte count at the time of the development of opportunistic disease. Can, candidal esophagitis; CMV, cytomegalovirus infection; Crp, cryptosporidiosis; Cry, cryptococcal meningitis; DEM, AIDS dementia complex; HSV, herpes simplex virus infection; HZos, herpes zoster; KS, Kaposi's sarcoma; MAC, *Mycobacterium avium* complex bacteremia; NHL, non-Hodgkin's lymphoma; PCP, primary *Pneumocystis jiroveci* pneumonia; PCP2, secondary *P. jiroveci* pneumonia; PML, progressive multifocal leukoencephalopathy; Tox, *Toxoplasma gondii* encephalitis; WS, wasting syndrome. (*From RD Moore, RE Chaisson: Ann Intern Med 124:633, 1996.*)

include skin lesions that resemble *molluscum contagiosum*, lymphadenopathy, palatal and glossal ulcers, arthritis, gastroenteritis, myocarditis, and prostatitis. The prostate gland may serve as a reservoir for smoldering cryptococcal infection. The diagnosis of cryptococcal meningitis is made by identification of organisms in spinal fluid with India ink examination or by the detection of cryptococcal antigen. A biopsy may be needed to make a diagnosis of CNS cryptococcoma. Treatment is with IV amphotericin B, at a dose of 0.7 mg/kg daily, or liposomal amphotericin 4-6 mg/kg daily, with flucytosine, 25 mg/kg qid for at least 2 weeks, and, if possible, until the CSF culture turns negative. This is followed by fluconazole, 400 mg/d PO for 8 weeks, and then fluconazole, 200 mg/d until the CD4+ T cell count has increased to >200 cells/μL for 6 months in response to cART. Repeated lumbar puncture may be required to manage increased intracranial pressure. Symptoms may recur with initiation of cART as an immune reconstitution syndrome. Other fungi that may cause meningitis in patients with HIV infection are *C. immitis* and *H. capsulatum*. Meningoencephalitis has also been reported due to *Acanthamoeba* or *Naegleria*.

Toxoplasmosis

Toxoplasmosis has been one of the most common causes of secondary CNS infections in patients with AIDS, but its incidence is decreasing in the era of cART. It is most common in patients from the Caribbean and from France, where the seroprevalence of *T. gondii* is around 50%. Toxoplasmosis is generally a late complication of HIV infection and usually occurs in patients with CD4+ T cell counts <200/μL. Cerebral toxoplasmosis is thought to represent a reactivation of latent tissue cysts. It is 10 times more common in patients with antibodies to the organism than in patients who are seronegative. Patients diagnosed with HIV infection should be screened for IgG antibodies to *T. gondii* during the time of their initial workup. Those who are seronegative should be counseled about ways to minimize the risk of primary infection including avoiding the consumption of undercooked meat and careful hand washing after contact with soil or changing the cat litter box. The most common clinical presentation of cerebral toxoplasmosis in patients with HIV infection is fever, headache, and focal neurologic deficits. Patients may present with seizure, hemiparesis, or aphasia as a manifestation of these focal deficits or with a picture more influenced by the accompanying cerebral edema and characterized by confusion, dementia, and lethargy, which can progress to coma. The diagnosis is usually suspected on the basis of MRI findings of multiple lesions in multiple locations, although in some cases only a single lesion is seen. Pathologically, these lesions generally exhibit inflammation and central necrosis and, as a result, demonstrate ring enhancement on contrast MRI **(Fig. 42-6)** or, if MRI is unavailable

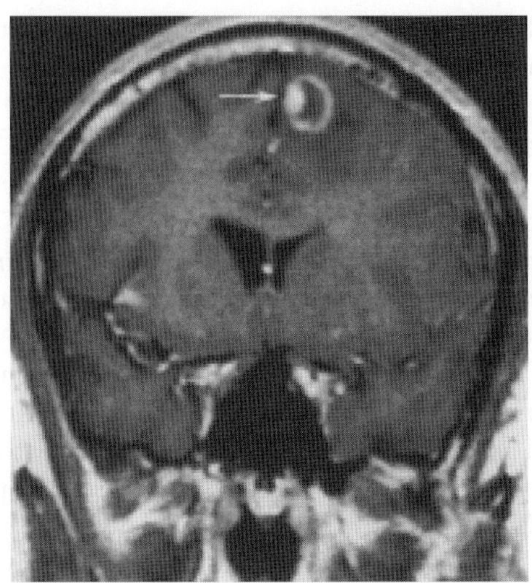

FIGURE 42-6

Central nervous system toxoplasmosis. A coronal post-contrast T1-weighted MR scan demonstrates a peripheral enhancing lesion in the left frontal lobe, associated with an eccentric nodular area of enhancement (*arrow*); this so-called eccentric target sign is typical of toxoplasmosis.

or contraindicated, on double-dose contrast CT. There is usually evidence of surrounding edema. In addition to toxoplasmosis, the differential diagnosis of single or multiple enhancing mass lesions in the HIV-infected patient includes primary CNS lymphoma and, less commonly, TB or fungal or bacterial abscesses. The definitive diagnostic procedure is brain biopsy. However, given the morbidity than can accompany this procedure, it is usually reserved for the patient who has failed 2–4 weeks of empiric therapy. If the patient is seronegative for *T. gondii*, the likelihood that a mass lesion is due to toxoplasmosis is <10%. In that setting, one may choose to be more aggressive and perform a brain biopsy sooner. Standard treatment is sulfadiazine and pyrimethamine with leucovorin as needed for a minimum of 4–6 weeks. Alternative therapeutic regimens include clindamycin in combination with pyrimethamine; atovaquone plus pyrimethamine; and azithromycin plus pyrimethamine plus rifabutin. Relapses are common, and it is recommended that patients with a history of prior toxoplasmic encephalitis receive maintenance therapy with sulfadiazine, pyrimethamine, and leucovorin as long as their CD4+ T cell counts remain <200 cells/μL. Patients with CD4+ T cell counts <100/μL and IgG antibody to *Toxoplasma* should receive primary prophylaxis for toxoplasmosis. Fortunately, the same daily regimen of a single double-strength tablet of TMP/SMX used for *P. jiroveci* prophylaxis provides adequate primary protection against toxoplasmosis. Secondary prophylaxis/maintenance therapy for toxoplasmosis may be discontinued in the setting of effective cART and increases in CD4+ T cell counts to >200/μL for 6 months.

Progressive multifocal leukoencephalopathy (PML)

JC virus, a human polyomavirus that is the etiologic agent of *progressive multifocal leukoencephalopathy* (PML), is an important opportunistic pathogen in patients with AIDS. While ~80% of the general adult population have antibodies to JC virus, indicative of prior infection, <10% of healthy adults show any evidence of ongoing viral replication. PML is the only known clinical manifestation of JC virus infection. It is a late manifestation of AIDS and is seen in ~4% of patients with AIDS. The lesions of PML begin as small foci of demyelination in subcortical white matter that eventually coalesce. The cerebral hemispheres, cerebellum, and brainstem may all be involved. Patients typically have a protracted course with multifocal neurologic deficits, with or without changes in mental status. Approximately 20% of patients experience seizures. Ataxia, hemiparesis, visual field defects, aphasia, and sensory defects may occur. MRI typically reveals multiple, non-enhancing white matter lesions that may coalesce and have a predilection for the occipital and parietal lobes. The lesions show signal hyperintensity on T2-weighted images and diminished signal on T1-weighted images. The measurement of JC virus DNA levels in CSF has a diagnostic sensitivity of 76% and a specificity of close to 100%. Prior to the availability of cART, the majority of patients with PML died within 3–6 months of the onset of symptoms. Paradoxical worsening of PML has been seen with initiation of cART as an immune reconstitution syndrome. There is no specific treatment for PML; however, a minimal median survival of 2 years and survival of >15 years have been reported in patients with PML treated with cART for their HIV disease. Unfortunately only ~50% of patients with HIV infection and PML show neurologic improvement with cART. Studies with other antiviral agents such as cidofovir have failed to show clear benefit. Factors influencing a favorable prognosis for PML in the setting of HIV infection include a CD4+ T cell count >100/μL at baseline and the ability to maintain an HIV viral load of <500 copies per milliliter. Baseline HIV-1 viral load does not have independent predictive value of survival. PML is one of the few opportunistic infections that continues to occur with some frequency despite the widespread use of cART.

Chagas' disease

Reactivation American trypanosomiasis may present as acute meningoencephalitis with focal neurologic signs, fever, headache, vomiting, and seizures. Accompanying cardiac disease in the form of arrhythmias or heart failure should increase the index of suspicion. The presence of antibodies to *Trypanosoma cruzi* supports the diagnosis. In South America, reactivation of *Chagas' disease* is considered to be an AIDS-defining condition and may be the initial AIDS-defining condition. The majority of cases occur in patients with CD4+ T cell counts <200 cells/μL. Lesions appear radiographically as single or multiple hypodense areas, typically with ring enhancement and edema. They are found predominantly in the subcortical areas, a feature that differentiates them from the deeper lesions of toxoplasmosis. *T. cruzi* amastigotes, or trypanosomes, can be identified from biopsy specimens or CSF. Other CSF findings include elevated protein and a mild (<100 cells/μL) lymphocytic pleocytosis. Organisms can also be identified by direct examination of the blood. Treatment consists of benzimidazole (2.5 mg/kg bid) or nifurtimox (2 mg/kg qid) for at least 60 days, followed by maintenance therapy for the duration of immunodeficiency with either drug at a dose of 5 mg/kg three times a week. As is the case with cerebral toxoplasmosis, successful therapy with antiretrovirals may allow discontinuation of therapy for Chagas' disease.

Specific neurologic presentations

Stroke

Stroke may occur in patients with HIV infection. In contrast to the other causes of focal neurologic deficits in patients with HIV infection, the symptoms of a stroke are sudden in onset. Patients with HIV infection have an increased prevalence of many classic risk factors associated with stroke, including smoking and diabetes. It also appears that HIV infection itself can lead to an increase in carotid artery stiffness. Among the secondary infectious diseases in patients with HIV infection that may be associated with stroke are vasculitis due to cerebral varicella zoster or neurosyphilis and septic embolism in association with fungal infection. Other elements of the differential diagnosis of stroke in the patient with HIV infection include atherosclerotic cerebral vascular disease, thrombotic thrombocytopenic purpura, and cocaine or amphetamine use.

Seizures

Seizures may be a consequence of opportunistic infections, neoplasms, or HIV-associated dementia. The seizure threshold is often lower than normal in patients with advanced HIV infection due to the frequent presence of electrolyte abnormalities. Seizures are seen in 15–40% of patients with cerebral toxoplasmosis, 15–35% of patients with primary CNS lymphoma, 8% of patients with cryptococcal meningitis, and 7–50% of patients with HIV-associated dementia. Seizures may also be seen in patients with CNS tuberculosis, aseptic meningitis, and progressive multifocal leukoencephalopathy. Seizures may be the presenting clinical symptom of HIV disease. In one study of 100 patients with HIV infection presenting with a first seizure, cerebral mass lesions were the most common cause, responsible for 32 of the 100 new-onset seizures. Of these 32 cases, 28 were due to toxoplasmosis and 4 to lymphoma. HIV-associated dementia accounted for an additional 24 new-onset seizures. Cryptococcal meningitis was the third most common diagnosis, responsible for 13 of the 100 seizures. In 23 cases, no cause could be found, and it is possible that these cases represent a subcategory of HIV-associated dementia. Of these 23 cases, 16 (70%) had two or more seizures, suggesting that anticonvulsant therapy is indicated in all patients with HIV infection and seizures unless a rapidly correctable cause is found. While phenytoin remains the initial treatment of choice, hypersensitivity reactions to this drug have been reported in >10% of patients with AIDS, and therefore the use of phenobarbital, valproic acid, or levetiracetam must be considered as an alternative. Due to a variety of drug-drug interactions between antiseizure medications and antiretrovirals, drug levels need to be monitored carefully.

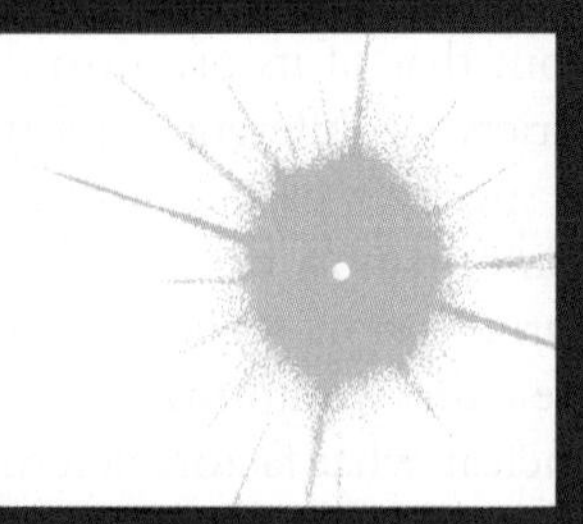

CHAPTER 43
PRION DISEASES

Stanley B. Prusiner ■ Bruce L. Miller

Prions are infectious proteins that cause degeneration of the central nervous system (CNS). Prion diseases are disorders of protein conformation, the most common of which in humans is called Creutzfeldt-Jakob disease (CJD). CJD typically presents with dementia and myoclonus, is relentlessly progressive, and generally causes death within a year of onset. Most CJD patients are between 50 and 75 years of age; however, patients as young as 17 and as old as 83 have been recorded.

In mammals, prions reproduce by binding to the normal, *c*ellular isoform of the *p*rion *p*rotein (PrP^C) and stimulating conversion of PrP^C into the di*s*ease-*c*ausing isoform (PrP^{Sc}). PrP^C is rich in α-helix and has little β-structure, while PrP^{Sc} has less α-helix and a high amount of β-structure (Fig. 43-1). This α-to-β structural transition in the prion protein (PrP) is the fundamental event underlying prion diseases (Table 43-1).

Four new concepts have emerged from studies of prions: (1) Prions are the only known infectious pathogens that are devoid of nucleic acid; all other infectious agents possess genomes composed of either RNA or DNA that direct the synthesis of their progeny. (2) Prion diseases may be manifest as infectious, genetic, and sporadic

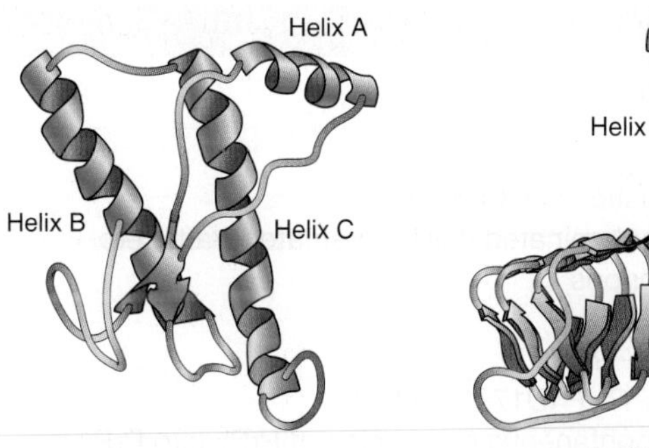

FIGURE 43-1

Structures of prion proteins. *A.* NMR structure of Syrian hamster recombinant (rec) PrP(90–231). Presumably, the structure of the α-helical form of recPrP(90–231) resembles that of PrP^C. recPrP(90–231) is viewed from the interface where PrP^{Sc} is thought to bind to PrP^C. Shown are: α-helices A (residues 144–157), B (172–193), and C (200–227). Flat ribbons depict β-strands S1 (129–131) and S2 (161–163). (***A,*** *from SB Prusiner: N Engl J Med 344:1516, 2001; with permission.*) ***B.*** Structural model of PrP^{Sc}. The 90–160 region has been modeled onto a β-helical architecture while the COOH terminal helices B and C are preserved as in PrP^C. (*Image prepared by C. Govaerts.*)

TABLE 43-1

GLOSSARY OF PRION TERMINOLOGY	
Prion	*Pro*teinaceous *in*fectious particle that lacks nucleic acid. Prions are composed entirely of PrP^{Sc} molecules. They can cause scrapie in sheep and goats, and related neurodegenerative diseases of humans such as Creutzfeldt-Jakob disease (CJD).
PrP^{Sc}	Disease-causing isoform of the prion protein. This protein is the only identifiable macromolecule in purified preparations of scrapie prions.
PrP^C	*C*ellular isoform of the prion protein. PrP^C is the precursor of PrP^{Sc}.
PrP 27-30	A fragment of PrP^{Sc}, generated by truncation of the NH_2-terminus by limited digestion with proteinase K. PrP 27-30 retains prion infectivity and polymerizes into amyloid.
PRNP	PrP gene located on human chromosome 20.
Prion rod	An aggregate of prions composed largely of PrP 27-30 molecules. Created by detergent extraction and limited proteolysis of PrP^{Sc}. Morphologically and histochemically indistinguishable from many amyloids.
PrP amyloid	Amyloid containing PrP in the brains of animals or humans with prion disease; often accumulates as plaques.

disorders; no other group of illnesses with a single etiology presents with such a wide spectrum of clinical manifestations. (3) Prion diseases result from the accumulation of PrP^{Sc}, the conformation of which differs substantially from that of its precursor, PrP^{C}. (4) PrP^{Sc} can exist in a variety of different conformations, each of which seems to specify a particular disease phenotype. How a specific conformation of a PrP^{Sc} molecule is imparted to PrP^{C} during prion replication to produce nascent PrP^{Sc} with the same conformation is unknown. Additionally, it is unclear what factors determine where in the CNS a particular PrP^{Sc} molecule will be deposited.

SPECTRUM OF PRION DISEASES

The sporadic form of CJD is the most common prion disorder in humans. Sporadic CJD (sCJD) accounts for ~85% of all cases of human prion disease, while inherited prion diseases account for 10–15% of all cases (Table 43-2). Familial CJD (fCJD), Gerstmann-Sträussler-Scheinker (GSS) disease, and fatal familial insomnia (FFI) are all dominantly inherited prion diseases that are caused by mutations in the PrP gene.

Although infectious prion diseases account for <1% of all cases and infection does not seem to play an important role in the natural history of these illnesses, the transmissibility of prions is an important biologic feature. *Kuru* of the Fore people of New Guinea is thought to have resulted from the consumption of brains from dead relatives during ritualistic cannibalism. With the cessation of ritualistic cannibalism in the late 1950s, kuru has nearly disappeared, with the exception of a few recent patients exhibiting incubation periods of >40 years. Iatrogenic CJD (iCJD) seems to be the result of the accidental inoculation of patients with prions. Variant CJD (vCJD) in teenagers and young adults in Europe is the result of exposure to tainted beef from cattle with bovine spongiform encephalopathy (BSE).

Six diseases of animals are caused by prions (Table 43-2). Scrapie of sheep and goats is the prototypic prion disease. Mink encephalopathy, BSE, feline spongiform encephalopathy, and exotic ungulate encephalopathy are all thought to occur after the consumption of prion-infected foodstuffs. The BSE epidemic emerged in Britain in the late 1980s and was shown to be due to industrial cannibalism. Whether BSE began as a sporadic case of BSE in a cow or started with scrapie in sheep is unknown. The origin of chronic wasting disease (CWD), a prion disease endemic in deer and elk in regions of North America, is uncertain. In contrast to other prion diseases, CWD is highly communicable. Feces from asymptomatic, infected cervids contain prions that are likely to be responsible for the spread of CWD.

EPIDEMIOLOGY

CJD is found throughout the world. The incidence of sCJD is approximately one case per million population, and thus it accounts for about 1 in every 10,000 deaths.

TABLE 43-2

THE PRION DISEASES

DISEASE	HOST	MECHANISM OF PATHOGENESIS
Human		
Kuru	Fore people	Infection through ritualistic cannibalism
iCJD	Humans	Infection from prion-contaminated hGH, duramater grafts, etc.
vCJD	Humans	Infection from bovine prions
fCJD	Humans	Germ-line mutations in *PRNP*
GSS	Humans	Germ-line mutations in *PRNP*
FFI	Humans	Germ-line mutation in *PRNP* (D178N, M129)
sCJD	Humans	Somatic mutation or spontaneous conversion of PrP^{C} into PrP^{Sc}?
sFI	Humans	Somatic mutation or spontaneous conversion of PrP^{C} into PrP^{Sc}?
Animal		
Scrapie	Sheep, goats	Infection in genetically susceptible sheep
BSE	Cattle	Infection with prion-contaminated MBM
TME	Mink	Infection with prions from sheep or cattle
CWD	Mule deer, elk	Unknown
FSE	Cats	Infection with prion-contaminated beef
Exotic ungulate encephalopathy	Greater kudu, nyala,or oryx	Infection with prion-contaminated MBM

Abbreviations: BSE, bovine spongiform encephalopathy; CJD, Creutzfeldt-Jakob disease; CWD, chronic wasting disease; fCJD, familial Creutzfeldt-Jakob disease; FFI, fatal familial insomnia; FSE, feline spongiform encephalopathy; GSS, Gerstmann-Sträussler-Scheinker disease; hGH, human growth hormone; iCJD, iatrogenic Creutzfeldt-Jakob disease; MBM, meat and bone meal; sCJD, sporadic Creutzfeldt-Jakob disease; sFI, sporadic fatal insomnia; TME, transmissible mink encephalopathy; vCJD, variant Creutzfeldt-Jakob disease.

Because sCJD is an age-dependent neurodegenerative disease, its incidence is expected to increase steadily as older segments of populations in developed and developing countries continue to expand. Although many geographic clusters of CJD have been reported, each has been shown to segregate with a PrP gene mutation. Attempts to identify common exposure to some etiologic agent have been unsuccessful for both the sporadic and familial cases. Ingestion of scrapie-infected sheep or goat meat as a cause of CJD in humans has not been demonstrated by epidemiologic studies, although speculation about this potential route of inoculation continues. Of particular interest are deer hunters who develop CJD, because up to 90% of culled deer in some game herds have been shown to harbor CWD prions. Whether prion disease in deer or elk has passed to cows, sheep, or directly to humans remains unknown. Studies with rodents demonstrate that oral infection with prions can occur, but the process is inefficient compared to intracerebral inoculation.

PATHOGENESIS

The human prion diseases were initially classified as neurodegenerative disorders of unknown etiology on the basis of pathologic changes being confined to the CNS. With the transmission of kuru and CJD to apes, investigators began to view these diseases as infectious CNS illnesses caused by slow viruses. Even though the familial nature of a subset of CJD cases was well described, the significance of this observation became more obscure with the transmission of CJD to animals. Eventually the meaning of heritable CJD became clear with the discovery of mutations in the *PRNP* gene of these patients. The prion concept explains how a disease can manifest as a heritable as well as an infectious illness. Moreover, the hallmark of all prion diseases, whether sporadic, dominantly inherited, or acquired by infection, is that they involve the aberrant metabolism of PrP.

A major feature that distinguishes prions from viruses is the finding that both PrP isoforms are encoded by a chromosomal gene. In humans, the PrP gene is designated *PRNP* and is located on the short arm of chromosome 20. Limited proteolysis of PrP^{Sc} produces a smaller, protease-resistant molecule of ~142 amino acids designated PrP 27-30; PrP^{C} is completely hydrolyzed under the same conditions (Fig. 43-2). In the presence of detergent, PrP 27-30 polymerizes into amyloid. Prion rods formed by limited proteolysis and detergent extraction are indistinguishable from the filaments that aggregate to form PrP amyloid plaques in the CNS. Both the rods and the PrP amyloid filaments found in brain tissue exhibit similar ultrastructural morphology and green-gold birefringence after staining with Congo red dye.

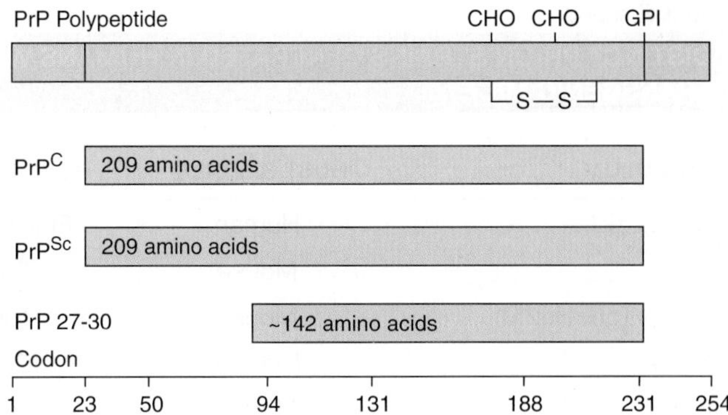

FIGURE 43-2

Prion protein isoforms. Bar diagram of Syrian hamster PrP, which consists of 254 amino acids. After processing of the NH_2 and COOH termini, both PrP^{C} and PrP^{Sc} consist of 209 residues. After limited proteolysis, the NH_2 terminus of PrP^{Sc} is truncated to form PrP 27–30 composed of ~142 amino acids.

Prion strains

The existence of prion strains raised the question of how heritable biologic information can be enciphered in a molecule other than nucleic acid. Various strains of prions have been defined by incubation times and the distribution of neuronal vacuolation. Subsequently, the patterns of PrP^{Sc} deposition were found to correlate with vacuolation profiles, and these patterns were also used to characterize prion strains.

Persuasive evidence that strain-specific information is enciphered in the tertiary structure of PrP^{Sc} comes from transmission of two different inherited human prion diseases to mice expressing a chimeric human-mouse PrP transgene. In FFI, the protease-resistant fragment of PrP^{Sc} after deglycosylation has a molecular mass of 19 kDa, whereas in fCJD and most sporadic prion diseases, it is 21 kDa (Table 43-3). This difference in molecular mass was shown to be due to different sites of proteolytic cleavage at the NH_2 termini of the two human PrP^{Sc} molecules, reflecting different tertiary structures. These distinct conformations were not unexpected because the amino acid sequences of the PrPs differ.

Extracts from the brains of patients with FFI transmitted disease into mice expressing a chimeric human-mouse PrP transgene and induced formation of the 19-kDa PrP^{Sc}, whereas brain extracts from fCJD and sCJD patients produced the 21-kDa PrP^{Sc} in mice expressing the same transgene. On second passage, these differences were maintained, demonstrating that chimeric PrP^{Sc} can exist in two different conformations based on the sizes of the protease-resistant fragments, even though the amino acid sequence of PrP^{Sc} is invariant.

This analysis was extended when patients with sporadic fatal insomnia (sFI) were identified. Although they did not carry a *PRNP* gene mutation, the patients demonstrated a clinical and pathologic phenotype that

TABLE 43-3

DISTINCT PRION STRAINS GENERATED IN HUMANS WITH INHERITED PRION DISEASES AND TRANSMITTED TO TRANSGENIC MICE[a]

INOCULUM	HOST SPECIES	HOST PrP GENOTYPE	INCUBATION TIME [DAYS ± SEM] (n/n_0)	PrP^{Sc}(kDa)
None	Human	FFI(D178N, M129)		19
FFI	Mouse	Tg(MHu2M)	206 ± 7 (7/7)	19
FFI → Tg(MHu2M)	Mouse	Tg(MHu2M)	136 ± 1 (6/6)	19
None	Human	fCJD(E200K)		21
fCJD	Mouse	Tg(MHu2M)	170 ± 2 (10/10)	21
fCJD → Tg(MHu2M)	Mouse	Tg(MHu2M)	167 ± 3 (15/15)	21

[a]Tg(MHu2M) mice express a chimeric mouse-human PrP gene.

Notes: Clinicopathologic phenotype is determined by the conformation of PrP^{Sc} in accord with the results of the transmission of human prions from patients with FFI to transgenic mice. fCJD, familial Creutzfeldt-Jakob disease; FFI, fatal familial insomnia.

was indistinguishable from that of patients with FFI. Furthermore, 19-kDa PrP^{Sc} was found in their brains, and on passage of prion disease to mice expressing a chimeric human-mouse PrP transgene, 19-kDa PrP^{Sc} was also found. These findings indicate that the disease phenotype is dictated by the conformation of PrP^{Sc} and not the amino acid sequence. PrP^{Sc} acts as a template for the conversion of PrP^C into nascent PrP^{Sc}. On the passage of prions into mice expressing a chimeric hamster-mouse PrP transgene, a change in the conformation of PrP^{Sc} was accompanied by the emergence of a new strain of prions.

Many new strains of prions were generated using recombinant (rec) PrP produced in bacteria; recPrP was polymerized into amyloid fibrils and inoculated into transgenic mice expressing high levels of wild-type mouse PrP^C; about 500 days later, the mice died of prion disease. The incubation times of the "synthetic prions" in mice were dependent on the conditions used for polymerization of the amyloid fibrils. Highly stable amyloids gave rise to stable prions with long incubation times; low-stability amyloids led to prions with short incubation times. Amyloids of intermediate stability gave rise to prions with intermediate stabilities and intermediate incubation times. Such findings are consistent with earlier studies showing that the incubation times of synthetic and naturally occurring prions are directly proportional to the stability of the prion.

Species barrier

Studies on the role of the primary and tertiary structures of PrP in the transmission of prion disease have given new insights into the pathogenesis of these maladies. The amino acid sequence of PrP encodes the species of the prion, and the prion derives its PrP^{Sc} sequence from the last mammal in which it was passaged. While the primary structure of PrP is likely to be the most important or even sole determinant of the tertiary structure of PrP^C, PrP^{Sc} seems to function as a template in determining the tertiary structure of nascent PrP^{Sc} molecules as they are formed from PrP^C. In turn, prion diversity appears to be enciphered in the conformation of PrP^{Sc}, and thus prion strains seem to represent different conformers of PrP^{Sc}.

In general, transmission of prion disease from one species to another is inefficient, in that not all intracerebrally inoculated animals develop disease, and those that fall ill do so only after long incubation times that can approach the natural life span of the animal. This "species barrier" to transmission is correlated with the degree of similarity between the amino acid sequences of PrP^C in the inoculated host and of PrP^{Sc} in the prion inoculum. The importance of sequence similarity between the host and donor PrP argues that PrP^C directly interacts with PrP^{Sc} in the prion conversion process.

SPORADIC AND INHERITED PRION DISEASES

Several different scenarios might explain the initiation of sporadic prion disease: (1) A somatic mutation may be the cause and thus follow a path similar to that for germ-line mutations in inherited disease. In this situation, the mutant PrP^{Sc} must be capable of targeting wild-type PrP^C, a process known to be possible for some mutations but less likely for others. (2) The activation energy barrier separating wild-type PrP^C from PrP^{Sc} could be crossed on rare occasions when viewed in the context of a population. Most individuals would be spared while presentations in the elderly with an incidence of ~1 per million would be seen. (3) PrP^{Sc} may be present at low levels in some normal cells, where it performs some important, as yet unknown, function. The level of PrP^{Sc} in such cells is hypothesized to be sufficiently low as to be not detected by routine bioassay. In some altered metabolic states, the cellular mechanisms for clearing PrP^{Sc} might become compromised and the rate of PrP^{Sc} formation would then begin to exceed the capacity of the cell to clear it. The third possible mechanism is attractive since it suggests PrP^{Sc} is not simply a misfolded protein, as proposed for the first and second mechanisms, but that it is an alternatively folded molecule with a function. Moreover, the multitude of conformational states that PrP^{Sc} can adopt, as described earlier, raises the possibility that PrP^{Sc} or another prion-like protein might function in a process like short-term memory where information storage occurs in the absence of new protein synthesis.

More than 40 different mutations resulting in nonconservative substitutions in the human *PRNP* gene have been found to segregate with inherited human prion diseases. Missense mutations and expansions in the octapeptide repeat region of the gene are responsible for familial forms of prion disease. Five different mutations of the *PRNP* gene have been linked genetically to heritable prion disease.

Although phenotypes may vary dramatically within families, specific phenotypes tend to be observed with certain mutations. A clinical phenotype indistinguishable from typical sCJD is usually seen with substitutions at codons 180, 183, 200, 208, 210, and 232. Substitutions at codons 102, 105, 117, 198, and 217 are associated with the GSS variant of prion disease. The normal human PrP sequence contains five repeats of an eight-amino-acid sequence. Insertions from two to nine extra octarepeats frequently cause variable phenotypes ranging from a condition indistinguishable from sCJD to a slowly progressive dementing illness of many years' duration to an early-age-of-onset disorder that is similar to Alzheimer's disease. A mutation at codon 178 resulting in substitution of asparagine for aspartic acid produces FFI if a methionine is encoded at the polymorphic 129 residue on the same allele. Typical CJD is seen if the D178N mutation occurs with a valine encoded at position 129 of the same allele.

HUMAN *PRNP* GENE POLYMORPHISMS

Polymorphisms influence the susceptibility to sporadic, inherited, and infectious forms of prion disease. The methionine/valine polymorphism at position 129 not only modulates the age of onset of some inherited prion diseases but can also determine the clinical phenotype. The finding that homozygosity at codon 129 predisposes to sCJD supports a model of prion production that favors PrP interactions between homologous proteins.

Substitution of the basic residue lysine at position 218 in mouse PrP produced dominant-negative inhibition of prion replication in transgenic mice. This same lysine at position 219 in human PrP has been found in 12% of the Japanese population, and this group appears to be resistant to prion disease. Dominant-negative inhibition of prion replication was also found with substitution of the basic residue arginine at position 171; sheep with arginine are resistant to scrapie prions but are susceptible to BSE prions that were inoculated intracerebrally.

INFECTIOUS PRION DISEASES

IATROGENIC CJD

Accidental transmission of CJD to humans appears to have occurred with corneal transplantation, contaminated electroencephalogram (EEG) electrode implantation, and surgical procedures. Corneas from donors with inapparent CJD have been transplanted to apparently healthy recipients who developed CJD after prolonged incubation periods. The same improperly decontaminated EEG electrodes that caused CJD in two young patients with intractable epilepsy caused CJD in a chimpanzee 18 months after their experimental implantation.

Surgical procedures may have resulted in accidental inoculation of patients with prions, presumably because some instrument or apparatus in the operating theater became contaminated when a CJD patient underwent surgery. Although the epidemiology of these studies is highly suggestive, no proof for such episodes exists.

Dura mater grafts

More than 160 cases of CJD after implantation of dura mater grafts have been recorded. All of the grafts were thought to have been acquired from a single manufacturer whose preparative procedures were inadequate to inactivate human prions. One case of CJD occurred after repair of an eardrum perforation with a pericardium graft.

Human growth hormone and pituitary gonadotropin therapy

The transmission of CJD prions from contaminated human growth hormone (hGH) preparations derived from human pituitaries has been responsible for fatal cerebellar disorders with dementia in >180 patients ranging in age from 10 to 41 years. These patients received injections of hGH every 2–4 days for 4–12 years. If it is thought that these patients developed CJD from injections of prion-contaminated hGH preparations, the possible incubation periods range from 4 to 30 years. Only recombinant hGH is now used therapeutically so that possible contamination with prions is no longer an issue. Four cases of CJD have occurred in women receiving human pituitary gonadotropin.

VARIANT CJD

The restricted geographic occurrence and chronology of vCJD raised the possibility that BSE prions had been transmitted to humans through the consumption of tainted beef. More than 190 cases of vCJD have occurred, with >90% of these in Britain. vCJD has also been reported in people either living in or originating from France, Ireland, Italy, Netherlands, Portugal, Spain, Saudi Arabia, United States, Canada, and Japan.

The steady decline in the number of vCJD cases over the past decade argues that there will not be a prion disease epidemic in Europe, similar to those seen for BSE and kuru. What is certain is that prion-tainted meat should be prevented from entering the human food supply.

The most compelling evidence that vCJD is caused by BSE prions was obtained from experiments in mice expressing the bovine PrP transgene. Both BSE and vCJD prions were efficiently transmitted to these transgenic mice and with similar incubation periods. In contrast to sCJD prions, vCJD prions did not transmit disease efficiently to mice expressing a chimeric human-mouse PrP transgene. Earlier studies with nontransgenic mice suggested that vCJD and BSE might be derived from the same source because both inocula transmitted disease with similar but very long incubation periods.

Attempts to determine the origin of BSE and vCJD prions have relied on passaging studies in mice, some of which are described earlier, as well as studies of the conformation and glycosylation of PrP^{Sc}. One scenario suggests that a particular conformation of bovine PrP^{Sc} was selected for heat resistance during the rendering process and was then reselected multiple times as cattle infected by ingesting prion-contaminated meat and bone meal (MBM) were slaughtered and their offal rendered into more MBM.

NEUROPATHOLOGY

Frequently the brains of patients with CJD have no recognizable abnormalities on gross examination. Patients who survive for several years have variable degrees of cerebral atrophy.

On light microscopy, the pathologic hallmarks of CJD are spongiform degeneration and astrocytic gliosis. The lack of an inflammatory response in CJD and other prion diseases is an important pathologic feature of these degenerative disorders. Spongiform degeneration is characterized by many 1- to 5-μm vacuoles in the neuropil between nerve cell bodies. Generally the spongiform changes occur in the cerebral cortex, putamen, caudate nucleus, thalamus, and molecular layer of the cerebellum. Astrocytic gliosis is a constant but nonspecific feature of prion diseases. Widespread proliferation of fibrous astrocytes is found throughout the gray matter of brains infected with CJD prions. Astrocytic processes filled with glial filaments form extensive networks.

Amyloid plaques have been found in ~10% of CJD cases. Purified CJD prions from humans and animals exhibit the ultrastructural and histochemical characteristics of amyloid when treated with detergents during limited proteolysis. In first passage from some human Japanese CJD cases, amyloid plaques have been found in mouse brains. These plaques stain with antibodies raised against PrP.

The amyloid plaques of GSS disease are morphologically distinct from those seen in kuru or scrapie. GSS plaques consist of a central dense core of amyloid surrounded by smaller globules of amyloid. Ultrastructurally, they consist of a radiating fibrillar network of amyloid fibrils, with scant or no neuritic degeneration. The plaques can be distributed throughout the brain but are most frequently found in the cerebellum. They are often located adjacent to blood vessels. Congophilic angiopathy has been noted in some cases of GSS disease.

In vCJD, a characteristic feature is the presence of "florid plaques." These are composed of a central core of PrP amyloid, surrounded by vacuoles in a pattern suggesting petals on a flower.

CLINICAL FEATURES

Nonspecific prodromal symptoms occur in about a third of patients with CJD and may include fatigue, sleep disturbance, weight loss, headache, anxiety, vertigo, malaise, and ill-defined pain. Most patients with CJD present with deficits in higher cortical function. These deficits almost always progress over weeks or months to a state of profound dementia characterized by memory loss, impaired judgment, and a decline in virtually all aspects of intellectual function. A few patients present with either visual impairment or cerebellar gait and coordination deficits. Frequently the cerebellar deficits are rapidly followed by progressive dementia. Visual problems often begin with blurred vision and diminished acuity, rapidly followed by dementia.

Other symptoms and signs include extrapyramidal dysfunction manifested as rigidity, masklike facies, or (less commonly) choreoathetoid movements; pyramidal signs (usually mild); seizures (usually major motor) and, less commonly, hypoesthesia; supranuclear gaze palsy; optic atrophy; and vegetative signs such as changes in weight, temperature, sweating, or menstruation.

Myoclonus

Most patients (~90%) with CJD exhibit myoclonus that appears at various times throughout the illness. Unlike other involuntary movements, myoclonus persists during sleep. Startle myoclonus elicited by loud sounds or bright lights is frequent. It is important to stress that myoclonus is neither specific nor confined to CJD and tends to occur later in the course of CJD. Dementia with myoclonus can also be due to Alzheimer's disease (AD) (Chap. 29), dementia with Lewy bodies (Chap. 29), corticobasal degeneration (Chap. 29), cryptococcal encephalitis, or the myoclonic epilepsy disorder Unverricht-Lundborg disease (Chap. 26).

Clinical course

In documented cases of accidental transmission of CJD to humans, an incubation period of 1.5–2 years preceded the development of clinical disease. In other cases, incubation periods of up to 40 years have been suggested. Most patients with CJD live 6–12 months after the onset of clinical signs and symptoms, whereas some live for up to 5 years.

DIAGNOSIS

The constellation of dementia, myoclonus, and periodic electrical bursts in an afebrile 60-year-old patient generally indicates CJD. Clinical abnormalities in CJD are confined to the CNS. Fever, elevated sedimentation rate, leukocytosis in blood, or a pleocytosis in cerebrospinal fluid (CSF) should alert the physician to another etiology to explain the patient's CNS dysfunction.

Variations in the typical course appear in inherited and transmitted forms of the disease. fCJD has an earlier mean age of onset than sCJD. In GSS disease, ataxia is usually a prominent and presenting feature, with dementia occurring late in the disease course. GSS disease typically presents earlier than CJD (mean age 43 years) and is typically more slowly progressive than CJD; death usually occurs within 5 years of onset. FFI is characterized by insomnia and dysautonomia; dementia occurs only in the terminal phase of the illness. Rare sporadic cases have been identified. vCJD has an unusual clinical course, with a prominent psychiatric prodrome that may include visual hallucinations and early ataxia, while frank dementia is usually a late sign of vCJD.

DIFFERENTIAL DIAGNOSIS

Many conditions may mimic CJD superficially. Dementia with Lewy bodies (Chap. 29) is the most common disorder to be mistaken for CJD. It can present in a subacute fashion with delirium, myoclonus, and extrapyramidal features. Other neurodegenerative disorders (Chap. 29) to consider include AD, frontotemporal dementia, corticobasal degeneration, progressive supranuclear palsy, ceroid lipofuscinosis, and myoclonic epilepsy with Lafora bodies (Chap. 26). The absence of abnormalities on diffusion-weighted and fluid-attenuated inversion recovery (FLAIR) MRI will almost always distinguish these dementing conditions from CJD.

Hashimoto's encephalopathy, which presents as a subacute progressive encephalopathy with myoclonus and periodic triphasic complexes on the EEG, should be excluded in every case of suspected CJD. It is diagnosed by the finding of high titers of antithyroglobulin or antithyroid peroxidase (antimicrosomal) antibodies in the blood and improves with glucocorticoid therapy. Unlike CJD, fluctuations in severity typically occur in Hashimoto's encephalopathy.

Intracranial vasculitides may produce nearly all of the symptoms and signs associated with CJD, sometimes without systemic abnormalities. Myoclonus is exceptional with cerebral vasculitis, but focal seizures may confuse the picture. Prominent headache, absence of myoclonus, stepwise change in deficits, abnormal CSF, and focal white matter changes on MRI or angiographic abnormalities all favor vasculitis.

Paraneoplastic conditions, particularly limbic encephalitis and cortical encephalitis, can also mimic CJD. In many of these patients, dementia appears prior to the diagnosis of a tumor, and in some, no tumor is ever found. Detection of the paraneoplastic antibodies is often the only way to distinguish these cases from CJD.

Other diseases that can simulate CJD include neurosyphilis, AIDS dementia complex (Chap. 42), progressive multifocal leukoencephalopathy (Chap. 40), subacute sclerosing panencephalitis, progressive rubella panencephalitis, herpes simplex encephalitis (Chap. 40), diffuse intracranial tumor (gliomatosis cerebri; Chap. 37), anoxic encephalopathy, dialysis dementia, uremia, hepatic encephalopathy, voltage-gated potassium channel (VGkC) autoimmune encephalopathy, and lithium or bismuth intoxication.

LABORATORY TESTS

The only specific diagnostic tests for CJD and other human prion diseases measure PrP^{Sc}. The most widely used method involves limited proteolysis that generates PrP 27-30, which is detected by immunoassay after denaturation. The conformation-dependent immunoassay (CDI) is based on immunoreactive epitopes that are exposed in PrP^{C} but buried in PrP^{Sc}. In humans, the diagnosis of CJD can be established by brain biopsy if PrP^{Sc} is detected. If no attempt is made to measure PrP^{Sc}, but the constellation of pathologic changes frequently found in CJD is seen in a brain biopsy, then the diagnosis is reasonably secure (see "Neuropathology," earlier in the chapter). The high sensitivity and specificity of cortical ribboning and basal ganglia hyperintensity on FLAIR and diffusion-weighted MRI for the diagnosis of CJD have greatly diminished the need for brain biopsy in patients with suspected CJD. Because PrP^{Sc} is not uniformly distributed throughout the CNS, the apparent absence of

PrP^{Sc} in a limited sample such as a biopsy does not rule out prion disease. At autopsy, sufficient brain samples should be taken for both PrP^{Sc} immunoassay, preferably by CDI, and immunohistochemistry of tissue sections.

To establish the diagnosis of either sCJD or familial prion disease, sequencing the *PRNP* gene must be performed. Finding the wild-type *PRNP* gene sequence permits the diagnosis of sCJD if there is no history to suggest infection from an exogenous source of prions. The identification of a mutation in the *PRNP* gene sequence that encodes a nonconservative amino acid substitution argues for familial prion disease.

CT may be normal or show cortical atrophy. MRI is valuable for distinguishing sCJD from most other conditions. On FLAIR sequences and diffusion-weighted imaging, ~90% of patients show increased intensity in the basal ganglia and cortical ribboning (Fig. 43-3). This pattern is not seen with other neurodegenerative disorders but has been seen infrequently with viral encephalitis, paraneoplastic syndromes, or seizures. When the typical MRI pattern is present, in the proper clinical setting, diagnosis is facilitated. However, some cases of sCJD do not show this typical pattern, and other early diagnostic approaches are still needed.

CSF is nearly always normal but may show protein elevation and, rarely, mild pleocytosis. Although the stress protein 14-3-3 is elevated in the CSF of some patients with CJD, similar elevations of 14-3-3 are found in patients with other disorders; thus this elevation is not specific. Similarly, elevations of CSF neuron-specific enolase and tau occur in CJD but lack specificity for diagnosis.

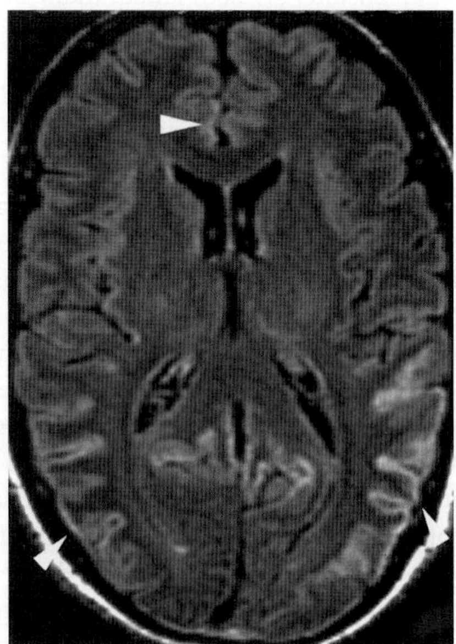

FIGURE 43-3
T2-weighted (FLAIR) MRI showing hyperintensity in the cortex in a patient with sporadic CJD. This so-called "cortical ribboning" along with increased intensity in the basal ganglia on T2 or diffusion-weighted imaging can aid in the diagnosis of CJD.

The EEG is often useful in the diagnosis of CJD, although only about 60% of individuals show the typical pattern. During the early phase of CJD, the EEG is usually normal or shows only scattered theta activity. In most advanced cases, repetitive, high-voltage, triphasic, and polyphasic sharp discharges are seen, but in many cases their presence is transient. The presence of these stereotyped periodic bursts of <200 ms duration, occurring every 1–2 s, makes the diagnosis of CJD very likely. These discharges are frequently but not always symmetric; there may be a one-sided predominance in amplitude. As CJD progresses, normal background rhythms become fragmentary and slower.

CARE OF CJD PATIENTS

Although CJD should not be considered either contagious or communicable, it is transmissible. The risk of accidental inoculation by aerosols is very small; nonetheless, procedures producing aerosols should be performed in certified biosafety cabinets. Biosafety level 2 practices, containment equipment, and facilities are recommended by the Centers for Disease Control and Prevention and the National Institutes of Health. The primary problem in caring for patients with CJD is the inadvertent infection of health care workers by needle and stab wounds. Electroencephalographic and electromyographic needles should not be reused after studies on patients with CJD have been performed.

There is no reason for pathologists or other morgue employees to resist performing autopsies on patients whose clinical diagnosis was CJD. Standard microbiologic practices outlined here, along with specific recommendations for decontamination, seem to be adequate precautions for the care of patients with CJD and the handling of infected specimens.

DECONTAMINATION OF CJD PRIONS

Prions are extremely resistant to common inactivation procedures, and there is some disagreement about the optimal conditions for sterilization. Some investigators recommend treating CJD-contaminated materials once with 1 *N* NaOH at room temperature, but we believe this procedure may be inadequate for sterilization. Autoclaving at 134°C for 5 h or treatment with 2 *N* NaOH for several hours is recommended for sterilization of prions. The term *sterilization* implies complete destruction of prions; any residual infectivity can be hazardous. Recent studies show that sCJD prions bound to stainless steel surfaces are resistant to inactivation by autoclaving at 134°C for 2 h; exposure of bound prions to an acidic detergent solution prior to autoclaving rendered prions susceptible to inactivation.

PREVENTION AND THERAPEUTICS

There is no known effective therapy for preventing or treating CJD. The finding that phenothiazines and acridines inhibit PrP^{Sc} formation in cultured cells led to clinical studies of quinacrine in CJD patients. Unfortunately, quinacrine failed to slow the rate of cognitive decline in CJD, possibly because therapeutic concentrations in the brain were not achieved. Although inhibition of the P-glycoprotein (Pgp) transport system resulted in substantially increased quinacrine levels in the brains of mice, the prion incubation times were not extended by treatment with the drug. Whether such an approach can be used to treat CJD remains to be established.

Like the acridines, anti-PrP antibodies have been shown to eliminate PrP^{Sc} from cultured cells. Additionally, such antibodies in mice, either administered by injection or produced from a transgene, have been shown to prevent prion disease when prions are introduced by a peripheral route, such as intraperitoneal inoculation. Unfortunately, the antibodies were ineffective in mice inoculated intracerebrally with prions. Several drugs, including pentosan polysulfate as well as porphyrin and phenylhydrazine derivatives, delay the onset of disease in animals inoculated intracerebrally with prions if the drugs are given intracerebrally beginning soon after inoculation.

PRION-LIKE PROTEINS CAUSING OTHER NEURODEGENERATIVE DISEASES

There is mounting evidence that prion-like changes in protein conformation underlie Alzheimer's (AD), Parkinson's (PD), and Huntington's (HD) diseases as well as the frontotemporal dementias (FTDs) and amyotrophic lateral sclerosis (ALS). Experimental studies have shown that transgenic mice expressing mutant amyloid precursor protein (APP) develop amyloid plaques containing fibrils composed of the amyloid beta (Aβ) peptide about a year after inoculation with extracts prepared from the brains of patients with AD. Mutant tau aggregates in transgenic mice and cultured cells can trigger the aggregation of wild-type tau into fibrils that resemble those in neurofibrillary tangles and Pick bodies that have been found in AD, FTDs, Pick's disease, and some cases of posttraumatic head injury. In patients with advanced PD who received grafts of fetal substantia nigral neurons, Lewy bodies containing β-sheet–rich α-synuclein have been identified in grafted cells about 10 years after transplantation. These findings argue for the axonal transport of misfolded α-synuclein crossing into grafted neurons, where it initiates aggregation of nascent α-synuclein into fibrils that coalesce to form Lewy bodies.

Taken together, a wealth of data argues that all neurodegenerative diseases are caused by proteins that undergo aberrant processing, which results in their assembly into amyloid fibrils. In each degenerative brain disease, prion-like protein processing is responsible for the accumulation of a particular protein in an altered state that leads to neurodegeneration. Interestingly, once these aberrant, prion-like proteins have polymerized into amyloid fibrils, they are probably inert. Amyloid plaques containing PrP^{Sc} are a nonobligatory feature of prion disease in humans and animals. Furthermore, amyloid plaques in AD do not correlate with the level of dementia; however, the level of soluble (oligomeric) Aβ peptide does correlate with memory loss and other intellectual deficits.

CHAPTER 44

PARANEOPLASTIC NEUROLOGIC SYNDROMES

Josep Dalmau ■ Myrna R. Rosenfeld

Paraneoplastic neurologic disorders (PNDs) are cancer-related syndromes that can affect any part of the nervous system (Table 44-1). They are caused by mechanisms other than metastasis or by any of the complications of cancer such as coagulopathy, stroke, metabolic and nutritional conditions, infections, and side effects of cancer therapy. In 60% of patients the neurologic symptoms precede the cancer diagnosis. Clinically disabling PNDs occur in 0.5–1% of all cancer patients, but they affect 2–3% of patients with neuroblastoma or small cell lung cancer (SCLC) and 30–50% of patients with thymoma or sclerotic myeloma.

TABLE 44-1

PARANEOPLASTIC SYNDROMES OF THE NERVOUS SYSTEM

CLASSIC SYNDROMES: USUALLY OCCUR WITH CANCER ASSOCIATION	NONCLASSIC SYNDROMES: MAY OCCUR WITH AND WITHOUT CANCER ASSOCIATION
Encephalomyelitis	Brainstem encephalitis
Limbic encephalitis	Stiff-person syndrome
Cerebellar degeneration (adults)	Necrotizing myelopathy
Opsoclonus-myoclonus	Motor neuron disease
Subacute sensory neuronopathy	Guillain-Barré syndrome
Gastrointestinal paresis or pseudo-obstruction	Subacute and chronic mixed sensory-motor neuropathies
Dermatomyositis (adults)	Neuropathy associated with plasma cell dyscrasias and lymphoma
Lambert-Eaton myasthenic syndrome	Vasculitis of nerve
Cancer or melanoma associated retinopathy	Pure autonomic neuropathy
	Acute necrotizing myopathy
	Polymyositis
	Vasculitis of muscle
	Optic neuropathy
	BDUMP

Abbreviation: BDUMP, bilateral diffuse uveal melanocytic proliferation.

PATHOGENESIS

Most PNDs are mediated by immune responses triggered by neuronal proteins (onconeuronal antigens) expressed by tumors. In PNDs of the central nervous system (CNS), many antibody-associated immune responses have been identified (Table 44-2). These antibodies react with the patient's tumor, and their detection in serum or cerebrospinal fluid (CSF) usually predicts the presence of cancer. When the antigens are intracellular, most syndromes are associated with extensive infiltrates of CD4+ and CD8+ T cells, microglial activation, gliosis, and variable neuronal loss. The infiltrating T cells are often in close contact with neurons undergoing degeneration, suggesting a primary pathogenic role. T cell–mediated cytotoxicity may contribute directly to cell death in these PNDs. Thus both humoral and cellular immune mechanisms participate in the pathogenesis of many PNDs. This complex immunopathogenesis may underlie the resistance of many of these conditions to therapy.

In contrast to the disorders associated with immune responses against intracellular antigens, those associated with antibodies to antigens expressed on the neuronal cell surface of the CNS or at neuromuscular synapses are more responsive to immunotherapy (Table 44-3, Fig. 44-1). These disorders occur with and without a cancer association, and there is increasing evidence that they are mediated by the antibodies.

Other PNDs are likely immune-mediated, although their antigens are unknown. These include several syndromes of inflammatory neuropathies and myopathies. In addition, many patients with typical PND syndromes are antibody-negative.

For still other PNDs, the cause remains quite obscure. These include, among others, several neuropathies that occur in the terminal stages of cancer and a number of neuropathies associated with plasma cell

TABLE 44-2

ANTIBODIES TO INTRACELLULAR ANTIGENS, SYNDROMES, AND ASSOCIATED CANCERS

ANTIBODY	ASSOCIATED NEUROLOGIC SYNDROME(S)	TUMORS
Anti-Hu	Encephalomyelitis, subacute sensory neuronopathy	SCLC
Anti-Yo	Cerebellar degeneration	Ovary, breast
Anti-Ri	Cerebellar degeneration, opsoclonus	Breast, gynecologic, SCLC
Anti-Tr	Cerebellar degeneration	Hodgkin lymphoma
Anti-CV_2/CRMP5	Encephalomyelitis, chorea, optic neuritis, uveitis, peripheral neuropathy	SCLC, thymoma, other
Anti-Ma proteins	Limbic, hypothalamic, brainstem encephalitis	Testicular (Ma2), other (Ma)
Anti-amphiphysin	Stiff-person syndrome, encephalomyelitis	Breast, SCLC
Recoverin, bipolar cell antibodies, others[a]	Cancer-associated retinopathy (CAR) Melanoma-associated retinopathy (MAR)	SCLC (CAR), melanoma (MAR)
Anti-GAD	Stiff-person, cerebellar syndromes	Infrequent tumor association (thymoma)

[a]A variety of target antigens have been identified.
Abbreviations: CRMP, collapsing response-mediator protein; SCLC, small cell lung cancer.

dyscrasias or lymphoma without evidence of inflammatory infiltrates or deposits of immunoglobulin, cryoglobulin, or amyloid.

APPROACH TO THE PATIENT

Paraneoplastic Neurologic Disorders

Three key concepts are important for the diagnosis and management of PNDs. First, it is common for symptoms to appear before the presence of a tumor is known; second, the neurologic syndrome usually develops rapidly, producing severe deficits in a short period of time; and third, there is evidence that prompt tumor control improves the neurologic outcome. Therefore, the major concern of the physician is to recognize a disorder promptly as paraneoplastic to identify and treat the tumor.

PND OF THE CENTRAL NERVOUS SYSTEM AND DORSAL ROOT GANGLIA When symptoms involve brain, spinal cord, or dorsal root ganglia, the suspicion of PND is usually based on a combination of clinical, radiologic, and CSF findings. In these cases, a biopsy of the affected tissue is often difficult to obtain, and although useful to rule out other disorders

TABLE 44-3

ANTIBODIES TO CELL SURFACE OR SYNAPTIC ANTIGENS, SYNDROMES, AND ASSOCIATED TUMORS

ANTIBODY	NEUROLOGIC SYNDROME	TUMOR TYPE WHEN ASSOCIATED
Anti-AChR (muscle)[a]	Myasthenia gravis	Thymoma
Anti-AChR (neuronal)[a]	Autonomic neuropathy	SCLC
Anti-VGKC-related proteins[b] (LGI1, Caspr2)	Neuromyotonia, limbic encephalitis	Thymoma, SCLC
Anti-VGCC[c]	LEMS, cerebellar degeneration	SCLC
Anti-NMDAR[d]	Anti-NMDAR encephalitis	Teratoma
Anti-AMPAR[d]	Limbic encephalitis with relapses	SCLC, thymoma, breast
Anti-$GABA_BR$[d]	Limbic encephalitis, seizures	SCLC, neuroendocrine
Glycine receptor[d]	Encephalomyelitis with rigidity, stiff-person syndrome	Lung cancer

[a]A direct pathogenic role of these antibodies has been demonstrated.
[b]Anti-VGKC-related proteins are pathogenic for some types of neuromyotonia.
[c]Anti-VGCC antibodies are pathogenic for LEMS.
[d]These antibodies are strongly suspected to be pathogenic.
Abbreviations: AChR, acetylcholine receptor; AMPAR, α-amino-3-hydroxy-5-methylisoxazole-4-propionic acid receptor; $GABA_BR$, gamma-aminobutyric acid B receptor; GAD, glutamic acid decarboxylase; LEMS, Lambert-Eaton myasthenic syndrome; NMDAR, *N*-methyl-D-aspartate receptor; SCLC, small cell lung cancer; VGCC, voltage-gated calcium channel; VGKC, voltage-gated potassium channel.

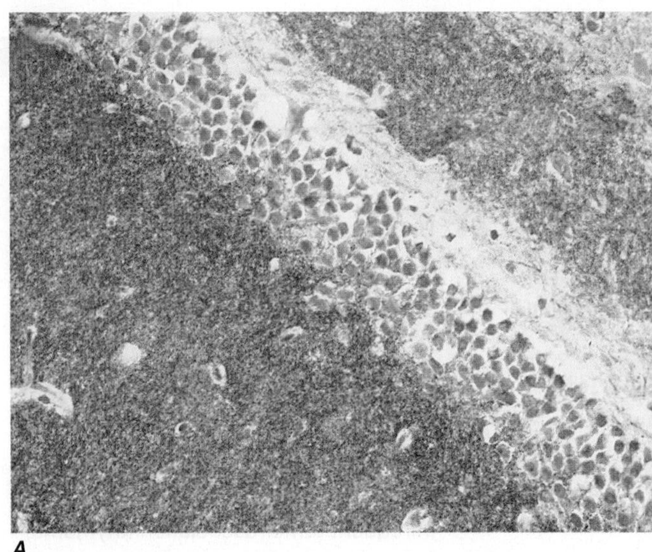

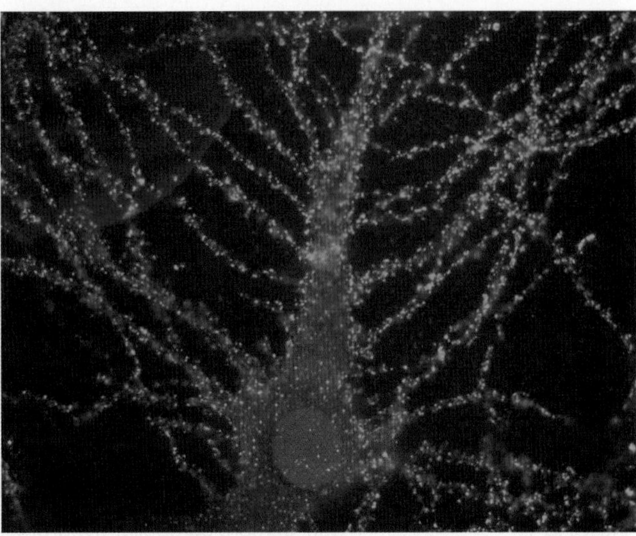

FIGURE 44-1

Antibodies to NR1/NR2 subunits of the NMDA receptor in a patient with paraneoplastic encephalitis and ovarian teratoma. ***Panel A*** is a section of dentate gyrus of rat hippocampus immunolabeled (brown staining) with the patient's antibodies. The reactivity predominates in the molecular layer, which is highly enriched in dendritic processes. ***Panel B*** shows the antibody reactivity with cultures of rat hippocampal neurons; the intense green immunolabeling is due to the antibodies against the NR1 subunits of NMDA receptors.

(e.g., metastasis, infection), neuropathologic findings are not specific for PND. Furthermore, there are no specific radiologic or electrophysiologic tests that are diagnostic of PND. The presence of antineuronal antibodies (Tables 44-2 and 44-3) may help in the diagnosis, but only 60–70% of PNDs of the CNS and less than 20% of those involving the peripheral nervous system have neuronal or neuromuscular antibodies that can be used as diagnostic tests.

MRI and CSF studies are important to rule out neurologic complications due to the direct spread of cancer, particularly metastatic and leptomeningeal disease. In most PNDs the MRI findings are nonspecific. Paraneoplastic limbic encephalitis is usually associated with characteristic MRI abnormalities in the mesial temporal lobes (discussed later), but similar findings can occur with other disorders (e.g., nonparaneoplastic autoimmune limbic encephalitis, and human herpesvirus type 6 [HHV-6] encephalitis) (Fig. 44-2). The CSF profile of patients with PND of the CNS or dorsal root ganglia typically consists of mild to moderate pleocytosis (<200 mononuclear cells, predominantly lymphocytes), an increase in the protein concentration, intrathecal synthesis of IgG, and a variable presence of oligoclonal bands.

PND OF NERVE AND MUSCLE If symptoms involve peripheral nerve, neuromuscular junction, or muscle, the diagnosis of a specific PND is usually established on clinical, electrophysiologic, and pathologic grounds. The clinical history, accompanying symptoms (e.g., anorexia, weight loss), and type of syndrome dictate the studies and degree of effort needed to demonstrate a neoplasm. For example, the frequent association of Lambert-Eaton myasthenic syndrome (LEMS) with SCLC should lead to a chest and abdomen CT or body positron emission tomography (PET) scan and, if negative, periodic tumor screening for at least 3 years

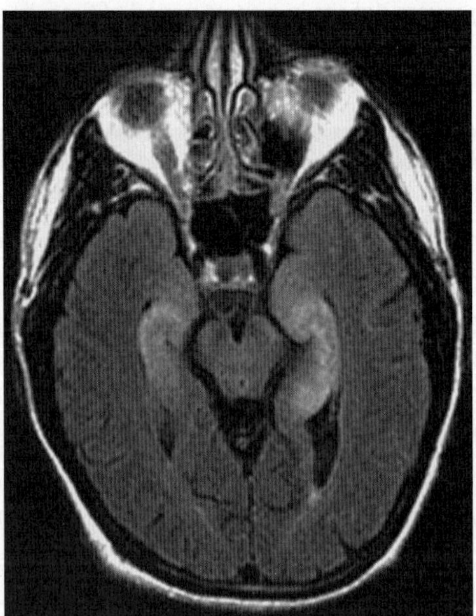

FIGURE 44-2

Fluid-attenuated inversion recovery sequence MRI of a patient with limbic encephalitis and LGI1 antibodies. Note the abnormal hyperintensity involving the medial aspect of the temporal lobes.

after the neurologic diagnosis. In contrast, the weak association of polymyositis with cancer calls into question the need for repeated cancer screenings in this situation. Serum and urine immunofixation studies should be considered in patients with peripheral neuropathy of unknown cause; detection of a monoclonal gammopathy suggests the need for additional studies to uncover a B cell or plasma cell malignancy. In paraneoplastic neuropathies, diagnostically useful antineuronal antibodies are limited to anti-CV_2/CRMP5 and anti-Hu.

For any type of PND, if antineuronal antibodies are negative, the diagnosis relies on the demonstration of cancer and the exclusion of other cancer-related or independent neurologic disorders. Combined CT and PET scans often uncover tumors undetected by other tests. For germ-cell tumors of the testis and teratomas of the ovary ultrasound and MRI may reveal tumors undetectable by PET.

SPECIFIC PARANEOPLASTIC NEUROLOGIC SYNDROMES

PARANEOPLASTIC ENCEPHALOMYELITIS AND FOCAL ENCEPHALITIS

The term *encephalomyelitis* describes an inflammatory process with multifocal involvement of the nervous system, including brain, brainstem, cerebellum, and spinal cord. It is often associated with dorsal root ganglia and autonomic dysfunction. For any given patient, the clinical manifestations are determined by the areas predominantly involved, but pathologic studies almost always reveal abnormalities beyond the symptomatic regions. Several clinicopathologic syndromes may occur alone or in combination: (1) *cortical encephalitis*, which may present as "epilepsia partialis continua"; (2) *limbic encephalitis*, characterized by confusion, depression, agitation, anxiety, severe short-term memory deficits, partial complex seizures, and sometimes dementia (the MRI usually shows unilateral or bilateral medial temporal lobe abnormalities, best seen with T2 and fluid-attenuated inversion recovery sequences, and occasionally enhancing with gadolinium); (3) *brainstem encephalitis*, resulting in eye movement disorders (nystagmus, opsoclonus, supranuclear or nuclear paresis), cranial nerve paresis, dysarthria, dysphagia, and central autonomic dysfunction; (4) *cerebellar gait and limb ataxia*; (5) *myelitis*, which may cause lower or upper motor neuron symptoms, myoclonus, muscle rigidity, and spasms; and (6) *autonomic dysfunction* as a result of involvement of the neuraxis at multiple levels, including hypothalamus, brainstem, and autonomic nerves (see autonomic neuropathy). Cardiac arrhythmias, postural hypotension, or central hypoventilation are frequent causes of death in patients with encephalomyelitis.

Paraneoplastic encephalomyelitis and focal encephalitis are usually associated with SCLC, but many other cancers have also been reported. Patients with SCLC and these syndromes usually have anti-Hu antibodies in serum and CSF. Anti-CV_2/CRMP5 antibodies occur less frequently; some of these patients may develop chorea, uveitis, or optic neuritis. Antibodies to Ma proteins are associated with limbic, hypothalamic, and brainstem encephalitis and occasionally with cerebellar symptoms (Fig. 44-3); some patients develop hypersomnia, cataplexy, and severe hypokinesia. MRI abnormalities are frequent, including those described with limbic encephalitis and variable involvement of the hypothalamus, basal ganglia, or upper brainstem. The oncologic associations of these antibodies are shown in Table 44-2.

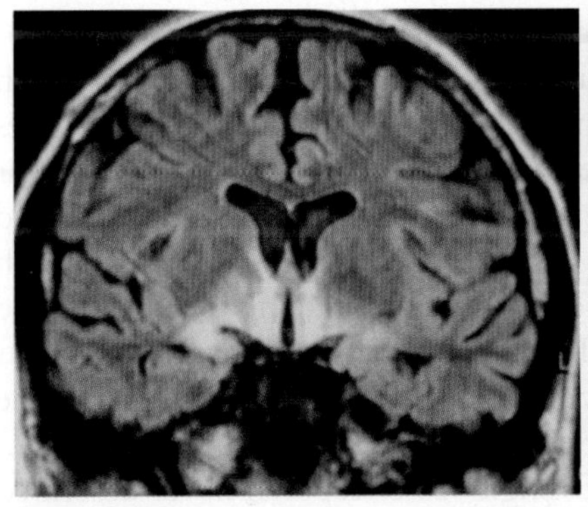

A

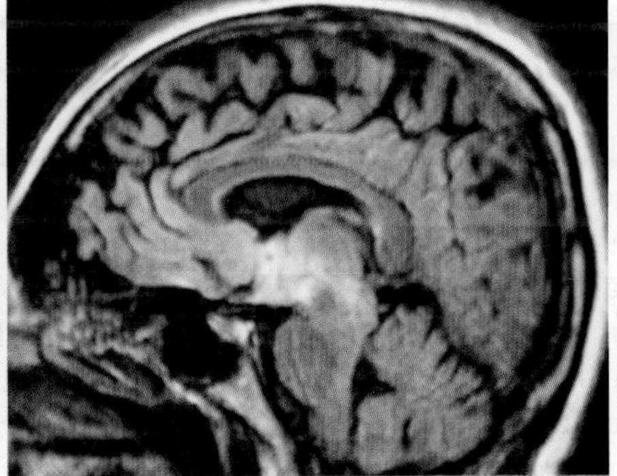

B

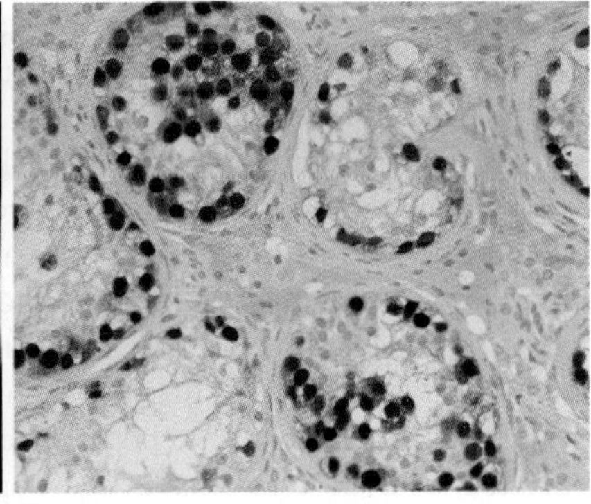

C

FIGURE 44-3

MRI and tumor of a patient with anti-Ma2-associated encephalitis. Panels *A* and *B* are fluid-attenuated inversion recovery MRI sequences showing abnormal hyperintensities in the medial temporal lobes, hypothalamus, and upper brainstem. ***Panel C*** corresponds to a section of the patient's orchiectomy incubated with a specific marker (Oct4) of germ-cell tumors. The positive (brown) cells correspond to an intratubular germ-cell neoplasm.

TREATMENT Encephalomyelitis and Focal Encephalitis

Most types of paraneoplastic encephalitis and encephalomyelitis respond poorly to treatment. Stabilization of symptoms or partial neurologic improvement may occasionally occur, particularly if there is a satisfactory response of the tumor to treatment. The roles of plasma exchange, intravenous immunoglobulin (IVIg), and immunosuppression have not been established. Approximately 30% of patients with anti-Ma2-associated encephalitis respond to treatment of the tumor (usually a germ-cell neoplasm of the testis) and immunotherapy.

ENCEPHALITIDES WITH ANTIBODIES TO CELL-SURFACE OR SYNAPTIC PROTEINS (TABLE 44-3)

These disorders are important for three reasons: (1) they can occur with and without tumor association, (2) some syndromes predominate in young individuals and children, and (3) despite the severity of the symptoms, patients usually respond to treatment of the tumor, if found, and immunotherapy (glucocorticoids, plasma exchange, IVIg, rituximab, or cyclophosphamide).

Encephalitis with antibodies to voltage-gated potassium channel (VGKC)-related proteins (LGI1, Caspr2) predominates in men and frequently presents with memory loss and seizures (limbic encephalopathy), along with hyponatremia and sleep and autonomic dysfunction. Less commonly, patients develop neuromyotonia or a mixed clinical picture (Morvan's syndrome). Approximately 20% of patients with antibodies to VGKC-related proteins have an underlying tumor, usually SCLC or thymoma.

Encephalitis with N*-methyl-*D*-aspartate (NMDA) receptor antibodies* (Fig. 44-1) usually occurs in young women and children, but men and older patients of both sexes can be affected. The disorder has a characteristic pattern of symptom progression that includes a prodrome resembling a viral process, followed in a few days by the onset of severe psychiatric symptoms, memory loss, seizures, decreased level of consciousness, abnormal movements (orofacial, limb, and trunk dyskinesias, dystonic postures), autonomic instability, and frequent hypoventilation. The syndrome is often misdiagnosed as a viral or idiopathic encephalitis, neuroleptic malignant syndrome, or encephalitis lethargica, and many patients are initially evaluated by psychiatrists with the suspicion of drug abuse or an acute psychosis. The detection of an associated ovarian teratoma is age-dependant; 50% of female patients older than age 18 have uni- or bilateral ovarian teratomas, while less than 9% of girls younger than 14 years have a teratoma. In male patients the detection of a tumor is rare.

Encephalitis with α-amino-3-hydroxy-5-methylisoxazole-4-propionate (AMPA) receptor antibodies affects middle-aged women, who develop acute limbic dysfunction or less frequently prominent psychiatric symptoms; 70% of the patients have an underlying tumor in the lung, breast, or thymus. The neurologic disorder responds to treatment of the tumor and immunotherapy. Neurologic relapses may occur; these also respond to immunotherapy and are not necessarily associated with tumor recurrence.

Encephalitis with γ-aminobutyric acid type B ($GABA_B$) receptor antibodies usually presents with limbic encephalitis and seizures; 50% of the patients have SCLC or a neuroendocrine tumor of the lung. Neurologic symptoms often respond to immunotherapy and treatment of the tumor if found. Patients may have additional antibodies to glutamic acid decarboxylase (GAD), of unclear significance. Other antibodies to nonneuronal proteins are often found in these patients as well as in patients with AMPA receptor antibodies, indicating a general tendency to autoimmunity.

PARANEOPLASTIC CEREBELLAR DEGENERATION

This disorder is often preceded by a prodrome that may include dizziness, oscillopsia, blurry or double vision, nausea, and vomiting. A few days or weeks later, patients develop dysarthria, gait and limb ataxia, and variable dysphagia. The examination usually shows downbeating nystagmus and, rarely, opsoclonus. Brainstem dysfunction, upgoing toes, or a mild neuropathy may occur, but more often the clinical features are restricted to the cerebellum. Early in the course, MRI studies are usually normal; later, the MRI typically reveals cerebellar atrophy. The disorder results from extensive degeneration of Purkinje cells, with variable involvement of other cerebellar cortical neurons, deep cerebellar nuclei, and spinocerebellar tracts. The tumors more frequently involved are SCLC, cancer of the breast and ovary, and Hodgkin lymphoma.

Anti-Yo antibodies in patients with breast and gynecologic cancers and anti-Tr antibodies in patients with Hodgkin lymphoma are the two immune responses typically associated with prominent or pure cerebellar degeneration. Antibodies to P/Q-type voltage-gated calcium channels (VGCC) occur in some patients with SCLC and cerebellar dysfunction; only some of these patients develop LEMS. A variable degree of cerebellar dysfunction can be associated with virtually any of the antibodies and PND of the CNS shown in Table 44-2.

A number of single case reports have described neurologic improvement after tumor removal, plasma exchange, IVIg, cyclophosphamide, rituximab, or glucocorticoids. However, large series of patients with antibody-positive paraneoplastic cerebellar degeneration show that this disorder rarely improves with any treatment.

PARANEOPLASTIC OPSOCLONUS-MYOCLONUS SYNDROME

Opsoclonus is a disorder of eye movement characterized by involuntary, chaotic saccades that occur in all directions of gaze; it is frequently associated with myoclonus and ataxia. Opsoclonus-myoclonus may be cancer-related or idiopathic. When the cause is paraneoplastic, the tumors involved are usually cancer of the lung and breast in adults and neuroblastoma in children. The pathologic substrate of opsoclonus-myoclonus is unclear, but studies suggest that disinhibition of the fastigial nucleus of the cerebellum is involved. Most patients do not have detectable antineuronal antibodies. A small subset of patients with ataxia, opsoclonus, and other eye-movement disorders develop anti-Ri antibodies; in rare instances muscle rigidity, autonomic dysfunction, and dementia also occur. The tumors most frequently involved in anti-Ri-associated syndromes are breast and ovarian cancer. If the tumor is not successfully treated, the neurologic syndrome in adults often progresses to encephalopathy, coma, and death. In addition to treating the tumor, symptoms may respond to immunotherapy (glucocorticoids, plasma exchange, and/or IVIg).

At least 50% of children with opsoclonus-myoclonus have an underlying neuroblastoma. Hypotonia, ataxia, behavioral changes, and irritability are frequent accompanying symptoms. Neurologic symptoms often improve with treatment of the tumor and glucocorticoids, adrenocorticotropic hormone (ACTH), plasma exchange, IVIg, and rituximab. Many patients are left with psychomotor retardation and behavioral and sleep problems.

PARANEOPLASTIC SYNDROMES OF THE SPINAL CORD

The number of reports of paraneoplastic spinal cord syndromes, such as *subacute motor neuronopathy* and *acute necrotizing myelopathy*, has decreased in recent years. This may represent a true decrease in incidence, due to improved and prompt oncologic interventions, or the identification of nonparaneoplastic etiologies.

Some patients with cancer develop *upper* or *lower motor neuron dysfunction* or both, resembling amyotrophic lateral sclerosis. It is unclear whether these disorders have a paraneoplastic etiology or simply coincide with the presence of cancer. There are isolated case reports of cancer patients with motor neuron dysfunction who had neurologic improvement after tumor treatment. A search for lymphoma should be undertaken in patients with a rapidly progressive motor neuron syndrome and a monoclonal protein in serum or CSF.

Paraneoplastic myelitis may present with upper or lower motor neuron symptoms, segmental myoclonus, and rigidity, and can be the first manifestation of encephalomyelitis.

Paraneoplastic myelopathy can also produce several syndromes characterized by prominent muscle stiffness and rigidity. The spectrum ranges from focal symptoms in one or several extremities (*stiff-limb syndrome* or *stiff-person syndrome*) to a disorder that also affects the brainstem (known as *encephalomyelitis with rigidity*) and likely has a different pathogenesis. Some patients with encephalomyelitis and rigidity have glycine receptor antibodies.

PARANEOPLASTIC STIFF-PERSON SYNDROME

This disorder is characterized by progressive muscle rigidity, stiffness, and painful spasms triggered by auditory, sensory, or emotional stimuli. Rigidity mainly involves the lower trunk and legs, but it can affect the upper extremities and neck. Symptoms improve with sleep and general anesthetics. Electrophysiologic studies demonstrate continuous motor unit activity. Antibodies associated with the stiff-person syndrome target proteins (GAD, amphiphysin) involved in the function of inhibitory synapses utilizing γ-aminobutyric acid (GABA) or glycine as neurotransmitters. Paraneoplastic stiff-person syndrome and amphiphysin antibodies are often related to SCLC and breast cancer. By contrast, antibodies to GAD may occur in some cancer patients but are much more frequently present in the nonparaneoplastic disorder.

TREATMENT Stiff-Person Syndrome

Optimal treatment of stiff-person syndrome requires therapy of the underlying tumor, glucocorticoids, and symptomatic use of drugs that enhance GABA-ergic transmission (diazepam, baclofen, sodium valproate, tiagabine, vigabatrin). A benefit of IVIg has been demonstrated for the nonparaneoplastic disorder but remains to be established for the paraneoplastic syndrome.

PARANEOPLASTIC SENSORY NEURONOPATHY OR DORSAL ROOT GANGLIONOPATHY

This syndrome is characterized by sensory deficits that may be symmetric or asymmetric, painful dysesthesias, radicular pain, and decreased or absent reflexes. All modalities of sensation and any part of the body including face and trunk can be involved. Specialized sensations such as taste and hearing can also be affected. Electrophysiologic studies show decreased or absent sensory nerve potentials with normal or near-normal motor conduction velocities. Symptoms result from an inflammatory, likely immune-mediated, process that targets the dorsal root ganglia, causing neuronal loss, proliferation of satellite cells, and secondary degeneration of the posterior columns of the spinal cord. The dorsal and less frequently the anterior nerve roots and peripheral nerves may also be involved. This disorder often precedes or is associated with encephalomyelitis and autonomic dysfunction and has the same immunologic and oncologic associations, e.g., anti-Hu antibodies and SCLC.

TREATMENT Sensory Neuronopathy

As with anti-Hu-associated encephalomyelitis, the therapeutic approach focuses on prompt treatment of the tumor. Glucocorticoids occasionally produce clinical stabilization or improvement. The benefit of IVIg and plasma exchange is not proved.

PARANEOPLASTIC PERIPHERAL NEUROPATHIES

These disorders may develop any time during the course of the neoplastic disease. Neuropathies occurring at late stages of cancer or lymphoma usually cause mild to moderate sensorimotor deficits due to axonal degeneration of unclear etiology. These neuropathies are often masked by concurrent neurotoxicity from chemotherapy and other cancer therapies. In contrast, the neuropathies that develop in the early stages of cancer frequently show a rapid progression, sometimes with a relapsing and remitting course, and evidence of inflammatory infiltrates and axonal loss or demyelination in biopsy studies. If demyelinating features predominate (Chap. 45), IVIg, plasma exchange, or glucocorticoids may improve symptoms. Occasionally anti-CV_2/CRMP5 antibodies are present; detection of anti-Hu suggests concurrent dorsal root ganglionitis.

Guillain-Barré syndrome and *brachial plexitis* have occasionally been reported in patients with lymphoma, but there is no clear evidence of a paraneoplastic association.

Malignant monoclonal gammopathies include: (1) multiple myeloma and sclerotic myeloma associated with IgG or IgA monoclonal proteins; and (2) Waldenström's macroglobulinemia, B cell lymphoma, and chronic B cell lymphocytic leukemia associated with IgM monoclonal proteins. These disorders may cause neuropathy by a variety of mechanisms, including compression of roots and plexuses by metastasis to vertebral bodies and pelvis, deposits of amyloid in peripheral nerves, and paraneoplastic mechanisms. The paraneoplastic variety has several distinctive features. Approximately half of patients with sclerotic myeloma develop a sensorimotor neuropathy with predominantly motor deficits, resembling a chronic inflammatory demyelinating neuropathy (Chap. 46); some patients develop elements of the POEMS syndrome (*p*olyneuropathy, *o*rganomegaly, *e*ndocrinopathy, *M* protein, *s*kin changes). Treatment of the plasmacytoma or sclerotic lesions usually improves the neuropathy. In contrast, the sensorimotor or sensory neuropathy associated with multiple myeloma rarely responds to treatment. Between 5 and 10% of patients with Waldenström's macroglobulinemia develop a distal symmetric sensorimotor neuropathy with predominant involvement of large sensory fibers. These patients may have IgM antibodies in their serum against myelin-associated glycoprotein and various gangliosides (Chap. 46). In addition to treating the Waldenström's macroglobulinemia, other therapies may improve the neuropathy, including plasma exchange, IVIg, chlorambucil, cyclophosphamide, fludarabine, or rituximab.

Vasculitis of the nerve and muscle causes a painful symmetric or asymmetric distal axonal sensorimotor neuropathy with variable proximal weakness. It predominantly affects elderly men and is associated with an elevated erythrocyte sedimentation rate and increased CSF protein concentration. SCLC and lymphoma are the primary tumors involved. Glucocorticoids and cyclophosphamide often result in neurologic improvement.

Peripheral nerve hyperexcitability (*neuromyotonia,* or *Isaacs' syndrome*) is characterized by spontaneous and continuous muscle fiber activity of peripheral nerve origin. Clinical features include cramps, muscle twitching (fasciculations or myokymia), stiffness, delayed muscle relaxation (pseudomyotonia), and spontaneous or evoked carpal or pedal spasms. The involved muscles may be hypertrophic, and some patients develop paresthesias and hyperhidrosis. CNS dysfunction, including mood changes, sleep disorder, or hallucinations, may occur. The electromyogram (EMG) shows fibrillations; fasciculations; and doublet, triplet, or multiplet single-unit (myokymic) discharges that have a high intraburst frequency. Approximately 20% of patients have serum antibodies to Caspr2-related proteins. The disorder often occurs without cancer; if paraneoplastic, benign, and malignant thymomas and SCLC are the usual tumors. Phenytoin, carbamazepine, and plasma exchange improve symptoms.

Paraneoplastic autonomic neuropathy usually develops as a component of other disorders, such as LEMS and encephalomyelitis. It may rarely occur as a pure or predominantly autonomic neuropathy with adrenergic or cholinergic dysfunction at the pre- or postganglionic levels. Patients can develop several life-threatening complications, such as gastrointestinal paresis with pseudoobstruction, cardiac dysrhythmias, and postural hypotension. Other clinical features include abnormal pupillary responses, dry mouth, anhidrosis, erectile dysfunction, and problems in sphincter control. The disorder occurs in association with several tumors, including SCLC, cancer of the pancreas or testis, carcinoid tumors, and lymphoma. Because autonomic symptoms can be the presenting feature of encephalomyelitis, serum anti-Hu and anti-CV_2/CRMP5 antibodies should be sought. Antibodies to ganglionic (alpha3-type) neuronal acetylcholine receptors are the cause of autoimmune autonomic ganglionopathy, a disorder that frequently occurs without cancer association (Chap. 33).

LAMBERT-EATON MYASTHENIC SYNDROME

LEMS is discussed in Chap. 47.

MYASTHENIA GRAVIS

Myasthenia gravis is discussed in Chap. 47.

POLYMYOSITIS-DERMATOMYOSITIS

Polymyositis and dermatomyositis are discussed in detail in Chap. 49.

ACUTE NECROTIZING MYOPATHY

Patients with this syndrome develop myalgias and rapid progression of weakness involving the extremities and the pharyngeal and respiratory muscles, often resulting in death. Serum muscle enzymes are elevated, and muscle biopsy shows extensive necrosis with minimal or absent inflammation and sometimes deposits of complement. The disorder occurs as a paraneoplastic manifestation of a variety of cancers including SCLC and cancer of the gastrointestinal tract, breast, kidney, and prostate, among others. Glucocorticoids and treatment of the underlying tumor rarely control the disorder.

PARANEOPLASTIC VISUAL SYNDROMES

This group of disorders involves the retina and, less frequently, the uvea and optic nerves. The term *cancer-associated retinopathy* is used to describe paraneoplastic cone and rod dysfunction characterized by photosensitivity, progressive loss of vision and color perception, central or ring scotomas, night blindness, and attenuation of photopic and scotopic responses in the electroretinogram (ERG). The most commonly associated tumor is SCLC. Melanoma-associated retinopathy affects patients with metastatic cutaneous melanoma. Patients develop acute onset of night blindness and shimmering, flickering, or pulsating photopsias that often progress to visual loss. The ERG shows reduced b waves with normal dark adapted a waves. Paraneoplastic optic neuritis and uveitis are very uncommon and can develop in association with encephalomyelitis. Some patients with paraneoplastic uveitis harbor anti-CV_2/CRMP5 antibodies.

Some paraneoplastic retinopathies are associated with serum antibodies that specifically react with the subset of retinal cells undergoing degeneration, supporting an immune-mediated pathogenesis (Table 44-2). Paraneoplastic retinopathies usually fail to improve with treatment, although rare responses to glucocorticoids, plasma exchange, and IVIg have been reported.

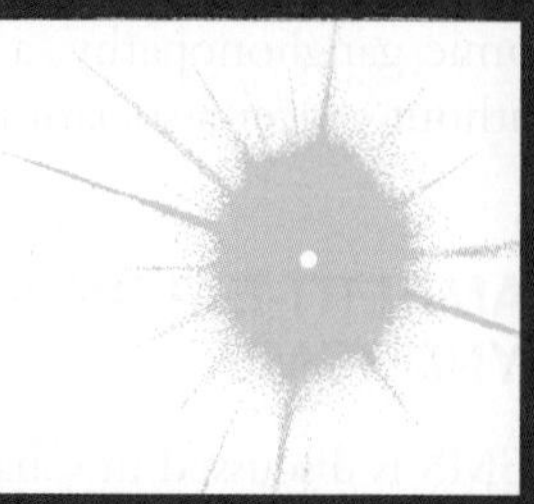

CHAPTER 45

PERIPHERAL NEUROPATHY

Anthony A. Amato ■ Richard J. Barohn

Peripheral nerves are composed of sensory, motor, and autonomic elements. Diseases can affect the cell body of a neuron or its peripheral processes, namely the axons or the encasing myelin sheaths. Most peripheral nerves are mixed and contain sensory and motor as well as autonomic fibers. Nerves can be subdivided into three major classes: large myelinated, small myelinated, and small unmyelinated. Motor axons are usually large myelinated fibers that conduct rapidly (approximately 50 m/s). Sensory fibers may be any of the three types. Large-diameter sensory fibers conduct proprioception and vibratory sensat ion to the brain, while the smaller-diameter myelinated and unmyelinated fibers transmit pain and temperature sensation. Autonomic nerves are also small in diameter. Thus, peripheral neuropathies can impair sensory, motor, or autonomic function, either singly or in combination. Peripheral neuropathies are further classified into those that primarily affect the cell body (e.g., neuronopathy or ganglionopathy), myelin (myelinopathy), and the axon (axonopathy). These different classes of peripheral neuropathies have distinct clinical and electrophysiologic features. This chapter discusses the clinical approach to a patient suspected of having a peripheral neuropathy, as well as specific neuropathies, including hereditary and acquired neuropathies. The inflammatory neuropathies are discussed in Chap. 46.

GENERAL APPROACH

In approaching a patient with a neuropathy, the clinician has three main goals: (1) identify where the lesion is, (2) identify the cause, and (3) determine the proper treatment. The first goal is accomplished by obtaining a thorough history, neurologic examination, and electrodiagnostic and other laboratory studies (Fig. 45-1). While gathering this information, seven key questions are asked (Table 45-1), the answers to which can usually identify the category of pathology that is present (Table 45-2). Despite an extensive evaluation, in approximately half of patients no etiology is ever found; these patients typically have a predominately sensory polyneuropathy and have been labeled as having idiopathic or cryptogenic sensory polyneuropathy (CSPN).

INFORMATION FROM THE HISTORY AND PHYSICAL EXAMINATION: SEVEN KEY QUESTIONS (TABLE 45-1)

1. What systems are involved?

It is important to determine if the patient's symptoms and signs are motor, sensory, autonomic, or a combination of these. If the patient has only weakness without any evidence of sensory or autonomic dysfunction, a motor neuropathy, neuromuscular junction abnormality, or myopathy should be considered. Some peripheral neuropathies are associated with significant autonomic nervous system dysfunction. Symptoms of autonomic involvement include fainting spells or orthostatic lightheadedness; heat intolerance; or any bowel, bladder, or sexual dysfunction (Chap. 33). There will typically be an orthostatic fall in blood pressure without an appropriate increase in heart rate. Autonomic dysfunction in the absence of diabetes should alert the clinician to the possibility of amyloid polyneuropathy. Rarely, a pandysautonomic syndrome can be the only manifestation of a peripheral neuropathy without other motor or sensory findings. The majority of neuropathies are predominantly sensory in nature.

2. What is the distribution of weakness?

Delineating the pattern of weakness, if present, is essential for diagnosis, and in this regard two additional questions should be answered: (1) Does the weakness only involve the distal extremity or is it both proximal

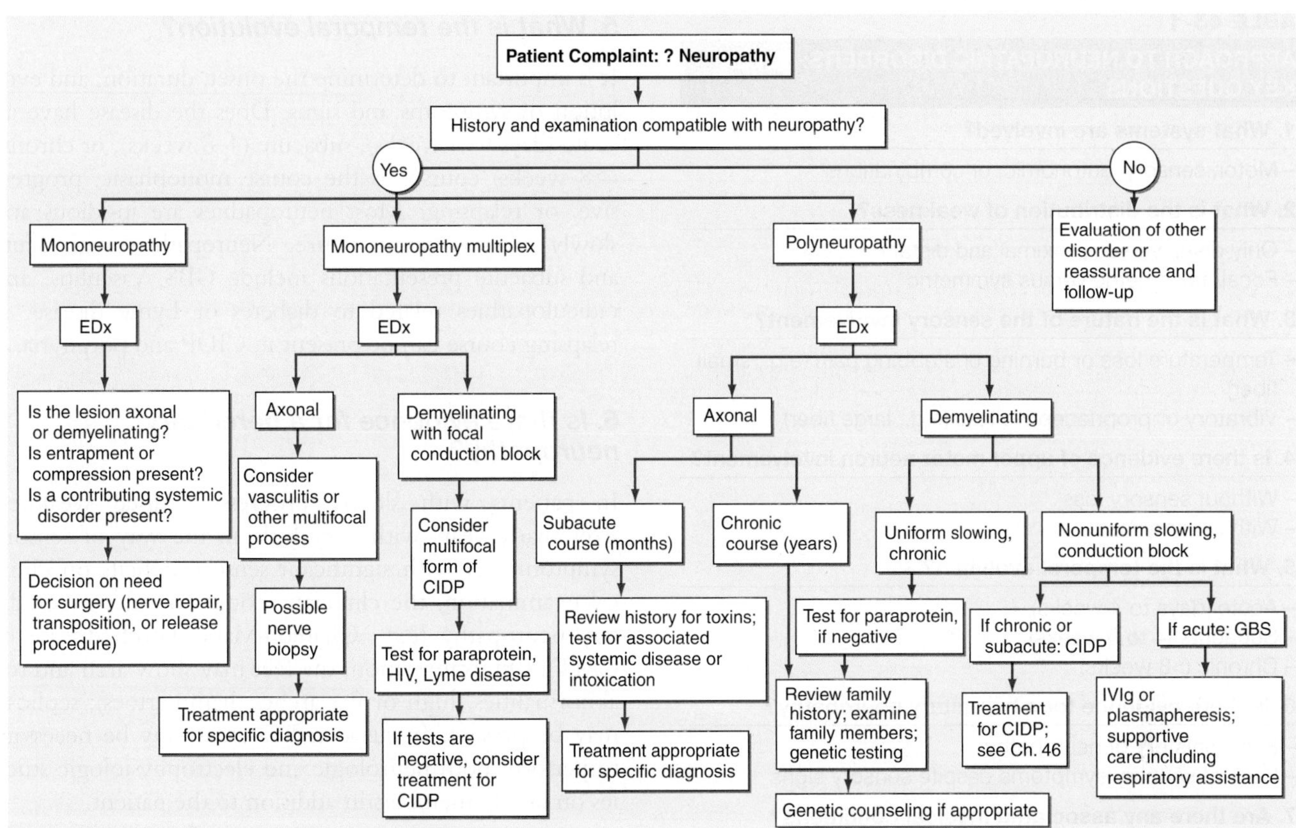

FIGURE 45-1
Approach to the evaluation of peripheral neuropathies. CIDP, chronic inflammatory demyelinating polyradiculoneuropathy; GBS, Guillain-Barré syndrome.

and distal? and (2) Is the weakness focal and asymmetric or is it symmetric? Symmetric proximal and distal weakness is the hallmark of acquired immune demyelinating polyneuropathies, both the acute form (acute inflammatory demyelinating polyneuropathy [AIDP] also known as Guillain-Barré syndrome [GBS]) and the chronic form (chronic inflammatory demyelinating polyneuropathy [CIDP]). The importance of finding symmetric proximal and distal weakness in a patient who presents with both motor and sensory symptoms cannot be overemphasized because this identifies the important subset of patients who may have a treatable acquired demyelinating neuropathic disorder (i.e., AIDP or CIDP).

Findings of an asymmetric or multifocal pattern of weakness narrows the differential diagnosis. Some neuropathic disorders may present with unilateral extremity weakness. In the absence of sensory symptoms and signs, such weakness evolving over weeks or months would be worrisome for motor neuron disease (e.g., amyotrophic lateral sclerosis [ALS]), but it would be important to exclude multifocal motor neuropathy that may be treatable (Chap. 32). In a patient presenting with asymmetric subacute or acute sensory and motor symptoms and signs, radiculopathies, plexopathies, compressive mononeuropathies, or multiple mononeuropathies (e.g., mononeuropathy multiplex) must be considered.

3. What is the nature of the sensory involvement?

The patient may have loss of sensation (numbness), altered sensation to touch (hyperpathia or allodynia), or uncomfortable spontaneous sensations (tingling, burning, or aching) (Chap. 15). Neuropathic pain can be burning, dull, and poorly localized (protopathic pain), presumably transmitted by polymodal C nociceptor fibers, or sharp and lancinating (epicritic pain), relayed by A-delta fibers. If pain and temperature perception are lost, while vibratory and position sense are preserved along with muscle strength, deep tendon reflexes, and normal nerve conduction studies, a small-fiber neuropathy is likely. This is important, as the most likely cause of small-fiber neuropathies, when one is identified, is diabetes mellitus or glucose intolerance. Amyloid neuropathy should be considered as well in such cases, but most of these small-fiber neuropathies remain idiopathic in nature despite extensive evaluation.

Severe proprioceptive loss also narrows the differential diagnosis. Affected patients will note imbalance,

TABLE 45-1

APPROACH TO NEUROPATHIC DISORDERS: SEVEN KEY QUESTIONS

1. What systems are involved?
– Motor, sensory, autonomic, or combinations
2. What is the distribution of weakness?
– Only distal versus proximal and distal – Focal/asymmetric versus symmetric
3. What is the nature of the sensory involvement?
– Temperature loss or burning or stabbing pain (e.g., small fiber) – Vibratory or proprioceptive loss (e.g., large fiber)
4. Is there evidence of upper motor neuron involvement?
– Without sensory loss – With sensory loss
5. What is the temporal evolution?
– Acute (days to 4 weeks) – Subacute (4 to 8 weeks) – Chronic (>8 weeks)
6. Is there evidence for a hereditary neuropathy?
– Family history of neuropathy – Lack of sensory symptoms despite sensory signs
7. Are there any associated medical conditions?
– Cancer, diabetes mellitus, connective tissue disease or other autoimmune diseases, infection (e.g., HIV, Lyme disease, leprosy) – Medications including over-the-counter drugs that may cause a toxic neuropathy – Preceding events, drugs, toxins

especially in the dark. A neurologic examination revealing a dramatic loss of proprioception with vibration loss and normal strength should alert the clinician to consider a sensory neuronopathy/ganglionopathy (Table 45-2, Pattern 8). In particular, if this loss is asymmetric or affects the arms more than the legs, this pattern suggests a non-length-dependent process as seen in sensory neuronopathies.

4. Is there evidence of upper motor neuron involvement?

If the patient presents with symmetric distal sensory symptoms and signs suggestive of a distal sensory neuropathy, but there is additional evidence of symmetric upper motor neuron involvement (Chap. 12), the physician should consider a disorder such as combined system degeneration with neuropathy. The most common cause for this pattern is vitamin B_{12} deficiency, but other causes of combined system degeneration with neuropathy should be considered (e.g., copper deficiency, HIV infection, severe hepatic disease, adrenomyeloneuropathy).

5. What is the temporal evolution?

It is important to determine the onset, duration, and evolution of symptoms and signs. Does the disease have an acute (days to 4 weeks), subacute (4–8 weeks), or chronic (>8 weeks) course? Is the course monophasic, progressive, or relapsing? Most neuropathies are insidious and slowly progressive in nature. Neuropathies with acute and subacute presentations include GBS, vasculitis, and radiculopathies related to diabetes or Lyme disease. A relapsing course can be present in CIDP and porphyria.

6. Is there evidence for a hereditary neuropathy?

In patients with slowly progressive distal weakness over many years with very little in the way of sensory symptoms yet with significant sensory deficits on clinical examination, the clinician should consider a hereditary neuropathy (e.g., Charcot-Marie-Tooth disease or CMT). On examination, the feet may show arch and toe abnormalities (high or flat arches, hammertoes); scoliosis may be present. In suspected cases, it may be necessary to perform both neurologic and electrophysiologic studies on family members in addition to the patient.

7. Does the patient have any other medical conditions?

It is important to inquire about associated medical conditions (e.g., diabetes mellitus, systemic lupus erythematosus); preceding or concurrent infections (e.g. diarrheal illness preceding GBS); surgeries (e.g., gastric bypass and nutritional neuropathies); medications (toxic neuropathy), including over-the-counter vitamin preparations (B_6), alcohol; dietary habits; and use of dentures (e.g., fixatives contain zinc that can lead to copper deficiency).

PATTERN RECOGNITION APPROACH TO NEUROPATHIC DISORDERS

Based upon the answers to the seven key questions, neuropathic disorders can be classified into several patterns based on the distribution or pattern of sensory, motor, and autonomic involvement (Table 45-2). Each pattern has a limited differential diagnosis. A final diagnosis is established by utilizing other clues such as the temporal course, presence of other disease states, family history, and information from laboratory studies.

ELECTRODIAGNOSTIC STUDIES

The electrodiagnostic (EDx) evaluation of patients with a suspected peripheral neuropathy consists of nerve conduction studies (NCS) and needle electromyography (EMG). In addition, studies of autonomic function can

TABLE 45-2

PATTERNS OF NEUROPATHIC DISORDERS

Pattern 1: Symmetric proximal and distal weakness with sensory loss
Consider: inflammatory demyelinating polyneuropathy (GBS and CIDP)
Pattern 2: Symmetric distal sensory loss with or without distal weakness
Consider: cryptogenic or idiopathic sensory polyneuropathy (CSPN), diabetes mellitus and other metabolic disorders, drugs, toxins, hereditary (Charcot-Marie-Tooth, amyloidosis, and others)
Pattern 3: Asymmetric distal weakness with sensory loss
With involvement of multiple nerves
Consider: multifocal CIDP, vasculitis, cryoglobulinemia, amyloidosis, sarcoid, infectious (leprosy, Lyme, hepatitis B or C, HIV, CMV), hereditary neuropathy with liability to pressure palsies (HNPP), tumor infiltration
With involvement of single nerves/regions
Consider: may be any of the above but also could be compressive mononeuropathy, plexopathy, or radiculopathy
Pattern 4: Asymmetric proximal and distal weakness with sensory loss
Consider: polyradiculopathy or plexopathy due to diabetes mellitus, meningeal carcinomatosis or lymphomatosis, hereditary plexopathy (HNPP, HNA), idiopathic
Pattern 5: Asymmetric distal weakness without sensory loss
With upper motor neuron findings
Consider: motor neuron disease
Without upper motor neuron findings
Consider: progressive muscular atrophy, juvenile monomelic amyotrophy (Hirayama disease), multifocal motor neuropathy, multifocal acquired motor axonopathy
Pattern 6: Symmetric sensory loss and distal areflexia with upper motor neuron findings
Consider: Vitamin B_{12}, vitamin E, and copper deficiency with combined system degeneration with peripheral neuropathy, hereditary leukodystrophies (e.g., adrenomyeloneuropathy)
Pattern 7: Symmetric weakness without sensory loss
With proximal and distal weakness
Consider: spinal muscular atrophy
With distal weakness
Consider: hereditary motor neuropathy ("distal" SMA) or atypical CMT
Pattern 8: Asymmetric proprioceptive sensory loss without weakness
Consider causes of a sensory neuronopathy (ganglionopathy):
Cancer (paraneoplastic)
Sjögren's syndrome
Idiopathic sensory neuronopathy (possible GBS variant)
Cisplatin and other chemotherapeutic agents
Vitamin B_6 toxicity
HIV-related sensory neuronopathy
Pattern 9: Autonomic symptoms and signs
Consider neuropathies associated with prominent autonomic dysfunction:
Hereditary sensory and autonomic neuropathy
Amyloidosis (familial and acquired)
Diabetes mellitus
Idiopathic pandysautonomia (may be a variant of Guillain-Barré syndrome)
Porphyria
HIV-related autonomic neuropathy
Vincristine and other chemotherapeutic agents

Abbreviations: CIDP, chronic inflammatory demyelinating polyneuropathy; CMT, Charcot-Marie-Tooth disease; CMV, cytomegalovirus; GBS, Guillain-Barré syndrome; HIV, human immunodeficiency virus; HNA, hereditary neuralgic amyotrophy; SMA, spinal muscular atrophy.

be valuable. The electrophysiologic data provides additional information about the distribution of the neuropathy that will support or refute the findings from the history and physical examination; it can confirm whether the neuropathic disorder is a mononeuropathy, multiple mononeuropathy (mononeuropathy multiplex), radiculopathy, plexopathy, or generalized polyneuropathy. Similarly, EDx evaluation can ascertain whether the process involves only sensory fibers, motor fibers, autonomic fibers, or a combination of these. Finally, the electrophysiologic data can help distinguish axonopathies from myelinopathies as well as axonal degeneration secondary to ganglionopathies from the more common length-dependent axonopathies.

NCS are most helpful in classifying a neuropathy as being due to axonal degeneration or segmental demyelination (Table 45-3). In general, low-amplitude potentials with relatively preserved distal latencies, conduction velocities, and late potentials, along with fibrillations on needle EMG, suggest an axonal neuropathy. On the other hand, slow conduction velocities, prolonged distal latencies and late potentials, relatively preserved amplitudes, and the absence of fibrillations on needle EMG imply a primary demyelinating neuropathy. The presence of nonuniform slowing of conduction velocity, conduction block, or temporal dispersion further suggests an acquired demyelinating neuropathy (e.g., GBS or CIDP) as opposed to a hereditary demyelinating neuropathy (e.g., CMT type 1).

Autonomic studies are used to assess small myelinated (A-delta) or unmyelinated (C) nerve fiber involvement. Such testing includes heart rate response to deep breathing, heart rate, and blood pressure response to both the Valsalva maneuver and tilt-table testing, and quantitative sudomotor axon reflex testing (Chap. 33). These studies are particularly useful in patients who have pure small-fiber neuropathy or autonomic neuropathy in which routine NCS are normal.

OTHER IMPORTANT LABORATORY INFORMATION

In patients with generalized symmetric peripheral neuropathy, a standard laboratory evaluation should include a complete blood count, basic chemistries including serum electrolytes and tests of renal and hepatic function, fasting blood glucose (FBS), HbA_{1c}, urinalysis, thyroid function tests, B_{12}, folate, erythrocyte sedimentation rate (ESR), rheumatoid factor, antinuclear antibodies (ANA), serum protein electrophoresis (SPEP), and urine for Bence Jones protein. An oral glucose tolerance test is indicated in patients with painful

TABLE 45-3

ELECTROPHYSIOLOGIC FEATURES: AXONAL DEGENERATION VS. SEGMENTAL DEMYELINATION

	AXONAL DEGENERATION	SEGMENTAL DEMYELINATION
Motor Nerve Conduction Studies		
CMAP amplitude	Decreased	Normal (except with CB)
Distal latency	Normal	Prolonged
Conduction velocity	Normal	Slow
Conduction block	Absent	Present
Temporal dispersion	Absent	Present
F wave	Normal or absent	Prolonged or absent
H reflex	Normal or absent	Prolonged or absent
Sensory Nerve Conduction Studies		
SNAP amplitude	Decreased	Normal
Distal latency	Normal	Prolonged
Conduction velocity	Normal	Slow
Needle EMG		
Spontaneous activity		
Fibrillations	Present	Absent
Fasciculations	Present	Absent
Motor unit potentials		
Recruitment	Decreased	Decreased
Morphology	Long duration/polyphasic	Normal

Abbreviations: CB, conduction block; CMAP, compound motor action potential; EMG, electromyography; SNAP, sensory nerve action potential.

sensory neuropathies even if FBS and HbA_{1c} are normal, as the test is abnormal in about one-third of such patients. Serum and urine immunofixation electrophoresis (IFE) are necessary, rather than just an SPEP, in patients with a demyelinating neuropathy or if one suspects amyloidosis (e.g., severe autonomic symptoms) as an IFE is more sensitive at identifying a monoclonal gammopathy. A skeletal survey should be performed in patients with acquired demyelinating neuropathies and M-spikes to look for osteosclerotic or lytic lesions. Patients with monoclonal gammopathy should also be referred to a hematologist for consideration of a bone marrow biopsy. In addition to the previously mentioned tests, patients with a mononeuropathy multiplex pattern of involvement should have a vasculitis workup, including antineutrophil cytoplasmic antibodies (ANCA), cryoglobulins, hepatitis serology, Western blot for Lyme disease, HIV, and occasionally a cytomegalovirus (CMV) titer.

There are many autoantibody panels (various antiganglioside antibodies) marketed for screening routine neuropathy patients for a treatable condition. These autoantibodies have no proven clinical utility or added benefit beyond the information obtained from a complete clinical examination and detailed EDx. A heavy metal screen is also not necessary as a screening procedure, unless there is a history of possible exposure or suggestive features on examination (e.g., severe painful sensorimotor and autonomic neuropathy and alopecia—thallium; severe painful sensorimotor neuropathy with or without GI disturbance and Mee's lines—arsenic; wrist or finger extensor weakness and anemia with basophilic stippling of red blood cells—lead).

In patients with suspected GBS or CIDP, a lumbar puncture is indicated to look for an elevated cerebral spinal fluid (CSF) protein. In idiopathic cases of GBS and CIDP, there should not be pleocytosis in the CSF. If cells are present, one should consider HIV infection, Lyme disease, sarcoidosis, or lymphomatous or leukemic infiltration of nerve roots. Some patients with GBS and CIDP have abnormal liver function tests. In these cases, it is important to also check for hepatitis B and C, HIV, CMV, and Epstein-Barr virus (EBV) infection. In patients with an axonal GBS (by EMG/NCS) or those with a suspicious coinciding history (e.g., unexplained abdominal pain, psychiatric illness, significant autonomic dysfunction), it is reasonable to screen for porphyria.

In patients with a severe sensory ataxia, a sensory ganglionopathy or neuronopathy should be considered. The most common causes of sensory ganglionopathies are Sjögren's syndrome and a paraneoplastic neuropathy. Neuropathy can be the initial manifestation of Sjögren's syndrome. Thus, one should always inquire about dry eyes and mouth in patients with sensory signs and symptoms. Further, some patients can manifest sicca complex without full-blown Sjögren's syndrome. Thus, patients with sensory ataxia should have an senile systemic amyloidosis (SSA) and single strand binding (SSB) in addition to the routine ANA. To workup a possible paraneoplastic sensory ganglionopathy, anti-neuronal nuclear antibodies (e.g., anti-Hu antibodies) should be obtained (Chap. 44). These antibodies are most commonly seen in patients with small cell carcinoma of the lung but are seen also in breast, ovarian, lymphoma, and other cancers. Importantly, the paraneoplastic neuropathy can precede the detection of the cancer, and detection of these autoantibodies should lead to a search for malignancy.

NERVE BIOPSIES

Nerve biopsies are now rarely indicated for evaluation of neuropathies. The primary indication for nerve biopsy is suspicion for amyloid neuropathy or vasculitis. In most instances, the abnormalities present on biopsies do not help distinguish one form of peripheral neuropathy from another (beyond what is already apparent by clinical examination and the NCS). Nerve biopsies should only be done if the NCS studies are abnormal. The sural nerve is most commonly biopsied because it is a pure sensory nerve and biopsy will not result in loss of motor function. In suspected vasculitis, a combination biopsy of a superficial peroneal nerve (pure sensory) and the underlying peroneus brevis muscle obtained from a single small incision increases the diagnostic yield. Tissue can be analyzed by frozen section and paraffin section to assess the supporting structures for evidence of inflammation, vasculitis, or amyloid deposition. Semithin plastic sections, teased fiber preparations, and electron microscopy are used to assess the morphology of the nerve fibers and to distinguish axonopathies from myelinopathies.

SKIN BIOPSIES

Skin biopsies are sometimes used to diagnose a small-fiber neuropathy. Following a punch biopsy of the skin in the distal lower extremity, immunologic staining can be used to measure the density of small unmyelinated fibers. The density of these nerve fibers is reduced in patients with small-fiber neuropathies in whom nerve conduction studies and routine nerve biopsies are often normal. This technique may allow for an objective measurement in patients with mainly subjective symptoms. However, it adds little to what one already knows from the clinical examination and EDx.

SPECIFIC DISORDERS

HEREDITARY NEUROPATHIES

Charcot-Marie-Tooth (CMT) disease is the most common type of hereditary neuropathy. Rather than one disease, CMT is a syndrome of several genetically distinct disorders (Table 45-4). The various subtypes of CMT are classified according to the nerve conduction velocities and predominant pathology (e.g., demyelination or axonal degeneration), inheritance pattern (autosomal dominant, recessive, or X-linked), and the specific mutated genes. Type 1 CMT (or CMT1) refers to inherited demyelinating sensorimotor neuropathies, while the axonal sensory neuropathies are classified as CMT2. By definition, motor conduction velocities in the arms are slowed to less than 38 m/s in CMT1 and are greater than 38 m/s in CMT2. However, most cases of CMT1 actually have motor nerve conduction velocities (NCVs) between 20 and 25 m/s. CMT1 and CMT2 usually begin in childhood or early adult life; however, onset later in life can occur, particularly in CMT2. Both are associated with autosomal dominant inheritance, with a few exceptions. CMT3 is an autosomal dominant neuropathy that appears in infancy and is associated with severe demyelination or hypomyelination. CMT4 is an autosomal recessive neuropathy that typically begins in childhood or early adult life. There are no medical therapies for any of the CMTs, but physical and occupational therapy can be beneficial as can bracing (e.g., ankle-foot orthotics for footdrop) and other orthotic devices.

CMT1

CMT1 is the most common form of hereditary neuropathy, with the ratio of CMT1:CMT2 being approximately 2:1. Affected individuals usually present in the first to third decade of life with distal leg weakness (e.g., footdrop), although patients may remain asymptomatic even late in life. People with CMT generally do not complain of numbness or tingling, which can be helpful in distinguishing CMT from acquired forms of neuropathy in which sensory symptoms usually predominate. Although usually asymptomatic in this regard, reduced sensation to all modalities is apparent on examination. Muscle stretch reflexes are unobtainable or reduced throughout. There is often atrophy of the muscles below the knee (particularly the anterior compartment), leading to so-called inverted champagne bottle legs.

TABLE 45-4

CLASSIFICATION OF CHARCOT-MARIE-TOOTH DISEASE AND RELATED NEUROPATHIES

NAME	INHERITANCE	GENE LOCATION	GENE PRODUCT
CMT1			
CMT1A	AD	17p11.2	PMP-22 (usually duplication of gene)
CMT1B	AD	1q21-23	MPZ
CMT1C	AD	16p13.1-p12.3	LITAF
CMT1D	AD	10q21.1-22.1	ERG2
CMT1E (with deafness)	AD	17p11.2	Point mutations in PMP 22 gene
CMT1F	AD	8p13-21	Neurofilament light chain
CMT1X	X-linked dominant	Xq13	Connexin-32
HNPP	AD	17p11.2 1q21-23	PMP-22 MPZ
CMT2			
CMT2A2 (allelic to HMSN VI with optic atrophy)	AD	1p36.2	MFN2
CMT2B	AD	3q13-q22	RAB7
CMT2B1 (allelic to LGMD 1B)	AR	1q21.2	Lamin A/C
CMT2B2	AR and AD	19q13	MED25 for AR Unknown for AD
CMT2C (with vocal cord and diaphragm paralysis)	AD	12q23-24	TRPV4
CMT2D (allelic to distal SMA5)	AD	7p14	Glycine tRNA synthetase
CMT2E (allelic to CMT 1F)	AD	8p21	Neurofilament light chain
CMT2F	AD	7q11-q21	Heat-shock 27-kDa protein-1

(continued)

TABLE 45-4

CLASSIFICATION OF CHARCOT-MARIE-TOOTH DISEASE AND RELATED NEUROPATHIES (*CONTINUED*)

NAME	INHERITANCE	GENE LOCATION	GENE PRODUCT
CMT2G (may be allelic to CMT4H)	AD	12q12-q13	? (Frabin)
CMT2H	AD	8q21.3	? (may be GDAP1)
CMT2I (allelic to CMT1B)	AD	1q22	MPZ
CMT2J	AD	1q22	MPZ
CMT2K (allelic to CMT4A)	AD	8q13-q21	GDAP1
CMT2L (allelic to distal hereditary motor neuropathy type 2)	AD	12q24	Heat-shock protein 8
CMT2M	AD	16q22	Dynamin-2
CMT2X	X-linked	Xq22-24	PRPS1
CMT3 (Dejerine-Sottas disease, congenital hypomyelinating neuropathy)	AD AD AR AR	17p11.2 1q21-23 10q21.1-22.1 19q13	PMP-22 MPZ ERG2 Periaxon
CMT4			
CMT4A	AR	8q13-21.1	GDAP1
CMT4B1 CMT4B2	AR AR	11q23 11p15	MTMR2 MTMR13
CMT4C	AR	5q23-33	SH3TC2
CMT4D (HMSN-Lom)	AR	8q24	NDRG1
CMT4E (Congenital hypomyelinating neuropathy)	AR	-	Probably includes PMP22, MPZ, and ERG-2
CMT4F	AR AR	19q13.1-13.3	Periaxin
CMT4G	AR	10q23.2	HKI
CMT4H	AR	12q12-q13	Frabin
CMT4J	AR	6q21	FIG4
HNA	AD	17q24	SEPT9
HMSN-P	AD	3q13-q14	?
HSAN1	AD; Rare AR and X-linked cases also reported	9q22	SPTLC1
HSAN2	AR	12p13.33	PRKWNK1
HSAN3	AR	9q21	IKAP
HSAN4	AR	3q	trkA/NGF receptor
HSAN5	AD or AR	1p11.2-p13.2	NGFb

Abbreviations: AARS, alanyl-tRNA synthetase; AD, autosomal dominant; AR, autosomal recessive; CMT, Charcot-Marie-Tooth; ERG2, early growth response-2 protein; FIG4, FDG1-related F actin–binding protein; GDAP1, ganglioside-induced differentiation-associated protein-1; HK1, hexokinase 1; HMSN-P, hereditary motor and sensory neuropathy-proximal; HNA, hereditary neuralgic amyotrophy; HNPP, hereditary neuropathy with liability to pressure palsies; HSAN; hereditary sensory and autonomic neuropathy; IKAP, $_{\kappa}$B kinase complex-associated protein; LGMD, limb girdle muscular dystrophy; LITAF, lipopolysaccharide-induced tumor necrosis factor α factor; MED25, mediator 25; MFN2, mitochondrial fusion protein mitofusin 2 gene; MPZ, myelin protein zero protein; MTMR2, myotubularin-related protein-2; NDRG1, N-myc downstream regulated 1; PMP-22, peripheral myelin protein-22; PRKWNK1, protein kinase, lysine deficient 1; PRPS1, phosphoribosylpyrophosphate synthetase 1; RAB7, Ras-related protein 7; SEPT9, Septin 9; SH3TC2, SH3 domain and tetratricopeptide repeats 2; SMA, spinal muscular atrophy; SPTLC1, serine palmitoyltransferase long-chain base 1; TrkA/NGF, tyrosine kinase A/nerve growth factor; tRNA, transfer ribonucleic acid; TRPV4, transient receptor potential cation channel, subfamily V, member 4.

Source: Modified from AA Amato, J Russell: *Neuromuscular Disease*. New York, McGraw-Hill, 2008.

Motor NCVs are usually in the 20–25 m/s range. Nerve biopsies usually are not performed on patients suspected of having CMT1, as the diagnosis usually can be made by less invasive testing (e.g., NCS and genetic studies). However, when done, the biopsies reveal reduction of myelinated nerve fibers with a predilection for the loss of the large-diameter fibers and Schwann cell proliferation around thinly or demyelinated fibers, forming so-called onion bulbs.

CMT1A is the most common subtype of CMT1, representing 70% of cases, and is caused by a 1.5-megabase (Mb) duplication within chromosome 17p11.2-12 wherein the gene for peripheral myelin protein-22 (PMP-22) lies. This results in patients having three copies of the PMP-22 gene rather than two. This protein accounts for 2–5% of myelin protein and is expressed in compact portions of the peripheral myelin sheath. Approximately 20% of patients with CMT1 have CMT1B, which is caused by mutations in the myelin protein zero (MPZ). CMT1B is for the most part clinically, electrophysiologically, and histologically indistinguishable from CMT1A. MPZ is an integral myelin protein and accounts for more than half of the myelin protein in peripheral nerves. Other forms of CMT1 are much less common and again indistinguishable from one another clinically and electrophysiologically.

CMT2

CMT2 tends to present later in life compared to CMT1. Affected individuals usually become symptomatic in the second decade of life; some cases present earlier in childhood, while others remain asymptomatic into late adult life. Clinically, CMT2 is for the most part indistinguishable from CMT1. NCS are helpful in this regard; in contrast to CMT1, the velocities are normal or only slightly slowed. The most common cause of CMT2 is a mutation in the gene for mitofusin 2 (MFN2), which accounts for one-third of CMT2 cases overall. MFN2 localizes to the outer mitochondrial membrane, where it regulates the mitochondrial network architecture by fusion of mitochondria. The other genes associated with CMT2 are much less common.

CMT3

CMT3 was originally described by Dejerine and Sottas as a hereditary demyelinating sensorimotor polyneuropathy presenting in infancy or early childhood. Affected children are severely weak. Motor NCVs are markedly slowed, typically 5–10 m/s or less. Most cases of CMT3 are caused by point mutations in the genes for PMP-22, MPZ, or ERG-2, which are also the genes responsible for CMT1.

CMT4

CMT4 is extremely rare and is characterized by a severe, childhood-onset sensorimotor polyneuropathy that is usually inherited in an autosomal recessive fashion. Electrophysiologic and histologic evaluations can show demyelinating or axonal features. CMT4 is genetically heterogenic (Table 45-4).

CMT1X

CMT1X is an X-linked dominant disorder with clinical features similar to CMT1 and -2, except that the neuropathy is much more severe in men than in women. CMT1X accounts for approximately 10–15% of CMT overall. Men usually present in the first two decades of life with atrophy and weakness of the distal arms and legs, areflexia, pes cavus, and hammertoes. Obligate women carriers are frequently asymptomatic, but can develop signs and symptoms. Onset in women is usually after the second decade of life, and the neuropathy is milder in severity.

NCS reveal features of both demyelination and axonal degeneration that are more severe in men compared to women. In men, motor NCVs in the arms and legs are moderately slowed (in the low to mid 30-m/s range). About 50% of men with CMT1X have motor NCVs between 15 and 35 m/s with about 80% of these falling between 25 and 35 m/s (intermediate slowing). In contrast, about 80% of women with CMT1X have NCV in the normal range and 20% had MNCV in the intermediate range. CMT1X is caused by mutations in the connexin 32 gene. Connexins are gap junction structural proteins that are important in cell-to-cell communication.

Hereditary neuropathy with liability to pressure palsies (HNPP)

HNPP is an autosomal dominant disorder related to CMT1A. While CMT1A is usually associated with a 1.5-Mb duplication in chromosome 17p11.2 that results in an extra copy of PMP-22 gene, HNPP is caused by inheritance of the chromosome with the corresponding 1.5-Mb deletion of this segment, and thus affected individuals have only one copy of the PMP-22 gene. Patients usually manifest in the second or third decade of life with painless numbness and weakness in the distribution of single peripheral nerves, although multiple mononeuropathies can occur. Symptomatic mononeu ropathy or multiple mononeuropathies are often precipitated by trivial compression of nerve(s) as can occur with wearing a backpack, leaning on the elbows, or crossing one's legs for even a short period of time. These pressure-related mononeuropathies may take weeks or months to resolve. In addition, some affected individuals manifest with a progressive or relapsing, generalized and symmetric, sensorimotor peripheral neuropathy that resembles CMT.

Hereditary neuralgic amyotrophy (HNA)

HNA is an autosomal dominant disorder characterized by recurrent attacks of pain, weakness, and sensory loss in the distribution of the brachial plexus often beginning in childhood. These attacks are similar to those seen with idiopathic brachial plexitis (discussed later). Attacks may occur in the postpartum period, following surgery, or at other times of stress. Most patients recover over several weeks or months. Slightly dysmorphic features, including hypotelorism, epicanthal folds, cleft palate, syndactyly, micrognathia, and facial asymmetry, are evident in some individuals. EDx demonstrate an axonal process. HNA is caused by mutations in septin 9 (*SEPT9*). Septins may be important in formation of the neuronal cytoskeleton and have a role in cell division, but the mechanism of causing HNA is unclear.

Hereditary sensory and autonomic neuropathy (HSAN)

The HSANs are a very rare group of hereditary neuropathies in which sensory and autonomic dysfunction predominates over muscle weakness, unlike CMT, in which motor findings are most prominent (Table 45-4). Nevertheless, affected individuals can develop motor weakness and there can be overlap with CMT. There are no medical therapies available to treat these neuropathies, other than prevention and treatment of mutilating skin and bone lesions.

Of the HSANs, only HSAN1 typically presents in adults. The HSAN1 is the most common of the HSANs and is inherited in an autosomal dominant fashion. Affected individuals with HSAN1 usually manifest in the second through fourth decade of life. HSAN1 is associated with the degeneration of small myelinated and unmyelinated nerve fibers leading to severe loss of pain and temperature sensation, deep dermal ulcerations, recurrent osteomyelitis, Charcot joints, bone loss, gross foot and hand deformities, and amputated digits. Although most people with HSAN1 do not complain of numbness, they often describe burning, aching, or lancinating pains. Autonomic neuropathy is not a prominent feature, but bladder dysfunction and reduced sweating in the feet may occur. HSAN1A is caused by mutations in the serine palmitoyltransferase long-chain base 1 (*SPTLC1*) gene.

OTHER HEREDITARY NEUROPATHIES (TABLE 45-5)

FABRY DISEASE

Fabry disease (angiokeratoma corporis diffusum) is an X-linked dominant disorder. While men are more commonly and severely affected, women can also show severe signs of the disease. Angiokeratomas are reddish-purple maculopapular lesions that are usually found around the umbilicus, scrotum, inguinal region, and perineum. Burning or lancinating pain in the hands and feet often develops in males in late childhood or early adult life. However, the neuropathy is usually overshadowed by complications arising from the associated premature atherosclerosis (e.g., hypertension, renal failure, cardiac disease, and stroke) that often lead to death by the fifth decade of life. Some patients also manifest primarily with a dilated cardiomyopathy.

TABLE 45-5
RARE HEREDITARY NEUROPATHIES

Rare Hereditary Neuropathies
Hereditary Disorders of Lipid Metabolism
Metachromatic leukodystrophy
Krabbe disease (globoid cell leukodystrophy)
Fabry disease
Adrenoleukodystrophy/adrenomyeloneuropathy
Refsum disease
Tangier disease
Cerebrotendinous xanthomatosis
Hereditary Ataxias with Neuropathy
Friedreich ataxia
Vitamin E deficiency
Spinocerebellar ataxia
Abetalipoproteinemia (Bassen-Kornzweig disease)
Disorders of Defective DNA Repair
Ataxia-telangiectasia
Cockayne syndrome
Giant Axonal Neuropathy
Porphyria
Acute intermittent porphyria (AIP)
Hereditary coproporphyria (HCP)
Variegate porphyria (VP)
Familial Amyloid Polyneuropathy (FAP)
Transthyretin-related
Gelsolin-related
Apolipoprotein A1-related

Fabry disease is caused by mutations in the α-galactosidase gene that leads to the accumulation of ceramide trihexoside in nerves and blood vessels. A decrease in α-galactosidase activity is evident in leukocytes and cultured fibroblasts. Glycolipid granules may be appreciated in ganglion cells of the peripheral and sympathetic nervous systems and in perineurial cells. Enzyme replacement therapy with α-galactosidase B can improve the neuropathy if patients are treated early, before irreversible nerve fiber loss.

ADRENOLEUKODYSTROPHY/ ADRENOMYELONEUROPATHY

Adrenoleukodystrophy (ALD) and adrenomyeloneuropathy (AMN) are allelic X-linked dominant disorders caused by mutations in the peroxisomal transmembrane adenosine triphosphate-binding cassette (ABC) transporter gene. Patients with ALD manifest with CNS abnormalities. However, 30% with mutations in this gene present with the AMN phenotype that typically manifests in the third to fifth decade of life with mild to moderate peripheral neuropathy combined with progressive spastic paraplegia (Chap. 35). Rare patients present with an adult-onset spinocerebellar ataxia or only with adrenal insufficiency.

EDx is suggestive of a primary axonopathy with secondary demyelination. Nerve biopsies demonstrate a loss of myelinated and unmyelinated nerve fibers with lamellar inclusions in the cytoplasm of Schwann cells. Very long chain fatty acid (VLCFA) levels (C24, C25, and C26) are increased in the urine. Laboratory evidence of adrenal insufficiency is evident in approximately two-thirds of patients. The diagnosis can be confirmed by genetic testing.

Adrenal insufficiency is managed by replacement therapy; however, there is no proven effective therapy for the neurologic manifestations of ALD/AMN. Diets low in VLCFAs and supplemented with Lorenzo's oil (erucic and oleic acids) reduce the levels of VLCFAs and increase the levels of C22 in serum, fibroblasts, and liver; however, several large, open-label trials of Lorenzo's oil failed to demonstrate efficacy.

REFSUM DISEASE

Refsum disease can manifest in infancy to early adulthood with the classic tetrad of (1) peripheral neuropathy, (2) retinitis pigmentosa, (3) cerebellar ataxia, and (4) elevated CSF protein concentration. Most affected individuals develop progressive distal sensory loss and weakness in the legs leading to footdrop by their 20s. Subsequently, the proximal leg and arm muscles may become weak. Patients may also develop sensorineural hearing loss, cardiac conduction abnormalities, ichthyosis, and anosmia.

Serum phytanic acid levels are elevated. Sensory and motor NCS reveal reduced amplitudes, prolonged latencies, and slowed conduction velocities. Nerve biopsy demonstrates a loss of myelinated nerve fibers, with remaining axons often thinly myelinated and associated with onion bulb formation.

Refsum disease is genetically heterogeneous but autosomal recessive in nature. Classical Refsum disease with childhood or early adult onset is caused by mutations in the gene that encodes for phytanoyl-CoA α-hydroxylase (*PAHX*). Less commonly, mutations in the gene encoding peroxin 7 receptor protein (PRX 7) are responsible. These mutations lead to the accumulation of phytanic acid in the central and peripheral nervous systems. Refsum disease is treated by removing phytanic precursors (phytols: fish oils, dairy products, and ruminant fats) from the diet.

TANGIER DISEASE

Tangier disease is a rare autosomal recessive disorder that can present as (1) asymmetric multiple mononeuropathies, (2) a slowly progressive symmetric polyneuropathy predominantly in the legs, or (3) a pseudo-syringomyelia pattern with dissociated sensory loss (i.e., abnormal pain/temperature perception but preserved position/vibration in the arms [Chap. 35]). The tonsils may appear swollen and yellowish-orange in color, while there may also be splenomegaly and lymphadenopathy.

Tangier disease is caused by mutations in the ATP-binding cassette transporter 1 (ABC1) gene, which leads to markedly reduced levels of high-density lipoprotein (HDL) cholesterol levels while triacylglycerol levels are increased. Nerve biopsies reveal axonal degeneration with demyelination and remyelination. Electron microscopy demonstrates abnormal accumulation of lipid in Schwann cells, particularly those encompassing umyelinated and small myelinated nerves. There is no specific treatment.

PORPHYRIA

Porphyria is a group of inherited disorders caused by defects in heme biosynthesis. Three forms of porphyria are associated with peripheral neuropathy: acute intermittent porphyria (AIP), hereditary coproporphyria (HCP), and variegate porphyria (VP). The acute neurologic manifestations are similar in each, with the exception that a photosensitive rash is seen with HCP and VP but not in AIP. Attacks of porphyria can be precipitated by certain drugs (usually those metabolized by the P450 system), hormonal changes (e.g., pregnancy, menstrual cycle), and dietary restrictions.

An acute attack of porphyria may begin with sharp abdominal pain. Subsequently, patients may develop agitation, hallucinations, or seizures. Several days later, back and extremity pain followed by weakness ensues, mimicking GBS. Weakness can involve the arms or the legs and can be asymmetric, proximal, or distal in distribution, as well as affecting the face and bulbar musculature. Dysautonomia and signs of sympathetic overactivity are common (e.g., pupillary dilation, tachycardia, and hypertension). Constipation, urinary retention, and incontinence can also be seen.

The CSF protein is typically normal or mildly elevated. Liver function tests and hematologic parameters are usually normal. Some patients are hyponatremic due to inappropriate secretion of antidiuretic hormone. The urine may appear brownish in color secondary to the high concentration of porphyrin metabolites. Accumulation of intermediary precursors of heme (i.e., δ-aminolevulinic acid, porphobilinogen, uroporphobilinogen, coproporphyrinogen, and protoporphyrinogen) are found in urine. Specific enzyme activities can also be measured in erythrocytes and leukocytes. The primary abnormalities on EDx are marked reductions in CMAP amplitudes and signs of active axonal degeneration on needle EMG.

The porphyrias are inherited in an autosomal dominant fashion. AIP is associated with porphobilinogen deaminase deficiency, HCP is caused by defects in coproporphyrin oxidase, and VP is associated with protoporphyrinogen oxidase deficiency. The pathogenesis of the neuropathy is not completely understood. Treatment with glucose and hematin may reduce the accumulation of heme precursors. Intravenous glucose is started at a rate of 10–20 g/h. If there is no improvement within 24 h, intravenous hematin 2–5 mg/kg per day for 3–14 days should be given.

FAMILIAL AMYLOID POLYNEUROPATHY

Familial amyloid polyneuropathy (FAP) is phenotypically and genetically heterogeneous and is caused by mutations in the genes for transthyretin (TTR), apolipoprotein A1, or gelsolin. The majority of patients with FAP have mutations in the TTR gene. Amyloid deposition may be evident in abdominal fat pad, rectal, or nerve biopsies. The clinical features, histopathology, and EDx reveal abnormalities consistent with a generalized or multifocal, predominantly axonal but occasionally demyelinating, sensorimotor polyneuropathy.

Patients with TTR-related FAP usually develop insidious onset of numbness and painful paresthesias in the distal lower limbs in the third to fourth decade of life, although some patients develop the disorder later in life. Carpal tunnel syndrome (CTS) is common. Autonomic involvement can be severe, leading to postural hypotension, constipation or persistent diarrhea, erectile dysfunction, and impaired sweating. Amyloid deposition also occurs in the heart, kidneys, liver, and the corneas. Patients usually die 10–15 years after the onset of symptoms from cardiac failure or complications from malnutrition. Because the liver produces much of the body's TTR, liver transplantation has been used to treat FAP related to TTR mutations. Serum TTR levels decrease after transplantation, and improvement in clinical and EDx features have been reported.

Patients with apolipoprotein A1–related FAP (Van Allen type) usually present in the fourth decade with numbness and painful dysesthesias in the distal limbs. Gradually, the symptoms progress, leading to proximal and distal weakness and atrophy. Although autonomic neuropathy is not severe, some patients develop diarrhea, constipation, or gastroparesis. Most patients die from systemic complications of amyloidosis (e.g., renal failure) 12–15 years after the onset of the neuropathy.

Gelsolin-related amyloidosis (Finnish type) is characterized by the combination of lattice corneal dystrophy and multiple cranial neuropathies that usually begin in the third decade of life. Over time, a mild generalized sensorimotor polyneuropathy develops. Autonomic dysfunction does not occur.

ACQUIRED NEUROPATHIES

PRIMARY OR AL AMYLOIDOSIS

Besides FAP, amyloidosis can also be acquired. In primary or AL amyloidosis, the abnormal protein deposition is composed of immunoglobulin light chains. AL amyloidosis occurs in the setting of multiple myeloma, Waldenström's macroglobulinemia, lymphoma, other plasmacytomas, or lymphoproliferative disorders, or without any other identifiable disease.

Approximately 30% of patients with AL primary amyloidosis present with a polyneuropathy, most typically painful dysesthesias and burning sensations in the feet. However, the trunk can be involved and some manifest with a mononeuropathy multiplex pattern. CTS occurs in 25% of patients and may be the initial manifestation. The neuropathy is slowly progressive, and eventually weakness develops along with large-fiber sensory loss. Most patients develop autonomic involvement with postural hypertension, syncope, bowel and bladder incontinence, constipation, impotence, and impaired sweating. Patients generally die from their systemic illness (renal failure, cardiac disease).

The monoclonal protein may be composed of IgG, IgA, IgM, or only free light chain. Lambda (λ) is more common than κ light chain (>2:1) in AL amyloidosis. The CSF protein is often increased (with normal cell count), and thus the neuropathy may be mistaken for CIDP (Chap. 46). Nerve biopsies reveal axonal degeneration and amyloid deposition in either a globular or diffuse pattern infiltrating the perineurial, epineurial, and endoneurial connected tissue and in blood vessel walls.

The median survival of patients with primary amyloidosis is less than 2 years, with death usually from progressive congestive heart failure or renal failure. Chemotherapy with melphalan, prednisone, and colchicine, to reduce the concentration of monoclonal proteins, and autologous stem cell transplantation may prolong survival, but whether the neuropathy improves is controversial.

DIABETIC NEUROPATHY

Diabetes mellitus (DM) is the most common cause of peripheral neuropathy in developed countries. DM is associated with several types of polyneuropathy:

distal symmetric sensory or sensorimotor polyneuropathy, autonomic neuropathy, diabetic neuropathic cachexia, polyradiculoneuropathies, cranial neuropathies, and other mononeuropathies. Risk factors for the development of neuropathy include long-standing, poorly controlled DM and the presence of retinopathy and nephropathy.

Diabetic distal symmetric sensory and sensorimotor polyneuropathy (DSPN)

DSPN is the most common form of diabetic neuropathy and manifests as sensory loss beginning in the toes that gradually progresses over time up the legs and into the fingers and arms. When severe, a patient may develop sensory loss in the trunk (chest and abdomen), initially in the midline anteriorly and later extending laterally. Tingling, burning, deep aching pains may also be apparent. NCS usually show reduced amplitudes and mild to moderate slowing of conduction velocities (CVs). Nerve biopsy reveals axonal degeneration, endothelial hyperplasia, and, occasionally, perivascular inflammation. Tight control of glucose can reduce the risk of developing neuropathy or improve the underlying neuropathy. A variety of medications have been used with variable success to treat painful symptoms associated with DSPN, including antiepileptic medications, antidepressants, sodium channel blockers, and other analgesics (Table 45-6).

Diabetic autonomic neuropathy

Autonomic neuropathy is typically seen in combination with DSPN. The autonomic neuropathy can manifest as abnormal sweating, dysfunctional thermoregulation, dry eyes and mouth, pupillary abnormalities, cardiac

TABLE 45-6

TREATMENT OF PAINFUL SENSORY NEUROPATHIES

THERAPY	ROUTE	DOSE	SIDE EFFECTS
First-Line			
Lidoderm 5% patch	Apply to painful area	Up to 3 patches qd	Skin irritation
Tricyclic antidepressants (e.g., amitriptylin, nortriptyline)	p.o.	10–100 mg qhs	Cognitive changes, sedation, dry eyes and mouth, urinary retention, constipation
Gabapentin	p.o.	300–1200 mg TID	Cognitive changes, sedation, peripheral edema
Pregabalin	p.o.	50–100 mg TID	Cognitive changes, sedation, peripheral edema
Duloxetine	p.o.	30–60 mg qd	Cognitive changes, sedation, dry eyes, diaphoresis, nausea, diarrhea, constipation
Second-Line			
Carbamazepine	p.o.	200–400 mg q 6–8 h	Cognitive changes, dizziness, leukopenia, liver dysfunction
Phenytoin	p.o.	200–400 mg qhs	Cognitive changes, dizziness, liver dysfunction
Venlafaxine	po	37.5–150 mg/d	Asthenia, sweating, nausea, constipation, anorexia, vomiting, somnolence, dry mouth, dizziness, nervousness, anxiety, tremor, and blurred vision as well as abnormal ejaculation/orgasm and impotence
Tramadol	p.o.	50 mg qid	Cognitive changes, GI upset
Third-Line			
Mexiletine	p.o.	200–300 mg tid	Arrhythmias
Other Agents			
EMLA cream 2.5% lidocaine 2.5% prilocaine	Apply cutaneously	q.i.d.	Local erythema
Capsaicin 0.025%–0.075% cream	Apply cutaneously	q.i.d.	Painful burning skin

Source: Modified from AA Amato, J Russell: *Neuromuscular Disease*. New York, McGraw-Hill, 2008.

arrhythmias, postural hypotension, gastrointestinal abnormalities (e.g., gastroparesis, postprandial bloating, chronic diarrhea or constipation), and genitourinary dysfunction (e.g., impotence, retrograde ejaculation, incontinence). Tests of autonomic function are generally abnormal, including sympathetic skin responses and quantitative sudomotor axon reflex testing. Sensory and motor NCS generally demonstrate features described earlier with DSPN.

Diabetic radiculoplexus neuropathy (diabetic amyotrophy or Bruns-Garland syndrome)

Diabetic radiculoplexus neuropathy is the presenting manifestation of DM in approximately one-third of patients. Typically, patients present with severe pain in the low back, hip, and thigh in one leg. Rarely, the diabetic polyradiculoneuropathy begins in both legs at the same time. Atrophy and weakness of proximal and distal muscles in the affected leg become apparent within a few days or weeks. The neuropathy is often accompanied or heralded by severe weight loss. Weakness usually progresses over several weeks or months, but can continue to progress for 18 months or more. Subsequently, there is slow recovery but many are left with residual weakness, sensory loss, and pain. In contrast to the more typical lumbosacral radiculoplexus neuropathy, some patients develop thoracic radiculopathy or, even less commonly, a cervical polyradiculoneuropathy. CSF protein is usually elevated, while the cell count is normal. ESR is often increased. EDx reveals evidence of active denervation in affected proximal and distal muscles in the affected limbs and in paraspinal muscles. Nerve biopsies may demonstrate axonal degeneration along with perivascular inflammation. Patients with severe pain are sometimes treated in the acute period with glucocorticoids, although a randomized controlled trial has yet to be performed, and the natural history of this neuropathy is gradual improvement.

Diabetic mononeuropathies or multiple mononeuropathies

The most common mononeuropathies are median neuropathy at the wrist and ulnar neuropathy at the elbow, but peroneal neuropathy at the fibular head, and sciatic, lateral femoral, cutaneous, or cranial neuropathies also occur. In regard to cranial mononeuropathies, seventh nerve palsies are relatively common but may have other, nondiabetic etiologies. In diabetics, a third nerve palsy is most common, followed by sixth nerve, and, less frequently, fourth nerve palsies. Diabetic third nerve palsies are characteristically pupil-sparing (Chap. 21).

HYPOTHYROIDISM

Hypothyroidism is more commonly associated with a proximal myopathy, but some patients develop a neuropathy, most typically carpal tunnel syndrome. Rarely, a generalized sensory polyneuropathy characterized by painful paresthesias and numbness in both the legs and hands can occur. Treatment is correction of the hypothyroidism.

SJÖGREN'S SYNDROME

Sjögren's syndrome, characterized by the sicca complex of xerophthalmia, xerostomia, and dryness of other mucous membranes, can be complicated by neuropathy. Most common is a length-dependent axonal sensorimotor neuropathy characterized mainly by sensory loss in the distal extremities. A pure small-fiber neuropathy or a cranial neuropathy, particularly involving the trigeminal nerve, can also be seen. Sjögren's syndrome is also associated with sensory neuronopathy/ganglionopathy. Patients with sensory ganglionopathies develop progressive numbness and tingling of the limbs, trunk, and face in a non-length-dependent manner such that symptoms can involve the face or arms more than the legs. The onset can be acute or insidious. Sensory examination demonstrates severe vibratory and proprioceptive loss leading to sensory ataxia.

Patients with neuropathy due to Sjögren's syndrome may have antinuclear antibodies (ANA), SS-A/Ro, and SS-B/La antibodies in the serum but most do not. NCS demonstrate reduced amplitudes of sensory studies in the affected limbs. Nerve biopsy demonstrates axonal degeneration. Nonspecific perivascular inflammation may be present, but only rarely is there necrotizing vasculitis. There is no specific treatment for neuropathies related to Sjögren's syndrome. When vasculitis is suspected, immunosuppressive agents may be beneficial. Occasionally, the sensory neuronopathy/ganglionopathy stabilizes or improves with immunotherapy, such as IVIg.

RHEUMATOID ARTHRITIS

Peripheral neuropathy occurs in at least 50% of patients with rheumatoid arthritis (RA) and may be vasculitic in nature. Vasculitic neuropathy can present with a mononeuropathy multiplex, a generalized symmetric pattern of involvement, or a combination of these patterns. Neuropathies may also be due to drugs used to treat the RA (e.g., tumor necrosis blockers, leflunomide). Nerve biopsy often reveals thickening of the epineurial and endoneurial blood vessels as well as perivascular inflammation or vasculitis, with transmural inflammatory cell infiltration and fibrinoid necrosis of vessel walls. The neuropathy often is responsive to immunomodulating therapies.

SYSTEMIC LUPUS ERYTHEMATOSUS (SLE)

Between 2 and 27% of individuals with SLE develop a peripheral neuropathy. Affected patients typically present with a slowly progressive sensory loss beginning in the feet. Some patients develop burning pain and paresthesias with normal reflexes, and nerve conduction studies suggest a pure small-fiber neuropathy. Less common are multiple mononeuropathies presumably secondary to necrotizing vasculitis. Rarely, a generalized sensorimotor polyneuropathy meeting clinical, laboratory, electrophysiologic, and histologic criteria for either GBS or CIDP may occur. Immunosuppressive therapy is beneficial in SLE patients with neuropathy due to vasculitis. Immunosuppressive agents are less likely to be effective in patients with a generalized sensory or sensorimotor polyneuropathy without evidence of vasculitis. Patients with a GBS or CIDP-like neuropathy should be treated accordingly (Chap. 46).

SYSTEMIC SCLEROSIS (SCLERODERMA)

A distal symmetric, mainly sensory, polyneuropathy complicates 5–67% of scleroderma cases. Cranial mononeuropathies can also develop, most commonly of the trigeminal nerve, producing numbness and dysesthesias in the face. Multiple mononeuropathies also occur. The EDx and histologic features of nerve biopsy are those of an axonal sensory greater than motor polyneuropathy.

MIXED CONNECTIVE TISSUE DISEASE (MCTD)

A mild distal axonal sensorimotor polyneuropathy occurs in approximately 10% of patients with MCTD.

SARCOIDOSIS

The peripheral or central nervous systems are involved in about 5% of patients with sarcoidosis. The most common cranial nerve involved is the seventh nerve, which can be affected bilaterally. Some patients develop radiculopathy or polyradiculopathy. With a generalized root involvement, the clinical presentation can mimic GBS or CIDP. Patients can also present with multiple mononeuropathies or a generalized, slowly progressive, sensory greater than motor polyneuropathy. Some have features of a pure small-fiber neuropathy. EDx reveals an axonal neuropathy. Nerve biopsy can reveal noncaseating granulomas infiltrating the endoneurium, perineurium, and epineurium along with lymphocytic necrotizing angiitis. Neurosarcoidosis may respond to treatment with glucocorticoids or other immunosuppressive agents.

HYPEREOSINOPHILIC SYNDROME

Hypereosinophilic syndrome is characterized by eosinophilia associated with various skin, cardiac, hematologic, and neurologic abnormalities. A generalized peripheral neuropathy or a mononeuropathy multiplex occurs in 6–14% of patients.

CELIAC DISEASE (GLUTEN-INDUCED ENTEROPATHY OR NON-TROPICAL SPRUE)

Neurologic complications, particularly ataxia and peripheral neuropathy, are estimated to occur in 10% of patients with celiac disease. A generalized sensorimotor polyneuropathy, pure motor neuropathy, multiple mononeuropathies, autonomic neuropathy, small-fiber neuropathy, and neuromyotonia have all been reported in association with celiac disease or antigliadin/antiendomysial antibodies. Nerve biopsy may reveal a loss of large myelinated fibers. The neuropathy may be secondary to malabsorption of vitamins B_{12} and E. However, some patients have no appreciable vitamin deficiencies. The pathogenic basis for the neuropathy in these patients is unclear but may be autoimmune in etiology. The neuropathy does not appear to respond to a gluten-free diet. In patients with vitamin B_{12} or vitamin E deficiency, replacement therapy may improve or stabilize the neuropathy.

INFLAMMATORY BOWEL DISEASE

Ulcerative colitis and Crohn's disease may be complicated by GBS, CIDP, generalized axonal sensory or sensorimotor polyneuropathy, small-fiber neuropathy, or mononeuropathy. These neuropathies may be autoimmune, nutritional (e.g., vitamin B_{12} deficiency), treatment related (e.g., metronidazole), or idiopathic in nature. An acute neuropathy with demyelination resembling GBS may occur, particularly in patients treated with tumor necrosis factor α blockers.

UREMIC NEUROPATHY

Approximately 60% of patients with renal failure develop a polyneuropathy characterized by length-dependent numbness, tingling, allodynia, and mild distal weakness. Rarely, a rapidly progressive weakness and sensory loss very similar to GBS can occur that improves with an increase in the intensity of renal dialysis or with transplantation. Mononeuropathies can also occur, the most common of which is carpal tunnel syndrome. Ischemic monomelic neuropathy (discussed later) can complicate arteriovenous shunts created in the arm for dialysis. EDx in uremic patients reveals features of a length-dependent, primarily axonal, sensorimotor polyneuropathy. Sural nerve biopsies demonstrate a loss of nerve fibers (particularly large myelinated nerve fibers), active axonal degeneration, and segmental and paranodal demyelination. The sensorimotor polyneuropathy can be stabilized by hemodialysis and improved with successful renal transplantation.

CHRONIC LIVER DISEASE

A generalized sensorimotor neuropathy characterized by numbness, tingling, and minor weakness in the distal aspects of primarily the lower limbs commonly occurs in patients with chronic liver failure. EDx studies are consistent with a sensory greater than motor axonopathy. Sural nerve biopsy reveals both segmental demyelination and axonal loss. It is not known if hepatic failure in isolation can cause peripheral neuropathy, as the majority of patients have liver disease secondary to other disorders, such as alcoholism or viral hepatitis, which can also cause neuropathy.

CRITICAL ILLNESS POLYNEUROPATHY

The most common causes of acute generalized weakness leading to admission to a medical intensive care unit (ICU) are GBS and myasthenia gravis (Chap. 47). However, weakness developing in critically ill patients while in the ICU is usually caused by critical illness polyneuropathy (CIP) or critical illness myopathy (CIM), or much less commonly, by prolonged neuromuscular blockade. From a clinical and EDx standpoint, it can be quite difficult to distinguish these disorders. Most specialists suggest that CIM is more common. Both CIM and CIP develop as a complication of sepsis and multiple organ failure. They usually present as an inability to wean a patient from a ventilator. A coexisting encephalopathy may limit the neurologic exam, in particular the sensory examination. Muscle stretch reflexes are absent or reduced.

Serum creatine kinase (CK) is usually normal; an elevated serum CK would point to CIM as opposed to CIP. NCS reveal absent or markedly reduced amplitudes of motor and sensory studies in CIP, while sensory studies are relatively preserved in CIM. Needle EMG usually reveals profuse positive sharp waves and fibrillation potentials, and it is not unusual in patients with severe weakness to be unable to recruit motor unit action potentials. The pathogenic basis of CIP is not known. Perhaps circulating toxins and metabolic abnormalities associated with sepsis and multiorgan failure impair axonal transport or mitochondrial function, leading to axonal degeneration.

LEPROSY (HANSEN DISEASE)

Leprosy, caused by the acid-fast bacteria *Mycobacterium leprae*, is the most common cause of peripheral neuropathy in Southeast Asia, Africa, and South America. Clinical manifestations range from tuberculoid leprosy at one end to lepromatous leprosy at the other end of the spectrum, with borderline leprosy in between. Neuropathies are most common in patients with borderline leprosy. Superficial cutaneous nerves of the ears and distal limbs are commonly affected. Mononeuropathies, multiple mononeuropathies, or a slowly progressive symmetric sensorimotor polyneuropathy may develop. Sensory NCS are usually absent in the lower limb and are reduced in amplitude in the arms. Motor NCS may demonstrate reduced amplitudes in affected nerves but occasionally can reveal demyelinating features. Leprosy is usually diagnosed by skin lesion biopsy. Nerve biopsy can also be diagnostic, particularly when there are no apparent skin lesions. The tuberculoid form is characterized by granulomas, and bacilli are not seen. In contrast, with lepromatous leprosy, large numbers of infiltrating bacilli, T_H2 lymphocytes, and organism-laden, foamy macrophages with minimal granulomatous infiltration are evident. The bacilli are best appreciated using the Fite stain, where they can be seen as red-staining rods often in clusters free in the endoneurium, within macrophages, or within Schwann cells.

Patients are generally treated with multiple drugs: dapsone, rifampin, and clofazimine. Other medications that are employed include thalidomide, pefloxacin, ofloxacin, sparfloxacin, minocycline, and clarithromycin. Patients are generally treated for 2 years. Treatment is sometimes complicated by the so-called reversal reaction, particularly in borderline leprosy. The reversal reaction can occur at any time during treatment and develops because of a shift to the tuberculoid end of the spectrum, with an increase in cellular immunity during treatment. The cellular response is upregulated as evidenced by an increased release of tumor necrosis factor α, interferon γ, and interleukin 2, with new granuloma formation. This can result in an exacerbation of the rash and the neuropathy as well as in appearance of new lesions. High-dose glucocorticoids blunt this adverse reaction and may be used prophylactically at treatment onset in high-risk patients. Erythema nodosum leprosum (ENL) is also treated with glucocorticoids or thalidomide.

LYME DISEASE

Lyme disease is caused by infection with *Borrelia burgdorferi*, a spirochete usually transmitted by the deer tick *Ixodes dammini*. Neurologic complications may develop during the second and third stages of infection. Facial neuropathy is most common and is bilateral in about half of cases, which is rare for idiopathic Bell's palsy. Involvement of nerves is frequently asymmetric. Some patients present with a polyradiculoneuropathy or multiple mononeuropathies. EDx is suggestive of a primary axonopathy. Nerve biopsies can reveal axonal degeneration with perivascular inflammation. Treatment is with antibiotics.

DIPHTHERITIC NEUROPATHY

Diphtheria is caused by the bacteria *Corynebacterium diphtheriae*. Infected individuals present with flulike symptoms of generalized myalgias, headache, fatigue, low-grade fever, and irritability within a week to 10 days of the exposure. About 20–70% of patients develop a peripheral neuropathy caused by a toxin released by the bacteria. Three to 4 weeks after infection, patients may note decreased sensation in their throat and begin to develop dysphagia, dysarthria, hoarseness, and blurred vision due to impaired accommodation. A generalized polyneuropathy may manifest 2 or 3 months following the initial infection, characterized by numbness, paresthesias, and weakness of the arms and legs and occasionally ventilatory failure. CSF protein can be elevated with or without lymphocytic pleocytosis. EDx suggests a diffuse axonal sensorimotor polyneuropathy. Antitoxin and antibiotics should be given within 48 h of symptom onset. Although early treatment reduces the incidence and severity of some complications (i.e., cardiomyopathy), it does not appear to alter the natural history of the associated peripheral neuropathy. The neuropathy usually resolves after several months.

HUMAN IMMUNODEFICIENCY VIRUS (HIV)

HIV infection can result in a variety of neurologic complications, including peripheral neuropathies. Approximately 20% of HIV-infected individuals develop a neuropathy either as a direct result of the virus itself, other associated viral infections (e.g., cytomegalovirus), or neurotoxicity secondary to antiviral medications (discussed later). The major presentations of peripheral neuropathy associated with HIV infection include (1) distal symmetric polyneuropathy (DSP), (2) inflammatory demyelinating polyneuropathy (including both GBS and CIDP), (3) multiple mononeuropathies (e.g., vasculitis, CMV-related), (4) polyradiculopathy (usually CMV-related), (5) autonomic neuropathy, and (6) sensory ganglionitis.

HIV-related distal symmetric polyneuropathy (DSP)

DSP is the most common form of peripheral neuropathy associated with HIV infection and usually is seen in patients with AIDS. It is characterized by numbness and painful paresthesias involving the distal extremities. The pathogenic basis for DSP is unknown but is not due to actual infection of the peripheral nerves. The neuropathy may be immune mediated, perhaps caused by the release of cytokines from surrounding inflammatory cells. Vitamin B_{12} deficiency may contribute in some instances but is not a major cause of most cases of DSP. Some antiretroviral agents (e.g., dideoxycytidine, dideoxyinosine, stavudine) are also neurotoxic and can cause a painful sensory neuropathy.

HIV-related inflammatory demyelinating polyradiculoneuropathy

Both AIDP and CIDP can occur as a complication of HIV infection. AIDP usually develops at the time of seroconversion, while CIDP can occur any time in the course of the infection. Clinical and EDx features are indistinguishable from idiopathic AIDP or CIDP (discussed in next chapter). In addition to elevated protein levels, lymphocytic pleocytosis is evident in the CSF, a finding that helps distinguish this HIV-associated polyradiculoneuropathy from idiopathic AIDP/CIDP.

HIV-related progressive polyradiculopathy

An acute, progressive lumbosacral polyradiculoneuropathy usually secondary to cytomegalovirus (CMV) infection can develop in patients with AIDS. Patients present with severe radicular pain, numbness, and weakness in the legs, which is usually asymmetric. CSF is abnormal, demonstrating an increased protein along with reduced glucose concentration and notably a neutrophilic pleocytosis. EDx studies reveal features of active axonal degeneration. The polyradiculoneuropathy may improve with antiviral therapy.

HIV-related multiple mononeuropathies

Multiple mononeuropathies can also develop in patients with HIV infection, usually in the context of AIDS. Weakness, numbness, paresthesias, and pain occur in the distribution of affected nerves. Nerve biopsies can reveal axonal degeneration with necrotizing vasculitis or perivascular inflammation. Glucocorticoid treatment is indicated for vasculitis directly due to HIV infection.

HIV-related sensory neuronopathy/ganglionopathy

Dorsal root ganglionitis is a very rare complication of HIV infection, and neuronopathy can be the presenting manifestation. Patients develop sensory ataxia similar to idiopathic sensory neuronopathy/ganglionopathy. NCS reveal reduced amplitudes or absence of SNAPs.

HERPES VARICELLA-ZOSTER VIRUS

Peripheral neuropathy from herpes varicella-zoster (HVZ) infection results from reactivation of latent virus or from a primary infection. Two-thirds of infections in adults are characterized by dermal zoster in which severe pain and paresthesias develop in a dermatomal region followed within a week or two by a vesicular rash in the same distribution. Weakness in muscles innervated by roots corresponding to the dermatomal distribution of skin lesions occurs in 5–30% of patients.

Approximately 25% of affected patients have continued pain (postherpetic neuralgia, or PHN). A large clinical trial demonstrated that vaccination against zoster reduces the incidence of HZ among vaccine recipients by 51% and reduces the incidence of PHN by 67%. Treatment of postherpetic neuralgia is symptomatic (Table 45-6).

CYTOMEGALOVIRUS

CMV can cause an acute lumbosacral polyradiculopathy and multiple mononeuropathies in patients with HIV infection and in other immune deficiency conditions.

EPSTEIN-BARR VIRUS

Epstein-Barr virus (EBV) infection has been associated with GBS, cranial neuropathies, mononeuropathy multiplex, brachial plexopathy, lumbosacral radiculoplexopathy, and sensory neuronopathies.

HEPATITIS VIRUSES

Hepatitis B and C can cause multiple mononeuropathies related to vasculitis, AIDP, or CIDP.

NEUROPATHIES ASSOCIATED WITH MALIGNANCY

Patients with malignancy can develop neuropathies due to (1) a direct effect of the cancer by invasion or compression of the nerves, (2) remote or paraneoplastic effect, (3) a toxic effect of treatment, or (4) as a consequence of immune compromise caused by immunosuppressive medications. The most common associated malignancy is lung cancer, but neuropathies also complicate carcinoma of the breast, ovaries, stomach, colon, rectum, and other organs, including the lymphoproliferative system.

PARANEOPLASTIC SENSORY NEURONOPATHY/GANGLIONOPATHY

Paraneoplastic encephalomyelitis/sensory neuronopathy (PEM/SN) usually complicates small cell lung carcinoma (Chap. 44). Patients usually present with numbness and paresthesias in the distal extremities that are often asymmetric. The onset can be acute or insidiously progressive. Prominent loss of proprioception leads to sensory ataxia. Weakness can be present, usually secondary to an associated myelitis, motor neuronopathy, or concurrent Lambert-Eaton myasthenic syndrome (LEMS). Many patients also develop confusion, memory loss, depression, hallucinations or seizures, or cerebellar ataxia. Polyclonal antineuronal antibodies (IgG) directed against a 35- to 40-kD protein or complex of proteins, the so-called Hu antigen, are found in the sera or CSF in the majority of patients with paraneoplastic PEM/SN. CSF may be normal or may demonstrate mild lymphocytic pleocytosis and elevated protein. PEM/SN is probably the result of antigenic similarity between proteins expressed in the tumor cells and neuronal cells, leading to an immune response directed against both cell types. Treatment of the underlying cancer generally does not affect the course of PEM/SN. However, occasional patients may improve following treatment of the tumor. Unfortunately, plasmapheresis, intravenous immunoglobulin, and immunosuppressive agents have not shown benefit.

NEUROPATHY SECONDARY TO TUMOR INFILTRATION

Malignant cells, in particular leukemia and lymphoma, can infiltrate cranial and peripheral nerves, leading to mononeuropathy, mononeuropathy multiplex, polyradiculopathy, plexopathy, or even a generalized symmetric distal or proximal and distal polyneuropathy. Neuropathy related to tumor infiltration is often painful; it can be the presenting manifestation of the cancer or the heralding symptom of a relapse. The neuropathy may improve with treatment of the underlying leukemia or lymphoma or with glucocorticoids.

NEUROPATHY AS A COMPLICATION OF BONE MARROW TRANSPLANTATION

Neuropathies may develop in patients who undergo bone marrow transplantation (BMT) because of the toxic effects of chemotherapy, radiation, infection, or an autoimmune response directed against the peripheral nerves. Peripheral neuropathy in BMT is often associated with graft-versus-host disease (GVHD). Chronic GVHD shares many features with a variety of autoimmune disorders, and it is possible that an immune-mediated response directed against peripheral nerves is responsible. Patients with chronic GVHD may develop cranial neuropathies, sensorimotor polyneuropathies, multiple mononeuropathies, and severe generalized peripheral neuropathies resembling AIDP or CIDP. The neuropathy may improve by increasing the intensity of immunosuppressive or immunomodulating therapy and resolution of the GVHD.

LYMPHOMA

Lymphomas may cause neuropathy by infiltration or direct compression of nerves or by a paraneoplastic process. The neuropathy can be purely sensory or motor, but most commonly is sensorimotor. The pattern of involvement may be symmetric, asymmetric, or multifocal, and the course may be acute, gradually progressive, or relapsing and remitting. EDx can be compatible with either an axonal or demyelinating process. CSF may reveal lymphocytic pleocytosis and an elevated protein. Nerve biopsy may demonstrate endoneurial inflammatory cells in both the infiltrative and the paraneoplastic etiologies. A monoclonal population of cells favors lymphomatous invasion. The neuropathy may respond to treatment of the underlying lymphoma or immunomodulating therapies.

MULTIPLE MYELOMA

Multiple myeloma (MM) usually presents in the fifth to seventh decade of life with fatigue, bone pain, anemia, and hypercalcemia. Clinical and EDx features of neuropathy occur in as many as 40% of patients. The most common pattern is that of a distal, axonal, sensory, or sensorimotor polyneuropathy. Less frequently, a chronic demyelinating polyradiculoneuropathy may develop (see POEMS, Chap. 46). MM can be complicated by amyloid polyneuropathy and should be considered in patients with painful paresthesias, loss of pinprick and temperature discrimination, and autonomic dysfunction (suggestive of a small-fiber neuropathy) and carpal tunnel syndrome. Expanding plasmacytomas can compress cranial nerves and spinal roots as well. A monoclonal protein, usually composed of γ or μ heavy chains or κ light chains, may be identified in the serum or urine. EDx usually shows reduced amplitudes with normal or only mildly abnormal distal latencies and conduction velocities. A superimposed median neuropathy at the wrist is common. Abdominal fat pad, rectal, or sural nerve biopsy can be performed to look for amyloid deposition. Unfortunately, the treatment of the underlying MM does not usually affect the course of the neuropathy.

NEUROPATHIES ASSOCIATED WITH MONOCLONAL GAMMOPATHY OF UNCERTAIN SIGNIFICANCE (SEE CHAP. 33)

Toxic neuropathies secondary to chemotherapy

Many of the commonly used chemotherapy agents can cause a toxic neuropathy (Table 45-7). The mechanisms by which these agents cause toxic neuropathies vary as can the specific type of neuropathy produced. The risk of developing a toxic neuropathy or more severe neuropathy appears to be greater in patients with a preexisting neuropathy (e.g., Charcot-Marie-Tooth disease, diabetic neuropathy) and those who also take other potentially neurotoxic drugs (e.g., nitrofurantoin, isoniazid, disulfiram, pyridoxine). Chemotherapeutic agents usually cause a sensory greater than motor length-dependent axonal neuropathy or neuronopathy/ganglionopathy.

TABLE 45-7

TOXIC NEUROPATHIES SECONDARY TO CHEMOTHERAPY

DRUG	MECHANISM OF NEUROTOXICITY	CLINICAL FEATURES	NERVE HISTOPATHOLOGY	EMG/NCS
Vinca alkaloids (vincristine, vinblastine, vindesine, vinorelbine)	Interfere with axonal microtubule assembly; impairs axonal transport	Symmetric, S-M, large-/small-fiber PN; autonomic symptoms common; infrequent cranial neuropathies	Axonal degeneration of myelinated and unmyelinated fibers; regenerating clusters, minimal segmental demyelination	Axonal sensorimotor PN; distal denervation on EMG; abnormal QST, particularly vibratory perception
Cisplatin	Preferential damage to dorsal root ganglia: ?binds to and cross-links DNA ?inhibits protein synthesis ?impairs axonal transport	Predominant large-fiber sensory neuronopathy; sensory ataxia	Loss of large > small myelinated and unmyelinated fibers; axonal degeneration with small clusters of regenerating fibers; secondary segmental demyelination	Low-amplitude or unobtainable SNAPs with normal CMAPs and EMG; abnormal QST, particularly vibratory perception
Taxanes (paclitaxel, docetaxel)	Promotes axonal microtubule assembly; interferes with axonal transport	Symmetric, predominantly sensory, PN; large-fiber modalities affected more than small-fiber	Loss of large > small myelinated and unmyelinated fibers; axonal degeneration with small clusters of regenerating fibers; secondary segmental demyelination	Axonal sensorimotor PN; distal denervation on EMG; abnormal QST, particularly vibratory perception

(continued)

TABLE 45-7

TOXIC NEUROPATHIES SECONDARY TO CHEMOTHERAPY (*CONTINUED*)

DRUG	MECHANISM OF NEUROTOXICITY	CLINICAL FEATURES	NERVE HISTOPATHOLOGY	EMG/NCS
Suramin Axonal PN	Unknown; ?inhibition of neurotrophic growth factor binding; ?neuronal lysosomal storage	Symmetric, length-dependent, sensory-predominant, PN	None described	Abnormalities consistent with an axonal S-M PN
Demyelinating PN	Unknown; ?immunomodulating effects	Subacute, S-M PN with diffuse proximal and distal weakness; areflexia; increased CSF protein	Loss of large and small myelinated fibers with primary demyelination and secondary axonal degeneration; occasional epi- and endoneurial inflammatory cell infiltrates	Features suggestive of an acquired demyelinating sensorimotor PN (e.g., slow CVs, prolonged distal latencies and F-wave latencies, conduction block, temporal dispersion)
Ara-C	Unknown; ?selective Schwann cell toxicity; ?immunomodulating effects	GBS-like syndrome; pure sensory neuropathy; brachial plexopathy	Loss of myelinated nerve fibers; axonal degeneration; segmental demyelination; no inflammation	Axonal, demyelinating, or mixed S-M PN; denervation on EMG
Etoposide (VP-16)	Unknown; ?selective dorsal root ganglia toxicity	Length-dependent, sensory predominant PN; autonomic neuropathy	None described	Abnormalities consistent with an axonal S-M PN
Bortezomib (Velcade)	Unknown	Length-dependent, sensory, predominantly small-fiber, PN	Not reported	Abnormalities consistent with an axonal sensory neuropathy with early small-fiber involvement (abnormal autonomic studies)

Abbreviations: CSF, cerebrospinal fluid; CVs, conduction velocities; EMG, electromyography; GBS, Guillain-Barré syndrome; NCS, nerve conduction studies; PN, polyneuropathy; QST, quantitative sensory testing; S-M, sensorimotor.
Source: From AA Amato, J Russell: *Neuromuscular Disease*. New York, McGraw-Hill, 2008.

OTHER TOXIC NEUROPATHIES

Neuropathies can develop as complications of toxic effects of various drugs and other environmental exposures (Table 45-8). The more common neuropathies associated with these agents are discussed here.

CHLOROQUINE AND HYDROXYCHLOROQUINE

Chloroquine and hydroxychloroquine can cause a toxic myopathy characterized by slowly progressive, painless, proximal weakness and atrophy, which is worse in the legs than the arms. In addition, neuropathy can also develop with or without the myopathy leading to sensory loss and distal weakness. The "neuromyopathy" usually appears in patients taking 500 mg daily for a year or more but has been reported with doses as low as 200 mg/d. Serum CK levels are usually elevated due to the superimposed myopathy. NCS reveal mild slowing of motor and sensory nerve conduction velocities with a mild to moderate reduction in the amplitudes, although NCS may be normal in patients with only the myopathy. EMG demonstrates myopathic muscle action potentials (MUAPs), increased insertional activity in the form of positive sharp waves, fibrillation potentials, and occasionally myotonic potentials, particularly in the proximal muscles. Neurogenic MUAPs and reduced recruitment are found in more distal muscles. Nerve biopsy demonstrates autophagic vacuoles within Schwann cells. Vacuoles may also be evident in muscle biopsies. The pathogenic basis of the neuropathy is not known but may be related to the amphiphilic properties of the drug. These agents contain both hydrophobic and hydrophilic regions that allow them to interact with the anionic phospholipids of cell membranes and organelles. The drug-lipid complexes may be resistant to digestion by lysosomal enzymes, leading to the

TABLE 45-8

TOXIC NEUROPATHIES

DRUG	MECHANISM OF NEUROTOXICITY	CLINICAL FEATURES	NERVE HISTOPATHOLOGY	EMG/NCS
Misonidazole	Unknown	Painful paresthesias and loss of large- and small-fiber sensory modalities and sometimes distal weakness in length-dependent pattern	Axonal degeneration of large myelinated fibers; axonal swellings; segmental demyelination	Low-amplitude or unobtainable SNAPs with normal or only slightly reduced CMAPs amplitudes
Metronidazole	Unknown	Painful paresthesias and loss of large- and small-fiber sensory modalities and sometimes distal weakness in length-dependent pattern	Axonal degeneration	Low-amplitude or unobtainable SNAPs with normal CMAPs
Chloroquine and hydroxychloroquine	Amphiphilic properties may lead to drug-lipid complexes that are indigestible and result in accumulation of autophagic vacuoles	Loss of large- and small-fiber sensory modalities and distal weakness in length-dependent pattern; superimposed myopathy may lead to proximal weakness	Axonal degeneration with autophagic vacuoles in nerves as well as muscle fibers	Low-amplitude or unobtainable SNAPs with normal or reduced CMAPs amplitudes; distal denervation on EMG; irritability and myopathic-appearing MUAPs proximally in patients with superimposed toxic myopathy
Amiodarone	Amphiphilic properties may lead to drug-lipid complexes that are indigestible and result in accumulation of autophagic vacuoles	Paresthesias and pain with loss of large- and small-fiber sensory modalities and distal weakness in length-dependent pattern; superimposed myopathy may lead to proximal weakness	Axonal degeneration and segmental demyelination with myeloid inclusions in nerves and muscle fibers	Low-amplitude or unobtainable SNAPs with normal or reduced CMAPs amplitudes; can also have prominent slowing of CVs; distal denervation on EMG; irritability and myopathic-appearing MUAPs proximally in patients with superimposed toxic myopathy
Colchicine	Inhibits polymerization of tubulin in microtubules and impairs axoplasmic flow	Numbness and paresthesias with loss of large-fiber modalities in a length-dependent fashion; superimposed myopathy may lead to proximal in addition to distal weakness	Nerve biopsy demonstrates axonal degeneration; muscle biopsy reveals fibers with vacuoles	Low-amplitude or unobtainable SNAPs with normal or reduced CMAPs amplitudes; irritability and myopathic-appearing MUAPs proximally in patients with superimposed toxic myopathy
Podophyllin	Binds to microtubules and impairs axoplasmic flow	Sensory loss, tingling, muscle weakness, and diminished muscle stretch reflexes in length-dependent pattern; autonomic neuropathy	Axonal degeneration	Low-amplitude or unobtainable SNAPs with normal or reduced CMAPs amplitudes
Thalidomide	Unknown	Numbness, tingling, and burning pain and weakness in a length-dependent pattern	Axonal degeneration; autopsy studies reveal degeneration of dorsal root ganglia	Low-amplitude or unobtainable SNAPs with normal or reduced CMAPs amplitudes

(*continued*)

TABLE 45-8

TOXIC NEUROPATHIES (*CONTINUED*)

DRUG	MECHANISM OF NEUROTOXICITY	CLINICAL FEATURES	NERVE HISTOPATHOLOGY	EMG/NCS
Disulfiram	Accumulation of neurofilaments and impaired axoplasmic flow	Numbness, tingling, and burning pain in a length-dependent pattern	Axonal degeneration with accumulation of neurofilaments in the axons	Low-amplitude or unobtainable SNAPs with normal or reduced CMAPs amplitudes
Dapsone	Unknown	Distal weakness that may progress to proximal muscles; sensory loss	Axonal degeneration and segmental demyelination	Low-amplitude or unobtainable CMAPs with normal or reduced SNAP amplitudes
Leflunomide	Unknown	Paresthesias and numbness in a length-dependent pattern	Unknown	Low-amplitude or unobtainable SNAPs with normal or reduced CMAPs amplitudes
Nitrofurantoin	Unknown	Numbness, painful paresthesias, and severe weakness that may resemble GBS	Axonal degeneration; autopsy studies reveal degeneration of dorsal root ganglia and anterior horn cells	Low-amplitude or unobtainable SNAPs with normal or reduced CMAPs amplitudes
Pyridoxine (vitamin B_6)	Unknown	Dysesthesias and sensory ataxia; impaired large-fiber sensory modalities on examination	Marked loss of sensory axons and cell bodies in dorsal root ganglia	Reduced amplitudes or absent SNAPs
Isoniazid	Inhibits pyridoxal phosphokinase leading to pyridoxine deficiency	Dysesthesias and sensory ataxia; impaired large-fiber sensory modalities on examination	Marked loss of sensory axons and cell bodies in dorsal root ganglia and degeneration of the dorsal columns	Reduced amplitudes or absent SNAPs and to lesser extent CMAPs
Ethambutol	Unknown	Numbness with loss of large-fiber modalities on examination	Axonal degeneration	Reduced amplitudes or absent SNAPs
Antinucleosides	Unknown	Dysesthesia and sensory ataxia; impaired large-fiber sensory modalities on examination	Axonal degeneration	Reduced amplitudes or absent SNAPs
Phenytoin	Unknown	Numbness with loss of large-fiber modalities on examination	Axonal degeneration and segmental demyelination	Low-amplitude or unobtainable SNAPs with normal or reduced CMAPs amplitudes
Lithium	Unknown	Numbness with loss of large-fiber modalities on examination	Axonal degeneration	Low-amplitude or unobtainable SNAPs with normal or reduced CMAPs amplitudes
Acrylamide	Unknown; may be caused by impaired axonal transport	Numbness with loss of large-fiber modalities on examination; sensory ataxia; mild distal weakness	Degeneration of sensory axons in peripheral nerves and posterior columns, spinocerebellar tracts, mammillary bodies, optic tracts, and corticospinal tracts in the CNS	Low-amplitude or unobtainable SNAPs with normal or reduced CMAPs amplitudes

TABLE 45-8

TOXIC NEUROPATHIES (*CONTINUED*)

DRUG	MECHANISM OF NEUROTOXICITY	CLINICAL FEATURES	NERVE HISTOPATHOLOGY	EMG/NCS
Carbon disulfide	Unknown	Length-dependent numbness and tingling with mild distal weakness	Axonal swellings with accumulation of neurofilaments	Low-amplitude or unobtainable SNAPs with normal or reduced CMAPs amplitudes
Ethylene oxide	Unknown; may act as alkylating agent and bind DNA	Length-dependent numbness and tingling; may have mild distal weakness	Axonal degeneration	Low-amplitude or unobtainable SNAPs with normal or reduced CMAPs amplitudes
Organophosphates	Bind and inhibit neuropathy target esterase	Early features are those of neuromuscular blockade with generalized weakness; later axonal sensorimotor PN ensues	Axonal degeneration along with degeneration of gracile fasciculus and corticospinal tracts	Early: repetitive firing of CMAPs and decrement with repetitive nerve stimulation; late: axonal sensorimotor PN
Hexacarbons	Unknown; may lead to covalent cross-linking between neurofilaments	Acute, severe sensorimotor PN that may resemble GBS	Axonal degeneration and giant axons swollen with neurofilaments	Features of a mixed axonal and/or demyelinating sensorimotor axonal PN—reduced amplitudes, prolonged distal latencies, conduction block, and slowing of CVs
Lead	Unknown; may interfere with mitochondria	Encephalopathy; motor neuropathy (often resembles radial neuropathy with wrist and finger drop); autonomic neuropathy; bluish-black discoloration of gums	Axonal degeneration of motor axons	Reduction of CMAP amplitudes with active denervation on EMG
Mercury	Unknown; may combine with sulfhydryl groups	Abdominal pain and nephrotic syndrome; encephalopathy; ataxia; paresthesias	Axonal degeneration; degeneration of dorsal root ganglia, calcarine, and cerebellar cortex	Low-amplitude or unobtainable SNAPs with normal or reduced CMAPs amplitudes
Thallium	Unknown	Encephalopathy; painful sensory symptoms; mild loss of vibration; distal or generalized weakness may also develop; autonomic neuropathy; alopecia	Axonal degeneration	Low-amplitude or unobtainable SNAPs with normal or reduced CMAPs amplitudes
Arsenic	Unknown; may combine with sulfhydryl groups	Abdominal discomfort, burning pain and paresthesias; generalized weakness; autonomic insufficiency; can resemble GBS	Axonal degeneration	Low-amplitude or unobtainable SNAPs with normal or reduced CMAPs amplitudes; may have demyelinating features: prolonged distal latencies and slowing of CVs
Gold	Unknown	Distal paresthesias and reduction of all sensory modalities	Axonal degeneration	Low-amplitude or unobtainable SNAPs

Abbreviations: CMAP, compound motor action potential; CVs, conduction velocities; EMG, electromyography; GBS, Guillain-Barré syndrome; MUAP, muscle action potential; NCS, nerve conduction studies; PN, polyneuropathy; S-M, sensorimotor; SNAP, sensory nerve action potential.
Source: From AA Amato, J Russell: *Neuromuscular Disease*. New York, McGraw-Hill, 2008.

formation of autophagic vacuoles filled with myeloid debris that may in turn cause degeneration of nerves and muscle fibers. The signs and symptoms of the neuropathy and myopathy are usually reversible following discontinuation of medication.

AMIODARONE

Amiodarone can cause a neuromyopathy similar to chloroquine and hydroxychloroquine. The neuromyopathy typically appears after patients have taken the medication for 2–3 years. Nerve biopsy demonstrates a combination of segmental demyelination and axonal loss. Electron microscopy reveals lamellar or dense inclusions in Schwann cells, pericytes, and endothelial cells. The inclusions in muscle and nerve biopsies have persisted as long as 2 years following discontinuation of the medication.

COLCHICINE

Colchicine can also cause a neuromyopathy. Patients usually present with proximal weakness and numbness and tingling in the distal extremities. EDx reveals features of an axonal polyneuropathy. Muscle biopsy reveals a vacuolar myopathy, while sensory nerves demonstrate axonal degeneration. Colchicine inhibits the polymerization of tubulin into microtubules. The disruption of the microtubules probably leads to defective intracellular movement of important proteins, nutrients, and waste products in muscle and nerves.

THALIDOMIDE

Thalidomide is an immunomodulating agent used to treat multiple myeloma, GVHD, leprosy, and other autoimmune disorders. Thalidomide is associated with severe teratogenic effects as well as peripheral neuropathy that can be dose-limiting. Patients develop numbness, painful tingling, and burning discomfort in the feet and hands and less commonly muscle weakness and atrophy. Even after stopping the drug for 4–6 years, as many as 50% patients continue to have significant symptoms. NCS demonstrate reduced amplitudes or complete absence of sensory nerve action potentials (SNAPs), with preserved conduction velocities when obtainable. Motor NCS are usually normal. Nerve biopsy reveals a loss of large-diameter myelinated fibers and axonal degeneration. Degeneration of dorsal root ganglion cells has been reported at autopsy.

PYRIDOXINE (VITAMIN B_6) TOXICITY

Pyridoxine is an essential vitamin that serves as a coenzyme for transamination and decarboxylation. However, at high doses (116 mg/d), patients can develop a severe sensory neuropathy with dysesthesias and sensory ataxia. NCS reveal absent or markedly reduced SNAP amplitudes with relatively preserved CMAPs. Nerve biopsy reveals axonal loss of fiber at all diameters. Loss of dorsal root ganglion cells with subsequent degeneration of both the peripheral and central sensory tracts have been reported in animal models.

ISONIAZID

One of the most common side effects of isoniazid (INH) is peripheral neuropathy. Standard doses of INH (3–5 mg/kg per d) are associated with a 2% incidence of neuropathy, while neuropathy develops in at least 17% of patients taking in excess of 6 mg/kg per d. The elderly, malnourished, and "slow acetylators" are at increased risk for developing the neuropathy. INH inhibits pyridoxal phosphokinase, resulting in pyridoxine deficiency and the neuropathy. Prophylactic administration of pyridoxine 100 mg/d can prevent the neuropathy from developing.

ANTIRETROVIRAL AGENTS

The nucleoside analogues zalcitabine (dideoxycytidine or ddC), didanosine (dideoxyinosine or ddI), stavudine (d4T), lamivudine (3TC), and antiretroviral nucleoside reverse transcriptase inhibitor (NRTI) are used to treat HIV infection. One of the major dose-limiting side effects of these medications is a predominantly sensory, length-dependent, symmetrically painful neuropathy. Zalcitabine (ddC) is the most extensively studied of the nucleoside analogues and at doses greater than 0.18 mg/kg per d is associated with a subacute onset of severe burning and lancinating pains in the feet and hands. NCS reveal decreased amplitudes of the SNAPs with normal motor studies. The nucleoside analogues inhibit mitochondrial DNA polymerase, which is the suspected pathogenic basis for the neuropathy. Because of a "coasting effect," patients can continue to worsen even 2–3 weeks after stopping the medication. Following dose reduction, improvement in the neuropathy is seen in most patients after several months (mean time about 10 weeks).

HEXACARBONS (*n*-HEXANE, METHYL *n*-BUTYL KETONE)/GLUE SNIFFER'S NEUROPATHY

n-Hexane and methyl *n*-butyl ketone are water-insoluble industrial organic solvents that are also present in some glues. Exposure through inhalation, accidentally or intentionally (glue sniffing), or through skin absorption can lead to a profound subacute sensory and motor polyneuropathy. NCS demonstrate decreased amplitudes of the SNAPs and CMAPs with slightly slow CVs. Nerve biopsy reveals a loss of myelinated fibers and giant axons that are filled with 10-nm neurofilaments. Hexacarbon exposure leads to covalent cross-linking between axonal neurofilaments that result in their aggregation, impaired axonal transport, swelling of the axons, and eventual axonal degeneration.

LEAD

Lead neuropathy is uncommon, but it can be seen in children who accidentally ingest lead-based paints in older buildings and in industrial workers exposed to lead-containing products. The most common presentation of lead poisoning is an encephalopathy; however, symptoms and signs of a primarily motor neuropathy can also occur. The neuropathy is characterized by an insidious and progressive onset of weakness usually beginning in the arms, in particular involving the wrist and finger extensors, resembling a radial neuropathy. Sensation is generally preserved; however, the autonomic nervous system can be affected. Laboratory investigation can reveal a microcytic hypochromic anemia with basophilic stippling of erythrocytes, an elevated serum lead level, and an elevated serum coproporphyrin level. A 24-h urine collection demonstrates elevated levels of lead excretion. The NCS may reveal reduced CMAP amplitudes, while the SNAPs are typically normal. The pathogenic basis may be related to abnormal porphyrin metabolism. The most important principle of management is to remove the source of the exposure. Chelation therapy with calcium disodium ethylenediaminetetraacetic acid (EDTA), British anti-Lewisite (BAL), and penicillamine also demonstrates variable efficacy.

MERCURY

Mercury toxicity may occur as a result of exposure to either organic or inorganic mercurials. Mercury poisoning presents with paresthesias in hands and feet that progress proximally and may involve the face and tongue. Motor weakness can also develop. CNS symptoms often overshadow the neuropathy. EDx shows features of a primarily axonal sensorimotor polyneuropathy. The primary site of neuromuscular pathology appears to be the dorsal root ganglia. The mainstay of treatment is removing the source of exposure.

THALLIUM

Thallium can exist in a monovalent or trivalent form and is primarily used as a rodenticide. The toxic neuropathy usually manifests as burning paresthesias of the feet, abdominal pain, and vomiting. Increased thirst, sleep disturbances, and psychotic behavior may be noted. Within the first week, patients develop pigmentation of the hair, an acne-like rash in the malar area of the face, and hyperreflexia. By the second and third week, autonomic instability with labile heart rate and blood pressure may be seen. Hyporeflexia and alopecia also occur but may not be evident until the third or fourth week following exposure. With severe intoxication, proximal weakness and involvement of the cranial nerves can occur. Some patients require mechanical ventilation due to respiratory muscle involvement. The lethal dose of thallium is variable, ranging from 8 to 15 mg/kg body weight. Death can result in less than 48 h following a particularly large dose. NCS demonstrate features of a primarily axonal sensorimotor polyneuropathy. With acute intoxication, potassium ferric ferrocyanide II may be effective in preventing absorption of thallium from the gut. However, there may be no benefit once thallium has been absorbed. Unfortunately, chelating agents are not very efficacious. Adequate diuresis is essential to help eliminate thallium from the body without increasing tissue availability from the serum.

ARSENIC

Arsenic is another heavy metal that can cause a toxic sensorimotor polyneuropathy. The neuropathy manifests 5–10 days after ingestion of arsenic and progresses for several weeks, sometimes mimicking GBS. The presenting symptoms are typically an abrupt onset of abdominal discomfort, nausea, vomiting, pain, and diarrhea followed within several days by burning pain in the feet and hands. Examination of the skin can be helpful in the diagnosis as the loss of the superficial epidermal layer results in patchy regions of increased or decreased pigmentation on the skin several weeks after an acute exposure or with chronic low levels of ingestion. Mee's lines, which are transverse lines at the base of the fingernails and toenails, do not become evident until 1 or 2 months after the exposure. Multiple Mee's lines may be seen in patients with long fingernails who have had chronic exposure to arsenic. Mee's lines are not specific for arsenic toxicity as they can also be seen following thallium poisoning. Because arsenic is cleared from blood rapidly, the serum concentration of arsenic is not diagnostically helpful. However, arsenic levels are increased in the urine, hair, and fingernails of patients exposed to arsenic. Anemia with stippling of erythrocytes is common, and occasionally pancytopenia and aplastic anemia can develop. Increased CSF protein levels without pleocytosis can be seen; this can lead to misdiagnosis as GBS. NCS are usually suggestive of an axonal sensorimotor polyneuropathy; however, demyelinating features can be present. Chelation therapy with BAL has yielded inconsistent results; therefore, it is not generally recommended.

NUTRITIONAL NEUROPATHIES

COBALAMIN (VITAMIN B_{12})

Pernicious anemia is the most common cause of cobalamin deficiency. Other causes include dietary avoidance (vegetarians), gastrectomy, gastric bypass surgery, inflammatory bowel disease, pancreatic insufficiency, bacterial overgrowth, and possibly histamine-2 blockers and proton-pump inhibitors. An underappreciated cause of cobalamin deficiency is food-cobalamin malabsorption. This typically occurs in older individuals and results from an inability to adequately absorb cobalamin in food protein. No apparent cause of deficiency is identified in a significant number of patients with cobalamin deficiency. The use of nitrous oxide as an anesthetic agent or from recreational use can produce acute cobalamin deficiency neuropathy and subacute combined degeneration.

Complaints of numb hands typically appear before lower extremity paresthesias are noted. A preferential large-fiber sensory loss affecting proprioception and vibration with sparing of small-fiber modalities is present; an unsteady gait reflects sensory ataxia. These features, coupled with diffuse hyperreflexia and absent Achilles reflexes, should always focus attention on the possibility of cobalamin deficiency. Optic atrophy and, in severe cases, behavioral changes ranging from mild irritability and forgetfulness to severe dementia and frank psychosis may appear. The full clinical picture of subacute combined degeneration is uncommon. CNS manifestations, especially pyramidal tract signs, may be missing, and in fact some patients may only exhibit symptoms of peripheral neuropathy.

EDx shows an axonal sensorimotor neuropathy. CNS involvement produces abnormal somatosensory and visual evoked potential latencies. The diagnosis is confirmed by finding reduced serum cobalamin levels. In up to 40% of patients, anemia and macrocytosis are lacking. Serum methylmalonic acid and homocysteine, the metabolites that accumulate when cobalamin-dependent reactions are blocked, are elevated. Antibodies to intrinsic factor are present in approximately 60%, and antiparietal cell antibodies in about 90%, of individuals with pernicious anemia.

Cobalamin deficiency can be treated with various regimens of cobalamin. One typical regimen consists of 1000 μg cyanocobalamin IM weekly for 1 month and monthly thereafter. Patients with food cobalamin malabsorption can absorb free cobalamin and therefore can be treated with oral cobalamin supplementation. An oral cobalamin dose of 1000 μg per day should be sufficient. Treatment for cobalamin deficiency usually does not completely reverse the clinical manifestations, and at least 50% of patients exhibit some permanent neurologic deficit.

THIAMINE DEFICIENCY

Thiamine (vitamin B_1) deficiency is an uncommon cause of peripheral neuropathy in developed countries. It is now most often seen as a consequence of chronic alcohol abuse, recurrent vomiting, total parenteral nutrition, and bariatric surgery. Thiamine deficiency polyneuropathy can occur in normal, healthy young adults who do not abuse alcohol but who engage in inappropriately restrictive diets. Thiamine is water-soluble. It is present in most animal and plant tissues, but the greatest sources are unrefined cereal grains, wheat germ, yeast, soybean flour, and pork. Beriberi means "I can't, I can't" in Singhalese, the language of natives of what was once part of the Dutch East Indies (now Sri Lanka). *Dry beriberi* refers to neuropathic symptoms. The term *wet beriberi* is used when cardiac manifestations predominate (in reference to edema). Beriberi was relatively uncommon until the late 1800s when it became widespread among people for whom rice was a dietary mainstay. This epidemic was due to a new technique of processing rice that removed the germ from the rice shaft, rendering the so-called polished rice deficient in thiamine and other essential nutrients.

Symptoms of neuropathy follow prolonged deficiency. These begin with mild sensory loss and/or burning dysesthesias in the toes and feet and aching and cramping in the lower legs. Pain may be the predominant symptom. With progression, patients develop features of a nonspecific generalized polyneuropathy, with distal sensory loss in the feet and hands.

Blood and urine assays for thiamine are not reliable for diagnosis of deficiency. Erythrocyte transketolase activity and the percentage increase in activity (in vitro) following the addition of thiamine pyrophosphate (TPP) may be more accurate and reliable. EDx shows nonspecific findings of an axonal sensorimotor polyneuropathy. When a diagnosis of thiamine deficiency is made or suspected, thiamine replacement should be provided until proper nutrition is restored. Thiamine is usually given intravenously or intramuscularly at a dose of 100 mg/d. Although cardiac manifestations show a striking response to thiamine replacement, neurologic improvement is usually more variable and less dramatic.

VITAMIN E DEFICIENCY

The term *vitamin E* is usually used for α-tocopherol, the most active of the four main types of vitamin E. Because vitamin E is present in animal fat, vegetable oils, and various grains, deficiency is usually due to factors other than insufficient intake. Vitamin E deficiency usually occurs secondary to lipid malabsorption or in uncommon disorders of vitamin E transport. One hereditary disorder is abetalipoproteinemia, a rare autosomal dominant disorder characterized by steatorrhea, pigmentary retinopathy, acanthocytosis, and progressive ataxia. Patients with cystic fibrosis may also have vitamin E deficiency secondary to steatorrhea. There are genetic forms of isolated vitamin E deficiency not associated with lipid malabsorption. Vitamin E deficiency may also occur as a consequence of various cholestatic and hepatobiliary disorders as well as short-bowel syndromes resulting from the surgical treatment of intestinal disorders.

Clinical features may not appear until many years after the onset of deficiency. The onset of symptoms tends to be insidious, and progression is slow. The main clinical features are spinocerebellar ataxia and polyneuropathy, thus resembling Friedreich ataxia or other spinocerebellar ataxias. Patients manifest progressive ataxia and signs of posterior column dysfunction, such as impaired joint position and vibratory sensation. Because of the polyneuropathy, there is hyporeflexia, but plantar responses may be extensor as a result of the spinal cord involvement. Other neurologic manifestations may include ophthalmoplegia, pigmented retinopathy, night blindness, dysarthria, pseudoathetosis, dystonia, and tremor. Vitamin E deficiency may present as an isolated polyneuropathy, but this is very rare. The yield of checking serum vitamin E levels in patients with isolated polyneuropathy is extremely low, and this test should not be part of routine practice.

Diagnosis is made by measuring α-tocopherol levels in the serum. EDx shows features of an axonal neuropathy. Treatment is replacement with oral vitamin E, but high doses are not needed. For patients with isolated vitamin E deficiency, treatment consists of 1500–6000 IU/d in divided doses.

VITAMIN B_6 DEFICIENCY

Vitamin B_6, or pyridoxine, can produce neuropathic manifestations from both deficiency and toxicity. Vitamin B_6 toxicity was discussed earlier. Vitamin B_6 deficiency is most commonly seen in patients treated with isoniazid or hydralazine. The polyneuropathy of vitamin B_6 is nonspecific, manifesting as a generalized axonal sensorimotor polyneuropathy. Vitamin B_6 deficiency can be detected by direct assay. Vitamin B_6 supplementation with 50–100 mg/d is suggested for patients being treated with isoniazid or hydralazine. This same dose is appropriate for replacement in cases of nutritional deficiency.

PELLAGRA (NIACIN DEFICIENCY)

Pellagra is produced by deficiency of niacin. Although pellagra may be seen in alcoholics, this disorder has essentially been eradicated in most Western countries by means of enriching bread with niacin. Nevertheless, pellagra continues to be a problem in a number of underdeveloped regions, particularly in Asia and Africa, where corn is the main source of carbohydrate. Neurologic manifestations are variable; abnormalities can develop in the brain and spinal cord as well as peripheral nerves. When peripheral nerves are involved, the neuropathy is usually mild and resembles beriberi. Treatment is with niacin 40–250 mg/d.

COPPER DEFICIENCY

A syndrome that has only recently been described is myeloneuropathy secondary to copper deficiency. Most patients present with lower limb paresthesias, weakness, spasticity, and gait difficulties. Large-fiber sensory function is impaired, reflexes are brisk, and plantar responses are extensor. In some cases, light touch and pinprick sensation are affected, and nerve conduction studies indicate sensorimotor axonal polyneuropathy in addition to myelopathy.

Hematologic abnormalities are a known complication of copper deficiency; these can include microcytic anemia, neutropenia, and occasionally pancytopenia. Because copper is absorbed in the stomach and proximal jejunum, many cases of copper deficiency are in the setting of prior gastric surgery. Excess zinc is an established cause of copper deficiency. Zinc upregulates enterocyte production of metallothionine, which results in decreased absorption of copper. Excessive dietary zinc supplements or denture cream containing zinc can produce this clinical picture. Other potential causes of copper deficiency include malnutrition, prematurity, total parenteral nutrition, and ingestion of copper chelating agents.

Following oral or IV copper replacement, some patients show neurologic improvement, but this may take many months or not occur at all. Replacement consists of oral copper sulfate or gluconate 2 mg one to three times a day. If oral copper replacement is not effective, elemental copper in the copper sulfate or copper chloride forms can be given as 2 mg IV daily for 3–5 days, then weekly for 1–2 months until copper levels normalize. Thereafter, oral daily copper therapy can be resumed. In contrast to the neurologic manifestations, most of the hematologic indices completely normalize in response to copper replacement therapy.

NEUROPATHY ASSOCIATED WITH GASTRIC SURGERY

Polyneuropathy may occur following gastric surgery for ulcer, cancer, or weight reduction. This usually occurs in the context of rapid, significant weight loss and recurrent, protracted vomiting. The clinical picture is one of acute or subacute sensory loss and weakness. Neuropathy following weight loss surgery usually occurs in the first several months after surgery. Weight reduction surgical procedures include gastrojejunostomy, gastric stapling, vertical banded gastroplasty, and gastrectomy with Roux-en-Y anastomosis. The initial manifestations are usually numbness and paresthesias in the feet. In many cases, no specific nutritional deficiency factor is identified.

Management consists of parenteral vitamin supplementation, especially including thiamine. Improvement has been observed following supplementation, parenteral nutritional support, and reversal of the surgical bypass. The duration and severity of deficits before identification and treatment of neuropathy are important predictors of final outcome.

CRYPTOGENIC (IDIOPATHIC) SENSORY AND SENSORIMOTOR POLYNEUROPATHY

CSPN is a diagnosis of exclusion, established after a careful medical, family, and social history; neurologic examination; and directed laboratory testing. Despite extensive evaluation, the cause of polyneuropathy in as many as 50% of all patients is idiopathic. CSPN should be considered a distinct diagnostic subset of peripheral neuropathy. The onset of CSPN is predominantly in the sixth and seventh decades. Patients complain of distal numbness, tingling, and often burning pain that invariably begins in the feet and may eventually involve the fingers and hands. Patients exhibit a distal sensory loss to pinprick, touch, and vibration in the toes and feet, and occasionally in the fingers. It is uncommon to see significant proprioception deficits, even though patients may complain of gait unsteadiness. However, tandem gait may be abnormal in a minority of cases. Neither subjective nor objective evidence of weakness is a prominent feature. Most patients have evidence of both large- and small-fiber loss on neurologic exam and EDx. Approximately 10% of patients have only evidence of small-fiber involvement. The ankle muscle stretch reflex is frequently absent, but in cases with predominantly small-fiber loss, this may be preserved. The EDx findings range from isolated sensory nerve action potential abnormalities (usually with loss of amplitude), to evidence for an axonal sensorimotor neuropathy, to a completely normal study (if primarily small fibers are involved). Therapy primarily involves the control of neuropathic pain (Table 45-6) if present. These drugs should not be used if the patient has only numbness and tingling but no pain.

Although no treatment is available that can reverse an idiopathic distal peripheral neuropathy, the prognosis is good. Progression often does not occur or is minimal, with sensory symptoms and signs progressing proximally up to the knees and elbows. The disorder does not lead to significant motor disability over time. The relatively benign course of this disorder should be explained to patients.

MONONEUROPATHIES/PLEXOPATHIES/RADICULOPATHIES

MEDIAN NEUROPATHY

CTS is a compression of the median nerve in the carpal tunnel at the wrist. The median nerve enters the hand through the carpal tunnel by coursing under the transverse carpal ligament. The symptoms of CTS consist of numbness and paresthesias variably in the thumb, index, middle, and half of the ring finger. At times, the paresthesias can include the entire hand and extend into the forearm or upper arm or can be isolated to one or two fingers. Pain is another common symptom and can be located in the hand and forearm and, at times, in the proximal arm. CTS is common and often misdiagnosed as thoracic outlet syndrome. The signs of CTS are decreased sensation in the median nerve distribution; reproduction of the sensation of tingling when a percussion hammer is tapped over the wrist (Tinel's sign) or the wrist is flexed for 30–60 s (Phalen's sign); and weakness of thumb opposition and abduction. EDx is extremely sensitive and shows slowing of sensory and, to a lesser extent, motor median potentials across the wrist. Treatment options consist of avoidance of precipitating activities; control of underlying systemic-associated conditions if present; nonsteroidal anti-inflammatory medications; neutral (volar) position wrist splints, especially for night use; glucocorticoid/anesthetic injection into the carpal tunnel; and surgical decompression by dividing the transverse carpal ligament. The surgical option should be considered if there is a poor response to nonsurgical treatments; if there is thenar muscle atrophy and/or weakness; and if there are significant denervation potentials on EMG.

Other proximal median neuropathies are very uncommon and include the pronator teres syndrome and anterior interosseous neuropathy. These often occur as a partial form of brachial plexitis.

ULNAR NEUROPATHY AT THE ELBOW—"CUBITAL TUNNEL SYNDROME"

The ulnar nerve passes through the condylar groove between the medial epicondyle and the olecranon. Symptoms consist of paresthesias, tingling, and numbness in the medial hand and half of the fourth and the entire fifth fingers, pain at the elbow or forearm, and weakness. Signs consist of decreased sensation in an ulnar distribution, Tinel's sign at the elbow, and weakness and atrophy of ulnar-innervated hand muscles. The Froment sign indicates thumb adductor weakness and consists of flexion of the thumb at the interphalangeal joint when attempting to oppose the thumb against the lateral border of the second digit. EDx may show slowing of ulnar motor nerve conduction velocity across the elbow with prolonged ulnar sensory latencies. Treatment consists of avoiding aggravating factors, using elbow pads, and surgery to decompress the nerve in the cubital tunnel. Ulnar neuropathies can also rarely occur at the wrist in the ulnar (Guyon) canal or in the hand, usually after trauma.

RADIAL NEUROPATHY

The radial nerve winds around the proximal humerus in the spiral groove and proceeds down the lateral arm and enters the forearm, dividing into the posterior interosseous nerve and superficial nerve. The symptoms and signs consist of wristdrop; finger extension weakness; thumb abduction weakness; and sensory loss in the dorsal web between the thumb and index finger. Triceps and brachioradialis strength is often normal, and triceps reflex is often intact. Most cases of radial neuropathy are transient compressive (neuropraxic) injuries that recover spontaneously in 6–8 weeks. If there has been prolonged compression and severe axonal damage, it may take several months to recover. Treatment consists of cock-up wrist and finger splints, avoiding further compression, and physical therapy to avoid flexion contracture. If there is no improvement in 2–3 weeks, an EDx study is recommended to confirm the clinical diagnosis and determine the degree of severity.

LATERAL FEMORAL CUTANEOUS NEUROPATHY (MERALGIA PARESTHETICA)

The lateral femoral cutaneous nerve arises from the upper lumbar plexus (spinal levels L2/3), crosses through the inguinal ligament near its attachment to the iliac bone, and supplies sensation to the anterior lateral thigh. The neuropathy affecting this nerve is also known as meralgia paresthetica. Symptoms and signs consist of paresthesias, numbness, and occasionally pain in the lateral thigh. Symptoms are increased by standing or walking and are relieved by sitting. There is normal strength and knee reflexes are intact. The diagnosis is clinical, and further tests usually are not performed. EDx is only needed to rule out lumbar plexopathy, radiculopathy, or femoral neuropathy. If the symptoms and signs are classic, electromyography is not necessary. Symptoms often resolve spontaneously over weeks or months, but the patient may be left with permanent numbness. Treatment consists of weight loss and avoiding tight belts. Analgesics in the form of a lidocaine patch, nonsteroidal agents, and occasionally medications for neuropathic pain, can be used (Table 45-6). Rarely, locally injecting the nerve with an anesthetic can be tried. There is no role for surgery.

FEMORAL NEUROPATHY

Femoral neuropathies can arise as complications of retroperitoneal hematoma, lithotomy positioning, hip arthroplasty or dislocation, iliac artery occlusion, femoral arterial procedures, infiltration by hematogenous malignancy, penetrating groin trauma, pelvic surgery including hysterectomy and renal transplantation, and diabetes (a partial form of lumbosacral diabetic plexopathy); some cases are idiopathic. Patients with femoral neuropathy have difficulty extending their knee and flexing the hip. Sensory symptoms occurring either on the anterior thigh and/or medial leg occur in only half of reported cases. A prominent painful component is the exception rather than the rule, may be delayed, and is often self-limited in nature. The quadriceps (patellar) reflex is diminished.

SCIATIC NEUROPATHY

Sciatic neuropathies commonly complicate hip arthroplasty, pelvic procedures in which patients are placed in a prolonged lithotomy position, trauma, hematomas, tumor infiltration, and vasculitis. In addition, many sciatic neuropathies are idiopathic. Weakness may involve all motions of the ankles and toes as well as flexion of the leg at the knee; abduction and extension of the thigh at the hip is spared. Sensory loss occurs in the entire foot and the distal lateral leg. The ankle jerk and on occasion the internal hamstring reflex are diminished or more typically absent on the affected side. The peroneal subdivision of the sciatic nerve is typically involved disproportionately to the tibial counterpart. Thus, patients may have only ankle dorsiflexion and eversion weakness with sparing of knee flexion, ankle inversion, and plantar flexion; these features can lead to misdiagnosis of a common peroneal neuropathy.

PERONEAL NEUROPATHY

The sciatic nerve divides at the distal femur into the tibial and peroneal nerve. The common peroneal nerve passes posterior and laterally around the fibular head, under the fibular tunnel. It then divides into the superficial peroneal nerve, which supplies the ankle evertor muscles and sensation over the anterolateral distal leg and dorsum of the foot, and the deep peroneal nerve, which supplies ankle dorsiflexors and toe extensor muscles and a small area of sensation dorsally in the area of the first and second toes.

Symptoms and signs consist of footdrop (ankle dorsiflexion, toe extension, and ankle eversion weakness) and variable sensory loss, which may involve the superficial and deep peroneal pattern. There is usually no pain. Onset may be on awakening in the morning. Peroneal neuropathy needs to be distinguished from L5 radiculopathy. In L5 radiculopathy, ankle invertors and evertors are weak and needle electromyography reveals denervation. EDx can help localize the lesion. Peroneal motor conduction velocity shows slowing and amplitude drop across the fibular head. Management consists of rapid weight loss and avoiding leg crossing. Footdrop is treated with an ankle brace. A knee pad can be worn over the lateral knee to avoid further compression. Most cases spontaneously resolve over weeks or months.

RADICULOPATHIES

Radiculopathies are most often due to compression from degenerative joint disease and herniated disks, but there are a number of unusual etiologies (Table 45-9). Degenerative spine disease affects a number of different structures, which narrow the diameter of the neural foramen or canal of the spinal column and compromise nerve root integrity; these are discussed in detail in Chap. 9.

TABLE 45-9

CAUSES OF RADICULOPATHY
• Herniated nucleus pulposus
• Degenerative joint disease
• Rheumatoid arthritis
• Trauma
• Vertebral body compression fracture
• Pott's disease
• Compression by extradural mass (e.g., meningioma, metastatic tumor, hematoma, abscess)
• Primary nerve tumor (e.g., neurofibroma, schwannoma, neurinoma)
• Carcinomatous meningitis
• Perineurial spread of tumor (e.g., prostate cancer)
• Acute inflammatory demyelinating polyradiculopathy
• Chronic inflammatory demyelinating polyradiculopathy
• Sarcoidosis
• Amyloidoma
• Diabetic radiculopathy
• Infection (Lyme disease, herpes zoster, cytomegalovirus, syphilis, schistosomiasis, strongyloides)

PLEXOPATHIES

BRACHIAL PLEXUS

The brachial plexus is composed of three trunks (upper, middle, and lower), with two divisions (anterior and posterior) per trunk (Fig. 45-2). Subsequently, the trunks divide into three cords (medial, lateral, and posterior), and from these arise the multiple terminal nerves innervating the arm. The anterior primary rami of C5 and C6 fuse to form the upper trunk; the anterior primary ramus of C7 continues as the middle trunk, while the anterior rami of C8 and T1 join to form the lower trunk. There are several disorders commonly associated with brachial plexopathy.

Immune-mediated brachial plexus neuropathy

Immune-mediated brachial plexus neuropathy (IBPN) goes by various terms, including *acute brachial plexitis*, *neuralgic amyotrophy*, and *Parsonage-Turner syndrome*. IBPN usually presents with an acute onset of severe pain in the shoulder region. The intense pain usually lasts several days to a few weeks, but a dull ache can persist. Individuals who are affected may not appreciate weakness of the arm early in the course because the pain limits movement. However, as the pain dissipates, weakness and often sensory loss are appreciated. Attacks can occasionally recur.

Clinical findings are dependent on the distribution of involvement (e.g., specific trunk, divisions, cords, or terminal nerves). The most common pattern of IBPN involves the upper trunk or a single or multiple mononeuropathies primarily involving the suprascapular, long thoracic, or axillary nerves. Additionally, the phrenic and anterior interosseous nerves may be concomitantly affected. Any of these nerves may also be affected in isolation. EDx is useful to confirm and localize the site(s) of involvement. Empirical treatment of severe pain with glucocorticoids is often used in the acute period.

Brachial plexopathies associated with neoplasms

Neoplasms involving the brachial plexus may be primary nerve tumors, local cancers expanding into the plexus (e.g., Pancoast lung tumor or lymphoma), and metastatic tumors. Primary brachial plexus tumors are less common than the secondary tumors and include schwannomas, neurinomas, and neurofibromas. Secondary tumors affecting the brachial plexus are more common and are always malignant. These may arise from local tumors, expanding into the plexus. For example, a Pancoast tumor of the upper lobe of the lung may invade or compress the lower trunk, while

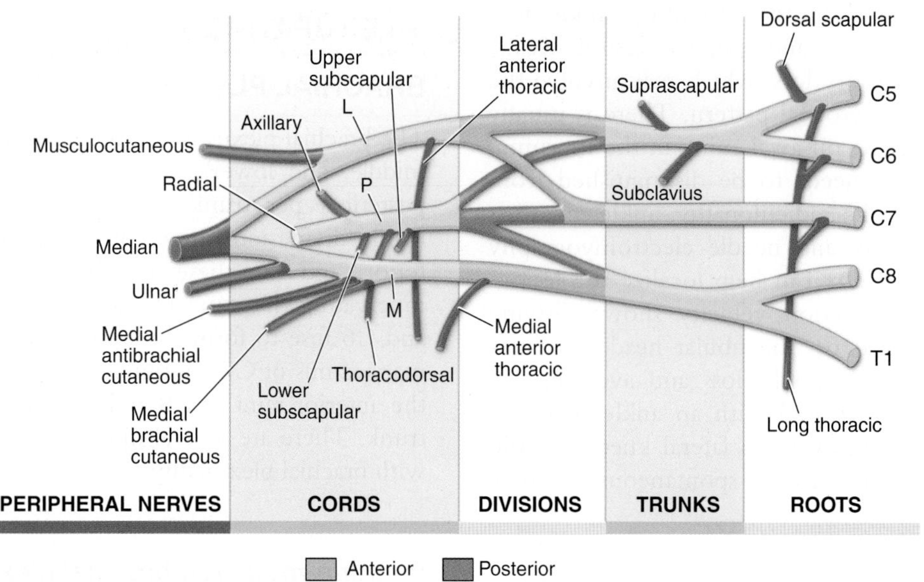

FIGURE 45-2

Brachial plexus anatomy. L, lateral; M, medial; P, posterior. *(From J Goodgold: Anatomical Correlates of Clinical Electromyography. Baltimore, Williams and Wilkins, 1974, p. 126, with permission.)*

a primary lymphoma arising from the cervical or axillary lymph nodes may also infiltrate the plexus. Pancoast tumors typically present as an insidious onset of pain in the upper arm, sensory disturbance in the medial aspect of the forearm and hand, and weakness and atrophy of the intrinsic hand muscles along with an ipsilateral Horner syndrome. Chest CT scans or MRI can demonstrate extension of the tumor into the plexus. Metastatic involvement of the brachial plexus may occur with spread of breast cancer into the axillary lymph nodes with local spread into the nearby nerves.

Perioperative plexopathies (median sternotomy)

The most common surgical procedures associated with brachial plexopathy as a complication are those that involve median sternotomies (e.g., open-heart surgeries and thoracotomies). Brachial plexopathies occur in as many as 5% of patients following a median sternotomy and typically affect the lower trunk. Thus, individuals manifest with sensory disturbance affecting the medial aspect of forearm and hand along with weakness of the intrinsic hand muscles. The mechanism is related to the stretch of the lower trunk, so most individuals who are affected recover within a few months.

LUMBOSACRAL PLEXUS

The lumbar plexus arises from the ventral primary rami of the first to the fourth lumbar spinal nerves (Fig. 45-3). These nerves pass downward and laterally from the vertebral column within the psoas major muscle. The femoral nerve derives from the dorsal branches of the second to the fourth lumbar ventral rami. The obturator nerve arises from the ventral branches of the same lumbar rami. The lumbar plexus communicates with the sacral plexus by the lumbosacral trunk, which contains some fibers from the fourth and all of those from the fifth lumbar ventral rami (Fig. 45-4).

The sacral plexus is the part of the lumbosacral plexus that is formed by the union of the lumbosacral trunk with the ventral rami of the first to fourth sacral nerves.

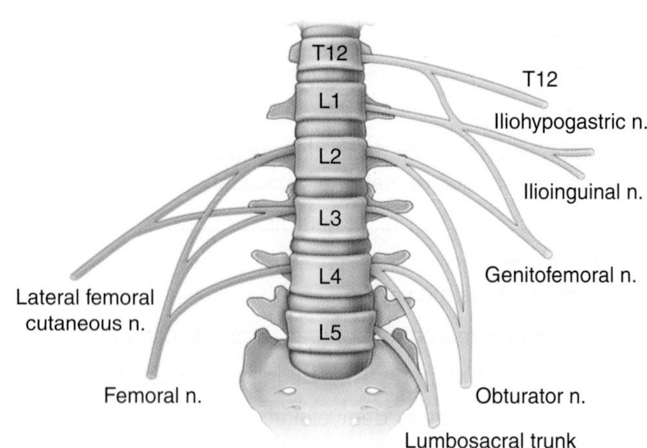

FIGURE 45-3

Lumbar plexus. Posterior divisions are in orange, anterior divisions are in yellow. *(From J Goodgold: Anatomical Correlates of Clinical Electromyography. Baltimore, Williams and Wilkins, 1974, p. 126, with permission.)*

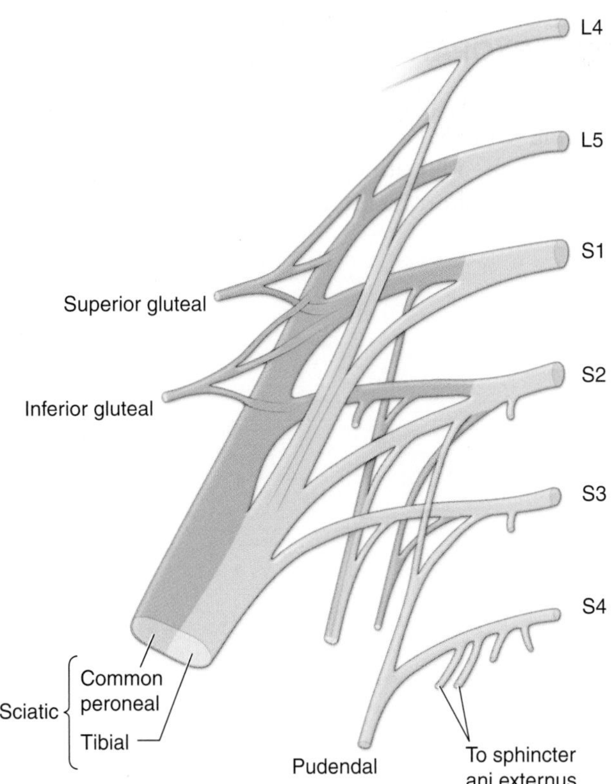

FIGURE 45-4

Lumbosacral plexus. Posterior divisions are in orange, anterior divisions are in yellow. *(From J Goodgold: Anatomical Correlates of Clinical Electromyography. Baltimore, Williams and Wilkins, 1974, p. 126, with permission.)*

The plexus lies on the posterior and posterolateral wall of the pelvis with its components converging toward the sciatic notch. The lateral trunk of the sciatic nerve (which forms the common peroneal nerve) arises from the union of the dorsal branches of the lumbosacral trunk (L4, L5) and the dorsal branches of the S1 and S2 spinal nerve ventral rami. The medial trunk of the sciatic nerve (which forms the tibial nerve) derives from the ventral branches of the same ventral rami (L4-S2).

LUMBOSACRAL PLEXOPATHIES

Plexopathies are typically recognized when motor, sensory, and if applicable, reflex deficits occur in multiple nerve and segmental distributions confined to one extremity. If localization within the lumbosacral plexus can be accomplished, designation as a lumbar plexopathy, a sacral plexopathy, a lumbosacral trunk lesion, or a pan-plexopathy is the best localization that can be expected. Although lumbar plexopathies may be bilateral, usually occurring in a stepwise and chronologically dissociated manner, sacral plexopathies are more likely to behave in this manner due to their closer anatomic proximity. The differential diagnosis of plexopathy includes disorders of the conus medullaris and cauda equina (polyradiculopathy). If there is a paucity of pain and sensory involvement, motor neuron disease should be considered as well.

TABLE 45-10

LUMBOSACRAL PLEXOPATHIES: ETIOLOGIES
• Retroperitoneal hematoma
• Psoas abscess
• Malignant neoplasm
• Benign neoplasm
• Radiation
• Amyloid
• Diabetic radiculoplexus neuropathy
• Idiopathic radiculoplexus neuropathy
• Sarcoidosis
• Aortic occlusion/surgery
• Lithotomy positioning
• Hip arthroplasty
• Pelvic fracture
• Obstetric injury

The causes of lumbosacral plexopathies are listed in Table 45-10. Diabetic radiculopathy (discussed earlier) is a fairly common cause of painful leg weakness. Lumbosacral plexopathies are a well-recognized complication of retroperitoneal hemorrhage. Various primary and metastatic malignancies can affect the lumbosacral plexus as well; these include carcinoma of the cervix, endometrium, and ovary; osteosarcoma; testicular cancer; multiple myeloma; lymphoma; acute myelogenous leukemia; colon cancer; squamous cell carcinoma of the rectum; adenocarcinoma of unknown origin; and intraneural spread of prostate cancer.

RECURRENT NEOPLASTIC DISEASE OR RADIATION-INDUCED PLEXOPATHY

The treatment for various malignancies is often radiation therapy, the field of which may include parts of the brachial plexus. It can be difficult in such situations to determine if a new brachial or lumbosacral plexopathy is related to tumor within the plexus or from radiation-induced nerve damage. Radiation can be associated with microvascular abnormalities and fibrosis of surrounding tissues, which can damage the axons and the Schwann cells. Radiation-induced plexopathy can develop months or years following therapy and is dose dependent.

Tumor invasion is usually painful and more commonly affects the lower trunk, while radiation injury is often painless and affects the upper trunk. Imaging studies such as MRI and CT scans are useful but can be misleading with small microscopic invasion of the plexus. EMG can be informative if myokymic discharges are appreciated, as this finding strongly suggests radiation-induced damage.

EVALUATION AND TREATMENT OF PLEXOPATHIES

Most patients with plexopathies will undergo both imaging with MRI and EDx evaluations. Severe pain from acute idiopathic lumbosacral plexopathy may respond to a short course of glucocorticoids.

CHAPTER 46

GUILLAIN-BARRÉ SYNDROME AND OTHER IMMUNE-MEDIATED NEUROPATHIES

Stephen L. Hauser ■ Anthony A. Amato

GUILLAIN-BARRÉ SYNDROME

Guillain-Barré syndrome (GBS) is an acute, frequently severe, and fulminant polyradiculoneuropathy that is autoimmune in nature. It occurs year-round at a rate of between 1 and 4 cases per 100,000 annually; in the United States, ~5000–6000 cases occur per year. Males are at slightly higher risk for GBS than females, and in Western countries adults are more frequently affected than children.

Clinical manifestations

GBS manifests as a rapidly evolving areflexic motor paralysis with or without sensory disturbance. The usual pattern is an ascending paralysis that may be first noticed as rubbery legs. Weakness typically evolves over hours to a few days and is frequently accompanied by tingling dysesthesias in the extremities. The legs are usually more affected than the arms, and facial diparesis is present in 50% of affected individuals. The lower cranial nerves are also frequently involved, causing bulbar weakness with difficulty handling secretions and maintaining an airway; the diagnosis in these patients may initially be mistaken for brainstem ischemia. Pain in the neck, shoulder, back, or diffusely over the spine is also common in the early stages of GBS, occurring in ~50% of patients. Most patients require hospitalization, and in different series up to 30% require ventilatory assistance at some time during the illness. The need for mechanical ventilation is associated with more severe weakness on admission, a rapid tempo of progression, and the presence of facial and/or bulbar weakness during the first week of symptoms. Fever and constitutional symptoms are absent at the onset and, if present, cast doubt on the diagnosis. Deep tendon reflexes attenuate or disappear within the first few days of onset. Cutaneous sensory deficits (e.g., loss of pain and temperature sensation) are usually relatively mild, but functions subserved by large sensory fibers, such as deep tendon reflexes and proprioception, are more severely affected. Bladder dysfunction may occur in severe cases but is usually transient. If bladder dysfunction is a prominent feature and comes early in the course, diagnostic possibilities other than GBS should be considered, particularly spinal cord disease. Once clinical worsening stops and the patient reaches a plateau (almost always within 4 weeks of onset), further progression is unlikely.

Autonomic involvement is common and may occur even in patients whose GBS is otherwise mild. The usual manifestations are loss of vasomotor control with wide fluctuation in blood pressure, postural hypotension, and cardiac dysrhythmias. These features require close monitoring and management and can be fatal. Pain is another common feature of GBS; in addition to the acute pain described earlier, a deep aching pain may be present in weakened muscles that patients liken to having overexercised the previous day. Other pains in GBS include dysesthetic pain in the extremities as a manifestation of sensory nerve fiber involvement. These pains are self-limited and often respond to standard analgesics (Chap. 7).

Several subtypes of GBS are recognized, as determined primarily by electrodiagnostic (Edx) and pathologic distinctions (Table 46-1). The most common variant is acute inflammatory demyelinating polyneuropathy (AIDP). Additionally, there are two axonal variants, which are often clinically severe—the acute motor axonal neuropathy (AMAN) and acute motor sensory axonal neuropathy (AMSAN) subtypes. In addition, a range of limited or regional GBS syndromes are also encountered. Notable among these is the Miller Fisher syndrome (MFS), which presents as rapidly evolving ataxia and areflexia of limbs without weakness, and ophthalmoplegia,

TABLE 46-1

SUBTYPES OF GUILLAIN-BARRÉ SYNDROME (GBS)

SUBTYPE	FEATURES	ELECTRODIAGNOSIS	PATHOLOGY
Acute inflammatory demyelinating polyneuropathy (AIDP)	Adults affected more than children; 90% of cases in Western world; recovery rapid; anti-GM1 antibodies (<50%)	Demyelinating	First attack on Schwann cell surface; widespread myelin damage, macrophage activation, and lymphocytic infiltration; variable secondary axonal damage
Acute motor axonal neuropathy (AMAN)	Children and young adults; prevalent in China and Mexico; may be seasonal; recovery rapid; anti-GD1a antibodies	Axonal	First attack at motor nodes of Ranvier; macrophage activation, few lymphocytes, frequent periaxonal macrophages; extent of axonal damage highly variable
Acute motor sensory axonal neuropathy (AMSAN)	Mostly adults; uncommon; recovery slow, often incomplete; closely related to AMAN	Axonal	Same as AMAN, but also affects sensory nerves and roots; axonal damage usually severe
Miller Fisher syndrome (MFS)	Adults and children; uncommon; ophthalmoplegia, ataxia, and areflexia; anti-GQ1b antibodies (90%)	Demyelinating	Few cases examined; resembles AIDP

often with pupillary paralysis. The MFS variant accounts for ~5% of all cases and is strongly associated with antibodies to the ganglioside GQ1b (see "Immunopathogenesis"). Other regional variants of GBS include (1) pure sensory forms; (2) ophthalmoplegia with anti-GQ1b antibodies as part of severe motor-sensory GBS; (3) GBS with severe bulbar and facial paralysis, sometimes associated with antecedent cytomegalovirus (CMV) infection and anti-GM2 antibodies; and (4) acute pandysautonomia (Chap. 33).

Antecedent events

Approximately 70% of cases of GBS occur 1–3 weeks after an acute infectious process, usually respiratory or gastrointestinal. Culture and seroepidemiologic techniques show that 20–30% of all cases occurring in North America, Europe, and Australia are preceded by infection or reinfection with *Campylobacter jejuni*. A similar proportion is preceded by a human herpes virus infection, often CMV or Epstein-Barr virus. Other viruses and also *Mycoplasma pneumoniae* have been identified as agents involved in antecedent infections, as have recent immunizations. The swine influenza vaccine, administered widely in the United States in 1976, is the most notable example. Influenza vaccines in use from 1992 to 1994, however, resulted in only one additional case of GBS per million persons vaccinated, and the more recent seasonal influenza vaccines appear to confer a GBS risk of <1 per million. A recent study demonstrated that there does not appear to be an increased risk of GBS with meningococcal vaccinations (Menactra) contrary to early reports. Older-type rabies vaccine, prepared in nervous system tissue, is implicated as a trigger of GBS in developing countries where it is still used; the mechanism is presumably immunization against neural antigens. GBS also occurs more frequently than can be attributed to chance alone in patients with lymphoma (including Hodgkin's disease), in HIV-seropositive individuals, and in patients with systemic lupus erythematosus (SLE). *C. jejuni* has also been implicated in summer outbreaks of AMAN among children and young adults exposed to chickens in rural China.

Immunopathogenesis

Several lines of evidence support an autoimmune basis for acute inflammatory demyelinating polyneuropathy (AIDP), the most common and best-studied type of GBS; the concept extends to all of the subtypes of GBS (Table 46-1).

It is likely that both cellular and humoral immune mechanisms contribute to tissue damage in AIDP. T cell activation is suggested by the finding that elevated levels of cytokines and cytokine receptors are present in serum (interleukin [IL] 2, soluble IL-2 receptor) and in cerebrospinal fluid (CSF) (IL-6, tumor necrosis factor α, interferon-γ). AIDP is also closely analogous to an experimental T cell–mediated immunopathy designated *experimental allergic neuritis* (EAN). EAN is induced in laboratory animals by immune sensitization against protein fragments derived from peripheral nerve proteins, and in particular against the P2 protein. Based on analogy to EAN, it was initially thought that AIDP was likely to be primarily a T cell–mediated disorder;

however, abundant data now suggest that autoantibodies directed against nonprotein determinants may be central to many cases.

Circumstantial evidence suggests that all GBS results from immune responses to nonself antigens (infectious agents, vaccines) that misdirect to host nerve tissue through a resemblance-of-epitope (molecular mimicry) mechanism (Fig. 46-1). The neural targets are likely to be glycoconjugates, specifically gangliosides (Table 46-2; Fig. 46-2). Gangliosides are complex glycosphingolipids that contain one or more sialic acid residues; various gangliosides participate in cell-cell interactions (including those between axons and glia), modulation of receptors, and regulation of growth. They are typically exposed on the plasma membrane of cells, rendering them susceptible to an antibody-mediated attack. Gangliosides and other glycoconjugates are present in large quantity in human nervous tissues and in key sites, such as nodes of Ranvier. Antiganglioside antibodies, most frequently to GM1, are common in GBS (20–50% of cases), particularly in those preceded by *C. jejuni* infection. Furthermore, isolates of *C. jejuni* from stool cultures of patients with GBS have surface glycolipid structures that antigenically cross react with gangliosides, including GM1, concentrated in human nerves. Sialic acid residues from pathogenic *C. jejuni* strains can also trigger activation of dendritic cells via signaling through a toll-like receptor (TLR4), promoting B-cell differentiation and further amplifying humoral autoimmunity. Another line of evidence is derived from experience in Europe with parenteral use of purified bovine brain gangliosides for treatment of various neuropathic disorders. Between 5 and 15 days after injection, some recipients developed acute motor axonal GBS with high titers of anti-GM1 antibodies that recognized epitopes at nodes of Ranvier and motor endplates. Experimentally, anti-GM1 antibodies can trigger complement-mediated injury at paranodal axon-glial junctions, disrupting the clustering of sodium channels and likely contributing to conduction block (see "Pathophysiology").

Anti-GQ1b IgG antibodies are found in >90% of patients with MFS (Table 46-2; Fig. 46-2), and titers

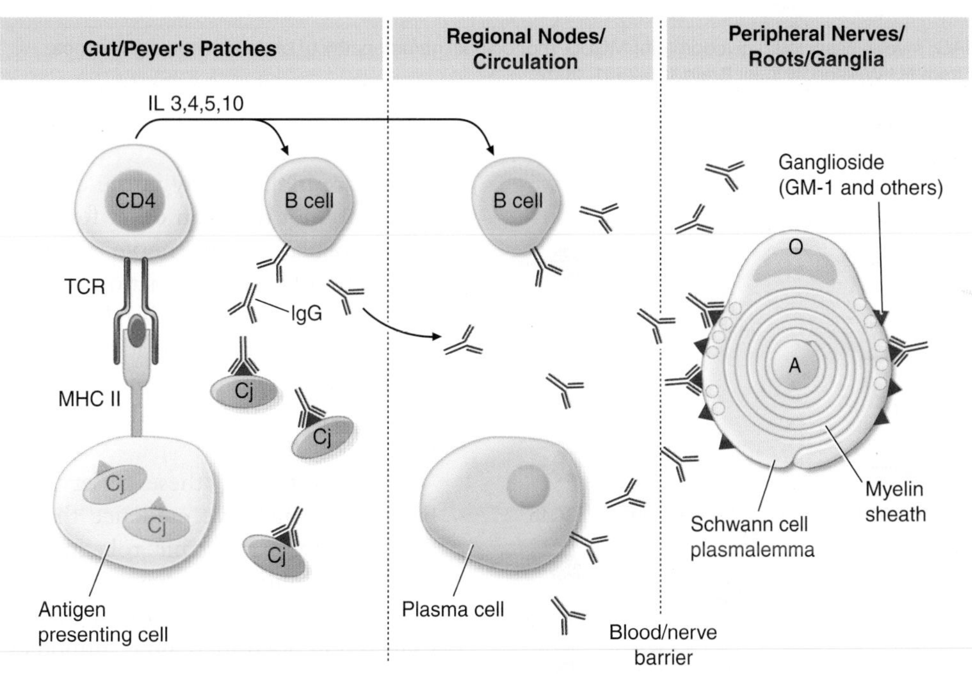

FIGURE 46-1

Postulated immunopathogenesis of GBS associated with *C. jejuni* infection. B cells recognize glycoconjugates on *C. jejuni* (Cj) (triangles) that cross-react with ganglioside present on Schwann cell surface and subjacent peripheral nerve myelin. Some B cells, activated via a T cell–independent mechanism, secrete primarily IgM (not shown). Other B cells (upper left side) are activated via a partially T cell–dependent route and secrete primarily IgG; T cell help is provided by CD4 cells activated locally by fragments of Cj proteins that are presented on the surface of antigen-presenting cells (APCs). A critical event in the development of GBS is the escape of activated B cells from Peyer's patches into regional lymph nodes. Activated T cells probably also function to assist in opening of the blood-nerve barrier, facilitating penetration of pathogenic autoantibodies. The earliest changes in myelin (right) consist of edema between myelin lamellae and vesicular disruption (shown as circular blebs) of the outermost myelin layers. These effects are associated with activation of the C5b-C9 membrane attack complex and probably mediated by calcium entry; it is possible that the macrophage cytokine tumor necrosis factor (TNF) also participates in myelin damage. B, B cell; MHC II, class II major histocompatibility complex molecule; TCR, T cell receptor; A, axon; O, oligodendrocyte.

TABLE 46-2

PRINCIPAL ANTI-GLYCOLIPID ANTIBODIES IMPLICATED IN IMMUNE NEUROPATHIES

CLINICAL PRESENTATION	ANTIBODY TARGET	USUAL ISOTYPE
Acute Immune Neuropathies (Guillain-Barré Syndrome)		
Acute inflammatory demyelinating polyneuropathy (AIDP)	No clear patterns	IgG (polyclonal)
Acute motor axonal neuropathy (AMAN)	GM1 most common GD1a, GM1, GM1b, GalNAc–GD1a (<50% for any)	IgG (polyclonal)
Miller Fisher syndrome (MFS)	GQ1b (>90%)	IgG (polyclonal)
Acute pharyngeal cervicobrachial neuropathy (APCBN)	GT1a (? Most)	IgG (polyclonal)
Chronic Immune Neuropathies		
Chronic inflammatory demyelinating polyneuropathy (CIDP) (75%)	Po in some	No clear pattern
CIDPa (MGUS associated) (25%)	Neural binding sites	IgG, IgA (monoclonal)
Chronic sensory > motor neuropathy	SPGP, SGLPG (on MAG) (50%)	IgM (monoclonal)
	Uncertain (50%)	IgM (monoclonal)
Multifocal motor neuropathy (MMN)	GM1, GalNAc–GD1a, others (25–50%)	IgM (polyclonal, monoclonal)
Chronic sensory ataxic neuropathy	GD1b, GQ1b, and other b-series gangliosides	IgM (monoclonal)

Abbreviations: MAG, myelin-associated glycoprotein; MGUS, monoclonal gammopathy of undetermined significance.
Source: Modified from HJ Willison, N Yuki: Brain 125:2591, 2002.

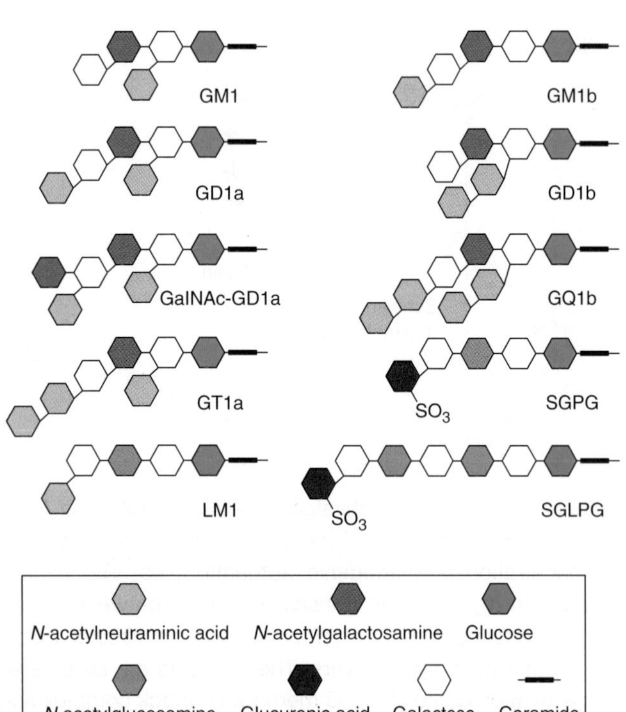

FIGURE 46-2

Glycolipids implicated as antigens in immune-mediated neuropathies. (*Modified from HJ Willison, N Yuki: Brain 125:2591, 2002.*)

of IgG are highest early in the course. Anti-GQ1b antibodies are not found in other forms of GBS unless there is extraocular motor nerve involvement. A possible explanation for this association is that extraocular motor nerves are enriched in GQ1b gangliosides in comparison to limb nerves. In addition, a monoclonal anti-GQ1b antibody raised against *C. jejuni* isolated from a patient with MFS blocked neuromuscular transmission experimentally.

Taken together, these observations provide strong but still inconclusive evidence that autoantibodies play an important pathogenic role in GBS. Although anti-ganglioside antibodies have been studied most intensively, other antigenic targets may also be important. One report identified IgG antibodies against Schwann cells and neurons (nerve growth cone region) in some GBS cases. Proof that these antibodies are pathogenic requires that they be capable of mediating disease following direct passive transfer to naïve hosts; this has not yet been demonstrated, although one case of possible maternal-fetal transplacental transfer of GBS has been described.

In AIDP, an early step in the induction of tissue damage appears to be complement deposition along the outer surface of the Schwann cell. Activation of complement initiates a characteristic vesicular disintegration of the myelin sheath, and also leads to recruitment of activated macrophages, which participate in damage to myelin and axons. In AMAN, the pattern is different in that complement is deposited along with IgG at the nodes of Ranvier along large motor axons. Interestingly, in cases of AMAN antibodies against GD1a appear to have a fine specificity that favors binding to motor rather than sensory nerve roots, even though this ganglioside is expressed on both fiber types.

Pathophysiology

In the demyelinating forms of GBS, the basis for flaccid paralysis and sensory disturbance is conduction block. This finding, demonstrable electrophysiologically, implies that the axonal connections remain intact. Hence, recovery can take place rapidly as remyelination occurs. In severe cases of demyelinating GBS, secondary axonal degeneration usually occurs; its extent can be estimated electrophysiologically. More secondary axonal degeneration correlates with a slower rate of recovery and a greater degree of residual disability. When a severe primary axonal pattern is encountered electrophysiologically, the implication is that axons have degenerated and become disconnected from their targets, specifically the neuromuscular junctions, and must therefore regenerate for recovery to take place. In motor axonal cases in which recovery is rapid, the lesion is thought to be localized to preterminal motor branches, allowing regeneration and reinnervation to take place quickly. Alternatively, in mild cases, collateral sprouting and reinnervation from surviving motor axons near the neuromuscular junction may begin to reestablish physiologic continuity with muscle cells over a period of several months.

Laboratory features

CSF findings are distinctive, consisting of an elevated CSF protein level (1–10 g/L [100–1000 mg/dL]) without accompanying pleocytosis. The CSF is often normal when symptoms have been present for ≤48 h; by the end of the first week, the level of protein is usually elevated. A transient increase in the CSF white cell count (10–100/μL) occurs on occasion in otherwise typical GBS; however, a sustained CSF pleocytosis suggests an alternative diagnosis (viral myelitis) or a concurrent diagnosis such as unrecognized HIV infection, leukemia or lymphoma with infiltration of nerves, or neurosarcoidosis. Edx features are mild or absent in the early stages of GBS and lag behind the clinical evolution. In AIDP, the earliest features are prolonged F-wave latencies, prolonged distal latencies and reduced amplitudes of compound muscle action potentials (CMAPs), probably owing to the predilection for involvement of nerve roots and distal motor nerve terminals early in the course. Later, slowing of conduction velocity, conduction block, and temporal dispersion may be appreciated (Table 46-1). Occasionally, sensory nerve action potentials (SNAPs) may be normal in the feet (e.g., sural nerve) when abnormal in the arms. This is also a sign that the patient does not have one of the more typical "length-dependent" polyneuropathies. In cases with primary axonal pathology, the principal Edx finding is reduced amplitude of CMAPs (and also SNAPS with AMSAN) without conduction slowing or prolongation of distal latencies.

Diagnosis

GBS is a descriptive entity. The diagnosis of AIDP is made by recognizing the pattern of rapidly evolving paralysis with areflexia, absence of fever or other systemic symptoms, and characteristic antecedent events (Table 46-3). Other disorders that may enter into the differential diagnosis include acute myelopathies (especially with prolonged back pain and sphincter disturbances); diphtheria (early oropharyngeal disturbances); Lyme polyradiculitis and other tick-borne paralyses; porphyria (abdominal pain, seizures, psychosis); vasculitic neuropathy (check erythrocyte sedimentation rate, described later); poliomyelitis (fever and meningismus common); West Nile virus; CMV polyradiculitis (in immunocompromised patients); critical illness neuropathy or myopathy; neuromuscular junction disorders such as myasthenia gravis and botulism (pupillary reactivity lost early); poisonings with organophosphates, thallium, or arsenic; paralytic shellfish poisoning; or severe hypophosphatemia (rare). Laboratory tests are helpful primarily to exclude mimics of GBS. Edx features may be minimal, and the CSF protein level may not rise until the end of the first week. If the diagnosis is strongly suspected, treatment should be initiated without waiting for evolution of the characteristic Edx and CSF findings to occur. Both tau and 14-3-3 protein levels are reported to be elevated early (during the first few days of symptoms) in some cases of GBS. Tau increases in CSF may reflect axonal damage and predict a residual deficit. GBS patients with risk factors for HIV or with CSF pleocytosis should have a serologic test for HIV.

TREATMENT Guillain-Barré Syndrome

In the vast majority of patients with GBS, treatment should be initiated as soon after diagnosis as possible. Each day counts; ~2 weeks after the first motor symptoms, it is not known whether immunotherapy is still effective. If the patient has already reached the plateau stage, then treatment probably is no longer

TABLE 46-3

DIAGNOSTIC FEATURES OF ACUTE INFLAMMATORY DEMYELINATING POLYNEUROPATHY (AIDP)

I. Required for Diagnosis
1. Progressive weakness of variable degree from mild paresis to complete paralysis
2. Generalized hypo- or areflexia

II. Supportive of Diagnosis
1. Clinical Features
   a. Symptom progression: Motor weakness rapidly progresses initially but ceases by 4 weeks. Nadir attained by 2 weeks in 50%, 3 weeks 80%, and 90% by 4 weeks.
   b. Demonstration of relative limb symmetry regarding paresis.
   c. Mild to moderate sensory signs.
   d. Frequent cranial nerve involvement: Facial (cranial nerve VII) 50% and typically bilateral but asymmetric; occasional involvement of cranial nerves XII, X, and occasionally III, IV, and VI as well as XI.
   e. Recovery typically begins 2–4 weeks following plateau phase.
   f. Autonomic dysfunction can include tachycardia, other arrhythmias, postural hypotension, hypertension, other vasomotor symptoms.
   g. A preceding gastrointestinal illness (e.g., diarrhea) or upper respiratory tract infection is common.
2. Cerebrospinal Fluid Features Supporting Diagnosis
   a. Elevated or serial elevation of CSF protein.
   b. CSF cell counts are <10 mononuclear cell/mm^3.
3. Electrodiagnostic Medicine Findings Supportive of Diagnosis
   a. 80% of patients have evidence of NCV slowing/conduction block at some time during disease process.
   b. Patchy reduction in NCV attaining values less than 60% of normal.
   c. Distal motor latency increase may reach 3 times normal values.
   d. F-waves indicate proximal NCV slowing.
   e. About 15–20% of patients have normal NCV findings.
   f. No abnormalities on nerve conduction studies may be seen for several weeks.

III. Findings Reducing Possibility of Diagnosis
1. Asymmetric weakness
2. Failure of bowel/bladder symptoms to resolve
3. Severe bowel/bladder dysfunction at initiation of disease
4. Greater than 50 mononuclear cells/mm^3 in CSF
5. Well-demarcated sensory level

IV. Exclusionary Criteria
1. Diagnosis of other causes of acute neuromuscular weakness (e.g., myasthenia gravis, botulism, poliomyelitis, toxic neuropathy).
2. Abnormal CSF cytology suggesting carcinomatous invasion of the nerve roots

Abbreviations: CSF, cerebrospinal fluid; NCV, nerve conduction velocity.
Source: AA Amato, D Dumitru, in D Dumitru et al (eds): *Electrodiagnostic Medicine*, 2nd ed. Philadelphia, Hanley & Belfus, 2002.

indicated, unless the patient has severe motor weakness and one cannot exclude the possibility that an immunologic attack is still ongoing. Either high-dose intravenous immune globulin (IVIg) or plasmapheresis can be initiated, as they are equally effective for typical GBS. A combination of the two therapies is not significantly better than either alone. IVIg is often the initial therapy chosen because of its ease of administration and good safety record. Anecdotal data has also suggested that IVIg may be preferable to PE for the AMAN and MFS variants of GBS. IVIg is administered as five daily infusions for a total dose of 2 g/kg body weight. There is some evidence that GBS autoantibodies are neutralized by anti-idiotypic antibodies present in IVIg preparations, perhaps accounting for the therapeutic effect. A course of plasmapheresis usually consists of ~40–50 mL/kg plasma exchange (PE) four to five times over a week. Meta-analysis of randomized clinical trials indicates that treatment reduces the need for mechanical ventilation by nearly half (from 27% to 14% with PE) and increases the likelihood of full recovery at 1 year (from 55% to 68%). Functionally significant improvement may occur toward the end of the first week of treatment, or may be delayed for several weeks. The lack of noticeable improvement following a course of IVIg or PE is not an indication to treat with the alternate treatment. However, there are occasional patients who are treated early in the course of GBS and improve, who then relapse within a month. Brief retreatment with the original therapy is usually effective in such cases. Glucocorticoids have not been found to be effective in GBS. Occasional patients with very mild forms of GBS, especially those who appear to have already reached a plateau when initially seen, may be managed conservatively without IVIg or PE.

In the worsening phase of GBS, most patients require monitoring in a critical care setting, with particular attention to vital capacity, heart rhythm, blood pressure, nutrition, deep vein thrombosis prophylaxis, cardiovascular status, early consideration (after 2 weeks of intubation) of tracheotomy, and chest physiotherapy. As noted, ~30% of patients with GBS require ventilatory assistance, sometimes for prolonged periods of time (several weeks or longer). Frequent turning and assiduous skin care are important, as are daily range-of-motion exercises to avoid joint contractures and daily reassurance as to the generally good outlook for recovery.

Prognosis and recovery

Approximately 85% of patients with GBS achieve a full functional recovery within several months to a year, although minor findings on examination (such as areflexia) may persist and patients often complain of continued symptoms, including fatigue. The mortality rate is <5% in optimal settings; death usually results from secondary pulmonary complications. The outlook is worst in patients with severe proximal motor and sensory axonal damage. Such axonal damage may be either primary or secondary in nature (see "Pathophysiology," earlier in the chapter), but in either case successful regeneration cannot occur. Other factors that worsen the outlook for recovery are advanced age, a fulminant or severe attack, and a delay in the onset of treatment. Between 5 and 10% of patients with typical GBS have one or more late relapses; such cases are then classified as chronic inflammatory demyelinating polyneuropathy (CIDP).

CHRONIC INFLAMMATORY DEMYELINATING POLYNEUROPATHY

CIDP is distinguished from GBS by its chronic course. In other respects, this neuropathy shares many features with the common demyelinating form of GBS, including elevated CSF protein levels and the Edx findings of acquired demyelination. Most cases occur in adults, and males are affected slightly more often than females. The incidence of CIDP is lower than that of GBS, but due to the protracted course the prevalence is greater.

Clinical manifestations

Onset is usually gradual over a few months or longer, but in a few cases the initial attack is indistinguishable from that of GBS. An acute-onset form of CIDP should be considered when GBS deteriorates >9 weeks after onset or relapses at least three times. Symptoms are both motor and sensory in most cases. Weakness of the limbs is usually symmetric but can be strikingly asymmetric in multifocal acquired demyelinating sensory and motor (MADSAM) neuropathy variant (Lewis-Sumner syndrome) in which discrete peripheral nerves are involved. There is considerable variability from case to case. Some patients experience a chronic progressive course, whereas others, usually younger patients, have a relapsing and remitting course. Some have only motor findings, and a small proportion present with a relatively pure syndrome of sensory ataxia. Tremor occurs in ~10% and may become more prominent during periods of subacute worsening or improvement. A small proportion have cranial nerve findings, including external ophthalmoplegia. CIDP tends to ameliorate over time with treatment; the result is that many years after onset, nearly 75% of patients have reasonable functional status. Death from CIDP is uncommon.

Diagnosis

The diagnosis rests on characteristic clinical, CSF, and electrophysiologic findings. The CSF is usually acellular with an elevated protein level, sometimes several times normal. As with GBS, a CSF pleocytosis should lead to the consideration of HIV infection, leukemia or lymphoma, and neurosarcoidosis. Edx findings reveal variable degrees of conduction slowing, prolonged distal latencies, distal and temporal dispersion of CMAPs, and conduction block as the principal features. In particular, the presence of conduction block is a certain sign of an acquired demyelinating process. Evidence of axonal loss, presumably secondary to demyelination, is present in >50% of patients. Serum protein electrophoresis with immunofixation is indicated to search for monoclonal gammopathy and associated conditions (see "Monoclonal Gammopathy of Undetermined Significance," later in the chapter). In all patients with presumptive CIDP, it is also reasonable to exclude vasculitis, collagen vascular disease (especially SLE), chronic hepatitis, HIV infection, amyloidosis, and diabetes mellitus. Other associated conditions include inflammatory bowel disease and lymphoma.

Pathogenesis

Although there is evidence of immune activation in CIDP, the precise mechanisms of pathogenesis are unknown. Biopsy typically reveals little inflammation and onion-bulb changes (imbricated layers of attenuated Schwann cell processes surrounding an axon) that result from recurrent demyelination and remyelination (Fig. 46-1). The response to therapy suggests that CIDP is immune-mediated; CIDP responds to glucocorticoids, whereas GBS does not. Passive transfer of demyelination into experimental animals has been accomplished using IgG purified from the serum of some patients with CIDP, lending support for a humoral autoimmune pathogenesis. Although the target antigen or antigens in CIDP have not yet been identified, the myelin protein Po has been implicated as a potential autoantigen in some patients. It is also of interest that a CIDP-like illness developed spontaneously in the nonobese diabetic (NOD) mouse when the immune co-stimulatory molecule B7-2 (CD86) was genetically deleted; this suggests that CIDP can result from altered triggering of T cells by antigen-presenting cells.

Approximately 25% of patients with clinical features of CIDP also have a monoclonal gammopathy of undetermined significance (MGUS). Cases associated with monoclonal IgA or IgG kappa usually respond to treatment as favorably as cases without a monoclonal gammopathy. Patients with IgM monoclonal gammopathy tend to have more sensory findings and a more protracted course, and usually have a less satisfactory response to treatment.

TREATMENT Chronic Inflammatory Demyelinating Polyneuropathy

Most authorities initiate treatment for CIDP when progression is rapid or walking is compromised. If the disorder is mild, management can be expectant, awaiting spontaneous remission. Controlled studies have shown that high-dose IVIg, PE, and glucocorticoids are all more effective than placebo. Initial therapy is usually with IVIg, administered as 2.0 g/kg body weight given in divided doses over 2–5 days; three monthly courses are generally recommended before concluding a patient is a treatment failure. If the patient responds, the infusion intervals can be gradually increased or the dosage decreased (e.g., 1 g/kg per month). PE, which appears to be as effective as IVIg, is initiated at two to three treatments per week for 6 weeks; periodic re-treatment may also be required. Treatment with glucocorticoids is another option (60–80 mg prednisone PO daily for 1–2 months, followed by a gradual dose reduction of 10 mg per month as tolerated), but long-term adverse effects including bone demineralization, gastrointestinal bleeding, and cushingoid changes are problematic. As many as one-third of patients with CIDP fail to respond adequately to the initial therapy chosen; a different treatment should then be tried. Patients who fail therapy with IVIg, PE, and glucocorticoids may benefit from treatment with immunosuppressive agents such as azathioprine, methotrexate, cyclosporine, and cyclophosphamide, either alone or as adjunctive therapy. Early experience with anti-CD20 (rituximab) has also shown promise. Use of these therapies requires periodic reassessment of their risks and benefits. In patients with a CIDP-like neuropathy who fail to respond to treatment it is important to evaluate for POEMS syndrome (polyneuropathy, organomegaly, endocrinopathy, monoclonal gammopathy, skin changes; discussed later).

MULTIFOCAL MOTOR NEUROPATHY

Multifocal motor neuropathy (MMN) is a distinctive but uncommon neuropathy that presents as slowly progressive motor weakness and atrophy evolving over years in the distribution of selected nerve trunks, associated with sites of persistent focal motor conduction block in the same nerve trunks. Sensory fibers are relatively spared. The arms are affected more frequently than the legs, and >75% of all patients are male. Some cases have been confused with lower motor neuron forms of amyotrophic lateral sclerosis (Chap. 32). Less than 50% of patients present with high titers of polyclonal IgM antibody to the ganglioside GM1. It is uncertain how this finding relates to the discrete foci of persistent motor conduction block, but high concentrations of GM1 gangliosides are normal constituents of nodes of Ranvier in peripheral nerve fibers. Pathology reveals demyelination and mild inflammatory changes at the sites of conduction block.

Most patients with MMN respond to high-dose IVIg (dosages as for CIDP, discussed earlier); periodic re-treatment is required (usually at least monthly) to maintain the benefit. Some refractory patients have responded to rituximab or cyclophosphamide. Glucocorticoids and PE are not effective.

NEUROPATHIES WITH MONOCLONAL GAMMOPATHY

MULTIPLE MYELOMA

Clinically overt polyneuropathy occurs in ~5% of patients with the commonly encountered type of multiple myeloma, which exhibits either lytic or diffuse osteoporotic bone lesions. These neuropathies are sensorimotor, are usually mild and slowly progressive but may be severe, and generally do not reverse with successful suppression of the myeloma. In most cases, Edx and pathologic features are consistent with a process of axonal degeneration.

In contrast, myeloma with osteosclerotic features, although representing only 3% of all myelomas, is associated with polyneuropathy in one-half of cases. These neuropathies, which may also occur with solitary plasmacytoma, are distinct because they (1) are usually demyelinating in nature and resemble CIDP; (2) often respond to radiation therapy or removal of the primary lesion; (3) are associated with different monoclonal proteins and light chains (almost always lambda as opposed to primarily kappa in the lytic type of multiple myeloma); (4) are typically refractory to standard treatments of CIDP; and (5) may occur in association with other systemic findings including thickening of the skin, hyperpigmentation, hypertrichosis, organomegaly, endocrinopathy, anasarca, and clubbing of fingers. These are features of the POEMS syndrome (*p*olyneuropathy, *o*rganomegaly, *e*ndocrinopathy, *M* protein, and *s*kin changes). Levels of vascular endothelial growth factor (VEGF) are increased in the serum, and this factor is felt to somehow play a pathogenic role in this syndrome. Treatment of the neuropathy is best directed at the osteosclerotic myeloma using surgery, radiotherapy, chemotherapy, or autologous peripheral blood stem cell transplantation.

Neuropathies are also encountered in other systemic conditions with gammopathy, including Waldenström's macroglobulinemia, primary systemic amyloidosis, and cryoglobulinemic states (mixed essential cryoglobulinemia, some cases of hepatitis C).

MONOCLONAL GAMMOPATHY OF UNDETERMINED SIGNIFICANCE

Chronic polyneuropathies occurring in association with MGUS are usually associated with the immunoglobulin isotypes IgG, IgA, and IgM. Most patients present with isolated sensory symptoms in their distal extremities and have Edx features of an axonal sensory or sensorimotor polyneuropathy. These patients otherwise resemble idiopathic sensory polyneuropathy and the MGUS might just be coincidental. They usually do not respond to immunotherapies designed to reduce the concentration of the monoclonal protein. Some patients, however, present with generalized weakness and sensory loss and Edx studies indistinguishable from CIDP without monoclonal gammopathy (see "Chronic Inflammatory Demyelinating Polyneuropathy," earlier in the chapter), and their response to immunosuppressive agents is also similar. An exception is the syndrome of IgM kappa monoclonal gammopathy associated with an indolent, longstanding, sometimes static sensory neuropathy, frequently with tremor and sensory ataxia. Most patients are male and older than age 50 years. In the majority, the monoclonal IgM immunoglobulin binds to a normal peripheral nerve constituent, myelin-associated glycoprotein (MAG), found in the paranodal regions of Schwann cells. Binding appears to be specific for a polysaccharide epitope that is also found in other normal peripheral nerve myelin glycoproteins, P0 and PMP22, and also in other normal nerve-related glycosphingolipids (Fig. 46-1). In the MAG-positive cases, IgM paraprotein is incorporated into the myelin sheaths of affected patients and widens the spacing of the myelin lamellae, thus producing a distinctive ultrastructural pattern. Demyelination and remyelination are the hallmarks of the lesions. The chronic demyelinating neuropathy appears to result from a destabilization of myelin metabolism rather than activation of an immune response. Therapy with chlorambucil, or cyclophosphamide combined with glucocorticoids or PE, often results in improvement of the neuropathy associated with a prolonged reduction in the levels in the circulating paraprotein; chronic use of these alkylating agents is associated with significant risks. In a small proportion of patients (30% at 10 years), MGUS will in time evolve into frankly malignant conditions such as multiple myeloma or lymphoma.

VASCULITIC NEUROPATHY

Peripheral nerve involvement is common in polyarteritis nodosa (PAN), appearing in half of all cases clinically and in 100% of cases at postmortem studies. The most common pattern is multifocal (asymmetric) motor-sensory neuropathy (mononeuropathy multiplex) due to ischemic lesions of nerve trunks and roots; however, some cases of vasculitic neuropathy present as a distal, symmetric sensorimotor polyneuropathy. Symptoms of neuropathy are a common presenting complaint in patients with PAN. The Edx findings are those of an axonal process. Small- to medium-sized arteries of the vasa nervorum, particularly the epineural vessels, are affected in PAN, resulting in a widespread ischemic neuropathy. A high frequency of neuropathy occurs in allergic angiitis and granulomatosis (Churg-Strauss syndrome).

Systemic vasculitis should always be considered when a subacute or chronically evolving mononeuropathy multiplex occurs in conjunction with constitutional symptoms (fever, anorexia, weight loss, loss of energy, malaise, and nonspecific pains). Diagnosis of suspected vasculitic neuropathy is made by a combined nerve and muscle biopsy, with serial section or skip-serial techniques.

Approximately one-third of biopsy-proven cases of vasculitic neuropathy are "nonsystemic" in that the vasculitis appears to affect only peripheral nerves. Constitutional symptoms are absent, and the course is more indolent than that of PAN. The erythrocyte sedimentation rate may be elevated, but other tests for systemic disease are negative. Nevertheless, clinically silent involvement of other organs is likely, and vasculitis is frequently found in muscle biopsied at the same time as nerve.

Vasculitic neuropathy may also be seen as part of the vasculitis syndrome occurring in the course of other connective tissue disorders. The most frequent is rheumatoid arthritis, but ischemic neuropathy due to involvement of vasa nervorum may also occur in mixed cryoglobulinemia, Sjögren's syndrome, granulomatosis with polyangiitis (Wegener's), hypersensitivity angiitis, systemic lupus erythematosus, and progressive systemic sclerosis. Management of these neuropathies, including the "nonsystemic" vasculitic neuropathy, consists of treatment of the underlying condition as well as the aggressive use of glucocorticoids and other immunosuppressant drugs. Use of these regimens has resulted in dramatic improvements in outcome, with 5-year survival rates now greater than 80%. One reasonable starting regimen is daily prednisone (initial dose 1 mg/kg per day PO with a gradual taper after 1 month) plus IV pulse (or daily oral) cyclophosphamide for 3–6 months.

ANTI-Hu PARANEOPLASTIC NEUROPATHY

This uncommon immune-mediated disorder manifests as a sensory neuronopathy (i.e., selective damage to sensory nerve bodies in dorsal root ganglia).

The onset is often asymmetric with dysesthesias and sensory loss in the limbs that soon progress to affect all limbs, the torso, and face. Marked sensory ataxia, pseudoathetosis, and inability to walk, stand, or even sit unsupported are frequent features and are secondary to the extensive deafferentation. Subacute sensory neuronopathy may be idiopathic, but more than half of cases are paraneoplastic, primarily related to lung cancer, and most of those are small cell lung cancer (SCLC). Diagnosis of the underlying SCLC requires awareness of the association, paraneoplastic testing, and often PET scanning for the tumor. The target antigens are a family of RNA-binding proteins (HuD, HuC, and Hel-N1) that in normal tissues are only expressed by neurons. The same proteins are usually expressed by SCLC, triggering in some patients an immune response characterized by antibodies and cytotoxic T cells that cross-react with the Hu proteins of the dorsal root ganglion neurons, resulting in immune-mediated neuronal destruction. An encephalomyelitis may accompany the sensory neuronopathy and presumably has the same pathogenesis. Neurologic symptoms usually precede, by ≤6 months, the identification of SCLC. The sensory neuronopathy runs its course in a few weeks or months and stabilizes, leaving the patient disabled. Most cases are unresponsive to treatment with glucocorticoids, IVIg, PE, or immunosuppressant drugs.

CHAPTER 47

MYASTHENIA GRAVIS AND OTHER DISEASES OF THE NEUROMUSCULAR JUNCTION

Daniel B. Drachman

Myasthenia gravis (MG) is a neuromuscular disorder characterized by weakness and fatigability of skeletal muscles. The underlying defect is a decrease in the number of available acetylcholine receptors (AChRs) at neuromuscular junctions due to an antibody-mediated autoimmune attack. Treatment now available for MG is highly effective, although a specific cure has remained elusive.

PATHOPHYSIOLOGY

At the neuromuscular junction (Fig. 47-1), acetylcholine (ACh) is synthesized in the motor nerve terminal and stored in vesicles (quanta). When an action potential travels down a motor nerve and reaches the nerve terminal, ACh from 150 to 200 vesicles is released and combines with AChRs that are densely packed at the peaks of postsynaptic folds. The structure of the AChR has been fully elucidated; it consists of five subunits (2α, 1β, 1δ, and 1γ or ε) arranged around a central pore. When ACh combines with the binding sites on the α subunits of the AChR, the channel in the AChR opens, permitting the rapid entry of cations, chiefly sodium, which produces depolarization at the end-plate region of the muscle fiber. If the depolarization is sufficiently large, it initiates an action potential that is propagated along the muscle fiber, triggering muscle contraction. This process is rapidly terminated by hydrolysis of ACh by acetylcholinesterase (AChE), which is present within the synaptic folds, and by diffusion of ACh away from the receptor.

In MG, the fundamental defect is a decrease in the number of available AChRs at the postsynaptic muscle membrane. In addition, the postsynaptic folds are flattened,

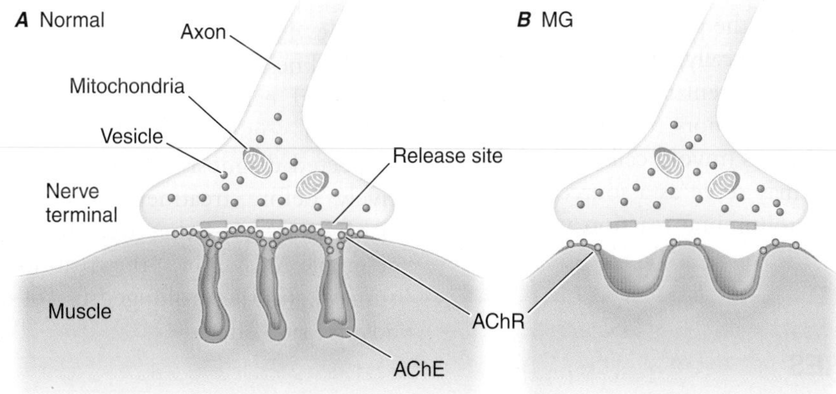

FIGURE 47-1

Diagrams of (*A*) normal and (*B*) myasthenic neuromuscular junctions. AChE, acetylcholinesterase. See text for description of normal neuromuscular transmission. The MG junction demonstrates a normal nerve terminal; a reduced number of AChRs (stippling); flattened, simplified postsynaptic folds; and a widened synaptic space. (*Modified from DB Drachman: N Engl J Med 330:1797, 1994; with permission.*)

or "simplified." These changes result in decreased efficiency of neuromuscular transmission. Therefore, although ACh is released normally, it produces small end-plate potentials that may fail to trigger muscle action potentials. Failure of transmission at many neuromuscular junctions results in weakness of muscle contraction.

The amount of ACh released per impulse normally declines on repeated activity (termed *presynaptic rundown*). In the myasthenic patient, the decreased efficiency of neuromuscular transmission combined with the normal rundown results in the activation of fewer and fewer muscle fibers by successive nerve impulses and hence increasing weakness, or *myasthenic fatigue*. This mechanism also accounts for the decremental response to repetitive nerve stimulation seen on electrodiagnostic testing.

The neuromuscular abnormalities in MG are brought about by an autoimmune response mediated by specific anti-AChR antibodies. The anti-AChR antibodies reduce the number of available AChRs at neuromuscular junctions by three distinct mechanisms: (1) accelerated turnover of AChRs by a mechanism involving cross-linking and rapid endocytosis of the receptors; (2) damage to the postsynaptic muscle membrane by the antibody in collaboration with complement; and (3) blockade of the active site of the AChR, i.e., the site that normally binds ACh. An immune response to muscle-specific kinase (MuSK), a protein involved in AChR clustering at neuromuscular junctions, can also result in myasthenia gravis, with reduction of AChRs demonstrated experimentally. The pathogenic antibodies are IgG, and are T cell-dependent. Thus, immunotherapeutic strategies directed against either the antibody-producing B cells or helper T cells are effective in this antibody-mediated disease.

How the autoimmune response is initiated and maintained in MG is not completely understood, but the thymus appears to play a role in this process. The thymus is abnormal in ~75% of patients with MG; in ~65% the thymus is "hyperplastic," with the presence of active germinal centers detected histologically, though the hyperplastic thymus is not necessarily enlarged. An additional 10% of patients have thymic tumors (thymomas). Muscle-like cells within the thymus (myoid cells), which bear AChRs on their surface, may serve as a source of autoantigen and trigger the autoimmune reaction within the thymus gland.

CLINICAL FEATURES

MG is not rare, having a prevalence of 2–7 in 10,000. It affects individuals in all age groups, but peaks of incidence occur in women in their twenties and thirties and in men in their fifties and sixties. Overall, women are affected more frequently than men, in a ratio of ~3:2. The cardinal features are *weakness* and *fatigability* of muscles. The weakness increases during repeated use (fatigue) or late in the day, and may improve following rest or sleep. The course of MG is often variable. Exacerbations and remissions may occur, particularly during the first few years after the onset of the disease. Remissions are rarely complete or permanent. Unrelated infections or systemic disorders can lead to increased myasthenic weakness and may precipitate "crisis" (discussed later).

The distribution of muscle weakness often has a characteristic pattern. The cranial muscles, particularly the lids and extraocular muscles, are typically involved early in the course of MG; diplopia and ptosis are common initial complaints. Facial weakness produces a "snarling" expression when the patient attempts to smile. Weakness in chewing is most noticeable after prolonged effort, as in chewing meat. Speech may have a nasal timbre caused by weakness of the palate, or a dysarthric "mushy" quality due to tongue weakness. Difficulty in swallowing may occur as a result of weakness of the palate, tongue, or pharynx, giving rise to nasal regurgitation or aspiration of liquids or food. Bulbar weakness is especially prominent in MuSK antibody–positive MG. In ~85% of patients, the weakness becomes generalized, affecting the limb muscles as well. If weakness remains restricted to the extraocular muscles for 3 years, it is likely that it will not become generalized, and these patients are said to have *ocular MG*. The limb weakness in MG is often proximal and may be asymmetric. Despite the muscle weakness, deep tendon reflexes are preserved. If weakness of respiration becomes so severe as to require respiratory assistance, the patient is said to be in *crisis*.

DIAGNOSIS AND EVALUATION

(Table 47-1) The diagnosis is suspected on the basis of weakness and fatigability in the typical distribution described earlier, without loss of reflexes or impairment of sensation or other neurologic function. The suspected diagnosis should always be confirmed definitively before treatment is undertaken; this is essential because (1) other treatable conditions may closely resemble MG and (2) the treatment of MG may involve surgery and the prolonged use of drugs with potentially adverse side effects.

Antibodies to AChR or MuSK

As noted earlier, anti-AChR antibodies are detectable in the serum of ~85% of all myasthenic patients but in only about 50% of patients with weakness confined to the ocular muscles. The presence of anti-AChR

TABLE 47-1

DIAGNOSIS OF MYASTHENIA GRAVIS (MG)

History
- Diplopia, ptosis, weakness
- Weakness in characteristic distribution
- Fluctuation and fatigue: worse with repeated activity, improved by rest
- Effects of previous treatments

Physical examination
- Ptosis, diplopia
- Motor power survey: quantitative testing of muscle strength
- Forward arm abduction time (5 min)
- Vital capacity
- Absence of other neurologic signs

Laboratory testing
- Anti-AChR radioimmunoassay: ~85% positive in generalized MG; 50% in ocular MG; definite diagnosis if positive; negative result does not exclude MG. ~40% of AChR antibody–negative patients with generalized MG have anti-MuSK antibodies.
- Repetitive nerve stimulation: decrement of >15% at 3 Hz: highly probable
- Single-fiber electromyography: blocking and jitter, with normal fiber density; confirmatory, but not specific
- Edrophonium chloride (Tensilon) 2 mg + 8 mg IV; highly probable diagnosis if unequivocally positive
- For ocular or cranial MG: exclude intracranial lesions by CT or MRI

Abbreviations: AChR, acetylcholine receptor; MuSK, muscle-specific tyrosine kinase.
Source: From RT Johnson, JW Griffin (eds): *Current Therapy in Neurologic Disease*, 4th ed. St. Louis, Mosby Year Book, 1994; with permission.

antibodies is virtually diagnostic of MG, but a negative test does not exclude the disease. The measured level of anti-AChR antibody does not correspond well with the severity of MG in different patients. However, in an individual patient, a treatment-induced fall in the antibody level often correlates with clinical improvement, while a rise in the level may occur with exacerbations. Antibodies to MuSK have been found to be present in ~40% of AChR antibody–negative patients with generalized MG, and their presence is a useful diagnostic test in these patients. MuSK antibodies are rarely present in AChR antibody–positive patients or in patients with MG limited to ocular muscles. These antibodies may interfere with clustering of AChRs at neuromuscular junctions, as MuSK is known to do during early development. There is also evidence that MG patients without antibodies demonstrable by standard AChR or MuSK tests may have either low-affinity antibodies, or other—as yet undefined—antibodies that impair neuromuscular transmission.

Electrodiagnostic testing

Repetitive nerve stimulation may provide helpful diagnostic evidence of MG. Anti-AChE medication is stopped 6–24 h before testing. It is best to test weak muscles or proximal muscle groups. Electric shocks are delivered at a rate of two or three per second to the appropriate nerves, and action potentials are recorded from the muscles. In normal individuals, the amplitude of the evoked muscle action potentials does not change at these rates of stimulation. However, in myasthenic patients there is a rapid reduction of >10–15% in the amplitude of the evoked responses.

Anticholinesterase test

Drugs that inhibit the enzyme AChE allow ACh to interact repeatedly with the limited number of AChRs in MG, producing improvement in muscle strength. Edrophonium is used most commonly for diagnostic testing because of the rapid onset (30 s) and short duration (~5 min) of its effect. An objective end-point must be selected to evaluate the effect of edrophonium, such as weakness of extraocular muscles, impairment of speech, or the length of time that the patient can maintain the arms in forward abduction. An initial IV dose of 2 mg of edrophonium is given. If definite improvement occurs, the test is considered positive and is terminated. If there is no change, the patient is given an additional 8 mg IV. The dose is administered in two parts because some patients react to edrophonium with side effects such as nausea, diarrhea, salivation, fasciculations, and rarely with severe symptoms of syncope or bradycardia. Atropine (0.6 mg) should be drawn up in a syringe, ready for IV administration if these symptoms become troublesome. The edrophonium test is now reserved for patients with clinical findings that are suggestive of MG but who have negative antibody and electrodiagnostic test results. False-positive tests occur in occasional patients with other neurologic disorders, such as amyotrophic lateral sclerosis, and in placebo-reactors. False-negative or equivocal tests may also occur. In some cases, it is helpful to use a longer-acting drug such as neostigmine (15 mg PO), since this permits more time for detailed evaluation of strength.

Inherited myasthenic syndromes

The congenital myasthenic syndromes (CMS) comprise a heterogeneous group of disorders of the neuromuscular junction that are not autoimmune but rather are due to genetic mutations in which virtually any component of the neuromuscular junction may be affected. Alterations in function of the presynaptic nerve terminal or in the various subunits of the AChR or AChE have been identified in the different forms of CMS.

TABLE 47-2

THE CONGENITAL MYASTHENIC SYNDROMES

TYPE	CLINICAL FEATURES	ELECTROPHYSIOLOGY	GENETICS	END-PLATE EFFECTS	TREATMENT
Slow channel	Most common; weak forearm extensors; onset 2nd to 3rd decade; variable severity	Repetitive muscle response on nerve stimulation; prolonged channel opening and MEPP duration	Autosomal dominant; α, β, ε AChR mutations	Excitotoxic end-plate myopathy; decreased AChRs; postsynaptic damage	Quinidine: decreases end-plate damage; made worse by anti-AChE
Low-affinity fast channel	Onset early; moderately severe; ptosis, EOM involvement; weakness and fatigue	Brief and infrequent channel openings; opposite of slow channel syndrome	Autosomal recessive; may be heteroallelic	Normal end-plate structure	3,4-DAP; anti-AChE
Severe AChR deficiencies	Early onset; variable severity; fatigue; typical MG features	Decremental response to repetitive nerve stimulation; decreased MEPP amplitudes	Autosomal recessive; ε mutations most common; many different mutations	Increased length of end plates; variable synaptic folds	Anti-AChE; ?3,4-DAP
AChE deficiency	Early onset; variable severity; scoliosis; may have normal EOM, absent pupillary responses	Decremental response to repetitive nerve stimulation	Mutant gene for AChE's collagen anchor	Small nerve terminals; degenerated junctional folds	Worse with anti-AChE drugs

Abbreviations: AChR, acetylcholine receptor; AChE, acetylcholinesterase; EOM, extraocular muscles; MEPP, miniature end-plate potentials; 3,4-DAP, 3,4-diaminopyridine.

These disorders share many of the clinical features of autoimmune MG, including weakness and fatigability of skeletal muscles, in some cases involving extraocular muscles (EOMs), lids, and proximal muscles, similar to the distribution in autoimmune MG. CMS should be suspected when symptoms of myasthenia have begun in infancy or childhood and AChR antibody tests are consistently negative. Features of four of the most common forms of CMS are summarized in Table 47-2. Although clinical features and electrodiagnostic and pharmacologic tests may suggest the correct diagnosis, molecular analysis is required for precise elucidation of the defect; this may lead to helpful treatment as well as genetic counseling. In the forms that involve the AChR, a wide variety of mutations have been identified in each of the subunits, but the ε subunit is affected in ~75% of these cases. In most of the recessively inherited forms of CMS, the mutations are heteroallelic; that is, different mutations affecting each of the two alleles are present.

Differential diagnosis

Other conditions that cause weakness of the cranial and/or somatic musculature include the nonautoimmune CMS discussed earlier, drug-induced myasthenia, Lambert-Eaton myasthenic syndrome (LEMS), neurasthenia, hyperthyroidism, botulism, intracranial mass lesions, and progressive external ophthalmoplegia. Treatment with penicillamine (used for scleroderma or rheumatoid arthritis) may result in true autoimmune MG, but the weakness is usually mild, and recovery occurs within weeks or months after discontinuing its use. Aminoglycoside antibiotics or procainamide can cause exacerbation of weakness in myasthenic patients; very large doses can cause neuromuscular weakness in normal individuals.

LEMS is a presynaptic disorder of the neuromuscular junction that can cause weakness similar to that of MG. The proximal muscles of the lower limbs are most commonly affected, but other muscles may be involved as well. Cranial nerve findings, including ptosis of the eyelids and diplopia, occur in up to 70% of patients and resemble features of MG. However, the two conditions are usually readily distinguished, since patients with LEMS have depressed or absent reflexes and experience autonomic changes such as dry mouth and impotence. Nerve stimulation produces an initial low-amplitude response and, at low rates of repetitive stimulation (2–3 Hz), decremental responses like those of MG; however, at high rates (50 Hz), or following exercise, incremental responses occur. LEMS is caused by autoantibodies directed against P/Q-type calcium channels at the motor nerve terminals, which can be detected in ~85% of LEMS patients by radioimmunoassay. These autoantibodies result in impaired release of ACh from nerve terminals. Most patients with LEMS have an associated malignancy, most commonly small cell carcinoma of the lung, which may express calcium channels that stimulate the autoimmune response. The diagnosis of LEMS may signal the presence of a tumor long before it would otherwise be detected, permitting early removal. Treatment of LEMS involves plasmapheresis and immunosuppression, as for MG. 3,4-Diaminopyridine (3,4-DAP) and pyridostigmine may also be symptomatically helpful. 3,4-DAP acts by blocking potassium channels, which results in prolonged depolarization of the motor nerve terminals and thus enhances ACh release. Pyridostigmine prolongs the action of ACh, allowing repeated interactions with AChRs.

Botulism is due to potent bacterial toxins produced by any of seven different strains of *Clostridium botulinum*. The toxins enzymatically cleave specific proteins essential for the release of acetylcholine from the motor nerve terminal, thereby interfering with neuromuscular transmission. Most commonly, botulism is caused by ingestion of improperly prepared food containing toxin. Rarely, the nearly ubiquitous spores of *C. botulinum* may germinate in wounds. In infants the spores may germinate in the GI tract, and release toxin, causing muscle weakness. Patients present with myasthenia-like bulbar weakness (e.g., diplopia, dysarthria, dysphagia) and lack sensory symptoms and signs. Weakness may generalize to the limbs and may result in respiratory failure. Reflexes are present early, but they may be diminished as the disease progresses. Mentation is normal. Autonomic findings include paralytic ileus, constipation, urinary retention, dilated or poorly reactive pupils, and dry mouth. The demonstration of toxin in serum by bioassay is definitive, but the results usually take a relatively long time to be completed and may be negative. Nerve stimulation studies reveal findings of presynaptic neuromuscular blockade with reduced compound muscle action potentials (CMAPs) that increase in amplitude following high-frequency repetitive stimulation. Treatment includes ventilatory support, and aggressive inpatient supportive care (e.g., nutrition, DVT prophylaxis) as needed. Antitoxin should be given as early as possible to be effective. A preventive vaccine is available for laboratory workers or other highly exposed individuals.

Neurasthenia is the historic term for a myasthenia-like fatigue syndrome without an organic basis. These patients may present with subjective symptoms of weakness and fatigue, but muscle testing usually reveals the "give-away weakness" characteristic of nonorganic disorders; the complaint of fatigue in these patients means tiredness or apathy rather than decreasing muscle power on repeated effort. Hyperthyroidism is readily diagnosed or excluded by tests of thyroid function, which should be carried out routinely in patients with suspected MG. Abnormalities of thyroid function (hyper- or hypothyroidism) may increase myasthenic weakness. Diplopia resembling that in MG may occasionally be due to an intracranial mass lesion that compresses nerves to the EOMs (e.g., sphenoid ridge meningioma), but MRI of the head and orbits usually reveals the lesion.

Progressive external ophthalmoplegia is a rare condition resulting in weakness of the EOMs, which may be accompanied by weakness of the proximal muscles of the limbs and other systemic features. Most patients with this condition have mitochondrial disorders that can be detected on muscle biopsy (Chap. 48).

Search for associated conditions

(Table 47-3) Myasthenic patients have an increased incidence of several associated disorders. Thymic abnormalities occur in ~75% of patients, as noted earlier. Neoplastic change (thymoma) may produce enlargement of the thymus, which is detected by CT scanning of the anterior mediastinum. A thymic shadow on CT scan may normally be present through young adulthood, but enlargement of the thymus in a patient aged >40 years is highly suspicious of thymoma. Hyperthyroidism occurs in 3–8% of patients and may aggravate the myasthenic weakness. Thyroid function tests should be obtained in all patients with suspected MG. Because

TABLE 47-3

DISORDERS ASSOCIATED WITH MYASTHENIA GRAVIS AND RECOMMENDED LABORATORY TESTS

Associated disorders
Disorders of the thymus: thymoma, hyperplasia
Other autoimmune disorders: Hashimoto's thyroiditis, Graves' disease, rheumatoid arthritis, lupus erythematosus, skin disorders, family history of autoimmune disorder
Disorders or circumstances that may exacerbate myasthenia gravis: hyperthyroidism or hypothyroidism, occult infection, medical treatment for other conditions (see Table 47-4)
Disorders that may interfere with therapy: tuberculosis, diabetes, peptic ulcer, gastrointestinal bleeding, renal disease, hypertension, asthma, osteoporosis, obesity
Recommended laboratory tests or procedures
CT or MRI of mediastinum
Tests for lupus erythematosus, antinuclear antibody, rheumatoid factor, antithyroid antibodies
Thyroid-function tests
PPD skin test
Chest radiography
Fasting blood glucose measurement, hemoglobin A1c
Pulmonary-function tests
Bone densitometry in older patients

Abbreviation: PPD, purified protein derivative.
Source: From RT Johnson, JW Griffin (eds): *Current Therapy in Neurologic Disease*, 4th ed. St. Louis, Mosby Year Book, 1993, p 379; with permission.

of the association of MG with other autoimmune disorders, blood tests for rheumatoid factor and antinuclear antibodies should also be carried out. Chronic infection of any kind can exacerbate MG and should be sought carefully. Finally, measurements of ventilatory function are valuable because of the frequency and seriousness of respiratory impairment in myasthenic patients.

Because of the side effects of glucocorticoids and other immunosuppressive agents used in the treatment of MG, a thorough medical investigation should be undertaken, searching specifically for evidence of chronic or latent infection (such as tuberculosis or hepatitis), hypertension, diabetes, renal disease, and glaucoma.

TREATMENT Myasthenia Gravis

The prognosis has improved strikingly as a result of advances in treatment. Nearly all myasthenic patients can be returned to full productive lives with proper therapy. The most useful treatments for MG include anticholinesterase medications, immunosuppressive agents, thymectomy, and plasmapheresis or intravenous immunoglobulin (IVIg) (Fig. 47-2).

ANTICHOLINESTERASE MEDICATIONS Anticholinesterase medication produces at least partial improvement in most myasthenic patients, although improvement is complete in only a few. Pyridostigmine is the most widely used anticholinesterase drug. The beneficial action of oral pyridostigmine begins within 15–30 min and lasts for 3–4 h, but individual responses vary. Treatment is begun with a moderate dose, e.g., 30–60 mg three to four times daily. The frequency and amount of the dose should be tailored to the patient's individual requirements throughout the day. For example, patients with weakness in chewing and swallowing may benefit by taking the medication before meals so that peak strength coincides with mealtimes. Long-acting pyridostigmine may occasionally be useful to get the patient through the night but should not be used for daytime medication because of variable absorption. The maximum useful dose of pyridostigmine rarely exceeds 120 mg every 4–6 h during daytime. Overdosage with anticholinesterase medication may cause increased weakness and other side effects. In some patients, muscarinic side effects of the anticholinesterase medication (diarrhea, abdominal cramps, salivation, nausea) may limit the dose tolerated. Atropine/diphenoxylate or loperamide is useful for the treatment of gastrointestinal symptoms.

THYMECTOMY Two separate issues should be distinguished: (1) surgical removal of thymoma, and (2) thymectomy as a treatment for MG. Surgical removal

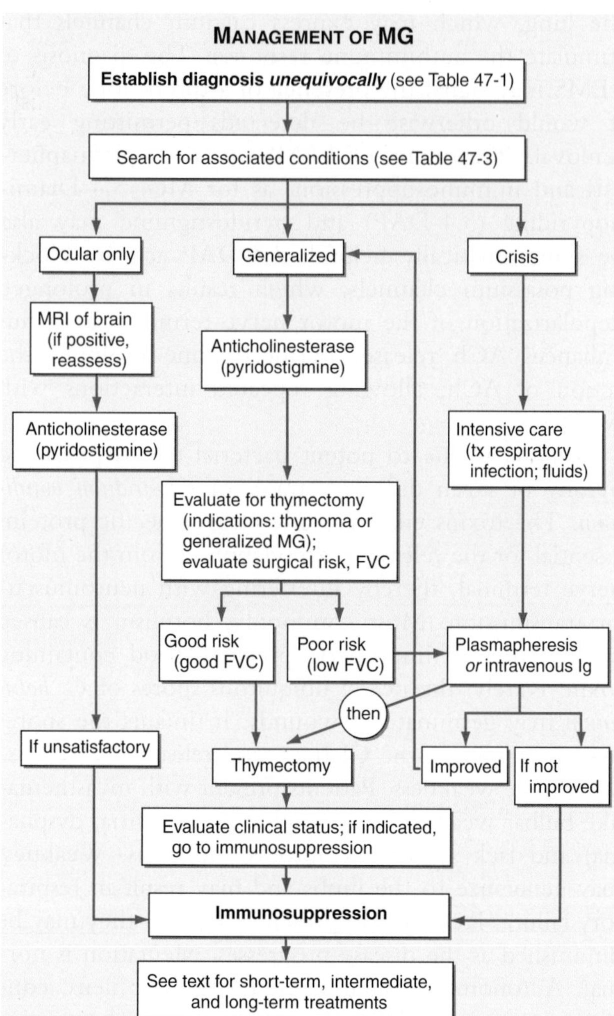

FIGURE 47-2
Algorithm for the management of myasthenia gravis. FVC, forced vital capacity.

of a thymoma is necessary because of the possibility of local tumor spread, although most thymomas are histologically benign. In the absence of a tumor, the available evidence suggests that up to 85% of patients experience improvement after thymectomy; of these, ~35% achieve drug-free remission. However, the improvement is typically delayed for months to years. The advantage of thymectomy is that it offers the possibility of long-term benefit, in some cases diminishing or eliminating the need for continuing medical treatment. In view of these potential benefits and of the negligible risk in skilled hands, thymectomy has gained widespread acceptance in the treatment of MG. It is the consensus that thymectomy should be carried out in all patients with generalized MG who are between the ages of puberty and at least 55 years. Whether thymectomy should be recommended in children, in adults >55 years of age, and in patients with weakness limited to the ocular muscles is still a matter of debate. There is also suggestive evidence that patients with MuSK antibody–positive MG may respond less well to thymectomy. Thymectomy must be carried out in a hospital where it is performed regularly and where the staff is experienced in the pre- and postoperative management, anesthesia, and surgical techniques of total thymectomy.

IMMUNOSUPPRESSION Immunosuppression using glucocorticoids, azathioprine, and other drugs is effective in nearly all patients with MG. The choice of drugs or other immunomodulatory treatments should be guided by the relative benefits and risks for the individual patient and the urgency of treatment. It is helpful to develop a treatment plan based on short-term, intermediate-term, and long-term objectives. For example, if immediate improvement is essential either because of the severity of weakness or because of the patient's need to return to activity as soon as possible, IVIg should be administered or plasmapheresis should be undertaken. For the intermediate term, glucocorticoids and cyclosporine or tacrolimus generally produce clinical improvement within a period of 1–3 months. The beneficial effects of azathioprine and mycophenolate mofetil usually begin after many months (as long as a year), but these drugs have advantages for the long-term treatment of patients with MG. For the occasional patient with MG that is genuinely refractory to optimal treatment with conventional immunosuppressive agents, a course of high-dose cyclophosphamide may induce long-lasting benefit by "rebooting" the immune system. At high doses, cyclophosphamide eliminates mature lymphocytes but spares hematopoietic precursors (stem cells), because they express the enzyme aldehyde dehydrogenase, which hydrolyzes cyclophosphamide. At present, this procedure is reserved for refractory patients and should be administered only in a facility fully familiar with this approach. We recommend maintenance immunotherapy after rebooting, to sustain the beneficial effect.

Glucocorticoid Therapy Glucocorticoids, when used properly, produce improvement in myasthenic weakness in the great majority of patients. To minimize adverse side effects, prednisone should be given in a single dose rather than in divided doses throughout the day. The initial dose should be relatively low (15–25 mg/d) to avoid the early weakening that occurs in about one-third of patients treated initially with a high-dose regimen. The dose is increased stepwise, as tolerated by the patient (usually by 5 mg/d at 2- to 3-day intervals), until there is marked clinical improvement or a dose of 50–60 mg/d is reached. This dose is maintained for 1–3 months and then is gradually modified to an alternate-day regimen over the course of an additional 1–3 months; the goal is to reduce the dose on the "off day" to zero or to a minimal level. Generally, patients begin to improve within a few weeks after reaching the maximum dose, and improvement continues to progress for months or years. The prednisone dosage may gradually be reduced, but usually months or years may be needed to determine the minimum effective dose, and close monitoring is required. Few patients are able to do without immunosuppressive agents entirely. Patients on long-term glucocorticoid therapy must be followed carefully to prevent or treat adverse side effects. The most common errors in glucocorticoid treatment of myasthenic patients include (1) insufficient persistence—improvement may be delayed and gradual; (2) tapering the dosage too early, too rapidly, or excessively; and (3) lack of attention to prevention and treatment of side effects.

Other Immunosuppressive Drugs Mycophenolate mofetil, azathioprine, cyclosporine, tacrolimus, and occasionally cyclophosphamide are effective in many patients, either alone or in various combinations.

Mycophenolate mofetil has become one of the most widely used drugs in the treatment of MG because of its effectiveness and relative lack of side effects. A dose of 1–1.5 g bid is recommended. Its mechanism of action involves inhibition of purine synthesis by the de novo pathway. Since lymphocytes lack the alternative salvage pathway that is present in all other cells, mycophenolate inhibits proliferation of lymphocytes but not proliferation of other cells. It does not kill or eliminate preexisting autoreactive lymphocytes, and therefore clinical improvement may be delayed for many months to a year, until the preexisting autoreactive lymphocytes die spontaneously. The advantage of mycophenolate lies in its relative lack of adverse side effects, with only occasional production of GI symptoms, rare development of leukopenia, and very small risks of malignancy or PML inherent in all immunosuppressive treatments. Although two published studies did not have positive outcomes, most experts attribute the negative results to flaws in the trial designs, and mycophenolate is widely used for long-term treatment of myasthenic patients. Until recently, azathioprine has been the most commonly used immunosuppressive agent for MG because of its relative safety in most patients and long track record. Its therapeutic effect may add to that of glucocorticoids and/or allow the glucocorticoid dose to be reduced. However, up to 10% of patients are unable to tolerate azathioprine because of idiosyncratic reactions consisting of flulike symptoms of fever and malaise, bone marrow suppression, or abnormalities of liver function. An initial dose of 50 mg/d should be used for several days to test for these side effects. If this dose is tolerated, it is increased gradually to about 2–3 mg/kg of total body weight, or until the white blood count falls to 3000 to 4000/μL. The beneficial effect of azathioprine takes 3–6 months to begin and even longer to peak. In patients taking azathioprine, allopurinol should never be used to treat hyperuricemia. Because the two drugs share a common degradation pathway; the result may be severe bone marrow suppression due to increased effects of the azathioprine.

The calcineurin inhibitors cyclosporine and tacrolimus (FK506) are approximately as effective as azathioprine and are being used increasingly in the management of MG. Their beneficial effect appears more rapidly than that of azathioprine. Either drug may be used alone, but they are usually used as an adjunct to glucocorticoids to permit reduction of the glucocorticoid dose. The usual dose of cyclosporine is 4–5 mg/kg per d, and the average dose of tacrolimus is 0.07–0.1 mg/kg per d, given in two equally divided doses (to minimize side effects). Side effects of these drugs include hypertension and nephrotoxicity, which must be closely monitored. "Trough" blood levels are measured 12 h after the evening dose. The therapeutic range for the trough level of cyclosporine is 150–200 ng/L, and for tacrolimus it is 5–15 ng/L.

Cyclophosphamide is reserved for occasional patients refractory to the other drugs (see earlier discussion of high-dose cyclophosphamide treatment). Rituximab, a monoclonal antibody that depletes CD20 B cells, has been used with variable—sometimes dramatic—success in the treatment of MG, especially in patients with anti-MuSK antibody.

PLASMAPHERESIS AND INTRAVENOUS IMMUNOGLOBULIN Plasmapheresis has been used therapeutically in MG. Plasma, which contains the pathogenic antibodies, is mechanically separated from the blood cells, which are returned to the patient. A course of five exchanges (3–4 L per exchange) is generally administered over a 10- to 14-day period. Plasmapheresis produces a short-term reduction in anti-AChR antibodies, with clinical improvement in many patients. It is useful as a temporary expedient in seriously affected patients or to improve the patient's condition prior to surgery (e.g., thymectomy).

The indications for the use of IVIg are the same as those for plasma exchange: to produce rapid improvement to help the patient through a difficult period of myasthenic weakness or prior to surgery. This treatment has the advantages of not requiring special equipment or large-bore venous access. The usual dose is 2 g/kg, which is typically administered over 5 days (400 mg/kg per d). If tolerated, the total dose of IVIg can be given over a 3- to 4-day period. Improvement occurs in ~70% of patients, beginning during treatment, or within a week, and continuing for weeks to months. The mechanism of action of IVIg is not known; the treatment has no consistent effect on the measurable amount of circulating AChR antibody. Adverse reactions are generally not serious but include headache, fluid overload, and rarely aseptic meningitis or renal failure. IVIg should rarely be used as a long-term treatment in place of rationally managed immunosuppressive therapy. Unfortunately, there is a tendency for physicians unfamiliar with immunosuppressive treatments to rely on repeated IVIg infusions, which usually produce only intermittent benefit, do not reduce the underlying autoimmune response, and are costly. The intermediate and long-term treatment of myasthenic patients requires other methods of therapy outlined earlier in this chapter.

MANAGEMENT OF MYASTHENIC CRISIS Myasthenic crisis is defined as an exacerbation of weakness sufficient to endanger life; it usually consists of respiratory failure caused by diaphragmatic and intercostal muscle weakness. Crisis rarely occurs in properly managed patients. Treatment should be carried out in intensive care units staffed with teams experienced in the management of MG, respiratory insufficiency, infectious disease, and fluid and electrolyte therapy. The possibility that deterioration could be due to excessive anticholinesterase medication ("cholinergic crisis") is best excluded by temporarily stopping anticholinesterase drugs. The most common cause of crisis is intercurrent infection. This should be treated immediately, because the mechanical and immunologic defenses of the patient can be assumed to be compromised. The myasthenic patient with fever and early infection should be treated like other immunocompromised patients. Early and effective antibiotic therapy, respiratory assistance (preferably noninvasive, using BiPap), and pulmonary physiotherapy are essentials of the treatment program. As discussed earlier, plasmapheresis or IVIg is frequently helpful in hastening recovery.

DRUGS TO AVOID IN MYASTHENIC PATIENTS Many drugs have been reported to exacerbate weakness in patients with MG (Table 47-4), but not all patients react adversely to all of these. Conversely, not all "safe" drugs can be used with impunity in patients with MG. As a rule, the listed drugs should be avoided *whenever possible*, and myasthenic patients should be followed closely when *any new drug* is introduced.

PATIENT ASSESSMENT

To evaluate the effectiveness of treatment as well as drug-induced side effects, it is important to assess the patient's clinical status systematically at baseline and on repeated interval examinations. Because of the variability of symptoms of MG, the interval history and

TABLE 47-4

DRUGS WITH INTERACTIONS IN MYASTHENIA GRAVIS (MG)

Drugs That May Exacerbate MG
Antibiotics
Aminoglycosides: e.g., streptomycin, tobramycin, kanamycin
Quinolones: e.g., ciprofloxacin, levofloxacin, ofloxacin, gatifloxacin
Macrolides: e.g., erythromycin, azithromycin,
Nondepolarizing muscle relaxants for surgery
D-Tubocurarine (curare), pancuronium, vecuronium, atracurium
Beta-blocking agents
Propranolol, atenolol, metoprolol
Local anesthetics and related agents
Procaine, Xylocaine in large amounts
Procainamide (for arrhythmias)
Botulinum toxin
Botox exacerbates weakness
Quinine derivatives
Quinine, quinidine, chloroquine, mefloquine (Lariam)
Magnesium
Decreases ACh release
Penicillamine
May cause MG
Drugs with Important Interactions In MG
Cyclosporine
Broad range of drug interactions, which may raise or lower cyclosporine levels.
Azathioprine
Avoid allopurinol—combination may result in myelosuppression.

physical findings on examination must be taken into account. The most useful clinical tests include forward arm abduction time (up to a full 5 min), forced vital capacity, range of eye movements, and time to development of ptosis on upward gaze. Manual muscle testing or, preferably, quantitative dynamometry of limb muscles, especially proximal muscles, is also important. An interval form can provide a succinct summary of the patient's status and a guide to treatment results; an abbreviated form is shown in Fig. 47-3. A progressive reduction in the patient's AChR antibody level also provides clinically valuable confirmation of the effectiveness of treatment; conversely, a rise in AChR antibody levels during tapering of immunosuppressive medication may predict clinical exacerbation. For reliable quantitative measurement of AChR antibody levels, it is best to compare antibody levels from prior frozen serum aliquots with current serum samples in simultaneously run assays.

Myasthenia Gravis Worksheet

History				
General	Normal	Good	Fair	Poor
Diplopia	None	Rare	Occasional	Constant
Ptosis	None	Rare	Occasional	Constant
Arms	Normal	Slightly limited	Some ADL impairment	Definitely limited
Legs	Normal	Walks/runs fatigues	Can walk limited distances	Minimal walking
Speech	Normal	Dysarthric	Severely dysarthric	Unintelligible
Voice	Normal	Fades	Impaired	Severely impaired
Chew	Normal	Fatigue on normal foods	Fatigue on soft foods	Feeding tube
Swallow	Normal	Normal foods	Soft foods only	Feeding tube
Respiration	Normal	Dyspnea on unusual effort	Dyspnea on any effort	Dyspnea at rest

Examination

BP _____ Pulse _____ Wt _____
Edema __________
Vital capacity __________
Cataracts? R _______ L _______
EOMS __________
Ptosis time __________
Face __________

Arm abduction time R_____ L_____
Deltoids R_____ L_____
Biceps R_____ L_____
Triceps R_____ L_____
Grip R_____ L_____
Iliopsoas R_____ L_____
Quadriceps R_____ L_____
Hamstrings R_____ L_____
Other R_____ L_____

FIGURE 47-3

Abbreviated interval assessment form for use in evaluating treatment for myasthenia gravis.

CHAPTER 48

MUSCULAR DYSTROPHIES AND OTHER MUSCLE DISEASES

Anthony A. Amato ■ Robert H. Brown, Jr.

Skeletal muscle diseases, or myopathies, are disorders with structural changes or functional impairment of muscle. These conditions can be differentiated from other diseases of the motor unit (e.g., lower motor neuron or neuromuscular junction pathologies) by characteristic clinical and laboratory findings.

Myasthenia gravis and related disorders are discussed in Chap. 47; dermatomyositis, polymyositis, and inclusion body myositis are discussed in Chap. 49.

CLINICAL FEATURES

Most myopathies present with proximal, symmetric limb weakness (arms or legs) with preserved reflexes and sensation. However, asymmetric and predominantly distal weakness can be seen in some myopathies. An associated sensory loss suggests injury to peripheral nerve or the central nervous system (CNS) rather than myopathy. On occasion, disorders affecting the motor nerve cell bodies in the spinal cord (anterior horn cell disease), the neuromuscular junction, or peripheral nerves can mimic findings of myopathy.

Muscle weakness

Symptoms of muscle weakness can be either intermittent or persistent. Disorders causing *intermittent weakness* (Fig. 48-1) include myasthenia gravis, periodic paralyses (hypokalemic, hyperkalemic, and paramyotonia congenita), and metabolic energy deficiencies of glycolysis (especially myophosphorylase deficiency), fatty acid utilization (carnitine palmitoyltransferase deficiency), and some mitochondrial myopathies. The states of energy deficiency cause activity-related muscle breakdown accompanied by myoglobinuria, appearing as light-brown- to dark-brown-colored urine.

Most muscle disorders cause *persistent weakness* (Fig. 48-2). In the majority of these, including most types of muscular dystrophy, polymyositis, and dermatomyositis, the proximal muscles are weaker than the distal and are symmetrically affected, and the facial muscles are spared, a pattern referred to as *limb-girdle*. The differential diagnosis is more restricted for other patterns of weakness. Facial weakness (difficulty with eye closure and impaired smile) and scapular winging (Fig. 48-3) are characteristic of facioscapulohumeral dystrophy (FSHD). Facial and distal limb weakness associated with hand grip myotonia is virtually diagnostic of myotonic dystrophy type 1. When other cranial nerve muscles are weak, causing ptosis or extraocular muscle weakness, the most important disorders to consider include neuromuscular junction disorders, oculopharyngeal muscular dystrophy, mitochondrial myopathies, or some of the congenital myopathies (Table 48-1). A pathognomonic pattern characteristic of inclusion body myositis is atrophy and weakness of the flexor forearm (e.g., wrist and finger flexors) and quadriceps muscles that is often asymmetric. Less frequently, but important diagnostically, is the presence of a dropped head syndrome indicative of selective neck extensor muscle weakness. The most important neuromuscular diseases associated with this pattern of weakness include myasthenia gravis, amyotrophic lateral sclerosis, late-onset nemaline myopathy, hyperparathyroidism, focal myositis, and some forms of inclusion body myopathy. A final pattern, recognized because of preferential distal extremity weakness, is typical of a unique category of muscular dystrophy, the distal myopathies.

It is important to examine functional capabilities to help disclose certain patterns of weakness (Table 48-2). The Gowers' sign (Fig. 48-4) is particularly useful. Observing the gait of an individual may disclose a lordotic posture caused by combined trunk and

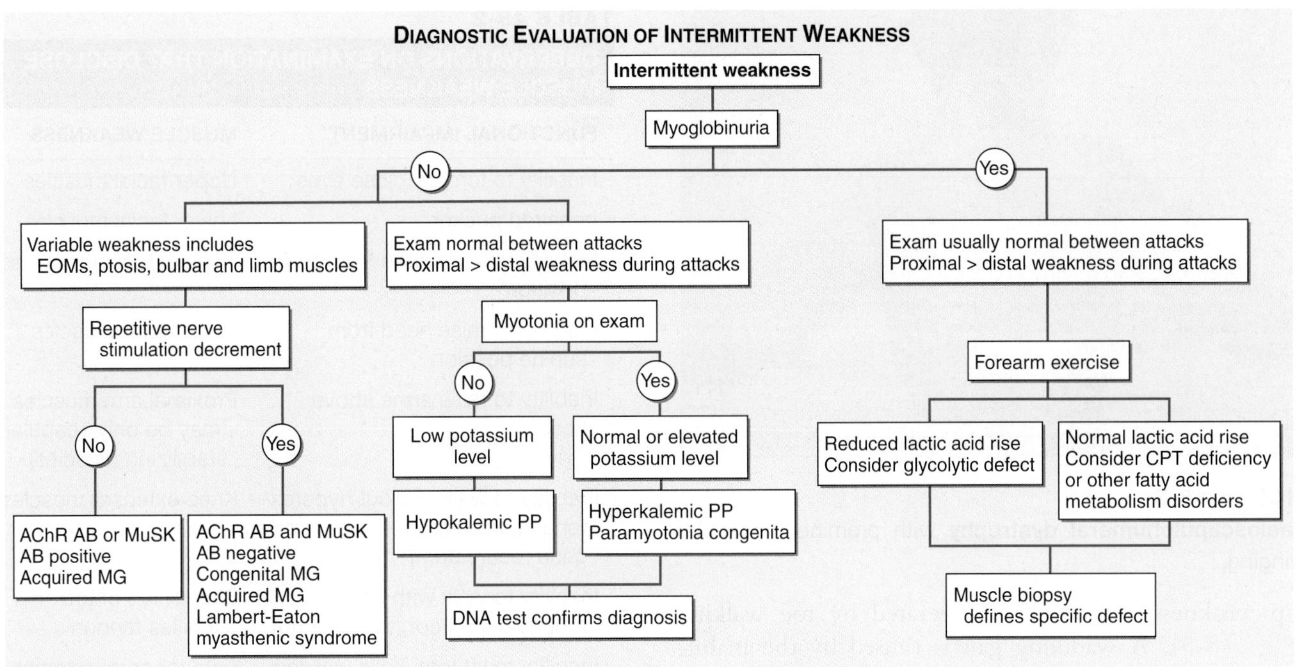

FIGURE 48-1

Diagnostic evaluation of intermittent weakness. AChR AB, acetylcholine receptor antibody; CPT, carnitine palmitoyltransferase; EOMs, extraocular muscles; MG, myasthenia gravis; PP, periodic paralysis.

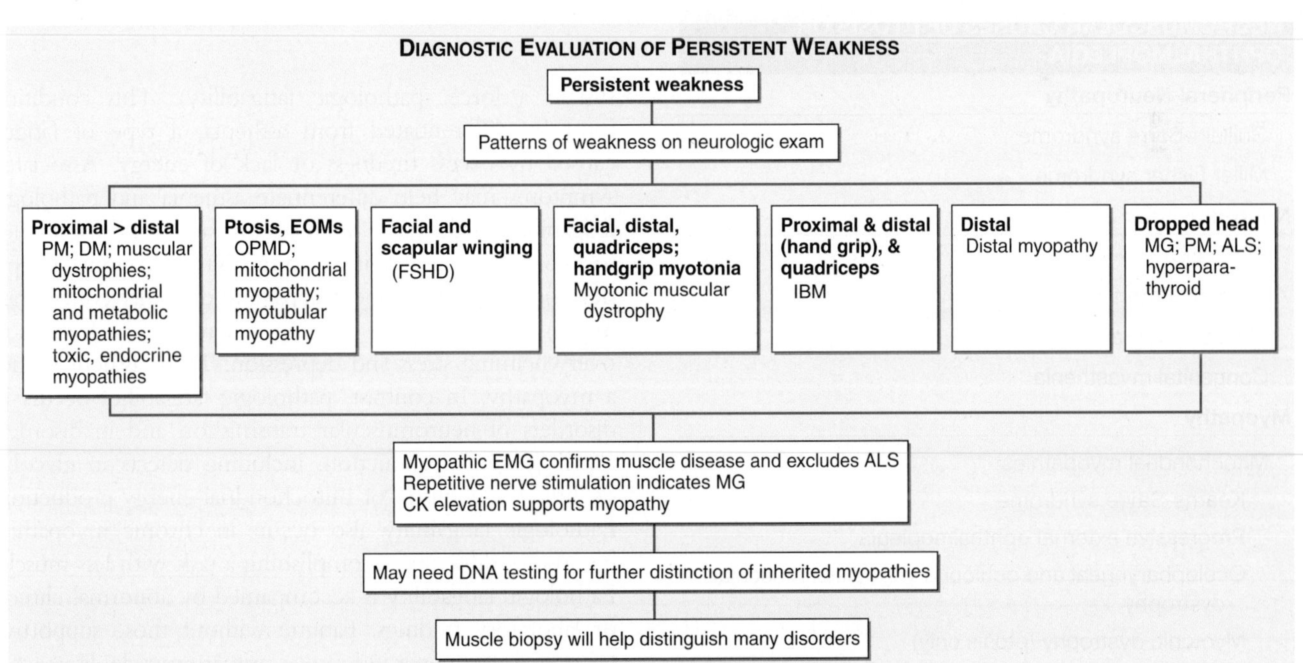

FIGURE 48-2

Diagnostic evaluation of persistent weakness. Examination reveals one of seven patterns of weakness. The pattern of weakness in combination with the laboratory evaluation leads to a diagnosis. EOMs, extraocular muscles; OPMD, oculopharyngeal muscular dystrophy; FSHD, facioscapulohumeral dystrophy; IBM, inclusion body myositis; DM, dermatomyositis; PM, polymyositis; MG, myasthenia gravis; ALS, amyotrophic lateral sclerosis; CK, creatine kinase; EMG, electromyography.

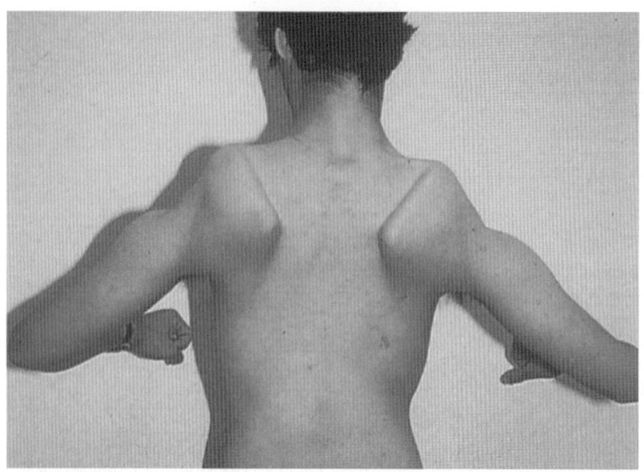

FIGURE 48-3
Facioscapulohumeral dystrophy with prominent scapular winging.

hip weakness, frequently exaggerated by toe walking (Fig. 48-5). A waddling gait is caused by the inability of weak hip muscles to prevent hip drop or hip dip. Hyperextension of the knee (genu recurvatum or back-kneeing) is characteristic of quadriceps muscle weakness; and a steppage gait, due to footdrop, accompanies distal weakness.

Any disorder causing muscle weakness may be accompanied by *fatigue*, referring to an inability to maintain or sustain a force (pathologic fatigability). This condition must be differentiated from asthenia, a type of fatigue caused by excess tiredness or lack of energy. Associated symptoms may help differentiate asthenia and pathologic fatigability. Asthenia is often accompanied by a tendency to avoid physical activities, complaints of daytime sleepiness, necessity for frequent naps, and difficulty concentrating on activities such as reading. There may be feelings of overwhelming stress and depression. Thus, asthenia is not a myopathy. In contrast, pathologic fatigability occurs in disorders of neuromuscular transmission and in disorders altering energy production, including defects in glycolysis, lipid metabolism, or mitochondrial energy production. Pathologic fatigability also occurs in chronic myopathies because of difficulty accomplishing a task with less muscle. Pathologic fatigability is accompanied by abnormal clinical or laboratory findings. Fatigue without those supportive features almost never indicates a primary muscle disease.

TABLE 48-1

NEUROMUSCULAR CAUSES OF PTOSIS OR OPHTHALMOPLEGIA

Peripheral Neuropathy
Guillain-Barré syndrome
Miller Fisher syndrome
Neuromuscular Junction
Botulism
Lambert-Eaton syndrome
Myasthenia gravis
Congenital myasthenia
Myopathy
Mitochondrial myopathies
Kearns-Sayre syndrome
Progressive external ophthalmoplegia
Oculopharyngeal and oculopharyngodistal muscular dystrophy
Myotonic dystrophy (ptosis only)
Congenital myopathy
Myotubular
Nemaline (ptosis only)
Hyperthyroidism/Graves' disease (ophthalmoplegia without ptosis)
Hereditary inclusion body myopathy type 3

TABLE 48-2

OBSERVATIONS ON EXAMINATION THAT DISCLOSE MUSCLE WEAKNESS

FUNCTIONAL IMPAIRMENT	MUSCLE WEAKNESS
Inability to forcibly close eyes	Upper facial muscles
Impaired pucker	Lower facial muscles
Inability to raise head from prone position	Neck extensor muscles
Inability to raise head from supine position	Neck flexor muscles
Inability to raise arms above head	Proximal arm muscles (may be only scapular stabilizing muscles)
Inability to walk without hyperextending knee (back-kneeing or genu recurvatum)	Knee extensor muscles
Inability to walk with heels touching the floor (toe walking)	Shortening of the Achilles tendon
Inability to lift foot while walking (steppage gait or footdrop)	Anterior compartment of leg
Inability to walk without a waddling gait	Hip muscles
Inability to get up from the floor without climbing up the extremities (Gowers' sign)	Hip, thigh, and trunk muscles
Inability to get up from a chair without using arms	Hip muscles

Muscle pain (myalgias), cramps, and stiffness

Muscle pain can be associated with cramps, spasms, contractures, and stiff or rigid muscles. In distinction, true myalgia (muscle aching), which can be localized or generalized, may be accompanied by weakness,

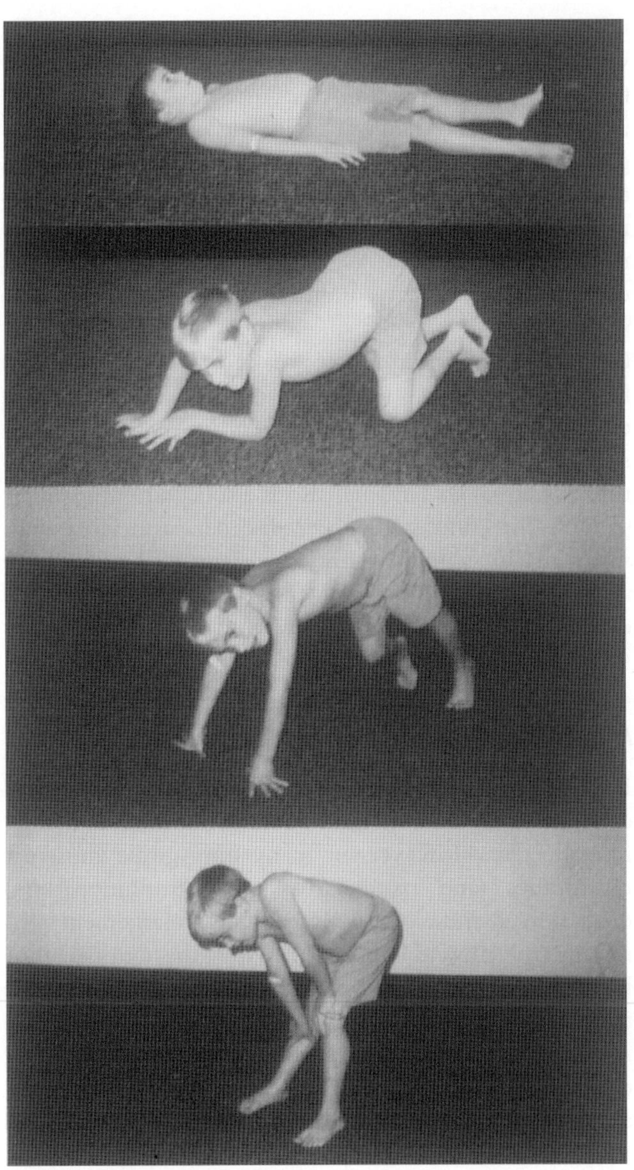

FIGURE 48-4
Gowers' sign showing a patient using arms to climb up the legs in attempting to get up from the floor.

tenderness to palpation, or swelling. Certain drugs cause true myalgia (Table 48-3).

There are two painful muscle conditions of particular importance, neither of which is associated with muscle weakness. *Fibromyalgia* is a common, yet poorly understood, type of myofascial pain syndrome. Patients complain of severe muscle pain and tenderness and have specific painful trigger points, sleep disturbances, and easy fatigability. Serum creatine kinase (CK), erythrocyte sedimentation rate (ESR), electromyography (EMG), and muscle biopsy are normal. *Polymyalgia rheumatica* occurs mainly in patients >50 years and is characterized by stiffness and pain in the shoulders, lower back, hips, and thighs. The ESR is elevated, while serum CK, EMG, and muscle biopsy are normal. Temporal arteritis, an inflammatory disorder of medium- and large-sized arteries, usually involving one or more

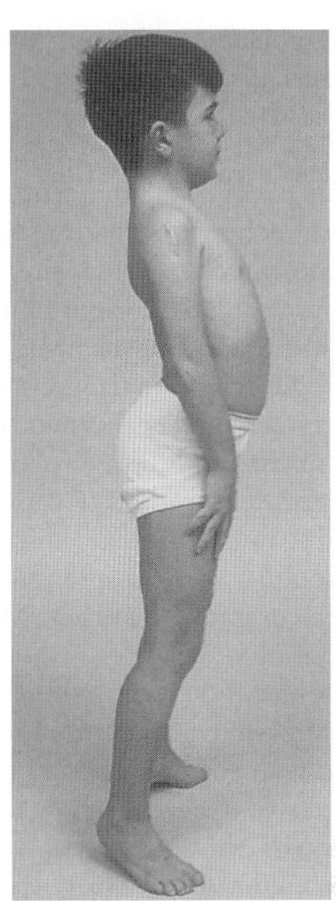

FIGURE 48-5
Lordotic posture, exaggerated by standing on toes, associated with trunk and hip weakness.

branches of the carotid artery, may accompany polymyalgia rheumatica. Vision is threatened by ischemic optic neuritis. Glucocorticoids can relieve the myalgias and protect against visual loss.

Localized muscle pain is most often traumatic. A common cause of sudden abrupt-onset pain is a ruptured tendon, which leaves the muscle belly appearing rounded and shorter in appearance compared to the

TABLE 48-3

DRUGS THAT CAUSE TRUE MYALGIA
Cimetidine
Cocaine
Cyclosporine
Danazol
Emetine
Gold
Heroin
Labetalol
Methadone
D-Penicillamine
Statins and other cholesterol-lowering agents
L-Tryptophan
Zidovudine

normal side. The biceps brachii and Achilles tendons are particularly vulnerable to rupture. Infection or neoplastic infiltration of the muscle is a rare cause of localized muscle pain.

A *muscle cramp* or *spasm* is a painful, involuntary, localized, muscle contraction with a visible or palpable hardening of the muscle. Cramps are abrupt in onset, short in duration, and may cause abnormal posturing of the joint. The EMG shows firing of motor units, reflecting an origin from spontaneous neural discharge. Muscle cramps often occur in neurogenic disorders, especially motor neuron disease (Chap. 32), radiculopathies, and polyneuropathies (Chap. 45), but are not a feature of most primary muscle diseases. Duchenne's muscular dystrophy is an exception since calf muscle complaints are a common complaint. Muscle cramps are also common during pregnancy.

A *muscle contracture* is different from a muscle cramp. In both conditions, the muscle becomes hard, but a contracture is associated with energy failure in glycolytic disorders. The muscle is unable to relax after an active muscle contraction. The EMG shows electrical silence. Confusion is created because contracture also refers to a muscle that cannot be passively stretched to its proper length (fixed contracture) because of fibrosis. In some muscle disorders, especially in Emery-Dreifuss muscular dystrophy and Bethlem's myopathy, fixed contractures occur early and represent distinctive features of the disease.

Muscle stiffness can refer to different phenomena. Some patients with inflammation of joints and periarticular surfaces feel stiff. This condition is different from the disorders of hyperexcitable motor nerves causing stiff or rigid muscles. In *stiff-person syndrome*, spontaneous discharges of the motor neurons of the spinal cord cause involuntary muscle contractions mainly involving the axial (trunk) and proximal lower extremity muscles. The gait becomes stiff and labored, with hyperlordosis of the lumbar spine. Superimposed episodic muscle spasms are precipitated by sudden movements, unexpected noises, and emotional upset. The muscles relax during sleep. Serum antibodies against glutamic acid decarboxylase are present in approximately two-thirds of cases. In *neuromyotonia* (*Isaac's syndrome*) there is hyperexcitability of the peripheral nerves manifesting as continuous muscle fiber activity. *Myokymia* (groups of fasciculations associated with continuous undulations of muscle) and impaired muscle relaxation are the result. Muscles of the leg are stiff, and the constant contractions of the muscle cause increased sweating of the extremities. This peripheral nerve hyperexcitability is mediated by antibodies that target voltage-gated potassium channels. The site of origin of the spontaneous nerve discharges is principally in the distal portion of the motor nerves.

Myotonia is a condition of prolonged muscle contraction followed by slow muscle relaxation. It always follows muscle activation (action myotonia), usually voluntary, but may be elicited by mechanical stimulation (percussion myotonia) of the muscle. Myotonia typically causes difficulty in releasing objects after a firm grasp. In myotonic muscular dystrophy type 1 (DM1), distal weakness usually accompanies myotonia, whereas in DM2 proximal muscles are more affected; thus the related term *proximal myotonic myopathy* (PROMM) is used to describe this condition. Myotonia also occurs with *myotonia congenita* (a chloride channel disorder), but in this condition muscle weakness is not prominent. Myotonia may also be seen in individuals with sodium channel mutations (*hyperkalemic periodic paralysis* or *potassium-sensitive myotonia*). Another sodium channelopathy, *paramyotonia congenita*, also is associated with muscle stiffness. In contrast to other disorders associated with myotonia in which the myotonia is eased by repetitive activity, paramyotonia congenita is named for a paradoxical phenomenon whereby the myotonia worsens with repetitive activity.

Muscle enlargement and atrophy

In most myopathies muscle tissue is replaced by fat and connective tissue, but the size of the muscle is usually not affected. However, in many limb-girdle muscular dystrophies (and particularly the dystrophinopathies) enlarged calf muscles are typical. The enlargement represents true muscle hypertrophy, thus the term pseudohypertrophy should be avoided when referring to these patients. The calf muscles remain very strong even late in the course of these disorders. Muscle enlargement can also result from infiltration by sarcoid granulomas, amyloid deposits, bacterial and parasitic infections, and focal myositis. In contrast, muscle atrophy is characteristic of other myopathies. In dysferlinopathies (LGMD2B), there is a predilection for early atrophy of the gastrocnemius muscles, particularly the medial aspect. Atrophy of the humeral muscles is characteristic of facioscapulohumeral dystrophy (FSHD).

LABORATORY EVALUATION

A limited battery of tests can be used to evaluate a suspected myopathy. Nearly all patients require serum enzyme level measurements and electrodiagnostic studies as screening tools to differentiate muscle disorders from other motor unit diseases. The other tests described—DNA studies, the forearm exercise test, and muscle biopsy—are used to diagnose specific types of myopathies.

Serum enzymes

CK is the preferred muscle enzyme to measure in the evaluation of myopathies. Damage to muscle causes the CK to leak from the muscle fiber to the serum. The MM isoenzyme predominates in skeletal muscle, while creatine kinase-myocardial bound (CK-MB) is the marker for cardiac muscle. Serum CK can be elevated in normal individuals without provocation, presumably on a genetic basis or after strenuous activity, minor trauma (including the EMG needle), a prolonged muscle cramp, or a generalized seizure. Aspartate aminotransferase (AST), alanine aminotransferase (ALT), aldolase, and lactic dehydrogenase (LDH) are enzymes sharing an origin in both muscle and liver. Problems arise when the levels of these enzymes are found to be elevated in a routine screening battery, leading to the erroneous assumption that liver disease is present when in fact muscle could be the cause. An elevated γ-glutamyl transferase (GGT) helps to establish a liver origin since this enzyme is not found in muscle.

Electrodiagnostic studies

EMG, repetitive nerve stimulation, and nerve conduction studies (Chap. 5) are essential methods for evaluation of the patient with suspected muscle disease. In combination, they provide the information necessary to differentiate myopathies from neuropathies and neuromuscular junction diseases. Routine nerve conduction studies are typically normal in myopathies but reduced amplitudes of compound muscle action potentials may be seen in atrophied muscles. The needle EMG may reveal irritability on needle placement suggestive of a necrotizing myopathy (inflammatory myopathies, dystrophies, toxic myopathies, myotonic myopathies), whereas a lack of irritability is characteristic of long-standing myopathic disorders (muscular dystrophies, endocrine myopathies, disuse atrophy, and many of the metabolic myopathies). In addition, the EMG may demonstrate myotonic discharges that will narrow the differential diagnosis (Table 48-4). Another important EMG finding is the presence of short-duration, small-amplitude, polyphasic motor unit action potentials (MUAPs). Such MUAPs can be seen in both myopathic and neuropathic disorders; however, the recruitment or firing pattern is different. In myopathies, the MUAPs fire early but at a normal rate to compensate for the loss of individual muscle fibers, whereas in neurogenic disorders the MUAPs fire faster. The EMG is usually normal in steroid or disuse myopathy, both of which are associated with type 2 fiber atrophy; this is because the EMG preferentially assesses the physiologic function of type 1 fibers. The EMG can also be invaluable in helping to choose an appropriately affected muscle to sample for biopsy.

DNA analysis

This serves as an important tool for the definitive diagnosis of many muscle disorders. Nevertheless, there are a number of limitations in currently available molecular diagnostics. For example, in Duchenne's and Becker's dystrophies, two-thirds of patients have deletion or duplication mutations that are easy to detect, while the remainder have point mutations that are much more difficult to find. For patients without identifiable gene defects, the muscle biopsy remains the main diagnostic tool.

TABLE 48-4

MYOTONIC DISORDERS
Myotonic dystrophy type 1
Myotonic dystrophy type 2/proximal myotonic myopathy
Myotonia congenita
Paramyotonia congenita
Hyperkalemic periodic paralysis
Chondrodystrophic myotonia (Schwartz-Jampel syndrome)
Centronuclear/myotubular myopathy[a]
Drug-induced
Cholesterol-lowering agents (statin medications, fibrates)
Cyclosporine
Chloroquine
Glycogen storage disorders[a] (Pompe's disease, debrancher deficiency, branching enzyme deficiency)
Myofibrillar myopathies[a]

[a]Associated with myotonic discharges on EMG but no clinical myotonia.

Forearm exercise test

In myopathies with intermittent symptoms, and especially those associated with myoglobinuria, there may be a defect in glycolysis. Many variations of the forearm exercise test exist. For safety, the test should not be performed under ischemic conditions to avoid an unnecessary insult to the muscle, causing rhabdomyolysis. The test is performed by placing a small indwelling catheter into an antecubital vein. A baseline blood sample is obtained for lactic acid and ammonia. The forearm muscles are exercised by asking the patient to vigorously open and close the hand for 1 min. Blood is then obtained at intervals of 1, 2, 4, 6, and 10 min for comparison with the baseline sample. A three- to fourfold rise of lactic acid is typical. The simultaneous measurement of ammonia serves as a control, since it should also rise with exercise. In patients with myophosphorylase deficiency or other glycolytic defects, the lactic acid rise will be absent or below normal, while the rise in ammonia will reach control values. If there is lack of effort, neither lactic acid nor ammonia will rise. Patients with selective failure to increase ammonia may have myoadenylate deaminase deficiency. This condition has been reported to be a cause of myoglobinuria, but deficiency of this enzyme in asymptomatic individuals makes interpretation controversial.

Muscle biopsy

Muscle biopsy is an important step in establishing the diagnosis of a suspected myopathy. The biopsy is usually obtained from a quadriceps or biceps brachii muscle, less commonly from a deltoid muscle. Evaluation includes a combination of techniques—light microscopy, histochemistry, immunocytochemistry with a battery of antibodies, and electron microscopy. Not all techniques are needed for every case. A specific diagnosis can be established in many disorders. Endomysial inflammatory cells surrounding and invading muscle fibers are seen in polymyositis; similar endomysial infiltrates associated with muscle fibers containing rimmed vacuoles, amyloid deposits within fibers, and TDP-43 inclusions are characteristic of inclusion body myositis; while perivascular, perimysial inflammation associated with perifascicular atrophy are features of dermatomyositis. In addition, the congenital myopathies have distinctive light and electron microscopy features essential for diagnosis. Mitochondrial and metabolic (e.g., glycogen and lipid storage diseases) myopathies also demonstrate distinctive histochemical and electron-microscopic profiles. Biopsied muscle tissue can be sent for metabolic enzyme or mitochondrial DNA analyses. A battery of antibodies is available for the identification of missing components of the dystrophin-glycoprotein complex and related proteins to help diagnose specific types of muscular dystrophies. Western blot analysis on muscle specimens can be performed to determine whether specific muscle proteins are reduced in quantity or are of abnormal size.

HEREDITARY MYOPATHIES

Muscular dystrophy refers to a group of hereditary progressive diseases each with unique phenotypic and genetic features (Tables 48-5, 48-6, and 48-7).

DUCHENNE'S MUSCULAR DYSTROPHY

This X-linked recessive disorder, sometimes also called *pseudohypertrophic muscular dystrophy*, has an incidence of ~30 per 100,000 live-born males.

Clinical features

Duchenne's dystrophy is present at birth, but the disorder usually becomes apparent between ages 3 and 5 years. The boys fall frequently and have difficulty keeping up with friends when playing. Running, jumping, and hopping are invariably abnormal. By age 5 years, muscle weakness is obvious by muscle testing. On getting up from the floor, the patient uses his hands to climb up himself (Gowers' maneuver [Fig. 48-4]). Contractures of the heel cords and iliotibial bands become apparent by age 6 years, when toe walking is associated with a lordotic posture. Loss of muscle strength is progressive, with predilection for proximal limb muscles and the neck flexors; leg involvement is more severe than arm involvement. Between ages 8 and 10 years, walking may require the use of braces; joint contractures and limitations of hip flexion, knee, elbow, and wrist extension are made worse by prolonged sitting. By age 12 years, most patients are wheelchair dependent. Contractures become fixed, and a progressive scoliosis often develops that may be associated with pain. The chest deformity with scoliosis impairs pulmonary function, which is already diminished by muscle weakness. By age 16–18 years, patients are predisposed to serious, sometimes fatal pulmonary infections. Other causes of death include aspiration of food and acute gastric dilation.

A cardiac cause of death is uncommon despite the presence of a cardiomyopathy in almost all patients. Congestive heart failure seldom occurs except with severe stress such as pneumonia. Cardiac arrhythmias are rare. The typical electrocardiogram (ECG) shows an increased net RS in lead V_1; deep, narrow Q waves in the precordial leads; and tall right precordial R waves in V_1. Intellectual impairment in Duchenne's dystrophy is common; the average intelligence quotient (IQ) is ~1 SD below the mean. Impairment of intellectual function appears to be nonprogressive and affects verbal ability more than performance.

Laboratory features

Serum CK levels are invariably elevated to between 20 and 100 times normal. The levels are abnormal at birth but decline late in the disease because of inactivity and loss of muscle mass. EMG demonstrates features typical of myopathy. The muscle biopsy shows muscle fibers of varying size as well as small groups of necrotic and regenerating fibers. Connective tissue and fat replace lost muscle fibers. A definitive diagnosis of Duchenne's dystrophy can be established on the basis of dystrophin deficiency in a biopsy of muscle tissue or mutation analysis on peripheral blood leukocytes, as discussed later.

Duchenne's dystrophy is caused by a mutation of the gene that encodes dystrophin, a 427-kDa protein localized to the inner surface of the sarcolemma of the muscle fiber. The dystrophin gene is >2000 kb in size and thus is one of the largest identified human genes. It is localized to the short arm of the X chromosome at

TABLE 48-5

PROGRESSIVE MUSCULAR DYSTROPHIES

TYPE	INHERITANCE	DEFECTIVE GENE/ PROTEIN	ONSET AGE	CLINICAL FEATURES	OTHER ORGAN SYSTEMS INVOLVED
Duchenne's	XR	Dystrophin	Before 5 years	Progressive weakness of girdle muscles	Cardiomyopathy
				Unable to walk after age 12	Mental impairment
				Progressive kyphoscoliosis	
				Respiratory failure in 2nd or 3rd decade	
Becker's	XR	Dystrophin	Early childhood to adult	Progressive weakness of girdle muscles	Cardiomyopathy
				Able to walk after age 15	
				Respiratory failure may develop by 4th decade	
Limb-girdle	AD/AR	Several (Tables 48-6, 48-7)	Early childhood to early adult	Slow progressive weakness of shoulder and hip girdle muscles	± Cardiomyopathy
Emery-Dreifuss	XR/AD	Emerin/Lamins A/C Nesprin-1, Nesprin 2, *TMEM43*	Childhood to adult	Elbow contractures, humeral and peroneal weakness	Cardiomyopathy
Congenital	AR	Several	At birth or within first few months	Hypotonia, contractures, delayed milestones	CNS abnormalities (hypomyelination, malformation)
				Progression to respiratory failure in some; static course in others	Eye abnormalities
Myotonic[a] (DM1, DM2)	AD	DM1: Expansion CTG repeat	Childhood to adult	Slowly progressive weakness of face, shoulder girdle, and foot dorsiflexion	Cardiac conduction defects
		DM2: Expansion CCTG repeat	Maybe infancy if mother affected (DM1 only)	Preferential proximal weakness in DM2	Mental impairment Cataracts
					Frontal baldness
					Gonadal atrophy
Facioscapulohumeral	AD	*DUX4* 4q	Childhood to adult	Slowly progressive weakness of face, shoulder girdle, and foot dorsiflexion	Deafness Coats' (eye) disease
Oculopharyngeal	AD	Expansion, poly-A RNA binding protein	5th to 6th decade	Slowly progressive weakness of extraocular, pharyngeal, and limb muscles	—

[a]Two forms of myotonic dystrophy, DM1 and DM2, have been identified. Many features overlap (see text).

Abbreviations: AD, autosomal dominant; AR, autosomal recessive; CNS, central nervous system; XR, X-linked recessive.

Xp21. The most common gene mutation is a deletion. The size varies but does not correlate with disease severity. Deletions are not uniformly distributed over the gene but rather are most common near the beginning (5′ end) and middle of the gene. Less often, Duchenne's dystrophy is caused by a gene duplication or point mutation. Identification of a specific mutation allows for an unequivocal diagnosis, makes possible accurate testing of potential carriers, and is useful for prenatal diagnosis.

A diagnosis of Duchenne's dystrophy can also be made by Western blot analysis of muscle biopsy specimens, revealing abnormalities on the quantity and molecular weight of dystrophin protein. In addition,

TABLE 48-6

AUTOSOMAL DOMINANT LIMB-GIRDLE MUSCULAR DYSTROPHIES (LGMDs)

DISEASE	CLINICAL FEATURES	LABORATORY FEATURES	LOCUS OR GENE
LGMD1A	Onset 3rd to 4th decade Muscle weakness affects distal limb muscles, vocal cords, and pharyngeal muscles	Serum CK 2 × normal EMG mixed myopathy/neuropathy NCS normal	Myotilin
LGMD1B	Onset 1st or 2nd decade Proximal lower limb weakness and cardiomyopathy with conduction defects Some cases indistinguishable from Emery-Dreifuss muscular dystrophy with joint contractures	Serum CK 3–5 × normal NCS normal EMG myopathic	Lamin A/C
LGMD1C	Onset in early childhood Proximal weakness Gowers' sign, calf hypertrophy Exercise-related muscle cramps	Serum CK 4–25 × normal NCS normal EMG myopathic	Caveolin-3
LGMD1D	Onset 3rd to 5th decade Proximal muscle weakness Cardiomyopathy and arrhythmias	Serum CK 2–4 × normal NCS normal EMG myopathic	Linked to chromosome 7q Gene unidentified
LGMD1E	Childhood onset Proximal muscle weakness	Serum CK usually normal NCS normal EMG myopathic	Linked to chromosome 6q23 Gene unidentified

Abbreviations: CK, creatine kinase; EMG, electromyography; NCS, nerve conduction studies.

immunocytochemical staining of muscle with dystrophin antibodies can be used to demonstrate absence or deficiency of dystrophin localizing to the sarcolemmal membrane. Carriers of the disease may demonstrate a mosaic pattern, butdystrophin analysis of muscle biopsy specimens for carrier detection is not reliable.

Pathogenesis

Dystrophin is part of a large complex of sarcolemmal proteins and glycoproteins (Fig. 48-6). Dystrophin binds to F-actin at its amino terminus and to β-dystroglycan at the carboxyl terminus. β-Dystroglycan complexes to α-dystroglycan, which binds to laminin in the extracellular matrix (ECM). Laminin has a heterotrimeric molecular structure arranged in the shape of a cross with one heavy chain and two light chains, β_1 and γ_1. The laminin heavy chain of skeletal muscle is designated laminin α_2. Collagen proteins IV and VI are also found in the ECM. Like β-dystroglycan, the transmembrane sarcoglycan proteins also bind to dystrophin; these five proteins (designated α- through ε-sarcoglycan) complex tightly with each other. More recently, other membrane proteins implicated in muscular dystrophy have been found to be loosely affiliated with constituents of the dystrophin complex. These include caveolin-3, α_7 integrin, and collagen VI.

Dystrophin localizes to the cytoplasmic face of the muscle cell membrane. It complexes with two transmembrane protein complexes, the dystroglycans and the sarcoglycans. The dystroglycans bind to the extracellular matrix protein merosin, which is also complexed with β_1 and α_7 integrins (Tables 48-5, 48-6, 48-7). Dysferlin complexes with caveolin-3 (which binds to neuronal nitric oxide synthase, or nNOS) but not with the dystrophin-associated proteins or the integrins. In some of the congenital dystrophies and limb-girdle muscular dystrophies (LGMDs), there is loss of function of different enzymes that glycosylate α-dystroglycan, which thereby inhibits proper binding to merosin: POMT1, POMT2, POMGnT1, Fukutin, Fukutin-related protein, and LARGE.

The dystrophin-glycoprotein complex appears to confer stability to the sarcolemma, although the function of each individual component of the complex is incompletely understood. Deficiency of one member of the complex may cause abnormalities in other components. For example, a primary deficiency of dystrophin (Duchenne's dystrophy) may lead to secondary loss of the sarcoglycans and dystroglycan. The primary loss of a single sarcoglycan (see "Limb-Girdle Muscular Dystrophy," later in the chapter) results in a secondary loss of other sarcoglycans in the membrane without uniformly affecting dystrophin. In either instance, disruption of the dystrophin-glycoprotein complexes weakens the sarcolemma, causing membrane tears and a cascade of events leading to muscle fiber necrosis. This sequence of events occurs repeatedly during the life of a patient with muscular dystrophy.

TABLE 48-7

AUTOSOMAL RECESSIVE LIMB-GIRDLE MUSCULAR DYSTROPHIES (LGMDs)

DISEASE	CLINICAL FEATURES	LABORATORY FEATURES	LOCUS OR GENE
LGMD2A	Onset 1st or 2nd decade Tight heel cords Contractures at elbows, wrists, and fingers; rigid spine in some Proximal and distal weakness	Serum CK 3–15 × normal NCS normal EMG myopathic	Calpain-3
LGMD2B	Onset 2nd or 3rd decade Proximal muscle weakness at onset, later distal (calf) muscles affected Miyoshi's myopathy is variant of LGMD2B with calf muscles affected at onset	Serum CK 3–100 × normal NCS normal EMG myopathic Inflammation on muscle biopsy may simulate polymyositis	Dysferlin
LGMD2C–F	Onset in childhood to teenage years Clinical condition similar to Duchenne's and Becker's muscular dystrophies Cardiomyopathy uncommon Cognitive function normal	Serum CK 5–100 × normal NCS normal EMG myopathic	γ, α, β, δ sarcoglycans
LGMD2G	Onset age 10 to 15 Proximal and distal muscle weakness	Serum CK 3–17 × normal NCS normal EMG myopathic	Telethonin
LGMD2H	Onset 1st to 3rd decade Proximal muscle weakness	Serum CK 2–25 × normal NCS normal EMG myopathic	TRIM32 gene
LGMD2I	Onset 1st to 3rd decade Clinical condition similar to Duchenne's or Becker's dystrophies Cardiomyopathy (some not all) Cognitive function normal	Serum CK 10–30 × normal NCS normal EMG myopathic	Fukutin-related protein
LGMD2J[a]	Onset 1st to 3rd decade Proximal lower limb weakness Mild distal weakness Progressive weakness causes loss of ambulation	Serum CK 1.5–2 × normal NCS normal EMG myopathic	Titin
LGMD2K	Usually presents in infancy as Walker-Warburg syndrome but can present in early adult life with proximal weakness and only minor CNS abnormalities	CK 10–20 × normal NCS normal EMG myopathic	POMT1
LGMD2IL	Presents in childhood or adult life May manifest with quadriceps atrophy and myalgia Some present with early involvement of the calves in the second decade of life, resembling Miyoshi's myopathy (dysferlinopathy)	CK normal to 50 × normal NCS normal EMG myopathic	Anoctamin 5
LGMD2M	Usually presents in infancy as Fukuyama congenital muscular dystrophy but can present in early adult life with proximal weakness and only minor CNS abnormalities	CK 10–50 × normal NCS normal EMG myopathic	Fukutin
LGMD2N	Usually presents in infancy as muscle-eye-brain disease but can present in early adult life with proximal weakness and only minor CNS abnormalities	CK 5–20 × normal NCS normal EMG myopathic	POMGnT1
LGMD2O	Usually presents in infancy as Walker-Warburg syndrome but can present in early adult life with proximal weakness and only minor CNS abnormalities	CK 5–20 × normal NCS normal EMG myopathic	POMT2

[a]Tibial muscular dystrophy is a form of titin deficiency with only distal muscle weakness (see Table 48-9).

Abbreviations: CK, creatine kinase; EMG, electromyography; NCS, nerve conduction studies; POMT1, protein-O-mannosyl transferase 1; POMT2, protein-O-mannosyltransferase 2; POMGnT1, O-linked mannose beta 1,2-*N*-acetylglucosaminyltransferase.

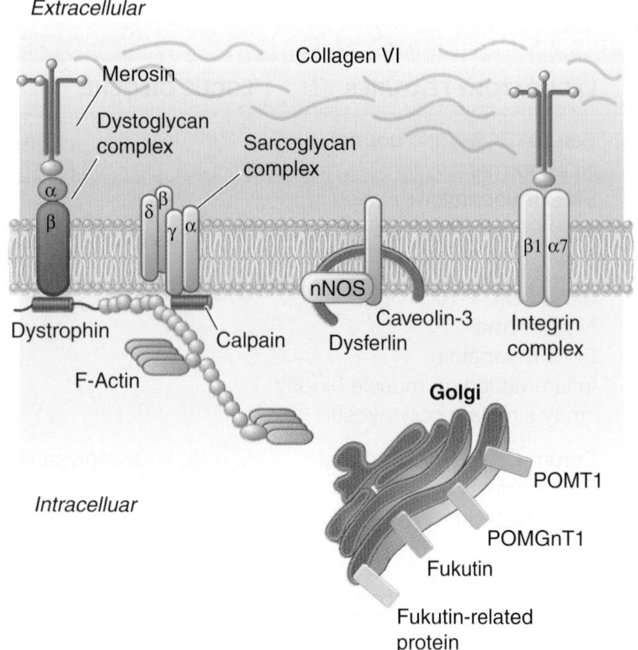

FIGURE 48-6

Selected muscular dystrophy–associated proteins in the cell membrane and Golgi complex.

TREATMENT Duchenne's Muscular Dystrophy

Glucocorticoids, administered as prednisone in a dose of 0.75 mg/kg per day, significantly slow progression of Duchenne's dystrophy for up to 3 years. Some patients cannot tolerate glucocorticoid therapy; weight gain and increased risk of fractures in particular represent a significant deterrent for some boys. As in other recessively inherited dystrophies presumed to arise from loss of function of a critical muscle gene, there is optimism that Duchenne's disease may benefit from novel therapies that either replace the defective gene or missing protein or implement downstream corrections (e.g., skipping mutated exons or reading through mutations that introduce stop codons).

BECKER'S MUSCULAR DYSTROPHY

This less severe form of X-linked recessive muscular dystrophy results from allelic defects of the same gene responsible for Duchenne's dystrophy. Becker's muscular dystrophy is ~10 times less frequent than Duchenne's, with an incidence of about 3 per 100,000 live-born males.

Clinical features

The pattern of muscle wasting in Becker's muscular dystrophy closely resembles that seen in Duchenne's. Proximal muscles, especially of the lower extremities, are prominently involved. As the disease progresses, weakness becomes more generalized. Significant facial muscle weakness is not a feature. Hypertrophy of muscles, particularly in the calves, is an early and prominent finding.

Most patients with Becker's dystrophy first experience difficulties between ages 5 and 15 years, although onset in the third or fourth decade or even later can occur. By definition, patients with Becker's dystrophy walk beyond age 15, while patients with Duchenne's dystrophy are typically in a wheelchair by the age of 12. Patients with Becker's dystrophy have a reduced life expectancy, but most survive into the fourth or fifth decade.

Mental retardation may occur in Becker's dystrophy, but it is not as common as in Duchenne's. Cardiac involvement occurs in Becker's dystrophy and may result in heart failure; some patients manifest with only heart failure. Other less common presentations are asymptomatic hyper-CK-emia, myalgias without weakness, and myoglobinuria.

Laboratory features

Serum CK levels, results of EMG, and muscle biopsy findings closely resemble those in Duchenne's dystrophy. The diagnosis of Becker's muscular dystrophy requires Western blot analysis of muscle biopsy samples, demonstrating a reduced amount or abnormal size of dystrophin or mutation analysis of DNA from peripheral blood leukocytes. Genetic testing reveals deletions or duplications of the dystrophin gene in 65% of patients with Becker's dystrophy, approximately the same percentage as in Duchenne's dystrophy. In both Becker's and Duchenne's dystrophies, the size of the DNA deletion does not predict clinical severity; however, in ~95% of patients with Becker's dystrophy, the DNA deletion does not alter the translational reading frame of messenger RNA. These "in-frame" mutations allow for production of some dystrophin, which accounts for the presence of altered rather than absent dystrophin on Western blot analysis.

TREATMENT Becker's Muscular Dystrophy

The use of glucocorticoids has not been adequately studied in Becker's dystrophy.

LIMB-GIRDLE MUSCULAR DYSTROPHY

The syndrome of LGMD represents more than one disorder. Both males and females are affected, with onset ranging from late in the first decade to the fourth decade. The LGMDs typically manifest with progressive weakness of pelvic and shoulder girdle musculature. Respiratory insufficiency from weakness of the diaphragm may occur, as may cardiomyopathy.

A systematic classification of LGMD is based on autosomal dominant (LGMD1) and autosomal recessive (LGMD2) inheritance. Superimposed on the backbone of LGMD1 and LGMD2, the classification employs a sequential alphabetical lettering system (LGMD1A, LGMD2A, etc.). Disorders receive letters in the order in which they are found to have chromosomal linkage. This results in an ever-expanding list of conditions. Presently there are 5 autosomal dominant and 10 autosomal recessive disorders, summarized in Tables 48-6 and 48-7. None of the conditions is as common as the dystrophinopathies; however, prevalence data for the LGMDs have not been systematically gathered for any large heterogeneous population. In referral-based clinical populations, Fukutin-related protein (FKRP) deficiency (LGMD2I), calpainopathies (LGMD2A), and to a lesser extent dysferlinopathies (LGMD2B) have emerged as the most common disorders.

EMERY-DREIFUSS MUSCULAR DYSTROPHY

There are at least five genetically distinct forms of Emery-Dreifuss muscular dystrophy (EDMD). Emerin mutations are the most common cause of X-linked EDMD, though mutations in *FHL1* may also be associated with a similar phenotype, which is X-linked as well. Mutations involving the gene for lamin A/C are the most common cause of autosomal dominant EDMD (also known as LGMD1B) and is also a common cause of hereditary cardiomyopathy. Less commonly, autosomal dominant EDMD has been reported with mutations in nesprin-1, nesprin-2, and *TMEM43*.

Clinical features

Prominent contractures can be recognized in early childhood and teenage years, often preceding muscle weakness. The contractures persist throughout the course of the disease and are present at the elbows, ankles, and neck. Muscle weakness affects humeral and peroneal muscles at first and later spreads to a limb-girdle distribution. The cardiomyopathy is potentially life threatening and may result in sudden death. A spectrum of atrial rhythm and conduction defects includes atrial fibrillation and paralysis and atrioventricular heart block. Some patients have a dilated cardiomyopathy. Female carriers of the X-linked variant may have cardiac manifestations that become clinically significant.

Laboratory features

Serum CK may be elevated two- to tenfold. EMG is myopathic. Muscle biopsy usually shows nonspecific dystrophic features, though cases associated with FHL1 mutations have features of myofibrillar myopathy. Immunohistochemistry reveals absent emerin staining of myonuclei in X-linked EDMD due to emerin mutations. ECGs demonstrate atrial and atrioventricular rhythm disturbances.

X-linked EDMD usually arises from defects in the emerin gene encoding a nuclear envelope protein. FHL1 mutations are also a cause of scapuloperoneal dystrophy, but can also present with an EDMD phenotype. The autosomal dominant disease can be caused by mutations in the *LMNA* gene encoding lamin A and C; in the synaptic nuclear envelope protein 1 (*SYNE1*) or 2 (*SYNE2*) encoding nesprin-1 and nesprin-2, respectively; and most recently in *TMEM43* encoding LUMA. These proteins are essential components of the filamentous network underlying the inner nuclear membrane. Loss of structural integrity of the nuclear envelope from defects in emerin, lamin A/C, nesprin-1, nesprin-2, and LUMA accounts for overlapping phenotypes (Fig. 48-7).

TREATMENT Emery-Dreifuss Muscular Dystrophy

Supportive care should be offered for neuromuscular disability, including ambulatory aids, if necessary. Stretching of contractures is difficult. Management of cardiomyopathy and arrhythmias (e.g., early use of a defibrillator or cardiac pacemaker) may be life saving.

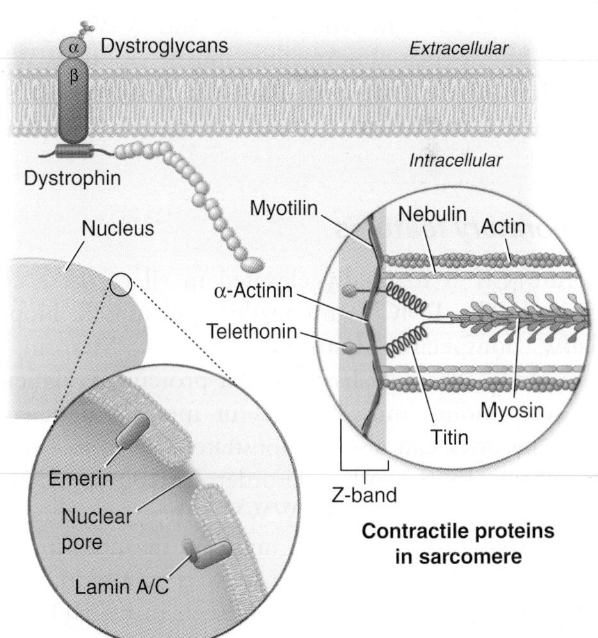

FIGURE 48-7

Selected muscular dystrophy–associated proteins in the nuclear membrane and sarcomere. As shown in the exploded view, emerin and lamin A/C are constituents of the inner nuclear membrane. Several dystrophy-associated proteins are represented in the sarcomere including titin, nebulin, calpain, telethonin, actinin, and myotilin. The position of the dystrophin-dystroglycan complex is also illustrated.

CONGENITAL MUSCULAR DYSTROPHY (CMD)

This is not one entity but rather a group of disorders with varying degrees of muscle weakness, CNS impairment, and eye abnormalities.

Clinical features

As a group, CMDs present at birth or in the first few months of life with hypotonia and proximal or generalized muscle weakness. Calf muscle hypertrophy is seen in some patients. Facial muscles may be weak, but other cranial nerve–innervated muscles are spared (e.g., extraocular muscles are normal). Most patients have joint contractures of varying degrees at elbows, hips, knees, and ankles. Contractures present at birth are referred to as *arthrogryposis*. Respiratory failure may be seen in some cases.

The CNS is affected in some forms of CMD. In merosin and FKRP deficiency, cerebral hypomyelination may be seen by MRI, though only a small number of patients have mental retardation and seizures. Three forms of congenital muscular dystrophy have severe brain impairment. These include Fukuyama congenital muscular dystrophy (FCMD), muscle-eye-brain (MEB) disease, and Walker-Warburg syndrome (WWS). Patients are severely disabled in all three of these conditions. In MEB disease and WWS, but not in FCMD, ocular abnormalities impair vision. WWS is the most severe congenital muscular dystrophy, causing death by 1 year of age.

Laboratory features

Serum CK is markedly elevated in all of these conditions. The EMG is myopathic and muscle biopsies show nonspecific dystrophic features. Merosin, or laminin α_2 chain (a basal lamina protein), is deficient in surrounding muscle fibers in merosin deficiency. Skin biopsies can also demonstrate defects in laminin α_2 chain. In the other disorders (FKRP deficiency, FCMD, MEB disease, WWS), there is abnormal α-dystroglycan staining in muscle. In merosin deficiency, cerebral hypomyelination is common, and a host of brain malformations are seen in FCMD, MEB disease, and WWS.

All forms of CMD are inherited as autosomal recessive disorders. Chromosomal linkage and specific gene defects are presented in Table 48-8. With the exception of merosin, the other gene defects affect posttranslational glycosylation of α-dystroglycan. This abnormality is thought to impair binding with merosin and leads to weakening of the dystrophin-glycoprotein complex, instability of the muscle membrane, and/or abnormalities in muscle contraction. CMDs with brain and eye phenotypes probably involve defective glycosylation of additional proteins, accounting for the more extensive phenotypes.

TREATMENT Congenital Muscular Dystrophy

There is no specific treatment for CMD. Proper wheelchair seating is important. Management of epilepsy and cardiac manifestations is necessary for some patients.

MYOTONIC DYSTROPHY

Myotonic dystrophy is also known as *dystrophia myotonica* (DM). The condition is composed of at least two clinical disorders with overlapping phenotypes and distinct molecular genetic defects: myotonic dystrophy type 1 (DM1), the classic disease originally described by Steinert, and myotonic dystrophy type 2 (DM2), also called *proximal myotonic myopathy* (PROMM).

Clinical features

The clinical expression of DM1 varies widely and involves many systems other than muscle. Affected patients have a typical "hatchet-faced" appearance due to temporalis, masseter, and facial muscle atrophy and weakness. Frontal baldness is also characteristic of the disease. Neck muscles, including flexors and sternocleidomastoids, and distal limb muscles are involved early. Weakness of wrist extensors, finger extensors, and intrinsic hand muscles impairs function. Ankle dorsiflexor weakness may cause footdrop. Proximal muscles remain stronger throughout the course, although preferential atrophy and weakness of quadriceps muscles occur in many patients. Palatal, pharyngeal, and tongue involvement produce a dysarthric speech, nasal voice, and swallowing problems. Some patients have diaphragm and intercostal muscle weakness, resulting in respiratory insufficiency.

Myotonia, which usually appears by age 5 years, is demonstrable by percussion of the thenar eminence, the tongue, and wrist extensor muscles. Myotonia causes a slow relaxation of hand grip after a forced voluntary closure. Advanced muscle wasting makes myotonia more difficult to detect.

Cardiac disturbances occur commonly in patients with DM1. ECG abnormalities include first-degree heart block and more extensive conduction system involvement. Complete heart block and sudden death can occur. Congestive heart failure occurs infrequently but may result from cor pulmonale secondary to respiratory failure. Mitral valve prolapse also occurs commonly. Other associated features include intellectual impairment, hypersomnia, posterior subcapsular cataracts, gonadal

TABLE 48-8

CONGENITAL MUSCULAR DYSTROPHIES[a]

DISEASE	CLINICAL FEATURES	LABORATORY FEATURES	LOCUS OR GENE
Merosin deficiency	Onset at birth with hypotonia, joint contractures, delayed milestones, generalized muscle weakness Cerebral hypomyelination, less often cortical dysplasia Normal intelligence usually, some with MR (~6%) and seizures (~8%) Partial deficiency leads to milder phenotype (LGMD picture)	Serum CK 5–35 × normal EMG myopathic NCS abnormal in some cases	Laminin α_2 chain
Fukitin-related protein deficiency[b]	Onset at birth or shortly after Hypotonia and feeding problems Weakness of proximal muscles, especially shoulder girdles Hypertrophy of leg muscles Joint contractures Cognition normal	Serum CK 10–50 × normal EMG myopathic NCS normal	Fukutin-related protein
Fukuyama congenital muscular dystrophy[b]	Onset at birth Hypotonia, joint contractures Generalized muscle weakness Hypertrophy of calf muscles Seizures, mental retardation Cardiomyopathy	Serum CK 10–50 × normal EMG myopathic NCS normal MRI shows hydrocephalus and periventricular and frontal hypomyelination	Fukutin
Muscle-eye-brain disease	Onset at birth, hypotonia Eye abnormalities include: progressive myopia, cataracts, and optic nerve, glaucoma, retinal pigmentary changes Progressive muscle weakness Joint contractures Seizures, mental retardation	Serum CK 5–20 × normal MRI shows hydrocephalus, cobblestone lissencephaly, corpus callosum and cerebellar hypoplasia, cerebral hypomyelination	*N*-acetyl-glucosaminyl transferase (POMGnT1)
Walker-Warburg syndrome[b]	Onset at birth, hypotonia Generalized muscle weakness Joint contractures Microphthalmos, retinal dysplasia, buphthalmos, glaucoma, cataracts Seizures, MR	Serum CK 5–20 × normal MRI shows cobblestone lissencephaly, hydrocephalus, encephalocele, absent corpus callosum	*O*-mannoxyl-transferase-1 (POMT1)

[a]All are inherited as recessive traits.
[b]There is phenotypic overlap between disorders related to defective glycosylation. In muscle, this is a consequence of altered glycosylation of dystroglycans; in brain/eye, other glycosylated proteins are involved. Clinically, Walker-Warburg syndrome is more severe, with death by 1 year.
Abbreviations: CK, creatine kinase; EMG, electromyography; LGMD, limb-girdle muscular dystrophy; MR, mental retardation; NCS, nerve conduction studies.

atrophy, insulin resistance, and decreased esophageal and colonic motility.

Congenital myotonic dystrophy is a more severe form of DM1 and occurs in ~25% of infants of affected mothers. It is characterized by severe facial and bulbar weakness, transient neonatal respiratory insufficiency, and mental retardation.

DM2, or PROMM, has a distinct pattern of muscle weakness affecting mainly proximal muscles. Other features of the disease overlap with DM1, including cataracts, testicular atrophy, insulin resistance, constipation, hypersomnia, and cognitive defects. Cardiac conduction defects occur but are less common, and the hatchet face and frontal baldness are less consistent features. A very striking difference is the failure to clearly identify a congenital form of DM2.

Laboratory features

The diagnosis of myotonic dystrophy can usually be made on the basis of clinical findings. Serum CK levels may be normal or mildly elevated. EMG evidence of myotonia is present in most cases of DM1 but may be more patchy in DM2. Muscle biopsy shows muscle atrophy, which selectively involves type 1 fibers in 50% of cases, and ringed fibers in DM1 but not in DM2. Typically, numerous internalized nuclei can be seen in individual muscle fibers as well as atrophic fibers with pyknotic nuclear clumps in both DM1 and DM2. Necrosis of muscle fibers and increased connective tissue, common in other muscular dystrophies, are less apparent in myotonic dystrophy.

DM1 and DM2 are both autosomal dominant disorders. New mutations do not appear to contribute to the pool of affected individuals. DM1 is transmitted by an intronic mutation consisting of an unstable expansion of a CTG trinucleotide repeat in a serine-threonine protein kinase gene (named *DMPK*) on chromosome 19q13.3. An increase in the severity of the disease phenotype in successive generations (genetic anticipation) is accompanied by an increase in the number of trinucleotide repeats. A similar type of mutation has been identified in fragile X syndrome. The unstable triplet repeat in myotonic dystrophy can be used for prenatal diagnosis. Congenital disease occurs almost exclusively in infants born to affected mothers; it is possible that sperm with greatly expanded triplet repeats do not function well.

DM2 is caused by a DNA expansion mutation consisting of a CCTG repeat in intron 1 of the *ZNF9* gene located at chromosome 3q13.3-q24. The gene is believed to encode an RNA-binding protein expressed in many different tissues, including skeletal and cardiac muscle.

The DNA expansions in DM1 and DM2 almost certainly impair muscle function by a toxic gain of function of the mutant mRNA. In both DM1 and DM2, the mutant RNA appears to form intranuclear inclusions composed of aberrant RNA. These RNA inclusions sequester RNA-binding proteins essential for proper splicing of a variety of other mRNAs. This leads to abnormal transcription of multiple proteins in a variety of tissues/organ systems, in turn causing the systemic manifestations of DM1 and DM2.

TREATMENT **Myotonic Dystrophy**

The myotonia in DM1 rarely warrants treatment, though some patients with DM2 are significantly bothered by the discomfort related to the associated muscle stiffness. Phenytoin and mexiletine are the preferred agents for the occasional patient who requires an antimyotonia drug; other agents, particularly quinine and procainamide, may worsen cardiac conduction. A cardiac pacemaker should be considered for patients with unexplained syncope, advanced conduction system abnormalities with evidence of second-degree heart block, or trifascicular conduction disturbances with marked prolongation of the PR interval. Molded ankle-foot orthoses help stabilize gait in patients with foot drop. Excessive daytime somnolence with or without sleep apnea is not uncommon. Sleep studies, noninvasive respiratory support (biphasic positive airway pressure, BiPAP), and treatment with modafinil may be beneficial.

FACIOSCAPULOHUMERAL (FSH) MUSCULAR DYSTROPHY

This form of muscular dystrophy has a prevalence of ~1 in 20,000. There are two forms of FSHD that have similar pathogenesis, as will be discussed. Most patients have FSHD type 1 (95%), while approximately 5% have FSHD2. FSHD1 and FSHD2 are clinically and histopathologically identical. FSHD is not to be confused with the genetically distinct scapuloperoneal dystrophies.

Clinical features

The condition typically has an onset in childhood or young adulthood. In most cases, facial weakness is the initial manifestation, appearing as an inability to smile, whistle, or fully close the eyes. Weakness of the shoulder girdles, rather than the facial muscles, usually brings the patient to medical attention. Loss of scapular stabilizer muscles makes arm elevation difficult. Scapular winging (Fig. 48-3) becomes apparent with attempts at abduction and forward movement of the arms. Biceps and triceps muscles may be severely affected, with relative sparing of the deltoid muscles. Weakness is invariably worse for wrist extension than for wrist flexion, and weakness of the anterior compartment muscles of the legs may lead to footdrop.

In most patients, the weakness remains restricted to facial, upper extremity, and distal lower extremity muscles. In 20% of patients, weakness progresses to involve the pelvic girdle muscles, and severe functional impairment and possible wheelchair dependency result.

Characteristically, patients with FSHD do not have involvement of other organ systems, although labile hypertension is common, and there is an increased incidence of nerve deafness. *Coats' disease*, a disorder consisting of telangiectasia, exudation, and retinal detachment, also occurs.

Laboratory features

The serum CK level may be normal or mildly elevated. EMG usually indicates a myopathic pattern. The muscle biopsy shows nonspecific features of a myopathy. A prominent inflammatory infiltrate, which is often multifocal in distribution, is present in some biopsy samples. The cause or significance of this finding is unknown.

An autosomal dominant inheritance pattern with almost complete penetrance has been established, but each family member should be examined for the presence of the disease, since ~30% of those affected are unaware of involvement. FSHD1 is associated with deletions of tandem 3.3-kb repeats at 4q35. The deletion reduces the number of repeats to a fragment of <35 kb in most patients. Within these repeats lies the *DUX4* gene, which usually is not expressed. In patients with FSHD1 these deletions in the setting of a specific polymorphism leads to hypomethylation of the region and toxic expression of the *DUX 4* gene. Interestingly, in patients with FSHD2, there is no deletion but in the setting of the same polymorphism there again is seen hypomethylation of the region and the permissive expression of the *DUX4* gene. In either instance, the permissive polymorphism introduces a polyadenylation signal that results in an aberrant, toxic *DUX4* transcript.

TREATMENT Facioscapulohumeral Muscular Dystrophy

No specific treatment is available; ankle-foot orthoses are helpful for footdrop. Scapular stabilization procedures improve scapular winging but may not improve function.

OCULOPHARYNGEAL DYSTROPHY

This form of muscular dystrophy represents one of several disorders characterized by progressive external ophthalmoplegia, which consists of slowly progressive ptosis and limitation of eye movements with sparing of pupillary reactions for light and accommodation. Patients usually do not complain of diplopia, in contrast to patients having conditions with a more acute onset of ocular muscle weakness (e.g., myasthenia gravis).

Clinical features

Oculopharyngeal muscular dystrophy has a late onset; it usually presents in the fourth to sixth decade with ptosis and/or dysphagia. The extraocular muscle impairment is less prominent in the early phase but may be severe later. The swallowing problem may become debilitating and result in pooling of secretions and repeated episodes of aspiration. Mild weakness of the neck and extremities also occurs.

Laboratory features

The serum CK level may be two to three times normal. Myopathic EMG findings are typical. On biopsy, muscle fibers are found to contain rimmed vacuoles, which by electron microscopy are shown to contain membranous whorls, accumulation of glycogen, and other nonspecific debris related to lysosomes. A distinct feature of oculopharyngeal dystrophy is the presence of tubular filaments, 8.5 nm in diameter, in muscle cell nuclei.

Oculopharyngeal dystrophy has an autosomal dominant inheritance pattern with complete penetrance. The incidence is high in French-Canadians and in Spanish-American families of the southwestern United States. Large kindreds of Italian and of eastern European Jewish descent have been reported. The molecular defect in oculopharyngeal muscular dystrophy is a subtle expansion of a modest polyalanine repeat tract in a poly-RNA-binding protein (PABP2) in muscle.

TREATMENT Oculopharyngeal Dystrophy

Dysphagia can lead to significant undernourishment and inanition, making oculopharyngeal muscular dystrophy a potentially life-threatening disease. Cricopharyngeal myotomy may improve swallowing, although it does not prevent aspiration. Eyelid crutches can improve vision when ptosis obstructs vision; candidates for ptosis surgery must be carefully selected—those with severe facial weakness are not suitable.

DISTAL MYOPATHIES

A group of muscle diseases, the distal myopathies, are notable for their preferential distal distribution of muscle weakness in contrast to most muscle conditions associated with proximal weakness. The major distal myopathies are summarized in Table 48-9.

Clinical features

Welander's, *Udd's*, and *Markesbery-Griggs distal myopathies* are all late onset, dominantly inherited disorders of distal limb muscles, usually beginning after age 40 years. Welander's distal myopathy preferentially involves the wrist and finger extensors, whereas the others are associated with anterior tibial weakness leading to progressive footdrop. *Laing's distal myopathy* is also a dominantly inherited disorder heralded by tibial weakness; however, it is distinguished by onset in childhood or early adult life. *Nonaka's distal myopathy* and *Miyoshi's myopathy* are distinguished by autosomal recessive inheritance and onset in the late teens or twenties. Nonaka's myopathy entails anterior tibial weakness, whereas Miyoshi's myopathy is unique in that gastrocnemius muscles are preferentially affected at onset. Finally, the *myofibrillar myopathies* (MFMs) are a clinically and genetically heterogeneous group of disorders that can be associated with prominent distal weakness; they can be inherited in an autosomal dominant or recessive pattern. Of note,

TABLE 48-9

DISTAL MYOPATHIES

DISEASE	CLINICAL FEATURES	LABORATORY FEATURES	INHERITANCE/LOCUS OR GENE
Welander's distal myopathy	Onset in 5th decade Weakness begins in hands Slow progression with spread to distal lower extremities Lifespan normal	Serum CK 2–3 × normal EMG myopathic NCS normal Muscle biopsy shows dystrophic features	AD Chromosome 2p13
Tibial muscular dystrophy (Udd's)	Onset 4th to 8th decade Distal lower extremity weakness (tibial distribution) Upper extremities usually normal Lifespan normal	Serum CK 2–4 × normal EMG myopathic NCS normal Muscle biopsy shows dystrophic features Titin absent in M-line of muscle	AD Titin AR (associated with more proximal weakness—LGMD2J)
Markesbery-Griggs distal myopathy	Onset 4th to 8th decade Distal lower extremity weakness (tibial distribution) with progression to distal arms and proximal muscles	Serum CK is usually mildly elevated EMG reveals irritative myopathy Muscle biopsies demonstrate rimmed vacuoles and features of myofibrillar myopathy	AD Z-band alternatively spliced PDX motif-containing protein (ZASP)
Laing's distal myopathy	Onset childhood to 3rd decade Distal lower extremity weakness (tibial distribution) and neck flexors affected early May have cardiomyopathy	Serum CK is normal or slightly elevated Muscle biopsies do not show rimmed vacuoles Large deposits of myosin heavy chain are seen in type 1 muscle fibers	AD Myosin heavy chain 7
Nonaka's distal myopathy (autosomal recessive hereditary inclusion body myopathy)	Onset: 2nd to 3rd decade Lower extremity distal weakness Mild distal upper limb weakness may be present early Progression to other muscles sparing quadriceps Ambulation may be lost in 10–15 y	Serum CK 3–10 × normal EMG myopathic NCS normal Dystrophic features on muscle biopsy plus rimmed vacuoles and 15- to 19-nm filaments within vacuoles	AR *GNE* gene: UDP-*N*-acetylglucosamine 2-epimerase/*N*-acetylmannosamine kinase Allelic to hereditary inclusion body myopathy
Miyoshi's myopathy	Onset: 2nd to 3rd decade Lower extremity weakness in posterior compartment muscles Progression leads to weakness in other muscle groups Ambulation lost after 10–15 y in about one-third of cases	Serum CK 20–100 × normal EMG myopathic NCS normal Muscle biopsy shows nonspecific dystrophic features often with prominent inflammatory cell infiltration; no rimmed vacuoles	AR Allelic to LGMD2B (see Table 48-7) Dysferlin
Myofibrillar myopathies	Onset from early childhood to late adult life Weakness may be distal, proximal, or generalized Cardiomyopathy and respiratory involvement is not uncommon	Serum CKs can be normal or moderately elevated EMG is myopathic and often associated with myotonic discharges Muscle biopsy demonstrates abnormal accumulation of desmin and other proteins, rimmed vacuoles, and myofibrillar degeneration	Genetically heterogeneous AD Myotilin (also known as LGMD 1A) ZASP (see Markesbery-Griggs distal myopathy) Filamin-C Desmin Alpha B crystallin Bag3 FHL-1 AR Desmin Selenoprotein N1

Markesbery-Griggs myopathy (caused by mutations in ZASP) and LGMD1B (caused by mutations in myotilin) are in fact subtypes of myofibrillar myopathy.

Laboratory features

Serum CK level is particularly helpful in diagnosing Miyoshi's myopathy since it is very elevated. In the other conditions, serum CK is only slightly increased. EMGs are myopathic. In the MFMs, myotonic or pseudomyotonic discharges are common. Muscle biopsy shows nonspecific dystrophic features and, with the exception of Laing's and Miyoshi's myopathies, often shows rimmed vacuoles. MFM is associated with the accumulation of dense inclusions, as well as amorphous material best seen on Gomori's trichrome and myofibrillar disruption on electron microscopy. Immune staining sometimes demonstrates accumulation of desmin and other proteins in MFM, large deposits of myosin heavy chain in the subsarcolemmal region of type 1 muscle fibers in Laing's myopathy, and reduced or absent dysferlin in Miyoshi's myopathy.

The affected genes and their gene products are listed in Table 48-9. The gene for Welander's disease awaits identification.

TREATMENT Distal Myopathies

Occupational therapy is offered for loss of hand function; ankle-foot orthoses can support distal lower limb muscles. The MFMs can be associated with cardiomyopathy (congestive heart failure or arrhythmias) and respiratory failure that may require medical management. Laing's-type distal myopathy can also be associated with a cardiomyopathy.

CONGENITAL MYOPATHIES

These rare disorders are distinguished from muscular dystrophies by the presence of specific histochemical and structural abnormalities in muscle. Although primarily disorders of infancy or childhood, three forms that may present in adulthood are described here: central core disease, nemaline (rod) myopathy, and centronuclear (myotubular) myopathy. Sarcotubular myopathy is caused by mutations in TRIM-32 and is identical to LGMD2H. Other types, such as minicore myopathy (multi-minicore disease), fingerprint body myopathy, and cap myopathy, are not discussed.

CENTRAL CORE DISEASE

Patients with central core disease may have decreased fetal movements and breech presentation. Hypotonia and delay in motor milestones, particularly in walking, are common. Later in childhood, patients develop problems with stair climbing, running, and getting up from the floor. On examination, there is mild facial, neck-flexor, and proximal-extremity muscle weakness. Legs are more affected than arms. Skeletal abnormalities include congenital hip dislocation, scoliosis, and pes cavus; clubbed feet also occur. Most cases are nonprogressive, but exceptions are well documented. Susceptibility to malignant hyperthermia must be considered as a potential risk factor for patients with central core disease.

The serum CK level is usually normal. Needle EMG demonstrates a myopathic pattern. Muscle biopsy shows fibers with single or multiple central or eccentric discrete zones (*cores*) devoid of oxidative enzymes. Cores occur preferentially in type 1 fibers and represent poorly aligned sarcomeres associated with Z disk streaming.

Autosomal dominant inheritance is characteristic; sporadic cases also occur. The disease is caused by point mutations of the ryanodine receptor gene on chromosome 19q, encoding the calcium-release channel of the sarcoplasmic reticulum of skeletal muscle; mutations of this gene also account for some cases of inherited malignant hyperthermia. Malignant hyperthermia is an allelic condition; C-terminal mutations of the *RYR1* gene predispose to this complication.

Specific treatment is not required, but establishing a diagnosis of central core disease is extremely important because these patients have a known predisposition to malignant hyperthermia during anesthesia.

NEMALINE MYOPATHY

The term *nemaline* refers to the distinctive presence in muscle fibers of rods or threadlike structures (Greek *nema*, "thread"). Nemaline myopathy is clinically heterogeneous. A severe neonatal form presents with hypotonia and feeding and respiratory difficulties, leading to early death. Nemaline myopathy usually presents in infancy or childhood with delayed motor milestones. The course is nonprogressive or slowly progressive. The physical appearance is striking because of the long, narrow facies, high-arched palate, and open-mouthed appearance due to a prognathous jaw. Other skeletal abnormalities include pectus excavatum, kyphoscoliosis, pes cavus, and clubfoot deformities. Facial and generalized muscle weakness, including respiratory muscle weakness, is common. An adult-onset disorder with progressive proximal weakness may be seen. Myocardial involvement is occasionally present in both the childhood and adult-onset forms. The serum CK level is usually normal or slightly elevated. The EMG demonstrates a myopathic pattern. Muscle biopsy shows clusters of small rods (nemaline bodies), which occur preferentially, but not exclusively, in the sarcoplasm of type 1 muscle fibers. Occasionally, the rods are also apparent in myonuclei. The muscle often shows type 1 muscle fiber predominance. Rods originate from the Z disk material of the muscle fiber.

Six genes have been associated with nemaline myopathy. Five of these code for thin filament–associated proteins, suggesting disturbed assembly or interplay of these structures as a pivotal mechanism. Mutations of the nebulin (*NEB*) gene account for most cases, including both severe neonatal and early childhood forms, inherited as autosomal recessive disorders. Neonatal and childhood cases, inherited as predominantly autosomal dominant disorders, are caused by mutations of the skeletal muscle α-actinin (*ACTA1*) gene. In milder forms of the disease with autosomal dominant inheritance, mutations have been identified in both the slow α-tropomyosin (*TPM3*) and β-tropomyosin (*TPM2*) genes accounting for <3% of cases. Muscle troponin T (*TNNT1*) gene mutations appear to be limited to the Amish population in North America. Mutations in a sixth nemaline myopathy gene, *NEM6*, have recently been reported; this gene encodes a putative BTB/Kelch protein. No specific treatment is available.

CENTRONUCLEAR (MYOTUBULAR) MYOPATHY

Three distinct variants of centronuclear myopathy occur. A neonatal form, also known as *myotubular myopathy*, presents with severe hypotonia and weakness at birth. The late infancy–early childhood form presents with delayed motor milestones. Later, difficulty with running and stair climbing becomes apparent. A marfanoid, slender body habitus, long narrow face, and high-arched palate are typical. Scoliosis and clubbed feet may be present. Most patients exhibit progressive weakness, some requiring wheelchairs. Progressive external ophthalmoplegia with ptosis and varying degrees of extraocular muscle impairment are characteristic of both the neonatal and the late-infantile forms. A third variant, the late childhood–adult form, has an onset in the second or third decade. Patients have full extraocular muscle movements and rarely exhibit ptosis. There is mild, slowly progressive limb weakness that may be distally predominant (some of these patients have been classified as having Charcot-Marie-Tooth disease type 2 [CMT2; Chap. 45]).

Normal or slightly elevated CK levels occur in each of the forms. Nerve conduction studies may reveal reduced amplitudes of distal compound muscle action potentials, in particular in adult-onset cases that resemble CMT2. EMG studies often give distinctive results, showing positive sharp waves and fibrillation potentials, complex and repetitive discharges, and rarely myotonic discharges. Muscle biopsy specimens in longitudinal section demonstrate rows of central nuclei, often surrounded by a halo. In transverse sections, central nuclei are found in 25–80% of muscle fibers.

A gene for the neonatal form of centronuclear myopathy has been localized to Xq28; this gene encodes myotubularin, a protein tyrosine phosphatase. Missense, frameshift, and splice-site mutations predict loss of myotubularin function in affected individuals. Carrier identification and prenatal diagnosis are possible. Autosomal recessive forms are caused by mutations in *BIB1* that encodes for amphyphysin-2, while some autosomal dominant cases, which are allelic to a form of CMT2, are associated with mutations in the gene that encodes dynamin-2. No specific medical treatments are available at this time.

DISORDERS OF MUSCLE ENERGY METABOLISM

There are two principal sources of energy for skeletal muscle—fatty acids and glucose. Abnormalities in either glucose or lipid utilization can be associated with distinct clinical presentations that can range from an acute, painful syndrome with rhabdomyolysis and myoglobinuria to a chronic, progressive muscle weakness simulating muscular dystrophy.

GLYCOGEN STORAGE AND GLYCOLYTIC DEFECTS

Disorders of glycogen storage causing progressive weakness

α-Glucosidase, or acid maltase, deficiency (Pompe's disease)

Three clinical forms of α-glucosidase, or acid maltase, deficiency (*type II glycogenosis*) can be distinguished. The infantile form is the most common, with onset of symptoms in the first 3 months of life. Infants develop severe muscle weakness, cardiomegaly, hepatomegaly, and respiratory insufficiency. Glycogen accumulation in motor neurons of the spinal cord and brainstem contributes to muscle weakness. Death usually occurs by 1 year of age. In the childhood form, the picture resembles muscular dystrophy. Delayed motor milestones result from proximal limb muscle weakness and involvement of respiratory muscles. The heart may be involved, but the liver and brain are unaffected. The adult form usually begins in the third or fourth decade but can present as late as the seventh decade. Respiratory failure and diaphragmatic weakness are often initial manifestations, heralding progressive proximal muscle weakness. The heart and liver are not involved.

The serum CK level is 2 to 10 times normal in infantile or childhood-onset Pompe's disease but can be normal in adult-onset cases. EMG examination demonstrates a myopathic pattern, but other features are especially distinctive, including myotonic discharges, trains of fibrillation and positive waves, and complex repetitive discharges. EMG discharges are very prominent in the paraspinal muscles. The muscle biopsy in infants typically reveals vacuoles containing glycogen and the lysosomal enzyme acid phosphatase. Electron microscopy reveals membrane-bound and free tissue glycogen. However, muscle biopsies in late-onset Pompe's disease may demonstrate only nonspecific abnormalities. Enzyme analysis of dried blood spots is a sensitive technique to screen for Pompe's disease. A definitive diagnosis is established by enzyme assay in muscle or cultured fibroblasts or by genetic testing.

Pompe's disease is inherited as an autosomal recessive disorder caused by mutations of the α-glucosidase gene. Enzyme replacement therapy (ERT) with IV recombinant human α-glucosidase has been shown to be beneficial in infantile-onset Pompe's disease. Clinical benefits in the infantile disease include reduced heart size, improved muscle function, reduced need for ventilatory support, and longer life. In late-onset cases, ERT has not been associated with the dramatic response that can be seen in classic infantile Pompe's disease, yet it appears to stabilize the disease process.

Other glycogen storage diseases with progressive weakness

In *debranching enzyme deficiency* (*type III glycogenosis*), a slowly progressive form of muscle weakness can develop after puberty. Rarely, myoglobinuria may be seen. Patients are usually diagnosed in infancy, however, because of hypotonia and delayed motor milestones, hepatomegaly, growth retardation, and hypoglycemia. *Branching enzyme deficiency* (*type IV glycogenosis*) is a rare and fatal glycogen storage disease characterized by failure to thrive and hepatomegaly. Hypotonia and muscle wasting may be present, but the skeletal muscle manifestations are minor compared to liver failure.

Disorders of glycolysis causing exercise intolerance

Several glycolytic defects are associated with recurrent myoglobinuria: *myophosphorylase deficiency* (*type V glycogenosis*), *phosphofructokinase deficiency* (*type VII glycogenosis*), *phosphoglycerate kinase deficiency* (*type IX glycogenosis*), *phosphoglycerate mutase deficiency* (*type X glycogenosis*), *lactate dehydrogenase deficiency* (*glycogenosis type XI*), and β-*enolase deficiency*. Myophosphorylase deficiency, also known as *McArdle's disease*, is by far the most common of the glycolytic defects associated with exercise intolerance. These glycolytic defects result in a common failure to support energy production at the initiation of exercise, although the exact site of energy failure remains controversial.

Clinical muscle manifestations in these conditions usually begin in adolescence. Symptoms are precipitated by brief bursts of high-intensity exercise such as running or lifting heavy objects. A history of myalgia and muscle stiffness usually precedes the intensely painful muscle contractures, which may be followed by myoglobinuria. Acute renal failure accompanies significant pigmenturia.

Certain features help distinguish some enzyme defects. In McArdle's disease, exercise tolerance can be enhanced by a slow induction phase (warm-up) or brief periods of rest, allowing for the start of the "second-wind" phenomenon (switching to utilization of fatty acids). Varying degrees of hemolytic anemia accompany deficiencies of both phosphofructokinase (mild) and phosphoglycerate kinase (severe). In phosphoglycerate kinase deficiency, the usual clinical presentation is a seizure disorder associated with mental retardation; exercise intolerance is an infrequent manifestation.

In all of these conditions, the serum CK levels fluctuate widely and may be elevated even during symptom-free periods. CK levels >100 times normal are expected, accompanying myoglobinuria. All patients with suspected glycolytic defects leading to exercise intolerance should undergo a forearm exercise test. An impaired rise in venous lactate is highly indicative of a glycolytic defect. In lactate dehydrogenase deficiency, venous levels of lactate do not increase, but pyruvate rises to normal. A definitive diagnosis of glycolytic disease is made by muscle biopsy and subsequent enzyme analysis or by genetic testing.

Myophosphorylase deficiency, phosphofructokinase deficiency, and phosphoglycerate mutase deficiency are inherited as autosomal recessive disorders. Phosphoglycerate kinase deficiency is X-linked recessive. Mutations can be found in the respective genes encoding the abnormal proteins in each of these disorders.

Training may enhance exercise tolerance, perhaps by increasing perfusion to muscle. Dietary intake of free glucose or fructose prior to activity may improve function but care must be taken to avoid obesity from ingesting too many calories.

LIPID AS AN ENERGY SOURCE AND ASSOCIATED DEFECTS

Lipid is an important muscle energy source during rest and during prolonged, submaximal exercise. Fatty acids are derived from circulating very low-density lipoprotein (VLDL) in the blood or from triglycerides stored in muscle fibers. Oxidation of fatty acids occurs in the mitochondria. To enter the mitochondria, a fatty acid must first be converted to an "activated fatty acid," acyl-CoA. The acyl-CoA must be linked with carnitine by the enzyme carnitine palmitoyltransferase (CPT) I for transport into the mitochondria. CPT I is present on the inner side of the outer mitochondrial membrane. Carnitine is removed by CPT II, an enzyme attached to the inside of the inner mitochondrial membrane, allowing transport of acyl-CoA into the mitochondrial matrix for β-oxidation.

Carnitine palmitoyltransferase deficiency

CPT II deficiency is the most common recognizable cause of recurrent myoglobinuria, more common than the glycolytic defects. Onset is usually in the teenage years or early twenties. Muscle pain and myoglobinuria typically occur after prolonged exercise but can also be precipitated by fasting or infections; up to 20% of patients do not exhibit myoglobinuria, however. Strength is normal between attacks. In contrast to disorders caused by defects in glycolysis, in which muscle cramps follow short, intense bursts of exercise, the muscle pain in CPT II deficiency does not occur until the limits of utilization have been exceeded and muscle breakdown has already begun. Episodes of rhabdomyolysis may produce severe weakness. In young children and newborns, CPT II deficiency can present with a very severe clinical picture including hypoketotic hypoglycemia, cardiomyopathy, liver failure, and sudden death.

Serum CK levels and EMG findings are both usually normal between episodes. A normal rise of venous lactate during forearm exercise distinguishes this condition from glycolytic defects, especially myophosphorylase deficiency. Muscle biopsy does not show lipid accumulation and is usually normal between attacks. The diagnosis requires direct measurement of muscle CPT or genetic testing.

CPT II deficiency is much more common in men than women (5:1); nevertheless, all evidence indicates autosomal recessive inheritance. A mutation in the gene for CPT II (chromosome 1p36) causes the disease in some individuals. Attempts to improve exercise tolerance with frequent meals and a low-fat, high-carbohydrate diet, or by substituting medium-chain triglycerides in the diet, have not proven to be beneficial.

Myoadenylate deaminase deficiency

The muscle enzyme myoadenylate deaminase converts adenosine-5′-monophosphate (5′-AMP) to inosine monophosphate (IMP) with liberation of ammonia. Myoadenylate deaminase may play a role in regulating adenosine triphosphate (ATP) levels in muscles. Most individuals with myoadenylate deaminase deficiency have no symptoms. There have been a few reports of patients with this disorder who have exercise-exacerbated myalgia and myoglobinuria. Many questions have been raised about the clinical effects of myoadenylate deaminase deficiency, and, specifically, its relationship to exertional myalgia and fatigability, but there is no consensus.

MITOCHONDRIAL MYOPATHIES

In 1972, Olson and colleagues recognized that muscle fibers with significant numbers of abnormal mitochondria could be highlighted with the modified trichrome stain; the term *ragged red fibers* was coined. By electron microscopy, the mitochondria in ragged red fibers are enlarged and often bizarrely shaped and have crystalline inclusions. Since that seminal observation, the understanding of these disorders of muscle and other tissues has expanded.

Mitochondria play a key role in energy production. Oxidation of the major nutrients derived from carbohydrate, fat, and protein leads to the generation of reducing equivalents. The latter are transported through the respiratory chain in the process known as *oxidative phosphorylation*. The energy generated by the oxidation-reduction reactions of the respiratory chain is stored in an electrochemical gradient coupled to ATP synthesis.

A novel feature of mitochondria is their genetic composition. Each mitochondrion possesses a DNA genome that is distinct from that of the nuclear DNA. Human mitochondrial DNA (mtDNA) consists of a double-strand, circular molecule comprising 16,569 base pairs. It codes for 22 transfer RNAs, 2 ribosomal RNAs, and 13 polypeptides of the respiratory chain enzymes. The genetics of mitochondrial diseases differ from the genetics of chromosomal disorders. The DNA of mitochondria is directly inherited from the cytoplasm of the gametes, mainly from the oocyte. The sperm contributes very little of its mitochondria to the offspring at the time of fertilization. Thus, mitochondrial genes are derived almost exclusively from the mother, accounting for maternal inheritance of some mitochondrial disorders.

Patients with mitochondrial myopathies have clinical manifestations that usually fall into three groups: chronic progressive external ophthalmoplegia (CPEO), skeletal muscle–CNS syndromes, and pure myopathy simulating muscular dystrophy or metabolic myopathy.

PROGRESSIVE EXTERNAL OPHTHALMOPLEGIA SYNDROMES WITH RAGGED RED FIBERS

The single most common sign of a mitochondrial myopathy is CPEO, occurring in >50% of all mitochondrial myopathies. Varying degrees of ptosis and weakness of extraocular muscles are seen, usually in the absence of diplopia, a point of distinction from disorders with fluctuating eye weakness (e.g., myasthenia gravis).

KEARNS-SAYRE SYNDROME (KSS)

KSS is a widespread multiorgan system disorder with a defined triad of clinical findings: onset before age 20, CPEO, and pigmentary retinopathy, plus one or more of the following features: complete heart block, cerebrospinal fluid (CSF) protein >1 g/L (100 mg/dL), or cerebellar ataxia. Some patients with CPEO and ragged red fibers may not fulfill all of the criteria for KSS. The cardiac disease includes syncopal attacks and cardiac arrest related to the abnormalities in the cardiac conduction system: prolonged intraventricular conduction time, bundle branch block, and complete atrioventricular block. Death attributed to heart block occurs in ~20% of the patients. Varying degrees of progressive limb muscle weakness and easy fatigability affect activities of daily living. Endocrine abnormalities are common, including gonadal dysfunction in both sexes with delayed puberty, short stature, and infertility. Diabetes mellitus is a cardinal sign of mitochondrial disorders and is estimated to occur in 13% of KSS patients. Other less common endocrine disorders include thyroid disease, hyperaldosteronism, Addison's disease, and hypoparathyroidism. Both mental retardation and dementia are common accompaniments to this disorder. Serum CK levels are normal or slightly elevated. Serum lactate and pyruvate levels may be elevated. EMG is myopathic. Nerve conduction studies may be abnormal related to an associated neuropathy. Muscle biopsies reveal ragged red fibers, highlighted in oxidative enzyme stains, many showing defects in cytochrome oxidase. By electron microscopy there are increased numbers of mitochondria that often appear enlarged and contain paracrystalline inclusions.

KSS is a sporadic disorder. The disease is caused by single mtDNA deletions presumed to arise spontaneously in the ovum or zygote. The most common deletion, occurring in about one-third of patients, removes 4,977 bp of contiguous mtDNA. Monitoring for cardiac conduction defects is critical. Prophylactic pacemaker implantation is indicated when ECGs demonstrate a bifascicular block. In KSS, no benefit has been shown for supplementary therapies, including multivitamins or coenzyme Q10. Of all the proposed options, exercise might be the most applicable but must be approached cautiously because of defects in the cardiac conduction system.

PROGRESSIVE EXTERNAL OPHTHALMOPLEGIA (PEO)

This condition is caused by nuclear DNA mutations affecting mtDNA copy number and integrity and is thus inherited in a Mendelian fashion. Onset is usually after puberty. Fatigue, exercise intolerance, and complaints of muscle weakness are typical. Some patients notice swallowing problems. The neurologic examination confirms the ptosis and ophthalmoplegia, usually asymmetric in distribution. A sensorineural hearing loss may be encountered. Mild facial, neck flexor, and proximal weakness are typical. Rarely, respiratory muscles may be progressively affected and may be the direct cause of death. Serum CK is normal or mildly elevated. The resting lactate level is normal or slightly elevated but may rise excessively after exercise. CSF protein is normal. The EMG is myopathic, and nerve conduction studies are usually normal. Ragged red fibers are prominently displayed in the muscle biopsy. Southern blots of muscle reveal a normal mtDNA band at 16.6 kb and several additional mtDNA deletion bands with genomes varying from 0.5 to 10 kb.

This autosomal dominant form of CPEO has been linked to loci on three chromosomes: 4q35, 10q24, and 15q22–26. In the chromosome 4q-related form of disease, mutations of the gene encoding the heart and skeletal muscle–specific isoform of the adenine nucleotide translocator 1 (*ANT1*) gene are found. This highly abundant mitochondrial protein forms a homodimeric inner mitochondrial channel through which adenosine diphosphate (ADP) enters and ATP leaves the mitochondrial matrix. In the chromosome 10q–related disorder, mutations of the gene *C10orf2* are found. Its gene product, *twinkle*, co-localizes with the mtDNA and is named for its punctate, starlike staining properties. The function of twinkle is presumed to be critical for lifetime maintenance of mitochondrial integrity. In the cases mapped to chromosome 15q, a mutation affects the gene encoding mtDNA polymerase (*POLG*), an enzyme important in mtDNA replication. Autosomal recessive PEO has also been described with mutations in the *POLG* gene. Point mutations have been identified within various mitochondrial tRNA (Leu, Ile, Asn, Trp) genes in families with maternal inheritance of PEO.

Exercise may improve function but will depend on the patient's ability to participate.

MITOCHONDRIAL DNA SKELETAL MUSCLE–CENTRAL NERVOUS SYSTEM SYNDROMES

Myoclonic epilepsy with ragged red fibers (MERRF)

The onset of MERRF is variable, ranging from late childhood to middle adult life. Characteristic features include myoclonic epilepsy, cerebellar ataxia, and progressive muscle weakness. The seizure disorder is an integral part of the disease and may be the initial symptom. Cerebellar ataxia precedes or accompanies epilepsy. It is slowly progressive and generalized. The third major feature of the disease is muscle weakness in a limb-girdle distribution. Other more variable features include dementia, peripheral neuropathy, optic atrophy, hearing loss, and diabetes mellitus.

Serum CK levels are normal or slightly increased. The serum lactate may be elevated. EMG is myopathic, and in some patients nerve conduction studies show a neuropathy. The electroencephalogram is abnormal, corroborating clinical findings of epilepsy. Typical ragged red fibers are seen on muscle biopsy. MERRF is caused by maternally inherited point mutations of mitochondrial tRNA genes. The most common mutation found in 80% of MERRF patients is an A to G substitution at nucleotide 8344 of tRNA lysine (A8344G tRNA^{lys}). Other tRNA^{lys} mutations include base-pair substitutions T8356C and G8363A. Only supportive treatment is possible, with special attention to epilepsy.

Mitochondrial myopathy, encephalopathy, lactic acidosis, and strokelike episodes (MELAS)

MELAS is the most common mitochondrial encephalomyopathy. The term *strokelike* is appropriate because the cerebral lesions do not conform to a strictly vascular distribution. The onset in the majority of patients is before age 20. Seizures, usually partial motor or generalized, are common and may represent the first clearly recognizable sign of disease. The cerebral insults that resemble strokes cause hemiparesis, hemianopia, and cortical blindness. A presumptive stroke occurring before age 40 should place this mitochondrial encephalomyopathy high in the differential diagnosis. Associated conditions include hearing loss, diabetes mellitus, hypothalamic pituitary dysfunction causing growth hormone deficiency, hypothyroidism, and absence of secondary sexual characteristics. In its full expression, MELAS leads to dementia, a bedridden state, and a fatal outcome. Serum lactic acid is typically elevated. The CSF protein is also increased but is usually ≤1 g/L (100 mg/dL). Muscle biopsies show ragged red fibers. Neuroimaging demonstrates basal ganglia calcification in a high percentage of cases. Focal lesions that mimic infarction are present predominantly in the occipital and parietal lobes. Strict vascular territories are not respected, and cerebral angiography fails to demonstrate lesions of the major cerebral blood vessels.

MELAS is caused by maternally inherited point mutations of mitochondrial tRNA genes. Most of the tRNA mutations are lethal, accounting for the paucity of multigeneration families with this syndrome. The A3243G point mutation in tRNA$^{Leu(UUR)}$ is the most common, occurring in ~80% of MELAS cases. About 10% of MELAS patients have other mutations of the tRNA$^{Leu(UUR)}$ gene, including 3252G, 3256T, 3271C, and 3291C. Other tRNA gene mutations have also been reported in MELAS, including G583A tRNA^{Phe}, G1642A tRNA^{Val}, G4332A tRNA^{Glu}, and T8316C tRNA^{Lys}. Mutations have also been reported in mtDNA polypeptide-coding genes. Two mutations were found in the ND5 subunit of complex I of the respiratory chain. A missense mutation has been reported at mtDNA position 9957 in the gene for subunit III of cytochrome C oxidase. No specific treatment is available. Supportive treatment is essential for the strokelike episodes, seizures, and endocrinopathies.

PURE MYOPATHY SYNDROMES

Muscle weakness and fatigue can be the predominant manifestations of mtDNA mutations. When the condition affects exclusively muscle (pure myopathy), the disorder becomes difficult to recognize. Occasionally, mitochondrial myopathies can present with recurrent myoglobinuria without fixed weakness and thus resemble a glycogen storage disorder or CPT deficiency.

Mitochondrial DNA depletion syndromes

Mitochondrial DNA depletion syndrome (MDS) is a heterogeneous group of disorders that are inherited in an autosomal recessive fashion and can present in infancy or adults. MDS can be caused by mutations in genes (*TK2, DGUOK, RRM2B, TYMP, SUCLA1,* and *SUCLA2*) that lead to depletion of pools of mitochondrial deoxyribonucleotide (dNTP) pools necessary for mtDNA replication The other major cause of MDS is a set of mutations in genes essential for mtDNA replication (e.g., *POLG1* and *C10orf2*). The clinical phenotypes associated with MDS vary. Patients may develop a severe encephalopathy (e.g., Leigh's syndrome), PEO, an isolated myopathy, myoneuro-gastrointestinal-encephalopathy (MNGIE), and a sensory neuropathy with ataxia.

DISORDERS OF MUSCLE MEMBRANE EXCITABILITY

Muscle membrane excitability is affected in a group of disorders referred to as *channelopathies*. The heart may also be involved, resulting in life-threatening complications (Table 48-10).

CALCIUM CHANNEL DISORDERS OF MUSCLE

Hypokalemic periodic paralysis (HypoKPP)

Onset occurs at adolescence. Men are more often affected because of decreased penetrance in women. Episodic weakness with onset after age 25 is almost never due to periodic paralyses, with the exception of thyrotoxic periodic paralysis (discussed later). Attacks are often

TABLE 48-10

CLINICAL FEATURES OF PERIODIC PARALYSIS AND NONDYSTROPHIC MYOTONIAS

	CALCIUM CHANNEL	SODIUM CHANNEL		POTASSIUM CHANNEL
FEATURE	HYPOKALEMIC PP	HYPERKALEMIC PP	PARAMYOTONIA CONGENITA	ANDERSEN-TAWIL SYNDROME[a]
Mode of inheritance	AD	AD	AD	AD
Age of onset	Adolescence	Early childhood	Early childhood	Early childhood
Myotonia[b]	No	Yes	Yes	No
Episodic weakness	Yes	Yes	Yes	Yes
Frequency of attacks of weakness	Daily to yearly	May be 2–3/d	With cold, usually rare	Daily to yearly
Duration of attacks of weakness	2–12 h	From 1–2 h to >1 d	2–24 h	2–24 h
Serum K^+ level during attacks of weakness	Decreased	Increased or normal	Usually normal	Variable
Effect of K^+ loading	No change	Increased myotonia, then weakness	Increased myotonia	No change
Effect of muscle cooling	No change	Increased myotonia	Increased myotonia, then weakness	No change
Fixed weakness	Yes	Yes	Yes	Yes

[a]Dysmorphic features and cardiac arrhythmias are distinguishing features (see text).
[b]May be paradoxical in paramyotonia congenita.
Abbreviations: AD, autosomal dominant; PP, periodic paralysis.

provoked by meals high in carbohydrates or sodium and may accompany rest following prolonged exercise. Weakness usually affects proximal limb muscles more than distal. Ocular and bulbar muscles are less likely to be affected. Respiratory muscles are usually spared but when they are involved, the condition may prove fatal. Weakness may take as long as 24 h to resolve. Life-threatening cardiac arrhythmias related to hypokalemia may occur during attacks. As a late complication, patients commonly develop severe, disabling proximal lower extremity weakness.

Attacks of thyrotoxic periodic paralysis resemble those of primary HypoKPP. Despite a higher incidence of thyrotoxicosis in women, men, particularly those of Asian descent, are more likely to manifest this complication. Attacks abate with treatment of the underlying thyroid condition.

A low serum potassium level during an attack, excluding secondary causes, establishes the diagnosis. Interattack muscle biopsies show the presence of single or multiple centrally placed vacuoles or tubular aggregates. Provocative tests with glucose and insulin to establish a diagnosis are usually not necessary and are potentially hazardous.

In the midst of an attack of weakness, motor conduction studies may demonstrate reduced amplitudes, whereas EMG may show electrical silence in severely weak muscles. In between attacks, the EMG and nerve conduction studies are normal, with the exception that myopathic MUAPs may be seen in patients with fixed weakness.

HypoKPP is caused by mutations in either of two genes. HypoKPP type 1, the most common form, is inherited as an autosomal dominant disorder with incomplete penetrance. These patients have mutations in the voltage-sensitive, skeletal muscle calcium channel gene, *CALCL1A3* (Fig. 48-8). Approximately 10% of cases are HypoKPP type 2, arising from mutations in the voltage-sensitive sodium channel gene (*SCN4A*). In either instance, the mutations lead to an abnormal gating pore current that predisposes the muscle cell to depolarize when potassium levels are low. It is also now recognized that some cases of thyrotoxic HypoKPP are caused by genetic variants in a potassium channel (Kir 2.6), whose expression is regulated by thyroid hormone.

The chloride channel is envisioned to have 10 membrane-spanning domains. The positions of mutations causing dominantly and recessively inherited myotonia congenita are indicated, along with mutations that cause this disease in mice and goats.

TREATMENT Hypokalemic Periodic Paralysis

The acute paralysis improves after the administration of potassium. Muscle strength and ECG should be monitored. Oral KCl (0.2–0.4 mmol/kg) should be given every

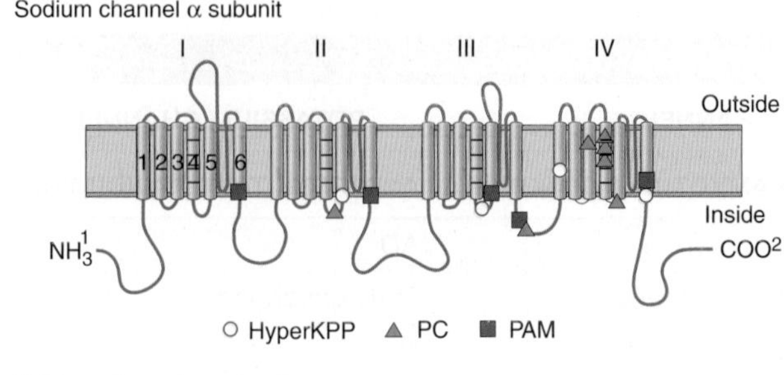

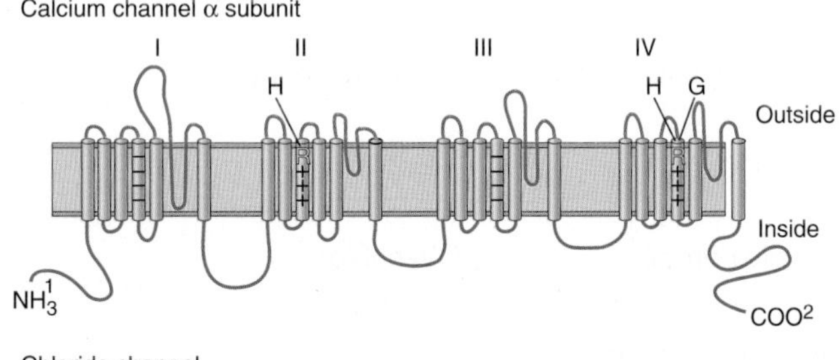

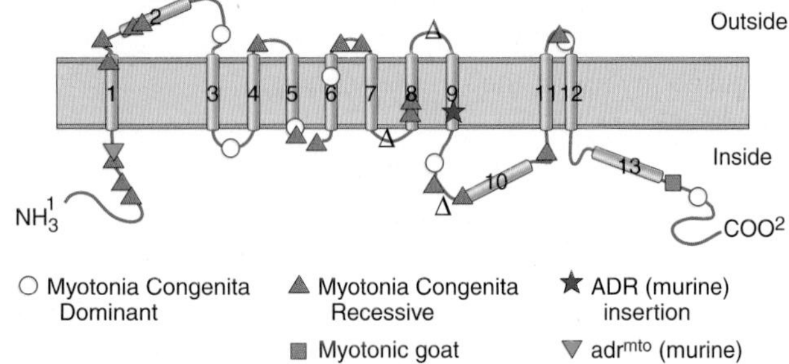

FIGURE 48-8

The sodium and calcium channels are depicted here as containing four homologous domains, each with six membrane-spanning segments. The fourth segment of each domain bears positive charges and acts as the "voltage sensor" for the channel. The association of the four domains is thought to form a pore through which ions pass. Sodium channel mutations are shown along with the phenotype that they confer. HyperKPP, hyperkalemic periodic paralysis; PC, paramyotonia congenita; PAM, potassium-aggravated myotonia. See text for details.

30 min. Only rarely is IV therapy necessary (e.g., when swallowing problems or vomiting is present). Administration of potassium in a glucose solution should be avoided because it may further reduce serum potassium levels. Mannitol is the preferred vehicle for administration of IV potassium. The long-term goal of therapy is to avoid attacks. This may reduce late-onset, fixed weakness. Patients should be made aware of the importance of a low-carbohydrate, low-sodium diet and consequences of intense exercise. Prophylactic administration of acetazolamide (125–1000 mg/d in divided doses) reduces or may abolish attacks in HypoKPP type 1. Paradoxically the potassium is lowered, but this is offset by the beneficial effect of metabolic acidosis. If attacks persist on acetazolamide, oral KCl should be added. Some patients require treatment with triamterine (25–100 mg/d) or spironolactone (25–100 mg/d). However, in patients with HypoKPP type 2, attacks of weakness can be exacerbated with acetazolamide.

SODIUM CHANNEL DISORDERS OF MUSCLE

Hyperkalemic periodic paralysis (HyperKPP)

The term *hyperkalemic* is misleading since patients are often normokalemic during attacks. The fact that attacks are precipitated by potassium administration best defines the disease. The onset is in the first decade; males and females are affected equally. Attacks are brief and mild, usually lasting 30 min to 4 h. Weakness affects proximal muscles, sparing bulbar muscles. Attacks are precipitated by rest following exercise and fasting. In a variant of this disorder, the predominant symptom is myotonia without weakness (*potassium-aggravated myotonia*). The symptoms are aggravated by cold, and myotonia makes the muscles stiff and painful. This disorder can be confused with paramyotonia congenita, myotonia congenita, and proximal myotonic myopathy (DM2).

Potassium may be slightly elevated but may also be normal during an attack. As in HypoKPP, nerve conduction studies in HyperKPP muscle may demonstrate reduced motor amplitudes and the EMG may be silent in very weak muscles. In between attacks of weakness, the conduction studies are normal. The EMG will often demonstrate myotonic discharges during and between attacks.

The muscle biopsy shows vacuoles that are smaller, less numerous, and more peripheral compared to the hypokalemic form or tubular aggregates. Provocative tests by administration of potassium can induce weakness but are usually not necessary to establish the diagnosis. HyperKPP and potassium-aggravated myotonia are inherited as autosomal dominant disorders. Mutations of the voltage-gated sodium channel *SCN4A* gene (Fig. 48-8) cause these conditions. For patients with frequent attacks, acetazolamide (125–1000 mg/d) is helpful. We have found mexiletine to be helpful in patients with significant myotonia.

Paramyotonia congenita

In paramyotonia congenita (PC), the attacks of weakness are cold-induced or occur spontaneously and are mild. Myotonia is a prominent feature but worsens with muscle activity (paradoxical myotonia). This is in contrast to classic myotonia in which exercise alleviates the condition. Attacks of weakness are seldom severe enough to require emergency room treatment. Over time patients develop interattack weakness as they do in other forms of periodic paralysis. PC is usually associated with normokalemia or hyperkalemia.

Serum CK is usually mildly elevated. Routine sensory and motor nerve conduction studies are normal. Cooling of the muscle often dramatically reduces the amplitude of the compound muscle action potentials. EMG reveals diffuse myotonic potentials in PC. Upon local cooling of the muscle, the myotonic discharges disappear as the patient becomes unable to activate MUAPs.

PC is inherited as an autosomal dominant condition; voltage-gated sodium channel mutations (Fig. 48-8) are responsible and thus this disorder is allelic with Hyper-KPP and potassium-aggravated myotonia. Patients with PC seldom seek treatment during attacks. Oral administration of glucose or other carbohydrates hastens recovery. Since interattack weakness may develop after repeated episodes, prophylactic treatment is usually indicated. Thiazide diuretics (e.g., chlorothiazide, 250–1000 mg/d) and mexiletine (slowly increase dose from 450 mg/d) are reported to be helpful. Patients should be advised to increase carbohydrates in their diet.

POTASSIUM CHANNEL DISORDERS

Andersen-Tawil syndrome

This rare disease is characterized by episodic weakness, cardiac arrhythmias, and dysmorphic features (short stature, scoliosis, clinodactyly, hypertelorism, small or prominent low-set ears, micrognathia, and broad forehead). The cardiac arrhythmias are potentially serious and life threatening. They include long QT, ventricular ectopy, bidirectional ventricular arrhythmias, and tachycardia. For many years the classification of this disorder was uncertain because episodes of weakness are associated with elevated, normal, or reduced levels of potassium during an attack. In addition, the potassium levels differ among kindreds but are consistent within a family. Inheritance is autosomal dominant, with incomplete penetrance and variable expressivity. The disease is caused by mutations of the inwardly rectifying potassium channel (*Kir 2.1*) gene that heighten muscle cell excitability. The treatment is similar to that for other forms of periodic paralysis and must include cardiac monitoring. The episodes of weakness may differ between patients because of potassium variability. Acetazolamide may decrease the attack frequency and severity.

CHLORIDE CHANNEL DISORDERS

Two forms of this disorder, autosomal dominant (*Thomsen's disease*) and autosomal recessive (*Becker's disease*), are related to the same gene abnormality. Symptoms are noted in infancy and early childhood. The severity lessens in the third to fourth decade. Myotonia is worsened by cold and improved by activity. The gait may appear slow and labored at first but improves with walking. In Thomsen's disease muscle strength is normal, but in Becker's disease, which is usually more severe, there may be muscle weakness. Muscle hypertrophy is usually present. Myotonic discharges are prominently displayed by EMG recordings.

Serum CK is normal or mildly elevated. The muscle biopsy shows hypertrophied fibers. The disease is inherited as dominant or recessive and is caused by mutations of the chloride channel gene (Fig. 48-8) that increase muscle cell excitability. Many patients will not require treatment and learn that the symptoms improve with activity. Medications that can be used to decrease myotonia include quinine, phenytoin, and mexiletine.

ENDOCRINE AND METABOLIC MYOPATHIES

Many endocrine disorders cause weakness. Muscle fatigue is more common than true weakness. The cause of weakness in these disorders is not well defined. It is not even clear that weakness results from disease of muscle as opposed to another part of the motor unit, since the serum CK level is often normal (except in hypothyroidism) and the muscle histology is characterized by atrophy rather than destruction of muscle fibers. Nearly all endocrine myopathies respond to treatment.

THYROID DISORDERS

Abnormalities of thyroid function can cause a wide array of muscle disorders. These conditions relate to the important role of thyroid hormones in regulating the metabolism of carbohydrates and lipids as well as the rate of protein synthesis and enzyme production. Thyroid hormones also stimulate calorigenesis in muscle, increase muscle demand for vitamins, and enhance muscle sensitivity to circulating catecholamines.

Hypothyroidism

Patients with hypothyroidism have frequent muscle complaints, and proximal muscle weakness occurs in about one-third of them. Muscle cramps, pain, and stiffness are common. Some patients have enlarged muscles. Features of slow muscle contraction and relaxation occur in 25% of patients; the relaxation phase of muscle stretch reflexes is characteristically prolonged and best observed at the ankle or biceps brachii reflexes. The serum CK level is often elevated (up to 10 times normal), even when there is minimal clinical evidence of muscle disease. EMG is typically normal. The cause of muscle enlargement has not been determined, and muscle biopsy shows no distinctive morphologic abnormalities.

Hyperthyroidism

Patients who are thyrotoxic commonly have proximal muscle weakness and atrophy on examination, but they rarely complain of myopathic symptoms. Activity of deep tendon reflexes may be enhanced. Bulbar, respiratory, and even esophageal muscles may occasionally be affected, causing dysphagia, dysphonia, and aspiration. When bulbar involvement occurs, it is usually accompanied by chronic proximal limb weakness, but occasionally it presents in the absence of generalized thyrotoxic myopathy. Fasciculations may be apparent and, when coupled with increased muscle stretch reflexes, may lead to an erroneous diagnosis of ALS. Other neuromuscular disorders occur in association with hyperthyroidism, including acquired hypokalemic periodic paralysis, myasthenia gravis, and a progressive ocular myopathy associated with proptosis (*Graves' ophthalmopathy*). Serum CK levels are not elevated in thyrotoxic myopathy, the EMG is normal, and muscle histology usually shows only atrophy of muscle fibers.

PARATHYROID DISORDERS

Hyperparathyroidism

Muscle weakness is an integral part of primary and secondary hyperparathyroidism. Proximal muscle weakness, muscle wasting, and brisk muscle stretch reflexes are the main features of this endocrinopathy. Some patients develop neck extensor weakness (part of the dropped head syndrome). Serum CK levels are usually normal or slightly elevated. Serum parathyroid hormone levels are elevated. Serum calcium and phosphorus levels show no correlation with the clinical neuromuscular manifestations. Muscle biopsies show only varying degrees of atrophy without muscle fiber degeneration.

Hypoparathyroidism

An overt myopathy due to hypocalcemia rarely occurs. Neuromuscular symptoms are usually related to localized or generalized tetany. Serum CK levels may be increased secondary to muscle damage from sustained tetany. Hyporeflexia or areflexia is usually present and contrasts with the hyperreflexia in hyperparathyroidism.

ADRENAL DISORDERS

Conditions associated with glucocorticoid excess cause a myopathy; in fact, steroid myopathy is the most commonly diagnosed endocrine muscle disease. Glucocorticoid excess, either endogenous or exogenous (see "Drug-Induced Myopathies"), produces various degrees of proximal limb weakness. Muscle wasting may be striking. A cushingoid appearance usually accompanies clinical signs of myopathy. Histologic sections demonstrate muscle fiber atrophy, preferentially affecting type 2b fibers, rather than degeneration or necrosis of muscle fibers. Adrenal insufficiency commonly causes muscle fatigue. The degree of weakness may be difficult to assess but is typically mild. In primary hyperaldosteronism (*Conn's syndrome*), neuromuscular complications are due to potassium depletion. The clinical picture is one of persistent muscle weakness. Long-standing hyperaldosteronism may lead to proximal limb weakness and wasting. Serum CK levels may be elevated, and a muscle biopsy may demonstrate degenerating fibers, some with vacuoles. These changes relate to hypokalemia and are not a direct effect of aldosterone on skeletal muscle.

PITUITARY DISORDERS

Patients with acromegaly usually have mild proximal weakness without muscle atrophy. Muscles often appear enlarged but exhibit decreased force generation. The duration of acromegaly, rather than the serum growth hormone levels, correlates with the degree of myopathy.

DIABETES MELLITUS

Neuromuscular complications of diabetes mellitus are most often related to neuropathy, with cranial and peripheral nerve palsies or distal sensorimotor polyneuropathy. *Diabetic amyotrophy* is a clumsy term since the condition represents a neuropathy affecting the proximal major nerve trunks and lumbosacral plexus. More appropriate terms for this disorder include *diabetic proximal neuropathy* and *lumbosacral radiculoplexus neuropathy*.

The only notable myopathy of diabetes mellitus is ischemic infarction of leg muscles, usually involving one of the thigh muscles but on occasion affecting the distal leg. This condition occurs in patients with poorly controlled diabetes and presents with abrupt onset of pain, tenderness, and edema of one thigh. The area of muscle infarction is hard and indurated. The muscles most often affected include the vastus lateralis, thigh adductors, and biceps femoris. CT or MRI can demonstrate focal abnormalities in the affected muscle. Diagnosis by imaging is preferable to muscle biopsy, if possible, as hemorrhage into the biopsy site can occur.

VITAMIN DEFICIENCY

Vitamin D deficiency due to either decreased intake, decreased absorption, or impaired vitamin D metabolism (as occurs in renal disease) may lead to chronic muscle weakness. Pain reflects the underlying bone disease (*osteomalacia*). Vitamin E deficiency may result from malabsorption. Clinical manifestations include ataxic neuropathy due to loss of proprioception and myopathy with proximal weakness. Progressive external ophthalmoplegia is a distinctive finding. It has not been established that deficiency of other vitamins causes a myopathy.

MYOPATHIES OF SYSTEMIC ILLNESS

Systemic illnesses such as chronic respiratory, cardiac, or hepatic failure are frequently associated with severe muscle wasting and complaints of weakness. Fatigue is usually a more significant problem than weakness, which is typically mild.

Myopathy may be a manifestation of chronic renal failure (CRF), independent of the better known uremic polyneuropathy. Abnormalities of calcium and phosphorus homeostasis and bone metabolism in chronic renal failure result from a reduction in 1,25-dihydroxyvitamin D, leading to decreased intestinal absorption of calcium. Hypocalcemia, further accentuated by hyperphosphatemia due to decreased renal phosphate clearance, leads to secondary hyperparathyroidism. Renal osteodystrophy results from the compensatory hyperparathyroidism, which leads to osteomalacia from reduced calcium availability and to osteitis fibrosa from the parathyroid hormone excess. The clinical picture of the myopathy of CRF is identical to that of primary hyperparathyroidism and osteomalacia. There is proximal limb weakness with bone pain.

Gangrenous calcification represents a separate, rare, and sometimes fatal complication of CRF. In this condition, widespread arterial calcification occurs and results in ischemia. Extensive skin necrosis may occur, along with painful myopathy and even myoglobinuria.

DRUG-INDUCED MYOPATHIES

Drug-induced myopathies are relatively uncommon in clinical practice with the exception of those caused by the cholesterol-lowering agents and glucocorticoids. Others impact practice to a lesser degree but are important to consider in specific situations. Table 48-11 provides a comprehensive list of drug-induced myopathies with their distinguishing features.

TABLE 48-11

DRUG-INDUCED MYOPATHIES

DRUGS	MAJOR TOXIC REACTION
Lipid-lowering agents Fibric acid derivatives HMG-CoA reductase inhibitors Niacin (nicotinic acid)	Drugs belonging to all three of the major classes of lipid-lowering agents can produce a spectrum of toxicity: asymptomatic serum creatine kinase elevation, myalgias, exercise-induced pain, rhabdomyolysis, and myoglobinuria.
Glucocorticoids	Acute, high-dose glucocorticoid treatment can cause acute quadriplegic myopathy. These high doses of steroids are often combined with nondepolarizing neuromuscular blocking agents, but the weakness can occur without their use. Chronic steroid administration produces predominantly proximal weakness.
Nondepolarizing neuromuscular blocking agents	Acute quadriplegic myopathy can occur with or without concomitant glucocorticoids.
Zidovudine	Mitochondrial myopathy with ragged red fibers.
Drugs of abuse Alcohol Amphetamines Cocaine Heroin Phencyclidine Meperidine	All drugs in this group can lead to widespread muscle breakdown, rhabdomyolysis, and myoglobinuria. Local injections cause muscle necrosis, skin induration, and limb contractures.
Autoimmune toxic myopathy D-Penicillamine	Use of this drug may cause polymyositis and myasthenia gravis.
Amphophilic cationic drugs Amiodarone Chloroquine Hydroxychloroquine	All amphophilic drugs have the potential to produce painless, proximal weakness associated with autophagic vacuoles in the muscle biopsy.
Antimicrotubular drugs Colchicine	This drug produces painless, proximal weakness especially in the setting of renal failure. Muscle biopsy shows autophagic vacuoles.

MYOPATHY FROM LIPID-LOWERING AGENTS

All classes of lipid-lowering agents have been implicated in muscle toxicity, including fibrates (clofibrate, gemfibrozil), HMG-CoA reductase inhibitors (referred to as *statins*), niacin (nicotinic acid), and ezetimibe. Myalgia, malaise, and muscle tenderness are the most common manifestations. Muscle pain may be related to exercise. Patients may exhibit proximal weakness. Varying degrees of muscle necrosis are seen, and in severe reactions rhabdomyolysis and myoglobinuria occur. Concomitant use of statins with fibrates and cyclosporine is more likely to cause adverse reactions than use of one agent alone. Elevated serum CK is an important indication of toxicity. Muscle weakness is accompanied by a myopathic EMG, and muscle necrosis is observed by muscle biopsy. Severe myalgias, muscle weakness, significant elevations in serum CK (>three times baseline), and myoglobinuria are indications for stopping the drug. Patients usually improve with drug cessation, although this may take several weeks. Rare cases continue to progress after the offending agent is discontinued. It is possible that in such cases the statin may have triggered an immune-mediated necrotizing myopathy, as these individuals require immunotherapy (e.g., prednisone and sometimes other agents) to improve and often relapse when these therapies are discontinued. Interestingly, antibodies directed against the 100-kD HMG-CoA reductase receptor on muscle fibers has been identified in many of these cases.

GLUCOCORTICOID-RELATED MYOPATHIES

Glucocorticoid myopathy occurs with chronic treatment or as "acute quadriplegic" myopathy secondary to high-dose IV glucocorticoid use. Chronic administration produces proximal weakness accompanied by cushingoid manifestations, which can be quite debilitating; the chronic use of prednisone at a daily dose of ≥30 mg/d is most often associated with toxicity. Patients taking fluorinated glucocorticoids (triamcinolone, betamethasone, dexamethasone) appear to be at especially high risk for myopathy. In chronic steroid myopathy, the serum CK is usually normal. Serum potassium may be low. The muscle biopsy in chronic cases shows preferential type 2 muscle fiber atrophy; this is not reflected in the EMG, which is usually normal.

Patients receiving high-dose IV glucocorticoids for status asthmaticus, chronic obstructive pulmonary disease, organ transplantation, or other indications may develop severe generalized weakness (critical illness myopathy). This myopathy, also known as acute quadriplegic myopathy, can also occur in the setting of sepsis. Involvement of the diaphragm and intercostal muscles causes respiratory failure and requires ventilatory support. In these settings, the use of glucocorticoids in combination with nondepolarizing neuromuscular blocking agents potentiate this complication. In critical illness myopathy, the muscle biopsy is abnormal, showing a distinctive loss of thick filaments (myosin) by electron microscopy. By light microscopy, there is focal loss of ATPase staining in central or paracentral areas of the muscle fiber. Calpain stains show diffusely reactive atrophic fibers. Withdrawal of glucocorticoids will improve the chronic myopathy. In acute quadriplegic myopathy, recovery is slow. Patients require supportive care and rehabilitation.

DRUG-INDUCED MITOCHONDRIAL MYOPATHY

Zidovudine, used in the treatment of HIV infection, is a thymidine analogue that inhibits viral replication by interrupting reverse transcriptase. Myopathy is a well-established complication of this agent. Patients present with myalgias, muscle weakness, and atrophy affecting the thigh and calf muscles. The complication occurs in about 17% of patients treated with doses of 1200 mg/d for 6 months. The introduction of protease inhibitors for treatment of HIV infection has led to lower doses of zidovudine therapy and a decreased incidence of myopathy. Serum CK is elevated and EMG is myopathic. Muscle biopsy shows ragged red fibers with minimal inflammation; the lack of inflammation serves to distinguish zidovudine toxicity from HIV-related myopathy. If the myopathy is thought to be drug related, the medication should be stopped or the dosage reduced.

DRUGS OF ABUSE AND RELATED MYOPATHIES

Myotoxicity is a potential consequence of addiction to alcohol and illicit drugs. Ethanol is one of the most commonly abused substances with potential to damage muscle. Other potential toxins include cocaine, heroin, and amphetamines. The most deleterious reactions occur from overdosing leading to coma and seizures, causing rhabdomyolysis, myoglobinuria, and renal failure. Direct toxicity can occur from cocaine, heroin, and amphetamines causing muscle breakdown and varying degrees of weakness. The effects of alcohol are more controversial. Direct muscle damage is less certain, since toxicity usually occurs in the setting of poor nutrition and possible contributing factors such as hypokalemia and hypophosphatemia. Alcoholics are also prone to neuropathy (Chap. 56).

Focal myopathies from self-administration of meperidine, heroin, and pentazocine can cause pain, swelling, muscle necrosis, and hemorrhage. The cause is multifactorial; needle trauma, direct toxicity of the drug or vehicle, and infection may all play a role. When severe, there may be overlying skin induration and contractures with replacement of muscle by connective tissue. Elevated serum CK and myopathic EMG are characteristic of these reactions. The muscle biopsy shows widespread or focal areas of necrosis. In conditions leading to rhabdomyolysis, patients need adequate hydration to reduce serum myoglobin and protect renal function. In all of these conditions, counseling is essential to limit drug abuse.

DRUG-INDUCED AUTOIMMUNE MYOPATHIES

The most consistent drug-related inflammatory or antibody-mediated myopathy is caused by D-penicillamine. This drug chelates copper and is used in the treatment of Wilson's disease. It is also used to treat other disorders including scleroderma, rheumatoid arthritis, and primary biliary cirrhosis. Adverse events include drug-induced polymyositis, indistinguishable from the spontaneous disease. The incidence of this inflammatory muscle disease is about 1%. Myasthenia gravis is also induced by D-penicillamine, with a higher incidence estimated at 7%. These disorders resolve with drug withdrawal, although immunosuppressive therapy may be warranted in severe cases.

Scattered reports of other drugs causing an inflammatory myopathy are rare and include a heterogeneous group of agents: cimetidine, phenytoin, procainamide, and propylthiouracil. In most cases, a cause-and-effect relationship is uncertain. A complication of interest was related to L-tryptophan. In 1989 an epidemic of eosinophilia-myalgia syndrome (EMS) in the United States was caused by a contaminant in the product from one manufacturer. The product was withdrawn, and incidence of EMS diminished abruptly following this action.

OTHER DRUG-INDUCED MYOPATHIES

Certain drugs produce painless, largely proximal, muscle weakness. These drugs include the amphophilic cationic drugs (amiodarone, chloroquine, hydroxychloroquine) and antimicrotubular drugs (colchicine) (Table 48-11). Muscle biopsy can be useful in the identification of toxicity since autophagic vacuoles are prominent pathologic features of these toxins.

CHAPTER 49

POLYMYOSITIS, DERMATOMYOSITIS, AND INCLUSION BODY MYOSITIS

Marinos C. Dalakas

The inflammatory myopathies represent the largest group of acquired and potentially treatable causes of skeletal muscle weakness. They are classified into three major groups: polymyositis (PM), dermatomyositis (DM), and inclusion body myositis (IBM).

CLINICAL FEATURES

The prevalence of the inflammatory myopathies is estimated at 1 in 100,000. PM as a stand-alone entity is a rare disease. DM affects both children and adults and women more often than men. IBM is three times more frequent in men than in women, more common in whites than blacks, and is most likely to affect persons aged >50 years.

These disorders present as progressive and symmetric muscle weakness except for IBM, which can have an asymmetric pattern. Patients usually report increasing difficulty with everyday tasks requiring the use of proximal muscles, such as getting up from a chair, climbing steps, stepping onto a curb, lifting objects, or combing hair. Fine-motor movements that depend on the strength of distal muscles, such as buttoning a shirt, sewing, knitting, or writing, are affected only late in the course of PM and DM, but fairly early in IBM. Falling is common in IBM because of early involvement of the quadriceps muscle, with buckling of the knees. Ocular muscles are spared, even in advanced, untreated cases; if these muscles are affected, the diagnosis of inflammatory myopathy should be questioned. Facial muscles are unaffected in PM and DM, but mild facial muscle weakness is common in patientswith IBM. In all forms of inflammatory myopathy, pharyngeal and neck-flexor muscles are often involved, causing dysphagia or difficulty in holding up the head (*head drop*). In advanced and rarely in acute cases, respiratory muscles may also be affected. Severe weakness, if untreated, is almost always associated with muscle wasting. Sensation remains normal. The tendon reflexes are preserved but may be absent in severely weakened or atrophied muscles, especially in IBM, where atrophy of the quadriceps and the distal muscles is common. Myalgia and muscle tenderness may occur in a small number of patients, usually early in the disease, and particularly in DM associated with connective tissue disorders. Weakness in PM and DM progresses subacutely over a period of weeks or months and rarely acutely; by contrast, IBM progresses very slowly, over years, simulating a late-life muscular dystrophy (Chap. 48) or slowly progressive motor neuron disorder (Chap. 32).

SPECIFIC FEATURES

(Table 49-1)

Polymyositis

The actual onset of PM is often not easily determined, and patients typically delay seeking medical advice for several weeks or even months. This is in contrast to DM, in which the rash facilitates early recognition (discussed later). PM mimics many other myopathies and is a diagnosis of exclusion. It is a subacute inflammatory myopathy affecting adults, and rarely children, who *do not have* any of the following: rash, involvement of the extraocular and facial muscles, family history of a neuromuscular disease, history of exposure to myotoxic drugs or toxins, endocrinopathy, neurogenic disease, muscular dystrophy, biochemical muscle disorder (deficiency of a muscle enzyme), or IBM as excluded by muscle biopsy analysis (discussed later). As an isolated entity, PM is a rare (and overdiagnosed) disorder; more commonly, PM occurs in association with a systemic autoimmune or connective tissue disease, or with a known viral or

TABLE 49-1

FEATURES ASSOCIATED WITH INFLAMMATORY MYOPATHIES

CHARACTERISTIC	POLYMYOSITIS	DERMATOMYOSITIS	INCLUSION BODY MYOSITIS
Age at onset	>18 years	Adulthood and childhood	>50 years
Familial association	No	No	Yes, in some cases
Extramuscular manifestations	Yes	Yes	Yes
Associated conditions			
Connective tissue diseases	Yes[a]	Scleroderma and mixed connective tissue disease (overlap syndromes)	Yes, in up to 20% of cases[a]
Systemic autoimmune diseases[b]	Frequent	Infrequent	Infrequent
Malignancy	No	Yes, in up to 15% of cases	No
Viruses	Yes[c]	Unproven	Yes[c]
Drugs[d]	Yes	Yes, rarely	No
Parasites and bacteria[e]	Yes	No	No

[a]Systemic lupus erythematosus, rheumatoid arthritis, Sjögren's syndrome, systemic sclerosis, mixed connective tissue disease.
[b]Crohn's disease, vasculitis, sarcoidosis, primary biliary cirrhosis, adult celiac disease, chronic graft-versus-host disease, discoid lupus, ankylosing spondylitis, Behçet's syndrome, myasthenia gravis, acne fulminans, dermatitis herpetiformis, psoriasis, Hashimoto's disease, granulomatous diseases, agammaglobulinemia, monoclonal gammopathy, hypereosinophilic syndrome, Lyme disease, Kawasaki's disease, autoimmune thrombocytopenia, hypergammaglobulinemic purpura, hereditary complement deficiency, IgA deficiency.
[c]HIV (human immunodeficiency virus) and HTLV-I (human T cell lymphotropic virus type I).
[d]Drugs include penicillamine (dermatomyositis and polymyositis), zidovudine (polymyositis), and contaminated tryptophan (dermatomyositis-like illness). Other myotoxic drugs may cause myopathy but not an inflammatory myopathy (see text for details).
[e]Parasites (protozoa, cestodes, nematodes), tropical and bacterial myositis (pyomyositis).

bacterial infection. Drugs, especially D-penicillamine, statins, or zidovudine (AZT), may also trigger an inflammatory myopathy similar to PM.

Dermatomyositis

DM is a distinctive entity identified by a characteristic rash accompanying, or more often preceding, muscle weakness. The rash may consist of a blue-purple discoloration on the upper eyelids with edema (heliotrope rash), a flat red rash on the face and upper trunk, and erythema of the knuckles with a raised violaceous scaly eruption (*Gottron's sign*). The erythematous rash can also occur on other body surfaces, including the knees, elbows, malleoli, neck and anterior chest (often in a *V sign*), or back and shoulders (*shawl sign*), and may worsen after sun exposure. In some patients, the rash is pruritic, especially on the scalp, chest, and back. Dilated capillary loops at the base of the fingernails are also characteristic. The cuticles may be irregular, thickened, and distorted, and the lateral and palmar areas of the fingers may become rough and cracked, with irregular, "dirty" horizontal lines, resembling *mechanic's hands*. The weakness can be mild, moderate, or severe enough to lead to quadriparesis. At times, the muscle strength appears normal, hence the term *dermatomyositis sine myositis*. When muscle biopsy is performed in such cases, however, significant perivascular and perimysial inflammation is often seen.

DM usually occurs alone but may overlap with scleroderma and mixed connective tissue disease. Fasciitis and thickening of the skin, similar to that seen in chronic cases of DM, have occurred in patients with the *eosinophilia-myalgia syndrome* associated with the ingestion of contaminated L-tryptophan.

Inclusion body myositis

In patients ≥50 years of age, IBM is the most common of the inflammatory myopathies. It is often misdiagnosed as PM and is suspected only later when a patient with presumed PM does not respond to therapy. Weakness and atrophy of the distal muscles, especially foot extensors and deep finger flexors, occur in almost all cases of IBM and may be a clue to early diagnosis. Some patients present with falls because their knees collapse due to early quadriceps weakness. Others present with weakness in the small muscles of the hands, especially finger flexors, and complain of inability to hold objects such as golf clubs or perform tasks such as turning keys or tying knots. On occasion, the weakness and accompanying atrophy can be asymmetric and selectively involve the quadriceps, iliopsoas, triceps, biceps, and finger flexors, resembling a lower motor neuron disease. Dysphagia is common, occurring in up to 60% of IBM patients, and may lead to episodes of choking. Sensory examination is generally normal; some patients have mildly diminished vibratory sensation at the ankles that presumably is age-related. The pattern of distal weakness, which superficially resembles motor neuron or peripheral nerve disease, results from the myopathic process affecting distal muscles selectively. Disease progression is slow but steady, and most patients require an assistive device such as cane, walker, or wheelchair within several years of onset.

In at least 20% of cases, IBM is associated with systemic autoimmune or connective tissue diseases. Familial aggregation of typical IBM may occur; such cases have been designated as *familial inflammatory IBM.* This disorder is distinct from *hereditary inclusion body myopathy* (h-IBM), which describes a heterogeneous group of recessive, and less frequently dominant, inherited syndromes; the h-IBMs are noninflammatory myopathies. A subset of h-IBM that spares the quadriceps muscles has emerged as a distinct entity. This disorder, originally described in Iranian Jews and now seen in many ethnic groups, is linked to chromosome 9p1 and results from mutations in the UDP-*N*-acetylglucosamine 2-epimerase/*N*-acetylmannosamine kinase (*GNE*) gene.

ASSOCIATED CLINICAL FINDINGS

Extramuscular manifestations

These may be present to a varying degree in patients with PM or DM, and include:

1. *Systemic symptoms*, such as fever, malaise, weight loss, arthralgia, and Raynaud's phenomenon, especially when inflammatory myopathy is associated with a connective tissue disorder.
2. *Joint contractures*, mostly in DM and especially in children.
3. *Dysphagia and gastrointestinal symptoms*, due to involvement of oropharyngeal striated muscles and upper esophagus, especially in DM and IBM.
4. *Cardiac disturbances*, including atrioventricular conduction defects, tachyarrhythmias, dilated cardiomyopathy, a low ejection fraction, and congestive heart failure, may rarely occur, either from the disease itself or from hypertension associated with long-term use of glucocorticoids.
5. *Pulmonary dysfunction*, due to weakness of the thoracic muscles, interstitial lung disease, or drug-induced pneumonitis (e.g., from methotrexate), which may cause dyspnea, nonproductive cough, and aspiration pneumonia. Interstitial lung disease may precede myopathy or occur early in the disease and develops in up to 10% of patients with PM or DM, most of whom have antibodies to t-RNA synthetases, as described later.
6. *Subcutaneous calcifications*, in DM, sometimes extruding on the skin and causing ulcerations and infections.
7. *Arthralgias*, synovitis, or deforming arthropathy with subluxation in the interphalangeal joints can occur in some patients with DM and PM who have Jo-1 antibodies (discussed later).

Association with malignancies

Although all the inflammatory myopathies can have a chance association with malignant lesions, especially in older age groups, the incidence of malignant conditions appears to be specifically increased only in patients with DM and not in those with PM or IBM. The most common tumors associated with DM are ovarian cancer, breast cancer, melanoma, colon cancer, and non-Hodgkin's lymphoma. The extent of the search that should be conducted for an occult neoplasm in adults with DM depends on the clinical circumstances. Tumors in these patients are usually uncovered by abnormal findings in the medical history and physical examination and not through an extensive blind search. The weight of evidence argues against performing expensive, invasive, and nondirected tumor searches. A complete annual physical examination with pelvic, breast (mammogram, if indicated), and rectal examinations (with colonoscopy according to age and family history); urinalysis; complete blood count; blood chemistry tests; and a chest film should suffice in most cases. In Asians, nasopharyngeal cancer is common, and a careful examination of ears, nose, and throat is indicated. If malignancy is clinically suspected, screening with whole-body PET scan should be considered.

Overlap syndromes

These describe the association of inflammatory myopathies with connective tissue diseases. A well-characterized overlap syndrome occurs in patients with DM who also have manifestations of systemic sclerosis or mixed connective tissue disease, such as sclerotic thickening of the dermis, contractures, esophageal hypomotility, microangiopathy, and calcium deposits (Table 49-1). By contrast, signs of rheumatoid arthritis, systemic lupus erythematosus, or Sjögren's syndrome are very rare in patients with DM. Patients with the overlap syndrome of DM and systemic sclerosis may have a specific antinuclear antibody, the anti-PM/Scl, directed against a nucleolar-protein complex.

PATHOGENESIS

An autoimmune etiology of the inflammatory myopathies is indirectly supported by an association with other autoimmune or connective tissue diseases; the presence of various autoantibodies; an association with specific major histocompatibility complex (MHC) genes; demonstration of T cell–mediated myocytotoxicity or complement-mediated microangiopathy; and a response to immunotherapy.

Autoantibodies and immunogenetics

Various autoantibodies against nuclear antigens (antinuclear antibodies) and cytoplasmic antigens are found in up to 20% of patients with inflammatory myopathies. The antibodies to cytoplasmic antigens are directed against ribonucleoproteins involved in protein synthesis (antisynthetases) or translational transport (anti-signal-recognition particles). The antibody directed against the histidyl-transfer RNA synthetase, called *anti-Jo-1*, accounts for 75% of all the antisynthetases and is clinically useful because up to 80% of patients with anti-Jo-1 antibodies have interstitial lung disease. Some patients with the anti-Jo-1 antibody also have Raynaud's phenomenon, nonerosive arthritis, and the MHC molecules DR3 and DRw52. DR3 haplotypes (molecular designation DRB1*0301, DQB1*0201) occur in up to 75% of patients with PM and IBM, whereas in juvenile DM there is an increased frequency of DQA1*0501.

Immunopathologic mechanisms

In DM, humoral immune mechanisms are implicated, resulting in a microangiopathy and muscle ischemia (Fig. 49-1). Endomysial inflammatory infiltrates are composed of B cells located in proximity to CD4 T cells, plasmacytoid dendritic cells, and macrophages; there is a relative absence of lymphocytic invasion of nonnecrotic muscle fibers. Activation of the complement C5b-9 membranolytic attack complex is thought to be a critical early event that triggers release of proinflammatory cytokines and chemokines, induces expression of vascular cell

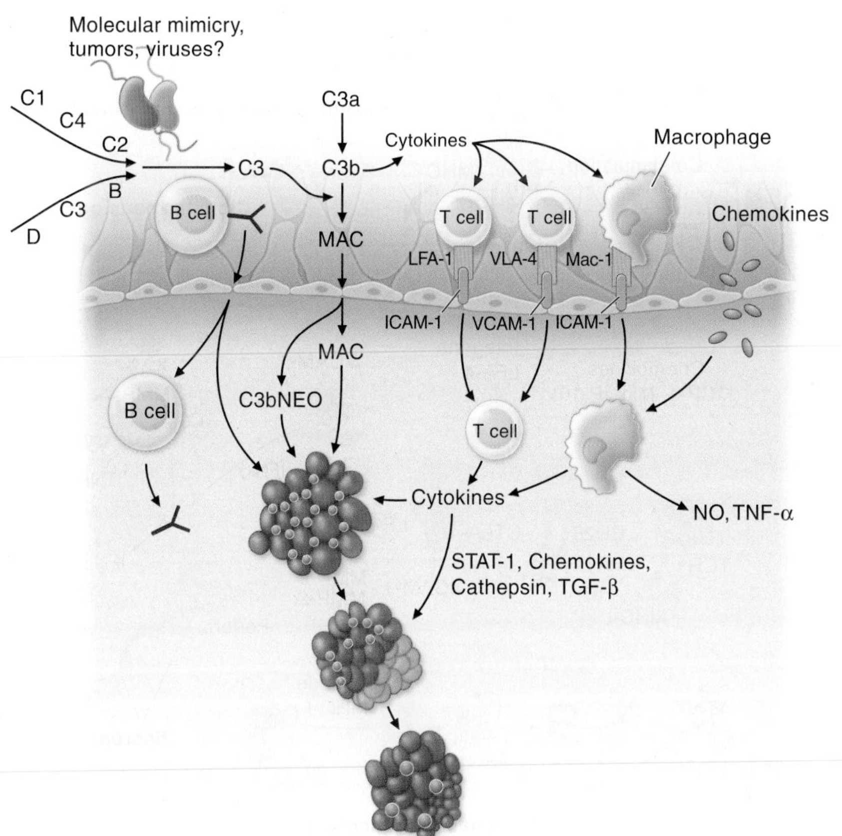

FIGURE 49-1

Immunopathogenesis of dermatomyositis. Activation of complement, possibly by autoantibodies (Y), against endothelial cells and formation of C3 via the classic or alternative pathway. Activated C3 leads to formation of C3b, C3bNEO, and membrane attack complexes (MAC), which are deposited in and around the endothelial cell wall of the endomysial capillaries. Deposition of MAC leads to destruction of capillaries, ischemia, or microinfarcts, most prominent in the periphery of the fascicles, and perifascicular atrophy. B cells, plasmacytoid dendritic cells, CD4 T cells, and macrophages traffic from the circulation to the muscle. Endothelial expression of vascular cell adhesion molecule (VCAM) and intercellular adhesion molecule (ICAM) is induced by cytokines released by the mononuclear cells. Integrins, specifically very late activation antigen (VLA)-4 and lymphocyte function–associated antigen (LFA)-1, bind VCAM and ICAM and promote T cell and macrophage infiltration of muscle through the endothelial cell wall.

adhesion molecule (VCAM) 1 and intercellular adhesion molecule (ICAM) 1 on endothelial cells, and facilitates migration of activated lymphoid cells to the perimysial and endomysial spaces. Necrosis of the endothelial cells, reduced numbers of endomysial capillaries, ischemia, and muscle-fiber destruction resembling microinfarcts occur. The remaining capillaries often have dilated lumens in response to the ischemic process. Larger intramuscular blood vessels may also be affected in the same pattern. Residual perifascicular atrophy reflects the endofascicular hypoperfusion that is prominent in the periphery of muscle fascicles. Increased expression of type I interferon-inducible proteins is also noted in these regions.

By contrast, in PM and IBM a mechanism of T cell–mediated cytotoxicity is likely. CD8 T cells, along with macrophages, initially surround and eventually invade and destroy healthy, nonnecrotic muscle fibers that aberrantly express class I MHC molecules. MHC-I expression, absent from the sarcolemma of normal muscle fibers, is probably induced by cytokines secreted by activated T cells and macrophages. The CD8/MHC-I complex is characteristic of PM and IBM; its detection can aid in confirming the histologic diagnosis of PM, as discussed later. The cytotoxic CD8 T cells contain perforin and granzyme granules directed toward the surface of the muscle fibers and capable of inducing myonecrosis. Analysis of T cell receptor molecules expressed by the infiltrating CD8 cells has revealed clonal expansion and conserved sequences in the antigen-binding region, both suggesting an antigen-driven T cell response. Whether the putative antigens are endogenous (e.g., muscle) or exogenous (e.g., viral) sequences is unknown. Viruses have not been identified within the muscle fibers. Co-stimulatory molecules and their counterreceptors, which are fundamental for T cell activation and antigen recognition, are strongly upregulated in PM and IBM. Key molecules involved in T cell–mediated cytotoxicity are depicted in Fig. 49-2.

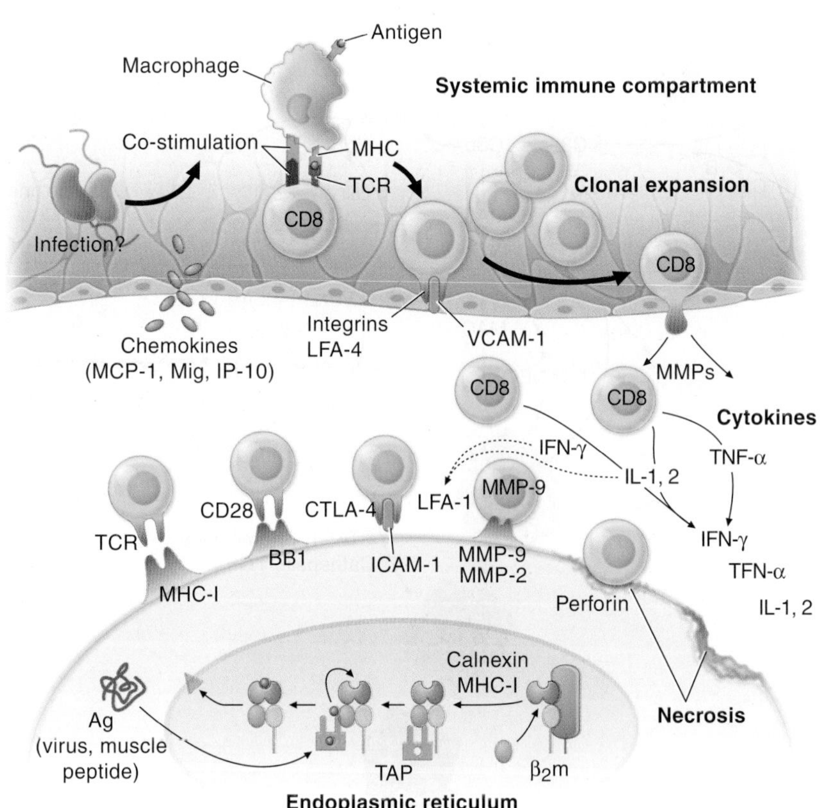

FIGURE 49-2

Cell-mediated mechanisms of muscle damage in polymyositis (PM) and inclusion body myositis (IBM). Antigen-specific CD8 cells are expanded in the periphery, cross the endothelial barrier, and bind directly to muscle fibers via T cell receptor (TCR) molecules that recognize aberrantly expressed MHC-I. Engagement of co-stimulatory molecules (BB1 and ICOSL) with their ligands (CD28, CTLA-4, and ICOS), along with ICAM-1/LFA-1, stabilize the CD8–muscle fiber interaction. Metalloproteinases (MMPs) facilitate the migration of T cells and their attachment to the muscle surface. Muscle fiber necrosis occurs via perforin granules released by the autoaggressive T cells. A direct myocytotoxic effect exerted by the cytokines interferon (IFN) γ, interleukin (IL) 1, or tumor necrosis factor (TNF) α may also play a role. Death of the muscle fiber is mediated by necrosis. MHC class I molecules consist of a heavy chain and a light chain [β_2 microglobulin (β_2m)] complexed with an antigenic peptide that is transported into the endoplasmic reticulum by TAP proteins.

The role of nonimmune factors in IBM

In IBM, the presence of Congo red–positive amyloid deposits within some vacuolated muscle fibers and abnormal mitochondria with cytochrome oxidase–negative fibers suggest that, in addition to the autoimmune component, there is also a degenerative process. Similar to Alzheimer's disease, the intracellular amyloid deposits in IBM are immunoreactive against amyloid precursor protein (APP), β-amyloid, chymotrypsin, apolipoprotein E, presenilin, ubiquitin, and phosphorylated tau, but it is unclear whether these deposits, which are also seen in other vacuolar myopathies, are directly pathogenic or represent secondary phenomena. The same is true for the mitochondrial abnormalities, which may also be secondary to the effects of aging or a bystander effect of upregulated cytokines. Expression of cytokines and upregulation of MHC class I by the muscle fibers may cause an endoplasmic reticulum stress response resulting in intracellular accumulation of stressor molecules or misfolded glycoproteins and activation of nuclear factor κB (NF-κB), leading to further cytokine activation.

Association with viral infections and the role of retroviruses

Several viruses, including coxsackieviruses, influenza, paramyxoviruses, mumps, cytomegalovirus, and Epstein-Barr virus, have been indirectly associated with myositis. For the coxsackieviruses, an autoimmune myositis triggered by molecular mimicry has been proposed because of structural homology between histidyl-transfer RNA synthetase that is the target of the Jo-1 antibody (discussed earlier) and genomic RNA of an animal picornavirus, the encephalomyocarditis virus. Sensitive polymerase chain reaction (PCR) studies, however, have repeatedly failed to confirm the presence of such viruses in muscle biopsies.

The best evidence of a viral connection in PM and IBM is with the retroviruses. Some individuals infected with HIV or with human T cell lymphotropic virus I (HTLV-I) develop PM or IBM; a similar disorder has been described in nonhuman primates infected with the simian immunodeficiency virus. The inflammatory myopathy may occur as the initial manifestation of a retroviral infection, or myositis may develop later in the disease course. Retroviral antigens have been detected only in occasional endomysial macrophages and not within the muscle fibers themselves, suggesting that persistent infection and viral replication within the muscle do not occur. Histologic findings are identical to retroviral-negative PM or IBM. The infiltrating T cells in the muscle are clonally driven and a number of them are retroviral-specific. This disorder should be distinguished from a toxic myopathy related to long-term therapy with AZT, characterized by fatigue, myalgia, mild muscle weakness, and mild elevation of creatine kinase (CK). AZT-induced myopathy, which generally improves when the drug is discontinued, is a mitochondrial disorder characterized histologically by "ragged-red" fibers. AZT inhibits γ-DNA polymerase, an enzyme found solely in the mitochondrial matrix.

DIFFERENTIAL DIAGNOSIS

The clinical picture of the typical skin rash and proximal or diffuse muscle weakness has few causes other than DM. However, proximal muscle weakness without skin involvement can be due to many conditions other than PM or IBM.

Subacute or chronic progressive muscle weakness

This may be due to denervating conditions such as the spinal muscular atrophies or amyotrophic lateral sclerosis (Chap. 32). In addition to the muscle weakness, upper motor neuron signs in the latter and signs of denervation detected by electromyography (EMG) aid in the diagnosis. The muscular dystrophies (Chap. 48) may be additional considerations; however, these disorders usually develop over years rather than weeks or months and rarely present after the age of 30 years. It may be difficult, even with a muscle biopsy, to distinguish chronic PM from a rapidly advancing muscular dystrophy. This is particularly true of facioscapulohumeral muscular dystrophy, dysferlin myopathy, and the dystrophinopathies where inflammatory cell infiltration is often found early in the disease. Such doubtful cases should always be given an adequate trial of glucocorticoid therapy and undergo genetic testing to exclude muscular dystrophy. Identification of the MHC/CD8 lesion by muscle biopsy is helpful to identify cases of PM. Some metabolic myopathies, including glycogen storage disease due to myophosphorylase or acid maltase deficiency, lipid storage myopathies due to carnitine deficiency, and mitochondrial diseases produce weakness that is often associated with other characteristic clinical signs; diagnosis rests upon histochemical and biochemical studies of the muscle biopsy. The endocrine myopathies such as those due to hypercorticosteroidism, hyper- and hypothyroidism, and hyper- and hypoparathyroidism require the appropriate laboratory investigations for diagnosis. Muscle wasting in patients with an underlying neoplasm may be due to disuse, cachexia, or rarely to a paraneoplastic neuromyopathy (Chap. 44).

Diseases of the neuromuscular junction, including myasthenia gravis or the Lambert-Eaton myasthenic syndrome, cause fatiguing weakness that also affects ocular and other cranial muscles (Chap. 47). Repetitive nerve stimulation and single-fiber EMG studies aid in diagnosis.

Acute muscle weakness

This may be caused by an acute neuropathy such as Guillain-Barré syndrome (Chap. 46), transverse myelitis (Chap. 35), a neurotoxin (Chap. 48), or a neurotropic viral infection such as poliomyelitis or West Nile virus (Chap. 40). When acute weakness is associated with very high levels of serum creatine kinase (CK) (often in the thousands), painful muscle cramps, rhabdomyolysis, and myoglobinuria, it may be due to a viral infection or a metabolic disorder such as myophosphorylase deficiency or carnitine palmitoyltransferase deficiency (Chap. 48). Several animal parasites, including protozoa (*Toxoplasma*, *Trypanosoma*), cestodes (cysticerci), and nematodes (trichinae), may produce a focal or diffuse inflammatory myopathy known as *parasitic polymyositis*. *Staphylococcus aureus*, *Yersinia*, *Streptococcus*, or anaerobic bacteria may produce a suppurative myositis, known as *tropical polymyositis*, or *pyomyositis*. Pyomyositis, previously rare in the West, is now occasionally seen in AIDS patients. Other bacteria, such as *Borrelia burgdorferi* (Lyme disease) and *Legionella pneumophila* (Legionnaire's disease), may infrequently cause myositis.

Patients with periodic paralysis experience recurrent episodes of acute muscle weakness without pain, always beginning in childhood. Chronic alcoholics may develop painful myopathy with myoglobinuria after a bout of heavy drinking. Acute painless muscle weakness with myoglobinuria may occur with prolonged hypokalemia, or hypophosphatemia and hypomagnesemia, usually in chronic alcoholics or in patients on nasogastric suction receiving parenteral hyperalimentation.

Myofasciitis

This distinctive inflammatory disorder affecting muscle and fascia presents as diffuse myalgias, skin induration, fatigue, and mild muscle weakness; mild elevations of serum CK are usually present. The most common form is eosinophilic myofasciitis characterized by peripheral blood eosinophilia and eosinophilic infiltrates in the endomysial tissue. In some patients, the eosinophilic myositis/fasciitis occurs in the context of parasitic infections, vasculitis, mixed connective tissue disease, hypereosinophilic syndrome, or toxic exposures (e.g., toxic oil syndrome, contaminated L-tryptophan) or with mutations in the calpain gene. A distinct subset of myofasciitis is characterized by pronounced infiltration of the connective tissue around the muscle by sheets of periodic acid–Schiff-positive macrophages and occasional CD8 T cells (macrophagic myofasciitis). Such histologic involvement is focal and limited to sites of previous vaccinations, which may have been administered months or years earlier. This disorder, which to date has not been observed outside of France, has been linked to an aluminum-containing substrate in vaccines. Most patients respond to glucocorticoid therapy, and the overall prognosis seems favorable.

Necrotizing myositis

This is an increasingly recognized entity that has distinct features, even though it is often labeled as PM. It presents often in the fall or winter as an acute or subacute onset of symmetric muscle weakness; CK is typically extremely high. The weakness can be severe. Coexisting interstitial lung disease and cardiomyopathy may be present. The disorder may develop after a viral infection or in association with cancer. Some patients have antibodies against signal recognition particle (SRP). The muscle biopsy demonstrates necrotic fibers infiltrated by macrophages but only rare, if any, T cell infiltrates. Muscle MHC-I expression is only slightly and focally upregulated. The capillaries may be swollen with hyalinization, thickening of the capillary wall, and deposition of complement. Some patients respond to immunotherapy, but others are resistant.

Hyperacute necrotizing fasciitis/myositis (flesh-eating disease)

This a fulminant infectious disease, seen most often in the tropics or in conditions with poor hygiene, characterized by widespread necrosis of the superficial fascia and muscle of a limb; if the scrotum, perineum, and abdominal wall are affected, the condition is referred to as Fournier's gangrene. It may be caused by group A β-hemolytic streptococcus, methicillin-sensitive *S. aureus*, *Pseudomonas aeruginosa*, *Vibrio vulnificus*, clostridial species (gas gangrene), or polymicrobial infection with anaerobes and facultative bacteria; toxins from these bacteria may act as superantigens. The port of bacterial entry is usually a trivial cut or skin abrasion and the source is contact with carriers of the organism. Individuals with diabetes mellitus, immunodeficiency states, or systemic illnesses such as liver failure are most susceptible. Systemic varicella is a predisposing factor in children.

The disease presents with swelling, pain, and redness in the involved area followed by a rapid tissue necrosis of fascia and muscle that progresses at an estimated rate of 3 cm/h. Emergency debridement, antibiotics, as well as IVIg, or even hyperbaric oxygen have been recommended. In progressive or advanced cases, amputation of the affected limb may be necessary to avoid a fatal outcome.

Drug-induced myopathies

D-Penicillamine, procainamide, and statins may produce a true myositis resembling PM, and a DM-like illness had been associated with the contaminated preparations of L-tryptophan. As noted earlier, AZT causes a mitochondrial myopathy. Other drugs may elicit a toxic noninflammatory myopathy that is histologically different from DM, PM, or IBM. These include cholesterol-lowering agents such as clofibrate, lovastatin, simvastatin, or provastatin, especially when combined with cyclosporine, amiodarone, or gemfibrozil. Statin-induced necrotizing myopathy or asymptomatic elevations of CK usually improve after discontinuation of the drug. In rare patients, however, muscle weakness continues to progress even after the statin is withdrawn; in these cases, a diagnostic muscle biopsy is indicated, and if evidence of inflammation and MHC-I upregulation is present, immunotherapy for PM should be considered. Rhabdomyolysis and myoglobinuria have been rarely associated with amphotericin B, ε-aminocaproic acid, fenfluramine, heroin, and phencyclidine. The use of amiodarone, chloroquine, colchicine, carbimazole, emetine, etretinate, ipecac syrup, chronic laxative or licorice use resulting in hypokalemia, and glucocorticoids or growth hormone administration have also been associated with myopathic muscle weakness. Some neuromuscular blocking agents such as pancuronium, in combination with glucocorticoids, may cause an acute critical illness myopathy. A careful drug history is essential for diagnosis of these drug-induced myopathies, which do not require immunosuppressive therapy except when an autoimmune myopathy has been triggered, as noted earlier.

"Weakness" due to muscle pain and muscle tenderness

A number of conditions including *polymyalgia rheumatica* and arthritic disorders of adjacent joints may enter into the differential diagnosis of inflammatory myopathy, even though they do not cause myositis. The muscle biopsy is either normal or discloses type II muscle fiber atrophy. Patients with *fibrositis* and *fibromyalgia* complain of focal or diffuse muscle tenderness, fatigue, and aching, which is sometimes poorly differentiated from joint pain. Some patients, however, have muscle tenderness, painful muscles on movement, and signs suggestive of a collagen vascular disorder, such as an increased erythrocyte sedimentation rate, C-reactive protein, antinuclear antibody, or rheumatoid factor, along with modest elevation of the serum CK and aldolase. They demonstrate a "breakaway" pattern of weakness with difficulty sustaining effort but not true muscle weakness. The muscle biopsy is usually normal or nonspecific. Many such patients show some response to nonsteroidal anti-inflammatory agents or glucocorticoids, though most continue to have indolent complaints. An indolent fasciitis in the setting of an ill-defined connective tissue disorder may be present, and these patients should not be labeled as having a psychosomatic disorder. *Chronic fatigue syndrome*, which may follow a viral infection, can present with debilitating fatigue, fever, sore throat, painful lymphadenopathy, myalgia, arthralgia, sleep disorder, and headache (Chap. 52). These patients do not have muscle weakness, and the muscle biopsy is normal.

DIAGNOSIS

The clinically suspected diagnosis of PM, DM, or IBM is confirmed by analysis of serum muscle enzymes, EMG findings, and muscle biopsy (Table 49-2).

The most sensitive enzyme is CK, which in active disease can be elevated as much as fiftyfold. Although the CK level usually parallels disease activity, it can be normal in some patients with active IBM or DM, especially when associated with a connective tissue disease. The CK is always elevated in patients with active PM. Along with the CK, the serum glutamic-oxaloacetic and glutamate pyruvate transaminases, lactate dehydrogenase, and aldolase may be elevated.

Needle EMG shows myopathic potentials characterized by short-duration, low-amplitude polyphasic units on voluntary activation and increased spontaneous activity with fibrillations, complex repetitive discharges, and positive sharp waves. Mixed potentials (polyphasic units of short and long duration) indicating a chronic process and muscle fiber regeneration are often present in IBM. These EMG findings are not diagnostic of an inflammatory myopathy but are useful to identify the presence of active or chronic myopathy and to exclude neurogenic disorders.

MRI is not routinely used for the diagnosis of PM, DM, or IBM. However, it may provide information or guide the location of the muscle biopsy in certain clinical settings.

Muscle biopsy—in spite of occasional variability in demonstrating all of the typical pathologic findings—is the most sensitive and specific test for establishing the diagnosis of inflammatory myopathy and for excluding other neuromuscular diseases. Inflammation is the histologic hallmark for these diseases; however, additional features are characteristic of each subtype (Figs. 49-3, 49-4, and 49-5).

In PM the inflammation is *primary*, a term used to indicate that the inflammation is not reactive and the T cell infiltrates, located primarily within the muscle fascicles (endomysially), surround individual, healthy muscle fibers and result in phagocytosis and necrosis (Fig. 49-3). The MHC-I molecule is ubiquitously expressed on the

TABLE 49-2

CRITERIA FOR DIAGNOSIS OF INFLAMMATORY MYOPATHIES

CRITERION	POLYMYOSITIS: DEFINITE	POLYMYOSITIS: PROBABLE	DERMATOMYOSITIS	INCLUSION BODY MYOSITIS
Myopathic muscle weakness[a]	Yes	Yes	Yes[b]	Yes; slow onset, early involvement of distal muscles, frequent falls
Electromyographic findings	Myopathic	Myopathic	Myopathic	Myopathic with mixed potentials
Muscle enzymes	Elevated (up to fiftyfold)	Elevated (up to fiftyfold)	Elevated (up to fiftyfold) or normal	Elevated (up to tenfold) or normal
Muscle biopsy findings[c]	"Primary" inflammation with the CD8/MHC-I complex and no vacuoles	Ubiquitous MHC-I expression but minimal inflammation and no vacuoles[d]	Perifascicular, perimysial, or perivascular infiltrates, perifascicular atrophy	Primary inflammation with CD8/MHC-I complex; vacuolated fibers with β-amyloid deposits; cytochrome oxygenase–negative fibers; signs of chronic myopathy[e]
Rash or calcinosis	Absent	Absent	Present[f]	Absent

[a]Myopathic muscle weakness, affecting proximal muscles more than distal ones and sparing eye and facial muscles, is characterized by a subacute onset (weeks to months) and rapid progression in patients who have no family history of neuromuscular disease, no endocrinopathy, no exposure to myotoxic drugs or toxins, and no biochemical muscle disease (excluded on the basis of muscle-biopsy findings).

[b]In some cases with the typical rash, the muscle strength is seemingly normal (dermatomyositis sine myositis); these patients often have new onset of easy fatigue and reduced endurance. Careful muscle testing may reveal mild muscle weakness.

[c]See text for details.

[d]An adequate trial of prednisone or other immunosuppressive drugs is warranted in probable cases. If, in retrospect, the disease is unresponsive to therapy, another muscle biopsy should be considered to exclude other diseases or possible evolution in inclusion body myositis.

[e]If the muscle biopsy does not contain vacuolated fibers but shows chronic myopathy with hypertrophic fibers, primary inflammation with the CD8/MHC-I complex and cytochrome oxygenase–negative fibers, the diagnosis is probable inclusion body myositis.

[f]If rash is absent but muscle biopsy findings are characteristic of dermatomyositis, the diagnosis is probable dermatomyositis.

sarcolemma, even in fibers not invaded by CD8+ cells. The CD8/MHC-I lesion is characteristic and essential to confirm or establish the diagnosis and to exclude disorders with secondary, nonspecific, inflammation, such as in some muscular dystrophies. When the disease is chronic, connective tissue is increased and may react positively with alkaline phosphatase.

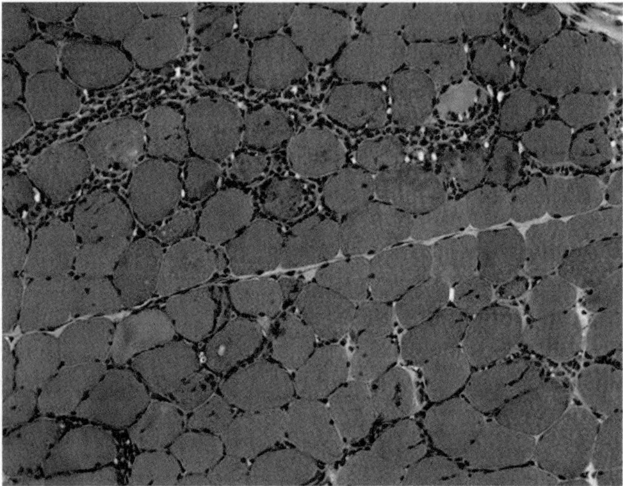

FIGURE 49-3

Cross-section of a muscle biopsy from a patient with polymyositis demonstrates scattered inflammatory foci with lymphocytes invading or surrounding muscle fibers. Note lack of chronic myopathic features (increased connective tissue, atrophic or hypertrophic fibers) as seen in inclusion body myositis.

In DM the endomysial inflammation is predominantly perivascular or in the interfascicular septae and around—rather than within—the muscle fascicles (Fig. 49-4). The intramuscular blood vessels show endothelial hyperplasia with tubuloreticular profiles, fibrin thrombi, and obliteration of capillaries. The muscle fibers undergo necrosis, degeneration, and phagocytosis, often in groups involving a portion of a muscle fasciculus in a wedgelike shape or at the periphery of the fascicle, due to microinfarcts within the muscle. This results in perifascicular atrophy, characterized by 2–10 layers of atrophic fibers at the periphery of the fascicles. The presence of perifascicular atrophy is diagnostic of DM, *even in the absence of inflammation.*

In IBM (Fig. 49-5), there is endomysial inflammation with T cells invading MHC-I-expressing nonvacuolated muscle fibers; basophilic granular deposits distributed around the edge of slitlike vacuoles (rimmed vacuoles); loss of fibers, replaced by fat and connective tissue, hypertrophic fibers, and angulated or round fibers; rare eosinophilic cytoplasmic inclusions; abnormal mitochondria characterized by the presence of ragged-red

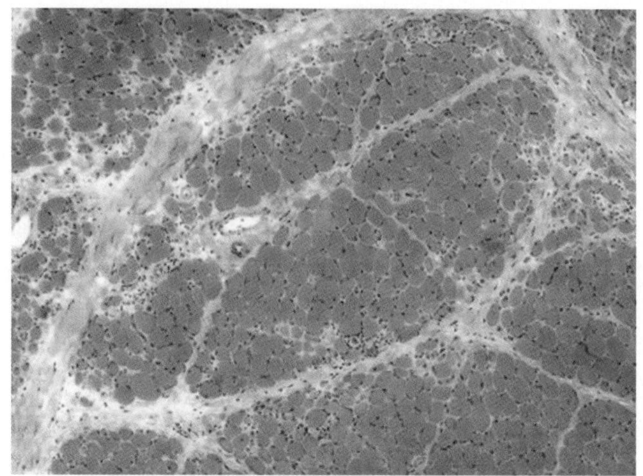

FIGURE 49-4
Cross-section of a muscle biopsy from a patient with dermatomyositis demonstrates atrophy of the fibers at the periphery of the fascicle (perifascicular atrophy).

fibers or cytochrome oxidase–negative fibers; and amyloid deposits within or next to the vacuoles best visualized with crystal violet or Congo-red staining viewed with fluorescent optics. Electron microscopy demonstrates filamentous inclusions in the vicinity of the rimmed vacuoles. In at least 15% of patients with the typical clinical phenotype of IBM, no vacuoles or amyloid deposits can be identified in muscle biopsy, leading to an erroneous diagnosis of PM. Close clinicopathologic correlations are essential; if uncertain, a repeat muscle biopsy from another site is often helpful.

TREATMENT Therapy of Inflammatory Myopathies

The goal of therapy is to improve muscle strength, thereby improving function in activities of daily living, and ameliorate the extramuscular manifestations (rash,

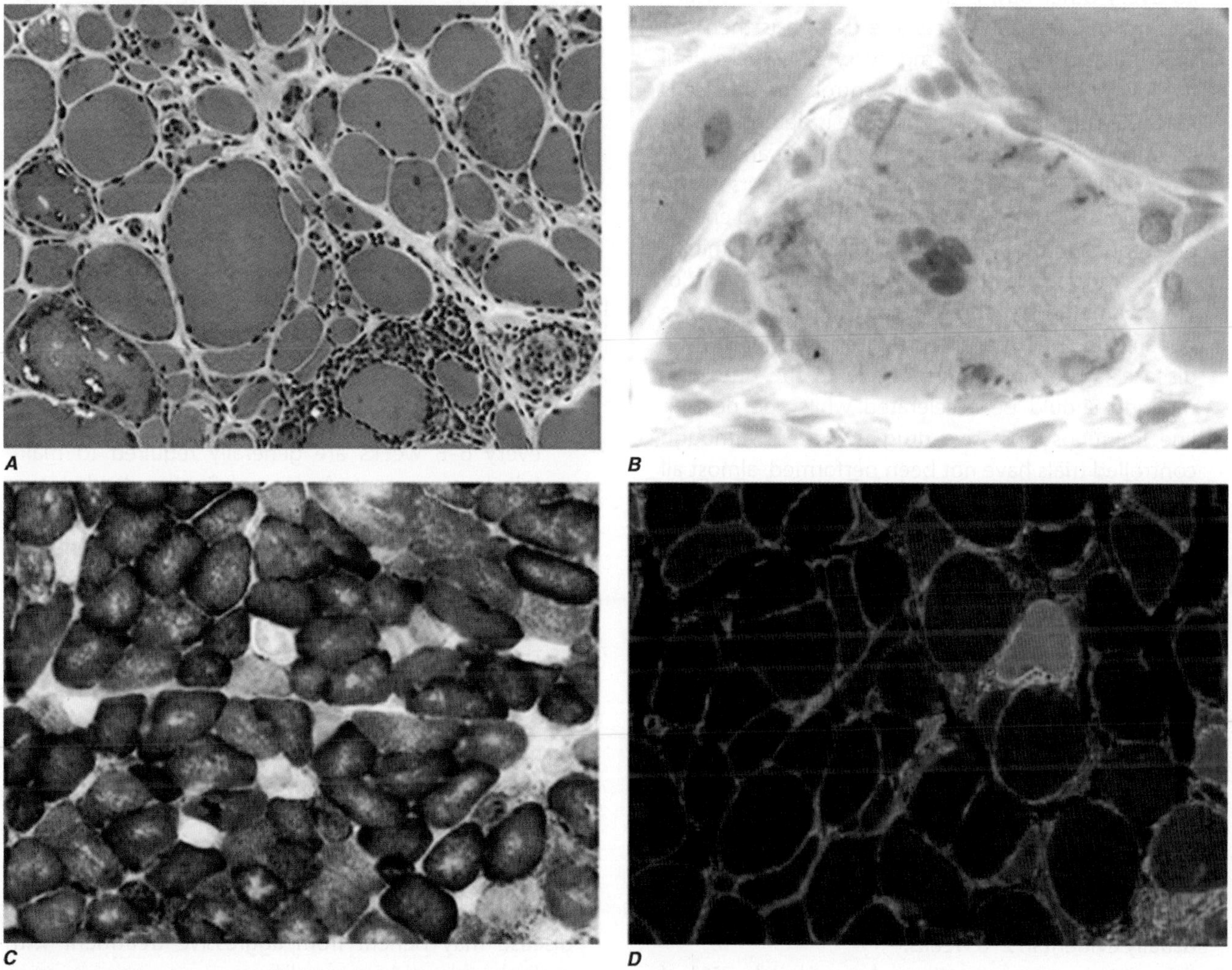

A

B

C

D

FIGURE 49-5
Cross-sections of a muscle biopsy from a patient with inclusion body myositis demonstrate the typical features of vacuoles with lymphocytic infiltrates surrounding nonvacuolated or necrotic fibers (***A***), tiny endomysial deposits of amyloid visualized with crystal violet (***B***), cytochrome oxidase–negative fibers, indicative of mitochondrial dysfunction (***C***), and ubiquitous MHC-I expression at the periphery of all fibers (***D***).

dysphagia, dyspnea, fever). When strength improves, the serum CK falls concurrently; however, the reverse is not always true. Unfortunately, there is a common tendency to "chase" or treat the CK level instead of the muscle weakness, a practice that has led to prolonged and unnecessary use of immunosuppressive drugs and erroneous assessment of their efficacy. It is prudent to discontinue these drugs if, after an adequate trial, there is no objective improvement in muscle strength whether or not CK levels are reduced. Agents used in the treatment of PM and DM include the following:

1. *Glucocorticoids*. Oral prednisone is the initial treatment of choice; the effectiveness and side effects of this therapy determine the future need for stronger immunosuppressive drugs. High-dose prednisone, at least 1 mg/kg per day, is initiated as early in the disease as possible. After 3–4 weeks, prednisone is tapered slowly over a period of 10 weeks to 1 mg/kg every other day. If there is evidence of efficacy and no serious side effects, the dosage is then further reduced by 5 or 10 mg every 3–4 weeks until the lowest possible dose that controls the disease is reached. The efficacy of prednisone is determined by an objective increase in muscle strength and activities of daily living, which almost always occurs by the third month of therapy. A feeling of increased energy or a reduction of the CK level without a concomitant increase in muscle strength is not a reliable sign of improvement. If prednisone provides no objective benefit after ~3 months of high-dose therapy, the disease is probably unresponsive to the drug and tapering should be accelerated while the next-in-line immunosuppressive drug is started. Although controlled trials have not been performed, almost all patients with true PM or DM respond to glucocorticoids to *some degree and for some period of time*; in general, DM responds better than PM.

   The long-term use of prednisone may cause increased weakness associated with a normal or unchanged CK level; this effect is referred to as *steroid myopathy*. In a patient who previously responded to high doses of prednisone, the development of new weakness may be related to steroid myopathy or to disease activity that either will respond to a higher dose of glucocorticoids or has become glucocorticoid-resistant. In uncertain cases, the prednisone dosage can be steadily increased or decreased as desired: the cause of the weakness is usually evident in 2–8 weeks.
2. *Other immunosuppressive drugs*. Approximately 75% of patients ultimately require additional treatment. This occurs when a patient fails to respond adequately to glucocorticoids after a 3-month trial, the patient becomes glucocorticoid-resistant, glucocorticoid-related side effects appear, attempts to lower the prednisone dose repeatedly result in a new relapse, or rapidly progressive disease with evolving severe weakness and respiratory failure develops.

   The following drugs are commonly used but have never been tested in controlled studies: (1) *Azathioprine* is well tolerated, has few side effects, and appears to be as effective for long-term therapy as other drugs. The dose is up to 3 mg/kg daily. (2) *Methotrexate* has a faster onset of action than azathioprine. It is given orally starting at 7.5 mg weekly for the first 3 weeks (2.5 mg every 12 h for 3 doses), with gradual dose escalation by 2.5 mg per week to a total of 25 mg weekly. A rare side effect is methotrexate pneumonitis, which can be difficult to distinguish from the interstitial lung disease of the primary myopathy associated with Jo-1 antibodies (described earlier). (3) *Mycophenolate mofetil* also has a faster onset of action than azathioprine. At doses up to 2.5 or 3 g/d in two divided doses, it is well tolerated for long-term use. (4) Monoclonal anti-CD20 antibody (rituximab) has been shown in a small uncontrolled series to benefit patients with DM and PM. (5) *Cyclosporine* has inconsistent and mild benefit. (6) *Cyclophosphamide* (0.5–1 g/m^2 IV monthly for 6 months) has limited success and significant toxicity. (7) Tacrolimus (formerly known as Fk506) has been effective in some difficult cases of PM.
3. *Immunomodulation*. In a controlled trial of patients with refractory DM, intravenous immunoglobulin (IVIg) improved not only strength and rash but also the underlying immunopathology. The benefit is often short-lived (≤8 weeks), and repeated infusions every 6–8 weeks are generally required to maintain improvement. A dose of 2 g/kg divided over 2–5 days per course is recommended. Uncontrolled observations suggest that IVIg may also be beneficial for patients with PM. Neither plasmapheresis nor leukapheresis appears to be effective in PM and DM.

The following sequential empirical approach to the treatment of PM and DM is suggested: *Step 1*: high-dose prednisone; *Step 2*: azathioprine, mycophenolate, or methotrexate for steroid-sparing effect; *Step 3*: IVIg; *Step 4*: a trial, with guarded optimism, of one of the following agents, chosen according to the patient's age, degree of disability, tolerance, experience with the drug, and general health: rituximab, cyclosporine, cyclophosphamide, or tacrolimus. Patients with interstitial lung disease may benefit from aggressive treatment with cyclophosphamide or tacrolimus.

A patient with presumed PM who has not responded to any form of immunotherapy most likely has IBM or another disease, usually a metabolic myopathy, a muscular dystrophy, a drug-induced myopathy, or an endocrinopathy. In these cases, a repeat muscle biopsy and a renewed search for another cause of the myopathy is indicated.

Calcinosis, a manifestation of DM, is difficult to treat; however, new calcium deposits may be prevented if the primary disease responds to the available therapies. Bisphosphonates, aluminum hydroxide, probenecid, colchicine, low doses of warfarin, calcium blockers, and surgical excision have all been tried without success.

IBM is generally resistant to immunosuppressive therapies. Prednisone together with azathioprine or methotrexate is often tried for a few months in newly diagnosed patients, although results are generally disappointing. Because occasional patients may feel subjectively weaker after these drugs are discontinued, some clinicians prefer to maintain these patients on low-dose, every-other-day prednisone along with mycophenolate in an effort to slow disease progression, even though there is no objective evidence or controlled study to support this practice. In two controlled studies of IVIg in IBM, minimal benefit in up to 30% of patients was found; the strength gains, however, were not of sufficient magnitude to justify its routine use. Another trial of IVIg combined with prednisone was ineffective. Nonetheless, many experts believe that a 2- to 3-month trial with IVIg may be reasonable for selected patients with IBM who experience rapid progression of muscle weakness or choking episodes due to worsening dysphagia.

PROGNOSIS The 5-year survival rate for treated patients with PM and DM is ~95% and the 10-year survival rate is 84%; death is usually due to pulmonary, cardiac, or other systemic complications. The prognosis is worse for patients who are severely affected at presentation, when initial treatment is delayed, and in cases with severe dysphagia or respiratory difficulties. Older patients, and those with associated cancer also have a worse prognosis. DM responds more favorably to therapy than PM and thus has a better prognosis. Most patients improve with therapy, and many make a full functional recovery, which is often sustained with maintenance therapy. Up to 30% may be left with some residual muscle weakness. Relapses may occur at any time.

IBM has the least favorable prognosis of the inflammatory myopathies. Most patients will require the use of an assistive device such as a cane, walker, or wheelchair within 5–10 years of onset. In general, the older the age of onset in IBM, the more rapidly progressive is the course.

CHAPTER 50

SPECIAL ISSUES IN INPATIENT NEUROLOGIC CONSULTATION

S. Andrew Josephson ■ Martin A. Samuels

Inpatient neurologic consultations usually involve questions about specific disease processes or prognostication after various cerebral injuries. Common reasons for neurologic consultation include stroke (Chap. 27), seizures (Chap. 26), altered mental status (Chap. 16), headache (Chap. 8), and management of coma and other neurocritical care conditions (Chaps. 17 and 28). This chapter focuses on additional common reasons for consultation that are not addressed elsewhere in the text.

CONSULTATIONS REGARDING CENTRAL NERVOUS SYSTEM DYSFUNCTION

HYPERPERFUSION STATES

A group of neurologic disorders shares the common feature of hyperperfusion playing a key role in pathogenesis. These seemingly diverse syndromes include hypertensive encephalopathy, eclampsia, postcarotid endarterectomy syndrome, and toxicity from calcineurin-inhibitor medications. Modern imaging techniques and experimental models suggest that vasogenic edema is usually the primary process leading to neurologic dysfunction; therefore, prompt recognition and management of this condition should allow for clinical recovery if superimposed hemorrhage or infarction has not occurred.

The brain's autoregulatory capability successfully maintains a fairly stable cerebral blood flow in adults despite alterations in systemic mean arterial pressure (MAP) ranging from 50–150 mmHg. In patients with chronic hypertension, this cerebral autoregulation curve is shifted, resulting in autoregulation working over a much higher range of pressures (e.g., 70–175 mmHg). In these hypertensive patients, cerebral blood flow is kept steady at higher MAP, but a rapid lowering of pressure can more easily lead to ischemia on the lower end of the autoregulatory curve. This autoregulatory phenomenon is achieved through both myogenic and neurogenic influences causing small arterioles to contract and dilate. When the systemic blood pressure exceeds the limits of this mechanism, breakthrough of autoregulation occurs, resulting in hyperperfusion via increased cerebral blood flow, capillary leakage into the interstitium, and resulting edema. The predilection of all of the hyperperfusion disorders to affect the posterior rather than anterior portions of the brain may be due to a lower threshold for autoregulatory breakthrough in the posterior circulation.

While elevated or relatively elevated blood pressure is common in many of these disorders, some hyperperfusion states such as calcineurin-inhibitor toxicity occur with no apparent pressure rise. In these cases, vasogenic edema is likely due primarily to dysfunction of the capillary endothelium itself, leading to breakdown of the blood-brain barrier. It is useful to separate disorders of hyperperfusion into those caused primarily by increased pressure and those due mostly to endothelial dysfunction from a toxic or autoimmune etiology (Table 50-1). In reality, both of these pathophysiologic processes are likely playing some role in each of these disorders.

The clinical presentation of the hyperperfusion syndromes is similar with prominent headaches, seizures, or focal deficits. Headaches have no specific characteristics, range from mild to severe, and may be accompanied by alterations in consciousness ranging from confusion to coma. Seizures may be present, and these can be of multiple types depending on the severity and location of the edema. Nonconvulsive seizures have been described in hyperperfusion states; therefore, a low threshold for obtaining an electroencephalogram (EEG) in these

TABLE 50-1

SOME COMMON ETIOLOGIES OF HYPERPERFUSION SYNDROME

Disorders in which increased capillary pressure dominates the pathophysiology
Hypertensive encephalopathy, including secondary causes such as renovascular hypertension, pheochromocytoma, cocaine use, etc.
Postcarotid endarterectomy syndrome
Preeclampsia/eclampsia
High-altitude cerebral edema
Disorders in which endothelial dysfunction dominates the pathophysiology
Calcineurin-inhibitor toxicity
Chemotherapeutic agent toxicity (e.g., cytarabine, azathioprine, 5-fluorouracil, cisplatin, methotrexate)
Glucocorticoids
Erythropoietin
HELLP syndrome (*h*emolysis, *e*levated *l*iver enzyme levels, *l*ow *p*latelet count)
Thrombotic thrombocytopenic purpura (TTP)
Hemolytic uremic syndrome (HUS)
Systemic lupus erythematosus (SLE)
Granulomatosis with polyangiitis (Wegener's)

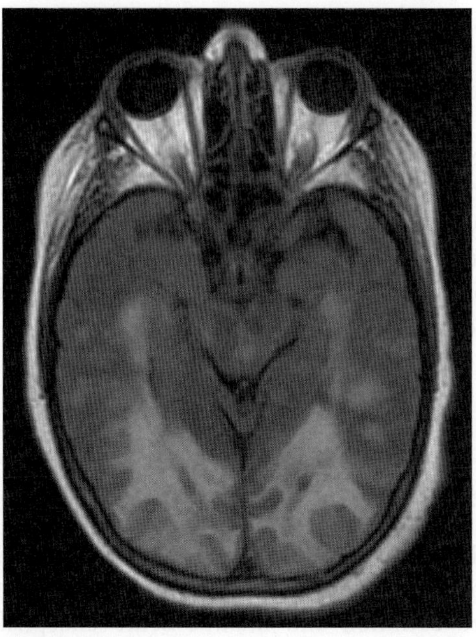

FIGURE 50-1
Axial fluid-attenuated inversion recovery (FLAIR) MRI of the brain in a patient taking cyclosporine after liver transplantation, who presented with seizures, headache, and cortical blindness. Increased signal is seen bilaterally in the occipital lobes predominantly involving the white matter, consistent with a hyperperfusion state secondary to calcineurin-inhibitor exposure.

patients should be maintained. The typical focal deficit in hyperperfusion states is cortical visual loss, given the tendency of the process to involve the occipital lobes. However, any focal deficit can occur depending on the area affected, as evidenced by patients who, after carotid endarterectomy, exhibit neurologic dysfunction in the ipsilateral newly reperfused hemisphere. In conditions where increased cerebral blood flow plays a role, examination of the inpatient vital signs record will usually reveal a systemic blood pressure that is increased above baseline. It appears as if the rapidity of rise rather than the absolute value of pressure is the most important risk factor.

The diagnosis in all of these conditions is clinical. The symptoms of these disorders are common and nonspecific, so a long differential diagnosis should be entertained, including consideration of other causes of confusion, focal deficits, headache, and seizures. MRI has improved the ability of clinicians to diagnose hyperperfusion syndromes, although cases have been reported with normal imaging. Patients classically exhibit the high T2 signal of edema primarily in the posterior occipital lobes, not respecting any single vascular territory (Fig. 50-1). Diffusion-weighted images are typically normal, emphasizing the vasogenic rather than cytotoxic nature of this edema. Imaging with CT is less sensitive but may show a pattern of patchy hypodensity in the involved territory. Previously this classic radiographic appearance had been termed *reversible posterior leukoencephalopathy* (RPLE). However, this term has fallen out of favor because none of its elements are completely accurate. The radiographic and clinical changes are not always reversible; the territory involved is not uniquely posterior; and gray matter may be affected as well, rather than purely white matter as the word "leukoencephalopathy" intimates. Other ancillary studies such as cerebrospinal fluid (CSF) analysis often yield nonspecific results. It should be noted that many of the substances that have been implicated, such as cyclosporine, can cause this syndrome even at low doses or after years of treatment. Therefore, normal serum levels of these medications do not exclude them as inciting agents.

In cases of hyperperfusion syndromes, treatment should commence urgently once the diagnosis is considered. Hypertension plays a key role commonly, and judicious lowering of the blood pressure with IV agents such as labetalol or nicardipine is advised along with continuous cardiac and blood pressure monitoring, often through an arterial line. It is reasonable to lower mean arterial pressure by ~20% initially, as further lowering of the pressure may cause secondary ischemia as pressure drops below the lower range of the patient's autoregulatory capability. In cases where there is an identified cause of the syndrome, these etiologies should be treated promptly, including discontinuation of offending substances such as calcineurin inhibitors in toxic processes, treatment of immune-mediated disorders such as thrombotic thrombocytopenic purpura (TTP), and prompt delivery of the fetus in eclampsia. Seizures must be identified and controlled, often necessitating continuous EEG monitoring. Anticonvulsants are effective, but in the special case of eclampsia, there is good evidence to support the use of magnesium sulfate for seizure control.

POST-CARDIAC BYPASS BRAIN INJURY

Central nervous system (CNS) injuries following open heart or coronary artery bypass grafting (CABG) surgery are common and include acute encephalopathy, stroke, and a chronic syndrome of cognitive impairment, which is now increasingly recognized. Hypoperfusion and embolic disease are frequently involved in the pathogenesis of these syndromes, although multiple mechanisms may be involved in these critically ill patients who are at risk for various metabolic and polypharmaceutical complications.

The frequency of hypoxic injury secondary to inadequate blood flow intraoperatively has been markedly decreased by the use of modern surgical and anesthetic techniques. Despite these advances, some patients still experience neurologic complications from cerebral hypoperfusion or may suffer focal ischemia from tight carotid or focal intracranial stenoses in the setting of regional hypoperfusion. Postoperative infarcts in the border zones between vascular territories commonly are blamed on systemic hypotension, although some have suggested that these infarcts can also result from embolic disease (Fig. 50-2).

Embolic disease is likely the predominant mechanism of cerebral injury during cardiac surgery as evidenced by diffusion-weighted MRI and intraoperative transcranial Doppler studies. It should be noted that some of the emboli that are found histologically in these patients are too small to be detected by standard imaging sequences; therefore, a negative MRI after surgery does not exclude the diagnosis of emboli-related complications. Thrombus in the heart itself as well as atheromas in the aortic arch can become dislodged during cardiac surgeries, releasing a shower of particulate matter into the cerebral circulation. Cross-clamping of the aorta, manipulation of the heart, extracorporeal circulation techniques ("bypass"), arrhythmias such as atrial fibrillation, and introduction of air through suctioning have all been implicated as potential sources of emboli. Histologic studies indicate that literally millions of tiny emboli may be released, even using modern surgical techniques.

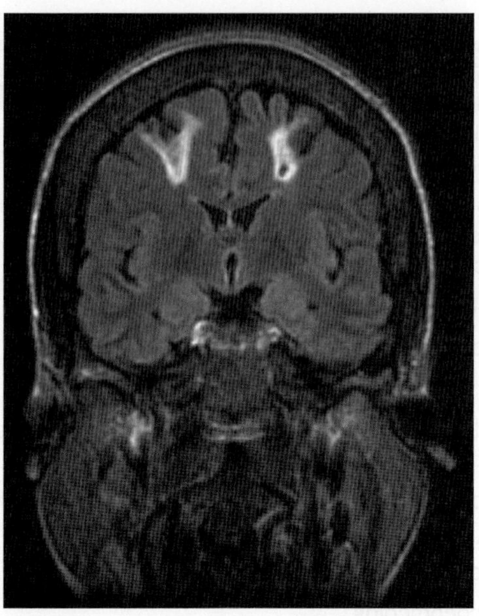

FIGURE 50-2
Coronal fluid-attenuated inversion recovery (FLAIR) MRI of the brain in a patient presenting with altered mental status after an episode of hypotension during coronary artery bypass grafting (CABG). Increased signal is seen in the border zones bilaterally between the middle cerebral artery and anterior cerebral artery territories. Diffusion-weighted MRI sequences demonstrated restricted diffusion in these same locations, suggesting acute infarction.

This shower of microemboli results in a number of clinical syndromes. Occasionally, a single large embolus leads to an isolated large-vessel stroke that presents with obvious clinical focal deficits. More commonly, the emboli released are multiple and smaller. When there is a high burden of these small emboli, an acute encephalopathy can occur postoperatively, presenting as either a hyperactive or hypoactive confusional state, the latter of which is frequently and incorrectly ascribed to depression. When the burden of microemboli is lower, no acute syndrome is recognized, but the patient may suffer a chronic cognitive deficit. Cardiac surgery can be viewed, like delirium, as a "stress test for the brain." Some patients with a low cerebral reserve due to underlying cerebrovascular disease or an early neurodegenerative process will develop a chronic, cognitive deficit, whereas others with higher reserves may remain asymptomatic despite a similar dose of microemboli. In this manner, cardiac surgery may serve to unmask the early manifestations of disorders such as vascular dementia and Alzheimer's disease.

Since modern techniques have successfully minimized hypoperfusion complications during these surgeries, much attention is now focused on reducing this inevitable shower of microemboli. Off-pump CABG surgeries have the advantages of reducing length of stay and perioperative complications; however, some recent data suggests that off-pump CABG does not preserve cognitive function compared with on-pump CABG. Filters placed in the aortic arch may have some promise in capturing these emboli, although convincing evidence is currently lacking. Development of successful endovascular operative approaches may provide a reasonable alternative to conventional CABG procedures, especially for patients at high risk of developing cognitive dysfunction after surgery due to advanced age, previous stroke, or severe atheromatous disease of the carotid arteries or aortic arch.

POST-SOLID ORGAN TRANSPLANT BRAIN INJURY

Patients who have undergone solid organ transplantation are at risk for neurologic injury in the postoperative period and for the months to years thereafter. Neurologic consultants should view these patients as a special population at risk for both unique neurologic complications as well as for the usual disorders found in any critically ill inpatient.

Immunosuppressive medications are administered in high doses to patients after solid organ transplant, and many of these compounds have well-described neurologic complications. In patients with headache, seizures, or focal neurologic deficits taking calcineurin inhibitors, the diagnosis of hyperperfusion syndrome should be considered, as discussed earlier. This neurotoxicity occurs mainly with cyclosporine and tacrolimus and can present even in the setting of normal serum drug levels. Treatment primarily involves lowering the drug dosage or discontinuing the drug. A related newer agent, sirolimus, has very few recorded cases of neurotoxicity and may be a reasonable alternative for some patients. Other examples of immunosuppressive medications and their neurologic complications include OKT3-associated akinetic mutism and the leukoencephalopathy seen with methotrexate, especially when it is administered intrathecally or with concurrent radiotherapy. In any solid organ transplant patient with neurologic complaints, a careful examination of the medication list is required to search for these possible drug effects.

Cerebrovascular complications of solid organ transplant are often first recognized in the immediate postoperative period. Border zone territory infarctions can occur, especially in the setting of systemic hypotension during cardiac transplant surgery. Embolic infarctions classically complicate cardiac transplantation, but all solid organ transplant procedures place patients at risk for systemic emboli. When cerebral embolization accompanies renal or liver transplantation surgery, a careful search for right-to-left shunting should include evaluation of the heart with agitated saline echocardiography, as well as looking for intrapulmonary shunting. Renal and some cardiac transplant patients often have advanced atherosclerosis, providing yet another mechanism for stroke. Imaging with CT or MRI with diffusion is advised when cerebrovascular complications are suspected to confirm the diagnosis and to exclude intracerebral hemorrhage, which most often occurs in the setting of coagulopathy secondary to liver failure or after cardiac bypass procedures.

Given that patients with solid organ transplants are chronically immunosuppressed, infections are a common concern. In any transplant patient with new CNS signs or symptoms such as seizure, confusion, or focal deficit, the diagnosis of a central nervous system infection should be considered and evaluated through imaging (usually MRI) and possibly lumbar puncture. The most common pathogens responsible for CNS infections in these patients vary based on time since transplant. In the first month posttransplant, common pathogens include the usual bacterial organisms associated with surgical procedures and indwelling catheters. Starting in the second month posttransplant, opportunistic infections of the CNS become more common, including *Nocardia* and *Toxoplasma* species as well as fungal infections such as aspergillosis. Viral infections that can affect the brain of the immunosuppressed patient, such as herpes simplex virus, cytomegalovirus, and varicella, also become more common after the first month posttransplant. After 6 months posttransplant, immunosuppressed patients still remain at risk for these opportunistic bacterial, fungal, and viral infections but can also suffer late CNS infectious complications such as progressive multifocal leukoencephalopathy (PML) associated with JC virus and Epstein-Barr virus–driven clonal expansions of B cells resulting in CNS lymphoma.

COMMON NEUROLOGIC COMPLICATIONS OF ELECTROLYTE DISTURBANCES

A wide variety of neurologic conditions can result from abnormalities in serum electrolytes, and consideration of electrolyte disturbances should be part of any inpatient neurologic consultation.

HYPERNATREMIA AND HYPEROSMOLALITY

The normal range of serum osmolality is around 275–295 mOsm/kg, but neurologic manifestations are usually seen only at levels >325 mOsm/kg. Hyperosmolality is usually due to hypernatremia, hyperglycemia, azotemia, or the addition of extrinsic osmoles such as mannitol, which is commonly used in critically ill neurologic patients. Hyperosmolality itself can lead to a generalized encephalopathy that is nonspecific and without focal findings; however, an underlying lesion such as a mass can become symptomatic under the metabolic stress of a hyperosmolar state, producing focal signs. Some patients with hyperosmolality from severe hyperglycemia can present, for unclear reasons, with generalized seizures or unilateral movement disorders, which usually respond to lowering of the serum glucose. The treatment of all forms of hyperosmolality involves calculation of apparent water losses and slow replacement so that the serum sodium declines no faster than 2 mmol/L (2 meq/L) per hour.

Hypernatremia leads to the loss of intracellular water, leading to cell shrinkage. In the cells of the brain, solutes such as glutamine and urea are generated under these conditions in order to minimize this shrinkage. Despite this corrective mechanism, when hypernatremia is severe (serum sodium >160 mmol/L [>160 meq/L]) or occurs rapidly, cellular metabolic processes fail and encephalopathy will result. There are many etiologies of hypernatremia including, most commonly, renal and extrarenal losses of water. Causes of neurologic relevance include central diabetes insipidus, where hyperosmolality is accompanied by submaximal urinary concentration due to inadequate release of arginine vasopressin (AVP) from the posterior pituitary, resulting often from pituitary injury in the setting of surgery, hemorrhage, infiltrative processes, or cerebral herniation.

HYPONATREMIA

Hyponatremia is commonly defined as a serum sodium <135 mmol/L (<135 meq/L). Neurologic symptoms occur at different levels of low sodium, depending not only on the absolute value but also on the rate of fall. In patients with hyponatremia that develops over hours, life-threatening seizures and cerebral edema may occur at values as high as 125 mmol/L. In contrast, some patients with more chronic hyponatremia that has slowly developed over months to years may be asymptomatic even with serum levels <110 mmol/L. Correction of hyponatremia, especially when chronic, must take place slowly in order to avoid additional neurologic complications. Cells in the brain swell in hypotonic hyponatremic states but may compensate over time by excreting solute into the extracellular space, leading to restoration of cell volume when water follows the solute out of the cells. If treatment of hyponatremia results in a rapid rise in serum sodium, cells in the brain may quickly shrink, leading to osmotic demyelination, a process that previously was thought to be limited exclusively to the brainstem (central pontine myelinolysis; see Fig. 28-6), but now has been described elsewhere in the CNS.

Treatment of hyponatremia is dependent on the cause. Hypertonic hyponatremia treatment focuses on the underlying condition, such as hyperglycemia. Isovolemic hyponatremia (syndrome of inappropriate antidiuretic hormone [SIADH]) is managed with water restriction or administration of AVP antagonists. The management of choice for patients with hypervolemic hypotonic hyponatremia is free-water restriction and treatment of the underlying edematous disorder, such as nephrotic syndrome or congestive heart failure. Finally, in hypovolemic hypotonic hyponatremia, volume is replaced with isotonic saline while underlying conditions of the kidneys, adrenals, and gastrointestinal tract are addressed.

One neurologic cause of hypovolemic hypotonic hyponatremia is the cerebral salt-wasting syndrome that accompanies subarachnoid hemorrhage and, less commonly, other cerebral processes such as meningitis or stroke. In these cases, the degree of renal sodium excretion can be remarkable, and large amounts of saline, hypertonic saline, or oral sodium may need to be given in a judicious fashion in order to avoid complications from cerebral edema.

HYPOKALEMIA

Hypokalemia, defined as a serum potassium level <3.5 mmol/L (<3.5 meq/L), occurs either because of excessive potassium losses (from the kidneys or gut) or due to an abnormal potassium distribution between the intracellular and extracellular spaces. At very low levels (<1.5 mmol/L), hypokalemia may be life threatening due to the risk of cardiac arrhythmia and may present neurologically with severe muscle weakness and paralysis. Hypokalemic periodic paralysis is a rare disorder caused by excessive intracellular potassium uptake in the setting of a calcium or sodium channel mutation. Treatment of hypokalemia is dependent on the etiology but usually includes replacement of potassium through oral or IV routes as well as correcting the cause of potassium balance problems (e.g., eliminating β_2-adrenergic agonist medications).

HYPERKALEMIA

Hyperkalemia is defined as a serum potassium level >5.5 mmol/L (>5.5 meq/L) and can neurologically present as muscle weakness with or without paresthesias. Hyperkalemia becomes life threatening when it produces electrocardiographic abnormalities such as peaked T waves or a widened QRS complex. In these cases, prompt treatment is essential and consists of strategies that protect the heart against arrhythmias (calcium gluconate administration); promote potassium redistribution into cells (with glucose, insulin, and β_2-agonist medications); and increase potassium removal (through sodium polystyrene sulfonate, loop diuretics, or hemodialysis).

CALCIUM DISTURBANCES

Hypercalcemia usually occurs in the setting of either hyperparathyroidism or systemic malignancy. Neurologic manifestations include encephalopathy as well as muscle weakness due to reduced neuromuscular excitability. Seizures can occur but are more common in states of low calcium.

Hypocalcemia in adults often follows surgical treatment of the thyroid or parathyroid. Seizures and altered mental status dominate the neurologic picture and usually resolve with calcium repletion. Tetany is due to spontaneous, repetitive action potentials in peripheral nerves and remains the classic sign of symptomatic hypocalcemia.

MAGNESIUM DISTURBANCES

Disorders of magnesium are difficult to correlate with serum levels because a very small amount of total-body magnesium is located in the extracellular space. Hypomagnesemia presents neurologically with seizures, tremor, and myoclonus. When intractable seizures occur in the setting of hypomagnesemia, only administration of magnesium will lead to resolution. High levels of magnesium, in contrast, lead to CNS depression. Hypermagnesemia usually only occurs in the setting of renal failure or magnesium administration and can lead to confusion and muscular paralysis when severe.

CONSULTATIONS REGARDING PERIPHERAL NERVOUS SYSTEM DYSFUNCTION

ENTRAPMENT NEUROPATHIES

Polyneuropathy is a common cause of outpatient neurologicconsultation (Chap. 45). In the inpatient setting, however, mononeuropathies are more frequent, especially the entrapment neuropathies that complicate many surgical procedures and medical conditions. Median neuropathy at the wrist (carpal tunnel syndrome) is the most frequent entrapment neuropathy by far, but it is rarely a cause for inpatient consultation. Mechanisms for perioperative mononeuropathy include traction, compression, and ischemia of the nerve. Imaging with MR neurography may allow these causes to be distinguished definitively. In all cases of mononeuropathy, the diagnosis can be made through the clinical examination and then confirmed with electrodiagnostic studies in the subacute period, if necessary. Treatment consists mainly of avoidance of repetitive trauma but may also include surgical approaches to relieve pressure on the nerve.

RADIAL NEUROPATHY

Radial nerve injury classically presents with weakness of extension of the wrist and fingers ("wrist drop") with or without more proximal weakness of extensor muscles of the upper extremity, depending on the site of injury. Sensory loss is in the distribution of the radial nerve, which includes the dorsum of the hand (Fig. 50-3*A*). Compression at the level of the axilla, e.g., resulting from use of crutches, includes weakness of the triceps, brachioradialis, and supinator muscles in addition to wrist drop. A more common site of compression occurs in the spiral groove of the upper arm in the setting of a humerus fracture or from sleeping with the arm draped over a bench or chair ("Saturday night palsy"). Sparing of the triceps is the rule when the nerve is injured in this location. Because extensors of the upper extremity are injured preferentially in radial nerve injury, these lesions may be mistaken for the pyramidal distribution of weakness that accompanies upper motor neuron lesions from brain or spinal cord processes.

ULNAR NEUROPATHY

Compression of the ulnar nerve is the second most common entrapment neuropathy after carpal tunnel syndrome. The most frequent site of compression is at the elbow where the nerve passes superficially in the ulnar groove. Symptoms usually begin with tingling in the ulnar distribution, including the fourth and fifth digits of the hand (Fig. 50-3*B*). Sensory symptoms may be worsened by elbow flexion due to increased pressure on the nerve, hence the tendency of patients to complain of increasing paresthesias at night when the arm is flexed at the elbow during sleep. Motor dysfunction can be disabling and involves most of the intrinsic hand muscles, limiting dexterity and strength of grasp and pinch. Etiologies of ulnar entrapment include trauma to the nerve (hitting the "funny bone"), malpositioning during anesthesia for surgical procedures, and chronic arthritis of the elbow. When a perioperative ulnar nerve injury is considered, stretch injury or trauma to the lower trunk of the brachial plexus should be entertained as well since its symptoms can mimic those of an ulnar neuropathy. If the clinical examination is equivocal, electrodiagnostic studies can definitively distinguish between plexus and ulnar nerve lesions a few weeks after the injury. Conservative methods of treatment are often the first step, but a variety of surgical approaches may be effective, including anterior ulnar

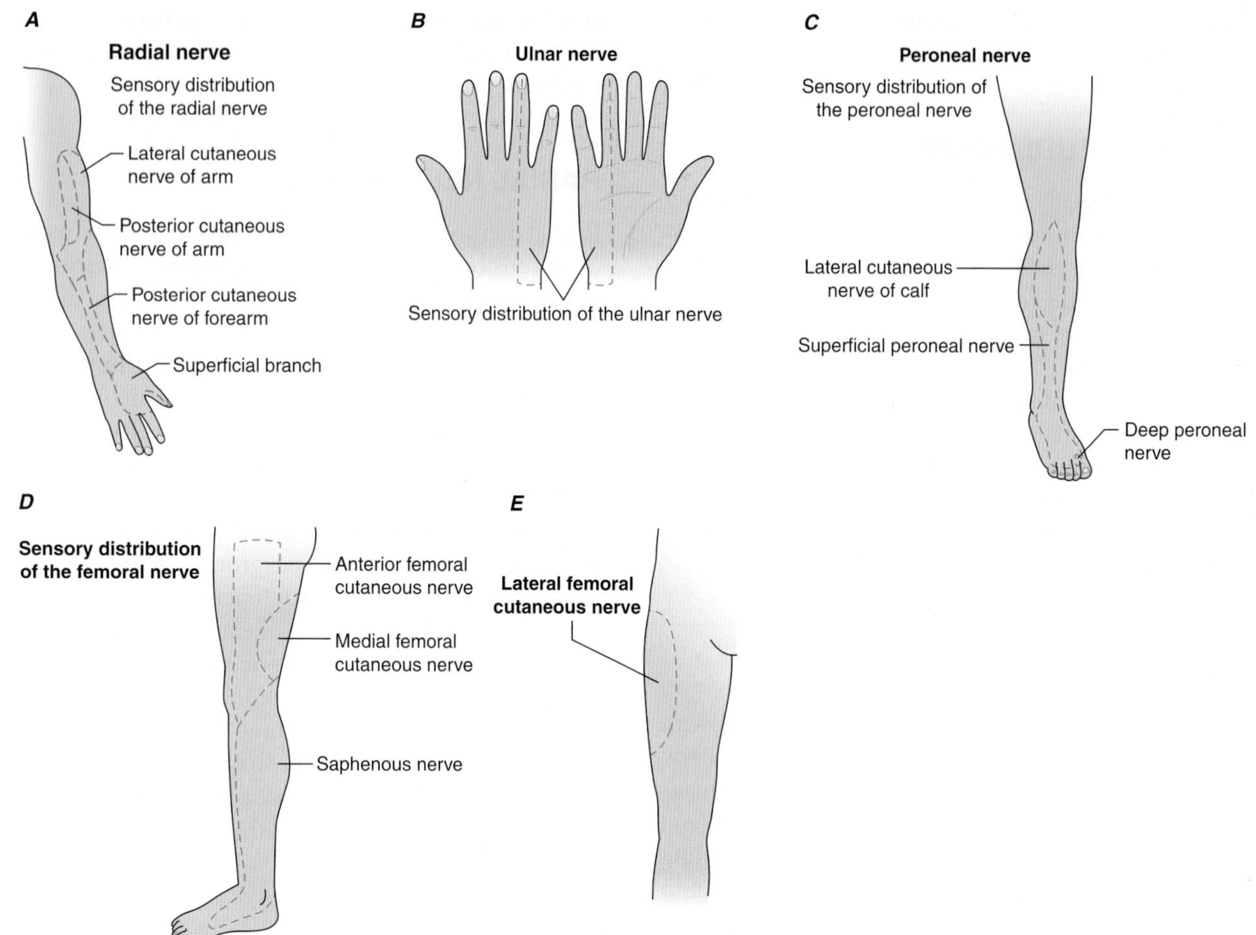

FIGURE 50-3
Sensory distribution of peripheral nerves commonly affected by entrapment neuropathies. ***A.*** Radial nerve. ***B.*** Ulnar nerve. ***C.*** Peroneal nerve. ***D.*** Femoral nerve. ***E.*** Lateral femoral cutaneous nerve.

nerve transposition and release of the flexor carpi ulnaris aponeurosis.

PERONEAL NEUROPATHY

The peroneal nerve winds around the head of the fibula in the leg below the lateral aspect of the knee, and its superficial location at this site makes it vulnerable to trauma. Patients present with weakness of foot dorsiflexion ("foot drop") as well as with weakness in eversion but not inversion at the ankle. Sparing of inversion, which is a function of muscles innervated by the tibial nerve, helps to distinguish peroneal neuropathies from L5 radiculopathies. Sensory loss involves the lateral aspect of the leg as well as the dorsum of the foot (Fig. 50-3*C*). Fractures of the fibular head may be responsible for peroneal neuropathies, but in the perioperative setting poorly applied braces exerting pressure on the nerve while the patient is unconscious are more often responsible. Tight-fitting stockings or casts of the upper leg can also cause a peroneal neuropathy, and thin individuals and those with recent weight loss are at increased risk.

PROXIMAL FEMORAL NEUROPATHY

Lesions of the proximal femoral nerve are relatively uncommon but may present dramatically with weakness of hip flexion, quadriceps atrophy, weakness of knee extension (often manifesting with leg-buckling falls), and an absent patellar reflex. Adduction of the thigh is spared as these muscles are supplied by the obturator nerve, thereby distinguishing a femoral neuropathy from a more proximal lumbosacral plexus lesion. The sensory loss found is in the distribution of the femoral nerve sensory branches on the anterior part of the thigh (Fig. 50-3*D*). Compressive lesions from retroperitoneal hematomas or masses are common, and a CT of the pelvis should be obtained in all cases of femoral neuropathy to exclude these conditions. Bleeding into the pelvis resulting in hematoma can occur spontaneously, following trauma, or after intrapelvic surgeries such as renal transplantation. In intoxicated or comatose patients, stretch injuries to the femoral nerve are seen following prolonged, extreme hip flexion or extension. Rarely, attempts at femoral vein or arterial puncture can be complicated by injury to this nerve.

LATERAL FEMORAL CUTANEOUS NERVE

The symptoms of lateral femoral cutaneous nerve entrapment, commonly known as "meralgia paresthetica," include sensory loss, pain, and dysesthesia in part of the area supplied by the nerve (Fig. 50-3*E*). There is no motor component to the nerve, and therefore weakness is not a part of this syndrome. Symptoms often are worsened by standing or walking. Compression of the nerve occurs where it enters the leg near the inguinal ligament, usually in the setting of tight-fitting belts, pants, corsets, or recent weight gain, including that of pregnancy. The differential diagnosis of these symptoms includes hip problems such as trochanteric bursitis.

OBSTETRIC NEUROPATHIES

Pregnancy and delivery place women at special risk for a variety of nerve injuries. Radiculopathy due to a herniated lumbar disc is not common during pregnancy, but compressive injuries of the lumbosacral plexus do occur secondary to either the fetal head passing through the pelvis or the use of forceps during delivery. These plexus injuries are more frequent with cephalopelvic disproportion and often present with a painless unilateral foot drop which must be distinguished from a peroneal neuropathy caused by pressure on the nerve while in lithotomy position during delivery. Other compressive mononeuropathies of pregnancy include meralgia paresthetica, carpal tunnel syndrome, femoral neuropathy when the thigh is abducted severely in an effort to facilitate delivery of the fetal shoulder, and obturator neuropathy during lithotomy positioning. The latter presents with medial thigh pain that may be accompanied by weakness of thigh adduction. There is also a clear association between pregnancy and an increased frequency of idiopathic facial palsy (Bell's palsy).

CHAPTER 51

ATLAS OF NEUROIMAGING

Andre Furtado ■ William P. Dillon

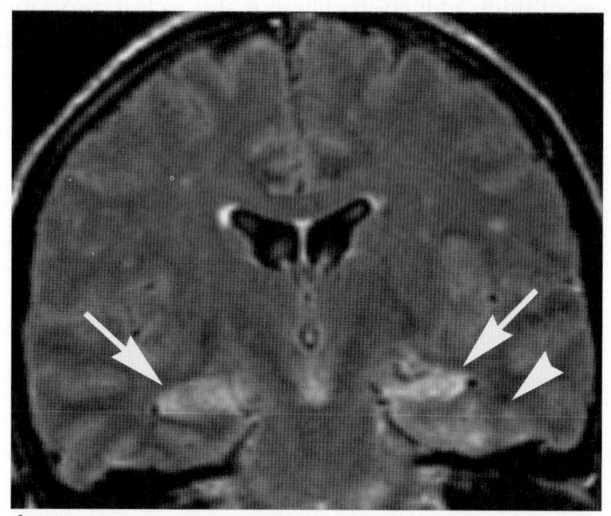

A

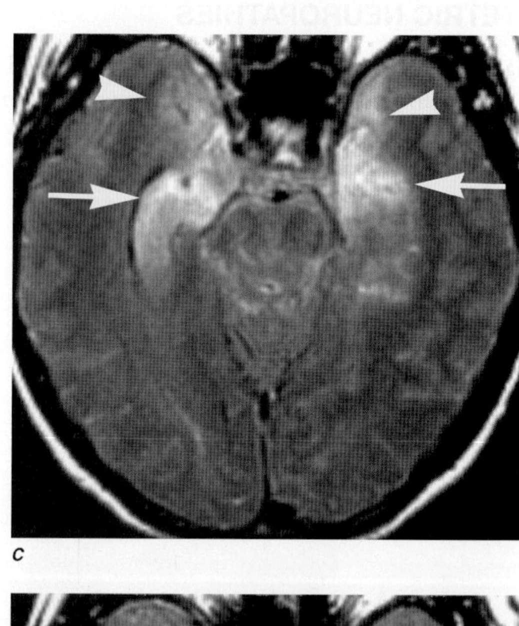

C

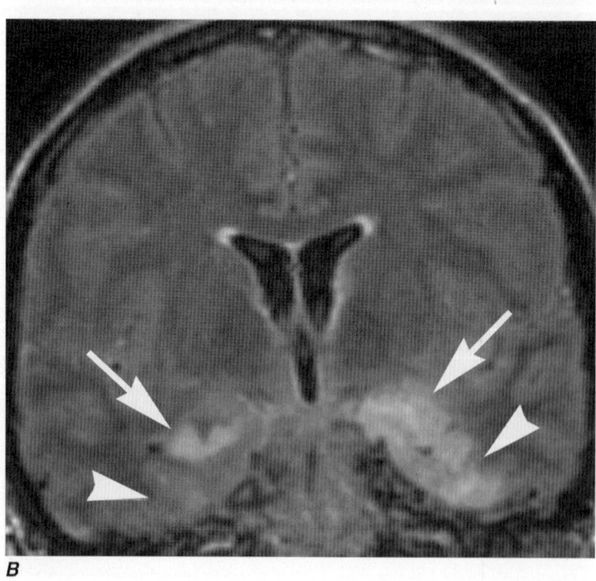

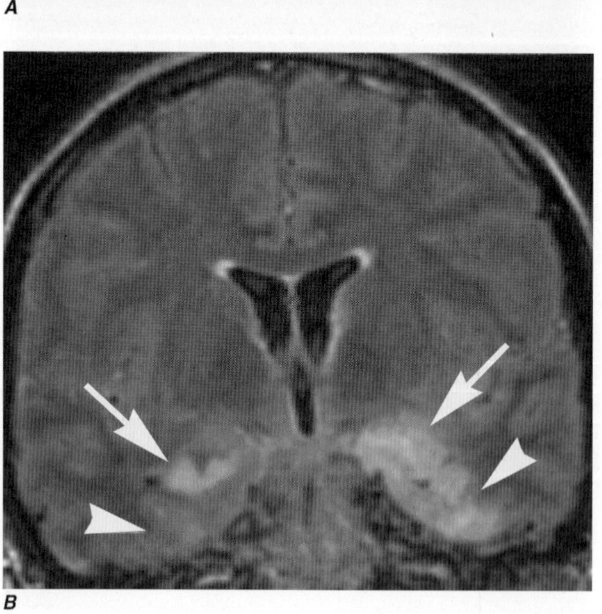

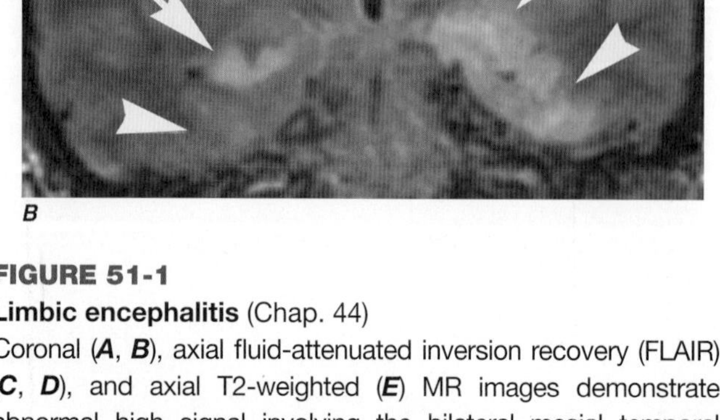

B

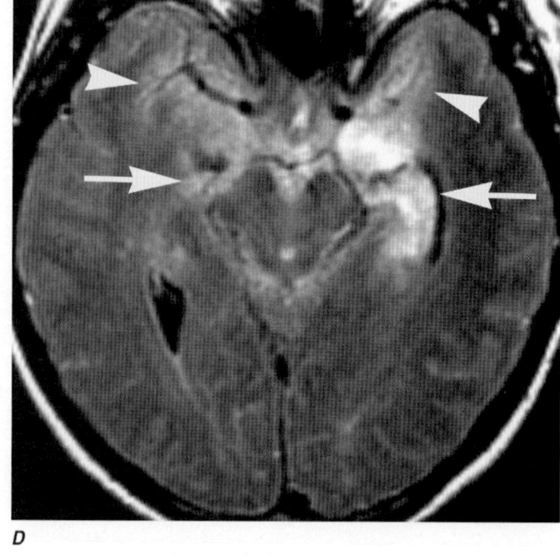

D

FIGURE 51-1

Limbic encephalitis (Chap. 44)

Coronal (***A***, ***B***), axial fluid-attenuated inversion recovery (FLAIR) (***C***, ***D***), and axial T2-weighted (***E***) MR images demonstrate abnormal high signal involving the bilateral mesial temporal lobes (*arrow-heads*) including the hippocampi (left greater than right) without significant mass effect (*arrows*). There was no enhancement on postgadolinium images (not shown).

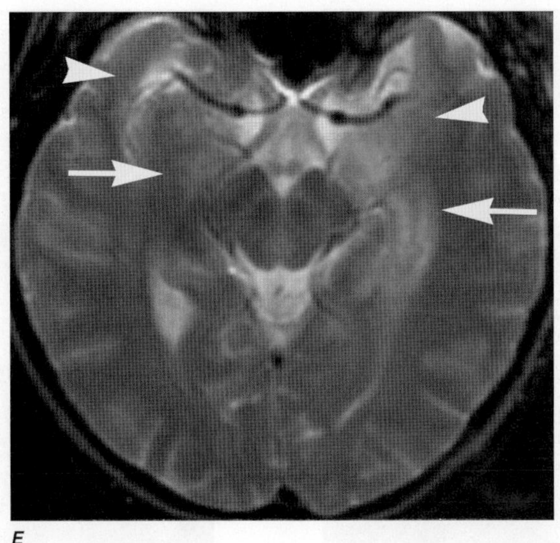

E

FIGURE 51-1
(*continued*)

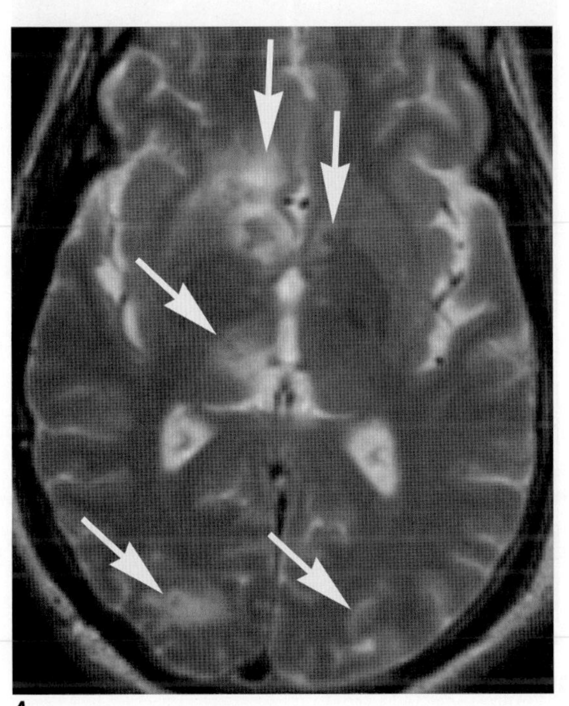

A

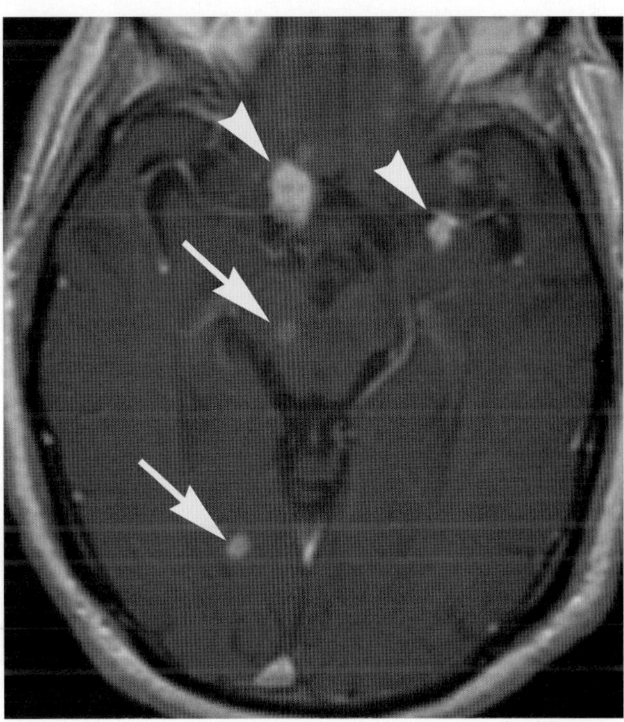

B

FIGURE 51-2
CNS tuberculosis
Axial T2-weighted MRI (***A***) demonstrates multiple lesions (*arrows*) with peripheral high signal and central low signal, located predominantly in the cortex and subcortical white matter, as well as in the basal ganglia.
Axial T1-weighted MR images postgadolinium (***B***, ***C***) demonstrate ring enhancement of the lesions (*arrows*) and additional lesions in the subarachnoid space (*arrowheads*).
Sagittal T2-weighted MR image of the cervical spine (***D***) demonstrates a hypointense lesion in the subarachnoid space at the level of T5 (*arrow*).
Sagittal T1-weighted MR image postgadolinium of the cervical spine (***E***) demonstrates enhancement of the lesion in the subarachnoid space at the level of T5 (*arrow*).

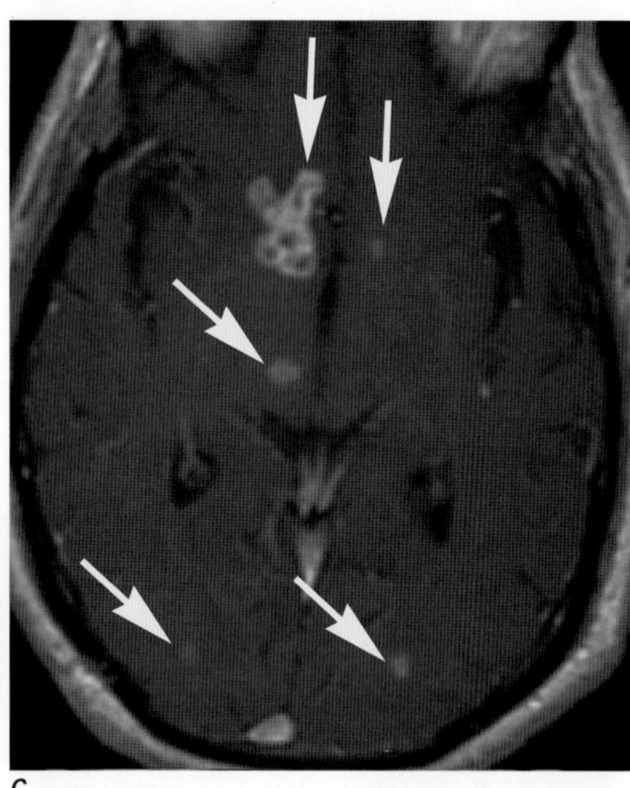

C

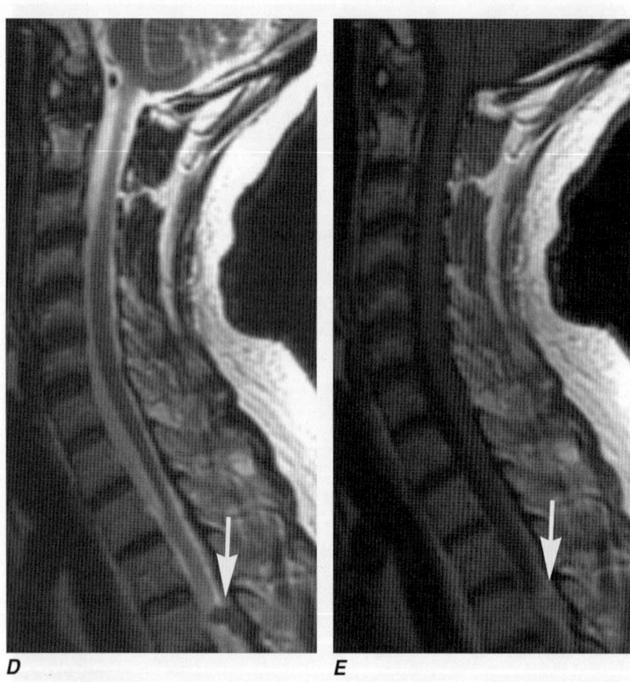

D *E*

FIGURE 51-2
(*continued*)

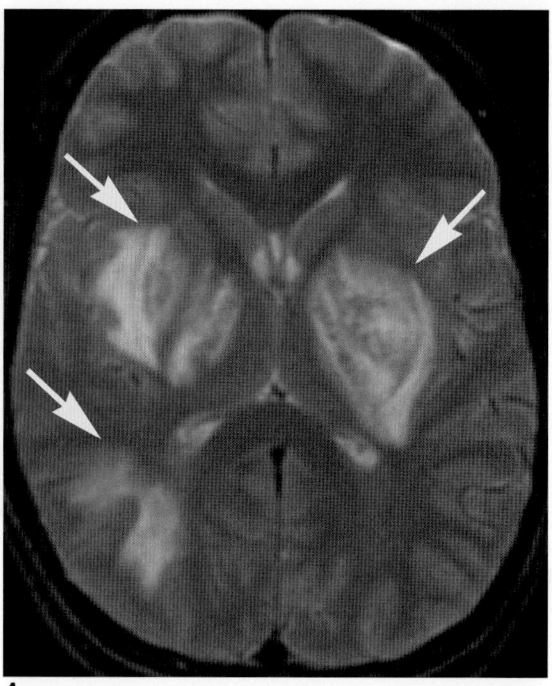

A

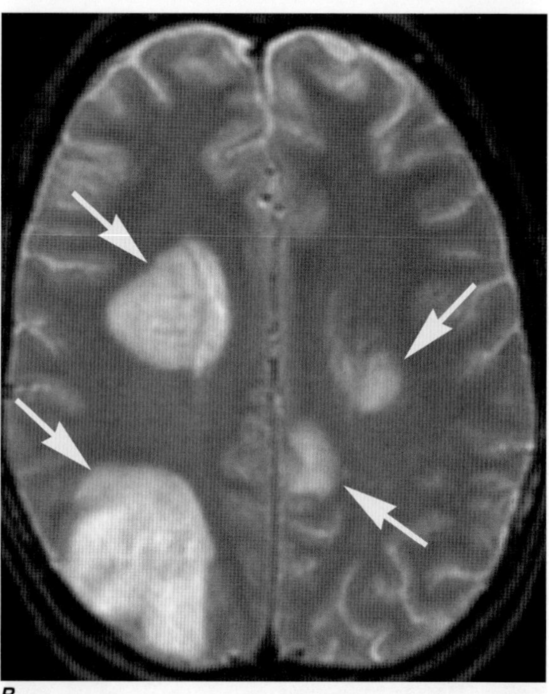

B

FIGURE 51-3
Neurosyphilis
Case I

Axial T2-weighted MR images (***A***, ***B***) demonstrate well-defined areas of abnormal high signal in the basal ganglia bilaterally and in a wedge-shaped distribution in the right parietal lobe (*arrows*).

Axial (***C***, ***D***) T1-weighted images postgadolinium.

Coronal (***E***, ***F***) T1-weighted images postgadolinium demonstrate irregular ring enhancement of the lesions (*arrows*).

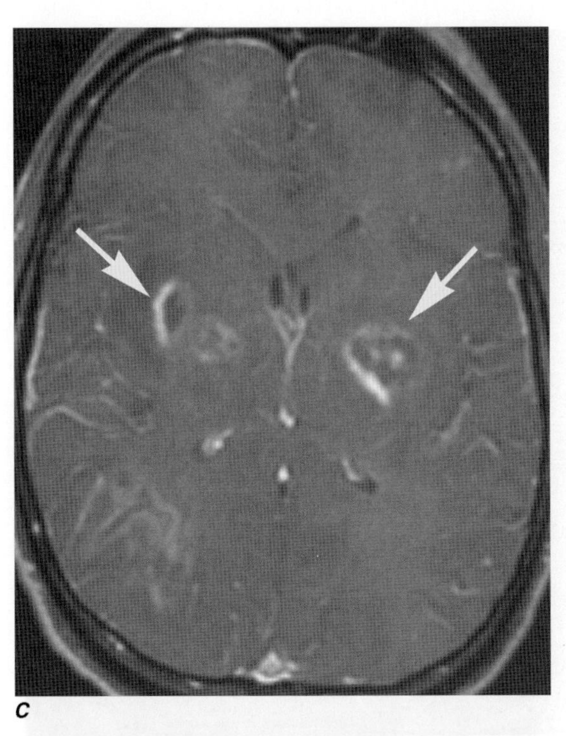

C

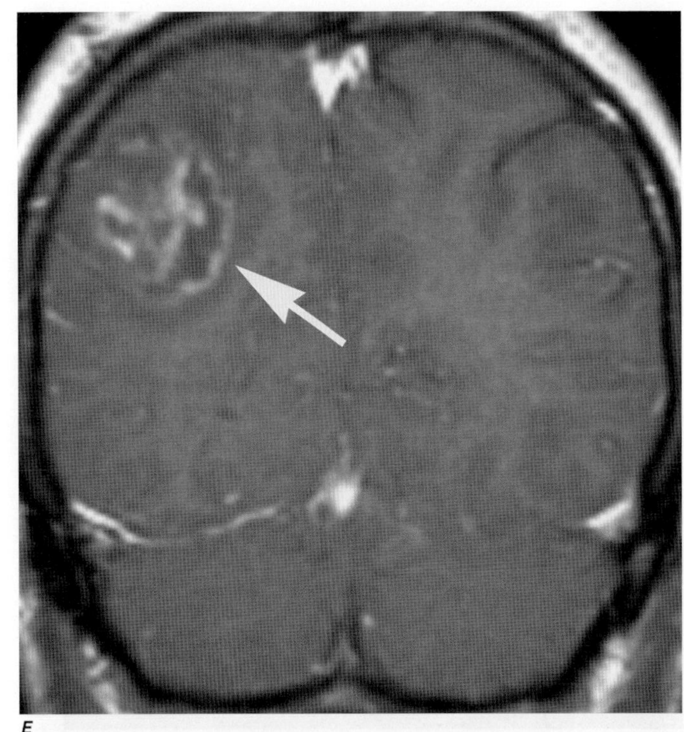

E

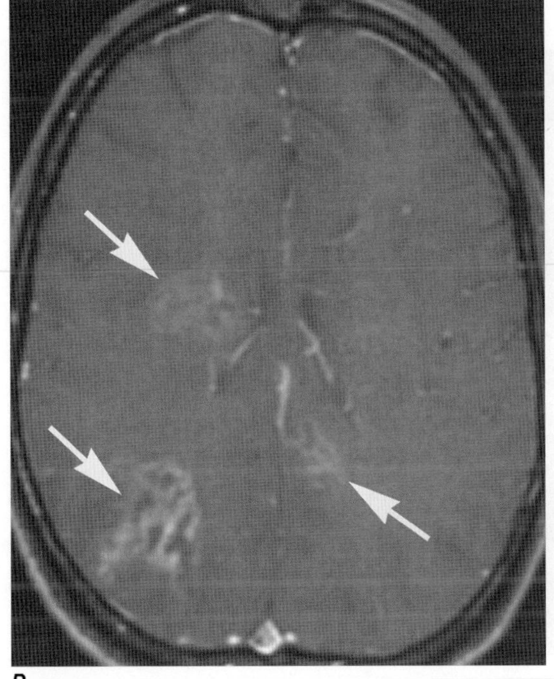

D

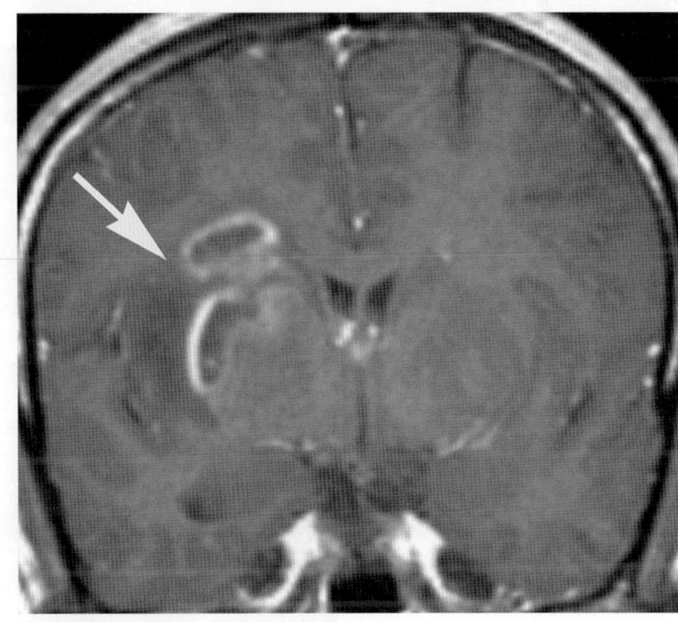

F

FIGURE 51-3
(continued)

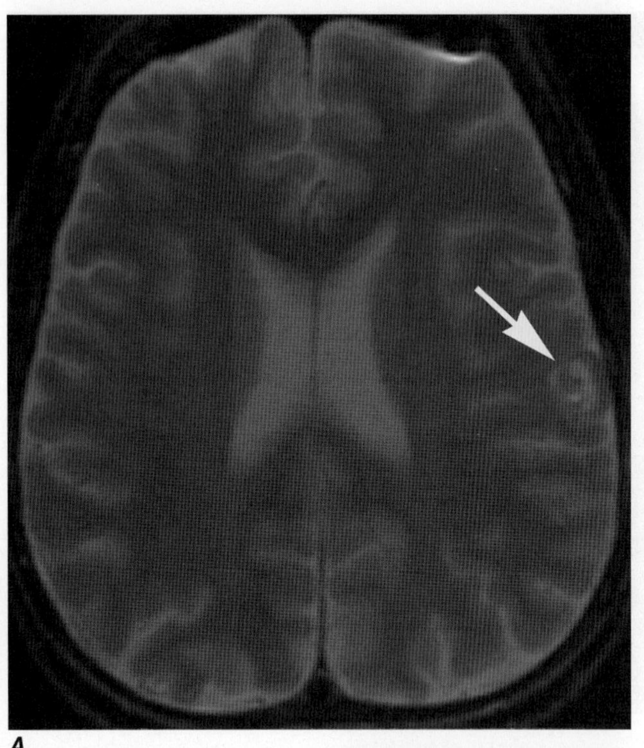

A

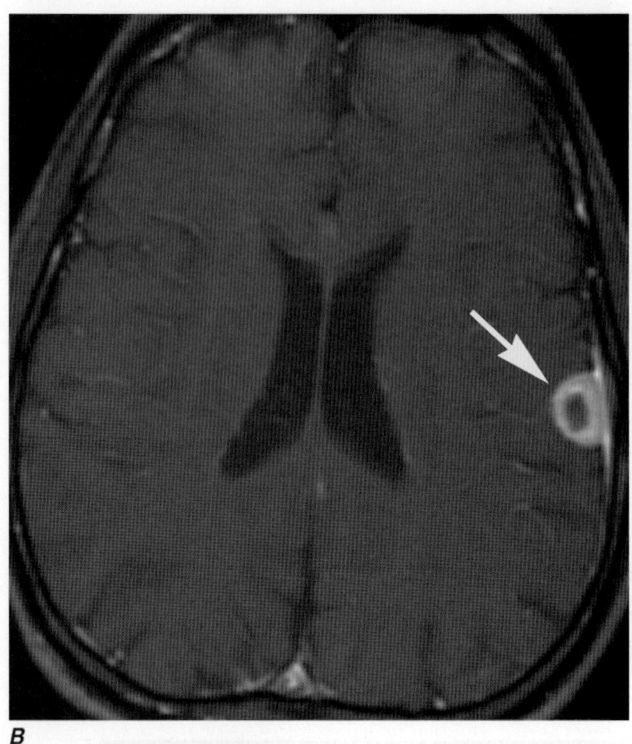

B

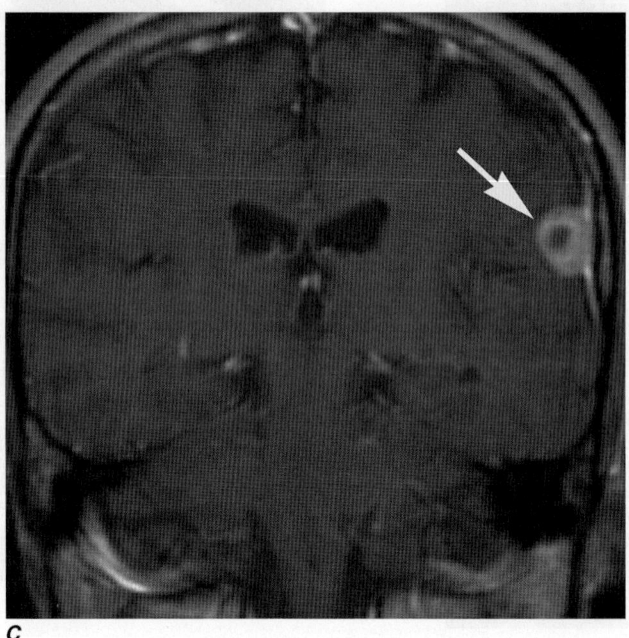

C

FIGURE 51-4
Neurosyphilis
Case II
Axial T2-weighted MRI (***A***) demonstrates a dural-based, peripherally hyperintense and centrally hypointense lesion located lateral to the left frontal lobe (*arrow*).

Axial (***B***) and coronal (***C***) T1-weighted MR images postgadolinium demonstrate peripheral enhancement of the lesion (*arrows*).

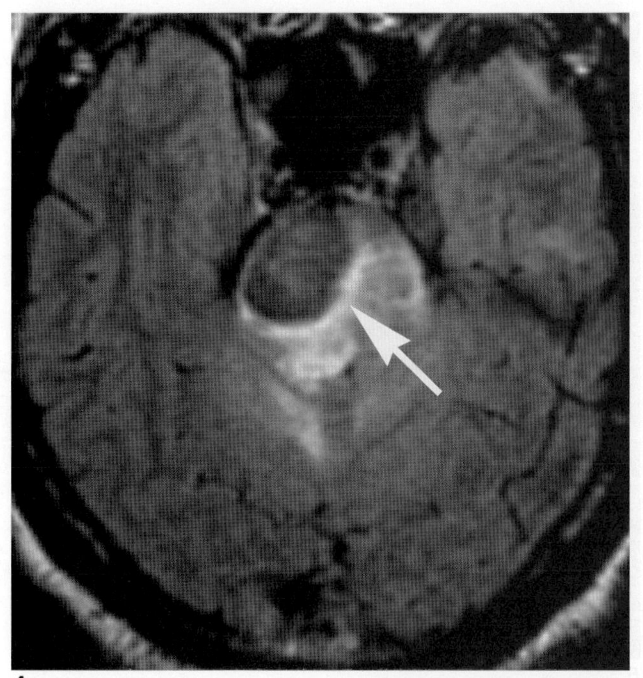

A

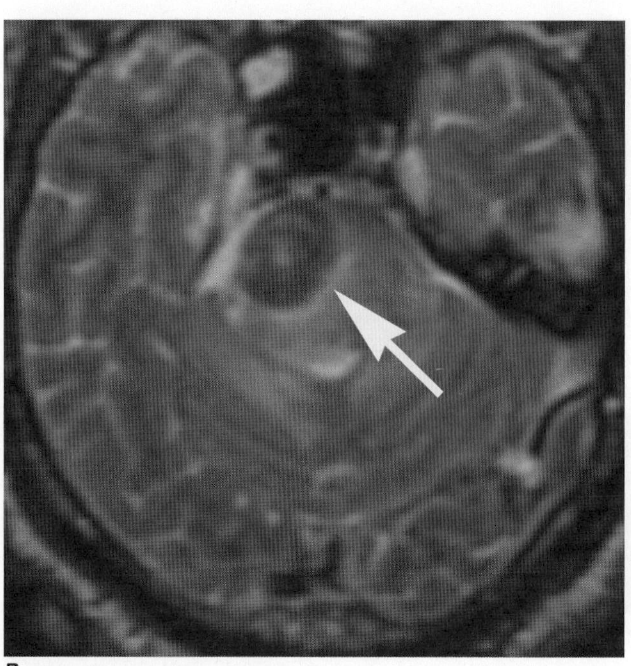

B

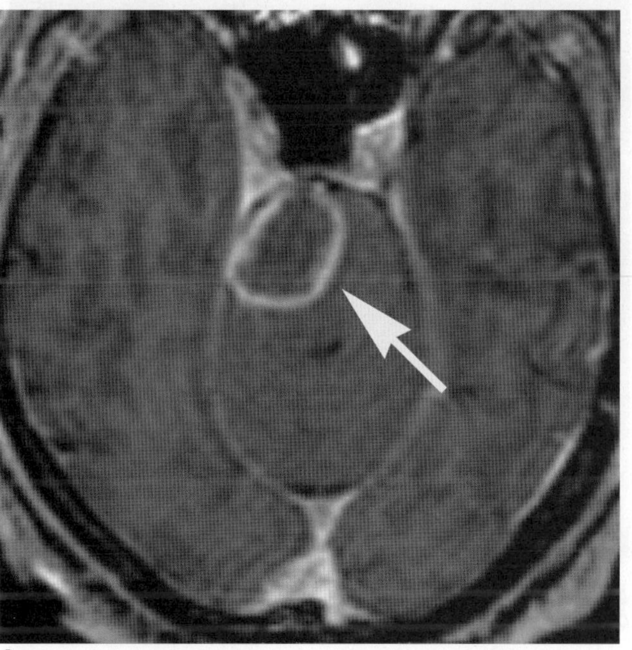

C

FIGURE 51-5

Histoplasmosis of the pons

Axial FLAIR (***A***) and T2-weighted (***B***) MR images demonstrate a low signal mass in the right pons (*arrows*) with surrounding vasogenic edema.

Axial T1-weighted MR image postgadolinium (***C***) demonstrates ring enhancement of the lesion in the right pons (*arrow*). Of note, there was no evidence of restricted diffusion (not shown).

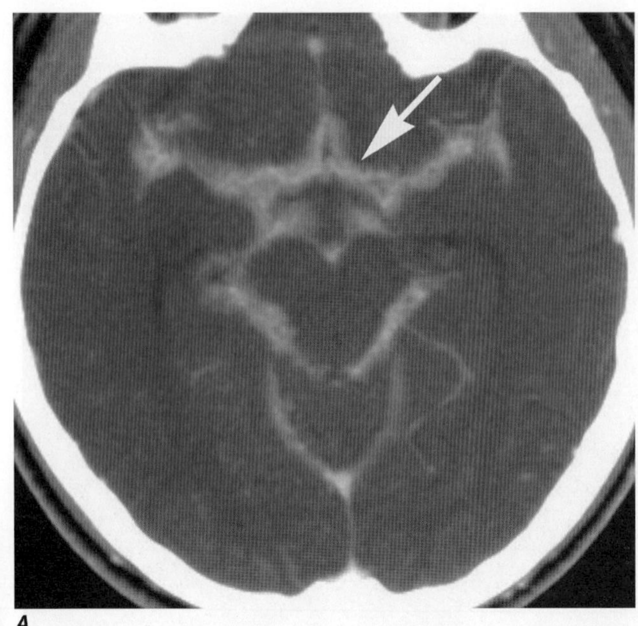

A

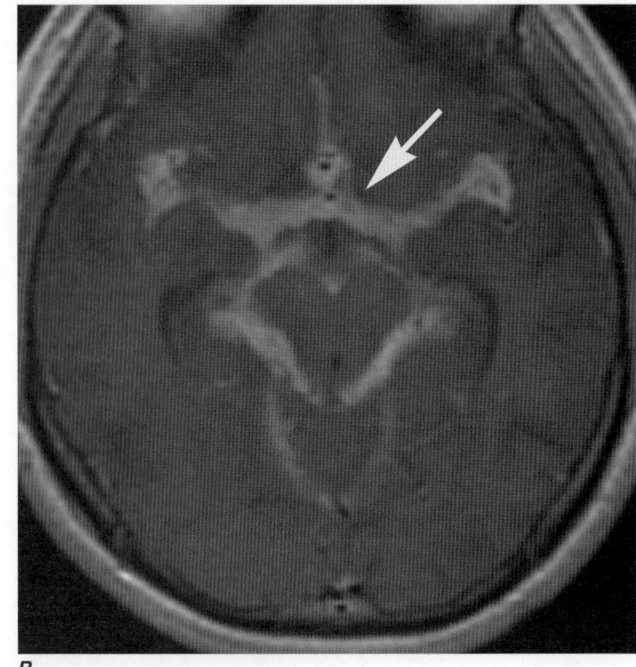

B

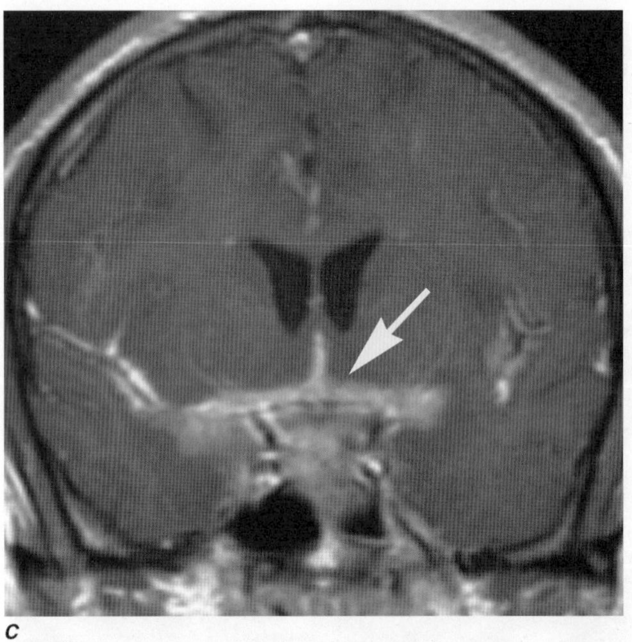

C

FIGURE 51-6
Coccidiomycosis meningitis
Axial postcontrast CT (***A***) and axial (***B***) and coronal (***C***) T1-weighted MR images postgadolinium demonstrate enhancement of the perimesencephalic cisterns (*arrows*), as well as the sylvian and interhemispheric fissures.

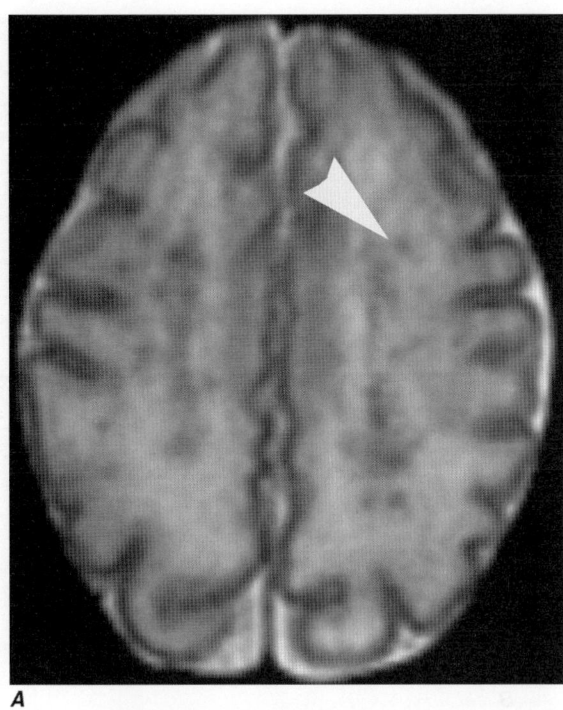
A

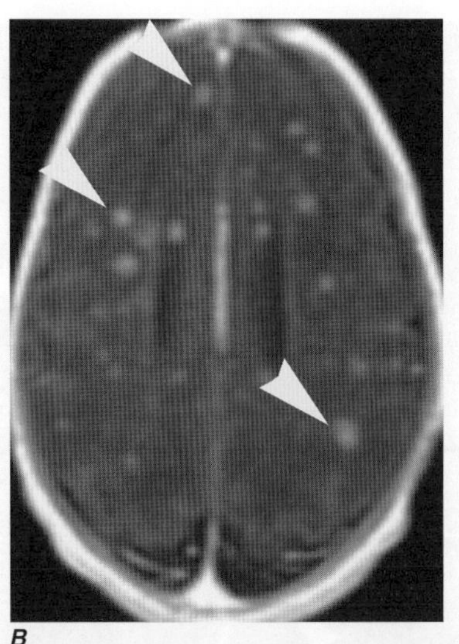
B

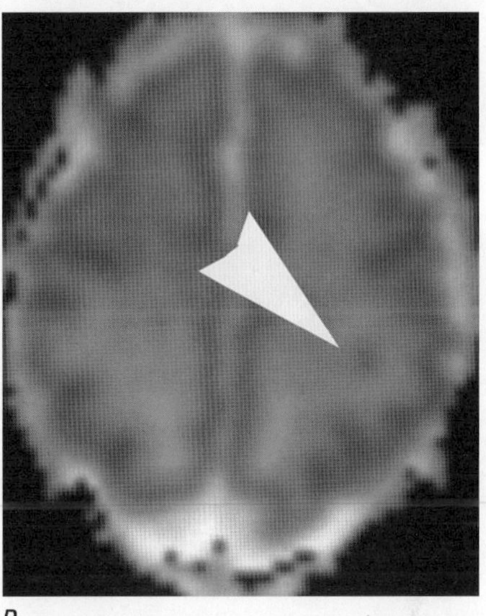
D

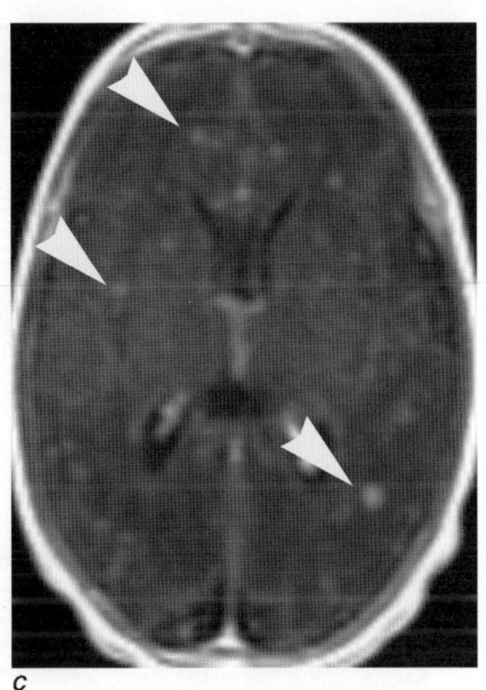
C

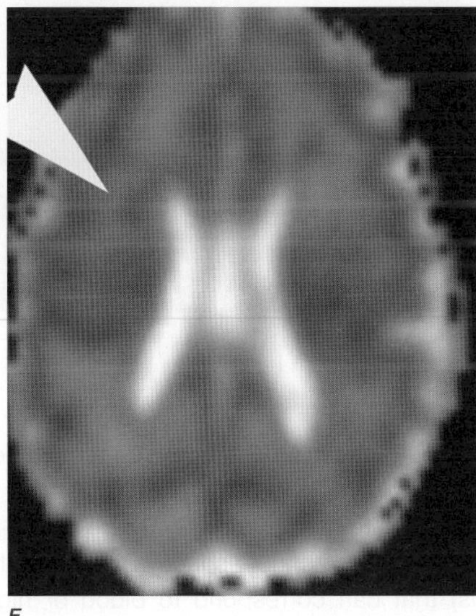
E

FIGURE 51-7

Candidiasis in a newborn

Axial T2-weighted MR image (***A***) demonstrates multiple punctate foci of low signal diffusely distributed in the brain parenchyma (*arrowhead*).

Axial T1-weighted MR images postgadolinium (***B***, ***C***) demonstrate marked enhancement of the lesions (*arrowheads*).

ADC map (***D***, ***E***) demonstrates restricted diffusion of water molecules in the lesions (*arrowheads*).

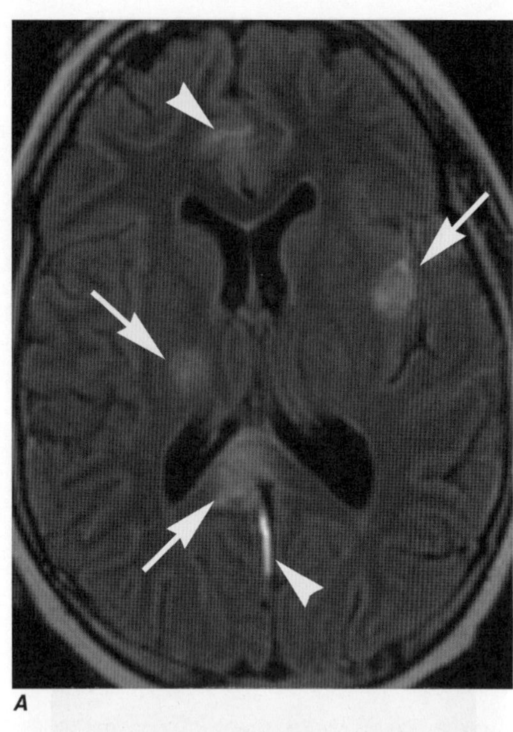

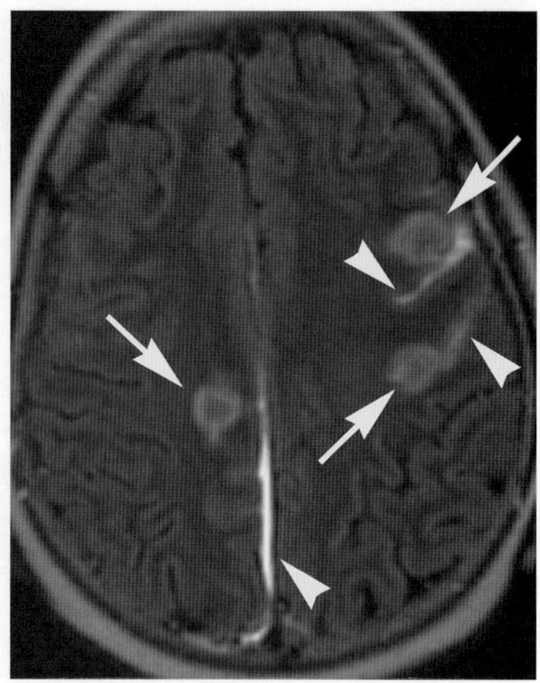

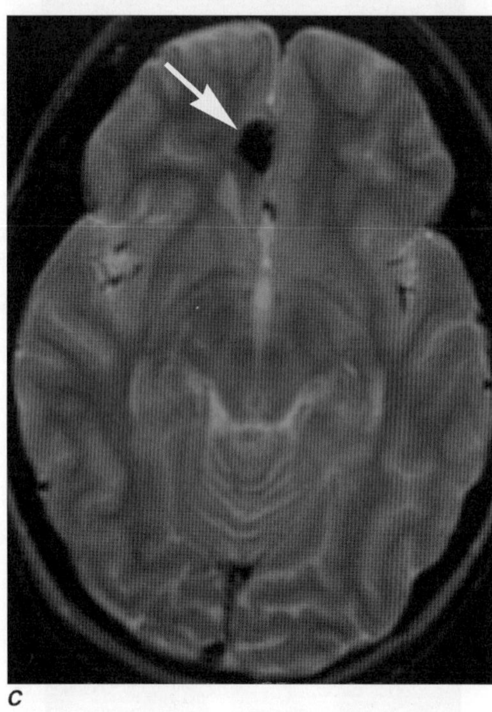

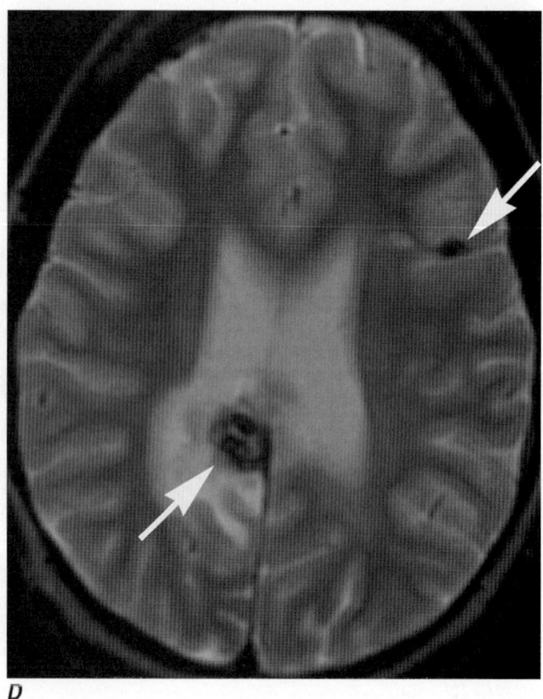

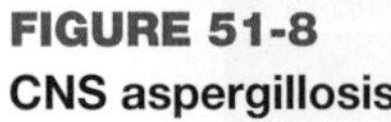

FIGURE 51-8
CNS aspergillosis
Axial FLAIR MR images (***A***, ***B***) demonstrate multiple areas of abnormal high signal in the basal ganglia as well as cortex and subcortical white matter (*arrows*). There is also abnormal high signal in the subarachnoid space adjacent to the lesions (*arrowheads*) that can correspond to blood or high protein content. Axial T2-weighted MR images (***C***, ***D***) demonstrate intrinsic low signal in the lesions (*arrows*), suggesting the presence of blood products. Some of the lesions also show vasogenic edema. Coronal (***E***) and axial (***F***) T1-weighted MR images postgadolinium demonstrate peripheral enhancement of the lesions (*arrows*).

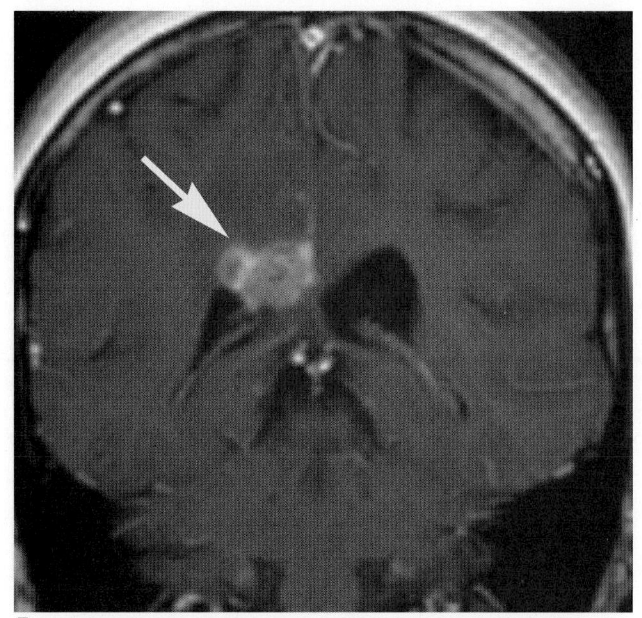

E

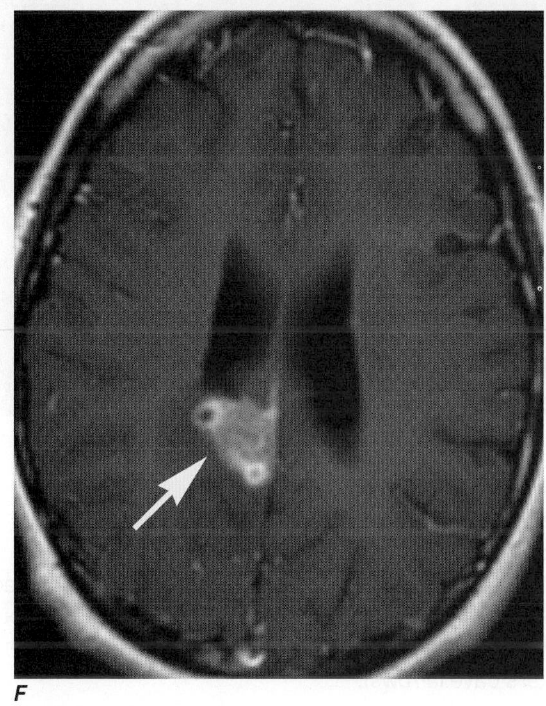

F

FIGURE 51-8
(continued)

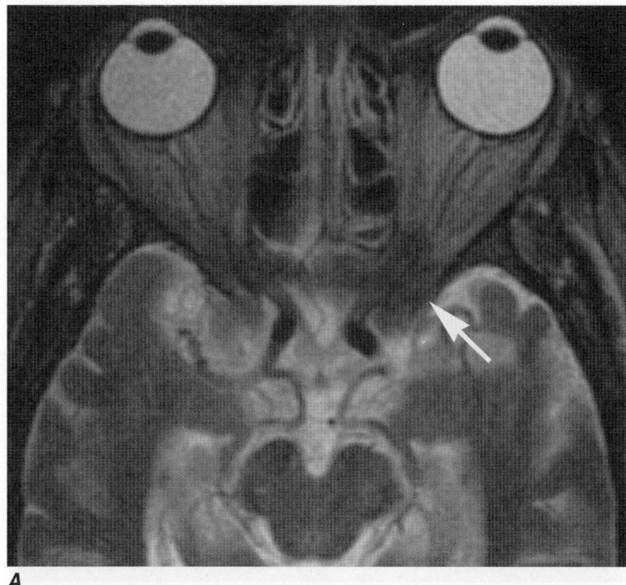

A

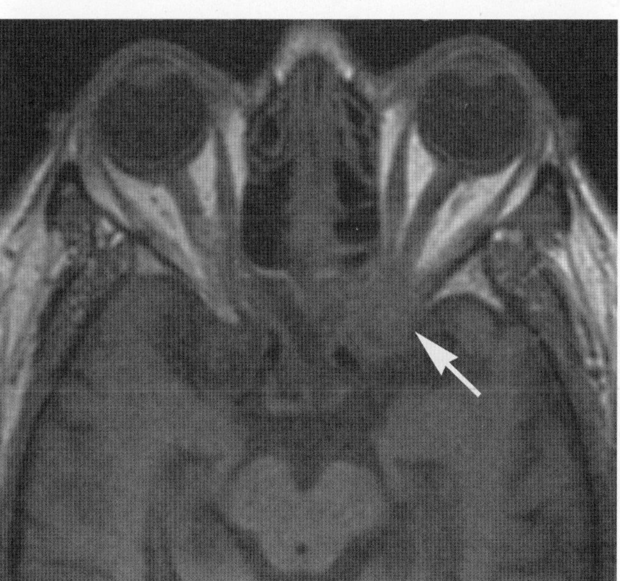

B

FIGURE 51-9
Invasive sinonasal aspergillosis
Axial T2-weighted MR image (***A***) demonstrates an irregularly shaped low signal lesion involving the left orbital apex (*arrow*).
B. T1-weighted image pregadolinium demonstrates low signal in left anterior clinoid process (*arrow*).
C. T1-weighted image postgadolinium demonstrates enhancement of lesion (*arrow*).

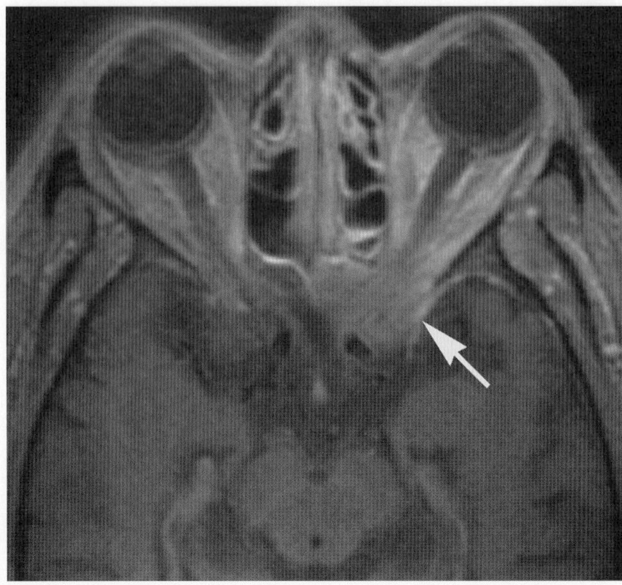

C

FIGURE 51-9
(*continued*)

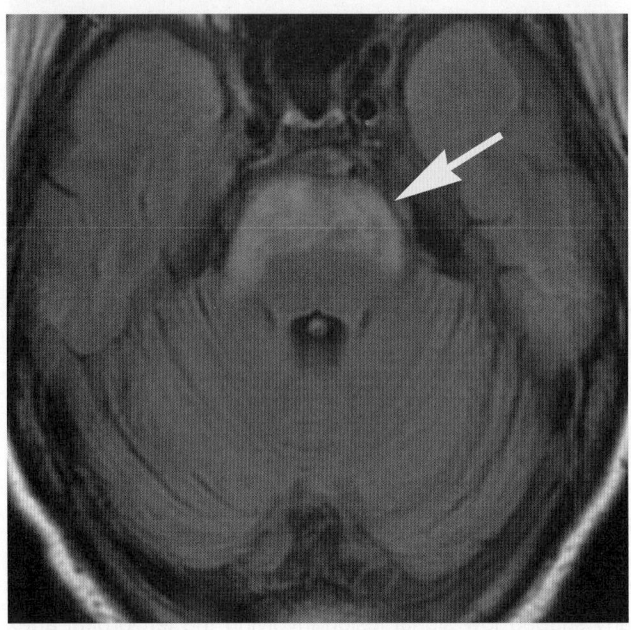

FIGURE 51-10
Behçet's disease
Axial FLAIR MRI demonstrates abnormal high signal involving the anterior pons (*arrow*); following gadolinium administration, the lesion was nonenhancing (not shown). Brainstem lesions are typical of Behçet's disease, caused primarily by vasculitis and in some cases demyelinating lesions.

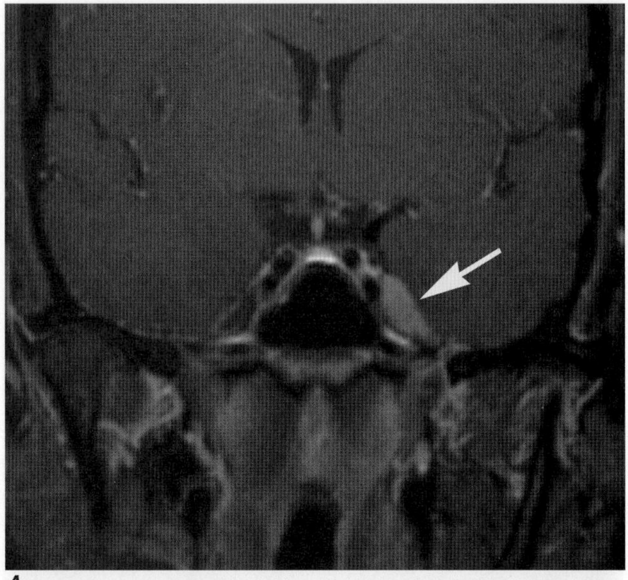

A

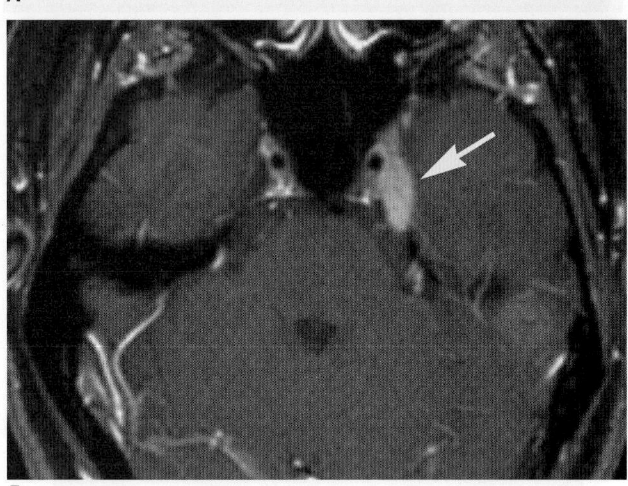

B

FIGURE 51-11
Neurosarcoid
Case I
Coronal (***A***) and axial (***B***) T1-weighted images postgadolinium with fat suppression demonstrate a homogeneously enhancing well-circumscribed mass centered in the left Meckel's cave (*arrows*).

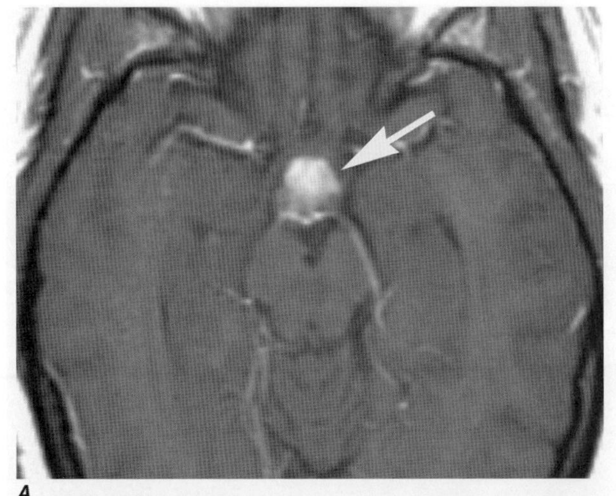

A

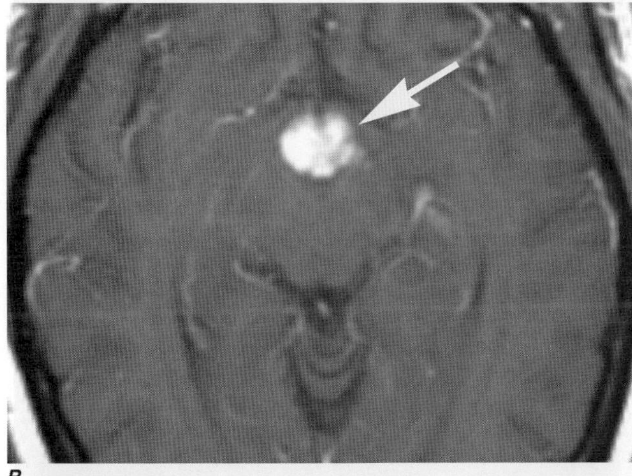

B

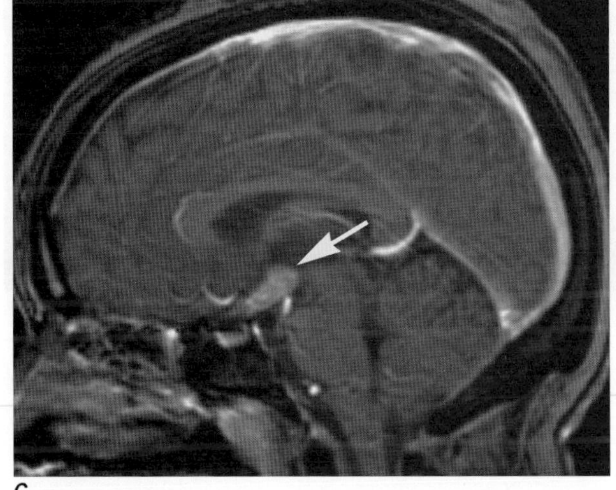

C

FIGURE 51-12
Neurosarcoid
Case II
Axial (***A***, ***B***) and sagittal (***C***) T1-weighted images postgadolinium with fat suppression demonstrate a homogeneously enhancing mass involving the hypothalamus and the pituitary stalk (*arrows*).

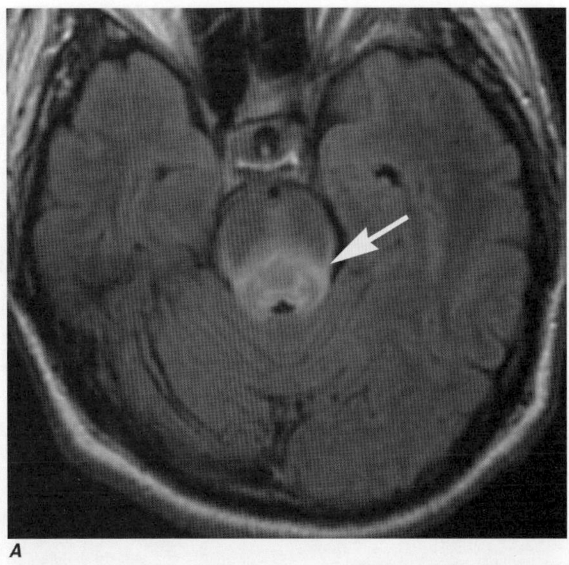

A

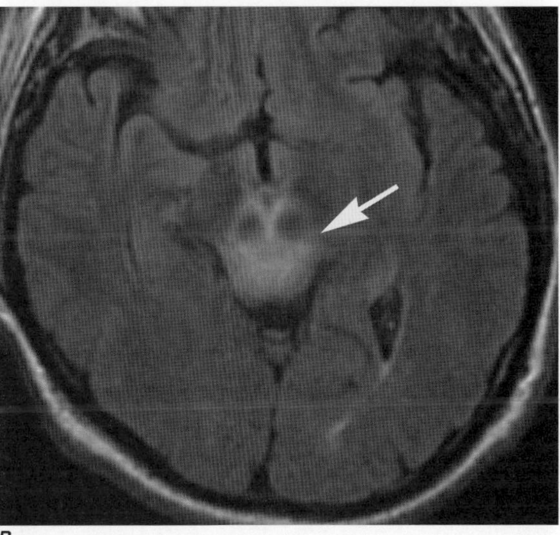

B

FIGURE 51-13
Neurosarcoid
Case III
Axial FLAIR images (***A–E***) demonstrate abnormal high signal and slight expansion in the midbrain, dorsal pons, and pineal region (*arrows*) without significant mass effect.
Sagittal T1-weighted images postgadolinium (***F***) with fat suppression demonstrate abnormal enhancement in the midbrain, dorsal pons, and pineal region (*arrows*).

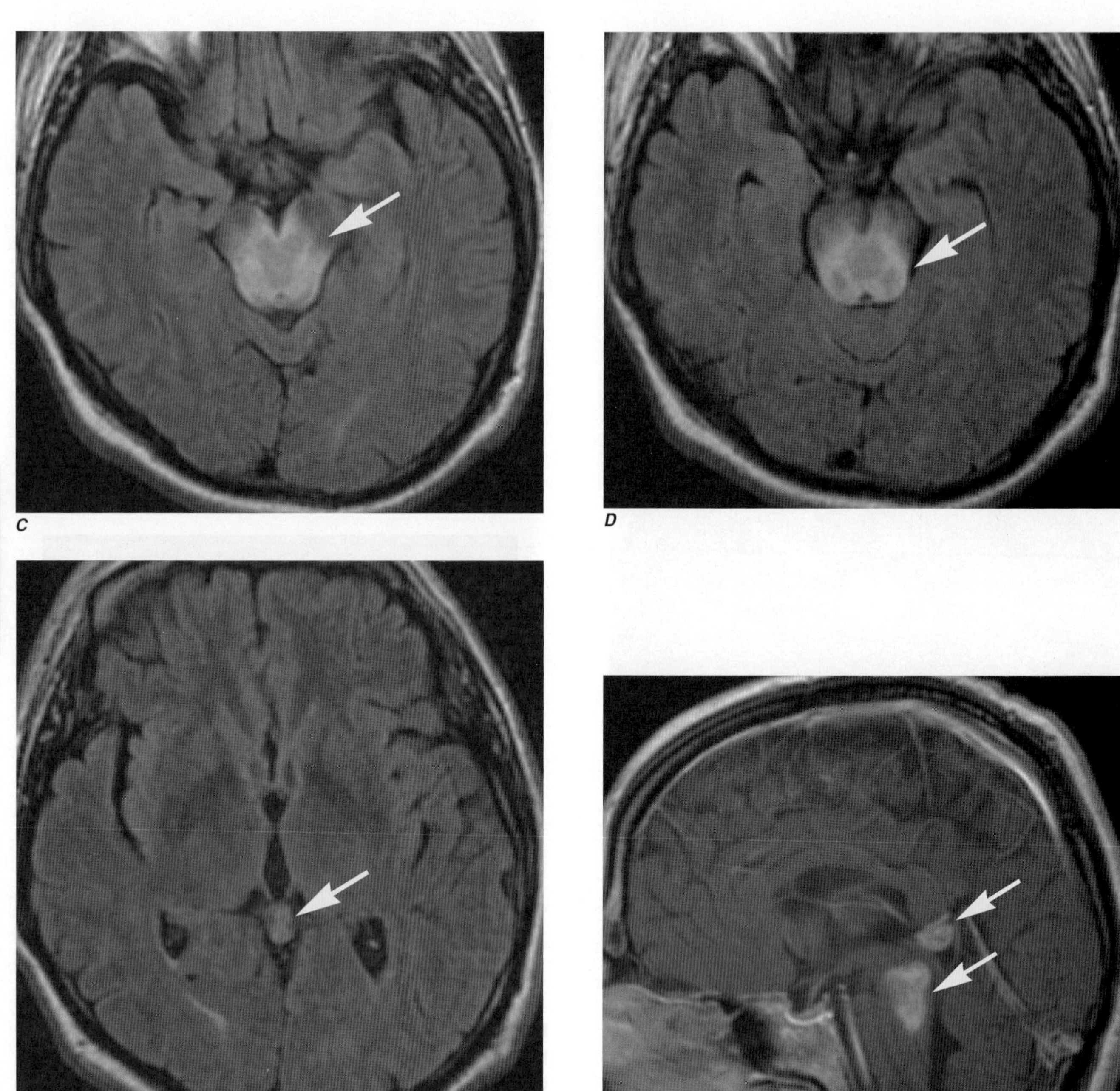

FIGURE 51-13
(*continued*)

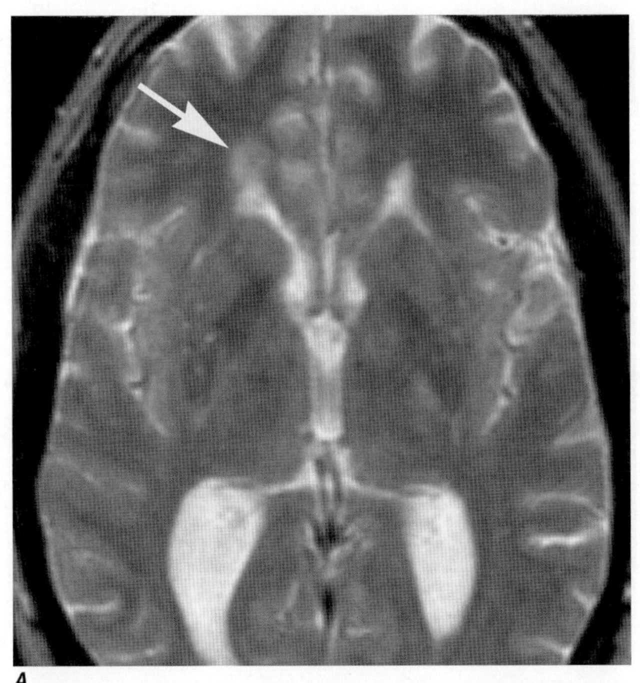

A

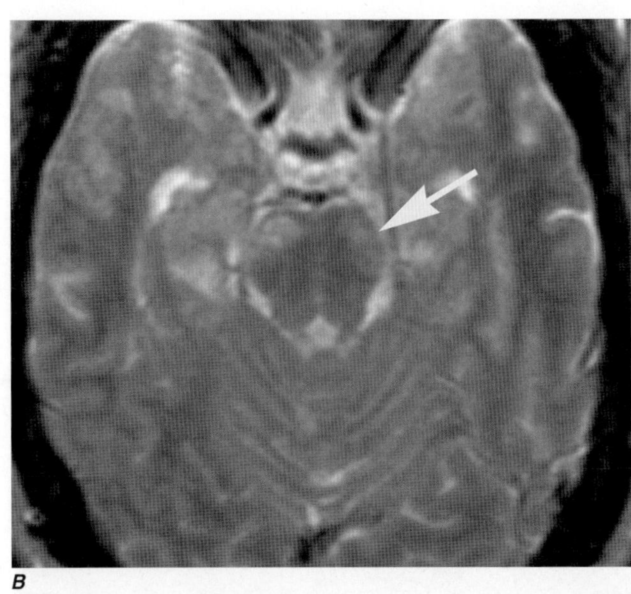

B

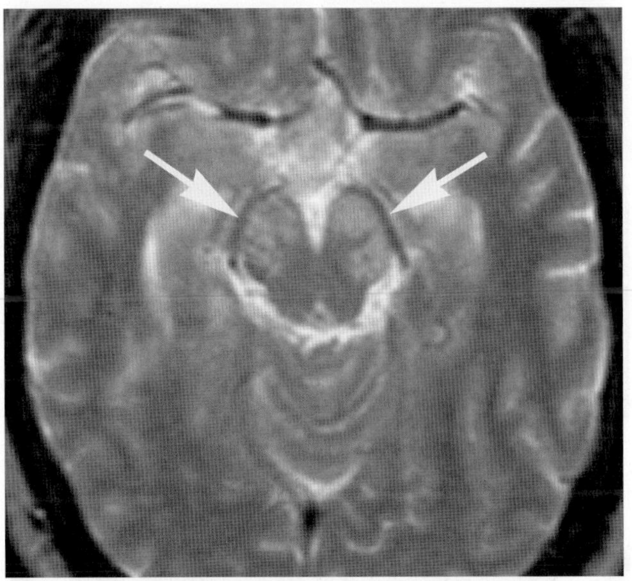

C

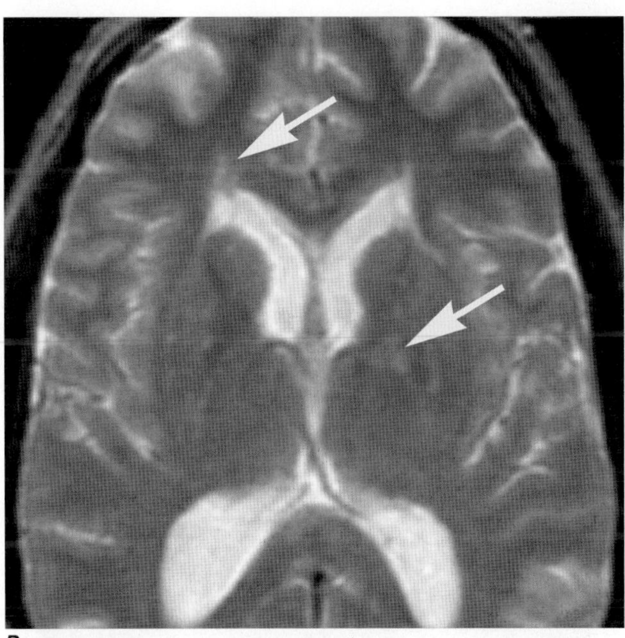

D

FIGURE 51-14
Neurosarcoid
Case IV
Axial T2-weighted images (***A–D***) demonstrate numerous areas of abnormal hyperintensity involving the corpus callosum, left internal capsule and globus pallidus, bilateral cerebral peduncles, bilateral gyrus rectus, right frontal lobe periventricular white matter, and patchy areas in bilateral temporal lobes.

T1-weighted images postgadolinium (***E–H***) demonstrate abnormal enhancement of those areas with high T2 signal.

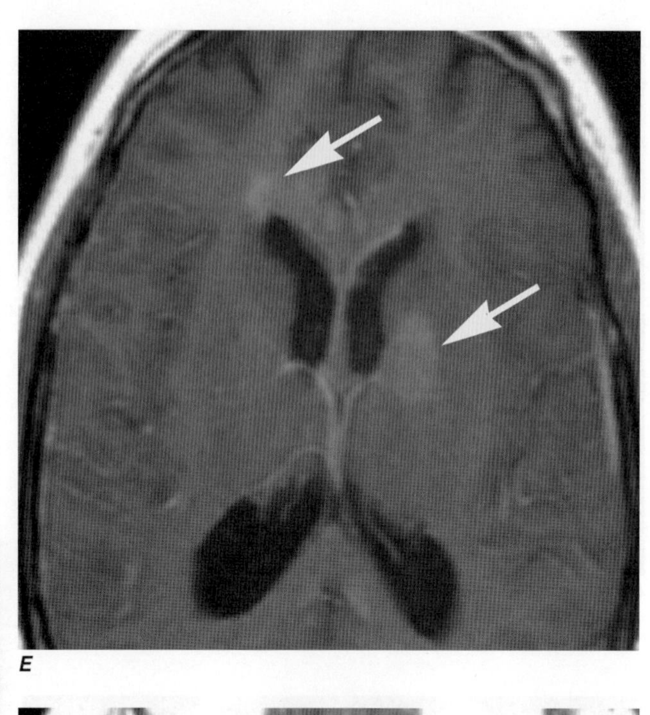

E

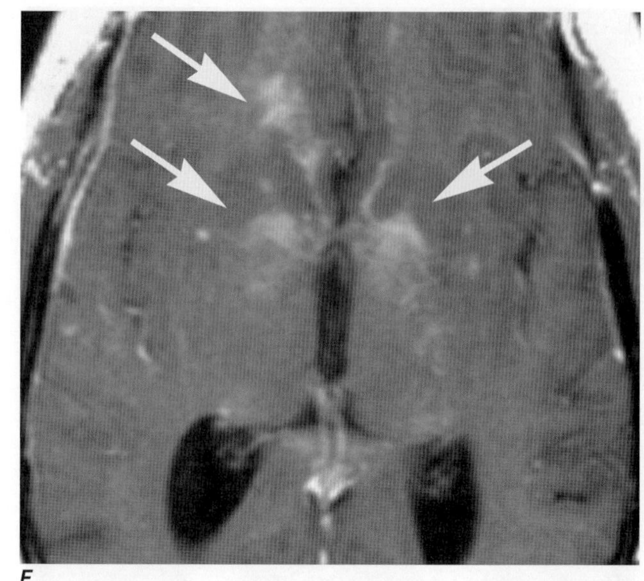

F

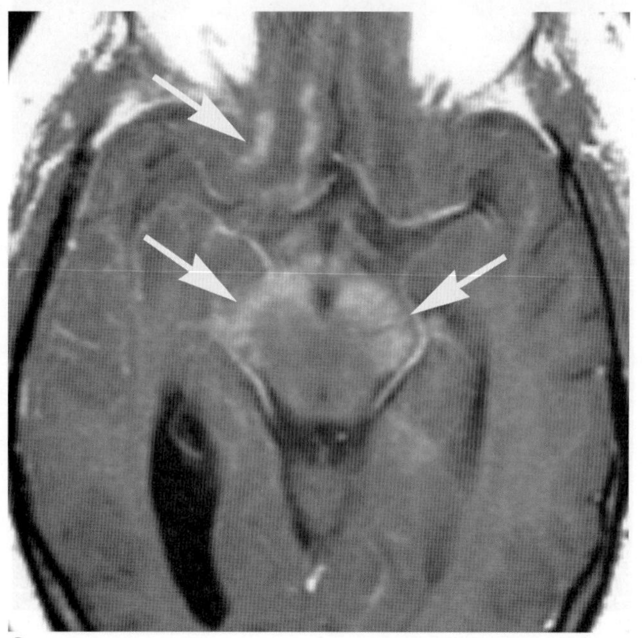

G

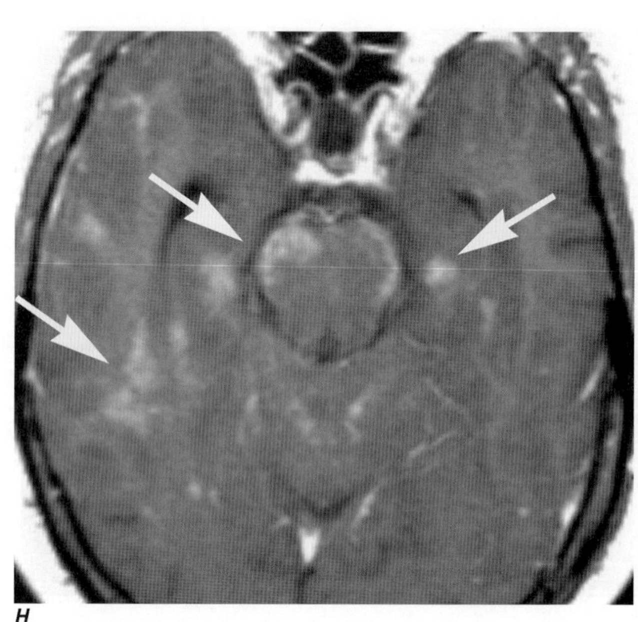

H

FIGURE 51-14
(*continued*)

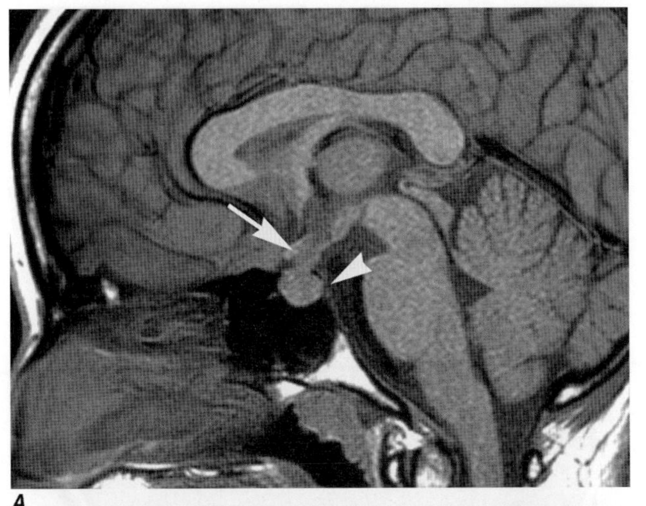

A

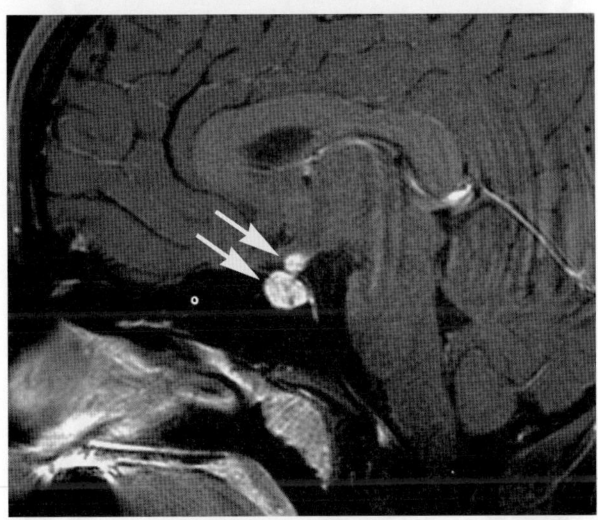

B

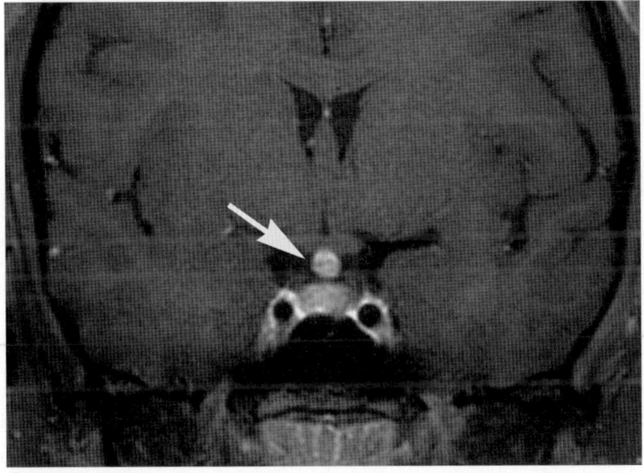

C

FIGURE 51-15

Histiocytosis

Sagittal T1-weighted image (***A***) demonstrates enlargement of the pituitary stalk (*arrow*) and absence of the posterior pituitary intrinsic T1 hyperintensity (*arrowhead*).

Sagittal and coronal T1-weighted images postgadolinium (***B***, ***C***) demonstrate enhancement of the pituitary stalk and infundibulum (*arrows*).

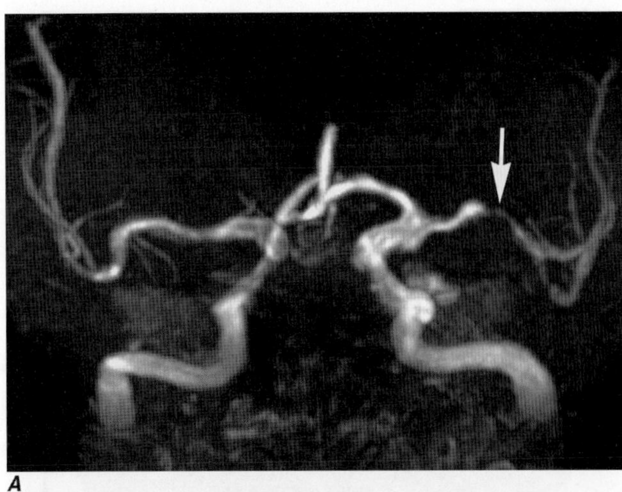

A

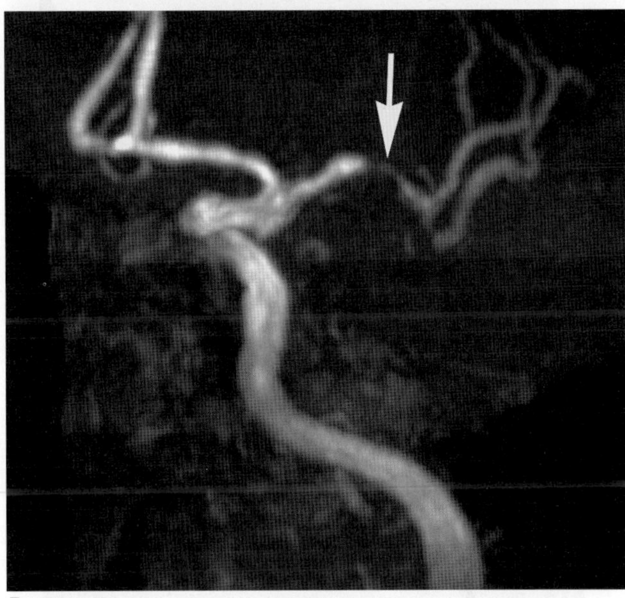

B

FIGURE 51-16

Middle cerebral artery stenosis (Chap. 27)

Time-of-flight (TOF) MR angiography (MRA) (***A***, ***B***) reveals narrowing within the left M1 segment that is likely secondary to atherosclerosis (*arrows*).

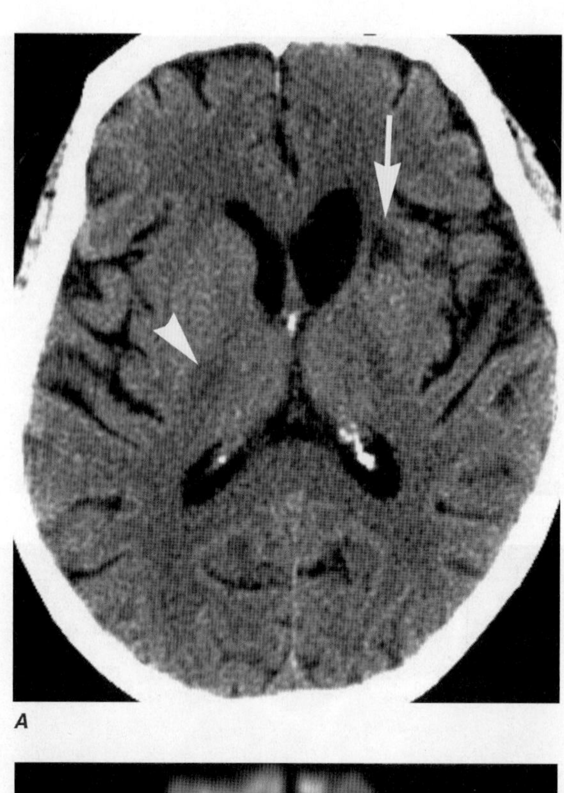

A

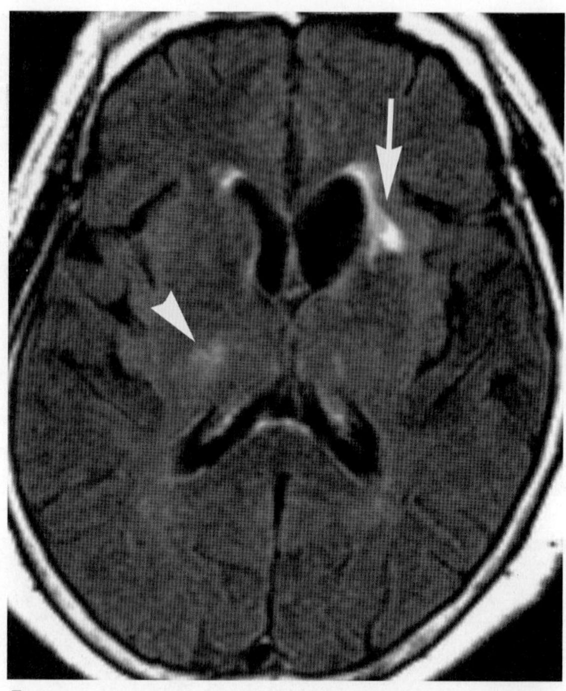

B

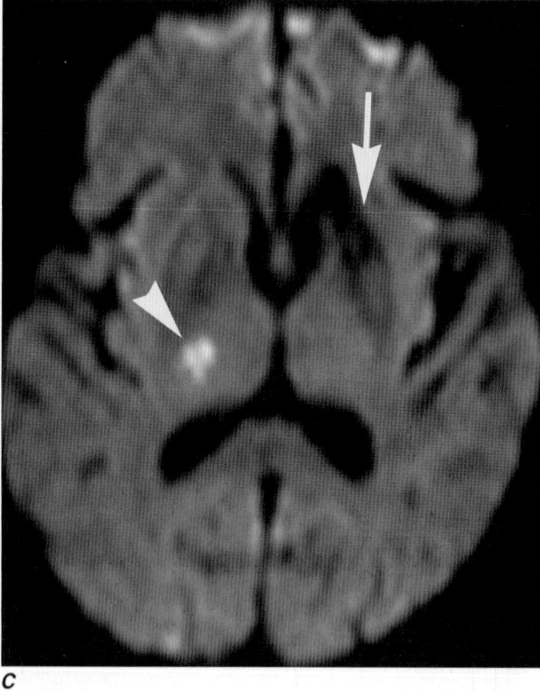

C

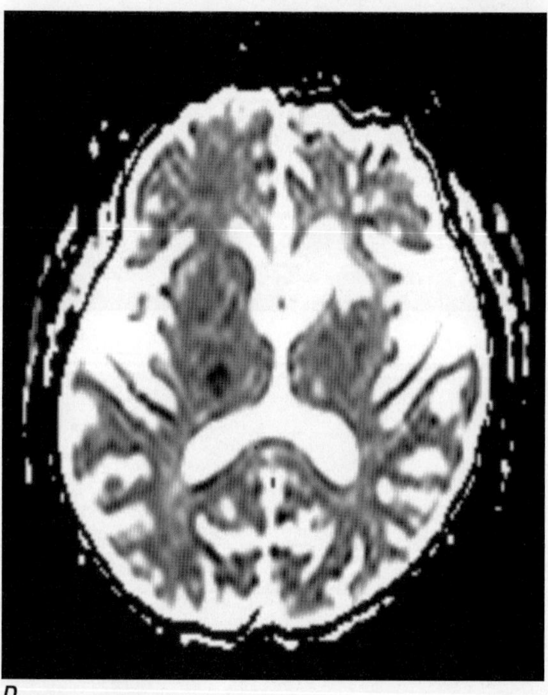

D

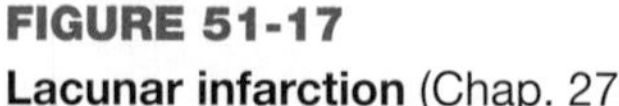

FIGURE 51-17

Lacunar infarction (Chap. 27)

Axial noncontrast CT (***A***) demonstrates abnormal hypodensity involving the left anterior putamen and anterior limb of internal capsule with ex-vacuo dilatation of the adjacent frontal horn of the left lateral ventricle, suggestive of an old infarction (*arrow*). A small area of slight hypodensity is also seen in the posterior limb of the right internal capsule that can correspond to an acute infarct (*arrowhead*).

Axial FLAIR MRI (***B***) demonstrates abnormal high signal involving the left anterior putamen and anterior limb of internal capsule with ex-vacuo dilatation of the adjacent frontal horn of the left lateral ventricle, suggestive of an old infarction (*arrow*). A small area of slight hyperintensity is also seen in the posterior limb of the right internal capsule that can correspond to an acute lacunar infarct (*arrowhead*).

Diffusion-weighted image (***C***) and apparent diffusion coefficient (ADC) map (***D***) demonstrate restricted water motion in the lesion of the posterior limb of the right internal capsule, strongly suggestive for an acute lacunar infarct (*arrowhead*). There is no evidence of restricted diffusion in the old infarct (*arrow*).

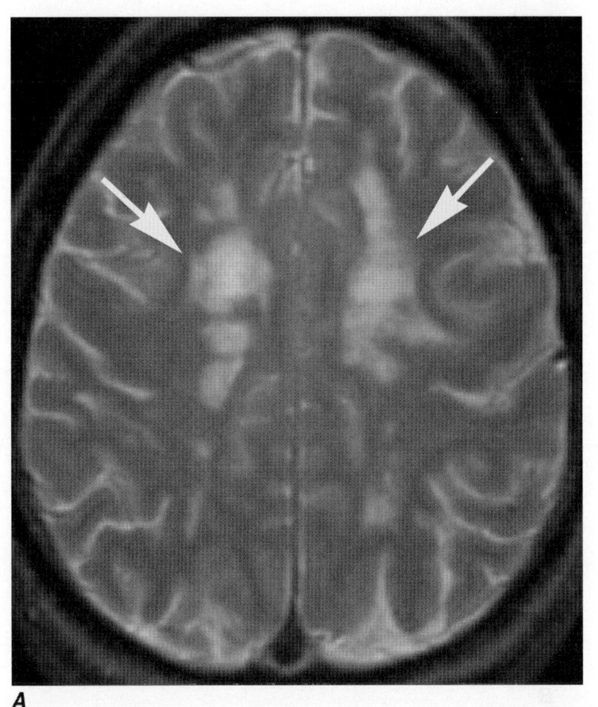

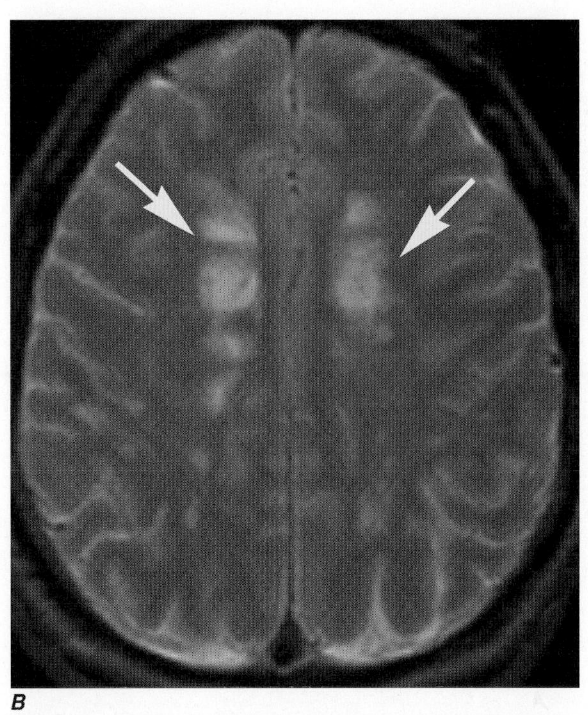

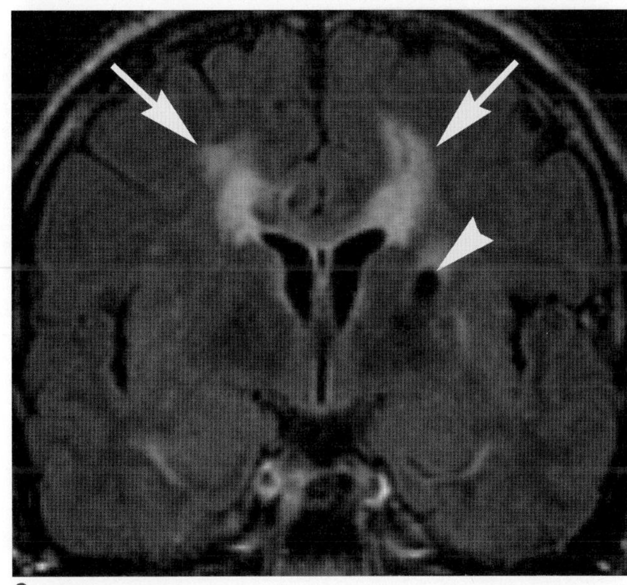

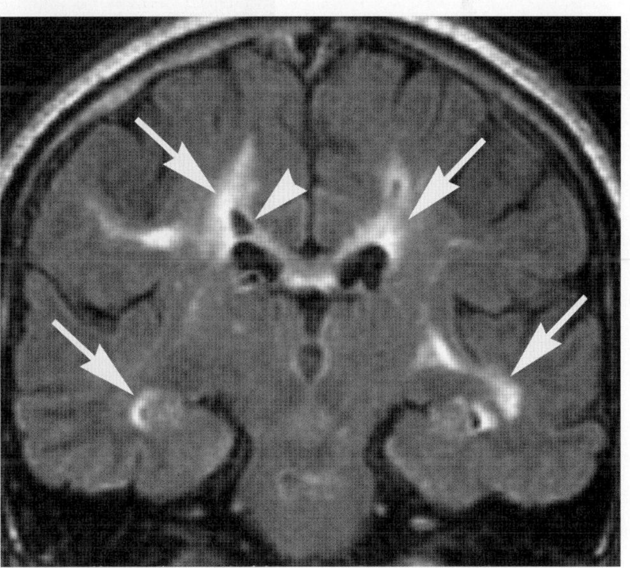

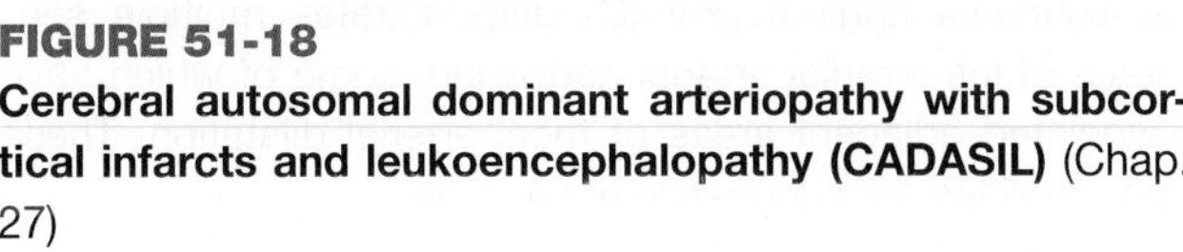

FIGURE 51-18

Cerebral autosomal dominant arteriopathy with subcortical infarcts and leukoencephalopathy (CADASIL) (Chap. 27)

Axial T2-weighted MR images (***A***, ***B***) demonstrate multiple patchy areas of abnormal high signal in the periventricular white matter (*arrows*). Coronal FLAIR MRI (***C***, ***D***) demonstrates multiple patchy areas of abnormal high signal in the periventricular white matter bilaterally, including the temporal lobes (*arrows*). In some of these areas, there are small areas of tissue loss (encephalomalacia) (*arrowheads*).

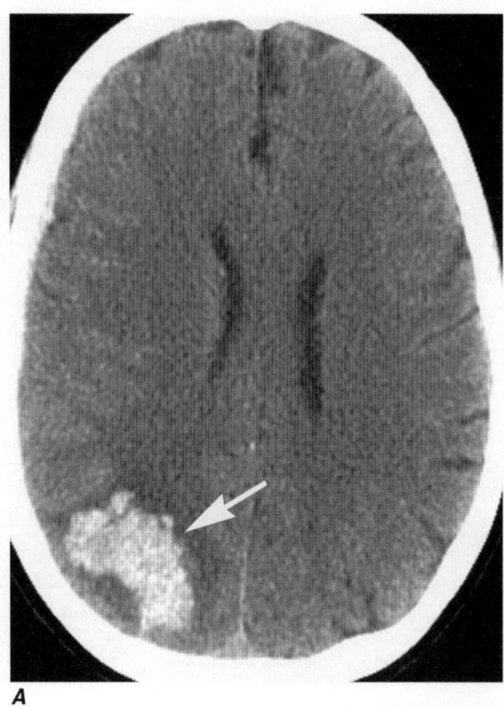
A

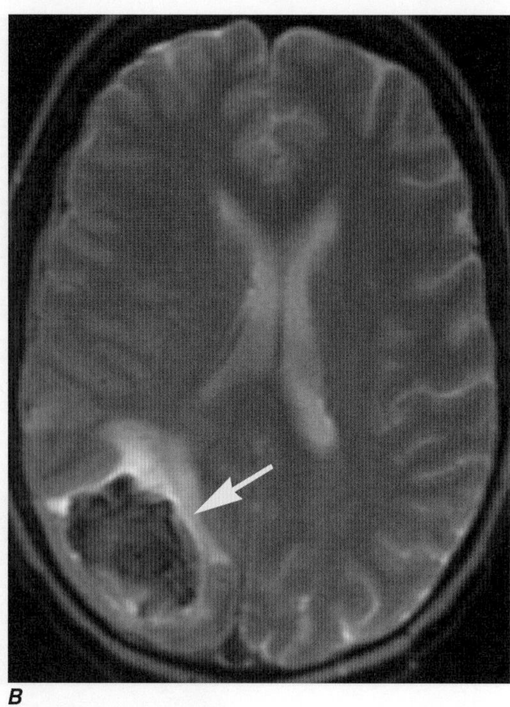
B

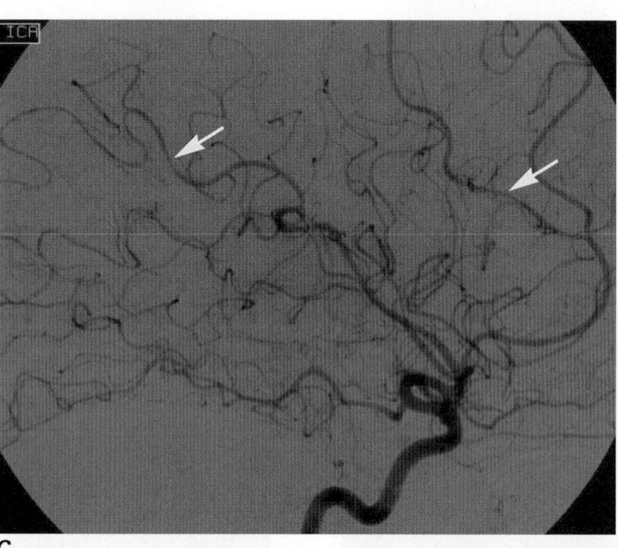

C

FIGURE 51-19

CNS vasculitis (Chap. 27)

Axial noncontrast CT (***A***) demonstrates a large hyperdense intraparenchymal hematoma surrounded by hypodense vasogenic edema in the right parietal lobe.

Axial T2-weighted MRI (***B***) demonstrates a large hypointense intraparenchymal hematoma surrounded by hyperintense vasogenic edema in the right parietal lobe.

Conventional angiography (***C***) demonstrates multiple segments of intracranial arterial narrowing, some of which have associated adjacent areas of focal arterial dilatation. These abnormalities are suggestive of vasculitis.

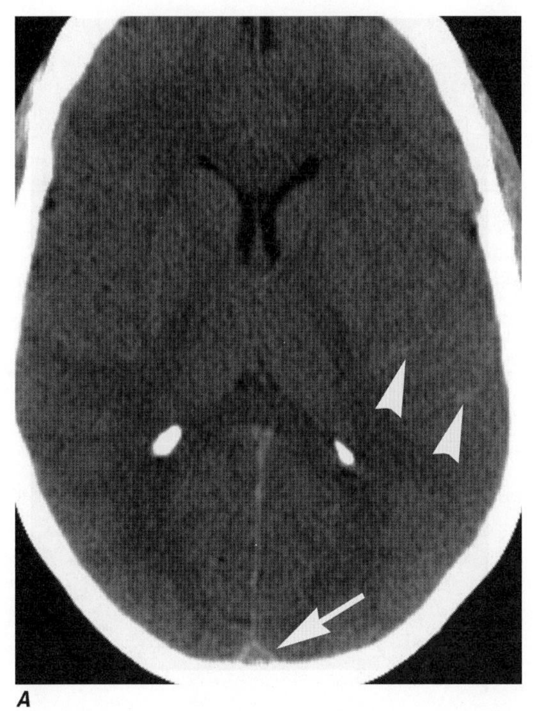

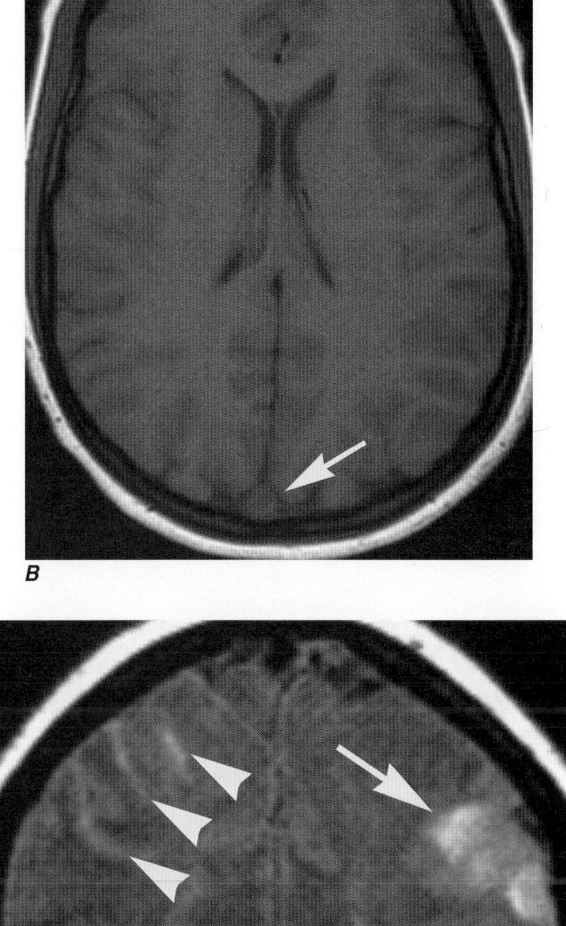

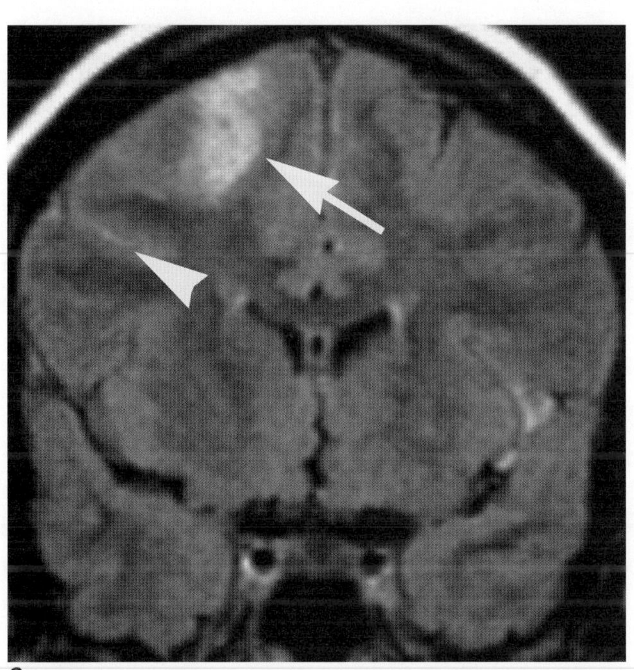

FIGURE 51-20

Superior sagittal sinus thrombosis (Chap. 27)

Noncontrast CT of the head (***A***) demonstrates increased density in the superior sagittal sinus, suggestive of thrombosis (*arrow*), and small linear hyperdensities in some temporal lobe sulci, suggestive of subarachnoid hemorrhage (*arrowheads*).

Axial T1-weighted MRI (***B***) demonstrates absence of flow void in the superior sagittal sinus, suggestive of thrombosis.

Coronal FLAIR images (***C***, ***D***) demonstrate areas of abnormal high signal involving the gray and the subcortical white matter of the right frontal and left parietal lobes, as well as the adjacent sulci. These findings are suggestive of vasogenic edema with subarachnoid hemorrhage (*arrowheads*).

Diffusion-weighted images (***E***, ***F***) and ADC maps (***G***, ***H***) demonstrate restricted diffusion of the abnormal areas on FLAIR, suggestive of infarct.

Phase-contrast venography of the brain (***I***) demonstrates absence of signal in the superior sagittal sinus down to the torcular herophili, and left transverse sinus and jugular vein.

Axial (***J***) and coronal (***K***) T1-weighted images postgadolinium demonstrate a filling defect in the superior sagittal sinus, suggestive of thrombosis.

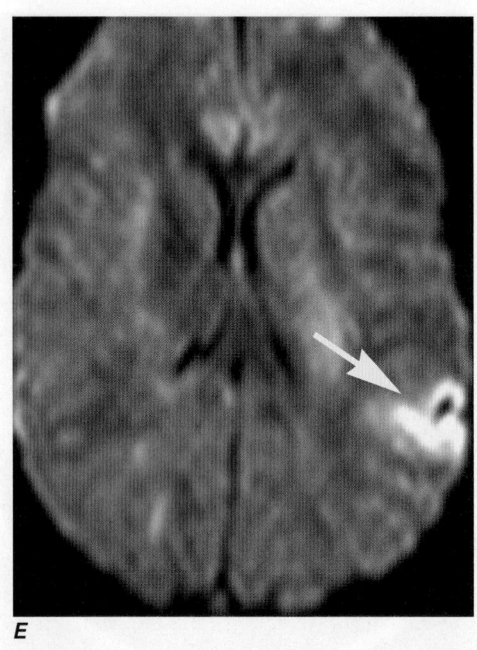
E

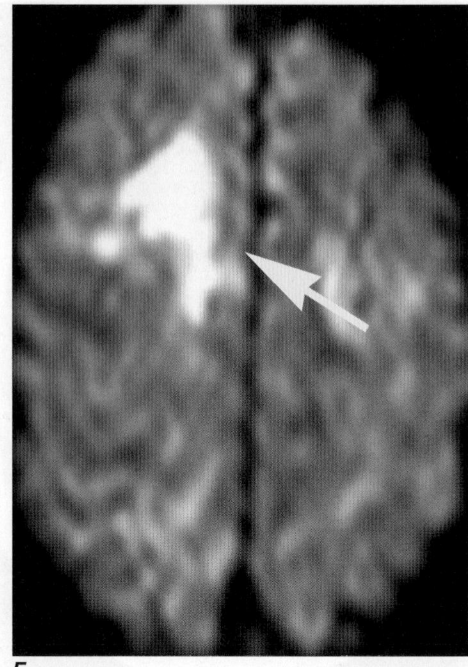
F

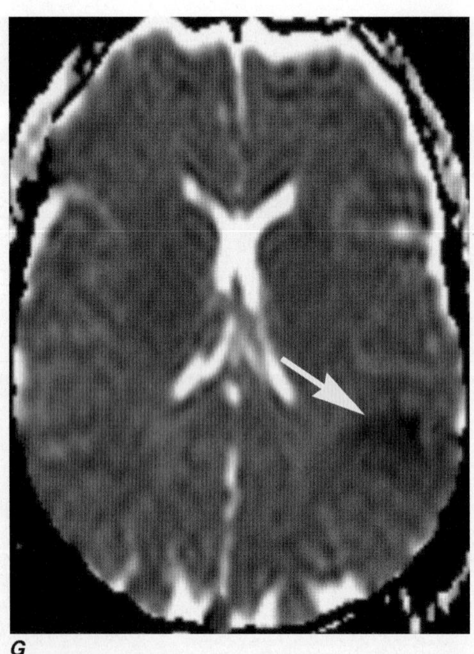
G

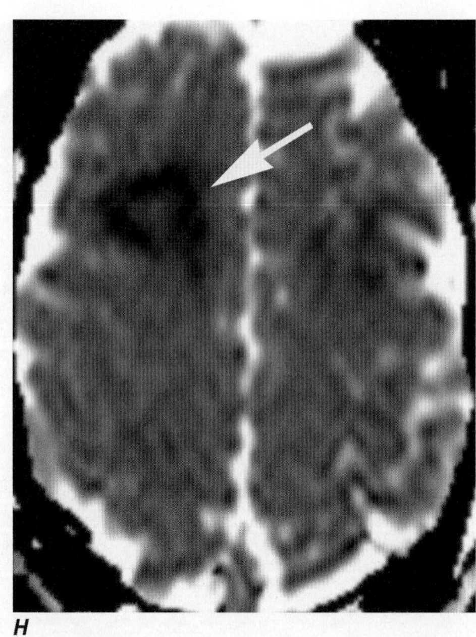
H

FIGURE 51-20
(continued)

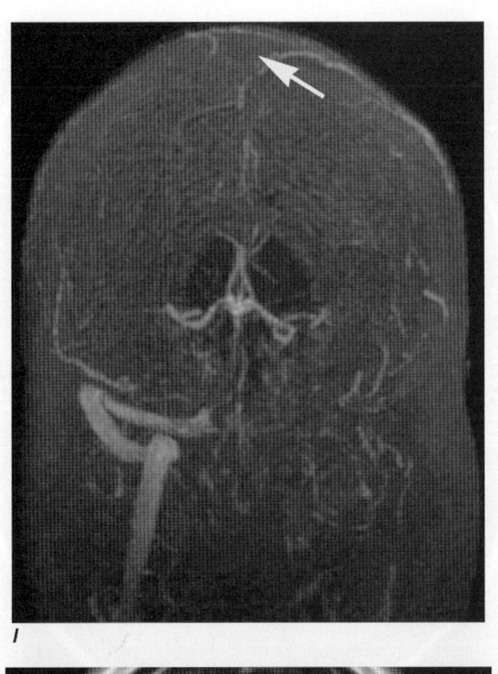

I

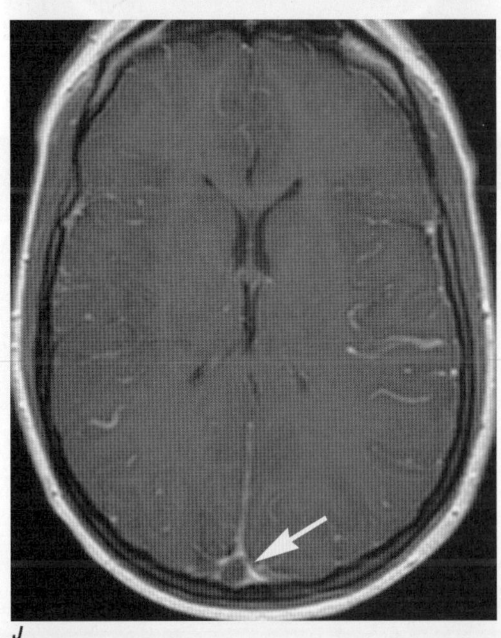

J

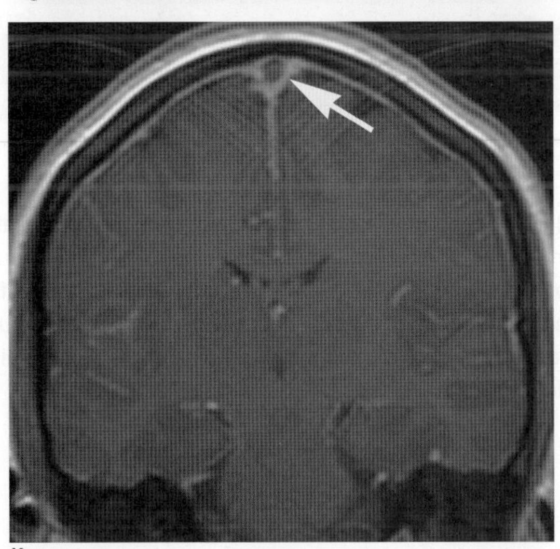

K

FIGURE 51-20
(*continued*)

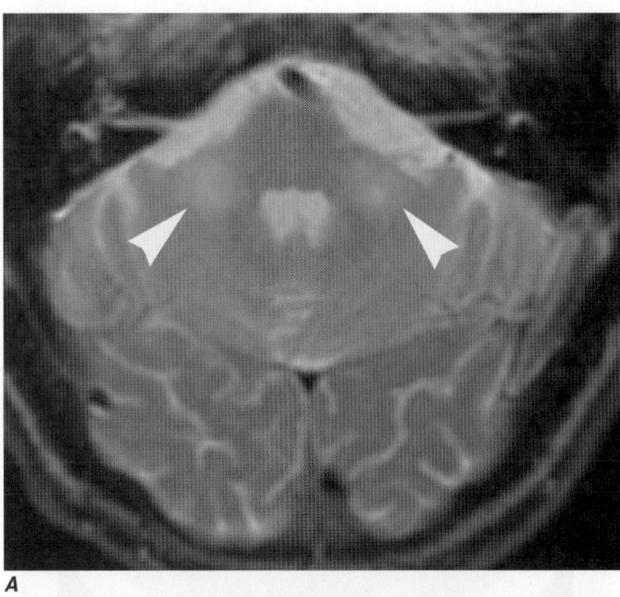

A

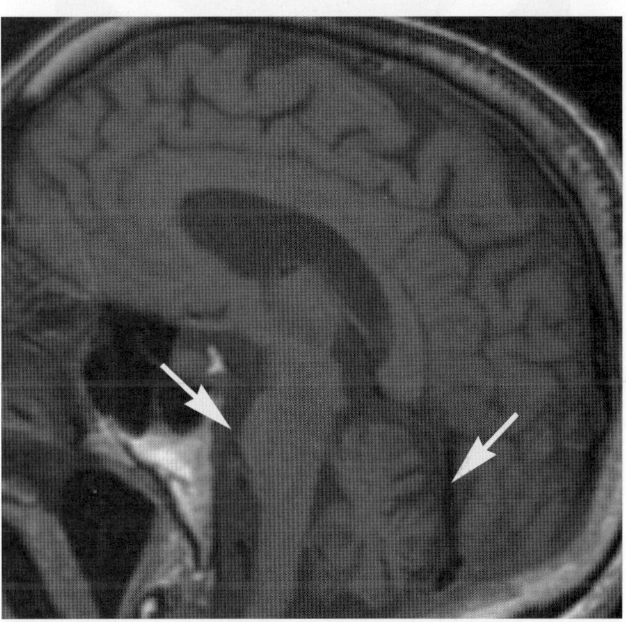

B

FIGURE 51-21
Multiple system atrophy (Chap. 30)
Axial T2-weighted MR image (***A***) reveals symmetric poorly circumscribed abnormal high signal in the middle cerebellar peduncles bilaterally (*arrowheads*).
Sagittal T1-weighted MR image (***B***) demonstrates pontine atrophy and enlarged cerebellar fissures as a result of cerebellar atrophy (*arrows*).

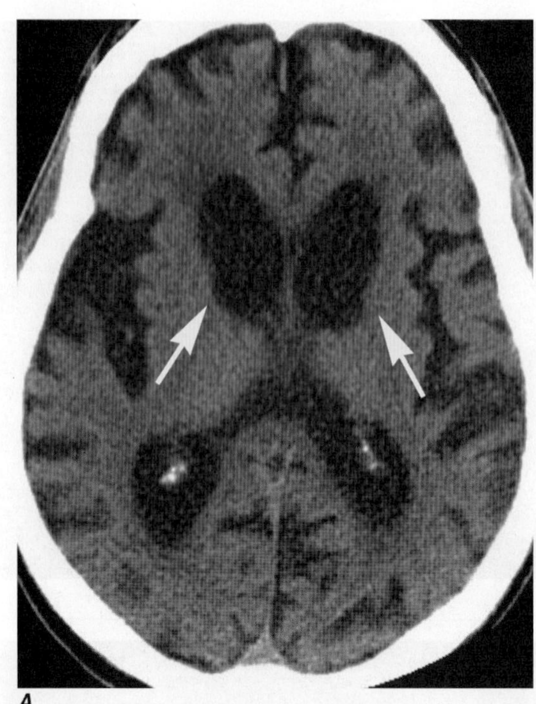

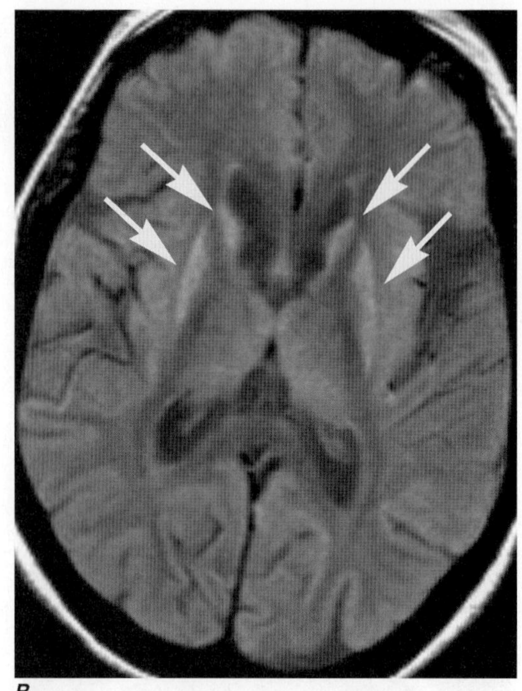

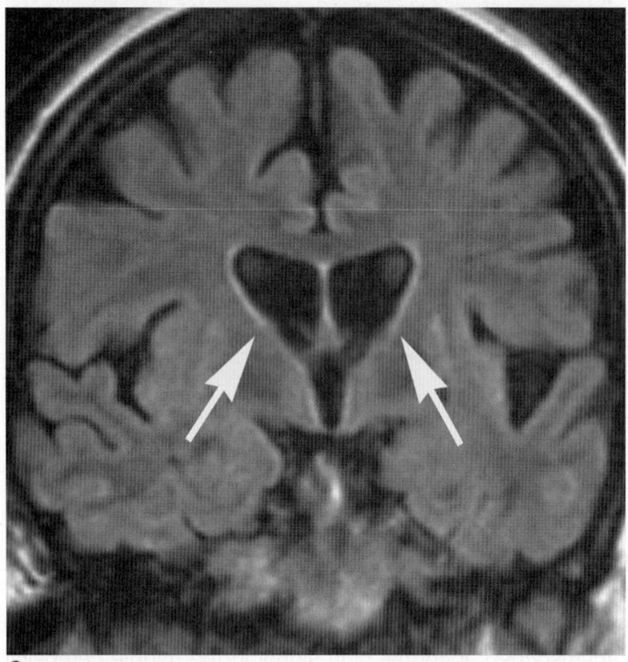

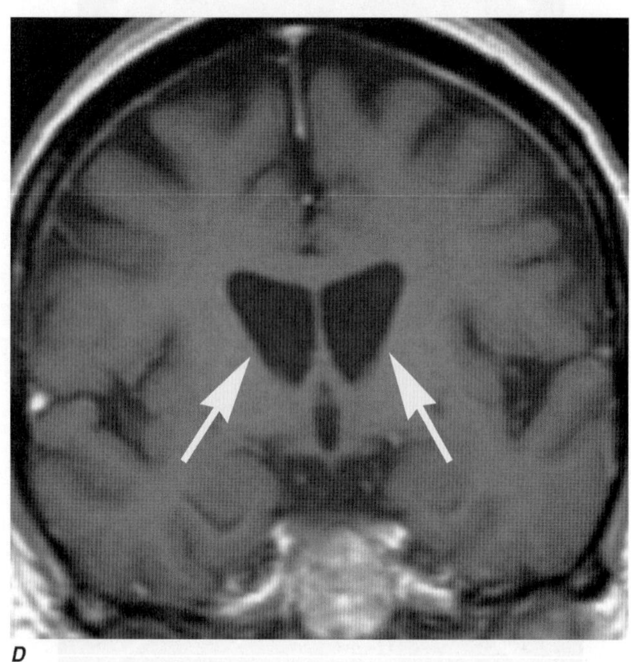

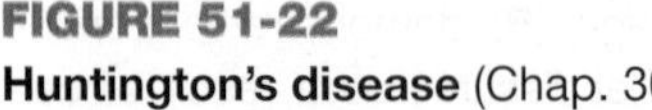

FIGURE 51-22

Huntington's disease (Chap. 30)

Axial noncontrast CT (***A***) demonstrates symmetric bilateral severe atrophy involving the caudate nuclei, putamen, and globus pallidi bilaterally with consequent enlargement of the frontal horns of the lateral ventricles (*arrows*). There is also diffuse prominence of the sulci indicating generalized cortical atrophy.

Axial (***B***) and coronal (***C***) FLAIR images demonstrate bilateral symmetric abnormal high signal in the caudate and putamen. Coronal T1-weighted image (***D***) demonstrates enlarged frontal horns with abnormal configuration. Also note diffusely decreased marrow signal, which could represent anemia or myeloproliferative disease.

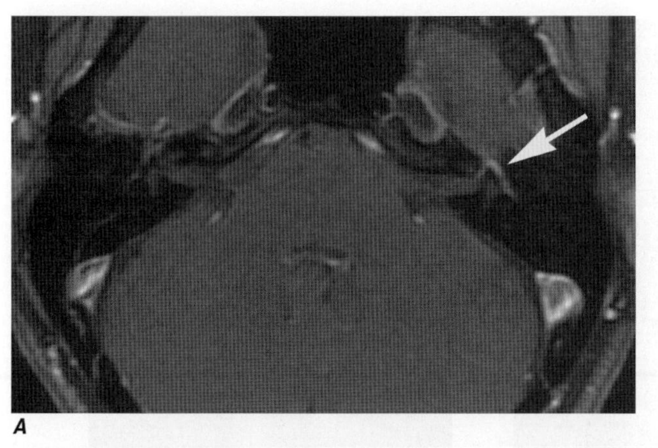

A

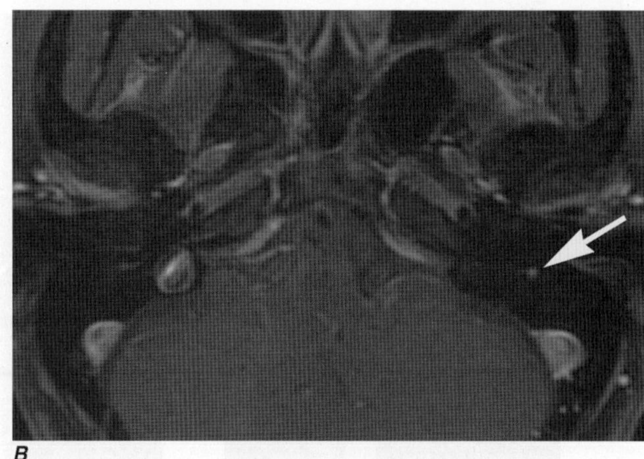

B

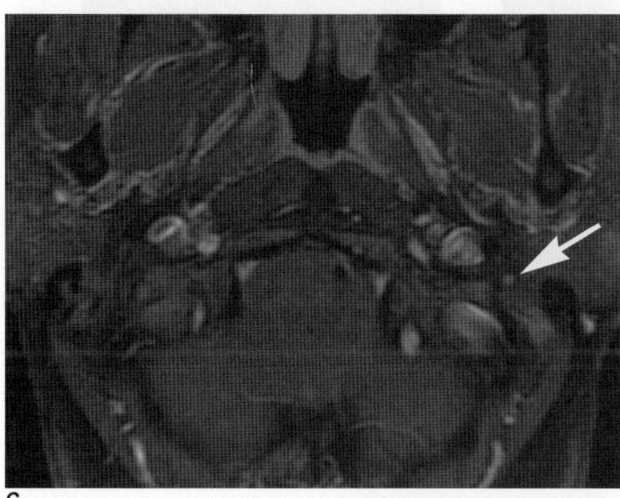

C

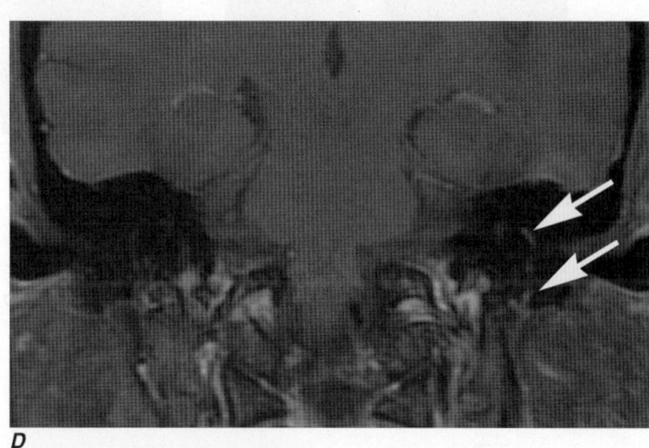

D

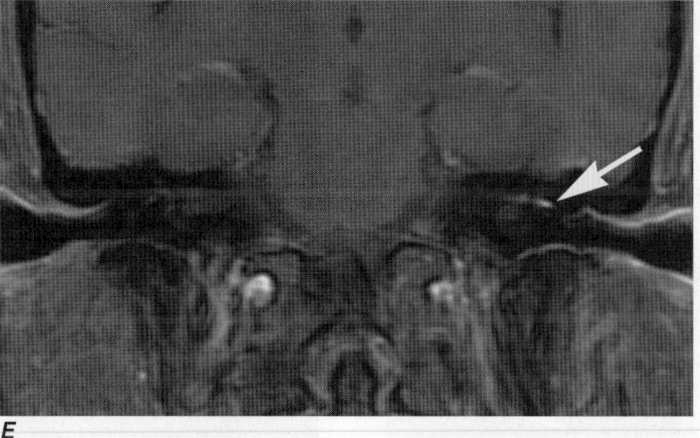

E

FIGURE 51-23

Bell's palsy (Chap. 34)

Axial T1-weighted images postgadolinium with fat suppression (***A–C***) demonstrate diffuse smooth linear enhancement along the left facial nerve, involving the second and third segments (genu, tympanic, and mastoid) within the temporal bone (*arrows*). Note that there is no evidence of a mass lesion. A potential pitfall for facial nerve enhancement in the stylomastoid foramen is the enhancement of the stylomastoid artery that enters the foramen and supplies the tympanic cavity, the tympanic antrum, mastoid cells, and the semicircular canals.

Coronal T1-weighted images postgadolinium with fat suppression (***D***, ***E***) demonstrate the course of the enhancing facial nerve (*arrows*). Although these findings are highly suggestive of Bell's palsy, the diagnosis is established on clinical grounds.

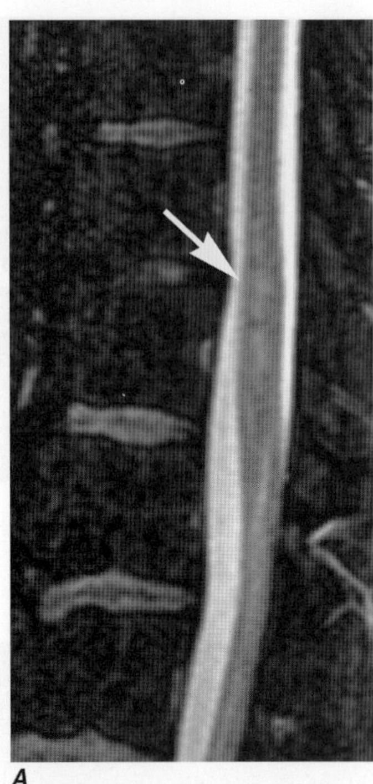

A

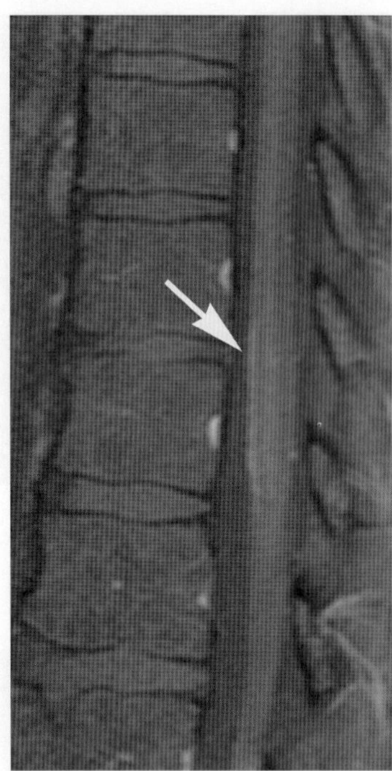

B

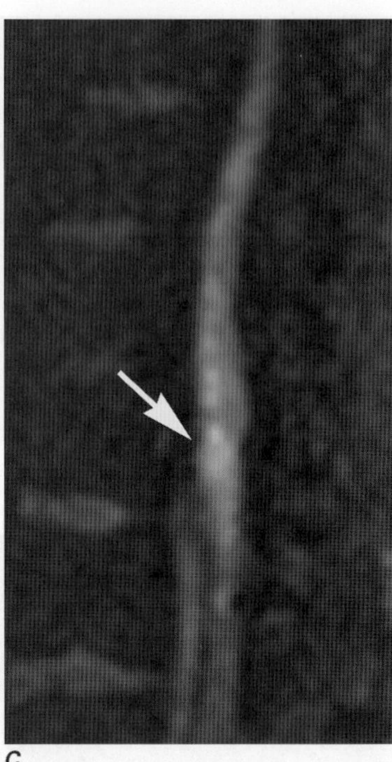

C

FIGURE 51-24

Spinal cord infarction (Chap. 35)

Sagittal T2-weighted MR image of the lumbar spine (***A***) demonstrates poorly defined areas of abnormal high signal in the conus medullaris and mild cord expansion (*arrow*). T1-weighted MR image of the lumbar spine postgadolinium (***B***) demonstrates mild enhancement (*arrow*). Sagittal diffusion-weighted MR image of the lumbar spine (***C***) demonstrates restricted diffusion (*arrow*) in the areas of abnormal high signal on the T2-weighted image (***A***).

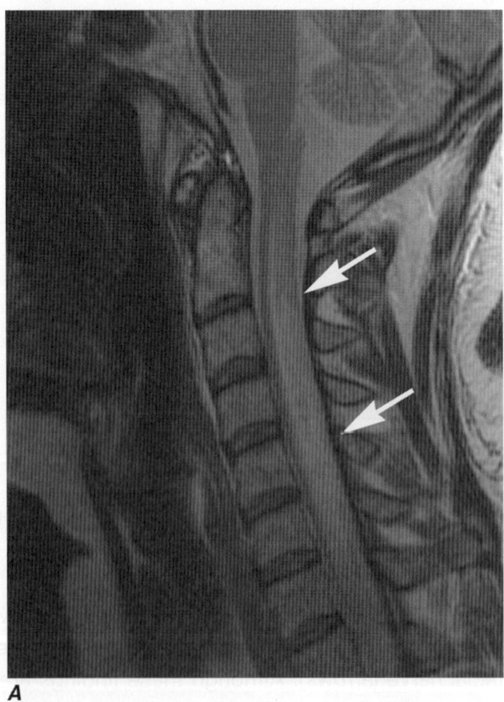

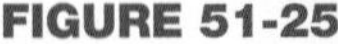

A

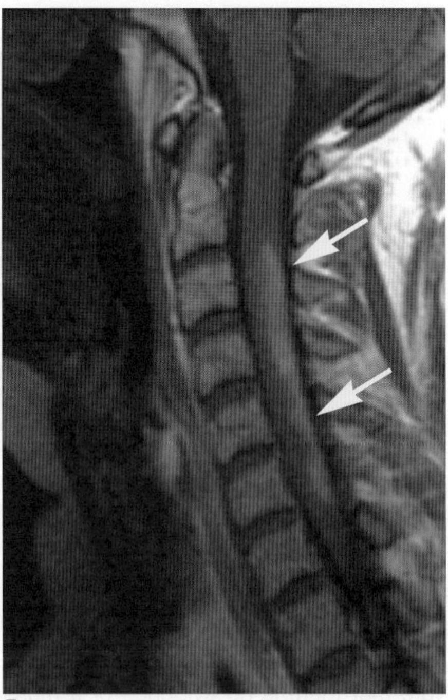

B

FIGURE 51-25

Acute transverse myelitis (Chap. 35)

Sagittal T2-weighted MR image (***A***) demonstrates abnormal high signal in the cervical cord extending from C1 to T1 with associated cord expansion (*arrows*). Sagittal T1-weighted MR image postgadolinium (***B***) demonstrates abnormal enhancement in the posterior half of the cord from C2 to T1 (*arrows*).

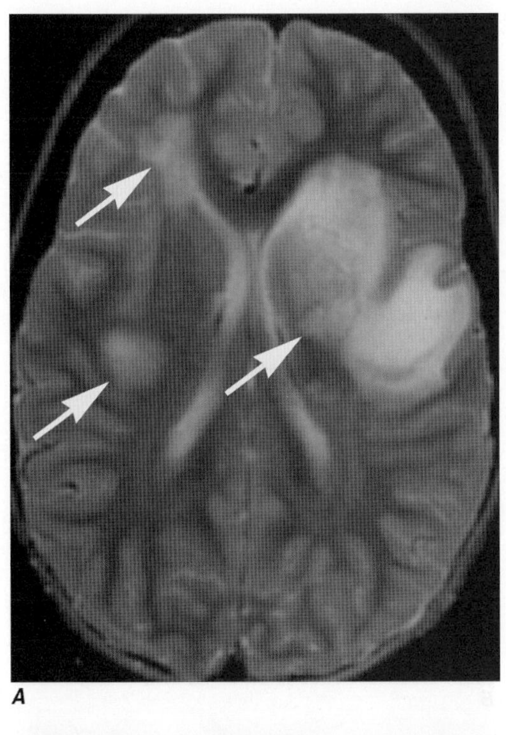

A

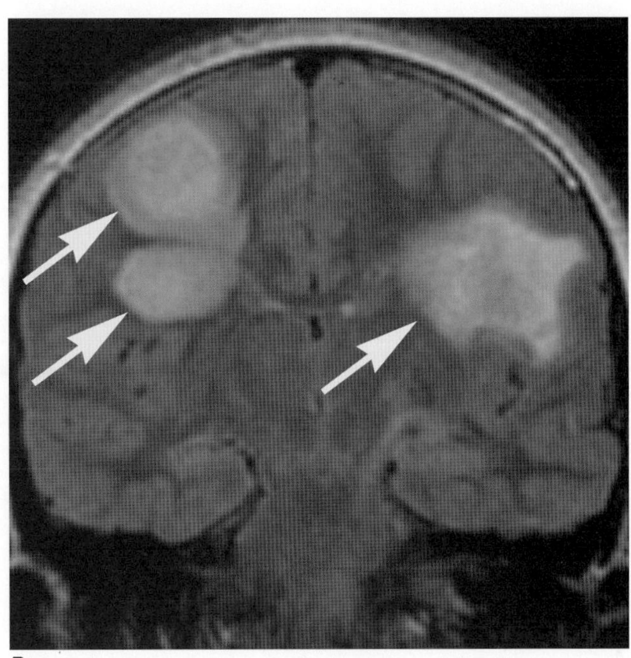

B

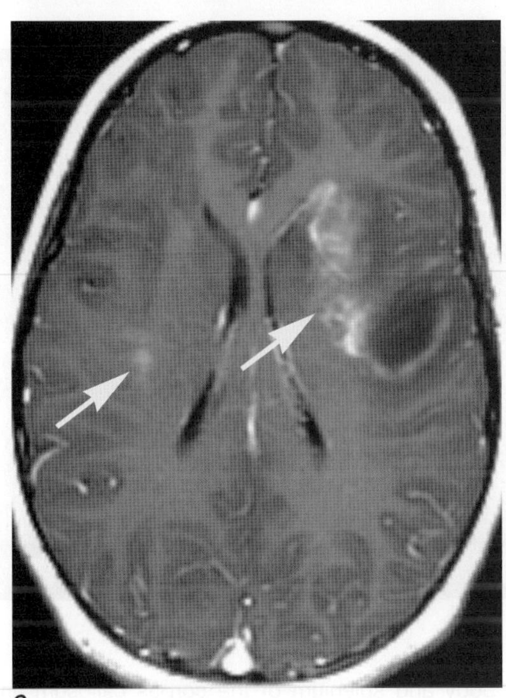

C

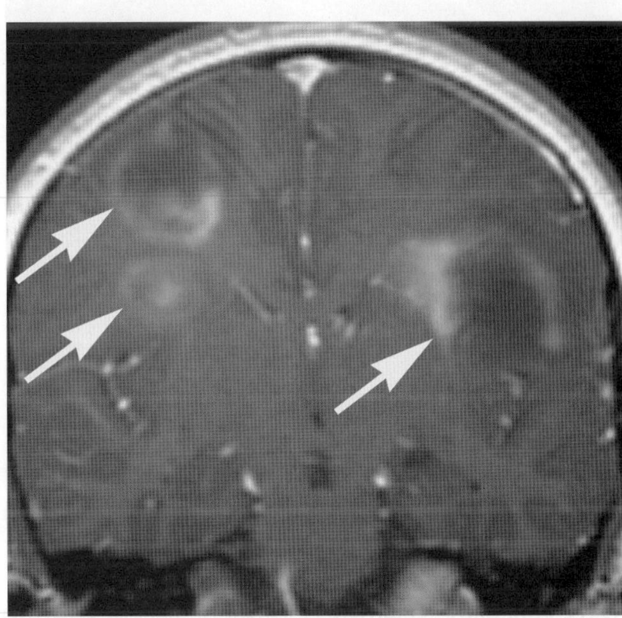

D

FIGURE 51-26

Acute disseminated encephalomyelitis (ADEM) (Chap. 39) Axial T2-weighted (***A***) and coronal FLAIR (***B***) images demonstrate abnormal areas of high signal involving predominantly the subcortical white matter of the frontal lobe bilaterally, and left caudate head. Following administration of gadolinium, corresponding axial (***C***) and coronal (***D***) T1-weighted images demonstrate irregular enhancement consistent with blood-brain barrier breakdown and inflammation; some lesions show incomplete rim enhancement, typical for demyelination.

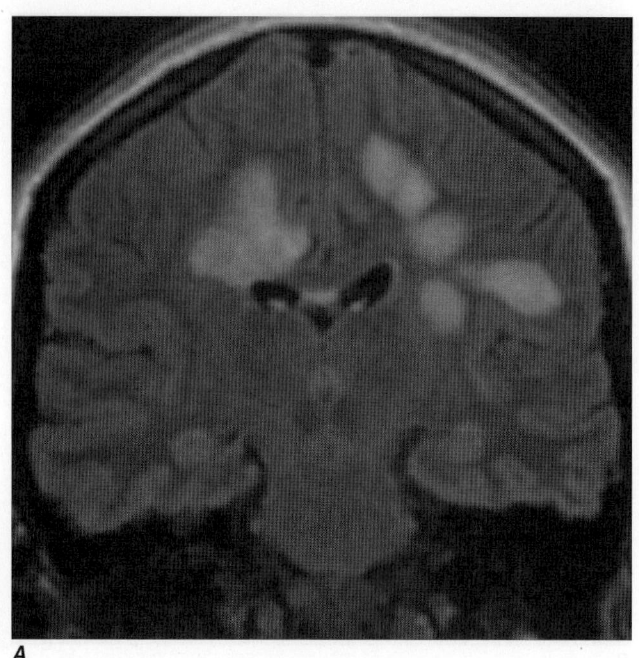

A

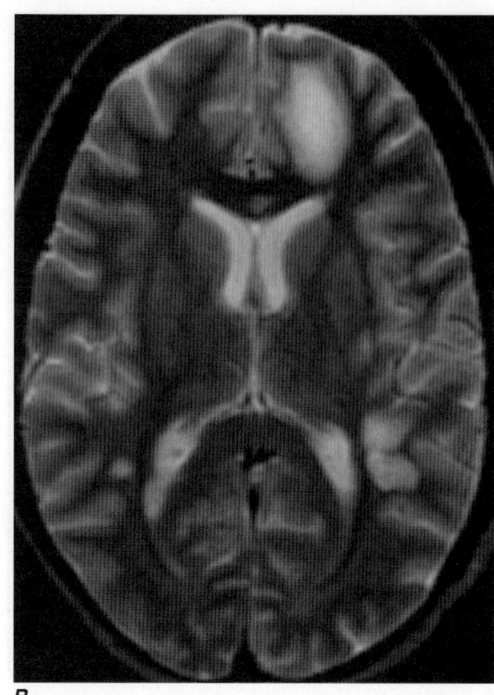

B

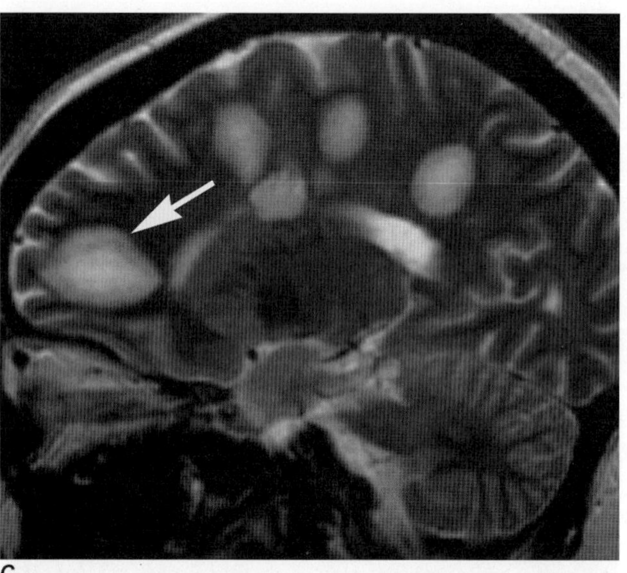

C

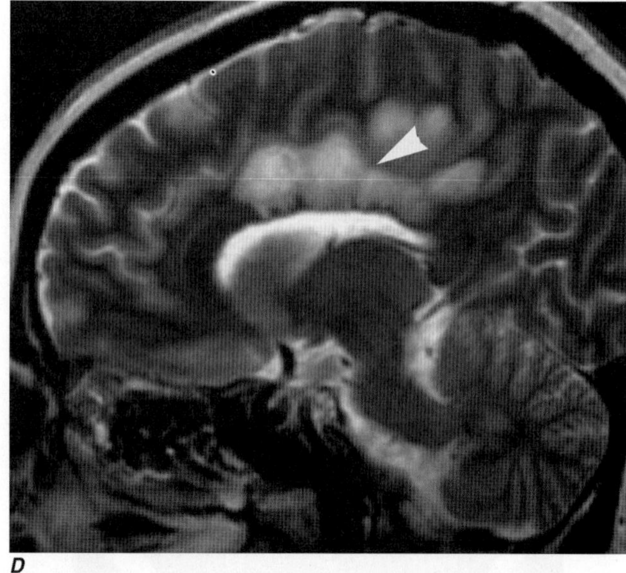

D

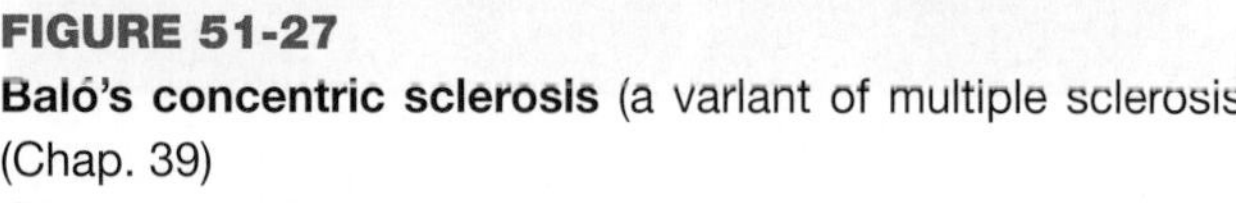

FIGURE 51-27

Baló's concentric sclerosis (a variant of multiple sclerosis) (Chap. 39)

Coronal FLAIR MRI (***A***) demonstrates multiple areas of abnormal high signal in the supratentorial white matter bilaterally. The lesions are ovoid in shape, perpendicular to the orientation of the lateral ventricles, and with little mass effect. Axial (***B***) and sagittal (***C–E***) T2-weighted MR images demonstrate multiple areas of abnormal high signal in the supratentorial white matter bilaterally, as well as the involvement of the body and splenium of the corpus callosum and the callosal-septal interface (*arrowhead*). Some of the lesions reveal concentric layers, typical of Baló's concentric sclerosis (*arrows*).

Sagittal (***F***) and axial (***G***, ***H***) T1-weighted MR images post-gadolinium demonstrate abnormal enhancement of all lesions with some of the lesions demonstrating concentric ring enhancement (*arrows*).

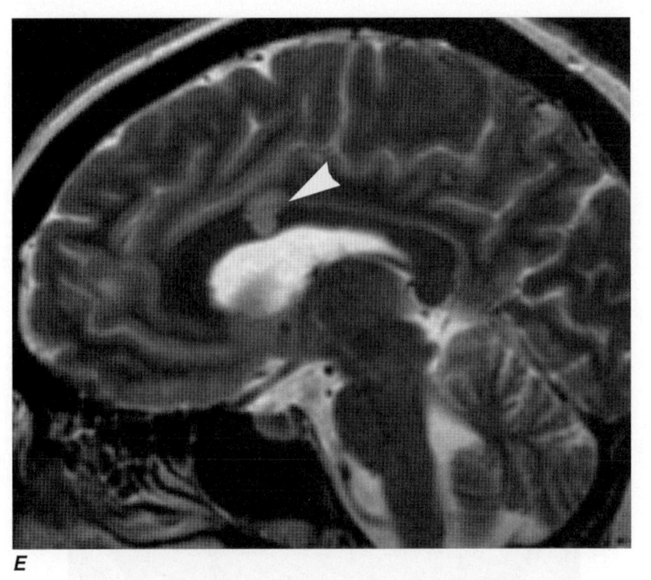
E

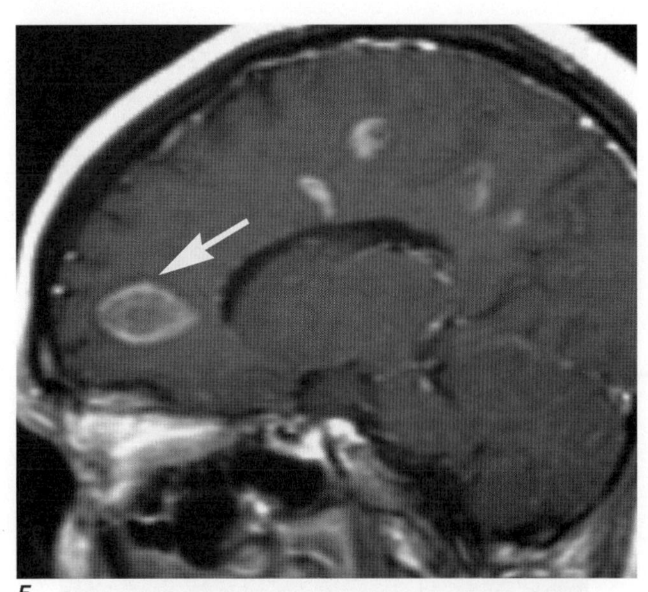
F

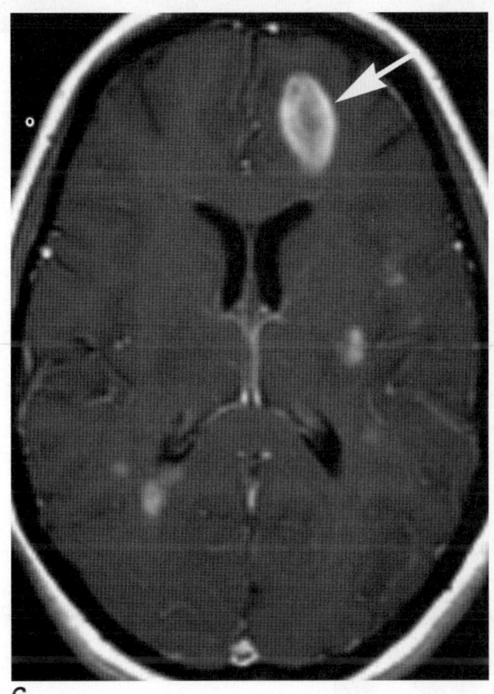
G

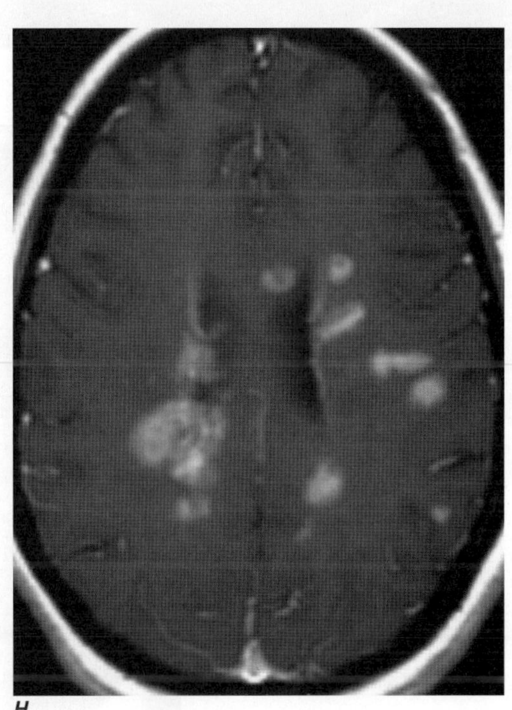
H

FIGURE 51-27
(*continued*)

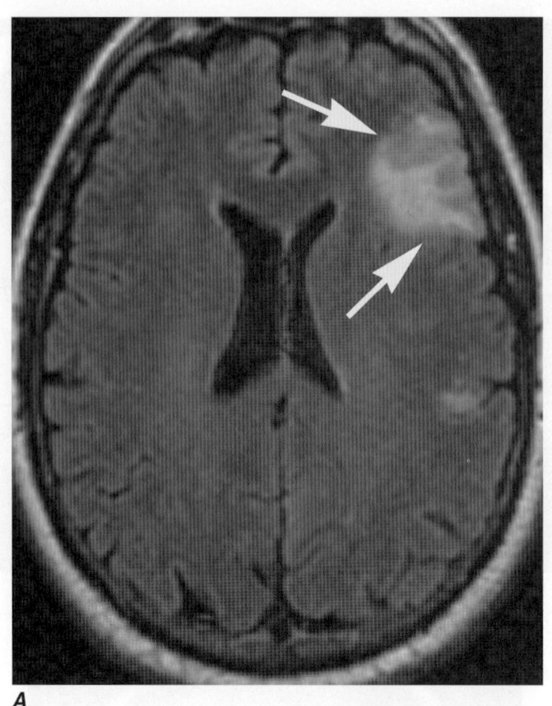
A

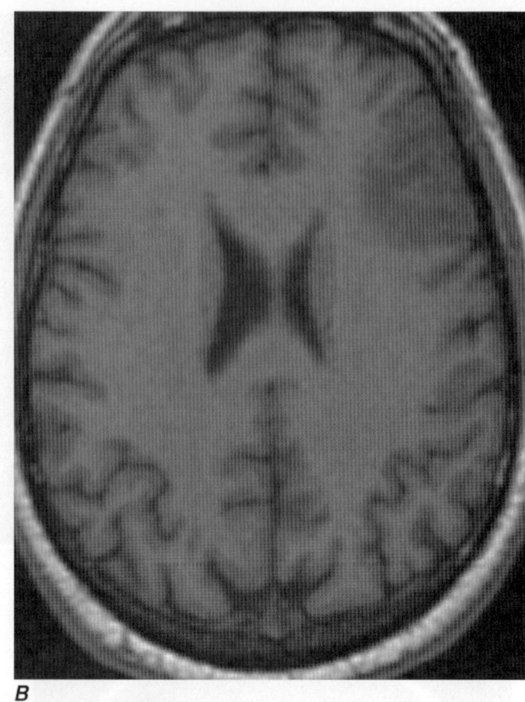
B

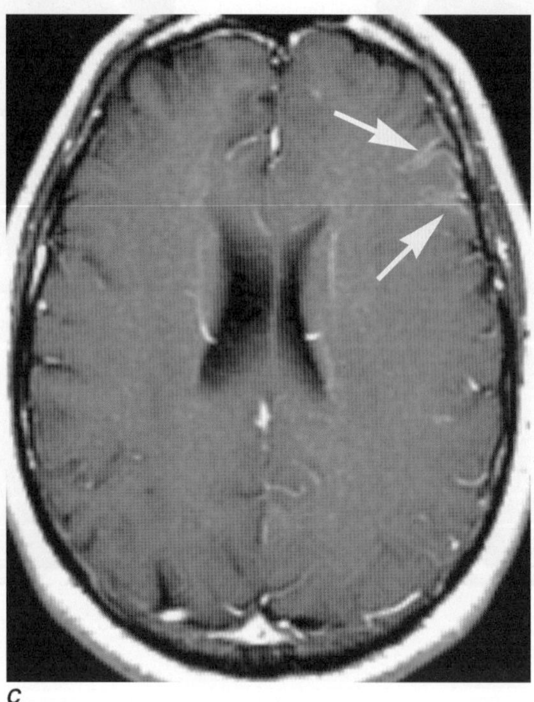
C

FIGURE 51-28

Hashimoto's encephalopathy (Chap. 40)
Axial FLAIR (***A***) demonstrates focal area of abnormal high signal involving the gray and white matter in the left frontal lobe. There is also a small area of abnormal high signal in the precentral gyrus.

Axial T1-weighted images (***B***, ***C***) pre- and postgadolinium demonstrate cortical/pial enhancement in the region of high signal on FLAIR.

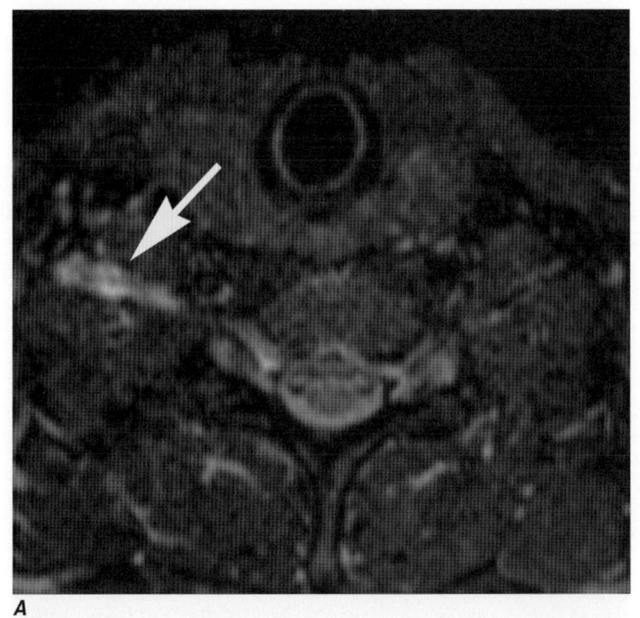

A

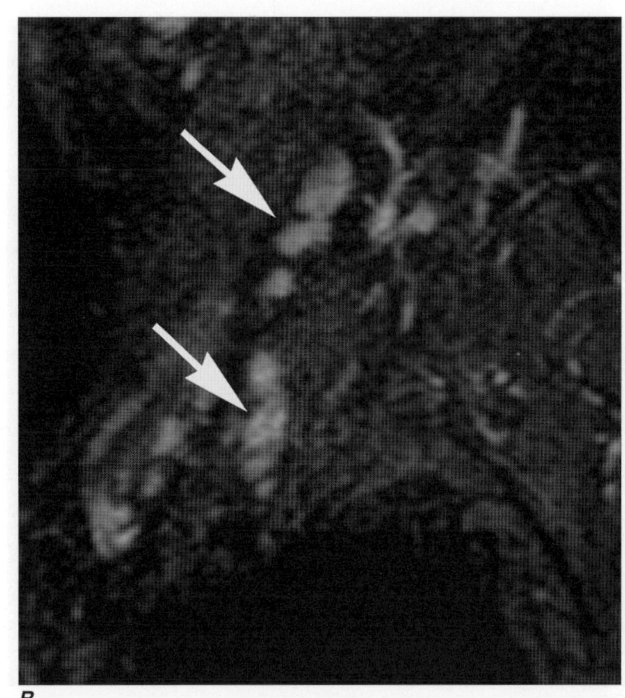

B

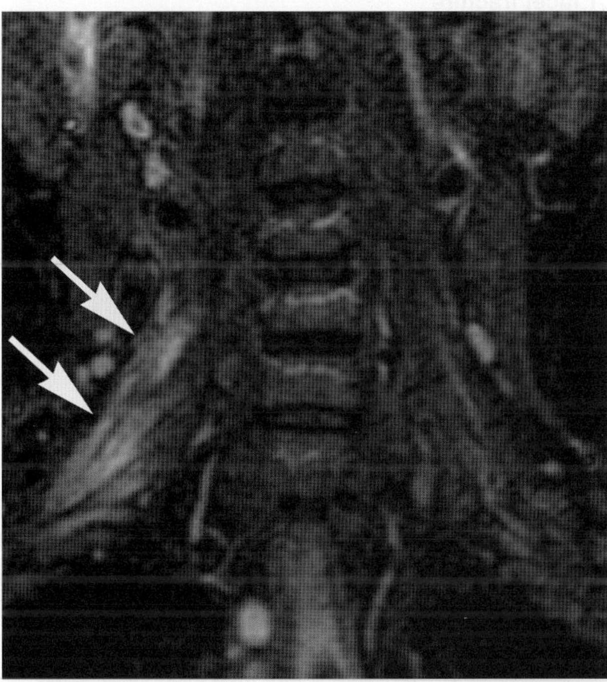

C

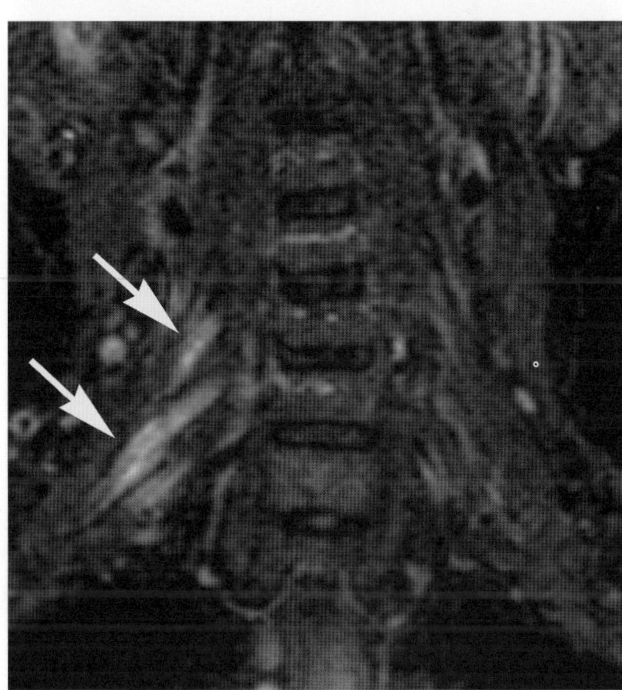

D

FIGURE 51-29
Brachial plexopathy (Chap. 45)
Axial (***A***), sagittal (***B***), and coronal (***C***, ***D***) short tau inversion recovery (STIR) MR images demonstrate abnormal enlargement and abnormal high signal involving the right C6, C7, and C8 nerve roots, and the trunks and divisions that originate from these roots *(arrows)*. Diffusion-weighted MR imaging (***E***) demonstrates abnormal reduced diffusion within the right C6, C7, and C8 nerve roots and their corresponding trunks and divisions (*arrow*). These findings are compatible with radiation-induced brachial plexopathy.

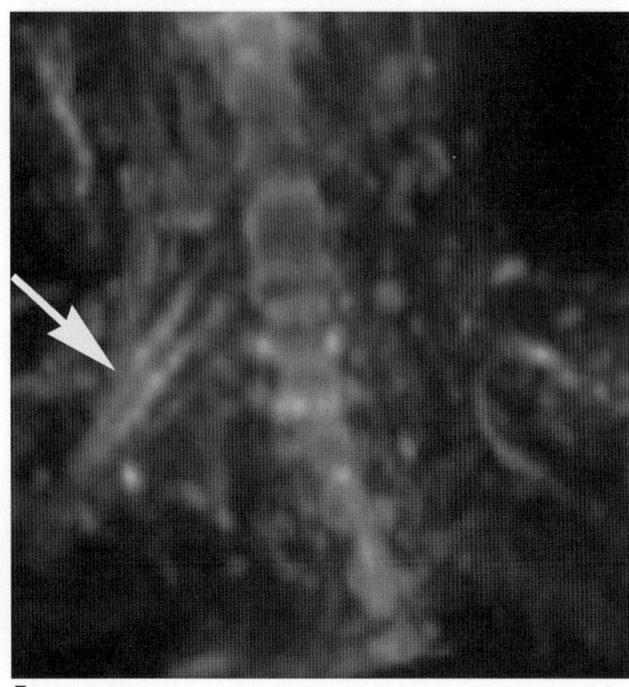

FIGURE 51-29
(*continued*)

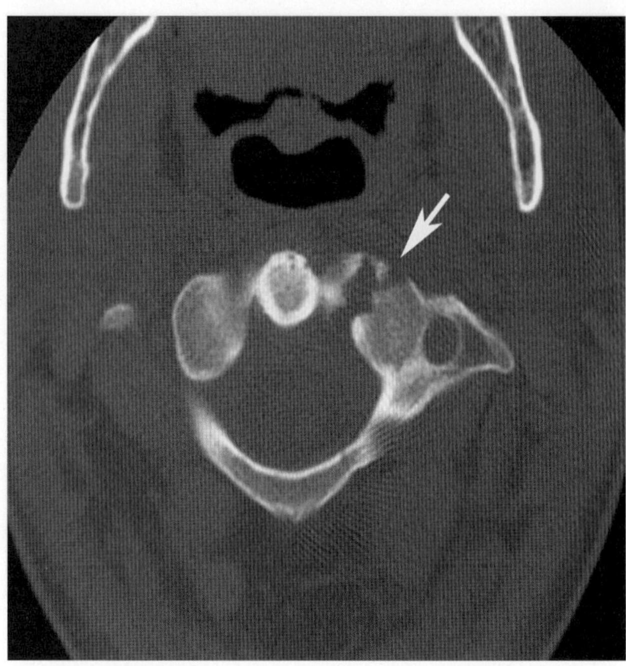

FIGURE 51-31
CT facet fracture
Axial CT demonstrates fracture line along the C2 facet (*arrow*).

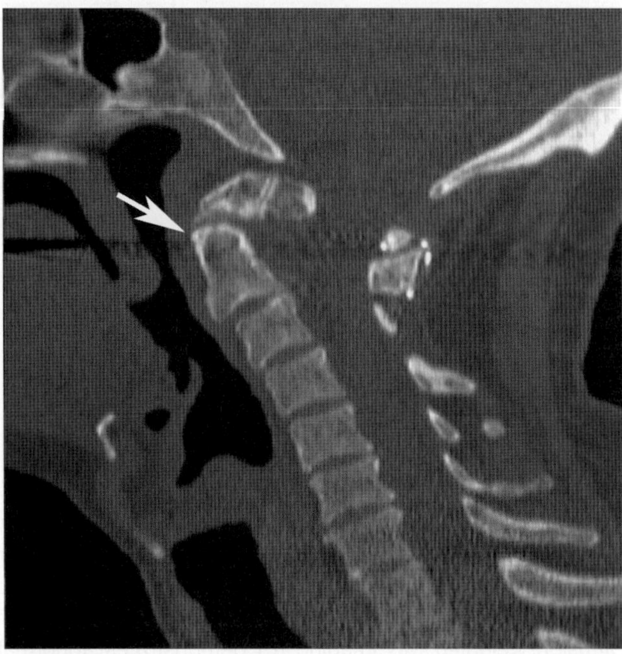

FIGURE 51-30
Anterior dens dislocation
Sagittal CT demonstrates the tip of the dens below the anterior arch of C2 (*arrow*), indicating anterior dislocation.

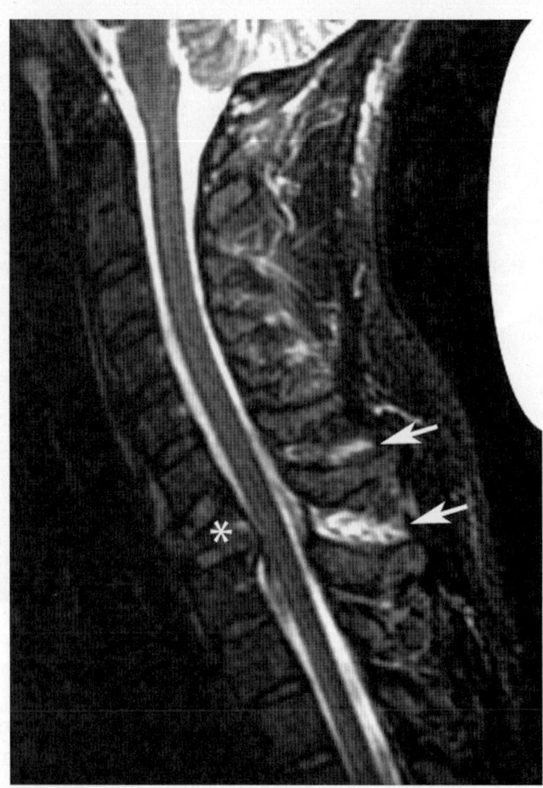

FIGURE 51-32
Compression fracture
Sagittal T2-weighted MRI demonstrates compression fracture of C7 (*) and high signal within the spinous processes of C6-C7 (*arrows*) and to a lesser degree C5-C6. This is suggestive of interspinous ligament injury. Note the pad under the patient's neck to maintain neck alignment during the scanning time.

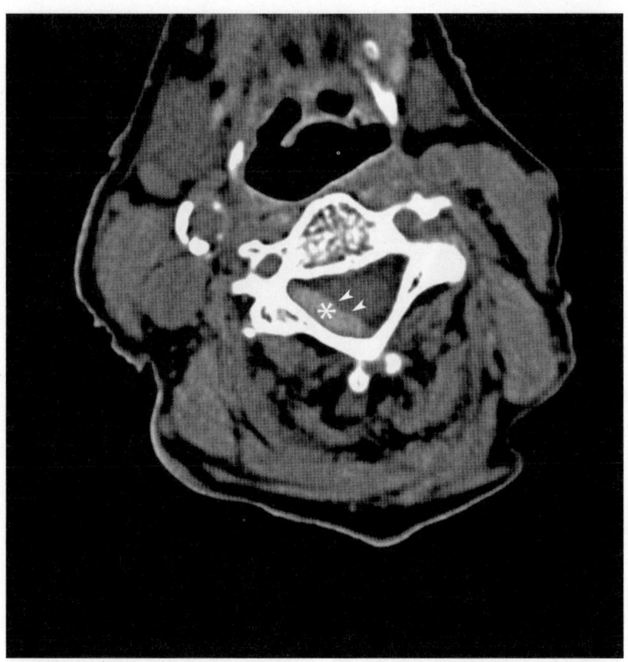

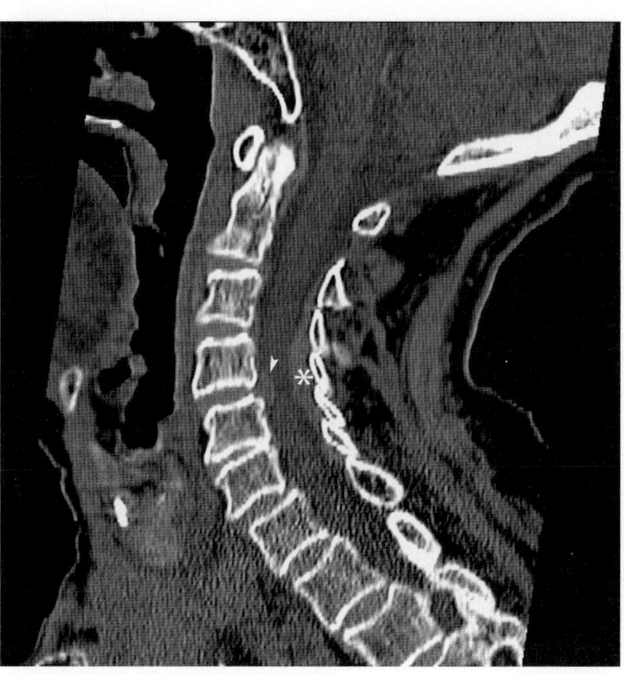

FIGURE 51-33
Epidural hematoma
Axial noncontrast CT (***A***) demonstrates a high-density epidural collection in the cervical spine (*), which is consistent with acute hemorrhage. Also noted is mass effect on the spinal cord (*arrowheads*). Sagittal reformatted CT image (***B***) demonstrates the extension of the acute epidural hematoma (*) and a disk bulge (*arrowhead*), which further contributes to spinal canal narrowing. CT is the imaging procedure of choice to detect acute hematoma.

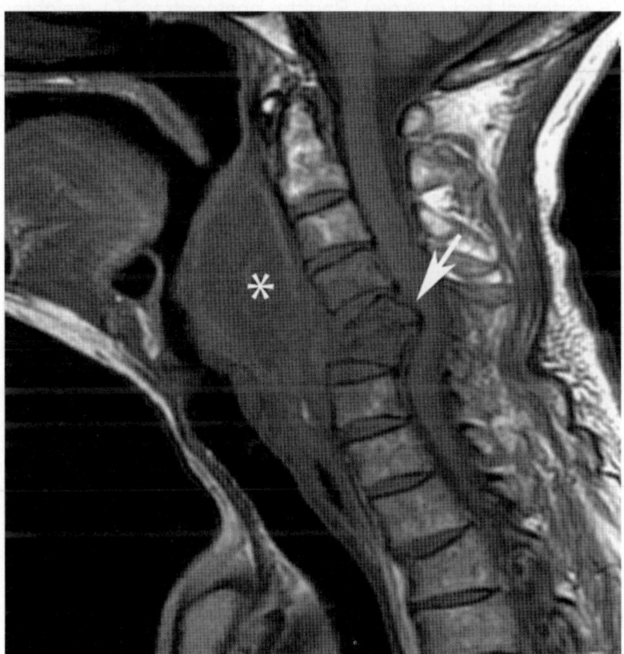

FIGURE 51-34
Retropharyngeal soft tissue mass
Sagittal T1-weighted MRI demonstrates a hyperflexion fracture with retropulsion of the posterior wall in the canal at C5 and C6 (*arrow*). There is also a large retropharyngeal hematoma (*). The distance from the posterior wall of the airway to the anterior wall of the vertebral body should not measure more than 6 mm at C2 or more than 20 mm at C6 (mnemonic "6 at 2 and 20 at 6").

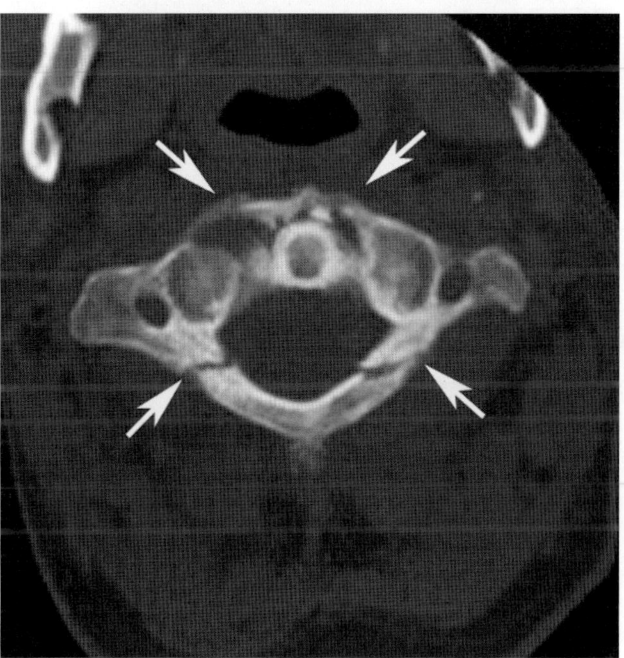

FIGURE 51-35
Jefferson fracture
Axial CT demonstrates four fracture lines (*arrows*) separating C1 in four parts. Jefferson fracture is usually caused by axial impact to the head such as diving in shallow water.

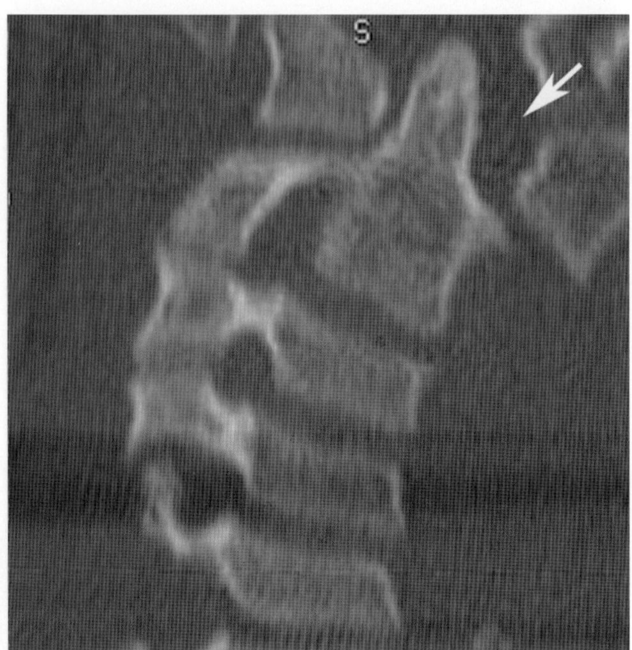

FIGURE 51-36
Ligament injury after trauma
Coronal CT reconstruction demonstrates abnormal asymmetry between the dens and the lateral masses of C1 indicating transverse ligament rupture.

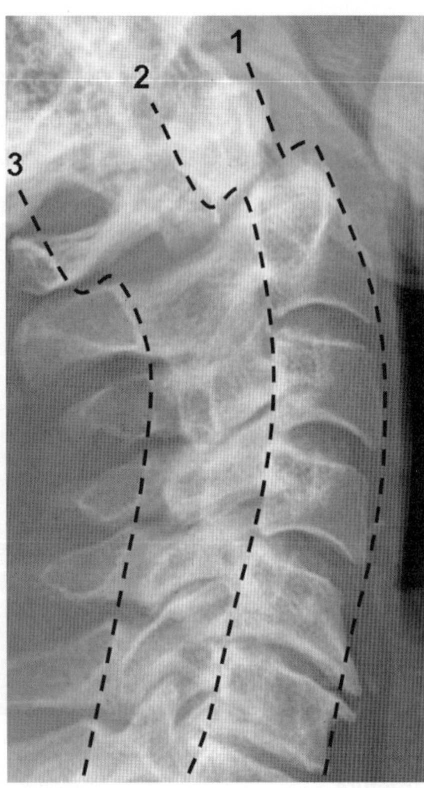

FIGURE 51-37
Odontoid fracture
Sagittal CT demonstrates disruption of the main reference cervical lines. 1: Anterior vertebral body line; 2: Posterior vertebral body line; 3: Spinolaminar line.

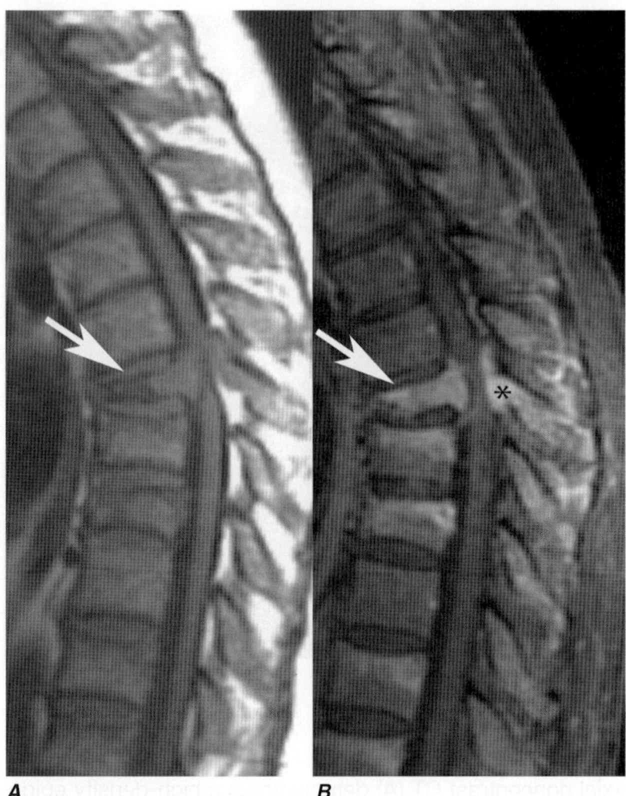

FIGURE 51-38
Pathologic fracture
Sagittal T1-weighted MRI (***A***) demonstrates wedge-shaped T6 vertebral body (*arrow*). Sagittal postcontrast T1-weighted MRI (***B***) depicts tumor extension into the epidural space and the involvement of the posterior arch (*), which are highly suggestive of metastatic or primary bone tumor.

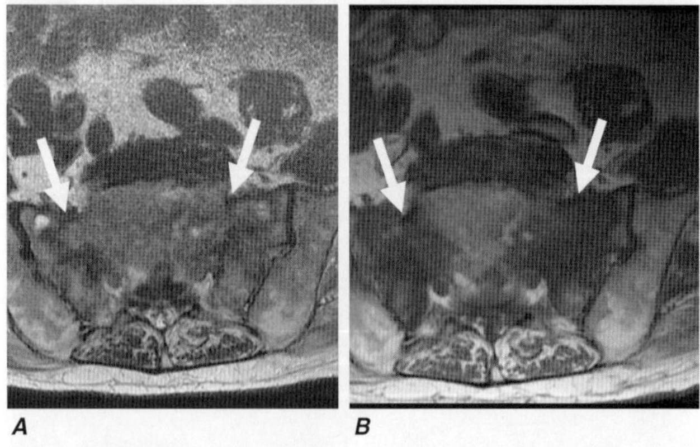

FIGURE 51-39
Sacral insufficiency fracture
Axial T2-weighted MRI (***A***) and T1-weighted MRI (***B***) demonstrate symmetric high T2 and low T1 signal involving the sacral alae longitudinally (*arrows*).

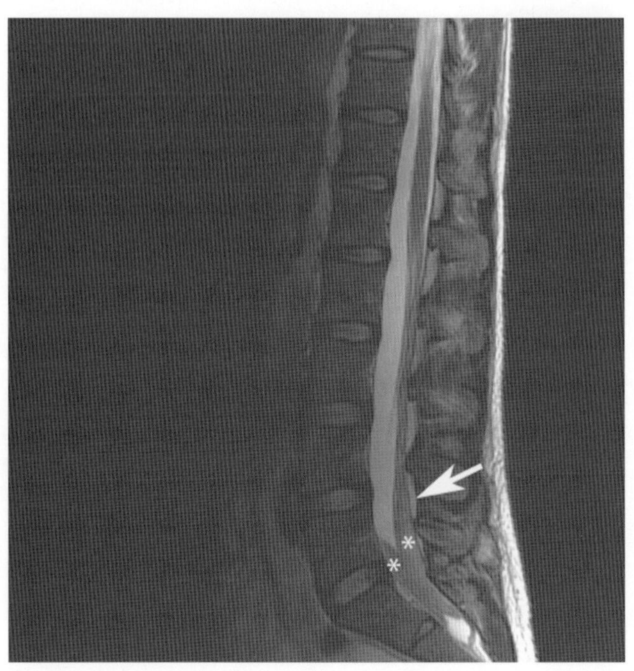

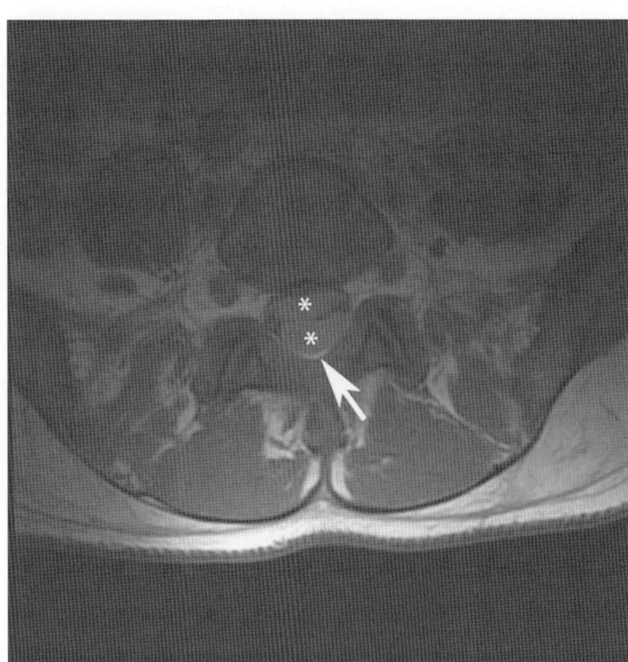

A *B*

FIGURE 51-40

Subdural hematoma

Sagittal T2-weighted MRI (***A***) and axial noncontrast T1-weighted MRI (***B***) demonstrate subdural collection in the lumbosacral region (**). Note that the epidural fat is compressed but not involved (*arrow*).

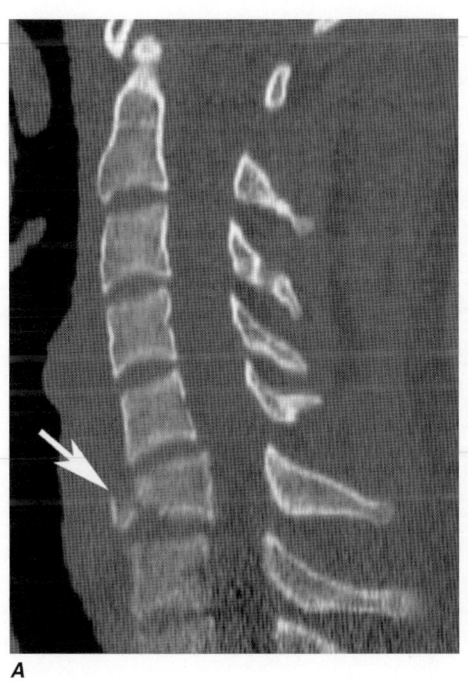

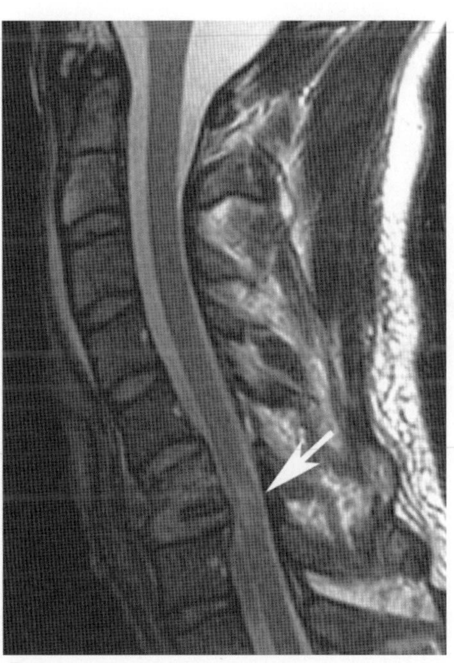

A *B*

FIGURE 51-41

Teardrop fracture

Sagittal CT (***A***) demonstrates fracture line separating the antero-inferior corner of C6 (*arrow*). Sagittal T2-weighted MRI (***B***) displays cord injury (*arrow*).

SECTION IV

CHRONIC FATIGUE SYNDROME

CHAPTER 52

CHRONIC FATIGUE SYNDROME

Gijs Bleijenberg ■ Jos W.M. van der Meer

DEFINITION

Chronic fatigue syndrome (CFS) is a disorder characterized by persistent and unexplained fatigue resulting in severe impairment in daily functioning. Besides intense fatigue, most patients with CFS report concomitant symptoms such as pain, cognitive dysfunction, and unrefreshing sleep. Additional symptoms can include headache, sore throat, tender lymph nodes, muscle aches, joint aches, feverishness, difficulty sleeping, psychiatric problems, allergies, and abdominal cramps. Criteria for the diagnosis of CFS have been developed by the U.S. Centers for Disease Control and Prevention (Table 52-1).

TABLE 52-1

DIAGNOSTIC CRITERIA FOR CHRONIC FATIGUE SYNDROME
Characterized by Persistent or Relapsing Unexplained Chronic Fatigue
Fatigue lasts for at least 6 months
Fatigue is of new or definite onset
Fatigue is not the result of an organic disease or of continuing exertion
Fatigue is not alleviated by rest
Fatigue results in a substantial reduction in previous occupational, educational, social, and personal activities
Four or more of the following symptoms, concurrently present for 6 months: impaired memory or concentration, sore throat, tender cervical or axillary lymph nodes, muscle pain, pain in several joints, new headaches, unrefreshing sleep, or malaise after exertion
Exclusion Criteria
Medical condition explaining fatigue
Major depressive disorder (psychotic features) or bipolar disorder
Schizophrenia, dementia, or delusional disorder
Anorexia nervosa, bulimia nervosa
Alcohol or substance abuse
Severe obesity (BMI >40)

EPIDEMIOLOGY

CFS is seen worldwide, with adult prevalence rates varying between 0.2 and 0.4%. In the United States, the prevalence is higher in women, members of minority groups (African and Native Americans), and individuals with lower levels of education and occupational status. Approximately 75% of all CFS patients are women. The mean age of onset is between 29 and 35 years. It is probable that many patients go undiagnosed and/or do not seek help.

ETIOLOGY

There are numerous hypotheses about the etiology of CFS; there is no definitively indentified cause. Distinguishing between predisposing, precipitating, and perpetuating factors in CFS helps to provide a framework for understanding this complex condition (Table 52-2).

Predisposing factors

Physical inactivity and trauma in childhood tend to increase the risk of CFS in adults. Neuroendocrine dysfunction may be associated with childhood trauma, reflecting a biological correlate of vulnerability. Psychiatric illness and physical hyperactivity in adulthood raise the risk of CFS in later life. Twin studies suggest a familial predisposition to CFS, but no causative genes have been identified.

Precipitating factors

Physical or psychological stress may elicit the onset of CFS. Most patients report an infection (usually a flu-like illness or infectious mononucleosis) as the trigger of their fatigue. Relatively high percentages of CFS follow Q fever and Lyme disease. However, no differences were

TABLE 52-2

PREDISPOSING, PRECIPITATING, AND PERPETUATING FACTORS IN CHRONIC FATIGUE SYNDROME

TIME
Predisposing Factors
Childhood trauma (sexual, physical, emotional abuse; emotional and physical neglect) Physical inactivity during childhood Premorbid psychiatric illness or psychopathology Premorbid hyperactivity ↓
Precipitating Factors
Somatic events: infection (mononucleosis, Q fever, Lyme disease), surgery, pregnancy Psychosocial stress, life events ↓
Perpetuating Factors
(Non)acknowledgement by physician Negative self-efficacy Strong physical attributions Strong focus on bodily symptoms Fear of fatigue (Lack of) social support Low physical activity pattern

found in Epstein-Barr virus load and immunologic reactivity in individuals who developed CFS and those who did not. While antecedent infections are associated with CFS, a direct microbial causality is unproven and unlikely. A recent study identified a murine leukemia virus-related retrovirus (XMRV); however, several subsequent studies have failed to confirm this result. Patients also often report other precipitating somatic events such as serious injury, surgery, pregnancy, or childbirth. Serious life events such as the loss of a loved one or a job, military combat, and other stressful situations may also precipitate CFS. A third of all patients cannot recall a trigger.

Perpetuating factors

Once CFS has developed, numerous factors may impede recovery. Physicians may contribute to chronicity by ordering unnecessary diagnostic procedures, by persistently suggesting psychological causes, and by not acknowledging CFS as a diagnosis.

A patient's focus on illness and avoidance of activities may perpetuate symptoms. A firm belief in a physical cause, a strong focus on bodily sensations, and a poor sense of control over symptoms may also prolong or exacerbate the fatigue and functional impairment. In most patients, inactivity is caused by negative illness perceptions rather than by poor physical fitness. Solicitous behavior of others may reinforce a patient's illness-related perceptions and behavior. A lack of social support is another known perpetuating factor.

PATHOPHYSIOLOGY

The pathophysiology of CFS is unclear. Neuroimaging studies have reported that CFS is associated with reduced gray matter volume, associated with a decline in physical activity; these changes were partially reversed following cognitive behavioral therapy (CBT). In addition, functional MRI data have suggested that abnormal patterns of activation correlate with self-reported problems with information processing. Neurophysiologic studies have shown altered CNS activation patterns during muscle contraction.

Evidence for immunologic dysfunction is inconsistent. Modest elevations in titers of antinuclear antibodies, reductions in immunoglobulin subclasses, deficiencies in mitogen-driven lymphocyte proliferation, reductions in natural killer cell activity, disturbances in cytokine production, and shifts in lymphocyte subsets have been described. None of these immune findings appear in most patients, nor do any correlate with the severity of CFS. In theory, symptoms of CFS could result from excessive production of a cytokine, such as interleukin 1, that induces asthenia and other flulike symptoms; however, compelling data in support of this hypothesis are lacking.

There is some evidence that CFS patients have mild hypocortisolism, the degree of which is associated with a poorer response to CBT.

Discrepancies in perceived and actual cognitive performance are a consistent finding in patients with CFS.

DIAGNOSIS

In addition to a thorough history, a systematic physical examination is warranted to exclude disorders causing fatigue (e.g., endocrine disorders, neoplasms, heart failure, etc.). The heart rate of CFS patients is often slightly above normal. Laboratory tests primarily serve to exclude other diagnoses; there is no test that can diagnose CFS. The following laboratory screen usually suffices: complete blood count; ESR, CRP; serum creatinine, electrolytes, calcium and iron; blood glucose; creatine kinase; liver function tests; TSH; anti-gliadin antibodies; urinalysis. Serology for viral or bacterial infections is usually not helpful. No specific abnormalities have been identified on MRI or CT scans. CFS is a constellation of symptoms without any pathognomonic features, and remains a diagnosis of exclusion.

Bipolar disorders, schizophrenia, and substance abuse exclude a diagnosis of CFS, as do eating disorders, unless these have been resolved 5 years or longer before symptom onset. Also, CFS is excluded if the chronic fatigue developed immediately after a depressive episode. Depression developing in the course of the fatigue, however, does not preclude CFS. Co-occurring psychiatric disorder, especially anxiety and mood disorders, is seen in 30–60% of all cases.

INITIAL MANAGEMENT

In cases of suspected CFS, the clinician should acknowledge the impact of the patient's symptoms on daily functioning. Disbelief or denial can provoke an exacerbation of genuine symptoms, which in turn strengthens the clinician's disbelief, leading to an unfortunate cycle of miscommunication. The possibility of CFS should be considered if a patient fulfils all criteria (Table 52-1) and if other diagnoses have been excluded.

The patient should be asked to describe the symptoms (fatigue and accompanying symptoms) and their duration as well as the consequences (reduction in daily activities). To assess symptom severity and the extent of daily-life impairment, the patient should describe a typical day, from waking to retiring, and to contrast this with an average day prior to symptom onset. Next, potential fatigue-precipitating factors are sought. The severity of fatigue is difficult to assess quantitatively; a brief questionnaire is often helpful (Fig. 52-1).

The patient should be informed of the current understanding of precipitating and perpetuating factors and effective treatments, and be offered general advice about disease management. If CBT for CFS is not available as an initial treatment option (see below) and depression and anxiety are present, these symptoms should be treated. For patients with headache, diffuse pain, and feverishness, nonsteroidal anti-inflammatory drugs may be helpful. Even modest improvements in symptoms can make an important difference in the patient's degree of self-sufficiency and ability to appreciate life's pleasures.

Controlled therapeutic trials have established that acyclovir, fludrocortisone, galantamine, modafinil, and IV immunoglobulin, among other agents, offer no significant benefit in CFS. Countless anecdotes circulate regarding other traditional and nontraditional therapies. It is important to guide patients away from those therapeutic modalities that are toxic, expensive, or unreasonable.

The patient should be encouraged to maintain regular sleep patterns, to remain as active as possible, and to gradually return to previous exercise and activity (work) levels.

TREATMENT Chronic Fatigue Syndrome

CBT and graded exercise therapy (GET) have been found to be the only beneficial interventions in CFS. Some patient groups argue against these approaches because of the implication that CFS is a purely mental disorder. CBT is a psychotherapeutic approach directed at changing condition-related cognitions and behaviors. CBT for CFS aims at changing a patient's perpetuating factors by exploiting various techniques and components.

How have you felt during the last two weeks?

Please rate all four statements and per statement check the box that reflects your situation best.

1. I feel tired	Yes, that is true								No, that is not true
2. I tire easily	Yes, that is true								No, that is not true
3. I feel fit	Yes, that is true								No, that is not true
4. Physically I feel exhausted	Yes, that is true								No, that is not true

Scoring:

1, 2 and 4:	Yes, that is true	7	6	5	4	3	2	1	No, that is not true	3: Reversed

Sum scores >18 indicate severe fatigue

FIGURE 52-1
Shortened fatigue questionnaire (SFQ).

It includes educating the patient about the etiologic model, setting goals, restoring fixed bedtime and wake-up time, challenging and changing fatigue- and activity-related cognitions, reducing symptom focusing, spreading activities evenly throughout the day, gradually increasing physical activity, planning a return to work, and resuming other activities. The intervention, which typically consists of 12–14 sessions spread over 6 months, helps CFS patients gain control over their symptoms.

GET is based on the model of deconditioning and exercise intolerance and usually involves a home exercise program that continues for 3–5 months. Walking or cycling is systematically increased, with set target heart rates. Evidence that deconditioning is the basis for symptoms in CFS is lacking, however. The primary component of CBT and GET that results in a reduction in fatigue is the change in the patient's perception of fatigue and focus on symptoms.

CBT is generally the more complex treatment, which might explain why CBT studies tend to yield better improvement rates than GET trials.

Not all patients benefit from CBT or GET. Predictors of poor outcome are somatic comorbidity, current disability claims, and severe pain. CBT offered in an early stage of the illness reduces the burden of CFS for the patient as well as society in terms of decreased medical and disability-related costs.

PROGNOSIS

Full recovery from untreated CFS is rare: the median annual recovery rate is 5% (range 0–31%) and the improvement rate 39% (range 8–63%). Patients with an underlying psychiatric disorder and those who continue to attribute their symptoms to an undiagnosed medical condition have poorer outcomes.

SECTION V

PSYCHIATRIC DISORDERS

CHAPTER 53

BIOLOGY OF PSYCHIATRIC DISORDERS

Robert O. Messing ■ John H. Rubenstein ■ Eric J. Nestler

Psychiatric disorders are central nervous system diseases characterized by disturbances in emotion, cognition, motivation, and socialization. As a result of their high prevalence, early onset, and persistence, they contribute substantially to the burden of illness worldwide. Most psychiatric disorders are heterogeneous syndromes that currently lack well-defined neuropathology and *bona fide* biological markers. Therefore, diagnoses continue to be made solely from clinical observations using criteria in the *Diagnostic and Statistical Manual of Mental Disorders* of the American Psychiatric Association (2000), 4th edition, text revision (DSM-IVTR). Recent advances in neuroimaging are beginning to provide evidence of brain pathology, which may one day be used for diagnosis and for following treatment. Family, twin, and adoption studies have shown that all common psychiatric syndromes are highly heritable, with genetic risk comprising 20–90% of disease vulnerability. The epidemiology, genetics, and biology of four common psychiatric disorders—autism, schizophrenia, mood disorders, and drug addiction—are presented in this chapter. A detailed discussion of the clinical manifestations and treatment of schizophrenia and mood disorders can be found in Chap. 54. Further discussion of alcoholism can be found in Chap. 56, opiate addiction in Chap. 57, and cocaine and other drugs of abuse in Chap. 58.

AUTISM SPECTRUM DISORDERS

The DSM-IVTR criteria for autism spectrum disorders (ASDs) require delays or abnormal functioning in social interactions, language as used in social communication, and symbolic or imaginative play, with onset prior to age 3. In addition to abnormal social behavior, ASDs are frequently, but not always, associated with reduced IQ and epilepsy. Individuals who exhibit some autism-like symptoms with relatively preserved cognitive functioning and language skills are described as having Asperger's syndrome.

EPIDEMIOLOGY

There has been a dramatic increase in the diagnosis of ASDs, from ~1/1000 (1950s–1990s) to a current level of ~1/150. Whether this increase reflects increased disease prevalence remains uncertain; ongoing studies are searching for genetic, environmental, and sociologic mechanisms that may have contributed to this change. In the 1950s–1960s, psychological factors were held to underlie autism. This conception was largely debunked by the 1970s, with the demonstration that prenatal rubella and phenylketonuria can cause ASDs, and with evidence for the genetic etiology of ASDs from twin studies. There is ongoing public concern that vaccines in general, or mercury-based preservatives in vaccines, can cause ASDs; however, large epidemiologic analyses have not supported this as an etiology. Whether environmental factors, such as perinatal infection and various toxins, for example, ethanol, illicit drugs, medications, and mutagenic agents, play a role is unclear.

NEUROPATHOLOGY AND NEUROIMAGING

ASDs show no defining neuroanatomic phenotype that would indicate neurodevelopmental abnormalities. However, structural neuroimaging and histologic studies of postmortem brain provide evidence for anatomic defects. There is a modest increase in cerebrum growth (~10%; affecting both the white and grey matter) during early childhood (years 1–3), with the largest effect in the frontal lobes; the growth rate then decreases with age. Cerebellar size is increased by about 7% in children under age 5 years, but is decreased in older patients, and there are reduced (~30%) numbers of cerebellar Purkinje neurons. Finally, there is reduced cell size and increased cell density in the limbic areas of the brain.

GENETICS

ASDs are highly heritable; concordance rates in monozygotic twins (~60–90%) are roughly tenfold higher than in dizygotic twins and siblings, and first-degree relatives show about fiftyfold increased risk for autism compared with prevalence in the general population. For unknown reasons, ASDs affect four times as many boys as girls. ASDs are also genetically heterogeneous. More than 20 known mutations, including copy number variations, account for about 10–20% of all cases, though none of these causes individually accounts for more than 1–2% (Table 53-1). Many of the genes linked to ASDs can also cause other illnesses. For instance, mutations in MeCP2,

TABLE 53-1

EXAMPLES OF GENES IMPLICATED IN AUTISM

GENE SYMBOL	GENE NAME	FUNCTION
PTEN	Phosphatase and tensin homolog	Signal transduction Synaptic function
TSC1	Tuberous sclerosis 1	Signal transduction Translation and protein stability Synaptic function
TSC2	Tuberous sclerosis 2	Signal transduction Translation and protein stability Synaptic function
FMR1	Fragile X mental retardation 1	Translation and protein stability Synaptic function
UBE3A	Ubiquitin protein ligase E3A	Translation and protein stability Synaptic function
CNTN3	Contactin 3	Synaptic function
CNTN4	Contactin 4	Synaptic function
CNTNAP2	Contactin-associated protein-like 2	Synaptic function
NLGN3	Neuroligin 3	Synaptic function
NLGN4	Neuroligin 4	Synaptic function
NRXN1	Neurexin 1	Synaptic function
PCDH10	Protocadherin 10	Synaptic function
SHANK3	Shank 3	Synaptic function
SLC6A4	Serotonin transporter	Neurotransmitter signaling
AVPR1	Arginine vasopressin receptor 1	Neurotransmitter signaling
OXTR	Oxytosin receptor	Neurotransmitter signaling
CACNA1C	Voltage-gated calcium channel–alpha 1C subunit	Ion channel
CACNA1H	Voltage-gated calcium channel–alpha 1H subunit	Ion channel
SCN1A	Sodium channel, voltage-gated, type I, alpha subunit	Ion channel
SCN2A	Sodium channel, voltage-gated, type II, alpha subunit	Ion channel
SLC9A9	Sodium/hydrogen exchanger	Ion channel
DHCR7	7-Dehydrocholesterol reductase	Metabolism
PAH	Phenylalanine hydroxylase	Metabolism
ARX	Arx transcription factor	Gene expression
En2	Engrailed 2 transcription factor	Gene expression
MeCP2	Methyl CpG-binding protein 2 (Rett syndrome)	Gene expression
RNF8	Ring finger protein 8	Gene expression

FMR1, and TSC1&2 (see Table 53-1 for abbreviations) can cause mental retardation without ASDs, and alleles of certain genes, for example, neurexin 1, are associated with both ASDs and schizophrenia. It is likely that many cases of ASDs result from more complex genetic mechanisms, including inheritance of multiple genetic variants or epigenetic modifications.

PATHOGENESIS

Despite the genetic heterogeneity of ASDs, there are some common themes that may explain pathogenesis. These include mutations in proteins involved in the formation and function of synapses, control over the size and projections of neurons, production and signaling of neurotransmitters and neuromodulators, the function of ion channels, general cell metabolism, gene expression, and protein synthesis (see Table 53-1). Many of these mutations have a clear relationship to activity-dependent neural responses and can affect the development of neural systems that underlie cognition and social behaviors. They may be detrimental by altering the balance of excitatory vs. inhibitory synaptic signaling in local and extended circuits, and by altering the mechanisms that control brain growth. Another class of mutations affects genes (e.g., PTEN and Tsc) that negatively regulate signaling from several types of extracellular stimuli, including those transduced by receptor tyrosine kinases. Their dysregulation can have pleiotropic effects, including altering brain and neuronal growth as well as synaptic development and function. With further understanding of pathogenesis and the definition of specific ASD subtypes, there is reason to believe that effective therapies will be identified, as in the case of dietary treatments for phenylketonuria. In addition, work in mouse models (e.g., with fragile X or Rett syndrome mutations) has suggested that autism-like behavioral abnormalities can be reversed even in fully developed adult animals by reversing the underlying pathology, which holds out hope for many affected individuals.

SCHIZOPHRENIA

Schizophrenia appears to be a heterogeneous collection of many distinct diseases, which remain poorly defined but linked by common clinical features. Three major symptom clusters are seen in schizophrenia: positive, negative, and cognitive symptoms. Positive symptoms include hallucinations and delusions, experiences that are not characteristic of normal mental life. Negative symptoms represent deficits in normal functions such as blunted affect, impoverished speech, asocial behavior, and diminished motivation. Cognitive symptoms include deficits in working memory and cognitive control of behavior that often prove extremely disabling. Current antipsychotic drugs are efficacious for positive symptoms only and generally lack efficacy for negative and cognitive symptoms.

EPIDEMIOLOGY

Schizophrenia is common, affecting males and females roughly equally, with a worldwide prevalence of approximately 1%. Environmental risks are thought to include prenatal exposure to viral infection (influenza), prenatal poor nutrition, perinatal hypoxia, psychotropic drug use (in particular, cannabis), and psychological stress. Advanced paternal age, birth order, and season of birth have also been implicated. However, none of these environmental influences has a specific or strong association with most cases of schizophrenia.

NEUROPATHOLOGY AND NEUROIMAGING

The best-established neuropathologic finding in schizophrenia is enlargement of the lateral ventricles of the cerebral hemispheres. This is accompanied by a reduction in cortical thickness. These abnormalities are not specific to schizophrenia and are seen in many other conditions, including many neurodegenerative disorders. However, there is a general consensus that the reduction in cortical thickness in schizophrenia is associated with increased cell packing density and reduced neuropil (defined as axons, dendrites, and glial cell processes) without an overt change in neuronal cell number. Specific classes of interneurons in prefrontal cortex consistently show reduced expression of the gene encoding the enzyme glutamic acid decarboxylase 1 (*GAD1*), which synthesizes γ-aminobutyric acid (GABA), the principal inhibitory neurotransmitter in the brain. Functional imaging studies, by positron emission tomography (PET) or functional magnetic resonance imaging (MRI), show evidence of reduced metabolic or neural activity in the dorsolateral prefrontal cortex at rest and when performing psychological tests of executive function, including working memory. Alleles of two candidate risk genes (catechol-*O*-methyltransferase [COMT] and metabotropic glutamate receptor 3 [mGluR3]) are reported to affect dorsolateral prefrontal cortex activity, but these findings need to be replicated in larger samples. Similar pathologic and brain imaging abnormalities are seen in several other brain regions, in particular, the hippocampus. There are also numerous reports of abnormalities in myelin and oligodendrocytes in the cerebral cortex of patients with schizophrenia.

GENETICS

Twins studies establish the heritability of schizophrenia, with co-inheritance at ~50% for monozygotic twins and ~10% for dizygotic twins. Genomewide linkage and association studies, and studies of copy number variation, have identified many regions and alleles that confer increased disease risk, particularly near genes on chromosome 22 (disrupted in schizophrenia 1 [DISC1], COMT, neuregulin 1, the neuregulin receptor ERBB4, and the DiGeorge [or velocardiofacial syndrome] region), and on chromosome 16p. The DiGeorge region deletions produce, in heterozygous form, a psychotic disorder with variable clinical features and a moderate to strong degree of penetrance. In contrast, the contribution of each of the individual genes to schizophrenia remains to be established with certainty. Moreover, the responsible genes within the DiGeorge region have not yet been identified. What is clear is that none of these other alleles produce schizophrenia with a high degree of penetrance. The current view in the field is that multiple rare alleles, many or most with limited penetrance, likely contribute to risk of schizophrenia. As for ASDs, the same allele may be a risk factor for multiple disorders. For instance, duplication of chromosome 16p is associated with both schizophrenia and autism, while DiGeorge region deletions and the *DISC1* locus on chromosome 22 are associated with schizophrenia, autism, and bipolar disorder.

PATHOGENESIS

There are several prevailing hypotheses about neurochemical mechanisms underlying schizophrenia. A reduction in the function of cortical and perhaps hippocampal GABAergic interneurons fits with reduced expression of glutamic acid decarboxylase. However, it is unknown whether this is a primary or compensatory feature of the disorder. Nevertheless, defects in parvalbumin-expressing GABAergic interneurons are known to reduce gamma-frequency activity on the EEG, which is a feature of many people with schizophrenia. Reduced excitatory neurotransmitter (glutamate) function is posited based on psychotic and cognitive symptoms generated in humans exposed to ketamine or phencyclidine, which are noncompetitive antagonists of the NMDA subtype of glutamate receptors. There are reports of altered levels of glutamate receptors or associated proteins in the brains of individuals with schizophrenia examined postmortem, but no findings have yet been widely replicated. Finally, overactivity of dopamine neurotransmission at D_2-type dopamine receptors is proposed based on the ability of D_2 antagonists (an action common to all current antipsychotic agents; see Chap. 54) to ameliorate the positive symptoms of schizophrenia. Excessive dopamine release in the striatum elicited by an acute dose of amphetamine has been demonstrated by PET imaging in some patients with schizophrenia. However, it is unclear whether this abnormality reflects the underlying illness or a lasting effect of antipsychotic medications. In contrast, reduced activity of dopamine at D_1 dopamine receptors in the prefrontal cortex has been implicated in working memory deficits based on the cognitive effects of D_1 receptor agonists and antagonists in the illness. Nevertheless, inferring something about disease pathogenesis from the actions of psychotropic drugs, for example, as with the glutamate and dopamine hypotheses, is fraught with artifact.

Efforts to understand how defects in these neurotransmitter systems might generate similar behavioral phenotypes have led to intriguing hypotheses. For instance, in the hippocampus, reduced glutamate transmission (based on a hypothesized deficit in glutamate release or glutamate receptors) onto GABAergic interneurons could lead to reduced glutamic acid decarboxylase expression, reduced gamma oscillations, and reduced inhibition onto excitatory neurons. These events in turn could lead to increased dopamine release from the ventral tegmental area, with dopamine antagonists thereby helping to reset the system to its nonpathologic state. It must be emphasized that these are working models only, and a true pathophysiology (or pathophysiologies) for schizophrenia remains to be established.

Overlaid on these neurotransmitter-based hypotheses is speculation as to how mutations in any of several genes implicated, however tentatively, in schizophrenia lead to the associated pathologic and behavioral abnormalities. DISC1 was originally discovered based on its association with schizophrenia in an Icelandic family. However, as stated earlier, DISC1 has since been variably associated with other neuropsychiatric conditions and its role in schizophrenia remains uncertain. The DISC1 protein has been implicated in several cellular functions, including neuronal growth and maturation, neurite outgrowth, and even the proliferation of new neurons during development. Neuregulin 1 (NRG1), a member of the EGF family of growth factors, and its receptor ERBB4 have also been implicated in schizophrenia in several genetic studies. Interestingly, NRG1 and ERBB4 play important roles in the maturation of GABAergic interneurons in cerebral cortex, and regulate dopamine transmission to several limbic brain regions. Moreover, loss of NRG1-ERBB4 in mice leads to reduced neuropil, thus phenocopying a pathologic finding in schizophrenia. Another gene of potential interest encodes Reelin, a secreted extracellular matrix serine protease. There are unconfirmed reports of association of schizophrenia with the Reelin locus on chromosome 7, and of reduced Reelin expression in the cerebral cortex of schizophrenic subjects, possibly related to increased methylation of the Reelin gene promoter.

Reelin is important during development in the migration of newly born neurons to their appropriate layers of cerebral cortex. In the adult brain, the protein is enriched in cortical GABAergic interneurons and has been implicated in regulating NMDA glutamate receptor function. It is, therefore, easy to imagine how abnormalities in DISC1, NRG1, or Reelin may be related to GABAergic, glutamatergic, and dopaminergic mechanisms in schizophrenia, and to associated pathologic abnormalities, but all such connections are currently speculative.

MOOD DISORDERS

Mood disorders are divided into depressive and bipolar disorders. Depressive disorders include the major depressive disorders, dysthymia, and more minor forms of depression. These disorders are heterogeneous syndromes, each composed of several diseases with presumably distinct pathophysiologies that remain to be elucidated.

EPIDEMIOLOGY

Mood disorders are common, with a prevalence of ~1–2% for bipolar disorder, ~5% for major depression, and ~15–20% for milder forms of depression. Between 40–50% of the risk for depression appears to be genetic. Nongenetic factors as diverse as stress and emotional trauma, viral infections, and even stochastic (random) processes during brain development have been implicated in the etiology. Depressive syndromes can occur in the context of general medical conditions such as endocrine disturbances (hyper- or hypocortisolemia, hyper- or hypothyroidism), autoimmune diseases, Parkinson's disease, traumatic brain injury, certain cancers, asthma, diabetes, and stroke. Depression and obesity/metabolic syndrome are important risk factors for each other. In predisposed individuals, stressful life events can lead to clear-cut depressive episodes, while severe stress can induce posttraumatic stress disorder (PTSD), instead of depression. Bipolar disorder is characterized by episodes of mania and depression and is one of the most heritable of psychiatric illnesses, with genetic risk of ~80%. Stress and disrupted circadian rhythms can promote the manic episodes, during which patients exhibit extremely elevated mood, abnormal thought patterns, and sometimes psychosis. Several of these clinical signs can resemble certain features of schizophrenia; indeed, recent epidemiologic and genetic research has questioned the DSM-IVTR designations of bipolar disorder, schizophrenia, and schizoaffective disorder as distinct syndromes.

NEUROPATHOLOGY AND NEUROIMAGING

Brain imaging studies in humans are defining the neural circuitry of mood within the brain's limbic system (Fig. 53-1). Integral to this system are the nucleus accumbens (important for brain reward—see later in the chapter under Substance Use Disorders), amygdala, hippocampus, and regions of prefrontal cortex. Given that many symptoms of depression (so-called neurovegetative symptoms) involve physiologic functions, a key role for the hypothalamus is also presumed. Depressed individuals show a small reduction in hippocampal size. PET and functional MRI have revealed increased activation of the amygdala by negative stimuli and reduced activation of the nucleus accumbens by rewarding stimuli. There is also evidence for altered activity in prefrontal cortex, for example, hyperactivity of subgenual area 25 in anterior cingulate cortex. Deep brain stimulation (DBS) of either the nucleus accumbens or subgenual area 25 elevates mood in normal and depressed individuals. While there are numerous reports of pathologic findings within these various regions postmortem, there is to date no defined neuropathology of depression.

GENETICS

Although depression and bipolar disorder are highly heritable, the specific genes that comprise this risk remain unknown. As noted earlier, some of the genes implicated in autism or schizophrenia seem to cause bipolar disorder in some families. Large genomewide association studies have identified genes for diacylglycerol kinase η (*DGKH*), ankyrin G (*ANK3*), an L-type voltage-gated calcium channel (*CACNA1C*), and a gene-rich region on chromosome 16p12 as being associated with bipolar disorder, but these findings await confirmation by additional studies. Numerous susceptibility genes have also been implicated in linkage and association studies, but none has yet been definitively established as a bona fide depression gene. However, a few genes with variants that may modify depression risk are worthy of mention since they may be linked to mechanisms of pathogenesis (discussed later). These include genes for the type 1 receptor for corticotrophin-releasing factor (*CRHR1*); the glucocorticoid receptor gene (*GR*); *FKBP5*, which encodes a chaperone protein for the glucocorticoid receptor; the serotonin transporter gene (*SLA6A4*); the catechol-*O*-methyltransferase gene (*COMT*); and brain-derived neurotrophic factor (*BDNF*).

PATHOGENESIS

Human and animal research in depression has focused on the long-term effects of chronic stress on the brain

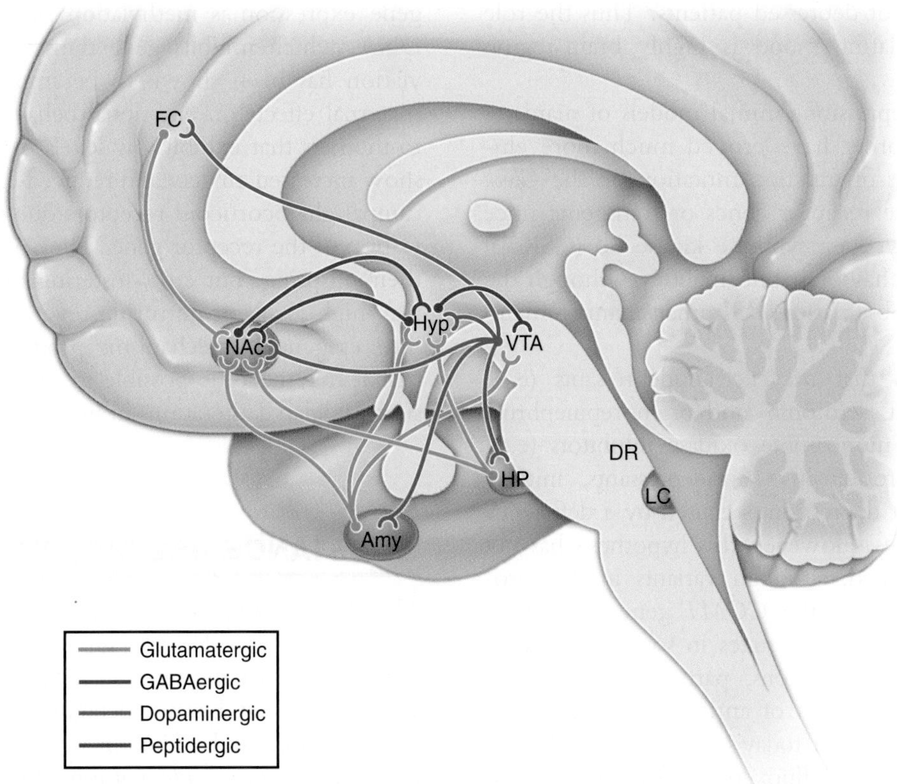

FIGURE 53-1
Neural circuitry of depression and addiction. The figure shows a simplified summary of a series of limbic circuits in brain that regulate mood and motivation and are implicated in depression and addiction. Shown in the figure are the hippocampus (HP) and amygdala (Amy), regions of prefrontal cortex, nucleus accumbens (NAc), and hypothalamus (Hyp). Only a subset of the known interconnections among these brain regions is shown. Also shown is the innervation of several of these brain regions by monoaminergic neurons. The ventral tegmental area (VTA) provides dopaminergic input to each of the limbic structures. Norepinephrine (from the locus coeruleus or LC) and serotonin (from the dorsal raphe [DR] and other raphe nuclei) innervate all of the regions shown. In addition, there are strong connections between the hypothalamus and the VTA-NAc pathway. Important peptidergic projections from the hypothalamus include those from the arcuate nucleus that release β-endorphin and melanocortin and from the lateral hypothalamus that release orexin.

and their reversal by antidepressant medications; prominent examples are discussed here. A subset of depressed patients show elevated levels of cortisol associated with increased production of corticotrophin-releasing factor from the hypothalamus and perhaps other brain regions (e.g., amygdala). In animals, sustained elevations in glucocorticoids impair hippocampal function, in part *via* direct damage to hippocampal neurons, which is consistent with reduced hippocampal volumes seen in some depressed humans. As the hippocampus exerts the major inhibitory influence over the hypothalamic-pituitary-adrenal axis, impairment of hippocampal function would lead to still further increases in glucocorticoid secretion, establishing a pathologic feed-forward loop.

Stress-induced damage to the hippocampus, and perhaps other limbic regions (e.g., amygdala), in animals is also mediated in part by reduced levels of BDNF and other growth factors and cytokines. Furthermore, stress leads to a decrease in the birth of new neurons in the adult hippocampus. Interestingly, antidepressant treatments reverse these effects of stress, and the antidepressant effects of these medications seem to depend, in part, on their ability to promote hippocampal neurogenesis in animal models of depression. The clinical ramifications of such observations are unproven, although similar regulation of adult hippocampal neurogenesis may be important for certain forms of learning and memory.

Another important target of stress in animals is the nucleus accumbens, where stress regulation of numerous signaling events (dopaminergic transmission and BDNF signaling are two examples) exert potent effects on depression-like behavioral abnormalities. While a reduction in BDNF in the hippocampus promotes depression-like behaviors, an induction of BDNF in the nucleus accumbens promotes depression; similar changes in BDNF expression have been observed in postmortem brains of depressed patients. Thus the role of BDNF in regulating mood is highly brain-region specific.

In contrast to depression, animal models of mania as well as bipolar disorder have proved much more elusive. Mice with loss-of-function mutations in the *Clock* or *GluR6* glutamate receptor genes or transgenic mice that overexpress glycogen synthase kinase 3β (GSK3β) show manic-like behavioral abnormalities, although the relevance of these observations to human mania remains unknown.

The observation that tricyclic antidepressants (e.g., imipramine) inhibit serotonin and/or norepinephrine reuptake, and that monoamine oxidase inhibitors (e.g., tranylcypromine) are effective antidepressants, initially led to the view that depression is caused by a deficiency of these monoamines. However, this hypothesis has not been well substantiated, although variants in the serotonin transporter, and in the *COMT* gene, have been associated with altered mood states in some individuals. Nevertheless, these medications, particularly the tricyclics, have formed the basis of antidepressant discovery efforts, with virtually all of today's marketed antidepressants being SSRIs (e.g., fluoxetine, sertraline, citalopram), serotonin, and norepinephrine reuptake inhibitors (SNRIs) (e.g., venlafaxine, duloxetine), or norepinephrine reuptake inhibitors (NRIs) (e.g., atomoxetine).

A cardinal feature of all antidepressant medications is that long-term administration is needed for their mood-elevating effects. This means that their short-term actions, namely promotion of serotonin or norepinephrine function, is not per se antidepressant but rather induces a cascade of adaptations in the brain that underlie their clinical effects. The nature of these therapeutic drug-induced adaptations has not been identified with certainty. Presumably, the rich innervation of the brain's limbic circuitry by serotonin and norepinephrine (Fig. 53-1) provide the anatomic basis of their therapeutic actions.

Lithium is a highly effective drug for bipolar disorder, and competes with magnesium to inhibit magnesium-dependent enzymes, including GSK3β and several enzymes involved in phosphoinositide signaling leading to activation of protein kinase C. These findings have led to discovery programs focused on developing GSK3 and PKC inhibitors as potential novel treatments for mood disorders. Another commonly prescribed drug for bipolar disorder is valproic acid, which has pleiotropic effects, including inhibition of histone deacetylases (HDACs). Histone acetylation promotes transcriptional activation through posttranslational modification of N-terminal lysine residues in histones and thereby causes chromatin decondensation. HDAC inhibitors have shown some antidepressant effects in animal models of depression. Another form of epigenetic control of gene expression is methylation of cytosine residues in DNA, which inhibits gene transcription. DNA methylation has been shown to be important for inherited maternal effects on emotional behavior. Thus, rats born to mothers that exhibit low levels of nurturing behavior show increased anxiety and reduced expression of hippocampal glucocorticoid receptors due to increased methylation of the receptor gene. They pass these traits on to their offspring, but cross-fostering by mothers that display high levels of nurturing reverses them. As research into epigenetic mechanisms progresses, there is hope that it may become possible to identify specific depression-associated alterations in human chromatin.

SUBSTANCE USE DISORDERS

The DSM-IVTR uses the terms *substance dependence* and *substance abuse* to describe substance use disorders. It is unfortunate that the term *substance dependence* instead of addiction is used, because dependence can develop without addiction, and addiction involves much more than dependence per se. *Physical dependence* develops through resetting of homeostatic cellular mechanisms to permit normal function despite the continued presence of a drug; when drug intake is terminated abruptly, a withdrawal syndrome emerges. Withdrawal from alcohol or other sedative-hypnotics causes nervous system hyperactivity, whereas withdrawal from psychostimulants produces fatigue and sedation. *Tolerance* is a reduction in response to a drug, which like dependence, develops after repeated use. It results from a change in drug metabolism (pharmacokinetic tolerance) or cell signaling (pharmacodynamic tolerance). It is important to recognize that many nonaddictive medications induce tolerance and physical dependence, including β-adrenergic antagonists (e.g., propranolol) and α_2-adrenergic agonists (e.g., clonidine).

What sets drugs of abuse apart is their unique ability to produce *euphoria*, a positive emotional state characterized by intensely pleasant feelings that are rewarding and *reinforcing* since they motivate users to take the drug repeatedly. Tolerance develops to the rewarding properties of most abused drugs during periods of heavy use, which promotes the use of higher drug doses. In addition, *psychological (or motivational) dependence* develops through the resetting of cellular mechanisms within reward-related regions of the brain and leads to negative emotional symptoms resembling depression during drug withdrawal. Addictive drugs can also cause *sensitization*, an increased drug effect upon repeated use, as exemplified by the paranoid psychosis induced by chronic use of cocaine or other psychostimulants (e.g., amphetamine). Addiction, therefore, results from drug-induced changes in reward-related regions of the brain that lead to a complex mixture of tolerance, sensitization, and motivational dependence, in addition to powerful conditioning effects of these drugs mediated by the brain's memory circuits.

EPIDEMIOLOGY

Substance use disorders, especially those involving alcohol and tobacco, are very prevalent. The World Health Organization (WHO) estimates that more than 76 million people worldwide have alcohol use disorders and ~1.3 billion people smoke tobacco products (~1 billion men, 250 million women). The most widely used illicit drug in the United States is marijuana, with ~17% of 18–25-year-olds reporting regular use. Estimates of the annual economic burden of substance use disorders in the United States, including health- and crime-related costs and losses in productivity, exceed $500 billion.

NEUROPATHOLOGY AND NEUROIMAGING

Imaging studies in humans demonstrate that addictive drugs, as well as craving for them, activate the brain's reward circuitry (discussed later). However, there is no established pathology associated with addiction risk. Patients who abuse alcohol or psychostimulants show reduced gray matter in the prefrontal cortex. Functional MRI or PET studies show reduced activity in anterior cingulate and orbitofrontal cortex during tasks of attention and inhibitory control. Damage to these cortical areas may contribute to addiction by impairing decision making and increasing impulsivity.

GENETICS

Substance use disorders are highly heritable, with genetic risk estimated to be 0.4 to 0.7; however, the specific genes that comprise this risk remain largely unknown. The best-established genetic contribution to addiction is the protective effect that mutations in alcohol-metabolizing enzymes have on risk for alcoholism. Mutations that increase alcohol dehydrogenase (ADH) activity and decrease aldehyde dehydrogenase (ALDH) activity are additive and promote accumulation of acetaldehyde following ingestion of alcohol. This produces intoxication at low doses and a flushing reaction that is unpleasant, resembling the reaction to disulfiram, a drug used to prevent relapse. These variants are common among people of East Asian descent, and individuals expressing these variants rarely abuse alcohol.

Genes that promote risk for addiction have begun to emerge from large family and population studies, but all genes identified to date represent only a very small fraction of the overall genetic risk for addiction. The best established susceptibility loci are regions on chromosomes 4 and 5 containing $GABA_A$ receptor gene clusters linked to alcohol use disorders and the nicotinic acetylcholine receptor gene cluster on chromosome 15 associated with nicotine and alcohol dependence. There are reports of numerous other addiction susceptibility genes (e.g., variants in COMT, the μ-opioid receptor, and the serotonin transporter), but further work is needed to validate these findings. In addition, several genes have been implicated in impulsivity, which is strongly associated with substance abuse. These include variants in genes for the D_4 dopamine receptor, the dopamine transporter, monoamine oxidase A, COMT, and the 5-HT1B serotonin receptor.

PATHOGENESIS

Work in rodents and nonhuman primates has established the brain's reward regions as key neural substrates for the acute actions of drugs of abuse and for addiction induced by repeated drug administration (Fig. 53-1). Midbrain dopamine neurons in the ventral tegmental area (VTA) function normally as rheostats of reward: They are activated by natural rewards (food, sex, social interaction) or even by the expectation of such rewards, and many are suppressed by the absence of an expected reward or by aversive stimuli. These neurons thereby transmit crucial survival signals to the rest of the limbic brain to promote reward-related behavior, including motor responses to seek and obtain the rewards (nucleus accumbens), memories of reward-related cues (amygdala, hippocampus), and executive control of obtaining rewards (prefrontal cortex).

Drugs of abuse alter neurotransmission through initial actions at different classes of ion channels, neurotransmitter receptors, or neurotransmitter transporters (**Table 53-2**). Although the initial targets differ, the actions of these drugs converge on the brain's reward circuitry by promoting dopamine neurotransmission in the nucleus accumbens and other limbic targets of the VTA. In addition, some drugs promote activation of opioid and cannabinoid receptors, which modulate this reward circuitry. By these mechanisms, drugs of abuse produce powerful rewarding signals, which, after repeated drug administration, corrupt the brain's reward circuitry in ways that promote addiction. Three major pathologic adaptations have been described. First, drugs produce tolerance and dependence in reward circuits, which promote escalating drug intake and a negative emotional state during drug withdrawal that promotes relapse. Second, sensitization to the rewarding effects of the drugs and associated cues is seen during prolonged abstinence and also triggers relapse. Third, executive function is impaired in such a way as to increase impulsivity and compulsivity, both of which promote relapse.

TABLE 53-2

INITIAL ACTIONS OF DRUGS OF ABUSE

DRUG	NEUROTRANSMITTER AFFECTED	DRUG TARGET (ACTION)
Opiates	Endorphins, enkephalins	μ- and δ-opioid receptors (agonist)
Psychostimulants (cocaine, amphetamine methamphetamine)	Dopamine	Dopamine transporter (antagonist—cocaine; reverse transport—amphetamine, methamphetamine)
Nicotine	Acetylcholine	Nicotinic cholinergic receptors (agonist)
Ethanol	GABA Glutamate Acetylcholine Serotonin —	$GABA_A$ receptors (positive allosteric modulator) NMDA glutamate receptors (antagonist) Nicotinic cholinergic receptors (allosteric modulator) 5HT-3 receptor (positive allosteric modulator) Calcium-activated K^+ channel (acivator)
Marijuana	Endocannabinoids (anandamide, 2-arachidonoylglycerol)	CB_1 receptor (agonist)
Phencyclidine	Glutamate	NMDA glutamate receptor (antagonist)

Repeated intake of abused drugs induces specific changes in cellular signal transduction, synaptic strength (long-term potentiation or depression), and neuronal structure (altered dendritic branching or cell soma size) within the brain's reward circuitry. These modifications are mediated in part by changes in gene expression, achieved by drug regulation of transcription factors (e.g., CREB [cAMP response element binding protein] and ΔFosB) and their target genes. Together, these drug-induced adaptations underlie alterations in numerous neurotransmitter systems (e.g., glutamate, GABA, dopamine), growth factors (e.g., BDNF), neuropeptides (e.g. corticotrophin releasing factor), and intracellular signaling cascades. These adaptations provide opportunities for developing treatments targeted to drug-addicted individuals. The fact that the spectrum of these adaptations partly differ depending on the particular addictive substance used creates opportunities for treatments that are specific for different classes of addictive drugs and that may, therefore, be less likely to disturb basic mechanisms that govern motivation and reward.

Increasingly, causal relationships are being established between individual molecular-cellular adaptations and specific behavioral abnormalities that characterize the addicted state. For example, acute activation of μ-opioid receptors by morphine or other opiates activates $G_{i/o}$ proteins leading to inhibition of adenylyl cyclase, resulting in reduced cAMP production, protein kinase A (PKA) activation, and activation of the transcription factor CREB. Repeated administration of these drugs (Fig. 53-2) evokes a homeostatic response resulting in upregulation of adenylyl cyclases, increased production of cAMP, and increased activation of PKA and CREB. Such upregulation of cAMP signaling has been identified in the locus coeruleus, periaqueductal gray, VTA, and nucleus accumbens and contributes to opiate craving and signs of opiate withdrawal. The fact that endogenous opioid peptides do not produce tolerance and dependence while morphine and heroin do may relate to the recent observation that, unlike endogenous opioids, morphine and heroin are weak inducers of μ-opioid receptor desensitization and endocytosis. Therefore, these drugs cause prolonged receptor activation and inhibition of adenylyl cyclases, which provides a powerful stimulus for the upregulation of cAMP signaling that characterizes the opiate-dependent state.

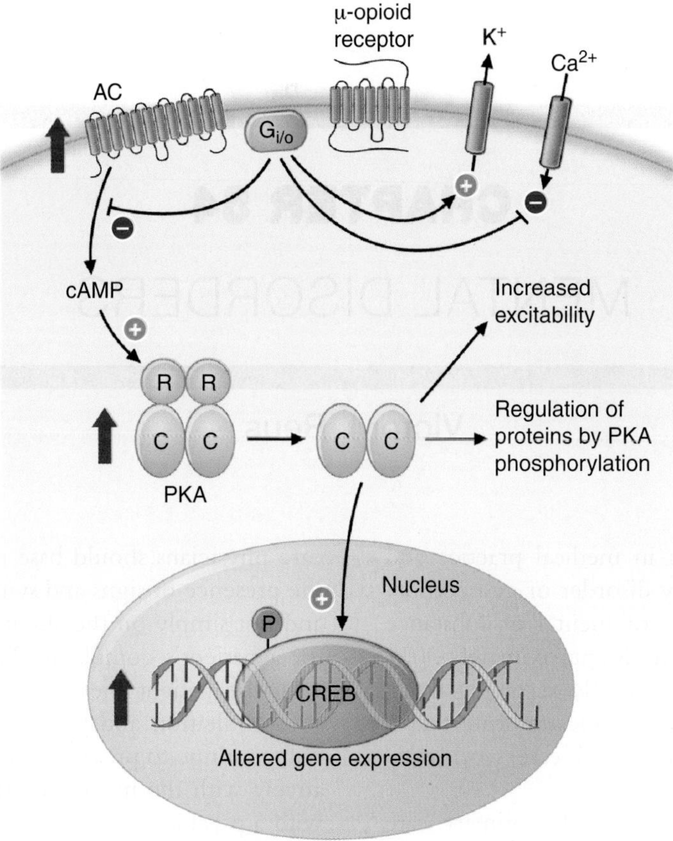

FIGURE 53-2

Opiate action in the locus coeruleus (LC). Binding of opiate agonists to μ-opioid receptors catalyzes nucleotide exchange on G_i and G_o proteins, leading to inhibition of adenylyl cyclase, neuronal hyperpolarization via activation of K^+ channels, and inhibition of neurotransmitter release *via* inhibition of $Ca^{2/+}$ channels. Activation of $G_{i/o}$ also inhibits adenylyl cyclase (AC), reducing protein kinase A (PKA) activity and phosphorylation of several PKA substrate proteins, thereby altering their function. For example, opiates reduce phosphorylation of the cAMP response element-binding protein (CREB), which appears to initiate long-term changes in neuronal function. Chronic administration of opiates increases levels of AC isoforms, PKA catalytic (C) and regulatory (R) subunits, and the phosphorylation of several proteins, including CREB (indicated by red arrows). These changes contribute to the altered phenotype of the drug-addicted state. For example, the excitability of LC neurons is increased by enhanced cAMP signaling, although the ionic basis of this effect remains unknown. Activation of CREB causes upregulation of AC isoforms and tyrosine hydroxylase, the rate-limiting enzyme in catecholamine biosynthesis.

CHAPTER 54

MENTAL DISORDERS

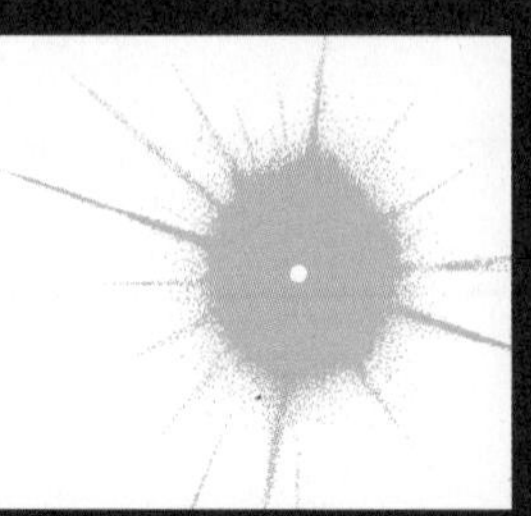

Victor I. Reus

Mental disorders are common in medical practice and may present either as a primary disorder or as a comorbid condition. The prevalence of mental or substance use disorders in the United States is approximately 30%, only one-third of whom are currently receiving treatment. Global burden of disease statistics indicate that 4 of the 10 most important causes of disease worldwide are psychiatric in origin.

The revised fourth edition for use by primary care physicians of the *Diagnostic and Statistical Manual* (DSM-IV-PC) provides a useful synopsis of mental disorders most likely to be seen in primary care practice. The current system of classification is multiaxial and includes the presence or absence of a major mental disorder (axis I), any underlying personality disorder (axis II), general medical condition (axis III), psychosocial and environmental problems (axis IV), and overall rating of general psychosocial functioning (axis V).

Changes in health care delivery underscore the need for primary care physicians to assume responsibility for the initial diagnosis and treatment of the most common mental disorders. Prompt diagnosis is essential to ensure that patients have access to appropriate medical services and to maximize the clinical outcome. Validated patient-based questionnaires have been developed that systematically probe for signs and symptoms associated with the most prevalent psychiatric diagnoses and guide the clinician into targeted assessment. Prime MD (and a self-report form, the PHQ) and the Symptom-Driven Diagnostic System for Primary Care (SDDS-PC) are inventories that require only 10 min to complete and link patient responses to the formal diagnostic criteria of anxiety, mood, somatoform, and eating disorders and to alcohol abuse or dependence.

A physician who refers patients to a psychiatrist should know not only when doing so is appropriate but also how to refer, since societal misconceptions and the stigma of mental illness impede the process. Primary care physicians should base referrals to a psychiatrist on the presence of signs and symptoms of a mental disorder and not simply on the absence of a physical explanation for a patient's complaint. The physician should discuss with the patient the reasons for requesting the referral or consultation and provide reassurance that he or she will continue to provide medical care and work collaboratively with the mental health professional. Consultation with a psychiatrist or transfer of care is appropriate when physicians encounter evidence of psychotic symptoms, mania, severe depression, or anxiety; symptoms of post-traumatic stress disorder (PTSD); suicidal or homicidal preoccupation; or a failure to respond to first-order treatment. The biology of psychiatric and addictive disorders is discussed in Chap. 53.

ANXIETY DISORDERS

Anxiety disorders, the most prevalent psychiatric illnesses in the general community, are present in 15–20% of medical clinic patients. Anxiety, defined as a subjective sense of unease, dread, or foreboding, can indicate a primary psychiatric condition or can be a component of, or reaction to, a primary medical disease. The primary anxiety disorders are classified according to their duration and course and the existence and nature of precipitants.

When evaluating the anxious patient, the clinician must first determine whether the anxiety antedates or postdates a medical illness or is due to a medication side effect. Approximately one-third of patients presenting with anxiety have a medical etiology for their psychiatric symptoms, but an anxiety disorder can also present with somatic symptoms in the absence of a diagnosable medical condition.

PANIC DISORDER

Clinical manifestations

Panic disorder is defined by the presence of recurrent and unpredictable panic attacks, which are distinct episodes of intense fear and discomfort associated with a variety of physical symptoms, including palpitations, sweating, trembling, shortness of breath, chest pain, dizziness, and a fear of impending doom or death (Table 54-1). Paresthesias, gastrointestinal distress, and feelings of unreality are also common. Diagnostic criteria require at least 1 month of concern or worry about the attacks or a change in behavior related to them. The lifetime prevalence of panic disorder is 1–3%. Panic attacks have a sudden onset, developing within 10 min and usually resolving over the course of an hour, and they occur in an unexpected fashion. The frequency and severity of panic attacks vary, ranging from once a week to clusters of attacks separated by months of well-being. The first attack is usually outside the home, and onset is typically in late adolescence to early adulthood. In some individuals, anticipatory anxiety develops over time and results in a generalized fear and a progressive avoidance of places or situations in which a panic attack might recur. *Agoraphobia*, which occurs commonly in patients with panic disorder, is an acquired irrational fear of being in places where one might feel trapped or unable to escape (Table 54-2). Typically, it leads the patient into a progressive restriction in lifestyle and, in a literal sense, in geography. Frequently, patients are embarrassed that they are housebound and dependent on the company of others to go out into the world and do not volunteer this information; thus physicians will fail to recognize the syndrome if direct questioning is not pursued.

TABLE 54-1

DIAGNOSTIC CRITERIA FOR PANIC ATTACK

A discrete period of intense fear or discomfort, in which four or more of the following symptoms developed abruptly and reached a peak within 10 min:

1. Palpitations, pounding heart, or accelerated heart rate
2. Sweating
3. Trembling or shaking
4. Sensations of shortness of breath or smothering
5. Feeling of choking
6. Chest pain or discomfort
7. Nausea or abdominal distress
8. Feeling dizzy, unsteady, lightheaded, or faint
9. Derealization (feelings of unreality) or depersonalization (being detached from oneself)
10. Fear of losing control or going crazy
11. Fear of dying
12. Paresthesias (numbness or tingling sensations)
13. Chills or hot flushes

Source: Reprinted with permission from the *Diagnostic and Statistical Manual of Mental Disorders*, Fourth Edition, Text Revision. Copyright © 2000 American Psychiatric Association.

TABLE 54-2

DIAGNOSTIC CRITERIA FOR AGORAPHOBIA

1. Anxiety about being in places or situations from which escape might be difficult (or embarrassing) or in which help may not be available in the event of having an unexpected or situationally predisposed panic attack or panic-like symptoms. Agoraphobic fears typically involve characteristic clusters of situations that include being outside the home alone; being in a crowd or standing in a line; being on a bridge; and traveling in a bus, train, or automobile.
2. The situations are avoided (e.g., travel is restricted) or else are endured with marked distress or with anxiety about having a panic attack or panic-like symptoms, or require the presence of a companion.
3. The anxiety or phobic avoidance is not better accounted for by another mental disorder such as social phobia (e.g., avoidance limited to social situations because of fear of embarrassment), specific phobia (e.g., avoidance limited to a single situation like elevators), obsessive-compulsive disorder (e.g., avoidance of dirt in someone with an obsession about contamination), posttraumatic stress disorder (e.g., avoidance of stimuli associated with a severe stressor), or separation anxiety disorder (e.g., avoidance of leaving home or relatives).

Source: Reprinted with permission from the *Diagnostic and Statistical Manual of Mental Disorders*, Fourth Edition, Text Revision. Copyright © 2000 American Psychiatric Association.

Differential diagnosis

A diagnosis of panic disorder is made after a medical etiology for the panic attacks has been ruled out. A variety of cardiovascular, respiratory, endocrine, and neurologic conditions can present with anxiety as the chief complaint. Patients with true panic disorder will often focus on one specific feature to the exclusion of others. For example, 20% of patients who present with syncope as a primary medical complaint have a primary diagnosis of a mood, anxiety, or substance-abuse disorder, the most common being panic disorder. The differential diagnosis of panic disorder is complicated by a high rate of comorbidity with other psychiatric conditions, especially alcohol and benzodiazepine abuse, which patients initially use in an attempt at self-medication. Some 75% of panic disorder patients will also satisfy criteria for major depression at some point in their illness.

When the history is nonspecific, physical examination and focused laboratory testing must be used to rule out anxiety states resulting from medical disorders such as pheochromocytoma, thyrotoxicosis, or hypoglycemia. Electrocardiogram (ECG) and echocardiogram may detect some cardiovascular conditions associated with panic such as paroxysmal atrial tachycardia and mitral valve prolapse. In two studies, panic disorder was the primary diagnosis in 43% of patients with chest pain who had normal coronary angiograms and was present in 9% of all outpatients referred for cardiac evaluation. Panic disorder has also been diagnosed in many patients referred for pulmonary function testing or with symptoms of irritable bowel syndrome.

Etiology and pathophysiology

The etiology of panic disorder is unknown but appears to involve a genetic predisposition, altered autonomic responsivity, and social learning. Panic disorder shows familial aggregation; the disorder is concordant in 30–45% of monozygotic twins, and genomewide screens have identified suggestive risk loci. Acute panic attacks appear to be associated with increased noradrenergic discharges in the locus coeruleus. Intravenous infusion of sodium lactate evokes an attack in two-thirds of panic disorder patients, as do the α_2-adrenergic antagonist yohimbine, cholecystokinin tetrapeptide (CCK-4), and carbon dioxide inhalation. It is hypothesized that each of these stimuli activates a pathway involving noradrenergic neurons in the locus coeruleus and serotonergic neurons in the dorsal raphe. Agents that block serotonin reuptake can prevent attacks. Panic-disorder patients have a heightened sensitivity to somatic symptoms, which triggers increasing arousal, setting off the panic attack; accordingly, therapeutic intervention involves altering the patient's cognitive interpretation of anxiety-producing experiences as well as preventing the attack itself.

TREATMENT Panic Disorder

Achievable goals of treatment are to decrease the frequency of panic attacks and to reduce their intensity. The cornerstone of drug therapy is antidepressant medication (Tables 54-3 through 54-5). Selective serotonin reuptake inhibitors (SSRIs) benefit the majority of panic disorder patients and do not have the adverse effects of tricyclic antidepressants (TCAs). Fluoxetine, paroxetine, sertraline, and the selective serotonin-norepinephrine reuptake inhibitor (SNRI) venlafaxine have received approval from the U.S. Food and Drug Administration (FDA) for this indication. These drugs should be started at one-third to one-half of their usual antidepressant dose (e.g., 5–10 mg fluoxetine, 25–50 mg sertraline, 10 mg paroxetine, 37.5 mg venlafaxine). Monoamine oxidase inhibitors (MAOIs) are also effective and may specifically benefit patients who have comorbid features of atypical depression (i.e., hypersomnia and weight gain). Insomnia, orthostatic hypotension, and the need to maintain a low-tyramine diet (avoidance of cheese and wine) have limited their use, however. Antidepressants typically take 2–6 weeks to become effective, and doses may need to be adjusted based upon the clinical response.

Because of anticipatory anxiety and the need for immediate relief of panic symptoms, benzodiazepines are useful early in the course of treatment and sporadically thereafter (Table 54-6). For example, alprazolam, starting at 0.5 mg qid and increasing to 4 mg/d in divided doses, is effective, but patients must be monitored closely, as some develop dependence and begin to escalate the dose of this medication. Clonazepam, at a final maintenance dose of 2–4 mg/d, is also helpful; its longer half-life permits twice-daily dosing, and patients appear less likely to develop dependence on this agent.

Early psychotherapeutic intervention and education aimed at symptom control enhances the effectiveness of drug treatment. Patients can be taught breathing techniques, be educated about physiologic changes that occur with panic, and learn to expose themselves voluntarily to precipitating events in a treatment program spanning 12–15 sessions. Homework assignments and monitored compliance are important components of successful treatment. Once patients have achieved a satisfactory response, drug treatment should be maintained for 1–2 years to prevent relapse. Controlled trials indicate a success rate of 75–85%, although the likelihood of complete remission is somewhat lower.

GENERALIZED ANXIETY DISORDER

Clinical manifestations

Patients with generalized anxiety disorder (GAD) have persistent, excessive, and/or unrealistic worry associated with muscle tension, impaired concentration, autonomic arousal, feeling "on edge" or restless, and insomnia (Table 54-7). Onset is usually before age 20 years, and a history of childhood fears and social inhibition may be present. The lifetime prevalence of GAD is 5–6%; the risk is higher in first-degree relatives of patients with the diagnosis. Interestingly, family studies indicate that GAD and panic disorder segregate independently. More than 80% of patients with GAD also suffer from major depression, dysthymia, or social phobia. Comorbid substance abuse is common in these patients, particularly alcohol and/or sedative/hypnotic abuse. Patients with GAD worry excessively over minor matters, with life-disrupting effects; unlike in panic disorder, complaints of shortness of breath, palpitations, and tachycardia are relatively rare.

TABLE 54-3

ANTIDEPRESSANTS

NAME	USUAL DAILY DOSE, mg	SIDE EFFECTS	COMMENTS
SSRIs			
Fluoxetine (Prozac) Sertraline (Zoloft) Paroxetine (Paxil) Fluvoxamine (Luvox) Citalopram (Celexa) Escitalopram (Lexapro)	10–80 50–200 20–60 100–300 20–60 10–30	Headache; nausea and other GI effects; jitteriness; insomnia; sexual dysfunction; can affect plasma levels of other medicines (except sertraline); akathisia rare	Once-daily dosing, usually in the morning; fluoxetine has very long half-life; must not be combined with MAOIs
TCAs			
Amitriptyline (Elavil) Nortriptyline (Pamelor) Imipramine (Tofranil) Desipramine (Norpramin) Doxepin (Sinequan) Clomipramine (Anafranil)	150–300 50–200 150–300 150–300 150–300 150–300	Anticholinergic (dry mouth, tachycardia, constipation, urinary retention, blurred vision); sweating; tremor; postural hypotension; cardiac conduction delay; sedation; weight gain	Once-daily dosing, usually qhs; blood levels of most TCAs available; can be lethal in O.D. (lethal dose = 2 g); nortriptyline best tolerated, especially by elderly
Mixed Norepinephrine/Serotonin Reuptake Inhibitors and Receptor Blockers			
Venlafaxine (Effexor)	75–375	Nausea; dizziness; dry mouth; headaches; increased blood pressure; anxiety and insomnia	Bid-tid dosing (extended release available); lower potential for drug interactions than SSRIs; contraindicated with MAOIs
Desvenlafaxine, (Pristiq)	50–400	Nausea, dizziness, insomnia	Primary metabolite of venlafaxine. No increased efficacy with higher dosing
Duloxetine (Cymbalta)	40–60	Nausea, dizziness, headache, insomnia, constipation	May have utility in treatment of neuropathic pain and stress incontinence
Mirtazapine (Remeron)	15–45	Somnolence; weight gain; neutropenia rare	Once daily dosing
Mixed-Action Drugs			
Bupropion (Wellbutrin)	250–450	Jitteriness; flushing; seizures in at-risk patients; anorexia; tachycardia; psychosis	Tid dosing, but sustained release also available; fewer sexual side effects than SSRIs or TCAs; may be useful for adult ADD
Trazodone (Desyrel)	200–600	Sedation; dry mouth; ventricular irritability; postural hypotension; priapism rare	Useful in low doses for sleep because of sedating effects with no anticholinergic side effects
Nefazodone (Serzone)	300–600	Sedation; headache; dry mouth; nausea; constipation	Discontinued sale in United States and several other countries due to risk of liver failure
Amoxapine (Asendin)	200–600	Sexual dysfunction	Lethality in overdose; EPS possible
MAOIs			
Phenelzine (Nardil) Tranylcypromine (Parnate) Isocarboxazid (Marplan)	45–90 20–50 20–60	Insomnia; hypotension; anorgasmia; weight gain; hypertensive crisis; toxic reactions with SSRIs; narcotics	May be more effective in patients with atypical features or treatment-refractory depression
Transdermal selegiline (Emsam)	6–12	Local skin reaction, hypertension	No dietary restrictions with 6 mg dose

Abbreviations: ADD, attention deficit disorder; EPS, extrapyramidal symptoms; MAOIs, monoamine oxidase inhibitors; SSRIs, selective serotonin reuptake inhibitors;TCAs, tricyclic antidepressants.

TABLE 54-4

MANAGEMENT OF ANTIDEPRESSANT SIDE EFFECTS

SYMPTOMS	COMMENTS AND MANAGEMENT STRATEGIES
Gastrointestinal	
Nausea, loss of appetite	Usually short-lived and dose-related; consider temporary dose reduction or administration with food and antacids
Diarrhea	Famotidine, 20–40 mg/d
Constipation	Wait for tolerance; try diet change, stool softener, exercise; avoid laxatives
Sexual dysfunction	Consider dose reduction; drug holiday
Anorgasmia/impotence; impaired ejaculation	Bethanechol, 10–20 mg, 2 h before activity, or cyproheptadine, 4–8 mg 2 h before activity, or bupropion, 100 mg bid or amantadine, 100 mg bid/tid
Orthostasis	Tolerance unlikely; increase fluid intake, use calf exercises/support hose; fludrocortisone, 0.025 mg/d
Anticholinergic	Wait for tolerance
Dry mouth, eyes	Maintain good oral hygiene; use artificial tears, sugar-free gum
Tremor/jitteriness	Antiparkinsonian drugs not effective; use dose reduction/slow increase; lorazepam, 0.5 mg bid, or propranolol, 10–20 mg bid
Insomnia	Schedule all doses for the morning; trazodone, 50–100 mg qhs
Sedation	Caffeine; schedule all dosing for bedtime; bupropion, 75–100 mg in afternoon
Headache	Evaluate diet, stress, other drugs; try dose reduction; amitriptyline, 50 mg/d
Weight gain	Decrease carbohydrates; exercise; consider fluoxetine
Loss of therapeutic benefit over time	Related to tolerance? Increase dose or drug holiday; add amantadine, 100 mg bid, buspirone, 10 mg tid, or pindolol, 2.5 mg bid

TABLE 54-5

POSSIBLE DRUG INTERACTIONS WITH SELECTIVE SEROTONIN REUPTAKE INHIBITORS

AGENT	EFFECT
Monoamine oxidase inhibitors	Serotonin syndrome—absolute contraindication
Serotonergic agonists, e.g., tryptophan, fenfluramine	Potential serotonin syndrome
Drugs that are metabolized by P450 isoenzymes: tricyclics, other SSRIs, antipsychotics, beta blockers, codeine, triazolobenzodiazepines, calcium channel blockers	Delayed metabolism resulting in increased blood levels and potential toxicity
Drugs that are bound tightly to plasma proteins, e.g., warfarin	Increased bleeding secondary to displacement
Drugs that inhibit the metabolism of SSRIs by P450 isoenzymes, e.g., quinidine	Increased SSRI side effects

Abbreviation: SSRIs, selective serotonin reuptake inhibitors.

Etiology and pathophysiology

All anxiogenic agents act on the γ-aminobutyric acid $(GABA)_A$ receptor/chloride ion channel complex, implicating this neurotransmitter system in the pathogenesis of anxiety and panic attacks. Benzodiazepines are thought to bind two separate $GABA_A$ receptor sites: type I, which has a broad neuroanatomic distribution, and type II, which is concentrated in the hippocampus, striatum, and neocortex. The antianxiety effects of the various benzodiazepines and side effects such as sedation and memory impairment are influenced by their relative binding to type I and type II receptor sites. Serotonin [5-hydroxytryptamine (5HT)] and 3α-reduced neuractive steroids (allosteric modulators of $GABA_A$) also appear to have a role in anxiety, and buspirone, a partial $5HT_{1A}$ receptor agonist, and certain $5HT_{2A}$ and $5HT_{2C}$ receptor antagonists (e.g., nefazodone) may have beneficial effects.

TREATMENT Generalized Anxiety Disorder

A combination of pharmacologic and psychotherapeutic interventions is most effective in GAD, but complete symptomatic relief is rare. A short course of a benzodiazepine is usually indicated, preferably lorazepam, oxazepam, or temazepam. (The first two of these agents are metabolized via conjugation rather than oxidation and thus do not accumulate if hepatic function is impaired.) Treatment should be initiated at the lowest dose possible and prescribed on an as-needed basis as symptoms warrant. Benzodiazepines differ in their milligram per kilogram potency, half-life, lipid solubility, metabolic pathways, and presence of active metabolites. Agents that are absorbed rapidly and are lipid soluble, such as diazepam, have a rapid onset of action and a higher abuse potential. Benzodiazepines should generally not be prescribed for >4–6 weeks because of

TABLE 54-6

ANXIOLYTICS

NAME	EQUIVALENT PO DOSE, mg	ONSET OF ACTION	HALF-LIFE, h	COMMENTS
Benzodiazepines				
Diazepam (Valium)	5	Fast	20–70	Active metabolites; quite sedating
Flurazepam (Dalmane)	15	Fast	30–100	Flurazepam is a prodrug; metabolites are active; quite sedating
Triazolam (Halcion)	0.25	Intermediate	1.5–5	No active metabolites; can induce confusion and delirium, especially in elderly
Lorazepam (Ativan)	1	Intermediate	10–20	No active metabolites; direct hepatic glucuronide conjugation; quite sedating
Alprazolam (Xanax)	0.5	Intermediate	12–15	Active metabolites; not too sedating; may have specific antidepressant and antipanic activity; tolerance and dependence develop easily
Chlordiazepoxide (Librium)	10	Intermediate	5–30	Active metabolites; moderately sedating
Oxazepam (Serax)	15	Slow	5–15	No active metabolites; direct glucuronide conjugation; not too sedating
Temazepam (Restoril)	15	Slow	9–12	No active metabolites; moderately sedating
Clonazepam (Klonopin)	0.5	Slow	18–50	No active metabolites; moderately sedating
Nonbenzodiazepines				
Buspirone (BuSpar)	7.5	2 weeks	2–3	Active metabolites; tid dosing—usual daily dose 10–20 mg tid; nonsedating; no additive effects with alcohol; useful for controlling agitation in demented or brain-injured patients

TABLE 54-7

DIAGNOSTIC CRITERIA FOR GENERALIZED ANXIETY DISORDER

A. Excessive anxiety and worry (apprehensive expectation), occurring more days than not for at least 6 months, about a number of events or activities (such as work or school performance).

B. The person finds it difficult to control the worry.

C. The anxiety and worry are associated with three (or more) of the following six symptoms (with at least some symptoms present for more days than not for the past 6 months): (1) restlessness or feeling keyed up or on edge; (2) being easily fatigued; (3) difficulty concentrating or mind going blank; (4) irritability; (5) muscle tension; (6) sleep disturbance (difficulty falling or staying asleep, or restless unsatisfying sleep).

D. The focus of the anxiety and worry is not confined to features of an axis I disorder [e.g., the anxiety or worry is not about having a panic attack (as in panic disorder), being embarrassed in public (as in social phobia), being contaminated (as in obsessive-compulsive disorder), being away from home or close relatives (as in separation anxiety disorder), gaining weight (as in anorexia nervosa), having multiple physical complaints (as in somatization disorder), or having a serious illness (as in hypochondriasis)], and the anxiety and worry do not occur exclusively during posttraumatic stress disorder.

E. The anxiety, worry, or physical symptoms cause clinically significant distress or impairment in social, occupational, or other important areas of functioning.

F. The disturbance is not due to the direct physiologic effects of a substance (e.g., a drug of abuse, a medication) or a general medical condition (e.g., hyperthyroidism) and does not occur exclusively during a mood disorder, a psychotic disorder, or a pervasive developmental disorder.

Source: Reprinted with permission from the *Diagnostic and Statistical Manual of Mental Disorders*, Fourth Edition, Text Revision. Copyright © 2000 American Psychiatric Association.

the development of tolerance and the risk of abuse and dependence. Withdrawal must be closely monitored as relapses can occur. It is important to warn patients that concomitant use of alcohol or other sedating drugs may be neurotoxic and impair their ability to function. An optimistic approach that encourages the patient to clarify environmental precipitants, anticipate his or her reactions, and plan effective response strategies is an essential element of therapy.

Adverse effects of benzodiazepines generally parallel their relative half-lives. Longer-acting agents, such as diazepam, chlordiazepoxide, flurazepam, and clonazepam, tend to accumulate active metabolites, with resultant sedation, impairment of cognition, and poor psychomotor performance. Shorter-acting compounds, such as alprazolam and oxazepam, can produce daytime anxiety, early morning insomnia, and, with discontinuation, rebound anxiety and insomnia. Although patients develop tolerance to the sedative effects of benzodiazepines, they are less likely to habituate to the adverse psychomotor effects. Withdrawal from the longer half-life benzodiazepines can be accomplished through gradual, stepwise dose reduction (by 10% every 1–2 weeks) over 6–12 weeks. It is usually more difficult to taper patients off shorter-acting benzodiazepines. Physicians may need to switch the patient to a benzodiazepine with a longer half-life or use an adjunctive medication such as a beta blocker or carbamazepine, before attempting to discontinue the benzodiazepine. Withdrawal reactions vary in severity and duration; they can include depression, anxiety, lethargy, diaphoresis, autonomic arousal, and, rarely, seizures.

Buspirone is a nonbenzodiazepine anxiolytic agent. It is nonsedating, does not produce tolerance or dependence, does not interact with benzodiazepine receptors or alcohol, and has no abuse or disinhibition potential. However, it requires several weeks to take effect and requires thrice-daily dosing. Patients who were previously responsive to a benzodiazepine are unlikely to rate buspirone as equally effective, but patients with head injury or dementia who have symptoms of anxiety and/or agitation may do well with this agent. Escitalopram, paroxetine, and venlafaxine are FDA approved for the treatment of GAD, usually at doses that are comparable to their efficacy in major depression. Benzodiazepines are contraindicated during pregnancy and breast-feeding.

Anticonvulsants with GABAergic properties may also be effective against anxiety. Gabapentin, oxcarbazepine, tiagabine, pregabalin, and divalproex have all shown some degree of benefit in a variety of anxiety-related syndromes. Agents that selectively target $GABA_A$ receptor subtypes are currently under development, and it is hoped that these will lack the sedating, memory-impairing, and addicting properties of benzodiazepines.

PHOBIC DISORDERS

Clinical manifestations

The cardinal feature of phobic disorders is a marked and persistent fear of objects or situations, exposure to which results in an immediate anxiety reaction. The patient avoids the phobic stimulus, and this avoidance usually impairs occupational or social functioning. Panic attacks may be triggered by the phobic stimulus or may occur spontaneously. Unlike patients with other anxiety disorders, individuals with phobias usually experience anxiety only in specific situations. Common phobias include fear of closed spaces (claustrophobia), fear of blood, and fear of flying. Social phobia is distinguished by a specific fear of social or performance situations in which the individual is exposed to unfamiliar individuals or to possible examination and evaluation by others. Examples include having to converse at a party, use public restrooms, and meet strangers. In each case, the affected individual is aware that the experienced fear is excessive and unreasonable given the circumstance. The specific content of a phobia may vary across gender, ethnic, and cultural boundaries.

Phobic disorders are common, affecting ~10% of the population. Full criteria for diagnosis are usually satisfied first in early adulthood, but behavioral avoidance of unfamiliar people, situations, or objects dating from early childhood is common.

In one study of female twins, concordance rates for agoraphobia, social phobia, and animal phobia were found to be 23% for monozygotic twins and 15% for dizygotic twins. A twin study of fear conditioning, a model for the acquisition of phobias, demonstrated a heritability of 35–45%, and a genomewide linkage scan identified a risk locus on chromosome 14 in a region previously implicated in a mouse model of fear. Animal studies of fear conditioning have indicated that processing of the fear stimulus occurs through the lateral nucleus of the amygdala, extending through the central nucleus and projecting to the periaqueductal gray region, lateral hypothalamus, and paraventricular hypothalamus.

TREATMENT Phobic Disorders

Beta blockers (e.g., propranolol, 20–40 mg orally 2 h before the event) are particularly effective in the treatment of "performance anxiety" (but not general social phobia) and appear to work by blocking the peripheral manifestations of anxiety such as perspiration, tachycardia, palpitations, and tremor. MAOIs alleviate social phobia independently of their antidepressant activity, and paroxetine, sertraline, and venlafaxine have received FDA approval for treatment of social anxiety. Benzodiazepines can be helpful in reducing fearful avoidance, but the chronic nature of phobic disorders limits their usefulness.

Behaviorally focused psychotherapy is an important component of treatment, as relapse rates are high when medication is used as the sole treatment. Cognitive-behavioral strategies are based upon the finding that distorted perceptions and interpretations of fear-producing stimuli play a major role in perpetuation of phobias. Individual and group therapy sessions teach the patient to identify specific negative thoughts associated with the anxiety-producing situation and help to reduce the patient's fear of loss of control. In desensitization therapy, hierarchies of feared situations are constructed and the patient is encouraged to pursue and master gradual exposure to the anxiety-producing stimuli.

Patients with social phobia, in particular, have a high rate of comorbid alcohol abuse, as well as of other psychiatric conditions (e.g., eating disorders), necessitating the need for parallel management of each disorder if anxiety reduction is to be achieved.

STRESS DISORDERS

Clinical manifestations

Patients may develop anxiety after exposure to extreme traumatic events such as the threat of personal death or injury or the death of a loved one. The reaction may occur shortly after the trauma (*acute stress disorder*) or be delayed and subject to recurrence (PTSD) (Table 54-8). In both syndromes, individuals experience associated symptoms of detachment and loss of emotional responsivity. The patient may feel depersonalized and unable to recall specific aspects of the trauma, though typically it is reexperienced through intrusions in thought, dreams, or flashbacks, particularly when cues of the original event are present. Patients often actively avoid stimuli that precipitate recollections of the trauma and demonstrate a resulting increase in vigilance, arousal, and startle response. Patients with stress disorders are at risk for the development of other disorders related to anxiety, mood, and substance abuse (especially alcohol). Between 5 and 10% of Americans will at some time in their life satisfy criteria for PTSD, with women more likely to be affected than men.

Risk factors for the development of PTSD include a past psychiatric history and personality characteristics of high neuroticism and extroversion. Twin studies show a substantial genetic influence on all symptoms associated with PTSD, with less evidence for an environmental effect.

Etiology and pathophysiology

It is hypothesized that in PTSD there is excessive release of norepinephrine from the locus coeruleus in

TABLE 54-8

DIAGNOSTIC CRITERIA FOR POSTTRAUMATIC STRESS DISORDER

A. The person has been exposed to a traumatic event in which both of the following were present:
   1. The person experienced, witnessed, or was confronted with an event or events that involved actual or threatened death or serious injury, or a threat to the physical integrity of self or others.
   2. The person's response involved intense fear, helplessness, or horror.

B. The traumatic event is persistently reexperienced in one (or more) of the following ways:
   1. Recurrent and intrusive distressing recollections of the event, including images, thoughts, or perceptions.
   2. Recurrent distressing dreams of the event.
   3. Acting or feeling as if the traumatic event were recurring (includes a sense of reliving the experience, illusions, hallucinations, and dissociative flashback episodes, including those that occur on awakening or when intoxicated).
   4. Intense psychological distress at exposure to internal or external cues that symbolize or resemble an aspect of the traumatic event.
   5. Physiologic reactivity on exposure to internal or external cues that symbolize or resemble an aspect of the traumatic event.

C. Persistent avoidance of stimuli associated with the trauma and numbing of general responsiveness (not present before the trauma), as indicated by three or more of the following:
   1. Efforts to avoid thoughts, feelings, or conversations associated with the trauma
   2. Efforts to avoid activities, places, or people that arouse recollections of the trauma
   3. Inability to recall an important aspect of the trauma
   4. Markedly diminished interest or participation in significant activities
   5. Feeling of detachment or estrangement from others
   6. Restricted range of affect (e.g., unable to have loving feelings)
   7. Sense of a foreshortened future (e.g., does not expect to have a career, marriage, children, or a normal life span)

D. Persistent symptoms of increased arousal (not present before the trauma), as indicated by two (or more) of the following:
   1. Difficulty falling or staying asleep
   2. Irritability or outbursts of anger
   3. Difficulty concentrating
   4. Hypervigilance
   5. Exaggerated startle response

E. Duration of the disturbance (symptoms in criteria B, C, and D) is more than 1 month

F. The disturbance causes clinically significant distress or impairment in social, occupational, or other important areas of functioning.

Source: Reprinted with permission from the *Diagnostic and Statistical Manual of Mental Disorders*, Fourth Edition, Text Revision. Copyright © 2000 American Psychiatric Association.

response to stress and increased noradrenergic activity at projection sites in the hippocampus and amygdala. These changes theoretically facilitate the encoding of fear-based memories. Greater sympathetic responses to cues associated with the traumatic event occur in PTSD, although pituitary adrenal responses are blunted.

TREATMENT Stress Disorders

Acute stress reactions are usually self-limited, and treatment typically involves the short-term use of benzodiazepines and supportive/expressive psychotherapy. The chronic and recurrent nature of PTSD, however, requires a more complex approach employing drug and behavioral treatments. PTSD is highly correlated with peritraumatic dissociative symptoms and the development of an acute stress disorder at the time of the trauma. TCAs such as imipramine and amitriptyline, the MAOI phenelzine, and the SSRIs can all reduce anxiety, symptoms of intrusion, and avoidance behaviors, as can prazosin, an α_1 antagonist. Propranolol and opiates such as morphine, given during the acute stress period may have beneficial effects in preventing the development of PTSD. Trazodone, a sedating antidepressant, is frequently used at night to help with insomnia (50–150 mg qhs). Carbamazepine, valproic acid, or alprazolam have also independently produced improvement in uncontrolled trials. Psychotherapeutic strategies for PTSD help the patient overcome avoidance behaviors and demoralization and master fear of recurrence of the trauma; therapies that encourage the patient to dismantle avoidance behaviors through stepwise focusing on the experience of the traumatic event are the most effective.

OBSESSIVE-COMPULSIVE DISORDER

Clinical manifestations

Obsessive-compulsive disorder (OCD) is characterized by obsessive thoughts and compulsive behaviors that impair everyday functioning. Fears of contamination and germs are common, as are handwashing, counting behaviors, and having to check and recheck such actions as whether a door is locked. The degree to which the disorder is disruptive for the individual varies, but in all cases obsessive-compulsive activities take up >1 h per day and are undertaken to relieve the anxiety triggered by the core fear. Patients often conceal their symptoms, usually because they are embarrassed by the content of their thoughts or the nature of their actions. Physicians must ask specific questions regarding recurrent thoughts and behaviors, particularly if physical clues such as chafed and reddened hands or patchy hair loss (from repetitive hair pulling, or trichotillomania) are present. Comorbid conditions are common, the most frequent being depression, other anxiety disorders, eating disorders, and tics. OCD has a lifetime prevalence of 2–3% worldwide. Onset is usually gradual, beginning in early adulthood, but childhood onset is not rare. The disorder usually has a waxing and waning course, but some cases may show a steady deterioration in psychosocial functioning.

Etiology and pathophysiology

A genetic contribution to OCD is suggested by twin studies. A genomewide association study (GWAS) reported linkage to chromosome 2p23.2; however, no susceptibility gene for OCD has been identified to date. Family studies show an aggregation of OCD with Tourette's disorder, and both are more common in males and in first-born children.

The anatomy of obsessive-compulsive behavior is thought to include the orbital frontal cortex, caudate nucleus, and globus pallidus. The caudate nucleus appears to be involved in the acquisition and maintenance of habit and skill learning, and interventions that are successful in reducing obsessive-compulsive behaviors also decrease metabolic activity measured in the caudate.

TREATMENT Obsessive-Compulsive Disorder

Clomipramine, fluoxetine, fluvoxamine, and sertraline are approved for the treatment of OCD. Clomipramine is a TCA that is often tolerated poorly owing to anticholinergic and sedative side effects at the doses required to treat the illness (25–250 mg/d); its efficacy in OCD is unrelated to its antidepressant activity. Fluoxetine (5–60 mg/d), fluvoxamine (25–300 mg/d), and sertraline (50–150 mg/d) are as effective as clomipramine and have a more benign side effect profile. Only 50–60% of patients with OCD show adequate improvement with pharmacotherapy alone. In treatment-resistant cases, augmentation with other serotonergic agents such as buspirone, or with a neuroleptic or benzodiazepine may be beneficial and in severe cases deep brain stimulation has been found to be effective. When a therapeutic response is achieved, long-duration maintenance therapy is usually indicated.

For many individuals, particularly those with time-consuming compulsions, behavior therapy will result in as much improvement as that afforded by medication. Effective techniques include the gradual increase in exposure to stressful situations, maintenance of a diary to clarify stressors, and homework assignments that substitute new activities for compulsive behaviors.

MOOD DISORDERS

Mood disorders are characterized by a disturbance in the regulation of mood, behavior, and affect. Mood disorders are subdivided into (1) depressive disorders, (2) bipolar disorders, and (3) depression in association with medical illness or alcohol and substance abuse (Chaps. 56 through 58). Major depressive disorder (MDD) is differentiated from bipolar disorder by the absence of a manic or hypomanic episode. The relationship between pure depressive syndromes and bipolar disorders is not well understood; MDD is more frequent in families of bipolar individuals, but the reverse is not true. In the Global Burden of Disease Study conducted by the World Health Organization, unipolar major depression ranked fourth among all diseases in terms of disability-adjusted life-years and was projected to rank second by the year 2020. In the United States, lost productivity directly related to mood disorders has been estimated at $55.1 billion per year.

DEPRESSION IN ASSOCIATION WITH MEDICAL ILLNESS

Depression occurring in the context of medical illness is difficult to evaluate. Depressive symptomatology may reflect the psychological stress of coping with the disease, may be caused by the disease process itself or by the medications used to treat it, or may simply coexist in time with the medical diagnosis.

Virtually every class of *medication* includes some agent that can induce depression. Antihypertensive drugs, anticholesterolemic agents, and antiarrhythmic agents are common triggers of depressive symptoms. Iatrogenic depression should also be considered in patients receiving glucocorticoids, antimicrobials, systemic analgesics, antiparkinsonian medications, and anticonvulsants. To decide whether a causal relationship exists between pharmacologic therapy and a patient's change in mood, it may sometimes be necessary to undertake an empirical trial of an alternative medication.

Between 20 and 30% of *cardiac* patients manifest a depressive disorder; an even higher percentage experience depressive symptomatology when self-reporting scales are used. Depressive symptoms following unstable angina, myocardial infarction, cardiac bypass surgery, or heart transplant impair rehabilitation and are associated with higher rates of mortality and medical morbidity. Depressed patients often show decreased variability in heart rate (an index of reduced parasympathetic nervous system activity), which may predispose individuals to ventricular arrhythmia and increased morbidity. Depression also appears to increase the risk of developing coronary heart disease, possibly through increased platelet aggregation. TCAs are contraindicated in patients with bundle branch block, and TCA-induced tachycardia is an additional concern in patients with congestive heart failure. SSRIs appear not to induce ECG changes or adverse cardiac events and thus are reasonable first-line drugs for patients at risk for TCA-related complications. SSRIs may interfere with hepatic metabolism of anticoagulants, however, causing increased anticoagulation.

In patients with *cancer*, the mean prevalence of depression is 25%, but depression occurs in 40–50% of patients with cancers of the pancreas or oropharynx. This association is not due to the effect of cachexia alone, as the higher prevalence of depression in patients with pancreatic cancer persists when compared to those with advanced gastric cancer. Initiation of antidepressant medication in cancer patients has been shown to improve quality of life as well as mood. Psychotherapeutic approaches, particularly group therapy, may have some effect on short-term depression, anxiety, and pain symptoms.

Depression occurs frequently in patients with *neurologic disorders*, particularly cerebrovascular disorders, Parkinson's disease, dementia, multiple sclerosis, and traumatic brain injury. One in five patients with left-hemisphere stroke involving the dorsolateral frontal cortex experiences major depression. Late-onset depression in otherwise cognitively normal individuals increases the risk of a subsequent diagnosis of Alzheimer's disease. Both TCA and SSRI agents are effective against these depressions, as are stimulant compounds and, in some patients, MAOIs.

The reported prevalence of depression in patients with *diabetes mellitus* varies from 8 to 27%, with the severity of the mood state correlating with the level of hyperglycemia and the presence of diabetic complications. Treatment of depression may be complicated by effects of antidepressive agents on glycemic control. MAOIs can induce hypoglycemia and weight gain, while TCAs can produce hyperglycemia and carbohydrate craving. SSRIs, like MAOIs, may reduce fasting plasma glucose, but they are easier to use and may also improve dietary and medication compliance.

Hypothyroidism is frequently associated with features of depression, most commonly depressed mood and memory impairment. Hyperthyroid states may also present in a similar fashion, usually in geriatric populations. Improvement in mood usually follows normalization of thyroid function, but adjunctive antidepressant medication is sometimes required. Patients with subclinical hypothyroidism can also experience symptoms of depression and cognitive difficulty that respond to thyroid replacement.

The lifetime prevalence of depression in *HIV-positive* individuals has been estimated at 22–45%. The relationship between depression and disease progression is multifactorial and likely to involve psychological and social factors, alterations in immune function, and central nervous system (CNS) disease. Chronic hepatitis C infection is also associated with depression, which may worsen with interferon-α treatment.

Some chronic disorders of uncertain etiology, such as chronic fatigue syndrome (Chap. 52) and fibromyalgia, are strongly associated with depression and anxiety; patients may benefit from antidepressant treatment or anticonvulsant agents such as pregabalin.

DEPRESSIVE DISORDERS

Clinical manifestations

Major depression is defined as depressed mood on a daily basis for a minimum duration of 2 weeks (Table 54-9). An episode may be characterized by sadness, indifference, apathy, or irritability and is usually associated with changes in sleep patterns, appetite, and weight; motor agitation or retardation; fatigue; impaired concentration and decision making; feelings of shame or guilt; and thoughts of death or dying. Patients with depression have a profound loss of pleasure in all enjoyable activities, exhibit early morning awakening, feel that the dysphoric mood state is qualitatively different from sadness, and often notice a diurnal variation in mood (worse in morning hours).

Approximately 15% of the population experiences a major depressive episode at some point in life, and 6–8% of all outpatients in primary care settings satisfy diagnostic criteria for the disorder. Depression is often undiagnosed, and, even more frequently, it is treated inadequately. If a physician suspects the presence of a major depressive episode, the initial task is to determine whether it represents unipolar or bipolar depression or is one of the 10–15% of cases that are secondary to general medical illness or substance abuse. Physicians should also assess the risk of suicide by direct questioning, as patients are often reluctant to verbalize such thoughts without prompting. If specific plans are uncovered or if significant risk factors exist (e.g., a past history of suicide attempts, profound hopelessness, concurrent medical illness, substance abuse, or social isolation), the patient must be referred to a mental health specialist for immediate care. The physician should specifically probe each of these areas in an empathic and hopeful manner, being sensitive to denial and possible minimization of distress. The presence of anxiety, panic, or agitation significantly increases near-term suicidal risk. Approximately 4–5% of all depressed patients will commit suicide; most will have sought help from physicians within 1 month of their deaths.

In some depressed patients, the mood disorder does not appear to be episodic and is not clearly associated with either psychosocial dysfunction or change from the individual's usual experience in life. *Dysthymic disorder* consists of a pattern of chronic (at least 2 years), ongoing, mild depressive symptoms that are less severe and less disabling than those found in major depression; the two conditions are sometimes difficult to separate, however, and can occur together ("double depression"). Many patients who exhibit a profile of pessimism, disinterest, and low self-esteem respond to antidepressant treatment. Dysthymic disorder exists in ~5% of primary care patients. The term *minor depression* is used for individuals who experience at least two depressive

TABLE 54-9

CRITERIA FOR A MAJOR DEPRESSIVE EPISODE

A. Five (or more) of the following symptoms have been present during the same 2-week period and represent a change from previous functioning; at least one of the symptoms is either (1) depressed mood or (2) loss of interest or pleasure. **Note**: Do not include symptoms that are clearly due to a general medical condition, or mood-incongruent delusions or hallucinations.
   1. Depressed mood most of the day, nearly every day, as indicated by either subjective report (e.g., feels sad or empty) or observation made by others (e.g., appears tearful)
   2. Markedly diminished interest or pleasure in all, or almost all, activities most of the day, nearly every day (as indicated by either subjective account or observation made by others)
   3. Significant weight loss when not dieting or weight gain (e.g., a change of >5% of body weight in a month), or decrease or increase in appetite nearly every day
   4. Insomnia or hypersomnia nearly every day
   5. Psychomotor agitation or retardation nearly every day (observable by others, not merely subjective feelings of restlessness or being slowed down)
   6. Fatigue or loss of energy nearly every day
   7. Feelings of worthlessness or excessive or inappropriate guilt (which may be delusional) nearly every day (not merely self-reproach or guilt about being sick)
   8. Diminished ability to think or concentrate, or indecisiveness, nearly every day (either by subjective account or as observed by others)
   9. Recurrent thoughts of death (not just fear of dying), recurrent suicidal ideation without a specific plan, or a suicide attempt or a specific plan for committing suicide

B. The symptoms do not meet criteria for a mixed episode

C. The symptoms cause clinically significant distress or impairment in social, occupational, or other important areas of functioning

D. The symptoms are not due to the direct physiologic effects of a substance (e.g., a drug of abuse, a medication) or a general medical condition (e.g., hypothyroidism)

E. The symptoms are not better accounted for by bereavement (i.e., after the loss of a loved one), the symptoms persist for >2 months or are characterized by marked functional impairment, morbid preoccupation with worthlessness, suicidal ideation, psychotic symptoms, or psychomotor retardation

Source: Reprinted with permission from the *Diagnostic and Statistical Manual of Mental Disorders*, Fourth Edition, Text Revision. Copyright © 2000 American Psychiatric Association.

symptoms for 2 weeks but who do not meet the full criteria for major depression. Despite its name, minor depression is associated with significant morbidity and disability and also responds to pharmacologic treatment.

Depression is approximately twice as common in women as in men, and the incidence increases with age in both sexes. Twin studies indicate that the liability to major depression of early onset (before age 25) is largely genetic in origin. Negative life events can precipitate and contribute to depression, but genetic factors influence the sensitivity of individuals to these stressful events. In most cases, both biologic and psychosocial factors are involved in the precipitation and unfolding of depressive episodes. The most potent stressors appear to involve death of a relative, assault, or severe marital or relationship problems.

Unipolar depressive disorders usually begin in early adulthood and recur episodically over the course of a lifetime. The best predictor of future risk is the number of past episodes; 50–60% of patients who have a first episode have at least one or two recurrences. Some patients experience multiple episodes that become more severe and frequent over time. The duration of an untreated episode varies greatly, ranging from a few months to ≤1 year. The pattern of recurrence and clinical progression in a developing episode are also variable. Within an individual, the nature of episodes (e.g., specific presenting symptoms, frequency and duration) may be similar over time. In a minority of patients, a severe depressive episode may progress to a psychotic state; in elderly patients, depressive symptoms may be associated with cognitive deficits mimicking dementia ("pseudodementia"). A seasonal pattern of depression, called *seasonal affective disorder*, may manifest with onset and remission of episodes at predictable times of the year. This disorder is more common in women, whose symptoms are anergy, fatigue, weight gain, hypersomnia, and episodic carbohydrate craving. The prevalence increases with distance from the equator, and improvement may occur by altering light exposure.

Etiology and pathophysiology

Although evidence for genetic transmission of unipolar depression is not as strong as in bipolar disorder, monozygotic twins have a higher concordance rate (46%) than dizygotic siblings (20%), with little support for any effect of a shared family environment.

Neuroendocrine abnormalities that reflect the neurovegetative signs and symptoms of depression include: (1) increased cortisol and corticotropin-releasing hormone (CRH) secretion, (2) an increase in adrenal size, (3) a decreased inhibitory response of glucocorticoids to dexamethasone, and (4) a blunted response of thyroid-stimulating hormone (TSH) level to infusion of thyroid-releasing hormone (TRH). Antidepressant treatment leads to normalization of these abnormalities. Major depression is also associated with an upregulation of proinflammatory cytokines, which also normalizes with antidepressant treatment.

Diurnal variations in symptom severity and alterations in circadian rhythmicity of a number of neurochemical and neurohumoral factors suggest that biologic differences may be secondary to a primary defect in regulation of biologic rhythms. Patients with major depression show consistent findings of a decrease in rapid eye movement (REM) sleep onset (REM latency), an increase in REM density, and, in some subjects, a decrease in stage IV delta slow-wave sleep.

Although antidepressant drugs inhibit neurotransmitter uptake within hours, their therapeutic effects typically emerge over several weeks, implicating adaptive changes in second messenger systems and transcription factors as possible mechanisms of action.

The pathogenesis of depression is discussed in detail in Chap. 53.

TREATMENT Depressive Disorders

Treatment planning requires coordination of short-term strategies to induce remission combined with longer term maintenance designed to prevent recurrence. The most effective intervention for achieving remission and preventing relapse is medication, but combined treatment, incorporating psychotherapy to help the patient cope with decreased self-esteem and demoralization, improves outcome (Fig. 54-1). Approximately 40% of primary care patients with depression drop out of treatment and discontinue medication if symptomatic improvement is not noted within a month, unless additional support is provided. Outcome improves with (1) increased intensity and frequency of visits during the first 4–6 weeks of treatment, (2) supplemental educational materials, and (3) psychiatric consultation as indicated. Despite the widespread use of SSRIs and other second-generation antidepressant drugs, there is no convincing evidence that this class of antidepressant is more efficacious than TCAs. Between 60 and 70% of all depressed patients respond to any drug chosen, if it is given in a sufficient dose for 6–8 weeks. There is no ideal antidepressant; no current compound combines rapid onset of action, moderate half-life, a meaningful relationship between dose and blood level, a low side effect profile, minimal interaction with other drugs, and safety in overdose.

A rational approach to selecting which antidepressant to use involves matching the patient's preference and medical history withthe metabolic and side effect profile of the drug (Tables 54-4 and 54-5). A previous response, or a family history of a positive response, to

MEDICAL MANAGEMENT OF MAJOR DEPRESSIVE DISORDER ALGORITHM

Determine whether there is a history of good response to a medication in the patient or a first-degree relative; if yes, consider treatment with this agent if compatible with considerations in step 2

↓

Evaluate patient characteristics and match to drug; consider health status, side effect profile, convenience, cost, patient preference, drug interaction risk, suicide potential, and medication compliance history.

↓

Begin new medication at 1/3 to 1/2 target dose if drug is a TCA, bupropion, venlafaxine, or mirtazapine, or full dose as tolerated if drug is an SSRI.

↓

If problem side effects occur, evaluate possibility of tolerance; consider temporary decrease in dose or adjunctive treatment.

↓

If unacceptable side effects continue, taper drug over 1 week and initiate new trial; consider potential drug interactions in choice.

↓

Evaluate response after 6 weeks at target dose; if response is inadequate, increase dose in stepwise fashion as tolerated.

↓

If inadequate response after maximal dose, consider tapering and switching to a new drug vs adjunctive treatment; if drug is a TCA, obtain plasma level to guide further treatment.

FIGURE 54-1

A guideline for the medical management of major depressive disorder. SSRI, selective serotonin reuptake inhibitor; TCA, tricyclic antidepressant.

a specific antidepressant often suggests that that drug be tried first. Before initiating antidepressant therapy, the physician should evaluate the possible contribution of comorbid illnesses and consider their specific treatment. In individuals with suicidal ideation, particular attention should be paid to choosing a drug with low toxicity if taken in overdose. The SSRIs, and other newer antidepressant drugs are distinctly safer in this regard; nevertheless, the advantages of TCAs have not been completely superseded. The existence of generic equivalents make TCAs relatively cheap, and for secondary tricyclics, particularly nortriptyline and desipramine, well-defined relationships among dose, plasma level, and therapeutic response exist. The steady-state plasma level achieved for a given drug dose can vary more than tenfold between individuals and plasma levels may help in interpreting apparent resistance to treatment and/or unexpected drug toxicity. The principal side effects of TCAs are antihistamine (sedation) and anticholinergic (constipation, dry mouth, urinary hesitancy, blurred vision). TCAs are contraindicated in patients with serious cardiovascular risk factors and overdoses of tricyclic agents can be lethal, with desipramine carrying the greatest risk. It is judicious to prescribe only a 10-day supply when suicide is a risk. Most patients require a daily dose of 150–200 mg of imipramine or amitriptyline or its equivalent to achieve a therapeutic blood level of 150–300 ng/mL and a satisfactory remission; some patients show a partial effect at lower doses. Geriatric patients may require a low starting dose and slow escalation. Ethnic differences in drug metabolism are significant, with Hispanic, Asian, and black patients generally requiring lower doses than whites to achieve a comparable blood level. P450 profiling using genetic chip technology may be clinically useful in predicting individual sensitivity.

Second-generation antidepressants include amoxapine, maprotiline, trazodone, and bupropion. Amoxapine is a dibenzoxazepine derivative that blocks norepinephrine and serotonin reuptake and has a metabolite that shows a degree of dopamine blockade. Long-term use of this drug carries a risk of tardive dyskinesia. Maprotiline is a potent noradrenergic reuptake blocker that has little anticholinergic effect but may produce seizures. Bupropion is a novel antidepressant whose mechanism of action is thought to involve enhancement of noradrenergic function. It has no anticholinergic, sedating, or orthostatic side effects and has a low incidence of sexual side effects. It may, however, be associated with stimulant-like side effects, may lower seizure threshold, and has an exceptionally short half-life, requiring frequent dosing. An extended-release preparation is available.

SSRIs such as fluoxetine, sertraline, paroxetine, citalopram, and escitalopram cause a lower frequency of anticholinergic, sedating, and cardiovascular side effects but a possibly greater incidence of gastrointestinal complaints, sleep impairment, and sexual dysfunction than do TCAs. Akathisia, involving an inner sense of restlessness and anxiety in addition to increased motor activity, may also be more common, particularly during the first week of treatment. One concern is the risk of "serotonin syndrome," thought to result from hyperstimulation of brainstem $5HT_{1A}$ receptors and characterized by myoclonus, agitation, abdominal cramping, hyperpyrexia, hypertension, and potentially death. Serotonergic agonists taken in combination should be monitored closely for this reason. Considerations such as half-life, compliance, toxicity, and drug-drug interactions may guide the choice of a particular SSRI. Fluoxetine and its principal active metabolite, norfluoxetine, for example, have a combined half-life of almost 7 days, resulting in a delay of 5 weeks before steady-state levels are achieved and a similar delay for complete drug excretion once its use is discontinued. All the SSRIs may impair sexual function, resulting in diminished libido, impotence, or difficulty in achieving orgasm. Sexual dysfunction frequently results in noncompliance and should be asked about specifically. Sexual dysfunction can sometimes be ameliorated by lowering the dose, by instituting weekend drug holidays (two or three times a month), or by treatment with amantadine (100 mg tid), bethanechol (25 mg tid), buspirone (10 mg tid), or bupropion (100–150 mg/d). Paroxetine appears to be more anticholinergic than either fluoxetine or sertraline, and sertraline carries a lower risk of producing an adverse drug interaction than the other two. Rare side effects of SSRIs include angina due to vasospasm and prolongation of the prothrombin time. Escitalopram is the most specific of currently available SSRIs and appears to have no specific inhibitory effects on the P450 system.

Venlafaxine, desvenlafaxine, and duloxetine block the reuptake of both norepinephrine and serotonin but produce relatively little in the way of traditional tricyclic side effects. Unlike the SSRIs, venlafaxine has a relatively linear dose-response curve. Patients should be monitored for a possible increase in diastolic blood pressure, and multiple daily dosing is required because of the drug's short half-life. An extended-release form is available and has a somewhat lower incidence of gastrointestinal side effects. Mirtazapine is a TCA that has a unique spectrum of activity. It increases noradrenergic and serotonergic neurotransmission through a blockade of central α_2-adrenergic receptors and postsynaptic $5HT_2$ and $5HT_3$ receptors. It is also strongly antihistaminic and, as such, may produce sedation.

With the exception of citalopram and escitalopram, each of the SSRIs may inhibit one or more cytochrome P450 enzymes. Depending on the specific isoenzyme involved, the metabolism of a number of concomitantly administered medications can be dramatically affected. Fluoxetine and paroxetine, for example, by inhibiting 2D6, can cause dramatic increases in the blood level of type 1C antiarrhythmics, while sertraline, by acting on 3A4, may alter blood levels of carbamazepine, or digoxin.

The MAOIs are highly effective, particularly in atypical depression, but the risk of hypertensive crisis following intake of tyramine-containing food or sympathomimetic drugs makes them inappropriate as first-line agents. Transdermal selegiline may avert this risk at low dose. Common side effects include orthostatic hypotension, weight gain, insomnia, and sexual dysfunction. MAOIs should not be used concomitantly with SSRIs, because of the risk of serotonin syndrome, or with TCAs, because of possible hyperadrenergic effects.

Electroconvulsive therapy is at least as effective as medication, but its use is reserved for treatment-resistant cases and delusional depressions. Transcranial magnetic stimulation (TMS) is approved for treatment-resistant depression and has been shown to have efficacy in several controlled trials. Vagus nerve stimulation (VNS) has also recently been approved for treatment-resistant depression, but its degree of efficacy is controversial. Deep brain stimulation is another treatment that is being used experimentally in treatment-resistant cases.

Regardless of the treatment undertaken, the response should be evaluated after ~2 months. Three-quarters of patients show improvement by this time, but if remission is inadequate the patient should be questioned about compliance and an increase in medication dose should be considered if side effects are not troublesome. If this approach is unsuccessful, referral to a mental health specialist is advised. Strategies for treatment then include selection of an alternative drug, combinations of antidepressants, and/or adjunctive treatment with other classes of drugs, including lithium, thyroid hormone, atypical antipsychotic agents, and dopamine agonists. A large randomized trial (STAR-D) was unable to show preferential efficacy, but the addition of atypical antipsychotic drugs has received FDA approval. Patients whose response to an SSRI wanes over time may benefit from the addition of buspirone (10 mg tid) or pindolol (2–5 mg tid) or small amounts of a TCA such as desipramine (25 mg bid or tid). Most patients will show some degree of response but aggressive treatment should be pursued until remission is achieved, and drug treatment should be continued for at least 6–9 more months to prevent relapse. In patients who have had two or more episodes of depression, indefinite maintenance treatment should be considered.

It is essential to educate patients both about depression and the benefits and side effects of medications they are receiving. Advice about stress reduction and cautions that alcohol may exacerbate depressive symptoms and impair drug response are helpful. Patients should be given time to describe their experience, their outlook, and the impact of the depression on them and their families. Occasional empathic silence may be as helpful for the treatment alliance as verbal reassurance. Controlled trials have shown that cognitive-behavioral and interpersonal therapies are effective in improving psychological and social adjustment and that a combined treatment approach is more successful than medication alone for many patients.

BIPOLAR DISORDER

Clinical manifestations

Bipolar disorder is characterized by unpredictable swings in mood from mania (or hypomania) to depression. Some patients suffer only from recurrent attacks of *mania*, which in its pure form is associated with increased psychomotor activity; excessive social extroversion; decreased need for sleep; impulsivity and impairment in judgment; and expansive, grandiose, and sometimes irritable mood (**Table 54-10**). In severe mania, patients may experience delusions and paranoid thinking indistinguishable from schizophrenia. One-half of patients with bipolar disorder present with a mixture of psychomotor agitation and activation with dysphoria,

TABLE 54-10

CRITERIA FOR A MANIC EPISODE

A. A distinct period of abnormally and persistently elevated, expansive, or irritable mood, lasting at least 1 week (or any duration if hospitalization is necessary)

B. During the period of mood disturbance, three (or more) of the following symptoms have persisted (four if the mood is only irritable) and have been present to a significant degree:
1. Inflated self-esteem or grandiosity
2. Decreased need for sleep (e.g., feels rested after only 3 h of sleep)
3. More talkative than usual or pressure to keep talking
4. Flight of ideas or subjective experience that thoughts are racing
5. Distractibility (i.e., attention too easily drawn to unimportant or irrelevant external stimuli)
6. Increase in goal-directed activity (either socially, at work or school, or sexually) or psychomotor agitation
7. Excessive involvement in pleasurable activities that have a high potential for painful consequences (e.g., engaging in unrestrained buying sprees, sexual indiscretions, or foolish business investments)

C. The symptoms do not meet criteria for a mixed episode.

D. The mood disturbance is sufficiently severe to cause marked impairment in occupational functioning or in usual social activities or relationships with others, or to necessitate hospitalization to prevent harm to self or others, or there are psychotic features.

E. The symptoms are not due to the direct physiologic effects of a substance (e.g., a drug of abuse, a medication, or other treatment) or a general medical condition (e.g., hyperthyroidism).

Note: Manic-like episodes that are clearly caused by somatic antidepressant treatment (e.g., medication, electroconvulsive therapy, light therapy) should not count toward a diagnosis of bipolar I disorder.
Source: Reprinted with permission from the *Diagnostic and Statistical Manual of Mental Disorders*, Fourth Edition, Text Revision. Copyright © 2000 American Psychiatric Association.

anxiety, and irritability. It may be difficult to distinguish *mixed mania* from *agitated depression*. In some bipolar patients (*bipolar II disorder*), the full criteria for mania are lacking, and the requisite recurrent depressions are separated by periods of mild activation and increased energy (hypomania). In *cyclothymic disorder*, there are numerous hypomanic periods, usually of relatively short duration, alternating with clusters of depressive symptoms that fail, either in severity or duration, to meet the criteria of major depression. The mood fluctuations are chronic and should be present for at least 2 years before the diagnosis is made.

Manic episodes typically emerge over a period of days to weeks, but onset within hours is possible, usually in the early morning hours. An untreated episode of either depression or mania can be as short as several weeks or last as long as 8–12 months, and rare patients have an unremitting chronic course. The term *rapid cycling* is used for patients who have four or more episodes of either depression or mania in a given year. This pattern occurs in 15% of all patients, almost all of whom are women. In some cases, rapid cycling is linked to an underlying thyroid dysfunction and, in others, it is iatrogenically triggered by prolonged antidepressant treatment. Approximately one-half of patients have sustained difficulties in work performance and psychosocial functioning, with depressive phases being more responsible for impairment than mania.

Bipolar disorder is common, affecting ~1.5% of the population in the United States. Onset is typically between 20 and 30 years of age, but many individuals report premorbid symptoms in late childhood or early adolescence. The prevalence is similar for men and women; women are likely to have more depressive and men more manic episodes over a lifetime.

Differential diagnosis

The differential diagnosis of mania includes secondary mania induced by stimulant or sympathomimetic drugs, hyperthyroidism, AIDS, neurologic disorders, such as Huntington's or Wilson's disease, and cerebrovascular accidents. Comorbidity with alcohol and substance abuse is common, either because of poor judgment and increased impulsivity or because of an attempt to self-treat the underlying mood symptoms and sleep disturbances.

Etiology and pathophysiology

Genetic predisposition to bipolar disorder is evident from family studies; the concordance rate for monozygotic twins approaches 80%. Patients with bipolar disorder also appear to have altered circadian rhythmicity, and lithium may exert its therapeutic benefit through a resynchronization of intrinsic rhythms keyed to the light/dark cycle. A detailed discussion of the pathogenesis of bipolar disorder is presented in Chap. 53.

TREATMENT Bipolar Disorder

(Table 54-11) Lithium carbonate is the mainstay of treatment in bipolar disorder, although sodium valproate and olanzapine are equally effective in acute mania, as is lamotrigine in the depressed phase. The response rate to lithium carbonate is 70–80% in acute mania, with beneficial effects appearing in 1–2 weeks. Lithium also has a prophylactic effect in prevention of recurrent mania and, to a lesser extent, in the prevention of recurrent depression. A simple cation, lithium is rapidly absorbed from the gastrointestinal tract and remains unbound to plasma or tissue proteins. Some 95% of a given dose is excreted unchanged through the kidneys within 24 h.

TABLE 54-11

CLINICAL PHARMACOLOGY OF MOOD STABILIZERS

AGENT AND DOSING	SIDE EFFECTS AND OTHER EFFECTS
Lithium	**Common Side Effects**
Starting dose: 300 mg bid or tid Therapeutic blood level: 0.8–1.2 meq/L	Nausea/anorexia/diarrhea, fine tremor, thirst, polyuria, fatigue, weight gain, acne, folliculitis, neutrophilia, hypothyroidism Blood level is increased by thiazides, tetracyclines, and NSAIDs Blood level is decreased by bronchodilators, verapamil, and carbonic anhydrase inhibitors *Rare side effects:* Neurotoxicity, renal toxicity, hypercalcemia, ECG changes
Valproic Acid	**Common Side Effects**
Starting dose: 250 mg tid Therapeutic blood level: 50–125 μg/mL	Nausea/anorexia, weight gain, sedation, tremor, rash, alopecia Inhibits hepatic metabolism of other medications *Rare side effects:* Pancreatitis, hepatotoxicity, Stevens-Johnson syndrome
Carbamazepine/ Oxcarbazepine	**Common Side Effects**
Starting dose: 200 mg bid for carbamazepine, 150 mg bid for oxcarbazepine Therapeutic blood level: 4–12 μg/mL for carbamazepine	Nausea/anorexia, sedation, rash, dizziness/ataxia Carbamazepine, but not oxcarbazepine, induces hepatic metabolism of other medications *Rare side effects:* Hyponatremia, agranulocytosis, Stevens-Johnson syndrome
Lamotrigine	**Common Side Effects**
Starting dose: 25 mg/d	Rash, dizziness, headache, tremor, sedation, nausea *Rare side effect:* Stevens-Johnson syndrome

Abbreviations: NSAIDs, nonsteroidal anti-inflammatory drugs; ECG, electrocardiogram.

Serious side effects from lithium are rare, but minor complaints such as gastrointestinal discomfort, nausea, diarrhea, polyuria, weight gain, skin eruptions, alopecia, and edema are common. Over time, urine-concentrating ability may be decreased, but significant nephrotoxicity does not usually occur. Lithium exerts an antithyroid effect by interfering with the synthesis and release of thyroid hormones. More serious side effects include tremor, poor concentration and memory, ataxia, dysarthria, and incoordination. There is suggestive, but not conclusive, evidence that lithium is teratogenic, inducing cardiac malformations in the first trimester.

In the treatment of acute mania, lithium is initiated at 300 mg bid or tid, and the dose is then increased by 300 mg every 2–3 days to achieve blood levels of 0.8–1.2 meq/L. Because the therapeutic effect of lithium may not appear until after 7–10 days of treatment, adjunctive usage of lorazepam (1–2 mg every 4 h) or clonazepam (0.5–1 mg every 4 h) may be beneficial to control agitation. Antipsychotics are indicated in patients with severe agitation who respond only partially to benzodiazepines. Patients using lithium should be monitored closely, since the blood levels required to achieve a therapeutic benefit are close to those associated with toxicity.

Valproic acid may be better than lithium for patients who experience rapid cycling (i.e., more than four episodes a year) or who present with a mixed or dysphoric mania. Tremor and weight gain are the most common side effects; hepatotoxicity and pancreatitis are rare toxicities.

Carbamazepine and oxcarbazepine, although not formally approved by the FDA for bipolar disorder, have clinical efficacy in the treatment of acute mania. Second-generation antipsychotic drugs (olanzapine, quetiapine, risperidone, ziprasidone, aripiprazole, and asenapine) have also been shown to be effective, either alone or in combination with a mood stabilizer. An increased risk of weight gain and other metabolic abnormalities is a concern with these agents.

The recurrent nature of bipolar mood disorder necessitates maintenance treatment. A sustained blood lithium level of at least 0.8 meq/L is important for optimal prophylaxis and has been shown to reduce risk of suicide, a finding not yet apparent for other mood stabilizers. Compliance is frequently an issue and often requires enlistment and education of concerned family members. Efforts to identify and modify psychosocial factors that may trigger episodes are important, as is an emphasis on lifestyle regularity. Antidepressant medications are sometimes required for the treatment of severe breakthrough depressions, but their use should generally be avoided during maintenance treatment because of the risk of precipitating mania or accelerating the cycle frequency. Loss of efficacy over time may be observed with any of the mood-stabilizing agents. In such situations, an alternative agent or combination therapy is usually helpful.

Consensus guidelines for the treatment of acute mania and bipolar depression are described in Table 54-12.

TABLE 54-12

CONSENSUS GUIDELINES ON THE DRUG TREATMENT OF ACUTE MANIA AND BIPOLAR DEPRESSION

CONDITION	PREFERRED AGENTS
Euphoric mania	Lithium
Mixed/dysphoric mania	Valproic acid
Mania with psychosis	Valproic acid with olanzapine, aripiprazole, conventional antipsychotic, or risperidone
Hypomania	Lithium, lamotrigine, or valproic acid alone
Severe depression with psychosis	Venlafaxine, bupropion, or paroxetine *plus* lithium *plus* olanzapine, *or* risperidone; consider ECT
Severe depression without psychosis	Bupropion, paroxetine, sertraline, venlafaxine, *or* citalopram *plus* lithium
Mild to moderate depression	Lithium *or* lamotrigine alone; add bupropion if needed

Abbreviation: ECT, electroconvulsive therapy.
Source: From GS Sachs et al: Postgrad Med April, 2000.

SOMATOFORM DISORDERS

CLINICAL MANIFESTATIONS

Patients with multiple somatic complaints that cannot be explained by a known medical condition or by the effects of alcohol or of recreational or prescription drugs are commonly seen in primary care practice; one survey indicated a prevalence of such complaints of 5%. In *somatization disorder*, the patient presents with multiple physical complaints referable to different organ systems (Table 54-13). Onset is usually before age 30 years, and the disorder is persistent. Formal diagnostic criteria require the recording of at least four pain, two gastrointestinal, one sexual, and one pseudoneurologic symptom. Patients with somatization disorder often present with dramatic complaints, but the complaints are inconsistent. Symptoms of comorbid anxiety and mood disorder are common and may be the result of drug interactions due to regimens initiated independently by different physicians. Patients with somatization disorder may be impulsive and demanding and frequently qualify for a formal comorbid psychiatric diagnosis. In *conversion disorder*, the symptoms focus on deficits that involve motor or sensory function and on psychological factors that initiate or exacerbate the medical presentation. Like somatization disorder, the deficit is not intentionally produced or simulated, as is the case in factitious disorder (malingering). In *hypochondriasis*, the essential feature is a belief

TABLE 54-13

DIAGNOSTIC CRITERIA FOR SOMATIZATION DISORDER

A. A history of many physical complaints beginning before age 30 years that occur over a period of several years and result in treatment being sought or significant impairment in social, occupational, or other important areas of functioning.
B. Each of the following criteria must have been met, with individual symptoms occurring at any time during the course of the disturbance:
   1. *Four pain symptoms:* a history of pain related to at least four different sites or functions (e.g., head, abdomen, back, joints, extremities, chest, rectum, during menstruation, during sexual intercourse, or during urination)
   2. *Two gastrointestinal symptoms:* a history of at least two gastrointestinal symptoms other than pain (e.g., nausea, bloating, vomiting other than during pregnancy, diarrhea, or intolerance of several different foods)
   3. *One sexual symptom:* a history of at least one sexual or reproductive symptom other than pain (e.g., sexual indifference, erectile or ejaculatory dysfunction, irregular menses, excessive menstrual bleeding, vomiting throughout pregnancy)
   4. *One pseudoneurologic symptom:* a history of at least one symptom or deficit suggesting a neurologic condition not limited to pain (conversion symptoms such as impaired coordination or balance, paralysis or localized weakness, difficulty swallowing or lump in throat, aphonia, urinary retention, hallucinations, loss of touch or pain sensation, double vision, blindness, deafness, seizures; dissociative symptoms such as amnesia; or loss of consciousness other than fainting)
C. Either of the following:
   1. After appropriate investigation, each of the symptoms in criterion B cannot be fully explained by a known general medical condition or the direct effects of a substance (e.g., a drug of abuse, a medication)
   2. When there is a related general medical condition, the physical complaints or resulting social or occupational impairment are in excess of what would be expected from the history, physical examination, or laboratory findings
D. The symptoms are not intentionally produced or feigned (as in factitious disorder or malingering).

Source: Reprinted with permission from the *Diagnostic and Statistical Manual of Mental Disorders*, Fourth Edition, Text Revision. Copyright © 2000 American Psychiatric Association.

of serious medical illness that persists despite reassurance and appropriate medical evaluation. As with somatization disorder, patients with hypochondriasis have a history of poor relationships with physicians stemming from their sense that they have been evaluated and treated inappropriately or inadequately. Hypochondriasis can be disabling in intensity and is persistent, with waxing and waning symptomatology.

In *factitious illnesses*, the patient consciously and voluntarily produces physical symptoms of illness. The term *Munchausen's syndrome* is reserved for individuals with particularly dramatic, chronic, or severe factitious illness. In true factitious illness, the sick role itself is gratifying. A variety of signs, symptoms, and diseases have been either simulated or caused by factitious behavior, the most common including chronic diarrhea, fever of unknown origin, intestinal bleeding or hematuria, seizures, and hypoglycemia. Factitious disorder is usually not diagnosed until 5–10 years after its onset, and it can produce significant social and medical costs. In *malingering*, the fabrication derives from a desire for some external reward such as a narcotic medication or disability reimbursement.

TREATMENT Somatoform Disorders

Patients with somatization disorders are frequently subjected to many diagnostic tests and exploratory surgeries in an attempt to find their "real" illness. Such an approach is doomed to failure and does not address the core issue. Successful treatment is best achieved through behavior modification, in which access to the physician is tightly regulated and adjusted to provide a sustained and predictable level of support that is less clearly contingent on the patient's level of presenting distress. Visits can be brief and should not be associated with a need for a diagnostic or treatment action. Although the literature is limited, some patients with somatization disorder may benefit from antidepressant treatment.

Any attempt to confront the patient usually creates a sense of humiliation and causes the patient to abandon treatment from that caregiver. A better strategy is to introduce psychological causation as one of a number of possible explanations and to include factitious illness as an option in the differential diagnoses that are discussed. Without directly linking psychotherapeutic intervention to the diagnosis, the patient can be offered a face-saving means by which the pathologic relationship with the health care system can be examined and alternative approaches to life stressors developed.

PERSONALITY DISORDERS

Clinical manifestations

Personality disorders are characteristic patterns of thinking, feeling, and interpersonal behavior that are relatively inflexible and cause significant functional impairment or subjective distress for the individual. The observed behaviors are not secondary to another mental disorder, nor are they precipitated by substance abuse or a general medical condition. This distinction is often difficult to make in clinical practice, as personality change may be the first sign of serious neurologic, endocrine, or other medical illness. Patients with frontal lobe tumors, for example, can present with changes in motivation and personality while the results of the neurologic examination remain within normal limits. Individuals with personality disorders are often regarded as "difficult patients" in clinical medical practice because they are seen as excessively demanding and/or unwilling to follow recommended treatment plans. Although DSM-IV portrays personality disorders as qualitatively distinct categories, there is an alternative perspective that personality characteristics vary as a continuum between normal functioning and formal mental disorder.

Personality disorders have been grouped into three overlapping clusters. *Cluster A* includes paranoid, schizoid, and schizotypal personality disorders. It includes individuals who are odd and eccentric and who maintain an emotional distance from others. Individuals have a restricted emotional range and remain socially isolated. Patients with schizotypal personality disorder frequently have unusual perceptual experiences and express magical beliefs about the external world. The essential feature of paranoid personality disorder is a pervasive mistrust and suspiciousness of others to an extent that is unjustified by available evidence. *Cluster B* disorders include antisocial, borderline, histrionic, and narcissistic types and describe individuals whose behavior is impulsive, excessively emotional, and erratic. *Cluster C* incorporates avoidant, dependent, and obsessive-compulsive personality types; enduring traits are anxiety and fear. The boundaries between cluster types are to some extent artificial, and many patients who meet criteria for one personality disorder also meet criteria for aspects of another. The risk of a comorbid major mental disorder is increased in patients who qualify for a diagnosis of personality disorder.

TREATMENT Personality Disorders

Dialectical behavior therapy (DBT) is a cognitive-behavioral approach that focuses on behavioral change while providing acceptance, compassion, and validation of the patient. Several randomized trials have demonstrated the efficacy of DBT in the treatment of personality disorders. Antidepressant medications and low-dose antipsychotic drugs have some efficacy in cluster A personality disorders, while anticonvulsant mood-stabilizing agents and MAOIs may be considered for patients with cluster B diagnoses who show marked mood reactivity, behavioral dyscontrol, and/or rejection hypersensitivity. Anxious or fearful cluster C patients often respond to medications used for axis I anxiety disorders (discussed earlier). It is important that the physician and the patient have reasonable expectations vis-à-vis the possible benefit of any medication used and its side effects. Improvement may be subtle and observable only over time.

SCHIZOPHRENIA

Clinical manifestations

Schizophrenia is a heterogeneous syndrome characterized by perturbations of language, perception, thinking, social activity, affect, and volition. There are no pathognomonic features. The syndrome commonly begins in late adolescence, has an insidious (and less commonly acute) onset, and, often, a poor outcome, progressing from social withdrawal and perceptual distortions to recurrent delusions and hallucinations. Patients may present with positive symptoms (such as conceptual disorganization, delusions, or hallucinations) or negative symptoms (loss of function, anhedonia, decreased emotional expression, impaired concentration, and diminished social engagement) and must have at least two of these for a 1-month period and continuous signs for at least 6 months to meet formal diagnostic criteria. As individuals age, positive psychotic symptoms tend to attenuate and some measure of social and occupational function may be regained. "Negative" symptoms predominate in one-third of the schizophrenic population and are associated with a poor long-term outcome and a poor response to drug treatment. However, marked variability in the course and individual character of symptoms is typical.

The four main subtypes of schizophrenia are catatonic, paranoid, disorganized, and residual. Many individuals have symptoms of more than one type. *Catatonic-type* describes patients whose clinical presentation is dominated by profound changes in motor activity, negativism, and echolalia or echopraxia. *Paranoid-type* describes patients who have a prominent preoccupation with a specific delusional system and who otherwise do not qualify as having *disorganized-type* disease, in which disorganized speech and behavior are accompanied by a superficial or silly affect. In *residual-type* disease, negative symptomatology exists in the absence of delusions, hallucinations, or motor disturbance. The term *schizophreniform disorder* describes patients who meet the symptom requirements but not the duration requirements for schizophrenia, and *schizoaffective disorder* is used for those who manifest symptoms of schizophrenia and independent periods of mood disturbance. Prognosis depends not on symptom severity but on the response to antipsychotic medication. A permanent remission without recurrence does occasionally occur. About 10% of schizophrenic patients commit suicide.

Schizophrenia is present in 0.85% of individuals worldwide, with a lifetime prevalence of ~1–1.5%. An estimated 300,000 episodes of acute schizophrenia occur annually in the United States, resulting in direct and indirect costs of $62.7 billion.

Differential diagnosis

The diagnosis is principally one of exclusion, requiring the absence of significant associated mood symptoms, any relevant medical condition, and substance abuse. Drug reactions that cause hallucinations, paranoia, confusion, or bizarre behavior may be dose-related or idiosyncratic; parkinsonian medications, clonidine, quinacrine, and procaine derivatives are the most common prescription medications associated with these symptoms. Drug causes should be ruled out in any case of newly emergent psychosis. The general neurologic examination in patients with schizophrenia is usually normal, but motor rigidity, tremor, and dyskinesias are noted in one-quarter of untreated patients.

Epidemiology and pathophysiology

Epidemiologic surveys identify several risk factors for schizophrenia, including genetic susceptibility, early developmental insults, winter birth, and increasing parental age. Genetic factors are involved in at least a subset of individuals who develop schizophrenia. Schizophrenia is observed in ~6.6% of all first-degree relatives of an affected proband. If both parents are affected, the risk for offspring is 40%. The concordance rate for monozygotic twins is 50%, compared to 10% for dizygotic twins. Schizophrenia-prone families are also at risk for other psychiatric disorders, including schizoaffective disorder and *schizotypal* and *schizoid personality disorders*, the latter terms designating individuals who show a lifetime pattern of social and interpersonal deficits characterized by an inability to form close interpersonal relationships, eccentric behavior, and mild perceptual distortions. The pathogenesis of schizophrenia is discussed in detail in Chap. 53.

TREATMENT Schizophrenia

Antipsychotic agents (Table 54-14) are the cornerstone of acute and maintenance treatment of schizophrenia and are effective in the treatment of hallucinations, delusions, and thought disorders, regardless of etiology. The mechanism of action involves, at least in part, binding to dopamine D_2/D_3 receptors in the ventral striatum; the clinical potencies of traditional antipsychotic drugs parallel their affinities for the D_2 receptor, and even the newer "atypical" agents exert some degree of D_2 receptor blockade. All neuroleptics induce expression of the immediate-early gene *c-fos* in the nucleus accumbens, a dopaminergic site connecting prefrontal and limbic

TABLE 54-14

ANTIPSYCHOTIC AGENTS

NAME	USUAL PO DAILY DOSE, mg	SIDE EFFECTS	SEDATION	COMMENTS
First-Generation Antipsychotics				
Low-potency				
Chlorpromazine (Thorazine)	100–1000	Anticholinergic effects; orthostasis; photosensitivity; cholestasis; QT prolongation	+ + +	EPSEs usually not prominent; can cause anticholinergic delirium in elderly patients
Thioridazine (Mellaril)	100–600			
Midpotency				
Trifluoperazine (Stelazine)	2–50	Fewer anticholinergic side effects	+ +	Well tolerated by most patients
Perphenazine (Trilafon)	4–64	Fewer EPSEs than with higher potency agents.	++	
Loxapine (Loxitane)	30–100	Frequent EPSEs	+ +	
Molindone (Moban)	30–100	Frequent EPSEs	0	Little weight gain
High potency				
Haloperidol (Haldol)	5–20	No anticholinergic side effects; EPSEs often prominent	0/+	Often prescribed in doses that are too high; long-acting injectable forms of haloperidol and fluphenazine available
Fluphenazine (Prolixin)	1–20	Frequent EPSEs	0/+	
Thiothixene (Navane)	2–50	Frequent EPSEs	0/+	
Second-Generation Antipsychotics				
Clozapine (Clozaril)	150–600	Agranulocytosis (1%); weight gain; seizures; drooling; hyperthermia	+ +	Requires weekly WBC count for first 6 months, then biweekly if stable
Risperidone (Risperdal)	2–8	Orthostasis	+	Requires slow titration; EPSEs observed with doses >6 mg qd
Olanzapine (Zyprexa)	10–30	Weight gain	+ +	Mild prolactin elevation
Quetiapine (Seroquel)	350–800	Sedation; weight gain; anxiety	+ + +	Bid dosing
Ziprasidone (Geodon)	120–200	Orthostatic hypotension	+/++	Minimal weight gain; increases QT interval
Aripiprazole (Abilify)	10–30	Nausea, anxiety, insomnia	0/+	Mixed agonist/antagonist
Paliperidone (Invega)	3–12	Restlessness, EPSEs	+	Active metabolite of risperidone
Iloperidone (Fanapt)	12–24	Dizziness, hypotension	0/+	Requires dose titration
Asenapine (Saphris)	10–20	Dizziness, EPSEs, weight gain	++	Sublingual tablets; bid dosing
Lurasidone (Latuda)	40–80	Nausea, EPSEs	++	Uses CYP3A4

Abbreviations: EPSEs, extrapyramidal side effects; WBC, white blood cell.

cortices. The clinical efficacy of newer atypical neuroleptics, however, may involve *N*-methyl-D-aspartate (NMDA) receptor blockade, α_1- and α_2-noradrenergic activity, altering the relationship between $5HT_2$ and D_2 receptor activity, as well as faster dissociation of D_2 binding and effects on neuroplasticity.

Conventional neuroleptics differ in their potency and side-effect profile. Older agents such as chlorpromazine and thioridazine, are more sedating and anticholinergic and more likely to cause orthostatic hypotension, while higher potency antipsychotics such as haloperidol, perphenazine, and thiothixene, are more likely to induce extrapyramidal side effects. The model "atypical" antipsychotic agent is *clozapine*, a dibenzodiazepine that has a greater potency in blocking the $5HT_2$ than the D_2 receptor and a much higher affinity for the D_4 than the D_2 receptor. Its principal disadvantage is a risk of blood dyscrasias. Paliperidone is a recently approved agent that is a metabolite of risperidone and shares many of its properties. Unlike other antipsychotics, clozapine does not cause a rise in prolactin level. Approximately 30% of patients who do not benefit from conventional antipsychotic agents will have a better response to this drug, which also has a demonstrated superiority to other antipsychotic agents in preventing suicide; however, its side-effect profile makes it most appropriate for treatment-resistant cases. *Risperidone*, a benzisoxazole derivative, is more potent at $5HT_2$ than D_2 receptor sites, like clozapine, but it also exerts significant α_2 antagonism, a property that may contribute to its perceived ability to improve mood and increase motor activity. Risperidone is not as effective as clozapine in treatment-resistant cases but does not carry a risk of blood dyscrasias. *Olanzapine* is similar neurochemically to clozapine but has a significant risk of inducing weight gain. *Quetiapine* is distinct in having a weak D_2 effect but potent α_1 and histamine blockade. *Ziprasidone* causes minimal weight gain and is unlikely to increase prolactin but may increase QT prolongation. *Aripiprazole* also has little risk of weight gain or prolactin increase but may increase anxiety, nausea, and insomnia as a result of its partial agonist properties.

Antipsychotic agents are effective in 70% of patients presenting with a first episode. Improvement may be observed within hours or days, but full remission usually requires 6–8 weeks. The choice of agent depends principally on the side effect profile and cost of treatment or on a past personal or family history of a favorable response to the drug in question. Atypical agents appear to be more effective in treating negative symptoms and improving cognitive function. An equivalent treatment response can usually be achieved with relatively low doses of any drug selected (i.e., 4–6 mg/d of haloperidol, 10–15 mg of olanzapine, or 4–6 mg/d of risperidone). Doses in this range result in >80% D_2 receptor blockade, and there is little evidence that higher doses increase either the rapidity or degree of response. Maintenance treatment requires careful attention to the possibility of relapse and monitoring for the development of a movement disorder. Intermittent drug treatment is less effective than regular dosing, but gradual dose reduction is likely to improve social functioning in many schizophrenic patients who have been maintained at high doses. If medications are completely discontinued, however, the relapse rate is 60% within 6 months. Long-acting injectable preparations (risperidone) are considered when noncompliance with oral therapy leads to relapses. In treatment-resistant patients, a transition to clozapine usually results in rapid improvement, but a prolonged delay in response in some cases necessitates a 6- to 9-month trial for maximal benefit to occur.

Antipsychotic medications can cause a broad range of side effects, including lethargy, weight gain, postural hypotension, constipation, and dry mouth. Extrapyramidal symptoms such as dystonia, akathisia, and akinesia are also frequent with first-generation agents and may contribute to poor adherence if not specifically addressed. Anticholinergic and parkinsonian symptoms respond well to trihexyphenidyl, 2 mg bid, or benztropine mesylate, 1–2 mg bid. Akathisia may respond to beta blockers. In rare cases, more serious and occasionally life-threatening side effects may emerge, including hyperprolactinemia, ventricular arrhythmias, gastrointestinal obstruction, retinal pigmentation, obstructive jaundice, and neuroleptic malignant syndrome (characterized by hyperthermia, autonomic dysfunction, muscular rigidity, and elevated creatine phosphokinase levels). The most serious adverse effects of clozapine are agranulocytosis, which has an incidence of 1%, and induction of seizures, which has an incidence of 10%. Weekly white blood cell counts are required, particularly during the first 3 months of treatment.

The risk of type 2 diabetes mellitus appears to be increased in schizophrenia, and second-generation agents as a group produce greater adverse effects on glucose regulation, independent of effects on obesity, than traditional agents. Clozapine, olanzapine, and quetiapine seem more likely to cause hyperglycemia, weight gain, and hypertriglyceridemia than other atypical antipsychotic drugs. Close monitoring of plasma glucose and lipid levels are indicated with the use of these agents.

A serious side effect of long-term use of first generation antipsychotic agents is *tardive dyskinesia*, characterized by repetitive, involuntary, and potentially irreversible movements of the tongue and lips (bucco-linguo-masticatory triad), and, in approximately half of cases, choreoathetosis. Tardive dyskinesia has an incidence of 2–4% per year of exposure, and a prevalence of 20% in chronically treated patients. The prevalence increases with age, total dose, and duration of drug administration. The risk associated with second-generation agents appears to be much lower. The cause may involve formation of free radicals and perhaps mitochondrial energy failure. Vitamin E may reduce abnormal involuntary movements if given early in the syndrome.

The CATIE study, a large-scale investigation of the effectiveness of antipsychotic agents in "real world" patients, revealed a high rate of discontinuation of treatment over 18 months. Olanzapine showed greater effectiveness than quetiapine, risperidone, perphenazine, or ziprasidone but also a higher discontinuation rate due to weight gain and metabolic effects. Surprisingly, perphenazine, a first-generation agent, showed little evidence of inferiority to newer drugs.

Drug treatment of schizophrenia is by itself insufficient. Educational efforts directed toward families and relevant community resources have proved to be necessary to maintain stability and optimize outcome. A treatment model involving a multidisciplinary case-management team that seeks out and closely follows the patient in the community has proved particularly effective.

ASSESSMENT AND EVALUATION OF VIOLENCE

Primary care physicians may encounter situations in which family, domestic, or societal violence is discovered or suspected. Such an awareness can carry legal and moral obligations; many state laws mandate reporting of child, spousal, and elder abuse. Physicians are frequently the first point of contact for both victim and abuser. Approximately 2 million older Americans and 1.5 million U.S. children are thought to experience some form of physical maltreatment each year. Spousal abuse is thought to be even more prevalent. An interview study of 24,000 women in 10 countries found a lifetime prevalence of physical or sexual violence that ranged from 15 to 71%; these individuals are more likely to suffer from depression, anxiety, somatization disorder, and substance abuse and to have attempted suicide. In addition, abused individuals frequently express low self-esteem, vague somatic symptomatology, social isolation, and a passive feeling of loss of control. Although it is essential to treat these elements in the victim, the first obligation is to ensure that the perpetrator has taken responsibility for preventing any further violence. Substance abuse and/or dependence and serious mental illness in the abuser may contribute to the risk of harm and require direct intervention. Depending on the situation, law enforcement agencies, community resources such as support groups and shelters, and individual and family counseling can be appropriate components of a treatment plan. A safety plan should be formulated with the victim, in addition to providing information about abuse, its likelihood of recurrence, and its tendency to increase in severity and frequency. Antianxiety and antidepressant medications may sometimes be useful in treating the acute symptoms, but only if independent evidence for an appropriate psychiatric diagnosis exists.

MENTAL HEALTH PROBLEMS IN THE HOMELESS

There is a high prevalence of mental disorders and substance abuse among homeless and impoverished individuals. Depending on the definition used, estimates of the total number of homeless individuals in the United States range from 800,000 to 2 million, one-third of whom qualify as having a serious mental disorder. Poor hygiene and nutrition, substance abuse, psychiatric illness, physical trauma, and exposure to the elements combine to make the provision of medical care challenging. Only a minority of these individuals receive formal mental health care; the main points of contact are outpatient medical clinics and emergency departments. Primary care settings represent a critical site in which housing needs, treatment of substance dependence, and evaluation and treatment of psychiatric illness can most efficiently take place. Successful intervention is dependent on breaking down traditional administrative barriers to health care and recognizing the physical constraints and emotional costs imposed by homelessness. Simplifying health care instructions and follow-up, allowing frequent visits, and dispensing medications in limited amounts that require ongoing contact are possible techniques for establishing a successful therapeutic relationship.

CHAPTER 55

NEUROPSYCHIATRIC ILLNESSES IN WAR VETERANS

Charles W. Hoge

Neuropsychiatric sequelae are common in combat veterans. Advances in personal protective body armor, armored vehicles, battlefield resuscitation, and the speed of evacuation to tertiary care have considerably improved the survivability of battlefield injuries, resulting in a greater awareness of the "silent wounds" associated with service in a combat zone. Although psychiatric and neurologic problems have been well documented in veterans of prior wars, the conflicts in Iraq and Afghanistan have been unique in terms of the level of commitment by the U.S. Department of Defense (DoD) and Department of Veterans Affairs (VA), Veterans Health Administration (VHA) to support research as the wars have unfolded, and to utilize that knowledge to guide population-level screening, evaluation, and treatment initiatives.

These conflicts, like previous ones, have produced hundreds of thousands of combat veterans, many of whom have received or will need care in government and civilian medical facilities. Studies have shown that service in the Iraq and Afghanistan theaters is associated with significantly elevated rates of mental disorders. Two conditions in particular have been labeled the signature injuries related to these wars: posttraumatic stress disorder (PTSD) and mild traumatic brain injury (mTBI)—also known as concussion. Although particular emphasis will be given in this chapter to PTSD and concussion/mTBI, it is important to understand that service in all wars is associated with a number of health concerns that coexist and overlap, and a multidisciplinary patient-centered approach to care is necessary.

EPIDEMIOLOGY OF WAR-RELATED PSYCHOLOGICAL AND NEUROLOGIC CONDITIONS

Service members from the current decade of war have faced multiple deployments to two very different high-intensity combat theaters, and the cumulative strain has negatively impacted marriages, parenting, educational goals, and civilian occupations. The stresses of service in these conflicts have led to a significant increase in the rate of suicide in personnel from the two branches of service involved in the greatest level of ground combat (army, marines).

Service in a war zone can involve extreme physical stress in austere environments, prolonged sleep deprivation, physical injury, exposure to highly life-threatening events and hazards such as explosive devices, sniper fire, ambushes, indirect fire from rockets and mortars, and chemical pollutants. Certain events such as loss of a close friend in combat, leave indelible scars. All of these experiences have additive effects on health, likely mediated through physiologic mechanisms involving dysregulation of neuroendocrine and autonomic nervous system (ANS) functions.

Veterans of virtually all wars have reported elevated rates of generalized and multisystem physical, cognitive, and psychological health concerns that often become the focus of treatment months or years after returning home. These multisystem health concerns include sleep disturbance, memory and concentration problems, headaches, musculoskeletal pain, gastrointestinal symptoms (including gastroesophageal reflux), residual effects of war-time injuries, fatigue, anger, hyperarousal symptoms, high blood pressure, rapid heart rate (sometimes associated with panic symptoms), sexual problems, and symptoms associated with PTSD and depression. In order to provide optimal care to veterans with these symptoms, it is important to understand how the symptoms interrelate, and to consider the possibility that there may be underlying combat-related physiologic effects.

POSTWAR SYMPTOMS

The overlapping and multisystem health symptoms reported by warriors from every generation have been given different labels, and have led to debates among medical professionals as to whether these are mediated primarily by physical or psychological causes. For example, World War I produced extensive debate about whether "shell shock," diagnosed in more than 80,000 British soldiers, was neurologic ("commotional" from the brain being shaken in the skull by concussive blasts) or psychological ("emotional" or "neurasthenia") in origin. World War II veterans were said to suffer from "battle fatigue," Korean War veterans developed "combat stress reactions," and Vietnam veterans developed the "post-Vietnam syndrome." The role of environmental exposure (e.g., agent orange) and psychological causes (alcohol addiction, drug addiction, and PTSD) continue to be debated.

Gulf War I led to extensive debates as to whether Gulf War syndrome, also known as multisystem illness, was best explained by environmental exposures (e.g., oil fires, depleted uranium, nerve gas, multiple vaccinations) or the psychological stress of deployment to a war zone where there was anticipation of high casualty rates from chemical and biologic weapons and stressful training exercises involving the use of impermeable full-body protective uniforms (made from rubber, vinyl, charcoal impregnated polyurethane, and other materials) in desert conditions under extreme temperatures. Although no clinical syndrome was ever definitively confirmed among the nearly 1 million service members who deployed in 1990–1991, studies consistently found that military personnel who served in the Gulf experienced elevations in generalized symptoms across all health domains (e.g. physical, cognitive, neurologic, psychological) compared with service members who deployed elsewhere or did not deploy. In addition, there is good evidence that deployment to the Persian Gulf region during this period was associated with subsequent development of PTSD; other psychiatric disorders including generalized anxiety disorder, depression, and substance abuse, particularly alcohol abuse (Chap. 56); functional gastrointestinal symptoms such as irritable bowel syndrome; and chronic fatigue syndrome (Chap. 52).

The conflicts in Iraq and Afghanistan have led to similar debates as to whether postwar symptoms such as headaches, irritability, sleep disturbance, dizziness, and concentration problems are best attributed to concussion/mTBI or to PTSD. Several studies have shown that either PTSD or depression explains the majority of the postdeployment "postconcussive" symptoms attributed to concussion/mTBI, a finding not well received by some experts in traumatic brain injury (TBI) but consistent with civilian studies on risk factors for developing persistent symptoms after concussion. As in past wars, it has taken years to understand how PTSD and concussion/mTBI interrelate with other deployment-related health concerns, and the implications for designing effective evaluation and treatment strategies.

Veterans understandably may become angry at the suggestion that their postwar health concerns are stress-related or psychological, and thus it is necessary for primary care professionals to be sensitive to this concern.

PTSD

PTSD is the most common mental disorder documented following war-zone service. Studies from the conflicts in Iraq and Afghanistan have found PTSD prevalence rates of 2–6% before deployment (comparable to civilian general population samples) and rates of 6–20% postdeployment, depending primarily on the level of combat frequency and intensity. Many other veterans experience subclinical PTSD symptoms after war-zone service, sometimes termed posttraumatic stress (PTS) or combat stress. These subclinical symptoms can contribute to distress and affect health, even if overall functioning is not as impaired as in the full disorder.

PTSD is defined by the American Psychiatric Association as persistent (>1 month) symptoms occurring after a life-threatening traumatic event in which there was an immediate response of fear, helplessness, or horror. The symptoms must be associated with significant distress or impairment in social or occupational functioning. Symptoms are grouped into three categories: (1) re-experiencing symptoms in which the person has nightmares, flashbacks, or intrusive thoughts and memories connected with the traumatic event; (2) hyperarousal symptoms in which the person is physiologically revved up, hyperalert, startles easily, and experiences sleep disturbance, anger, and/or concentration problems; and (3) avoidance symptoms where the person loses interest in things that previously brought enjoyment, and avoids places, situations, or other stimuli that serve as reminders of the traumatic event (e.g., a crowded mall that triggers heightened alertness to threat). Additional symptoms, currently categorized with the avoidance cluster, but which will likely become a fourth category in future definitions of PTSD, include emotional numbing, feeling distant or cutoff from others, and a foreshortened sense of future (Chap. 54). While PTSD is a clinical symptom-based case definition, it is best to think of PTSD not as an emotional or psychological/psychiatric condition, but rather as a physiologic-based response to life-threatening trauma that is associated with physical, cognitive, emotional, and psychological symptoms.

PTSD has strong biologic correlates, based in fear-conditioning responses to threat and responses to extreme stress involving neuroendocrine dysregulation and ANS reactivity. Numerous studies have shown that PTSD is highly correlated with generalized physical and cognitive symptoms—including hypertension, chronic pain, and cardiovascular disease—as well as cell-mediated immune dysfunction and shortened life expectancy. PTSD is frequently comorbid with other mental disorders such as major depressive disorder, generalized anxiety, substance use disorders (SUDs), as well as risky behaviors (e.g., aggression, accidents); it has been estimated that up to 80% of patients with PTSD exhibit one or more comorbid conditions. Misuse of alcohol or substances is most prevalent, often reflecting self-medication. PTSD is also associated with tolerance and withdrawal symptoms related to prescription pain and sleep medications, as well as nicotine dependence.

Clinicians should understand the limitations of the definition of PTSD when applied to responses to trauma occurring in the occupational context of military service (similar to police, firefighters, and other first responders). Service members are trained to respond to traumatic events, and relatively rarely report fear, helplessness, or horror, which are characteristic responses of civilian victims of trauma. In addition, the reactions that are labeled as symptoms of PTSD are based on the adaptive survival responses of warriors in a combat environment. For example, physiologic hyperarousal, use of anger, and being able to shut down other emotions are very useful skills in combat, and can be present prior to traumatic events when there is tough realistic training. These responses only become symptoms when they impair functioning after warriors return home.

CONCUSSION/mTBI

TBI (Chap. 36) gained increased recognition during the conflicts in Iraq and Afghanistan because of the widespread exposure of troops to improvised explosive devices. Contributing to heightened concern were high prevalence estimates of deployment-related TBI that did not distinguish concussion/mTBI from moderate or severe TBI; data from animal models of blast suggesting that explosions may cause a different kind of concussion associated with inflammatory changes; and speculation that repetitive blast exposure may lead to future dementia, based on case series of professional athletes (e.g., boxers, football players) exposed to highly repetitive injuries linked to chronic traumatic encephalopathy (previously termed *dementia pugilistica*). Many veterans of Iraq and Afghanistan reported experiencing multiple concussions during deployments, and many also reported ignoring concussions and not seeking treatment at the time of injury.

TBI includes closed and penetrating head injuries; closed head injuries are categorized as mild (mTBI or concussion), moderate, or severe based on the duration of loss of consciousness, duration of posttraumatic amnesia, and the Glasgow coma score (GCS) (Table 36-2). Several studies have estimated that 10–20% of all military personnel deployed to Iraq or Afghanistan sustained one or more concussion/mTBI events during deployment, most commonly from exposure to blasts.

Although there is a neurophysiologic continuum of injury, there are stark clinical and epidemiologic distinctions between concussion/mTBI and moderate or severe TBI **(Table 55-1)**. Concussion/mTBI is defined as a blow or jolt to the head that results in brief loss of consciousness (LOC) for <30 min (most commonly only a few seconds to minutes), posttraumatic amnesia (PTA) of <24 h (most commonly <1 h), or transient alteration in consciousness (AOC) without loss of consciousness. The majority of concussions in Iraq or Afghanistan have involved AOC without LOC or PTA (which soldiers may refer to as getting their "bell rung"). GCSs are usually normal (15 out of 15). Concussion is treated with rest to allow the brain time to heal, and almost never results in air-evacuation from the battlefield unless there are other injuries.

In contrast, moderate, severe, or penetrating TBI, which account for <1% of all battlefield head injuries in Iraq and Afghanistan, are characterized by LOC ≥30 min (up to permanent coma), PTA ≥24 h (also may be permanent), and GCSs as low as 3 (the minimum value). These virtually always result in air-evacuation from the battlefield and can result in severe long-term neurologic impairment and requirement for rehabilitative care.

Symptoms following concussion/mTBI can include headache; fatigue; concentration, memory, or attention problems; sleep disturbance; irritability; balance difficulties; and tinnitus, among other symptoms. Recovery is usually rapid, with symptoms usually resolving in a few hours to days, but in a small percentage of patients, symptoms may persist for a longer period or become chronic (referred to as persistent "postconcussive symptoms" or "PCS").

Establishing a clear causal connection between a deployment concussion injury and persistent PCS months or years after return from deployment is difficult and often confounded by other postwar conditions that cause similar symptoms, including injuries not involving the head, other medical disorders, sleep disorders, PTSD, depression, substance use disorders, chronic pain, and the general physiologic effects of wartime service. Contributing to the difficulty in establishing causation is the fact that the concussion/mTBI case definition refers only to the acute injury event and lacks symptoms, time-course or impairment; case definitions for persistent postconcussion syndrome are not well validated. Several studies found that PTSD was a much stronger predictor of postdeployment PCS after combat deployment than concussions/mTBIs, and one study even found that objective neuropsychological impairment after deployment was entirely explained by PTSD. These data do not minimize the importance of

TABLE 55-1

COMPARISON BETWEEN CONCUSSION/mTBI AND MODERATE/SEVERE TBI

	MILD TBI (CONCUSSION)	MOD/SEVERE TBI
Clinical case definition		
Loss of consciousness	<30 min (usually few seconds to minutes)	≥30 min to indefinite
Altered consciousness	<24 h (usually <30 min)	≥24 h to indefinite
Posttraumatic amnesia	<24 h (usually <30 min)	≥24 h to indefinite
Glasgow coma score	13–15 (usually 15)	As low as 3
Focal neurologic signs	None or transient	Frequently present
Traditional neuroimaging (CT/MRI)	Usually negative	Diagnostic
Clinical usefulness of neurocognitive testing after acute injury period	Usually inconclusive	Essential and valuable
Neuronal cell damage	Metabolic/ionic processes associated with axonal swelling, which can lead to disconnection	Direct injury effects plus metabolic/ionic effects
Sequelae, natural history, and recovery	Full recovery expected in majority of individuals; no consensus on natural history; the percentage who develop persistent symptoms is debated	Based directly on injury characteristics; may be severely disabling
Predictors of persistent postconcussive symptoms or disability	Intensely debated; risk factors found to be most predictive include psychiatric conditions (e.g., depression, PTSD) and negative expectations	Not debated, predictors are directly related to injury severity and clinical progress with rehabilitation treatment

concussion/mTBI, but highlight the complex interrelationships of war-related health problems.

Studies of veterans who sustained concussions in Iraq or Afghanistan have suggested that blast mechanisms produce similar clinical outcomes as nonblast mechanisms, in contrast to expectations based on animal models. An explosion can produce serious injury from rapid atmospheric pressure changes (primary blast wave mechanism), as well as from flying debris (secondary blast mechanism) or by being thrown into a hard object (tertiary blast mechanism). Secondary and tertiary mechanisms are similar to other mechanical mechanisms of concussions sustained during accidents. The possibility of a unique head injury from the primary blast wave in otherwise uninjured soldiers appears to be low, but cannot be discounted.

Multisystem health problems that lack clear case definitions do not lend themselves well to uniform public health strategies such as screening. Nevertheless, mass population screening for concussion/mTBI was mandated for all U.S. service members returning from Iraq or Afghanistan and all veterans presenting for care at VA health care facilities. These screening processes, which attempt to apply the acute concussion case definition (lacking symptoms, time-course, or impairment) months or years after injury, led to sharp criticism that they were encouraging clinicians to misattribute common postwar symptoms to concussion/mTBI.

Management is largely symptom-focused, and ideally carried out within primary-care based structures of care. Optimal care avoids unnecessary specialty referrals, use of nonevidence-based interventions, or poor communication that results in negative expectations. Concussion research has shown that negative expectations are one of the most important risk factors for persistent symptoms.

While many questions remain regarding the long-term health effects of concussions (particularly multiple concussions) sustained during deployment, these are important battlefield injuries that require careful attention. However, they need to be addressed within the context of all other war-related health concerns.

STIGMA AND BARRIERS TO CARE

Adding to the complexity of treating veterans is stigma and other barriers to care. Despite extensive education efforts among military leaders and service members, perceptions of stigma have shown little change over the many years of war; warriors are concerned that they will be perceived as weak by peers or leaders if they seek care. Studies showed that less than one-half of service members with serious mental health problems receive needed care. Many factors contribute to this, including the pervasive nature of stigma in society in general (particularly among men), the critical importance of group cohesiveness of military teams, the nature of avoidance symptoms in PTSD, and sometimes skepticism that mental health professionals will be able to help.

APPROACH TO THE PATIENT Evaluation of Veterans with Neuropsychiatric Health Concerns

Evaluation should begin with a careful occupational history as part of the routine medical evaluation; this includes the number of years served, military occupation, deployment locations and dates, illnesses or injuries resulting from service, and significant combat traumatic experiences that may be continuing to affect the individual (Table 55-2). The clinician should evaluate the degree to which the patient's current difficulties reflect the normal course of readjusting after the intense occupational experience of combat. It is helpful to reinforce the many strengths associated with being a professional in the military: courage, honor, service to country, resiliency in combat, leadership, ability to work as cohesive workgroup with peers, and demonstrated skills in handling extreme stress.

One of the challenges with current medical practice is that there may be multiple providers with different clinical perspectives. Care should be coordinated through the primary care clinician, with the assistance of a care manager if needed. It is particularly important to continually evaluate all medications prescribed by other practitioners and assess for possible long-term side effects, dependency, or drug-drug interactions. Particular attention should be given to the level of chronic pain and sleep disturbance, self-medication with alcohol or substances, chronic use of nonsteroidal anti-inflammatory agents (which can contribute to rebound headaches or pain), chronic use of sedative-hypnotic agents, chronic use of narcotic pain medications, and the impact of war-related health concerns on social and occupational functioning.

Screening for PTSD, depression, and alcohol misuse should be performed routinely in all combat veterans. Three screening tools, which are in the public domain, have been validated for use in primary care, and have been used frequently in veterans: the four-question Primary Care PTSD Screen (PC-PTSD), the two-question Patient Health Questionnaire (PHQ-2), and the three-question Alcohol Use Disorders Identification Test-Consumption module (AUDIT-C) (Table 55-3).

Since the clinical definition of an acute concussion/mTBI does not include symptoms, time-course, or impairment, there is currently no clinically validated screening process for use months or years after injury. However, it is important to gather information about all injuries sustained during deployment, including any that resulted in loss or alteration of consciousness or loss of memory around the time of the event. If concussion injuries have occurred, the clinician should assess the number of such injuries, the duration of time unconscious, and injury mechanisms. This should be followed by an assessment of any postconcussive symptoms immediately following the injury event (e.g., headaches, dizziness, tinnitus, nausea, irritability, insomnia, and concentration or memory problems), and the severity and duration of such symptoms.

TABLE 55-2

SPECIFIC CONSIDERATIONS IN THE MEDICAL EVALUATION OF VETERANS

Occupational context of health concerns	Deployment locations and dates, combat experiences or other deployment stressors, frequent moves, separations from family, impact of deployment on civilian occupation (for reservists)
Medical problems during deployment	History of deployment-related injuries (including concussions), environmental exposures, sleep pattern during deployment, use of caffeine/energy drinks, use of other substances
Current medical history	Current symptoms, level of chronic pain, sleep problems, evidence of persistent physiologic hyperarousal (hypertension, tachycardia, panic symptoms, concentration/memory problems, irritability/anger, sleep disturbance), chronic use of caffeine or energy drinks, chronic use of nonsteroidal anti-inflammatory medications, chronic use of narcotic pain medications, chronic use of nonbenzodiazepine sedative-hypnotic medications, chronic use of benzodiazepines for sleep or anxiety
Mental health assessment	Screen for PTSD, major depressive disorder. Ask about suicidal or homicidal ideation, intent, or plans, as well as access to firearms
Alcohol/substance use	Screen for alcohol and substance use disorders, quantity and frequency of use, and evidence of tolerance. Inquire about "self-medication" (e.g., use of alcohol for sleep or to "calm down" or "forget" war-zone experiences)
Functional impairment	Impact of current symptoms on social and occupational functioning. High-risk behaviors (e.g., drinking and driving, reckless driving, aggression)
Social support, impact of military service on marriage and family	Level of social support. Readjustment stress on spouse, children, or other family members

TABLE 55-3

PRIMARY CARE MENTAL HEALTH SCREENING TOOLS

PC-PTSD Screen

1. Have you ever had any experience that was so frightening, horrible, or upsetting that, in the past month, you:		
Have had nightmares about it or thought about it when you did not want to?	Yes	No
Tried hard not to think about it or went out of your way to avoid situations that remind you of it?	Yes	No
Were constantly on guard, watchful, or easily startled?	Yes	No
Felt numb or detached from others, activities, or your surroundings?	Yes	No

Note: Two or more "yes" responses (three or more a more specific cutoff) is considered a positive screen.
Source: A Prins et al: The Primary Care PTSD Screen (PC-PTSD): Development and operating characteristics. Prim Care Psychiatr 9:9, 2004.

PHQ-2 Depression Screen

2. Over the last 2 weeks, how often have you been bothered by any of the following problems?	**Not at all (0)**	**Few or several days (1)**	**More than half the days (2)**	**Nearly every day (3)**
Little interest or pleasure in doing things.	0	1	2	3
Feeling down, depressed, or hopeless.	0	1	2	3

Note: If either (or both) questions are marked 2 or 3 ("more than half the days or higher), this is considered a positive screen for depression.
Source: K Kroenke et al: The Patient Health Questionnaire-2: Validity of a two-item depression screener. Med Care 41:1284, 2003.

AUDIT-C Alcohol Screen

3a. How often do you have a drink containing alcohol?				
Never (0)	Monthly or less (1)	Two or four times a month (2)	Two to three times per week (3)	Four or more times a week (4)
3b. How many drinks containing alcohol do you have on a typical day when you are drinking?				
1 or 2 (0)	3 or 4 (1)	5 or 6 (2)	7 or 9 (3)	10 or more (4)
3c. How often do you have six or more drinks on one occasion?				
Never (0)	Less than Monthly (1)	Monthly (2)	Two to three times per week (3)	Four or more times a week (4)

Note: A positive AUDIT-C screen is defined as a total score for men ≥4; for women ≥3. A report of drinking 6 or more drinks on one occasion should prompt an in-depth assessment of drinking.
Source: K Bush et al: The AUDIT Alcohol Consumption Questions (AUDIT-C): An effective brief screening test for problem drinking. Arch Intern Med 158:1789, 1998.

TREATMENT Neuropsychiatric Illnesses in War Veterans

Given the interrelationship of postwar health concerns, care needs to be carefully coordinated. Specific techniques that have been found to be helpful include scheduling regular primary care visits instead of as needed visits, establishing care management, utilizing good risk-communication principles, establishing a consultative step care approach that draws on the expertise of specialists in a collaborative manner (instead of immediately referring the patient to a specialist and relying on the specialist to provide care), and having behavioral health support directly within primary care clinics (both for referrals and to provide education and support to primary care professionals prescribing treatment for depression or PTSD).

It is important not to implicitly or explicitly convey the message that physical or cognitive symptoms are psychological or due to stress. Even if depression or anxiety plays a large role in the etiology of physical health symptoms, the treatment approach should be designed within a patient-centered primary care structure, and referrals managed from within this framework. For example, it might help to explain that the primary goal of referral to a mental health professional is to improve sleep and reduce physiologic hyperarousal, which in turn will help with treatment of war-related chronic headaches, concentration problems, or chronic fatigue. If however, the primary care professional conveys the message that the cause of headaches or concentration problems is anxiety or depression, and this conflicts with the patient's own viewpoint, then this could damage therapeutic rapport and in turn exacerbate the symptoms.

Specific questions related to military service (Table 55-2) combined with screening for depression, PTSD, and alcohol use disorders (Table 55-3) should be a routine part of care for all veterans. A positive screen for depression or PTSD should prompt follow-up questions related to these disorders (or use of a longer screening tool such as the [PHQ-9] or National Center for PTSD Checklist), as well as risk assessment for suicide or homicide. It is important to assess the impact of depression or PTSD symptoms on occupational functioning and interpersonal relationships.

A positive screen for alcohol misuse should prompt a brief motivational intervention that includes bringing attention to the elevated level of drinking, informing the veteran about the effects of alcohol on health, recommending limiting use or abstaining, exploring and setting goals related to drinking behavior, and follow-up and referral to specialty care if needed. This type of brief primary care intervention has been found to be effective, and should be incorporated into routine practice. One way to facilitate dialogue about this topic with veterans is to point out how hyperarousal associated with combat service can lead to increased craving for alcohol as the body searches for ways to modulate this. Veterans may consciously or unconsciously drink more to help with sleep, reduce arousal, or avoid thinking about events that happened "downrange." A key educational strategy is to help the veteran to learn that drinking to get to sleep actually damages sleep architecture and makes sleep worse (e.g., reduces rapid eye movement [REM] sleep initially followed by rebound REM activity and early morning wakening).

SPECIFIC TREATMENT STRATEGIES FOR PTSD AND COMORBID DEPRESSION PTSD and depression are highly comorbid in combat veterans, and the evidence-based treatments are similar, involving either antidepressant medications, cognitive behavioral therapy (CBT), or both. Psychoeducation that assists veterans to understand that their symptoms of PTSD have a basis in adaptive survival mechanisms and skills they exhibited in combat can facilitate therapeutic rapport. Remaining hypervigilant to threat, being able to shut down emotions, being able to function on less sleep, and using anger to help focus and control fear are all adaptive beneficial survival skills in a combat environment. Therefore, PTSD for warriors is both a medical disorder and a set of reactions that have their roots in the physiologic adaptation and skills they successfully applied in combat.

It is important to know that combat is not the only important trauma in a war-zone environment. Rape, assault, and accidents also occur. Rape or assault by a fellow service member, which affects a greater number of women veterans, can be particularly devastating because it destroys the vital feeling of safety that individuals derive from their own unit peers in a war environment.

The treatments for PTSD considered by most consensus guideline committees to have an A level of evidence include CBTs and medications, specifically selective serotonin reuptake inhibitors (SSRIs) (of which paroxetine and sertraline received FDA approval for PTSD). Although lacking a specific FDA indication, there is increasing evidence that serotonin norepinephrine reuptake inhibitors (SNRIs) (e.g., venlafaxine and duloxetine) and mirtazapine are also effective. (See Table 54-3 for recommended dosages.)

CBT interventions include narrative therapy (often called "imaginal exposure"), in vivo exposure focused on retraining the body not to react to stimuli related to traumatic reminders (e.g., a crowded mall), and techniques to modulate physiologic hyperarousal (e.g., diaphragmatic breathing, progressive muscle relaxation). A number of complementary alternative medicine approaches including acupuncture, mindfulness meditation, yoga, and massage are also being tested in PTSD. Although not evidence-based treatments per se, if they facilitate a relaxation response and alleviation of hyperarousal symptoms, they can be considered useful adjunctive modalities.

There have been no head-to-head comparisons of medication compared with psychotherapy for treatment of PTSD. It is reasonable for primary care clinicians to consider initiating treatment for mild to moderate PTSD symptoms with an SSRI, and refer patients to a mental health professional if there are more severe symptoms, significant comorbidity, safety concerns, or limited response to initial treatment. All PTSD treatments are associated with a sizable proportion of individuals who fail to respond adequately, and it is often necessary to add modalities or switch treatment. SNRIs may be useful alternatives to SSRIs if there has been nonresponse, side effects, or if there is comorbid pain (duloxetine, in particular, has indications for pain). Both SSRIs and SNRIs can increase anxiety initially; patients should be warned about this possibility and treatment should be initiated with the lowest recommended dose (or even one-half of the lowest dose for a few days) and gradually increased thereafter. Mirtazapine use can cause drowsiness and weight gain. Antidepressants also are likely to be useful in comorbid depression, which is common in veterans with PTSD. All antidepressants have potential drug-drug interactions that must be considered.

Many other medications have been used in PTSD, including tricyclic antidepressants, benzodiazepines, atypical antipsychotics, and anticonvulsants. In general, these should be prescribed in conjunction with psychiatric consultation, because of their greater side effects and risks. Benzodiazepines, in particular, should be avoided in combat veterans. Studies have shown that they do not reduce core PTSD symptoms, are likely to exacerbate substance use disorders that are common in veterans with PTSD, and may produce significant rebound anxiety. Veterans with PTSD often report symptomatic relief upon initiation of a benzodiazepine, but this is generally short lived and associated with a high risk of tolerance and dependence that can worsen recovery. Atypical antipsychotics, which have gained widespread popularity as adjunctive treatment for depression, anxiety, or sleep problems, have significant long-term side effects, including metabolic effects (e.g., glucose dysregulation), weight gain, and cardiovascular risks.

Sleep disturbance should be addressed initially with sleep hygiene education, followed by consideration of an antihistamine, trazodone, or non-benzodiazepine sedative-hypnotic such as zolpidem, eszopiclone, or zaleplon. However, the non-benzodiazepine sedative-hypnotics should be used with caution in veterans as they can lead to tolerance and rebound sleep problems similar to those seen with benzodiazepine use.

TREATMENT STRATEGIES FOR CONCUSSION/mTBI AND POSTDEPLOYMENT POSTCONCUSSIVE SYMPTOMS Concussion/mTBI is best treated at the time of injury with education and rest to allow time for the brain to heal and protect against a second impact syndrome (a rare but life-threatening event involving brain swelling that can occur when a second concussion occurs before the brain has adequately healed from an initial event). Randomized trials have shown that education regarding concussion that informs the patient of what to expect and promotes the expectation of recovery is the most effective treatment in preventing persistent symptoms.

Once service members return from deployment and seek care for postwar health problems, treatment is largely symptom focused, following the principles of patient-centered and collaborative care models. Cognitive rehabilitation, which is very useful in moderate and severe TBI to improve memory, attention, and concentration, has generally not been shown to be effective for mTBI in randomized clinical studies, though consensus groups have supported its use.

General recommendations for the clinical management of persistent, chronic postconcussive symptoms include treating physical and cognitive health problems based on symptom presentation, coexisting health problems, and individual preferences; and addressing coexisting depression, PTSD, substance use disorders, or other factors that may be contributing to symptom persistence. Headache is the most common symptom associated with concussion/mTBI, and the evaluation and treatment of headache parallels those for other causes of headache (Chap. 8). Stimulant medications for alleviating neurocognitive effects attributed to concussion/mTBI are not recommended. Clinicians should be aware of the potential for cognitive or sedative side effects of certain medications that may be prescribed for depression, anxiety, sleep, or chronic pain.

Treatment of neuropsychiatric problems must be coordinated with care for other war-related health concerns, with the goal of treatment to reduce the severity of symptoms, improve social and occupational functioning, and prevent long-term disability. Understanding the occupational context of war-related health concerns is important in communicating with veterans and developing a comprehensive treatment strategy.

DISCLOSURE

This material has been reviewed by the Walter Reed Army Institute of Research. There is no objection to its presentation and/or publication. The opinions or assertions contained herein are the private views of the author and are not to be construed as official, or as reflecting true views of the Department of the Army or the Department of Defense.

SECTION VI

ALCOHOLISM AND DRUG DEPENDENCY

CHAPTER 56

ALCOHOL AND ALCOHOLISM

Marc A. Schuckit

INTRODUCTION

Alcohol (beverage ethanol) distributes throughout the body, affecting almost all systems and altering nearly every neurochemical process in the brain. This drug is likely to exacerbate most medical conditions, affect almost any medication metabolized in the liver, and temporarily mimic many medical (e.g., diabetes) and psychiatric (e.g., depression) conditions. Because ~80% of people in Western countries have consumed alcohol, and two-thirds have been drunk in the prior year, the lifetime risk for serious, repetitive alcohol problems is almost 20% for men and 10% for women, regardless of a person's education or income. While low doses of alcohol have some healthful benefits, the intake of more than three standard drinks per day on a regular basis enhances the risk for cancer and vascular disease, and alcohol use disorders decrease the life span by about 10 years. Unfortunately, most clinicians have had only limited education regarding these conditions. This chapter presents a brief overview of clinically useful information about alcohol use, abuse, and dependence.

PHARMACOLOGY AND NUTRITIONAL IMPACT OF ETHANOL

Blood levels of ethanol are expressed as milligrams or grams of ethanol per deciliter (e.g., 100 mg/dL = 0.10 g/dL), with values of ~0.02 g/dL resulting from the ingestion of one typical drink. In round figures, 340 mL (12 oz) of beer, 115 mL (4 oz) of nonfortified wine, and 43 mL (1.5 oz) (a shot) of 80-proof beverage such as whisky, gin, or vodka each contain ~10–15 g of ethanol and represent a standard drink; 0.5 L (1 pint) of 80-proof beverage contains ~160 g (about 16 standard drinks), and 750 mL of wine contains ~60 g of ethanol. These beverages also have additional components known as *congeners* that affect the drink's taste and might contribute to adverse effects on the body. Congeners include methanol, butanol, acetaldehyde, histamine, tannins, iron, and lead. Alcohol acutely decreases neuronal activity and has similar behavioral effects and cross-tolerance with other depressants, including benzodiazepines and barbiturates.

Alcohol is absorbed from mucous membranes of the mouth and esophagus (in small amounts), from the stomach and large bowel (in modest amounts), and from the proximal portion of the small intestine (the major site). The rate of absorption is increased by rapid gastric emptying (as can be induced by carbonated beverages); by the absence of proteins, fats, or carbohydrates (which interfere with absorption); and by dilution to a modest percentage of ethanol (maximum at ~20% by volume).

Between 2% (at low blood alcohol concentrations) and 10% (at high blood alcohol concentrations) of ethanol is excreted directly through the lungs, urine, or sweat, but the greater part is metabolized to acetaldehyde, primarily in the liver. The most important pathway occurs in the cell cytosol where alcohol dehydrogenase (ADH) produces acetaldehyde, which is then rapidly destroyed by aldehyde dehydrogenase (ALDH) in the cytosol and mitochondria (Fig. 56-1). A second pathway in the microsomes of the smooth endoplasmic reticulum (the microsomal ethanol-oxidizing system, or MEOS) is responsible for ≥10% of ethanol oxidation at high blood alcohol concentrations.

While alcohol supplies calories (a drink contains ~300 kJ, or 70–100 kcal), these are devoid of nutrients such as minerals, proteins, and vitamins. In addition, alcohol can also interfere with absorption of vitamins in the small intestine and decreases their storage in the liver with modest effects on folate (folacin or folic acid), pyridoxine (B_6), thiamine (B_1), nicotinic acid (niacin, B_3), and vitamin A.

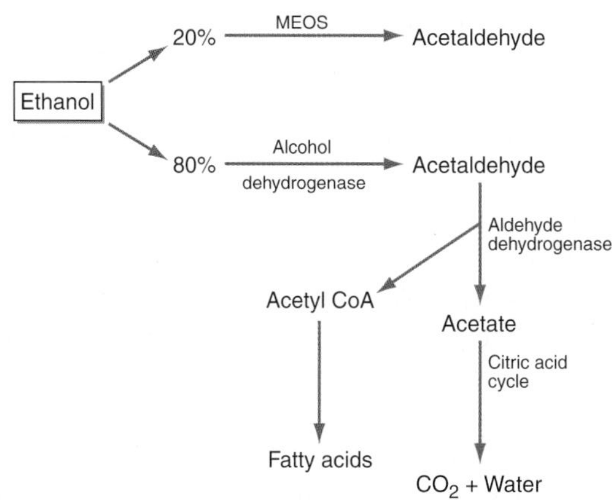

FIGURE 56-1

The metabolism of alcohol. MEOS, microsomal ethanol-oxidizing system.

A heavy ethanol load in a fasting, healthy individual is likely to produce transient hypoglycemia within 6–36 h, secondary to the acute actions of ethanol on gluconeogenesis. This can result in temporary abnormal glucose tolerance tests (with a resulting erroneous diagnosis of diabetes mellitus) until the alcoholic has abstained for 2–4 weeks. Alcohol ketoacidosis, probably reflecting a decrease in fatty acid oxidation coupled with poor diet or recurrent vomiting, can be misdiagnosed as diabetic ketosis. With the former, patients show an increase in serum ketones along with a mild increase in glucose but a large anion gap, a mild to moderate increase in serum lactate, and a β-hydroxybutyrate/lactate ratio of between 2:1 and 9:1 (with normal being 1:1).

In the brain, alcohol affects almost all neurotransmitter systems, with acute actions that are often the opposite of those seen following desistance after a period of heavy drinking. The most prominent actions relate to boosting gamma aminobutyric acid (GABA) activity, especially in $GABA_A$ receptors. Enhancement of this complex chloride channel system contributes to anticonvulsant, sleep-inducing, antianxiety, and muscle relaxation effects of all GABA-boosting drugs. Acutely administered alcohol produces a release of GABA, and continued use of this drug increases density of $GABA_A$ receptors, while alcohol withdrawal states are characterized by decreases in GABA-related activity. Equally important is the ability of acute alcohol to inhibit postsynaptic *N*-methyl-D-aspartate (NMDA) excitatory glutamate receptors, while chronic drinking and desistance are associated with an upregulation of these excitatory receptor subunits. The relationships between greater GABA and diminished NMDA receptor activity during acute intoxication and diminished GABA with enhanced NMDA actions during alcohol withdrawal explain much of intoxication and withdrawal phenomena.

As with all pleasurable activities, drinking alcohol acutely increases dopamine levels in the brain, especially in the ventral tegmentum and related brain regions, and this effect plays an important role in continued alcohol use, craving, and relapse. The changes in dopamine pathways are also linked to increases in "stress hormones," including cortisol and adrenocorticotropic hormone (ACTH) during intoxication and decreases in these hormones during withdrawal. Such alterations are likely to contribute to both feelings of reward during intoxication and depression during falling blood alcohol concentrations. Also closely linked to alterations in dopamine (especially in the nucleus accumbens) are alcohol-induced changes in opioid receptors, with acute alcohol also causing release of beta endorphins.

Additional important neurochemical changes include increases in synaptic levels of serotonin during acute intoxication, and subsequent upregulation of serotonin receptors. Acute increases in nicotinic acetylcholine systems also contribute to the impact of alcohol in the ventral tegmental region, which occur in concert with enhanced dopamine activity. In the same regions, alcohol impacts on cannabinol receptors, with resulting release of dopamine, GABA, and glutamate as well as subsequent effects on brain reward circuits.

BEHAVIORAL EFFECTS, TOLERANCE, AND DEPENDENCE

The acute effects of a drug depend on the dose, the rate of increase in plasma, the concomitant presence of other drugs, and the past experience with the agent. "Legal intoxication" with alcohol in most states requires a blood alcohol concentration of 0.08 g/dL, while levels of 0.04 or even lower are cited in other countries. However, behavioral, psychomotor, and cognitive changes are seen at levels as low as 0.02–0.03 g/dL (i.e., after one to two drinks) (Table 56-1). Deep but disturbed sleep can be seen at twice the legal intoxication level, and death can occur with levels between 0.30 and

TABLE 56-1

EFFECTS OF BLOOD ALCOHOL LEVELS IN THE ABSENCE OF TOLERANCE

BLOOD LEVEL, g/dL	USUAL EFFECT
0.02	Decreased inhibitions, a slight feeling of intoxication
0.08	Decrease in complex cognitive functions and motor performance
0.20	Obvious slurred speech, motor incoordination, irritability, and poor judgment
0.30	Light coma and depressed vital signs
0.40	Death

0.40 g/dL. Beverage alcohol is probably responsible for more overdose deaths than any other drug.

Repeated use of alcohol contributes to acquired tolerance, a complex phenomenon involving at least three types of compensatory mechanisms. (1) After 1–2 weeks of daily drinking, *metabolic or pharmacokinetic tolerance* can be seen, with up to 30% increase in the rate of hepatic ethanol metabolism. This alteration disappears almost as rapidly as it develops. (2) *Cellular or pharmacodynamic tolerance* develops through neurochemical changes that maintain relatively normal physiologic functioning despite the presence of alcohol. Subsequent decreases in blood levels contribute to symptoms of withdrawal. (3) Individuals learn to adapt their behavior so that they can function better than expected under influence of the drug (*learned or behavioral tolerance*).

The cellular changes caused by chronic ethanol exposure may not resolve for several weeks or longer following cessation of drinking. Rapid decreases in blood alcohol levels before that time can result in a withdrawal syndrome, which is most intense during the first 5 days, but some symptoms (e.g., disturbed sleep and anxiety) can take up to 4–6 months to resolve.

THE EFFECTS OF ETHANOL ON ORGAN SYSTEMS

Relatively low doses of alcohol (one or two drinks per day) have potential beneficial effects of increasing high-density lipoprotein cholesterol and decreasing aggregation of platelets, with a resulting decrease in risk for occlusive coronary disease and embolic strokes. Red wine has additional potential health-promoting qualities at relatively low doses due to flavinols and related substances, which may work by inhibiting platelet activation. Modest drinking might also decrease the risk for vascular dementia and, possibly, Alzheimer's disease. However, any potential healthful effects disappear with the regular consumption of three or more drinks per day, and knowledge about the deleterious effects of alcohol can both help the physician to identify patients with alcohol abuse and dependence, and to supply them with information that might help motivate a change in behavior.

NERVOUS SYSTEM

Approximately 35% of drinkers (and a much higher proportion of alcoholics) experience a *blackout*, an episode of temporary anterograde amnesia, in which the person forgets all or part of what occurred during a drinking evening. Another common problem, one seen after as few as one or two drinks shortly before bedtime, is disturbed sleep. Although alcohol might initially help a person to fall asleep, it disrupts sleep throughout the rest of the night. The stages of sleep are also altered, and time spent in rapid eye movement (REM) and deep sleep is reduced. Alcohol relaxes muscles in the pharynx, which can cause snoring and exacerbate sleep apnea; symptoms of the latter occur in 75% of alcoholic men older than age 60 years. Patients may also experience prominent and sometimes disturbing dreams. All of these sleep problems are more pronounced in alcoholics, and their persistence may contribute to relapse.

Another common consequence of alcohol use is impaired judgment and coordination, increasing the risk of accidents and injury. In the United States, ~40% of drinkers have at some time driven while intoxicated. Heavy drinking can also be associated with headache, thirst, nausea, vomiting, and fatigue the following day, a hangover syndrome that is responsible for much missed time and temporary cognitive deficits at work and school.

The effect of alcohol on the *nervous system* is even more pronounced among alcohol-dependent individuals. Chronic high doses cause *peripheral neuropathy* in ~10% of alcoholics: similar to diabetes, patients experience bilateral limb numbness, tingling, and paresthesias, all of which are more pronounced distally. Approximately 1% of alcoholics develop *cerebellar degeneration or atrophy*. This is a syndrome of progressive unsteady stance and gait often accompanied by mild nystagmus; neuroimaging studies reveal atrophy of the cerebellar vermis. Fortunately, very few alcoholics (perhaps as few as 1 in 500 for the full syndrome) develop *Wernicke's* (ophthalmoparesis, ataxia, and encephalopathy) and *Korsakoff's* (retrograde and anterograde amnesia) *syndromes*, although a higher proportion have one or more neuropathologic findings related to these syndromes. These occur as the result of low levels of thiamine, especially in predisposed individuals, e.g., those with transketolase deficiency. Alcoholics can manifest *cognitive problems* and temporary memory impairment lasting for weeks to months after drinking very heavily for days or weeks. Brain atrophy, evident as ventricular enlargement and widened cortical sulci on MRI and CT scans, occurs in ~50% of chronic alcoholics; these changes are usually reversible if abstinence is maintained. There is no single alcoholic dementia syndrome; rather, this label is used to describe patients who have apparently irreversible cognitive changes (possibly from diverse causes) in the context of chronic alcoholism.

Psychiatric comorbidity

As many as two-thirds of alcohol-dependent individuals meet the criteria for a psychiatric syndrome in the fourth edition of the *Diagnostic and Statistical Manual of Mental Disorders* (DSM-IV) of the American Psychiatric Association (Chap. 54). Half of these relate to a preexisting antisocial personality manifesting as impulsivity and disinhibition that contribute to both alcohol and drug dependence. The lifetime risk is 3% in males, and ≥80% of such individuals demonstrate alcohol and/or drug dependence. Another common comorbidity occurs with dependence on illicit substances. The remainder of alcoholics with psychiatric syndromes have preexisting conditions such as schizophrenia or manic-depressive disease and anxiety disorders such as panic disorder. The comorbidities of alcoholism with independent psychiatric disorders might represent an overlap in genetic vulnerabilities, impaired judgment in the use of alcohol from the independent psychiatric condition, or an attempt to use alcohol to alleviate some of the symptoms of the disorder or side effects of medications.

Many psychiatric syndromes can be seen *temporarily* during heavy drinking and subsequent withdrawal. These alcohol-induced conditions include an intense *sadness* lasting for days to weeks in the midst of heavy drinking seen in 40% of alcoholics, which tends to disappear over several weeks of abstinence (alcohol-induced mood disorder); temporary severe *anxiety* in 10–30% of alcoholics, often beginning during alcohol withdrawal, which can persist for a month or more after cessation of drinking (alcohol-induced anxiety disorder); and auditory *hallucinations* and/or paranoid delusions in a person who is alert and oriented, seen in 3–5% of alcoholics (*alcohol-induced psychotic disorder*).

Treatment of all forms of alcohol-induced psychopathology includes helping patients achieve abstinence and offering supportive care, as well as reassurance and "talk therapy" such as cognitive-behavioral approaches. However, with the exception of short-term antipsychotics or similar drugs for substance-induced psychoses, substance-induced psychiatric conditions only rarely require medications. Recovery is likely within several days to 4 weeks of abstinence. Conversely, because alcohol-induced conditions are temporary and do not indicate a need for long-term pharmacotherapy, a history of alcohol intake is an important part of the workup for any patient with one of these psychiatric symptoms.

THE GASTROINTESTINAL SYSTEM

Esophagus and stomach

Alcohol intake can result in inflammation of the esophagus and stomach causing epigastric distress and gastrointestinal bleeding, making alcohol one of the most common causes of hemorrhagic gastritis. Violent vomiting can produce severe bleeding through a Mallory-Weiss lesion, a longitudinal tear in the mucosa at the gastroesophageal junction.

Pancreas and liver

The incidence of acute pancreatitis (~25 per 1000 per year) is almost threefold higher in alcoholics than in the general population, accounting for an estimated 10% or more of the total cases. Alcohol impairs gluconeogenesis in the liver, resulting in a fall in the amount of glucose produced from glycogen, increased lactate production, and decreased oxidation of fatty acids. This contributes to an increase in fat accumulation in liver cells. In healthy individuals these changes are reversible, but with repeated exposure to ethanol, especially daily heavy drinking, more severe changes in the liver occur, including alcohol-induced hepatitis, perivenular sclerosis, and cirrhosis, with the latter observed in an estimated 15% of alcoholics. Perhaps through an enhanced vulnerability to infections, alcoholics have an elevated rate of hepatitis C, and drinking in the context of that disease is associated with more severe liver deterioration.

CANCER

As few as 1.5 drinks per day increases a woman's risk of breast cancer 1.4-fold. For both genders, four drinks per day increases the risk for oral and esophageal cancers approximately threefold and rectal cancers by a factor of 1.5; seven to eight or more drinks per day enhances approximately fivefold the risks for many cancers. These consequences may result directly from cancer-promoting effects of alcohol and acetaldehyde or indirectly by interfering with immune homeostasis.

HEMATOPOIETIC SYSTEM

Ethanol causes an increase in red blood cell size (mean corpuscular volume [MCV]), which reflects its effects on stem cells. If heavy drinking is accompanied by folic acid deficiency, there can also be hypersegmented neutrophils, reticulocytopenia, and a hyperplastic bone marrow; if malnutrition is present, sideroblastic changes can be observed. Chronic heavy drinking can decrease production of white blood cells, decrease granulocyte mobility and adherence, and impair delayed-hypersensitivity responses to novel antigens (with a possible false-negative tuberculin skin test). Associated immune deficiencies can contribute to vulnerability toward infections, including hepatitis and HIV, and interfere with their treatment. Finally, many alcoholics have mild thrombocytopenia, which usually resolves within a week of abstinence unless there is hepatic cirrhosis or congestive splenomegaly.

CARDIOVASCULAR SYSTEM

Acutely, ethanol decreases myocardial contractility and causes peripheral vasodilation, with a resulting mild decrease in blood pressure and a compensatory increase in cardiac output. Exercise-induced increases in cardiac oxygen consumption are higher after alcohol intake.

These acute effects have little clinical significance for the average healthy drinker but can be problematic when persisting cardiac disease is present.

The consumption of three or more drinks per day results in a dose-dependent increase in blood pressure, which returns to normal within weeks of abstinence. Thus, heavy drinking is an important factor in mild to moderate hypertension. Chronic heavy drinkers also have a sixfold increased risk for coronary artery disease, related, in part, to increased low-density lipoprotein cholesterol, and carry an increased risk for cardiomyopathy through direct effects of alcohol on heart muscle. Symptoms of the latter include unexplained arrhythmias in the presence of left ventricular impairment, heart failure, hypocontractility of heart muscle, and dilation of all four heart chambers with associated mural thrombi and mitral valve regurgitation. Atrial or ventricular arrhythmias, especially paroxysmal tachycardia, can also occur temporarily after heavy drinking in individuals showing no other evidence of heart disease—a syndrome known as the "holiday heart."

GENITOURINARY SYSTEM CHANGES, SEXUAL FUNCTIONING, AND FETAL DEVELOPMENT

Drinking in adolescence can affect normal sexual development and reproductive onset. At any age, modest ethanol doses (e.g., blood alcohol concentrations of 0.06 g/dL) can increase sexual drive but also decrease erectile capacity in men. Even in the absence of liver impairment, a significant minority of chronic alcoholic men show irreversible testicular atrophy with shrinkage of the seminiferous tubules, decreases in ejaculate volume, and a lower sperm count.

The repeated ingestion of high doses of ethanol by women can result in amenorrhea, a decrease in ovarian size, absence of corpora lutea with associated infertility, and an increased risk of spontaneous abortion. Heavy drinking during pregnancy results in the rapid placental transfer of both ethanol and acetaldehyde, which may have serious consequences for fetal development. One severe result is the *fetal alcohol syndrome* (FAS), seen in ~5% of children born to heavy-drinking mothers, which can include any of the following: facial changes with epicanthal eye folds; poorly formed ear concha; small teeth with faulty enamel; cardiac atrial or ventricular septal defects; an aberrant palmar crease and limitation in joint movement; and microcephaly with mental retardation. A less severe condition is the *fetal alcohol spectrum disorder* (FASD), which can include low birth weight, a lower IQ, hyperactive behavior, and some modest cognitive deficits. The amount of ethanol required and the time of vulnerability during pregnancy have not been defined, making it advisable for pregnant women to abstain completely.

OTHER EFFECTS

Between one-half and two-thirds of alcoholics have skeletal muscle weakness caused by acute *alcoholic myopathy*, a condition that improves but which might not fully remit with abstinence. Effects of repeated heavy drinking on the *skeletal system* include changes in calcium metabolism, lower bone density, and decreased growth in the epiphyses, leading to an increased risk for fractures and osteonecrosis of the femoral head. *Hormonal changes* include an increase in cortisol levels, which can remain elevated during heavy drinking; inhibition of vasopressin secretion at rising blood alcohol concentrations and enhanced secretion at falling blood alcohol concentrations (with the final result that most alcoholics are likely to be slightly overhydrated); a modest and reversible decrease in serum thyroxine (T_4); and a more marked decrease in serum triiodothyronine (T_3). Hormone irregularities should be reevaluated as they may disappear after a month of abstinence.

ALCOHOLISM (ALCOHOL ABUSE OR DEPENDENCE)

Because many drinkers occasionally imbibe to excess, temporary alcohol-related pathology is common in nonalcoholics, especially in the late teens to the late twenties. When repeated problems in multiple life areas develop, the individual is likely to meet criteria for alcohol abuse or dependence.

DEFINITIONS AND EPIDEMIOLOGY

Alcohol dependence is defined in DSM-IV as repeated alcohol-related difficulties in at least three of seven life areas that cluster together at about the same time (e.g., over the same 12-month period). Two of these seven items, tolerance and withdrawal, may have special importance as they are associated with a more severe clinical course. Dependence predicts a course of recurrent problems with the use of alcohol and the consequent shortening of the life span by a decade.

Alcohol abuse is defined as repetitive problems with alcohol in any one of four life areas—social, interpersonal, legal, and occupational—or repeated use in hazardous situations such as driving while intoxicated in an individual who is not alcohol dependent. About 50% of those with alcohol abuse continue to have alcohol problems 2–5 years later, but only ~10% of these patients—including adolescents—go on to develop alcohol dependence.

The lifetime risk for alcohol dependence in most Western countries is about 10–15% for men and 5–8% for women. Rates are generally similar in the United

States, Canada, Germany, Australia, and the United Kingdom; tend to be lower in most Mediterranean countries, such as Italy, Greece, and Israel; and may be higher in Ireland, France, and Scandinavia. An even higher lifetime prevalence has been reported for most native cultures, including American Indians, Eskimos, Maori groups, and aboriginal tribes of Australia. These differences reflect both cultural and genetic influences, as described later. In Western countries, the typical alcoholic is more often a blue- or white-collar worker or homemaker. The lifetime risk for alcoholism among physicians is similar to that of the general population.

GENETICS

Approximately 60% of the risk for alcohol use disorders is attributed to genes, as indicated by the fourfold higher risk for alcohol abuse and dependence in children of alcoholics (even if these children were adopted early in life and raised by nonalcoholics) and a higher risk in identical twins as compared to fraternal twins of alcoholics. The genetic variations appear to operate primarily through intermediate characteristics that subsequently relate to the environment in altering the risk for heavy drinking and alcohol problems. These include genes relating to a high risk for all substance use disorders that operate through impulsivity, schizophrenia, and bipolar disorder. Another characteristic, an intense flushing response when drinking, decreases the risk for only alcohol use disorders through gene variations for several alcohol-metabolizing enzymes, especially aldehyde dehydrogenase (a mutation only seen in Asians), and to a lesser extent, variations in alcohol dehydrogenase.

An additional genetically influenced characteristic, a low sensitivity to alcohol, affects the risk for heavy drinking and may operate, in part, through variations in genes relating to potassium channels, GABA, nicotinic, and serotonin systems. A low response per drink is observed early in the drinking career and before alcohol use disorders have developed. All follow-up studies have demonstrated that this need for higher doses of alcohol to achieve desired effects predicts future heavy drinking, alcohol problems, and alcohol use disorders. The impact of a low response to alcohol on adverse drinking outcomes is mediated, at least in part, by a range of environmental influences, including the selection of heavier-drinking friends, the development of more positive expectations of the effects of high doses of alcohol, and suboptimal ways of coping with stress.

NATURAL HISTORY

Although the age of the first drink (~15 years) is similar in most alcoholics and nonalcoholics, a slightly earlier onset of regular drinking and drunkenness, especially in the context of conduct problems, is associated with a higher risk for later alcohol use disorders. By the early to midtwenties, most nonalcoholic men and women moderate their drinking (perhaps learning from more minor problems), whereas alcoholics are likely to escalate their patterns of drinking despite difficulties. The first major life problem from alcohol often appears in the late teens to early twenties, and a pattern of multiple alcohol difficulties by the midtwenties. Once established, the course of alcoholism is likely to be one of exacerbations and remissions, with little difficulty in temporarily stopping or controlling alcohol use when problems develop, but without help, desistance usually gives way to escalations in alcohol intake and subsequent problems. Following treatment, between half and two-thirds of alcoholics maintain abstinence for years, and often permanently. Even without formal treatment or self-help groups there is also at least a 20% chance of spontaneous remission with long-term abstinence. However, should the alcoholic continue to drink, the life span is shortened by ~10 years on average, with the leading causes of death, heart disease, cancer, accidents, and suicide.

TREATMENT

The approach to treating alcohol-related conditions is relatively straightforward: (1) recognize that at least 20% of all patients have alcohol abuse or dependence; (2) learn how to identify and treat acute alcohol-related conditions; (3) know how to help patients begin to address their alcohol problems; and (4) know enough about treating alcoholism to appropriately refer patients for additional help.

IDENTIFICATION OF THE ALCOHOLIC

Even in affluent locales, ~20% of patients have an alcohol use disorder. These men and women can be identified by asking questions about *alcohol problems* and noting laboratory test results that are likely to be abnormal in the context of regular consumption of six to eight or more drinks per day. The two blood tests with ≥60% sensitivity and specificity for heavy alcohol consumption are γ-glutamyl transferase (GGT) (>35 U) and carbohydrate-deficient transferrin (CDT) (>20 U/L or >2.6%); the combination of the two is likely to be more accurate than either alone. The values for these serologic markers are likely to return toward normal within several weeks of abstinence. Other useful blood tests include high-normal MCVs (≥91 μm^3) and serum uric acid (>416 mol/L, or 7 mg/dL).

The diagnosis of alcohol abuse or dependence ultimately rests on the documentation of a pattern of repeated difficulties associated with alcohol use. Thus, in screening it is important to probe for marital or job problems, legal difficulties, histories of accidents, medical problems, evidence of tolerance, etc., and then attempt to tie in use of alcohol or another substance. Some standardized questionnaires can be helpful, including the 10-item Alcohol Use Disorders Identification Test (AUDIT) (Table 56-2), but these are only screening tools, and a face-to-face interview is still required for a meaningful diagnosis.

TABLE 56-2

THE ALCOHOL USE DISORDERS IDENTIFICATION TEST (AUDIT)[a]

ITEM	5-POINT SCALE (LEAST TO MOST)
1. How often do you have a drink containing alcohol?	Never (0) to 4+ per week (4)
2. How many drinks containing alcohol do you have on a typical day?	1 or 2 (0) to 10+ (4)
3. How often do you have six or more drinks on one occasion?	Never (0) to daily or almost daily (4)
4. How often during the last year have you found that you were not able to stop drinking once you had started?	Never (0) to daily or almost daily (4)
5. How often during the last year have you failed to do what was normally expected from you because of drinking?	Never (0) to daily or almost daily (4)
6. How often during the last year have you needed a first drink in the morning to get yourself going after a heavy drinking session?	Never (0) to daily or almost daily (4)
7. How often during the last year have you had a feeling of guilt or remorse after drinking?	Never (0) to daily or almost daily (4)
8. How often during the last year have you been unable to remember what happened the night before because you had been drinking?	Never (0) to daily or almost daily (4)
9. Have you or someone else been injured as a result of your drinking?	No (0) to yes, during the last year (4)
10. Has a relative, friend, doctor or other health worker been concerned about your drinking or suggested that you should cut down?	No (0) to yes, during the last year (4)

[a]The AUDIT is scored by summing the 10 values. A score >8 may indicate harmful alcohol use.

Source: Adapted from DF Reinert, GP Allen: *Alcoholism: Clinical & Experimental Research* 26:272, 2002, and from MA Schuckit: *Drug and Alcohol Abuse: A Clinical Guide to Diagnosis and Treatment*, 6th ed. New York, Springer 2006.

TREATMENT Alcohol-Related Conditions

Acute Intoxication The first priority in treating severe intoxication is to assess vital signs and manage respiratory depression, cardiac arrhythmia, or blood pressure instability, if present. The possibility of intoxication with other drugs should be considered by obtaining toxicology screens for opioids or other CNS depressants such as benzodiazepines. Aggressive behavior should be handled by offering reassurance but also by considering the possibility of a show of force with an intervention team. If the aggressive behavior continues, relatively low doses of a short-acting benzodiazepine such as lorazepam (e.g., 1–2 mg PO or IV) may be used and can be repeated as needed, but care must be taken not to destabilize vital signs or worsen confusion. An alternative approach is to use an antipsychotic medication (e.g., 0.5–5 mg of haloperidol PO or IM every 4–8 h as needed, or olanzapine 2.5–10 mg IM repeated at 2 and 6 h, if needed).

Intervention There are two main elements to intervention in a person with alcoholism: motivational interviewing and brief interventions. During motivational interviewing, the clinician helps the patient to think through the assets (e.g., comfort in social situations) and liabilities (e.g., health and interpersonal related problems) of the current pattern of drinking. The patient's responses are key, and the clinician should listen empathetically, helping to weigh options and encouraging the patient to take responsibility for changes that need to be made. Patients should be reminded that only they can decide to avoid the consequences that will occur without changes in drinking. The process of motivational interviewing has been summarized by the acronym FRAMES: Feedback to the patient; Responsibility to be taken by the patient; Advice, rather than orders, on what needs to be done; Menus of options that might be considered; Empathy for understanding of the patient's thoughts and feelings; and Self-efficacy, i.e., offering support for the capacity of the patient to succeed in making changes.

Once the patient begins to consider change, the emphasis shifts to brief interventions designed to help the patient understand more about potential action. Discussions focus on consequences of high alcohol consumption, suggested approaches to stopping drinking, and help in recognizing and avoiding situations likely to lead to heavy drinking. Both motivational interviewing and brief interventions can be carried out in 15-min sessions, but because patients do not always change behavior right away, multiple meetings are often required to explain the problem, discuss optimal treatments, and explain the benefits of abstinence.

Alcohol Withdrawal If the patient agrees to stop drinking, sudden decreases in alcohol intake can produce withdrawal symptoms, many of which are the opposite of those produced by intoxication. Features include tremor of the hands (shakes); agitation and anxiety; autonomic nervous system overactivity including an increase in pulse, respiratory rate, and body temperature; and insomnia. These symptoms usually begin within 5–10 h of decreasing ethanol intake, peak on day 2 or 3, and improve by day 4 or 5, although mild levels of these problems may persist for 4–6 months as a protracted abstinence syndrome.

About 2–5% of alcoholics experience a withdrawal seizure, with the risk increasing in the context of concomitant medical problems, misuse of additional drugs, and higher alcohol quantities. The same risk factors also contribute to a similar rate of *delirium tremens* (DTs), where the withdrawal includes delirium (mental confusion, agitation, and fluctuating levels of consciousness) associated with a tremor and autonomic overactivity (e.g., marked increases in pulse, blood pressure, and respirations). The risks for seizures and DTs can be diminished by identifying and treating any underlying medical conditions early in the course of withdrawal.

The first step in treating withdrawal is to perform a thorough physical examination in all alcoholics who are considering stopping drinking, including a search for evidence of liver failure, gastrointestinal bleeding, cardiac arrhythmia, infection, and glucose or electrolyte imbalance. It is also important to offer adequate nutrition and oral multiple B vitamins, including 50–100 mg of thiamine daily for a week or more. Because most alcoholics who enter withdrawal are either normally hydrated or mildly overhydrated, IV fluids should be avoided unless there is a relevant medical problem or significant recent bleeding, vomiting, or diarrhea.

The next step is to recognize that because withdrawal symptoms reflect the rapid removal of a CNS depressant, alcohol, the symptoms can be controlled by administering any depressant in doses that decrease the agitation and then gradually tapering the dose over 3–5 days. While most CNS depressants are effective, benzodiazepines (Chap. 54) have the highest margin of safety and lowest cost and are, therefore, the preferred class of drugs. Short-half-life benzodiazepines can be considered for patients with serious liver impairment or evidence of brain damage, but they must be given every 4 h to avoid abrupt blood-level fluctuations that may increase the risk for seizures. Therefore, most clinicians use drugs with longer half-lives (e.g., chlordiazepoxide), adjusting the dose if signs of withdrawal escalate, and withholding the drug if the patient is sleeping or has evidence of orthostatic hypotension. The average patient requires doses of 25–50 mg of chlordiazepoxide or 10 mg of diazepam given PO every 4–6 h on the first day, with doses then decreased to zero over the next 5 days. While alcohol withdrawal can be treated in a hospital, patients in good physical condition who demonstrate mild signs of withdrawal despite low blood alcohol concentrations and who have no prior history of DTs or withdrawal seizures can be considered for outpatient detoxification. These patients should return daily for evaluation of vital signs and can be hospitalized if signs and symptoms of withdrawal escalate.

Treatment of the patient with DTs can be challenging, and the condition is likely to run a course of 3–5 days regardless of the therapy employed. The focus of care is to identify and correct medical problems and to control behavior and prevent injuries. Many clinicians recommend the use of high doses of a benzodiazepine (as much as 800 mg/d of chlordiazepoxide has been reported), a treatment that will decrease agitation and raise the seizure threshold but probably does little to improve the confusion. Other clinicians recommend the use of antipsychotic medications, such as haloperidol or olanzapine as discussed earlier, although these drugs have not been directly evaluated for DTs. Antipsychotics are less likely to exacerbate confusion but may increase the risk of seizures; they have no place in the treatment of mild withdrawal symptoms.

Generalized withdrawal seizures rarely require more than giving an adequate dose of benzodiazepines. There is little evidence that anticonvulsants such as phenytoin or gabapentin are more effective in drug-withdrawal seizures, and the risk of seizures has usually passed by the time effective drug levels are reached. The rare patient with status epilepticus must be treated aggressively (Chap. 26).

REHABILITATION OF ALCOHOLICS

An Overview After completing alcoholic rehabilitation, ≥60% of alcoholics, especially middle-class patients, maintain abstinence for at least a year, and many achieve lifetime sobriety. The core of treatment uses cognitive-behavioral approaches to help patients recognize the need to change, while working with them to alter their behaviors to enhance compliance. A key step is to optimize motivation toward abstinence through education about alcoholism and instructions to family members to stop protecting the patient from problems caused by alcohol. After years of heavy drinking, patients also need counseling, vocational rehabilitation, and self-help groups such as Alcoholics Anonymous (AA) to help them learn how to deal with life's stresses while sober. A third component, *relapse prevention*, helps the patient to identify situations in which a return to drinking is likely, formulate ways of managing these risks, and develop coping strategies that increase the chances of a return to abstinence if a slip occurs.

While many patients can be treated as outpatients, more intense interventions work better, and some alcoholics do not respond to AA or outpatient groups. Whatever the setting, subsequent contact with outpatient treatment staff should be maintained for a minimum of 6 months and preferably a full year after abstinence. Counseling focuses on areas of improved functioning in the absence of alcohol (i.e., why it is a good idea to continue to abstain) and helping the patient to manage free time without alcohol, develop a nondrinking peer group, and handle stresses on the job.

The physician serves an important role in identifying the alcoholic, diagnosing and treating associated medical or psychiatric syndromes, overseeing detoxification, referring the patient to rehabilitation programs, providing counseling, and, if appropriate, selecting which (if any) medication might be needed. For insomnia, patients should be reassured that troubled sleep is normal after alcohol withdrawal and will improve over subsequent weeks. They should be taught the basic elements of "sleep hygiene" including maintaining consistent schedules for bedtime and awakening. Sleep medications have the danger of being misused and of rebound insomnia when stopped. Sedating antidepressants (e.g., trazodone) should not be used as they interfere with cognitive functioning the next morning and disturb the normal sleep architecture, but occasional use of over-the-counter sleeping medications (sedating antihistamines) can be considered. Anxiety can be addressed by helping the person to gain insight into the temporary nature of the symptoms and to develop strategies to achieve relaxation as well as by using forms of cognitive therapy.

Medications for Rehabilitation Several medications have modest benefits when used for the first 6 months of recovery. The opioid-antagonist, naltrexone, 50–150 mg/d orally, appears to shorten subsequent relapses, whether used in the oral form or as a once-per-month 380-mg injection, especially in individuals with the G allele of the AII8G polymorphism of the μ opioid receptor. By blocking opioid receptors, naltrexone may decrease activity in the dopamine-rich ventral tegmental reward system, and decrease the feeling of pleasure or reward if alcohol is imbibed. A second medication, acamprosate (Campral) at ~2 g/d divided into three oral doses, has similar modest effects; acamprosate inhibits NMDA receptors, decreasing mild symptoms of protracted withdrawal. Several trials of combined naltrexone and acamprosate using doses similar to those noted earlier have reported that the combination may be superior to either drug alone, although not all studies agree.

It is more difficult to establish the asset-to-liability ratio of a third drug, disulfiram, an ALDH inhibitor, used at doses of 250 mg/d. This drug produces vomiting and autonomic nervous system instability in the presence of alcohol as a result of rapidly rising blood levels of the first metabolite of alcohol, acetaldehyde. This reaction can be dangerous, especially for patients with heart disease, stroke, diabetes mellitus, or hypertension. The drug itself carries potential risks of depression, psychotic symptoms, peripheral neuropathy, and liver damage. Disulfiram is best given under supervision of another individual (such as a spouse), especially during discrete periods identified as representing high-risk drinking situations (such as the Christmas holiday). Other relevant drugs under investigation include the nicotinic receptor agonist varenicline, the serotonin antagonist ondansetron, the α-adrenergic agonist prazosin, the GABA-B receptor agonist baclofen, the anticonvulsant topiramate, and cannabinol receptor antagonists. At present, there are insufficient data to determine the asset-to-liability ratio for these medications in treating alcoholism and, therefore, no data to offer solid support for their use in clinical settings.

CHAPTER 57

OPIOID DRUG ABUSE AND DEPENDENCE

Thomas R. Kosten

INTRODUCTION

Opiate analgesics are some of the oldest and most common medications in clinical practice, but have also been abused since at least 300 B.C. Nepenthe (Greek "free from sorrow") helped the hero of the *Odyssey*, but widespread opium smoking in China and the Near East has caused harm for centuries. Since the first chemical isolation of opium and codeine 200 years ago, a wide range of synthetic opioids have been developed, and endogenous opioid peptides were discovered in 1995. Two of the most important adverse effects of all these agents are overdose and dependence. The 0.14% annual prevalence of heroin dependence in the United States is only about one-third the rate of prescription opiate abuse and is substantially lower than the 2% rate of morphine dependence in Southeast and Southwest Asia. While these rates are low relative to other abused substances, their disease burden is substantial, with high rates of morbidity and mortality; disease transmission; increased health care, crime, and law enforcement costs; and less tangible costs of family distress and lost productivity.

The diagnosis of opiate dependence in the *Diagnostic and Statistical Manual of Mental Disorders*, Fourth Edition (DSM-IV) requires the repeated use of the drug while producing problems in three or more areas in a 12-month period. The areas include tolerance, withdrawal, use of greater amounts of opiates than intended, and use despite adverse consequences. The abuse diagnosis is related to legal problems, inability to meet obligations, use in hazardous situations, and continued use despite problems. The most striking aspect of opiate abuse has been its marked increase as the gateway to illicit drugs in the United States. Since 2007, prescription opiates have surpassed marijuana as the most common illicit drug that adolescents initially abuse.

The most commonly abused opiates are diverted prescriptions for oxycodone, followed by heroin and morphine, and—among health professionals—meperidine and fentanyl. Two opiate maintenance treatment agents—methadone and buprenorphine—are also abused, but at substantially lower rates, and the partial opiate agonists such as butorphanol, tramadol, and pentazocine are infrequently abused. The chemistry and general pharmacology of these agents are covered in major pharmacology texts, and this chapter focuses on the neurobiology and pharmacology relevant to abuse, dependence, and their treatments.

NEUROBIOLOGY

During the past 30 years, substantial progress has been made in elucidating the neurobiology of opiates and their effects not only on the three types of opiate receptors (mu, kappa, and delta) but also on the cascade of second, third, and fourth intracellular messenger systems and on neuronal action potentials. The different functional activities of these three receptors are summarized in **Table 57-1**, and abuse liability is

TABLE 57-1

ACTIONS OF OPIOID RECEPTORS

RECEPTOR TYPE	ACTIONS
Mu (μ) (e.g., morphine)	Analgesia, reinforcement euphoria, cough and appetite suppression, decreased respirations, decreased GI motility, sedation, hormone changes, dopamine and acetylcholine release
Kappa (κ) (e.g., butorphanol)	Dysphoria, decreased GI motility, decreased appetite, decreased respiration, psychotic symptoms, sedation, diuresis, analgesia
Delta (Δ) (e.g., etorphine)	Hormone changes, appetite suppression, dopamine release

Abbreviation: GI, gastrointestinal.

primarily associated with the mu receptor. A fourth type of opiate receptor, the orphanin receptor, also modulates pain but is not affected by opiate drugs. These opiate receptors are all G protein–linked and coupled to the cyclic adenosine monophosphate (cyclic AMP) second messenger system and to potassium channels. Opiates are inhibitory and block the potassium channels from opening and depolarizing the neuron, which would produce an action potential. Thus, opiates acutely inhibit neuronal activity. Analgesia and sedation are induced through this inhibition of specific brain pathways, while the "high" from opiates involves an indirect activation of a different brain pathway—the mesolimbic dopamine pathway.

The various effects of opiates are related to the specific neuroanatomic locations of mu receptors. Reinforcing and euphoric effects of opiates occur in the dopaminegic pathway from the ventral tegmental area (VTA) to the nucleus accumbens, where opiates increase synaptic levels of dopamine. This increase is due to inhibition of GABAergic neurons that inhibit both the VTA and nucleus accumbens activity. However, the "high" only occurs when the *rate of change* in dopamine is fast. Large, rapidly administered doses of opiates block GABA inhibition and produce a burst of nucleus accumbens activity that is associated with "high" in all abused drugs. Therefore, routes of administration that slowly increase opiate blood and brain levels, such as oral and transdermal routes, are effective for analgesia and sedation but do not produce an opiate "high" that follows smoking and intravenous routes. Other acute effects such as analgesia and respiratory depression leading to overdose are due to stimulation of opiate receptors located in other areas such as the locus coeruleus.

Opiate dependence and withdrawal are chronic effects related to the cyclic AMP system. This second messenger phosphorylates various intracellular proteins and produces a cascade of changes reaching into the nucleus and DNA. Immediate early gene products such as c-*fos* and c-*jun* are activated followed by regulation of other genes with more sustained protein transcription such as *delta c-fos*. With these sustained gene activations, several receptor-level changes occur, including downregulation of receptor numbers, reduced neuronal cell-surface receptor trafficking, uncoupling of G proteins from the mu opiate receptors, and upregulation of cyclic AMP second messenger systems. These effects are also reflective of genetic risk factors for drug dependence, with estimates of up to 50% of the risk for dependence due to polygenic inheritance. Specific functional genetic polymorphisms in the mu opiate receptor gene appear associated with this risk for opiate abuse, including one producing a threefold increase in this receptor's affinity for opiates and the endogenous ligand beta endorphin. Epigenetic methylation changes also occur on the DNA of the mu receptor gene of opiate addicts. DNA methylation inhibits gene transcription.

This molecular cascade links acute intoxication and sedation to chronic opiate dependence and withdrawal within the specific neuroanatomic structure of the locus coeruleus. The locus coeruleus is the brain's largest concentration of noradrenergic neurons and is responsible for a large proportion of brain cortical activation. When large opiate doses saturate and activate all of its mu receptors, its steady rate of action potentials can cease due to the inactivation of potassium channels. When this direct inhibitory effect is sustained over weeks and months of opiate use, a secondary set of regulatory effects take place in the cyclic AMP system that leads to tolerance, dependence, and withdrawal symptoms.

Opiate withdrawal symptoms reflect overactivity of adrenergic neurons that are located in the locus ceruleus. Opiates suppress the activity of these neurons, and when this suppression continues chronically from daily opiate use, a secondary upregulation occurs in adenyl cyclase enzyme capacity and the production of cyclic AMP from ATP. This upregulation is a homeostatic response to the chronic opiate suppression, but when that suppression is terminated by discontinuing the opiate, this enhanced adenyl cyclase activity leads to a marked increase in cyclic AMP. The now very high levels of cyclic AMP activate the sodium-potassium channels and produce a high level of action potentials in these adrenergic neurons. This adrenergic arousal is one basis for the symptoms of opiate withdrawal and takes about 7 days to readjust to normal levels of adenyl cyclase activity and the associated resolution of opiate withdrawal symptoms. This molecular model of adrenergic neuronal activation during withdrawal has had important treatment implications, such as the use of clonidine for opioid withdrawal.

PHARMACOLOGY

Tolerance and withdrawal commonly occur with chronic daily use as quickly as 6–8 weeks depending on the dose and frequency of dosing. Tolerance appears to be primarily a pharmacodynamic rather than pharmacokinetic effect, with relatively limited induction of the cytochrome P450 or other liver enzymes. The metabolism of opiates occurs in the liver primarily through the cytochrome P450 systems of 2D6 and 3A4. They then are conjugated to glucuronic acid and excreted in small amounts in feces. The plasma half-lives generally range from 2.5 to 3 h for morphine and more than 22 h for methadone. The shortest half-lives of several minutes are for fentanyl-related opiates and the longest are for buprenorphine and its active metabolites, which can block opiate withdrawal for up to 3 days after a single dose. Tolerance to the mental effects of opioids leads to the need for ever-increasing amounts of drugs to sustain the desired euphoriant effects—as well as to avoid the discomfort of withdrawal. This combination has the expected consequence of strongly reinforcing dependence once it has started. The role of endogenous opioid peptides in opioid dependence is uncertain.

The clinical aspects of abuse are tied to route of administration and the rapidity of an opiate bolus in reaching the brain. Intravenous and smoked administration is routine not only because it is the most efficient route but also because it rapidly produces a bolus of high drug concentration in the brain. This bolus produces a "rush," followed by euphoria, a feeling of tranquility, and sleepiness ("the nod"). Heroin produces effects that last 3–5 h, and several doses a day are required to forestall manifestations of withdrawal in dependent persons. Symptoms of opioid withdrawal begin 8–10 h after the last dose. Many of these symptoms reflect increased activity of the autonomic nervous system. Lacrimation, rhinorrhea, yawning, and sweating appear first. Restless sleep followed by weakness, chills, gooseflesh ("cold turkey"), nausea and vomiting, muscle aches, and involuntary movements ("kicking the habit"), hyperpnea, hyperthermia, and hypertension occur in later stages of the withdrawal syndrome. The acute course of withdrawal may last 7–10 days. A secondary phase of protracted abstinence lasts for 26–30 weeks and is characterized by hypotension, bradycardia, hypothermia, mydriasis, and decreased responsiveness of the respiratory center to carbon dioxide.

Opioid effects on organs

Besides the brain effects of opioids on sedation and euphoria and the combined brain and peripheral nervous system effects on analgesia, a wide range of other organs can be affected. The cough reflex is inhibited through the brain, leading to the use of some opiates as an antitussive, and nausea and vomiting are due to brainstem effects on the medulla. The release of several hormones is inhibited including corticotropin-releasing factor (CRF) and luteinizing hormone, which reduce cortisol and sex hormone levels, respectively. The clinical manifestations of these reductions can involve poor responses to stress and reductions in sex drive. An increase in prolactin also contributes to the reduced sex drive in males. Two other hormones affected are decreased thyrotropin and increased growth hormone. Respiratory depression results from opiate-induced insensitivity of brainstem neurons to increases in carbon dioxide. This depression contributes to overdose, but in patients with pulmonary disease even opiate doses well below those typical of overdose can produce clinically significant complications. In overdoses, aspiration pneumonia is a common complication due to loss of the choking reflex. Opiates reduce gut motility, which is helpful for diarrhea, but can lead to nausea, constipation, and anorexia with weight loss. Deaths have occurred in early methadone maintenance programs due to severe constipation and toxic megacolon. Opiates may prolong QT intervals and lead to sudden death in some patients. Two opiates particularly noted for this complication are methadone and a long-acting form of methadone called LAAM that was withdrawn from the market. Orthostatic hypotension may occur due to histamine release and peripheral blood vessel dilation, which is an opiate effect usefully applied to managing acute myocardial infarction.

Heroin users in particular tend to use opiates intravenously and be polydrug users, also using alcohol, sedatives, cannabinoids, and stimulants. None of these other drugs serve as substitutes for opioids, but they have desired additive effects. One needs to be sure that the person undergoing a withdrawal reaction is not also withdrawing from alcohol or sedatives, which might be more dangerous and more difficult to manage.

Besides the ever-present risk of fatal overdose, hepatitis B and AIDS are among the many potential complications of sharing contaminated hypodermic syringes. Bacterial infections lead to septic complications such as meningitis, osteomyelitis, and abscesses in various organs. Attempts to illicitly manufacture meperidine in the 1980s resulted in the production of a highly specific neurotoxin, MPTP, which produced parkinsonism in users.

Toxicity and overdose

Lethal overdose is a relatively common complication of opiate dependence and must be rapidly recognized and treated because naloxone provides a highly specific reversal agent that is relatively free of complications. The diagnosis generally does not rely on blood or urine toxicology results but on clinical signs and symptoms. The presentation involves shallow and slow respirations, pupillary miosis (mydriasis does not occur until significant brain anoxia supervenes), bradycardia, hypothermia, and stupor or coma. If naloxone is not administered, progression to respiratory and cardiovascular collapse leading to death occurs. At autopsy, cerebral edema and sometimes frothy pulmonary edema are generally found, but those pulmonary effects are most likely from allergic reactions to adulterants mixed with the heroin. Opiates generally do not produce seizures except for unusual cases of mixed drug abuse with the opiate meperidine or with high doses of tramadol.

TREATMENT Opioid Overdose

Beyond the acute treatment of opiate overdose with naloxone, clinicians have two general treatment paths: opioid maintenance treatment or detoxification. Most opioid-dependent individuals engage in multiple episodes of all three categories of treatment during the course of their drug-using careers. Agonist and partial agonist medications are commonly utilized for both maintenance and detoxification purposes. Alpha-2-adrenergic agonists are primarily used for detoxification. Antagonists are used to accelerate detoxification and then continued postdetoxification to prevent relapse. Only the residential medication-free programs have had success that comes close to matching that of the medication-based programs. Success of the various treatment approaches is assessed as retention in treatment, reduced opioid and other drug use, as well as secondary outcomes such as HIV risk behaviors, crime, psychiatric symptoms, and medical comorbidity.

Stopping opiates is like stopping most drugs of abuse—it is much easier to stop than to prevent relapses. Long-term relapse prevention for opioid-dependent persons requires combined pharmacologic and psychosocial approaches. Chronic users tend to prefer pharmacologic approaches; those with shorter histories of drug abuse are more amenable to detoxification and psychosocial interventions.

Opiate Overdose Treatment Managing overdose requires naloxone and support of vital functions, including intubation if needed. The opiate antagonist naloxone is given at 0.4–2 mg IV or IM, with an expected response within 1–2 min. If the overdose is due to buprenorphine, then naloxone might be required at total doses of 10 mg or greater, but primary buprenorphine overdose is nearly impossible because this agent is a partial opiate agonist. Partial agonism means that as the dose of buprenorphine is increased, it has greater opiate antagonist than agonist activity. Thus, a 0.2-mg buprenorphine dose leads to analgesia and sedation, while a hundred times greater 20-mg dose produces profound opiate antagonism, precipitating opiate withdrawal in a person who was opiate dependent on morphine or methadone. When 10 mg of naloxone fails to produce arousal in the patient, another cause of toxicity must be found. Before reaching such large naloxone doses, however, it is important to recognize that the goal is to reverse the respiratory depression and not to administer so much naloxone that it precipitates opiate withdrawal. Because naloxone only lasts a few hours and most opiates last considerably longer, close monitoring and an IV naloxone drip is frequently employed to provide a continuous level of antagonism for 24–72 h depending on the opiate used in the overdose (e.g., morphine vs. methadone). Other sedative drugs that produce significant overdoses must also be considered if naloxone has only a limited effect. The most common are benzodiazepines, which have produced overdoses and deaths in combination with buprenorphine. A specific antagonist for benzodiazepines—flumazenil at 0.2 mg/min—can be given to a maximum of 3 g/h, but it may precipitate seizures and increase intracranial pressure. Like naloxone, administration for a prolonged period is usually required since most benzodiazepines remain active for considerably longer than flumazenil.

Support of vital functions may include oxygen and positive-pressure breathing, IV fluids, pressor agents for hypotension, and cardiac monitoring to detect QT prolongation, which might require treatment. Activated charcoal and gastric lavage may be helpful for oral ingestions, but intubation will be needed if the patient is stuporous.

Opiate Withdrawal Treatment The principles of detoxification are the same for all drugs: to substitute a longer-acting, orally active, pharmacologically equivalent drug for the abused drug, stabilize the patient on that drug, and then gradually withdraw the substituted drug. Methadone is admirably suited for such use in opioid-dependent persons, and the partial mu agonist buprenorphine is another option. Clonidine, a centrally acting sympatholytic agent, has also been used for detoxification. By reducing central sympathetic outflow, clonidine mitigates many of the signs of sympathetic overactivity. Clonidine has no narcotic action and is not addictive. Lofexidine, a clonidine analogue with less hypotensive effect, is being developed for use.

Methadone for Detoxification Methadone dose tapering regimens for detoxification range from 2 to 3 weeks to as long as 180 days, but this approach is controversial given the relative effectiveness of methadone maintenance and the low success rates of detoxification. Unfortunately, the vast majority of patients tend to relapse to heroin or other opiates during or after the detoxification period, indicative of the chronic and relapsing nature of opioid dependence.

Buprenorphine for Detoxification Because it is a partial agonist, buprenorphine produces fewer withdrawal symptoms and may allow briefer detoxifications compared with full agonists like methadone, but it does not appear to have better outcomes than methadone tapering. Buprenorphine is superior to the alpha-2-adrenergic agonist clonidine in reducing symptoms of withdrawal, retaining patients in a withdrawal protocol, and in treatment completion.

Alpha-2-Adrenergic Agonists for Detoxification Several alpha-2-adrenergic agonists have relieved opioid withdrawal by suppressing central noradrenergic hyperactivity. Alpha-2-adrenergic agonists moderate the symptoms of noradrenergic hyperactivity via actions in the central nervous system. Clonidine relieves some signs and symptoms of opiate withdrawal such as lacrimation, rhinorrhea, muscle pain, joint pain, restlessness, and gastrointestinal symptoms, but it is not a drug of abuse or dependence. Unfortunately, clonidine is associated with significant hypotension, which has stimulated investigation of lofexidine, guanfacine, and guanabenz acetate. Lofexidine can be dosed up to ~2 mg/d and appears to be associated with fewer adverse effects, and it is therefore likely to replace clonidine as the leading opioid withdrawal treatment in this drug class. Clonidine or lofexidine are typically administered orally, in three or four doses per day, with dizziness, sedation, lethargy, and dry mouth as the primary adverse side effects. Completion rates of managed withdrawal assisted with clonidine and other alpha-2-adrenergic agents vs. methadone have been comparable.

Rapid and Ultrarapid Opiate Detoxification

The opioid antagonist naltrexone typically combined with an alpha-2-adrenergic agonist has been purported to shorten the duration of withdrawal without significantly increasing patient discomfort. Another benefit to rapid opiate detoxification (ROD) is the reduced time between opioid use and the commencement of sustained naltrexone treatment for prevention of relapse (discussed later). ROD completion rates using naltrexone and clonidine range from 75 to 81% compared to 40 to 65% for methadone or clonidine alone. Buprenorphine in combination with naltrexone and clonidine reduced ROD from 3 days to 1 day of detoxification. Ultrarapid opiate detoxification is an extension of ROD using anesthetics, but is highly controversial due to the medical risks and mortality associated with it.

Agonist medications for opioid dependence

Methadone maintenance substitutes a once-daily oral opioid dose for three-to-four times daily heroin. Methadone saturates the opioid receptors, and by inducing a high level of opiate tolerance, blocks the desired euphoria from additional opiates. Buprenorphine, a partial opioid agonist, also can be given once daily at sublingual doses of 4–32 mg daily, and in contrast to methadone it can be given in an office-based primary care setting.

Methadone maintenance

Methadone's slow onset of action when taken orally, long elimination half-life (24–36 h), and production of cross-tolerance at doses from 80 to 150 mg are the basis for its efficacy in treatment retention and reductions in IV drug use, criminal activity, and HIV risk behaviors and mortality. Methadone can prolong the QT interval at rates as high as 16% above the rates in non-methadone-maintained, drug-injecting patients, but it has been used safely in the treatment of opioid dependence for 40 years.

Buprenorphine maintenance

While France and Australia have had sublingual buprenorphine maintenance since 1996, the USFDA approved it as a Schedule III drug in 2002 for managing opiate dependence. Unlike the full agonist methadone, buprenorphine is a partial agonist of mu-opioid receptors with a slow onset and long duration of action, allowing for alternate-day dosing. Its partial agonism reduces the risk of unintentional overdose but limits its efficacy to patients who need the equivalent of only 60–70 mg of methadone, and many patients in methadone maintenance require higher doses up to 150 mg daily. Buprenorphine is combined with naloxone at a 4:1 ratio in order to reduce its abuse liability. A subcutaneous buprenorphine implant has also been tested, but results are not yet available.

In the United States, the ability of primary care physicians to prescribe buprenorphine for opioid dependence presents an important and far-reaching opportunity to improve access and quality of treatment as well as reduce social harm. Europe, Asia, and Australia have found reduced opioid-related deaths and drug-injection-related medical morbidity with buprenorphine available in primary care. Retention in office-based buprenorphine treatment has been greater than 70% at 6-month follow-ups.

Antagonist medications for opioid dependence

The rationale for using narcotic antagonist therapy is that blocking the action of self-administered opioids should eventually extinguish the habit, but this therapy is poorly accepted by patients. Naltrexone, a long-acting orally active pure opioid antagonist, can be given three times a week at doses of 100–150 mg and a depot form for monthly administration is available. Because it is an antagonist, the patient must first be detoxified from opioid dependence before starting naltrexone. When taken chronically for even years, it is safe, associated with few side effects (headache, nausea, abdominal pain), and can be given to patients infected with hepatitis B or C without producing hepatotoxicity. However, most providers refrain from prescribing it if liver function tests are 3–5 times above normal levels. Naltrexone maintenance combined with psychosocial therapy is effective in reducing heroin use, but medication adherence is low. Depot injection formulations lasting up to 4 weeks markedly improve adherence, retention, and drug use. Subcutaneous naltrexone implants in Russia,

China, and Australia have doubled treatment retention and reduced relapse to half that of oral naltrexone.

Medication-free treatment

Most opiate addicts enter medication-free treatments in inpatient, residential, or outpatient settings, but 1- to 5-year outcomes are very poor compared to pharmacotherapy except for residential settings lasting 6 to 18 months. The residential programs require full immersion in a regimented system that has progressively increasing levels of independence and responsibility within a controlled community of fellow drug abusers. These medication-free programs, as well as the pharmacotherapy programs, also include counseling and behavioral treatments designed to teach interpersonal and cognitive skills for coping with stress and for avoiding situations leading to easy access to drugs or to craving. Relapse is prevented by having the individual very gradually reintroduced to greater responsibilities and to the working environment outside of the protected therapeutic community.

PREVENTION

Preventing opiate abuse represents a critically important challenge for physicians. Opiate prescriptions are the most common source of drugs accessed by adolescents who begin a pattern of illicit drug abuse; in the United States, 9000 adolescents become opiate abusers every day. The major sources of these drugs are family members, not drug dealers or the Internet. Pain management involves giving sufficient opiates to relieve the pain over as short a period of time as the pain warrants. The patient then needs to dispose of any remaining opiates, not save them in the medicine cabinet, because this behavior leads to diversion to adolescents. Finally, physicians should never prescribe opiates for themselves.

CHAPTER 58

COCAINE AND OTHER COMMONLY ABUSED DRUGS

Nancy K. Mello ■ Jack H. Mendelson[a]

The abuse of cocaine and other psychostimulant drugs reflects a complex interaction between the pharmacologic properties of each drug, the personality and expectations of the user, and the environmental context in which the drug is used. Polydrug abuse involving the concurrent use of several drugs with different pharmacologic effects is increasingly common. Some forms of polydrug abuse, such as the combined use of heroin and cocaine intravenously, are especially dangerous and are a major problem in hospital emergency rooms. Sometimes one drug is used to enhance the effects of another, as with the combined use of benzodiazepines and methadone, or cocaine and heroin in methadone-maintained patients.

Chronic cocaine and psychostimulant abuse may cause a number of adverse health consequences, and preexisting disorders such as hypertension and cardiac disease may be exacerbated by drug abuse. The combined use of two or more drugs may accentuate medical complications associated with abuse of one of them. Chronic drug abuse is often associated with immune system dysfunction and increased vulnerability to infections, which in turn contributes to the risk for HIV infection. In addition, concurrent use of cocaine and opiates (the "speedball") is frequently associated with needle sharing by IV drug users. Intravenous drug abusers continue to represent the largest single group of persons with HIV infection in several major metropolitan areas in the United States as well as in many parts of Europe and Asia.

COCAINE

Cocaine is a stimulant and a local anesthetic with potent vasoconstrictor properties. The leaves of the *coca* plant (*Erythroxylon coca*) contain ~0.5–1% cocaine. The drug produces physiologic and behavioral effects when administered orally, intranasally, intravenously, or via inhalation following pyrolysis (smoking). The reinforcing effects of cocaine appear to be related to activation of dopaminergic neurons in the mesolimbic system. Cocaine increases synaptic concentrations of the monamine neurotransmitters dopamine, norepinephrine, and serotonin by binding to transporter proteins in presynaptic neurons and blocking reuptake.

Prevalence of cocaine use

Cocaine is widely available throughout the United States, and cocaine abuse occurs in virtually all social and economic strata of society. The prevalence of cocaine abuse in the general population has been accompanied by an increase in cocaine abuse by heroin-dependent persons, including those in methadone maintenance programs. Intravenous cocaine is often used concurrently with IV heroin. This combination purportedly attenuates the postcocaine "crash" and substitutes a cocaine "high" for the heroin "high" blocked by methadone.

Acute and chronic intoxication

There has been an increase in both IV administration and inhalation of pyrolyzed cocaine via smoking. Following intranasal administration, changes in mood and sensation are perceived within 3–5 min, and peak effects occur at 10–20 min. The effects rarely last more than 1 h. Inhalation of pyrolyzed materials includes inhaling crack/cocaine or smoking coca paste, a product made by extracting cocaine preparations with flammable solvents, and cocaine free-base smoking. Free-base cocaine, including the freebase prepared with sodium bicarbonate (crack), has become increasingly

[a]Deceased.

popular because of the relative high potency of the compound and its rapid onset of action (8–10 s following smoking).

Cocaine produces a brief, dose-related stimulation and enhancement of mood and an increase in cardiac rate and blood pressure. Body temperature usually increases following cocaine administration, and high doses of cocaine may induce lethal pyrexia or hypertension. Because cocaine inhibits reuptake of catecholamines at adrenergic nerve endings, the drug potentiates sympathetic nervous system activity. Cocaine has a short plasma half-life of approximately 45–60 min. It is metabolized by plasma esterases, and cocaine metabolites are excreted in urine. The very short duration of the euphorigenic effects of cocaine observed in chronic abusers is probably due to both acute and chronic tolerance. Frequent self-administration of the drug (two to three times per hour) is often reported by chronic cocaine abusers. Alcohol is often used to modulate both the cocaine high and the dysphoria associated with the abrupt disappearance of cocaine's effects. A metabolite of cocaine, cocaethylene, has been detected in the blood and urine of persons who concurrently abuse alcohol and cocaine. Cocaethylene induces changes in cardiovascular function similar to those of cocaine alone, and the pathophysiologic consequences of alcohol abuse plus cocaine abuse may be additive when both are used together.

The prevalent assumption that cocaine inhalation or IV administration is relatively safe is contradicted by reports of death from respiratory depression, cardiac arrhythmias, and convulsions associated with cocaine use. In addition to generalized seizures, neurologic complications may include headache, ischemic or hemorrhagic stroke, or subarachnoid hemorrhage. Disorders of cerebral blood flow and perfusion in cocaine-dependent persons have been detected with magnetic resonance spectroscopy (MRS) studies. Severe pulmonary disease may develop in individuals who inhale crack cocaine; this effect is attributed both to the direct effects of cocaine and to residual contaminants in the smoked material. Hepatic necrosis may occur following chronic crack/cocaine use. Protracted cocaine abuse may also cause paranoid ideation and visual and auditory hallucinations, a state that resembles alcoholic hallucinosis.

Although men and women who abuse cocaine may report that the drug enhances libidinal drive, chronic cocaine use causes significant loss of libido and adversely affects sexual function. Impotence and gynecomastia have been observed in male cocaine abusers, and these abnormalities often persist for long periods following cessation of drug use. Women who abuse cocaine may have major derangements in menstrual cycle function, including galactorrhea, amenorrhea, and infertility. Chronic cocaine abuse may cause persistent hyperprolactinemia as a consequence of disordered dopaminergic inhibition of prolactin secretion by the anterior pituitary. Cocaine abuse by pregnant women, particularly crack smoking, has been associated with both an increased risk of congenital malformations in the fetus and perinatal cardiovascular and cerebrovascular disease in the mother. However, cocaine abuse per se is probably not the sole cause of these perinatal disorders, because maternal cocaine abuse is often associated with poor nutrition and prenatal health care as well as polydrug abuse that may contribute to the risk for perinatal disease.

Psychological dependence on cocaine, indicated by inability to abstain from frequent compulsive use, has also been reported. Although the occurrence of withdrawal syndromes involving psychomotor agitation and autonomic hyperactivity remains controversial, severe depression ("crashing") following cocaine intoxication may accompany drug withdrawal.

TREATMENT Cocaine Overdose and Chronic Abuse

Treatment of cocaine overdose is a medical emergency that is best managed in an intensive care unit. Cocaine toxicity produces a hyperadrenergic state characterized by hypertension, tachycardia, tonic-clonic seizures, dyspnea, and ventricular arrhythmias. Intravenous diazepam in doses up to 0.5 mg/kg administered over an 8-h period has been shown to be effective for control of seizures. Ventricular arrhythmias have been managed successfully by administration of 0.5–1 mg of propranolol IV. Since many instances of cocaine-related mortality have been associated with concurrent use of other illicit drugs (particularly heroin), the physician must be prepared to institute effective emergency treatment for multiple drug toxicities.

Treatment of chronic cocaine abuse requires the combined efforts of primary care physicians, psychiatrists, and psychosocial care providers. Early abstinence from cocaine use is often complicated by symptoms of depression and guilt, insomnia, and anorexia, which may be as severe as those observed in major affective disorders. Individual and group psychotherapy, family therapy, and peer group assistance programs are often useful for inducing prolonged remission from drug use. A number of medications used for the treatment of various medical and psychiatric disorders have been administered to reduce the duration and severity of cocaine abuse and dependence. The search for a medication that is both safe and highly effective for cocaine detoxification or maintenance of abstinence is continuing. Although psychotherapy may be effective, no specific form of psychotherapy or behavioral modification is uniquely beneficial.

MARIJUANA AND CANNABIS COMPOUNDS

Cannabis sativa contains >400 compounds in addition to the psychoactive substance, delta-9-tetrahydrocannabinol (THC). Marijuana cigarettes are prepared from the leaves and flowering tops of the plant, and a typical marijuana cigarette contains 0.5–1 g of plant material. The usual THC concentration varies between 10 and 40 mg, but concentrations >100 mg per cigarette have been detected. Hashish is prepared from concentrated resin of *C. sativa* and contains a THC concentration of between 8 and 12% by weight. "Hash oil," a lipid-soluble plant extract, may contain THC between 25 and 60% and may be added to marijuana or hashish to enhance its THC concentration. Smoking is the most common mode of marijuana or hashish use. During pyrolysis, >150 compounds in addition to THC are released in the smoke. Although most of these compounds do not have psychoactive properties, they may have physiologic effects.

THC is quickly absorbed from the lungs into blood, and then rapidly sequestered in tissues. THC is metabolized primarily in the liver, where it is converted to 11-hydroxy-THC, a psychoactive compound, and >20 other metabolites. Many THC metabolites are excreted through the feces at a relatively slow rate of clearance in comparison to most other psychoactive drugs.

Specific cannabinoid receptors (CB_1 and CB_2) have been identified in the central and peripheral nervous system. High densities of cannabinoid receptors have been found in the cerebral cortex, basal ganglia, and hippocampus. T and B lymphocytes also contain cannabinoid receptors, and these appear to mediate the anti-inflammatory and immunoregulatory properties of cannabinoids. A naturally occurring THC-like ligand has been identified and is widely distributed in the nervous system.

Prevalence of use

Marijuana is the most commonly used illegal drug in the United States, and its use is particularly prevalent among adolescents. Marijuana is relatively inexpensive and is often considered to be less hazardous than other controlled drugs and substances. Very potent forms of marijuana (sinsemilla) are now available in many locations, and concurrent use of marijuana with crack/cocaine and phencyclidine is not uncommon.

Acute and chronic intoxication

Acute intoxication from marijuana and cannabis compounds is related to both the dose of THC and the route of administration. THC is absorbed more rapidly from marijuana smoking than from orally ingested cannabis compounds. Acute marijuana intoxication may produce a perception of relaxation and mild euphoria resembling mild to moderate alcohol intoxication. This condition is usually accompanied by some impairment in thinking, concentration, and perceptual and psychomotor function. Higher doses of cannabis may produce more pronounced impairment in concentration and perception, as well as greater sedation. Although the acute effects of marijuana intoxication are relatively benign in normal users, the drug can precipitate severe emotional disorders in individuals who have antecedent psychotic or neurotic problems. Like other psychoactive compounds, both the user's expectations and the environmental context are important determinants of the type and severity of the effects of marijuana intoxication.

As with abuse of cocaine, opioids, and alcohol, chronic marijuana abusers may lose interest in common socially desirable goals and steadily devote more time to drug acquisition and use. However, THC does not cause a specific and unique "amotivational syndrome." The range of symptoms sometimes attributed to marijuana use is difficult to distinguish from mild to moderate depression and the maturational dysfunctions often associated with protracted adolescence. Chronic marijuana use has also been reported to increase the risk of psychotic symptoms in individuals with a past history of schizophrenia. Persons who initiate marijuana smoking before the age of 17 may exhibit more pronounced cognitive deficits and they may also be at higher risk for polydrug and alcohol abuse problems in later life, but the role of marijuana in this causal sequence is uncertain.

Physical effects

Conjunctival injection and tachycardia are the most frequent immediate physical concomitants of smoking marijuana. Tolerance for marijuana-induced tachycardia develops rapidly among regular users. However, marijuana smoking may precipitate angina in persons with a history of coronary insufficiency. Exercise-induced angina may be increased after marijuana use to a greater extent than after tobacco cigarette smoking. Patients with cardiac disease should be strongly advised not to smoke marijuana or use cannabis compounds.

Significant decrements in pulmonary vital capacity have been found in regular daily marijuana smokers. Because marijuana smoking typically involves deep inhalation and prolonged retention of marijuana smoke, marijuana smokers may develop chronic bronchial irritation. Impairment of single-breath carbon monoxide diffusion capacity (DL_{CO}) is greater in persons who smoke both marijuana and tobacco than in tobacco smokers.

Although marijuana has also been associated with a number of other adverse effects, many of these studies await replication and confirmation. A reported correlation between chronic marijuana use and decreased testosterone levels in males has not been confirmed. Decreased sperm count and sperm motility and morphologic abnormalities of spermatozoa following marijuana use have been reported. Prospective studies demonstrated a correlation between impaired fetal growth and development and heavy marijuana use during pregnancy. Marijuana has also been implicated in derangements of the immune system; in chromosomal abnormalities; and in inhibition of DNA, RNA, and protein synthesis; however, these findings have not been confirmed or related to any specific physiologic effect in humans.

Tolerance and physical dependence

Habitual marijuana users rapidly develop tolerance to the psychoactive effects of marijuana, then smoke more frequently and try to acquire more potent cannabis compounds. Tolerance for the physiologic effects of marijuana develops at different rates; e.g., tolerance develops rapidly for marijuana-induced tachycardia but more slowly for marijuana-induced conjunctival injection. Tolerance for both behavioral and physiologic effects of marijuana decreases rapidly upon cessation of marijuana use.

Withdrawal signs and symptoms have been reported in chronic cannabis users, and the severity of symptoms is related to dosage and duration of use. These symptoms typically reach their peak several days after cessation of chronic use and include irritability, anorexia, and sleep disturbances. Withdrawal signs and symptoms observed in chronic marijuana users are usually relatively mild in comparison to those observed in heavy opiate or alcohol users and rarely require medical or pharmacologic intervention. However, more severe and protracted abstinence syndromes may occur after sustained use of high-potency cannabis compounds.

Therapeutic use of marijuana

Marijuana, administered as cigarettes or as a synthetic oral cannabinoid (dronabinol), has been proposed to have a number of medicinal properties that may be clinically useful in some situations. These include antiemetic effects in chemotherapy recipients, appetite-promoting effects in AIDS patients, reduction of intraocular pressure in glaucoma, and reduction of spasticity in multiple sclerosis and other neurologic disorders. With the possible exception of AIDS-related cachexia, none of these attributes of marijuana compounds is clearly superior to other readily available therapies.

METHAMPHETAMINE

Methamphetamine is also referred to as "meth," "speed," "crank," "chalk," "ice," "glass," or "crystal." Methamphetamine is a mixed-action monoamine releaser with activity at dopamine, serotonin, and norepinephrine systems. Despite drug seizures, closures of clandestine laboratories that produce methamphetamine illegally, and an increase in methamphetamine abuse prevention programs, methamphetamine was considered second only to cocaine as a drug threat to society by the U.S. Department of Justice in 2009. Hospital admissions for methamphetamine treatment more than doubled between 1998 and 2007, and young adults (aged 18–25 years) have the highest use rates.

Methamphetamine can be used by smoking, snorting, IV injection, or oral administration. Methamphetamine abusers report that drug use induces feelings of euphoria and decreased fatigue. Adverse consequences of methamphetamine abuse include headache, difficulty concentrating, diminished appetite, abdominal pain, vomiting or diarrhea, disordered sleep, paranoid or aggressive behavior, and psychosis. Chronic methamphetamine abuse can result in severe dental caries, described as blackened, rotting, crumbling teeth. Severe, life-threatening methamphetamine toxicity may include hypertension, cardiac arrhythmia or cardiac failure, subarachnoid hemorrhage, ischemic stroke, intracerebral hemorrhage, convulsions, or coma. Methamphetamines increase the release of monoamine neurotransmitters (dopamine, norepinephrine, and serotonin) from presynaptic neurons. It is thought that the euphoric and reinforcing effects of this class of drugs are mediated through dopamine and the mesolimbic system, whereas the cardiovascular effects are related to norepinephrine. MRS studies of the brain suggest that chronic abusers have neuronal damage in the frontal areas and basal ganglia.

Therapy of acute methamphetamine overdose is largely symptomatic. Ammonium chloride may be useful to acidify the urine and enhance clearance of the drug. Hypertension may respond to sodium nitroprusside or α-adrenergic antagonists. Sedatives may reduce agitation and other signs of central nervous system hyperactivity. Treatment of chronic methamphetamine dependence may be accomplished in either an inpatient or outpatient setting using strategies similar to those described earlier for cocaine abuse.

MDMA (3,4-methylenedioxymethamphetamine), or *ecstasy*, is a derivative of methamphetamine. Ecstasy is usually taken orally but may be injected or inhaled; its effects last for 3–6 h. In addition to amphetamine-like effects, MDMA can induce hyperthermia and vivid hallucinations and other perceptual distortions. Recent studies have revealed that MDMA use is associated with cognitive and memory impairment and a mild withdrawal syndrome after cessation of use. The long-term consequences of recreational use of MDMA by young persons are poorly understood.

LYSERGIC ACID DIETHYLAMIDE (LSD)

The discovery of the psychedelic effects of LSD led to an epidemic of LSD abuse during the 1960s. Imposition of stringent constraints on the manufacture and distribution of LSD (classified as a Schedule I substance by the U.S. Food and Drug Administration), as well as public recognition that psychedelic experiences induced by LSD were a health hazard, have resulted in a reduction in LSD abuse. LSD still remains popular among adolescents and young adults, and there are indications that LSD use among young persons has been increasing in some areas in the United States.

LSD is a very potent hallucinogen; oral doses as low as 20 μg may induce profound psychological and physiologic effects. Tachycardia, hypertension, pupillary dilation, tremor, and hyperpyrexia occur within minutes following oral administration of 0.5–2 μg/kg. A variety of bizarre and often conflicting perceptual and mood changes, including visual illusions, synesthesias, and extreme lability of mood, usually occur within 30 min after LSD intake. These effects of LSD may persist for 12–18 h, even though the half-life of the drug is only 3 h.

The most frequent acute medical emergency associated with LSD use is a panic episode (the "bad trip"), which may persist up to 24 h. Management of this problem is best accomplished by supportive reassurance ("talking down") and, if necessary, administration of small doses of anxiolytic drugs. Adverse consequences of chronic LSD use include enhanced risk for schizophreniform psychosis and derangements in memory function, problem solving, and abstract thinking. Treatment of these disorders is best carried out in specialized psychiatric facilities.

Tolerance develops rapidly for LSD-induced changes in psychological function when the drug is used one or more times per day for >4 days. Abrupt abstinence following continued use does not produce withdrawal signs or symptoms. There have been no clinical reports of death caused by the direct effects of LSD.

PHENCYCLIDINE (PCP)

Phencyclidine (PCP), a cyclohexylamine derivative, is widely used in veterinary medicine to briefly immobilize large animals and is sometimes described as a dissociative anesthetic. PCP binds to ionotropic *N*-methyl-D-aspartate (NMDA) receptors in the nervous system, blocking ion current through these channels. PCP is easily synthesized; its abusers are primarily young people and polydrug users. It is used orally, by smoking, by snorting, or by IV injection. It is also used as an adulterant in THC, LSD, amphetamine, or cocaine. The most common street preparation, *angel dust*, is a white granular powder that contains 50–100% of the drug. Low doses (5 mg) produce agitation, excitement, impaired motor coordination, dysarthria, and analgesia. Physical signs of intoxication may include horizontal or vertical nystagmus, flushing, diaphoresis, and hyperacusis. Behavioral changes include distortions of body image, disorganization of thinking, and feelings of estrangement. Higher doses of PCP (5–10 mg) may produce profuse salivation, vomiting, myoclonus, fever, stupor, or coma. PCP doses of ≥10 mg cause convulsions, opisthotonus, and decerebrate posturing, which may be followed by prolonged coma.

The diagnosis of PCP overdose is difficult because the patient's initial symptoms (anxiety, paranoia, delusions, hallucinations) may suggest an acute schizophrenic reaction. Confirmation of PCP use is possible by determination of PCP levels in serum or urine. PCP assays are available at most toxicologic centers. PCP remains in urine for 1–5 days following high-dose intake.

PCP overdose requires life-support measures, including treatment of coma, convulsions, and respiratory depression in an intensive care unit. There is no specific antidote or antagonist for PCP. PCP excretion from the body can be enhanced by gastric lavage and acidification of urine. Death from PCP overdose may occur as a consequence of some combination of pharyngeal hypersecretion, hyperthermia, respiratory depression, severe hypertension, seizures, hypertensive encephalopathy, and intracerebral hemorrhage.

Acute psychosis associated with PCP use is a psychiatric emergency since patients may be at high risk for suicide or extreme violence toward others. Phenothiazines should not be used for treatment because these drugs potentiate PCP's anticholinergic effects. Haloperidol (5 mg IM) has been administered on an hourly basis to induce suppression of psychotic behavior. PCP, like LSD and mescaline, produces vasospasm of cerebral arteries at relatively low doses. Chronic PCP use has been shown to induce insomnia, anorexia, severe social and behavioral changes, and, in some cases, chronic schizophrenia.

OTHER DRUGS OF ABUSE

A number of other pharmacologically diverse drugs of abuse are often referred to as "club drugs" because these are frequently used in bars, at concerts, and rave parties. Commonly abused club drugs include flunitrazepam,

GHB, and ketamine and are described next. Methamphetamine, MDMA, and LSD are also considered club drugs and were described earlier in this chapter. Abuse of club drugs at high doses, especially in combination with alcohol, can be lethal and should be treated as a medical emergency. GHB and ketamine can be identified in blood, and flunitrazepam can be identified in urine and hair samples. Flunitrazepam and GHB toxicity can be treated with antagonists at benzodiazepine and $GABA_B$ receptors, respectively.

Flunitrazepam

Flunitrazepam (Rohypnol) is a benzodiazepine derivative primarily used for treatment of insomnia, but it has significant abuse potential because of its strong hypnotic, anxiolytic, and amnesia-producing effects. It is a club drug commonly referred to as a "date-rape drug" or "roofies." The drug enhances $GABA_A$ receptor activity, and overdose can be treated with flumazenil, a benzodiazepine receptor antagonist. Flunitrazepam is typically used orally but can be snorted or injected. Concomitant use of alcohol or opiates is common, and this enhances the sedative and hypnotic effects of flunitrazepam and also the risk of motor vehicle accidents. Overdose can produce life-threatening respiratory depression and coma. Abrupt cessation after chronic use may result in a benzodiazepine withdrawal syndrome consisting of anxiety, insomnia, disordered thinking, and seizures.

GHB

Gamma-hydroxybutyric acid (Xyrem) is a sedative drug that is FDA-approved for the treatment of narcolepsy. It is classified as a club drug, is sometimes used in combination with alcohol or other drugs of abuse, and has been implicated in cases of date rape. GHB is usually taken orally and has no distinctive color or odor. Its stimulant properties are attributed to agonist activity at the GHB receptor, but it also has sedative effects at high doses that reflect its activity at $GABA_B$ receptors. $GABA_B$ antagonists can reverse GHB's sedative effects, and opioid antagonists (naloxone, naltrexone) can attenuate GHB effects on dopamine release. Low doses of GHB may produce euphoria and disinhibition, whereas high doses result in nausea, agitation, convulsions, and sedation that can lead to unconsciousness and death from respiratory depression.

Ketamine

Ketamine (Ketaset, Ketalar) is a dissociative anesthetic, similar to phencyclidine (PCP). In veterinary medicine, it is used for brief immobilization. In clinical medicine, it is used for sedation, analgesia, and to supplement anesthesia. Ketamine increases heart rate and blood pressure, with less respiratory depression than other anesthetics. Ketamine's popularity as a club drug appears to reflect its ability to induce a dissociative state and feelings of depersonalization, accompanied by intense hallucinations and subsequent amnesia. It can be administered orally, by smoking (usually in combination with tobacco and/or marijuana), or by IV or IM injection. Like PCP, it binds to NMDA receptors and acts as an uncompetitive NMDA antagonist. Ketamine has a complex profile of action and appears to be useful as an antidepressant in treatment-resistant patients and as an analgesic in chronic-pain patients. The extent to which chronic recreational use leads to memory impairment remains controversial.

POLYDRUG ABUSE

Although some drug abusers may prefer a particular drug, the concurrent use of multiple drugs is often reported. Polydrug abuse often involves substances that may have different pharmacologic effects from the preferred drug. For example, concurrent use of such dissimilar compounds as stimulants and opiates or stimulants and alcohol is common. The diversity of reported drug use combinations suggests that achieving a subjective change in state, rather than any particular direction of change (stimulation or sedation), may be the primary reinforcer in polydrug abuse. There is also evidence that intoxication with alcohol, opiates, and cocaine is associated with increased tobacco smoking. There are relatively few controlled studies of multiple drug interactions. However, the combined use of cocaine, heroin, and alcohol increases the risk for toxic effects and adverse medical consequences. One determinant of polydrug use patterns is the relative availability and cost of the drugs. For example, alcohol abuse, with its attendant medical complications, is one of the most serious problems encountered in former heroin addicts participating in methadone maintenance programs.

The physician must recognize that perpetuation of polydrug abuse and drug dependence is not necessarily a symptom of an underlying emotional disorder. Neither alleviation of anxiety nor reduction of depression accounts for initiation and perpetuation of polydrug abuse. Severe depression and anxiety are the consequences of polydrug abuse as frequently as they are the antecedents. Interestingly, some adverse consequences of drug use may be reinforcing and contribute to the continuation of polydrug abuse.

Adequate treatment of polydrug abuse, as well as other forms of drug abuse, requires innovative intervention programs. The first step in successful treatment is detoxification, a process that may be difficult when several drugs with different pharmacologic actions (e.g., alcohol, opiates, and cocaine) have been abused. Since patients may not recall or may deny simultaneous multiple drug use, diagnostic evaluation should always include urinalysis for qualitative detection of psychoactive substances and their metabolites. Treatment of polydrug abuse often requires hospitalization or inpatient residential care during detoxification and the initial phase of drug abstinence. When possible, specialized facilities for the care and treatment of drug-dependent persons should be used. Outpatient detoxification of polydrug abuse patients is likely to be ineffective and may be dangerous.

Drug abuse disorders often respond to effective treatment, but episodes of relapse may occur unpredictably. The physician should continue to assist patients during relapse and recognize that occasional recurrent drug use is not unusual in this complex behavioral disorder.

APPENDIX

LABORATORY VALUES OF CLINICAL IMPORTANCE

Alexander Kratz ■ Michael A. Pesce ■ Robert C. Basner ■ Andrew J. Einstein

This Appendix contains tables of reference values for laboratory tests, special analytes, and special function tests. A variety of factors can influence reference values. Such variables include the population studied, the duration and means of specimen transport, laboratory methods and instrumentation, and even the type of container used for the collection of the specimen. The reference or "normal" ranges given in this appendix may therefore not be appropriate for all laboratories, and these values should only be used as general guidelines. Whenever possible, reference values provided by the laboratory performing the testing should be utilized in the interpretation of laboratory data. Values supplied in this Appendix reflect typical reference ranges in adults. Pediatric reference ranges may vary significantly from adult values.

In preparing the Appendix, the authors have taken into account the fact that the system of international units (SI, système international d'unités) is used in most countries and in some medical journals. However, clinical laboratories may continue to report values in "traditional" or conventional units. Therefore, both systems are provided in the Appendix. The dual system is also used in the text except for (1) those instances in which the numbers remain the same but only the terminology is changed (mmol/L for meq/L or IU/L for mIU/mL), when only the SI units are given; and (2) most pressure measurements (e.g., blood and cerebrospinal fluid pressures), when the traditional units (mmHg, mmH_2O) are used. In all other instances in the text the SI unit is followed by the traditional unit in parentheses.

REFERENCE VALUES FOR LABORATORY TESTS

TABLE 1

HEMATOLOGY AND COAGULATION

ANALYTE	SPECIMEN	SI UNITS	CONVENTIONAL UNITS
Activated clotting time	WB	70–180 s	70–180 s
Activated protein C resistance (factor V Leiden)	P	Not applicable	Ratio >2.1
ADAMTS13 activity	P	≥0.67	≥67%
ADAMTS13 inhibitor activity	P	Not applicable	≤0.4 U
ADAMTS13 antibody	P	Not applicable	≤18 U
$Alpha_2$ antiplasmin	P	0.87–1.55	87–155%
Antiphospholipid antibody panel			
PTT-LA (lupus anticoagulant screen)	P	Negative	Negative
Platelet neutralization procedure	P	Negative	Negative
Dilute viper venom screen	P	Negative	Negative
Anticardiolipin antibody	S		
IgG		0–15 arbitrary units	0–15 GPL
IgM		0–15 arbitrary units	0–15 MPL

(continued)

TABLE 1

HEMATOLOGY AND COAGULATION (*CONTINUED*)

ANALYTE	SPECIMEN	SI UNITS	CONVENTIONAL UNITS
Antithrombin III	P		
Antigenic		220–390 mg/L	22–39 mg/dL
Functional		0.7–1.30 U/L	70–130%
Anti-Xa assay (heparin assay)	P		
Unfractionated heparin		0.3–0.7 kIU/L	0.3–0.7 IU/mL
Low-molecular-weight heparin		0.5–1.0 kIU/L	0.5–1.0 IU/mL
Danaparoid (Orgaran)		0.5–0.8 kIU/L	0.5–0.8 IU/mL
Autohemolysis test	WB	0.004–0.045	0.4–4.50%
Autohemolysis test with glucose	WB	0.003–0.007	0.3–0.7%
Bleeding time (adult)		<7.1 min	<7.1 min
Bone marrow: See Table 7			
Clot retraction	WB	0.50–1.00/2 h	50–100%/2 h
Cryofibrinogen	P	Negative	Negative
D-dimer	P	220–740 ng/mL FEU	220–740 ng/mL FEU
Differential blood count	WB		
Relative counts:			
Neutrophils		0.40–0.70	40–70%
Bands		0.0–0.05	0–5%
Lymphocytes		0.20–0.50	20–50%
Monocytes		0.04–0.08	4–8%
Eosinophils		0.0–0.6	0–6%
Basophils		0.0–0.02	0–2%
Absolute counts:			
Neutrophils		$1.42–6.34 \times 10^9$/L	1420–6340/mm^3
Bands		$0–0.45 \times 10^9$/L	0–450/mm^3
Lymphocytes		$0.71–4.53 \times 10^9$/L	710–4530/mm^3
Monocytes		$0.14–0.72 \times 10^9$/L	140–720/mm^3
Eosinophils		$0–0.54 \times 10^9$/L	0–540/mm^3
Basophils		$0–0.18 \times 10^9$/L	0–180/mm^3
Erythrocyte count	WB		
Adult males		$4.30–5.60 \times 10^{12}$/L	$4.30–5.60 \times 10^6/mm^3$
Adult females		$4.00–5.20 \times 10^{12}$/L	$4.00–5.20 \times 10^6/mm^3$
Erythrocyte life span	WB		
Normal survival		120 days	120 days
Chromium labeled, half-life ($t_{1/2}$)		25–35 days	25–35 days
Erythrocyte sedimentation rate	WB		
Females		0–20 mm/h	0–20 mm/h
Males		0–15 mm/h	0–15 mm/h
Euglobulin lysis time	P	7200–14,400 s	120–240 min
Factor II, prothrombin	P	0.50–1.50	50–150%
Factor V	P	0.50–1.50	50–150%
Factor VII	P	0.50–1.50	50–150%
Factor VIII	P	0.50–1.50	50–150%
Factor IX	P	0.50–1.50	50–150%
Factor X	P	0.50–1.50	50–150%
Factor XI	P	0.50–1.50	50–150%
Factor XII	P	0.50–1.50	50–150 %
Factor XIII screen	P	Not applicable	Present
Factor inhibitor assay	P	<0.5 Bethesda Units	<0.5 Bethesda Units
Fibrin(ogen) degradation products	P	0–1 mg/L	0–1 μg/mL
Fibrinogen	P	2.33–4.96 g/L	233–496 mg/dL
Glucose-6-phosphate dehydrogenase (erythrocyte)	WB	<2400 s	<40 min
Ham's test (acid serum)	WB	Negative	Negative

(*continued*)

TABLE 1

HEMATOLOGY AND COAGULATION (*CONTINUED*)

ANALYTE	SPECIMEN	SI UNITS	CONVENTIONAL UNITS
Hematocrit	WB		
Adult males		0.388–0.464	38.8–46.4
Adult females		0.354–0.444	35.4–44.4
Hemoglobin			
Plasma	P	6–50 mg/L	0.6–5.0 mg/dL
Whole blood:	WB		
Adult males		133–162 g/L	13.3–16.2 g/dL
Adult females		120–158 g/L	12.0–15.8 g/dL
Hemoglobin electrophoresis	WB		
Hemoglobin A		0.95–0.98	95–98%
Hemoglobin A_2		0.015–0.031	1.5–3.1%
Hemoglobin F		0–0.02	0–2.0%
Hemoglobins other than A, A_2, or F		Absent	Absent
Heparin-induced thrombocytopenia antibody	P	Negative	Negative
Immature platelet fraction (IPF)	WB	0.011–0.061	1.1–6.1%
Joint fluid crystal	JF	Not applicable	No crystals seen
Joint fluid mucin	JF	Not applicable	Only type I mucin present
Leukocytes			
Alkaline phosphatase (LAP)	WB	0.2–1.6 μkat/L	13–100 μ/L
Count (WBC)	WB	$3.54–9.06 \times 10^9$/L	$3.54–9.06 \times 10^3/mm^3$
Mean corpuscular hemoglobin (MCH)	WB	26.7–31.9 pg/cell	26.7–31.9 pg/cell
Mean corpuscular hemoglobin concentration (MCHC)	WB	323–359 g/L	32.3–35.9 g/dL
Mean corpuscular hemoglobin of reticulocytes (CH)	WB	24–36 pg	24–36 pg
Mean corpuscular volume (MCV)	WB	79–93.3 fL	79–93.3 μm^3
Mean platelet volume (MPV)	WB	9.00–12.95 fL	9.00–12.95
Osmotic fragility of erythrocytes	WB		
Direct		0.0035–0.0045	0.35–0.45%
Indirect		0.0030–0.0065	0.30–0.65%
Partial thromboplastin time, activated	P	26.3–39.4 s	26.3–39.4 s
Plasminogen	P		
Antigen		84–140 mg/L	8.4–14.0 mg/dL
Functional		0.70–1.30	70–130%
Plasminogen activator inhibitor 1	P	4–43 μg/L	4–43 ng/mL
Platelet aggregation	PRP	Not applicable	>65% aggregation in response to adenosine diphosphate, epinephrine, collagen, ristocetin, and arachidonic acid
Platelet count	WB	$165–415 \times 10^9$/L	$165–415 \times 10^3/mm^3$
Platelet, mean volume	WB	6.4–11 fL	6.4–11.0 μm^3
Prekallikrein assay	P	0.50–1.5	50–150%
Prekallikrein screen	P		No deficiency detected
Protein C	P		
Total antigen		0.70–1.40	70–140%
Functional		0.70–1.30	70–130%
Protein S	P		
Total antigen		0.70–1.40	70–140%
Functional		0.65–1.40	65–140%
Free antigen		0.70–1.40	70–140%
Prothrombin gene mutation G20210A	WB	Not applicable	Not present
Prothrombin time	P	12.7–15.4 s	12.7–15.4 s

(*continued*)

TABLE 1

HEMATOLOGY AND COAGULATION (*CONTINUED*)

ANALYTE	SPECIMEN	SI UNITS	CONVENTIONAL UNITS
Protoporphyrin, free erythrocyte	WB	0.28–0.64 μmol/L of red blood cells	16–36 μg/dL of red blood cells
Red cell distribution width	WB	<0.145	<14.5%
Reptilase time	P	16–23.6 s	16–23.6 s
Reticulocyte count	WB		
Adult males		0.008–0.023 red cells	0.8–2.3% red cells
Adult females		0.008–0.020 red cells	0.8–2.0% red cells
Reticulocyte hemoglobin content	WB	>26 pg/cell	>26 pg/cell
Ristocetin cofactor (functional von Willebrand factor)	P		
Blood group O		0.75 mean of normal	75% mean of normal
Blood group A		1.05 mean of normal	105% mean of normal
Blood group B		1.15 mean of normal	115% mean of normal
Blood group AB		1.25 mean of normal	125% mean of normal
Serotonin release assay	S	<0.2 release	<20% release
Sickle cell test	WB	Negative	Negative
Sucrose hemolysis	WB	<0.1	<10% hemolysis
Thrombin time	P	15.3–18.5 s	15.3–18.5 s
Total eosinophils	WB	$150–300 \times 10^6$/L	$150–300/mm^3$
Transferrin receptor	S, P	9.6–29.6 nmol/L	9.6–29.6 nmol/L
Viscosity			
Plasma	P	1.7–2.1	1.7–2.1
Serum	S	1.4–1.8	1.4–1.8
von Willebrand factor (vWF) antigen (factor VIII:R antigen)			
Blood group O		0.75 mean of normal	75% mean of normal
Blood group A		1.05 mean of normal	105% mean of normal
Blood group B		1.15 mean of normal	115% mean of normal
Blood group AB		1.25 mean of normal	125% mean of normal
von Willebrand factor multimers	P	Normal distribution	Normal distribution
White blood cells: see "Leukocytes"			

Abbreviations: JF, joint fluid; P, plasma; PRP, platelet-rich plasma; S, serum; WB, whole blood.

TABLE 2

CLINICAL CHEMISTRY AND IMMUNOLOGY

ANALYTE	SPECIMEN	SI UNITS	CONVENTIONAL UNITS
Acetoacetate	P	49–294 μmol/L	0.5–3.0 mg/dL
Adrenocorticotropin (ACTH)	P	1.3–16.7 pmol/L	6.0–76.0 pg/mL
Alanine aminotransferase (ALT, SGPT)	S	0.12–0.70 μkat/L	7–41 U/L
Albumin	S	40–50 g/L	4.0–5.0 mg/dL
Aldolase	S	26–138 nkat/L	1.5–8.1 U/L
Aldosterone (adult)			
Supine, normal sodium diet	S, P	<443 pmol/L	<16 ng/dL
Upright, normal	S, P	111–858 pmol/L	4–31 ng/dL
Alpha fetoprotein (adult)	S	0–8.5 μg/L	0–8.5 ng/mL
$Alpha_1$ antitrypsin	S	1.0–2.0 g/L	100–200 mg/dL
Ammonia, as NH_3	P	11–35 μmol/L	19–60 μg/dL
Amylase (method dependent)	S	0.34–1.6 μkat/L	20–96 U/L

(continued)

TABLE 2

CLINICAL CHEMISTRY AND IMMUNOLOGY (*CONTINUED*)

ANALYTE	SPECIMEN	SI UNITS	CONVENTIONAL UNITS
Androstendione (adult)	S		
Males		0.81–3.1 nmol/L	23–89 ng/dL
Females			
Premenopausal		0.91–7.5 nmol/L	26–214 ng/dL
Postmenopausal		0.46–2.9 nmol/L	13–82 ng/dL
Angiotensin-converting enzyme (ACE)	S	0.15–1.1 μkat/L	9–67 U/L
Anion gap	S	7–16 mmol/L	7–16 mmol/L
Apolipoprotein A-1	S		
Male		0.94–1.78 g/L	94–178 mg/dL
Female		1.01–1.99 g/L	101–199 mg/dL
Apolipoprotein B	S		
Male		0.55–1.40 g/L	55–140 mg/dL
Female		0.55–1.25 g/L	55–125 mg/dL
Arterial blood gases	WB		
[HCO_3^-]		22–30 mmol/L	22–30 meq/L
P_{CO_2}		4.3–6.0 kPa	32–45 mmHg
pH		7.35–7.45	7.35–7.45
P_{O_2}		9.6–13.8 kPa	72–104 mmHg
Aspartate aminotransferase (AST, SGOT)	S	0.20–0.65 μkat/L	12–38 U/L
Autoantibodies	S		
Anti-centromere antibody IgG		≤29 AU/mL	≤29 AU/mL
Anti-double-strand (native) DNA		<25 IU/L	<25 IU/L
Anti-glomerular basement membrane antibodies			
Qualitative IgG, IgA		Negative	Negative
Quantitative IgG antibody		≤19 AU/mL	≤19 AU/mL
Anti-histone antibodies		<1.0 U	<1.0 U
Anti-Jo-1 antibody		≤29 AU/mL	≤29 AU/mL
Anti-mitochondrial antibody		Not applicable	<20 Units
Anti-neutrophil cytoplasmic autoantibodies		Not applicable	<1:20
Serine proteinase 3 antibodies		≤19 AU/mL	≤19 AU/mL
Myeloperoxidase antibodies		≤19 AU/mL	≤19 AU/mL
Antinuclear antibody		Not applicable	Negative at 1:40
Anti-parietal cell antibody		Not applicable	None detected
Anti-RNP antibody		Not applicable	<1.0 U
Anti-Scl 70 antibody		Not applicable	<1.0 U
Anti-Smith antibody		Not applicable	<1.0 U
Anti-smooth muscle antibody		Not applicable	<1.0 U
Anti-SSA antibody		Not applicable	<1.0 U
Anti-SSB antibody		Not applicable	Negative
Anti-thyroglobulin antibody		<40 kIU/L	<40 IU/mL
Anti-thyroid peroxidase antibody		<35 kIU/L	<35 IU/mL
B-type natriuretic peptide (BNP)	P	Age and gender specific: <100 ng/L	Age and gender specific: <100 pg/mL
Bence Jones protein, serum qualitative	S	Not applicable	None detected
Bence Jones protein, serum quantitative	S		
Free kappa		3.3–19.4 mg/L	0.33–1.94 mg/dL
Free lambda		5.7–26.3 mg/L	0.57–2.63 mg/dL
K/L ratio		0.26–1.65	0.26–1.65
Beta-2-microglobulin	S	1.1–2.4 mg/L	1.1–2.4 mg/L
Bilirubin	S		
Total		5.1–22 μmol/L	0.3–1.3 mg/dL
Direct		1.7–6.8 μmol/L	0.1–0.4 mg/dL
Indirect		3.4–15.2 μmol/L	0.2–0.9 mg/dL

(*continued*)

TABLE 2

CLINICAL CHEMISTRY AND IMMUNOLOGY (*CONTINUED*)

ANALYTE	SPECIMEN	SI UNITS	CONVENTIONAL UNITS
C peptide	S	0.27–1.19 nmol/L	0.8–3.5 ng/mL
C1-esterase-inhibitor protein	S	210–390 mg/L	21–39 mg/dL
CA 125	S	<35 kU/L	<35 U/mL
CA 19-9	S	<37 kU/L	<37 U/mL
CA 15-3	S	<33 kU/L	<33 U/mL
CA 27-29	S	0–40 kU/L	0–40 U/mL
Calcitonin	S		
Male		0–7.5 ng/L	0–7.5 pg/mL
Female		0–5.1 ng/L	0–5.1 pg/mL
Calcium	S	2.2–2.6 mmol/L	8.7–10.2 mg/dL
Calcium, ionized	WB	1.12–1.32 mmol/L	4.5–5.3 mg/dL
Carbon dioxide content (TCO_2)	P (sea level)	22–30 mmol/L	22–30 meq/L
Carboxyhemoglobin (carbon monoxide content)	WB		
Nonsmokers		0.0–0.015	0–1.5%
Smokers		0.04–0.09	4–9%
Loss of consciousness and death		>0.50	>50%
Carcinoembryonic antigen (CEA)	S		
Nonsmokers		0.0–3.0 µg/L	0.0–3.0 ng/mL
Smokers		0.0–5.0 µg/L	0.0–5.0 ng/mL
Ceruloplasmin	S	250–630 mg/L	25–63 mg/dL
Chloride	S	102–109 mmol/L	102–109 meq/L
Cholesterol: see Table 5			
Cholinesterase	S	5–12 kU/L	5–12 U/mL
Chromogranin A	S	0–50 µg/L	0–50 ng/mL
Complement	S		
C3		0.83–1.77 g/L	83–177 mg/dL
C4		0.16–0.47 g/L	16–47 mg/dL
Complement total		60–144 CAE units	60–144 CAE units
Cortisol			
Fasting, 8 A.M.–12 noon	S	138–690 nmol/L	5–25 µg/dL
12 noon–8 P.M.		138–414 nmol/L	5–15 µg/dL
8 P.M.–8 A.M.		0–276 nmol/L	0–10 µg/dL
C-reactive protein	S	<10 mg/L	<10 mg/L
C-reactive protein, high sensitivity	S	Cardiac risk Low: <1.0 mg/L Average: 1.0–3.0 mg/L High: >3.0 mg/L	Cardiac risk Low: <1.0 mg/L Average: 1.0–3.0 mg/L High: >3.0 mg/L
Creatine kinase (total)	S		
Females		0.66–4.0 µkat/L	39–238 U/L
Males		0.875.0 µkat/L	51–294 U/L
Creatine kinase-MB	S		
Mass		0.0–5.5 µg/L	0.0–5.5 ng/mL
Fraction of total activity (by electrophoresis)		0–0.04	0–4.0%
Creatinine	S		
Female		44–80 µmol/L	0.5–0.9 mg/dL
Male		53–106 µmol/L	0.6–1.2 mg/dL
Cryoglobulins	S	Not applicable	None detected
Cystatin C	S	0.5–1.0 mg/L	0.5–1.0 mg/L

(continued)

TABLE 2

CLINICAL CHEMISTRY AND IMMUNOLOGY (*CONTINUED*)

ANALYTE	SPECIMEN	SI UNITS	CONVENTIONAL UNITS
Dehydroepiandrosterone (DHEA) (adult)			
Male	S	6.2–43.4 nmol/L	180–1250 ng/dL
Female		4.5–34.0 nmol/L	130–980 ng/dL
Dehydroepiandrosterone (DHEA) sulfate	S		
Male (adult)		100–6190 μg/L	10–619 μg/dL
Female (adult, premenopausal)		120–5350 μg/L	12–535 μg/dL
Female (adult, postmenopausal)		300–2600 μg/L	30–260 μg/dL
11-Deoxycortisol (adult) (compound S)	S	0.34–4.56 nmol/L	12–158 ng/dL
Dihydrotestosterone			
Male	S, P	1.03–2.92 nmol/L	30–85 ng/dL
Female		0.14–0.76 nmol/L	4–22 ng/dL
Dopamine	P	0–130 pmol/L	0–20 pg/mL
Epinephrine	P		
Supine (30 min)		<273 pmol/L	<50 pg/mL
Sitting		<328 pmol/L	<60 pg/mL
Standing (30 min)		<491 pmol/L	<90 pg/mL
Erythropoietin	S	4–27 U/L	4–27 U/L
Estradiol	S, P		
Female			
Menstruating:			
Follicular phase		74–532 pmol/L	<20–145 pg/mL
Midcycle peak		411–1626 pmol/L	112–443 pg/mL
Luteal phase		74–885 pmol/L	<20–241 pg/mL
Postmenopausal		217 pmol/L	<59 pg/mL
Male		74 pmol/L	<20 pg/mL
Estrone	S, P		
Female			
Menstruating:			
Follicular phase		<555 pmol/L	<150 pg/mL
Luteal phase		<740 pmol/L	<200 pg/mL
Postmenopausal		11–118 pmol/L	3–32 pg/mL
Male		33–133 pmol/L	9–36 pg/mL
Fatty acids, free (nonesterified)	P	0.1–0.6 mmol/L	2.8–16.8 mg/dL
Ferritin	S		
Female		10–150 μg/L	10–150 ng/mL
Male		29–248 μg/L	29–248 ng/mL
Follicle-stimulating hormone (FSH)	S, P		
Female			
Menstruating:			
Follicular phase		3.0–20.0 IU/L	3.0–20.0 mIU/mL
Ovulatory phase		9.0–26.0 IU/L	9.0–26.0 mIU/mL
Luteal phase		1.0–12.0 IU/L	1.0–12.0 mIU/mL
Postmenopausal		18.0–153.0 IU/L	18.0–153.0 mIU/mL
Male		1.0–12.0 IU/L	1.0–12.0 mIU/mL
Fructosamine	S	<285 umol/L	<285 umol/L
Gamma glutamyltransferase	S	0.15–0.99 μkat/L	9–58 U/L
Gastrin	S	<100 ng/L	<100 pg/mL
Glucagon	P	40–130 ng/L	40–130 pg/mL

(*continued*)

TABLE 2

CLINICAL CHEMISTRY AND IMMUNOLOGY (*CONTINUED*)

ANALYTE	SPECIMEN	SI UNITS	CONVENTIONAL UNITS
Glucose	WB	3.6–5.3 mmol/L	65–95 mg/dL
Glucose (fasting)	P		
Normal		4.2–5.6 mmol/L	75–100 mg/dL
Increased risk for diabetes		5.6–6.9 mmol/L	100–125 mg/dL
Diabetes mellitus		Fasting >7.0 mmol/L A 2-hour level of >11.1 mmol/L during an oral glucose tolerance test A random glucose level of ≥11.1 mmol/L in patients with symptoms of hyperglycemia	Fasting >126 mg/dL A 2-hour level of ≥200 mg/dL during an oral glucose tolerance test A random glucose level of ≥200 mg/dL in patients with symptoms of hyperglycemia
Growth hormone	S	0–5 μg/L	0–5 ng/mL
Hemoglobin A_{1c}	WB	0.04–0.06 HgB fraction	4.0–5.6%
Pre-diabetes		0.057–0.064 HgB fraction	5.7–6.4%
Diabetes mellitus		A hemoglobin A_{1c} level of ≥0.065 Hgb fraction as suggested by the American Diabetes Association	A hemoglobin A_{1c} level of ≥6.5% as suggested by the American Diabetes Association
Hemoglobin A_{1c} with estimated average glucose (eAg)	WB	eAg mmoL/L = 1.59 × HbA_{1c} − 2.59	eAg (mg/dL) = 28.7 × HbA_{1c} − 46.7
High-density lipoprotein (HDL) (see Table 5)			
Homocysteine	P	4.4–10.8 μmol/L	4.4–10.8 μmol/L
Human chorionic gonadotropin (HCG)	S		
Nonpregnant female		<5 IU/L	<5 mIU/mL
1–2 weeks postconception		9–130 IU/L	9–130 mIU/mL
2–3 weeks postconception		75–2600 IU/L	75–2600 mIU/mL
3–4 weeks postconception		850–20,800 IU/L	850–20,800 mIU/mL
4–5 weeks postconception		4000–100,200 IU/L	4000–100,200 mIU/mL
5–10 weeks postconception		11,500–289,000 IU/L	11,500–289,000 mIU/mL
10–14 weeks post conception		18,300–137,000 IU/L	18,300–137,000 mIU/mL
Second trimester		1400–53,000 IU/L	1400–53,000 mIU/mL
Third trimester		940–60,000 IU/L	940–60,000 mIU/mL
β-Hydroxybutyrate	P	60–170 μmol/L	0.6–1.8 mg/dL
17-Hydroxyprogesterone (adult)	S		
Male		<4.17 nmol/L	<139 ng/dL
Female			
Follicular phase		0.45–2.1 nmol/L	15–70 ng/dL
Luteal phase		1.05–8.7 nmol/L	35–290 ng/dL
Immunofixation	S	Not applicable	No bands detected
Immunoglobulin, quantitation (adult)			
IgA	S	0.70–3.50 g/L	70–350 mg/dL
IgD	S	0–140 mg/L	0–14 mg/dL
IgE	S	1–87 kIU/L	1–87 IU/mL
IgG	S	7.0–17.0 g/L	700–1700 mg/dL
IgG_1	S	2.7–17.4 g/L	270–1740 mg/dL
IgG_2	S	0.3–6.3 g/L	30–630 mg/dL
IgG_3	S	0.13–3.2 g/L	13–320 mg/dL
IgG_4	S	0.11–6.2 g/L	11–620 mg/dL
IgM	S	0.50–3.0 g/L	50–300 mg/dL
Insulin	S, P	14.35–143.5 pmol/L	2–20 μU/mL
Iron	S	7–25 μmol/L	41–141 μg/dL

(*continued*)

TABLE 2

CLINICAL CHEMISTRY AND IMMUNOLOGY (*CONTINUED*)

ANALYTE	SPECIMEN	SI UNITS	CONVENTIONAL UNITS
Iron-binding capacity	S	45–73 μmol/L	251–406 μg/dL
Iron-binding capacity saturation	S	0.16–0.35	16–35%
Ischemia modified albumin	S	<85 kU/L	<85 U/mL
Joint fluid crystal	JF	Not applicable	No crystals seen
Joint fluid mucin	JF	Not applicable	Only type I mucin present
Ketone (acetone)	S	Negative	Negative
Lactate	P, arterial P, venous	0.5–1.6 mmol/L 0.5–2.2 mmol/L	4.5–14.4 mg/dL 4.5–19.8 mg/dL
Lactate dehydrogenase	S	2.0–3.8 μkat/L	115–221 U/L
Lipase	S	0.51–0.73 μkat/L	3–43 U/L
Lipids: see Table 5			
Lipoprotein (a)	S	0–300 mg/L	0–30 mg/dL
Low-density lipoprotein (LDL) (see Table 5)			
Luteinizing hormone (LH) Female Menstruating: Follicular phase Ovulatory phase Luteal phase Postmenopausal Male	S, P	 2.0–15.0 U/L 22.0–105.0 U/L 0.6–19.0 U/L 16.0–64.0 U/L 2.0–12.0 U/L	 2.0–15.0 mIU/mL 22.0–105.0 mIU/mL 0.6–19.0 mIU/mL 16.0–64.0 mIU/mL 2.0–12.0 mIU/mL
Magnesium	S	0.62–0.95 mmol/L	1.5–2.3 mg/dL
Metanephrine	P	<0.5 nmol/L	<100 pg/mL
Methemoglobin	WB	0.0–0.01	0–1%
Myoglobin Male Female	S	 20–71 μg/L 25–58 μg/L	 20–71 μg/L 25–58 μg/L
Norepinephrine Supine (30 min) Sitting Standing (30 min)	P	 650–2423 pmol/L 709–4019 pmol/L 739–4137 pmol/L	 110–410 pg/mL 120–680 pg/mL 125–700 pg/mL
N-telopeptide (cross-linked), NTx Female, premenopausal Male BCE = bone collagen equivalent	S	 6.2–19.0 nmol BCE 5.4–24.2 nmol BCE	 6.2–19.0 nmol BCE 5.4–24.2 nmol BCE
NT-Pro BNP	S, P	<125 ng/L up to 75 years <450 ng/L >75 years	<125 pg/mL up to 75 years <450 pg/mL >75 years
5′ Nucleotidase	S	0.00–0.19 μkat/L	0–11 U/L
Osmolality	P	275–295 mOsmol/kg serum water	275–295 mOsmol/kg serum water
Osteocalcin	S	11–50 μg/L	11–50 ng/mL
Oxygen content Arterial (sea level) Venous (sea level)	WB	 17–21 10–16	 17–21 vol% 10–16 vol%
Oxygen saturation (sea level) Arterial Venous, arm	WB	Fraction: 0.94–1.0 0.60–0.85	Percent: 94–100% 60–85%
Parathyroid hormone (intact)	S	8–51 ng/L	8–51 pg/mL

(*continued*)

TABLE 2

CLINICAL CHEMISTRY AND IMMUNOLOGY (*CONTINUED*)

ANALYTE	SPECIMEN	SI UNITS	CONVENTIONAL UNITS
Phosphatase, alkaline	S	0.56–1.63 µkat/L	33–96 U/L
Phosphorus, inorganic	S	0.81–1.4 mmol/L	2.5–4.3 mg/dL
Potassium	S	3.5–5.0 mmol/L	3.5–5.0 meq/L
Prealbumin	S	170–340 mg/L	17–34 mg/dL
Procalcitonin	S	<0.1 µg/L	<0.1 ng/mL
Progesterone	S, P		
Female: Follicular		<3.18 nmol/L	<1.0 ng/mL
Midluteal		9.54–63.6 nmol/L	3–20 ng/mL
Male		<3.18 nmol/L	<1.0 ng/mL
Prolactin	S		
Male		53–360 mg/L	2.5–17 ng/mL
Female		40–530 mg/L	1.9–25 ng/mL
Prostate-specific antigen (PSA)	S	0.0–4.0 µg/L	0.0–4.0 ng/mL
Prostate-specific antigen, free	S	With total PSA between 4 and 10 µg/L and when the free PSA is: >0.25 decreased risk of prostate cancer <0.10 increased risk of prostate cancer	With total PSA between 4 and 10 ng/mL and when the free PSA is: >25% decreased risk of prostate cancer <10% increased risk of prostate cancer
Protein fractions:	S		
Albumin		35–55 g/L	3.5–5.5 g/dL (50–60%)
Globulin		20–35 g/L	2.0–3.5 g/dL (40–50%)
$Alpha_1$		2–4 g/L	0.2–0.4 g/dL (4.2–7.2%)
$Alpha_2$		5–9 g/L	0.5–0.9 g/dL (6.8–12%)
Beta		6–11 g/L	0.6–1.1 g/dL (9.3–15%)
Gamma		7–17 g/L	0.7–1.7 g/dL (13–23%)
Protein, total	S	67–86 g/L	6.7–8.6 g/dL
Pyruvate	P	40–130 µmol/L	0.35–1.14 mg/dL
Rheumatoid factor	S	<15 kIU/L	<15 IU/mL
Serotonin	WB	0.28–1.14 umol/L	50–200 ng/mL
Serum protein electrophoresis	S	Not applicable	Normal pattern
Sex hormone–binding globulin (adult)	S		
Male		11–80 nmol/L	11–80 nmol/L
Female		30–135 nmol/L	30–135 nmol/L
Sodium	S	136–146 mmol/L	136–146 meq/L
Somatomedin-C (IGF-1) (adult)	S		
16 years		226–903 µg/L	226–903 ng/mL
17 years		193–731 µg/L	193–731 ng/mL
18 years		163–584 µg/L	163–584 ng/mL
19 years		141–483 µg/L	141–483 ng/mL
20 years		127–424 µg/L	127–424 ng/mL
21–25 years		116–358 µg/L	116–358 ng/mL
26–30 years		117–329 µg/L	117–329 ng/mL
31–35 years		115–307 µg/L	115–307 ng/mL
36–40 years		119–204 µg/L	119–204 ng/mL
41–45 years		101–267 µg/L	101–267 ng/mL
46–50 years		94–252 µg/L	94–252 ng/mL
51–55 years		87–238 µg/L	87–238 ng/mL
56–60 years		81–225 µg/L	81–225 ng/mL
61–65 years		75–212 µg/L	75–212 ng/mL

(*continued*)

TABLE 2

CLINICAL CHEMISTRY AND IMMUNOLOGY (*CONTINUED*)

ANALYTE	SPECIMEN	SI UNITS	CONVENTIONAL UNITS
66–70 years		69–200 μg/L	69–200 ng/mL
71–75 years		64–188 μg/L	64–188 ng/mL
76–80 years		59–177 μg/L	59–177 ng/mL
81–85 years		55–166 μg/L	55–166 ng/mL
Somatostatin	P	<25 ng/L	<25 pg/mL
Testosterone, free			
Female, adult	S	10.4–65.9 pmol/L	3–19 pg/mL
Male, adult		312–1041 pmol/L	90–300 pg/mL
Testosterone, total,	S		
Female		0.21–2.98 nmol/L	6–86 ng/dL
Male		9.36–37.10 nmol/L	270–1070 ng/dL
Thyroglobulin	S	1.3–31.8 μg/L	1.3–31.8 ng/mL
Thyroid-binding globulin	S	13–30 mg/L	1.3–3.0 mg/dL
Thyroid-stimulating hormone	S	0.34–4.25 mIU/L	0.34–4.25 μIU/mL
Thyroxine, free (fT4)	S	9.0–16 pmol/L	0.7–1.24 ng/dL
Thyroxine, total (T4)	S	70–151 nmol/L	5.4–11.7 μg/dL
Thyroxine index (free)	S	6.7–10.9	6.7–10.9
Transferrin	S	2.0–4.0 g/L	200–400 mg/dL
Triglycerides (see Table 5)	S	0.34–2.26 mmol/L	30–200 mg/dL
Triiodothyronine, free (fT3)	S	3.7–6.5 pmol/L	2.4–4.2 pg/mL
Triiodothyronine, total (T3)	S	1.2–2.1 nmol/L	77–135 ng/dL
Troponin I (method dependent)	S, P		
99th percentile of a healthy population		0–0.04 μg/L	0–0.04 ng/mL
Troponin T	S, P		
99th percentile of a healthy population		0–0.01 μg/L	0–0.01 ng/mL
Urea nitrogen	S	2.5–7.1 mmol/L	7–20 mg/dL
Uric acid	S		
Females		0.15–0.33 mmol/L	2.5–5.6 mg/dL
Males		0.18–0.41 mmol/L	3.1–7.0 mg/dL
Vasoactive intestinal polypeptide	P	0–60 ng/L	0–60 pg/mL
Zinc protoporphyrin	WB	0–400 μg/L	0–40 μg/dL
Zinc protoporphyrin (ZPP)-to-heme ratio	WB	0–69 μmol ZPP/mol heme	0–69 μmol ZPP/mol heme

Abbreviations: P, plasma; S, serum; WB, whole blood.

TABLE 3

TOXICOLOGY AND THERAPEUTIC DRUG MONITORING

DRUG	THERAPEUTIC RANGE SI UNITS	THERAPEUTIC RANGE CONVENTIONAL UNITS	TOXIC LEVEL SI UNITS	TOXIC LEVEL CONVENTIONAL UNITS
Acetaminophen	66–199 µmol/L	10–30 µg/mL	>1320 µmol/L	>200 µg/mL
Amikacin				
Peak	34–51 µmol/L	20–30 µg/mL	>60 µmol/L	>35 µg/mL
Trough	0–17 µmol/L	0–10 µg/mL	>17 µmol/L	>10 µg/mL
Amitriptyline/nortriptyline (total drug)	430–900 nmol/L	120–250 ng/mL	>1800 nmol/L	>500 ng/mL
Amphetamine	150–220 nmol/L	20–30 ng/mL	>1500 nmol/L	>200 ng/mL
Bromide	9.4–18.7 mmol/L	75–150 mg/dL	>18.8 mmol/L	>150 mg/dL
Mild toxicity			6.4–18.8 mmol/L	51–150 mg/dL
Severe toxicity			>18.8 mmol/L	>150 mg/dL
Lethal			>37.5 mmol/L	>300 mg/dL
Caffeine	25.8–103 µmol/L	5–20 µg/mL	>206 µmol/L	>40 µg/mL
Carbamazepine	17–42 µmol/L	4–10 µg/mL	>85 µmol/L	>20 µg/mL
Chloramphenicol				
Peak	31–62 µmol/L	10–20 µg/mL	>77 µmol/L	>25 µg/mL
Trough	15–31 µmol/L	5–10 µg/mL	>46 µmol/L	>15 µg/mL
Chlordiazepoxide	1.7–10 µmol/L	0.5–3.0 µg/mL	>17 µmol/L	>5.0 µg/mL
Clonazepam	32–240 nmol/L	10–75 ng/mL	>320 nmol/L	>100 ng/mL
Clozapine	0.6–2.1 µmol/L	200–700 ng/mL	>3.7 µmol/L	>1200 ng/mL
Cocaine			>3.3 µmol/L	>1.0 µg/mL
Codeine	43–110 nmol/mL	13–33 ng/mL	>3700 nmol/mL	>1100 ng/mL (lethal)
Cyclosporine				
Renal transplant				
0–6 months	208–312 nmol/L	250–375 ng/mL	>312 nmol/L	>375 ng/mL
6–12 months after transplant	166–250 nmol/L	200–300 ng/mL	>250 nmol/L	>300 ng/mL
>12 months	83–125 nmol/L	100–150 ng/mL	>125 nmol/L	>150 ng/mL
Cardiac transplant				
0–6 months	208–291 nmol/L	250–350 ng/mL	>291 nmol/L	>350 ng/mL
6–12 months after transplant	125–208 nmol/L	150–250 ng/mL	>208 nmol/L	>250 ng/mL
>12 months	83–125 nmol/L	100–150 ng/mL	>125 nmol/L	150 ng/mL
Lung transplant				
0–6 months	250–374 nmol/L	300–450 ng/mL	>374 nmol/L	>450 ng/mL
Liver transplant				
Initiation	208–291 nmol/L	250–350 ng/mL	>291 nmol/L	>350 ng/mL
Maintenance	83–166 nmol/L	100–200 ng/mL	>166 nmol/L	>200 ng/mL
Desipramine	375–1130 nmol/L	100–300 ng/mL	>1880 nmol/L	>500 ng/mL
Diazepam (and metabolite)				
Diazepam	0.7–3.5 µmol/L	0.2–1.0 µg/mL	>7.0 µmol/L	>2.0 µg/mL
Nordiazepam	0.4–6.6 µmol/L	0.1–1.8 µg/mL	>9.2 µmol/L	>2.5 µg/mL
Digoxin	0.64–2.6 nmol/L	0.5–2.0 ng/mL	>5.0 nmol/L	>3.9 ng/mL
Disopyramide	5.3–14.7 µmol/L	2–5 µg/mL	>20.6 µmol/L	>7 µg/mL
Doxepin and nordoxepin				
Doxepin	0.36–0.98 µmol/L	101–274 ng/mL	>1.8 µmol/L	>503 ng/mL
Nordoxepin	0.38–1.04 µmol/L	106–291 ng/mL	>1.9 µmol/L	>531 ng/mL
Ethanol				
Behavioral changes			>4.3 mmol/L	>20 mg/dL
Legal limit			≥17 mmol/L	≥80 mg/dL
Critical with acute exposure			>54 mmol/L	>250 mg/dL
Ethylene glycol				
Toxic			>2 mmol/L	>12 mg/dL
Lethal			>20 mmol/L	>120 mg/dL

(*continued*)

TABLE 3

TOXICOLOGY AND THERAPEUTIC DRUG MONITORING (*CONTINUED*)

	THERAPEUTIC RANGE		TOXIC LEVEL	
DRUG	**SI UNITS**	**CONVENTIONAL UNITS**	**SI UNITS**	**CONVENTIONAL UNITS**
Ethosuximide	280–700 µmol/L	40–100 µg/mL	>700 µmol/L	>100 µg/mL
Everolimus	3.13–8.35 nmol/L	3–8 ng/mL	>12.5 nmol/L	>12 ng/mL
Flecainide	0.5–2.4 µmol/L	0.2–1.0 µg/mL	>3.6 µmol/L	>1.5 µg/mL
Gentamicin				
Peak	10–21 µmol/mL	5–10 µg/mL	>25 µmol/mL	>12 µg/mL
Trough	0–4.2 µmol/mL	0–2 µg/mL	>4.2 µmol/mL	>2 µg/mL
Heroin (diacetyl morphine)			>700 µmol/L	>200 ng/mL (as morphine)
Ibuprofen	49–243 µmol/L	10–50 µg/mL	>970 µmol/L	>200 µg/mL
Imipramine (and metabolite)				
Desimipramine	375–1130 nmol/L	100–300 ng/mL	>1880 nmol/L	>500 ng/mL
Total imipramine + desimipramine	563–1130 nmol/L	150–300 ng/mL	>1880 nmol/L	>500 ng/mL
Lamotrigine	11.7–54.7 µmol/L	3–14 µg/mL	>58.7 µmol/L	>15 µg/mL
Lidocaine	5.1–21.3 µmol/L	1.2–5.0 µg/mL	>38.4 µmol/L	>9.0 µg/mL
Lithium	0.5–1.3 mmol/L	0.5–1.3 meq/L	>2 mmol/L	>2 meq/L
Methadone	1.0–3.2 µmol/L	0.3–1.0 µg/mL	>6.5 µmol/L	>2 µg/mL
Methamphetamine	0.07–0.34 µmol/L	0.01–0.05 µg/mL	>3.35 µmol/L	>0.5 µg/mL
Methanol			>6 mmol/L	>20 mg/dL
Methotrexate				
Low-dose	0.01–0.1 µmol/L	0.01–0.1 µmol/L	>0.1 mmol/L	>0.1 mmol/L
High-dose (24 h)	<5.0 µmol/L	<5.0 µmol/L	>5.0 µmol/L	>5.0 µmol/L
High-dose (48 h)	<0.50 µmol/L	<0.50 µmol/L	>0.5 µmol/L	>0.5 µmol/L
High-dose (72 h)	<0.10 µmol/L	<0.10 µmol/L	>0.1 µmol/L	>0.1 µmol/L
Morphine	232–286 µmol/L	65–80 ng/mL	>720 µmol/L	>200 ng/mL
Mycophenolic acid	3.1–10.9 µmol/L	1.0–3.5 ng/mL	>37 µmol/L	>12 ng/mL
Nitroprusside (as thiocyanate)	103–499 µmol/L	6–29 µg/mL	860 µmol/L	>50 µg/mL
Nortriptyline	190–569 nmol/L	50–150 ng/mL	>1900 nmol/L	>500 ng/mL
Phenobarbital	65–172 µmol/L	15–40 µg/mL	>258 µmol/L	>60 µg/mL
Phenytoin	40–79 µmol/L	10–20 µg/mL	>158 µmol/L	>40 µg/mL
Phenytoin, free	4.0–7.9 µg/mL	1–2 µg/mL	>13.9 µg/mL	>3.5 µg/mL
% Free	0.08–0.14	8–14%		
Primidone and metabolite				
Primidone	23–55 µmol/L	5–12 µg/mL	>69 µmol/L	>15 µg/mL
Phenobarbital	65–172 µmol/L	15–40 µg/mL	>215 µmol/L	>50 µg/mL
Procainamide				
Procainamide	17–42 µmol/L	4–10 µg/mL	>43 µmol/L	>10 µg/mL
NAPA (*N*-acetylprocainamide)	22–72 µmol/L	6–20 µg/mL	>126 µmol/L	>35 µg/mL
Quinidine	6.2–15.4 µmol/L	2.0–5.0 µg/mL	>19 µmol/L	>6 µg/mL
Salicylates	145–2100 µmol/L	2–29 mg/dL	>2900 µmol/L	>40 mg/dL
Sirolimus (trough level)				
Kidney transplant	4.4–15.4 nmol/L	4–14 ng/mL	>16 nmol/L	>15 ng/mL
Tacrolimus (FK506) (trough)				
Kidney and liver	12–19 nmol/L	10–15 ng/mL	>25 nmol/L	>20 ng/mL
Initiation				
Maintenance	6–12 nmol/L	5–10 ng/mL	>25 nmol/L	>20 ng/mL
Heart				
Initiation	19–25 nmol/L	15–20 ng/mL		
Maintenance	6–12 nmol/L	5–10 ng/mL		

(*continued*)

TABLE 3

TOXICOLOGY AND THERAPEUTIC DRUG MONITORING (*CONTINUED*)

DRUG	THERAPEUTIC RANGE		TOXIC LEVEL	
	SI UNITS	CONVENTIONAL UNITS	SI UNITS	CONVENTIONAL UNITS
Theophylline	56–111 μg/mL	10–20 μg/mL	>168 μg/mL	>30 μg/mL
Thiocyanate				
After nitroprusside infusion	103–499 μmol/L	6–29 μg/mL	860 μmol/L	>50 μg/mL
Nonsmoker	17–69 μmol/L	1–4 μg/mL		
Smoker	52–206 μmol/L	3–12 μg/mL		
Tobramycin				
Peak	11–22 μg/L	5–10 μg/mL	>26 μg/L	>12 μg/mL
Trough	0–4.3 μg/L	0–2 μg/mL	>4.3 μg/L	>2 μg/mL
Valproic acid	346–693 μmol/L	50–100 μg/mL	>693 μmol/L	>100 μg/mL
Vancomycin				
Peak	14–28 μmol/L	20–40 μg/mL	>55 μmol/L	>80 μg/mL
Trough	3.5–10.4 μmol/L	5–15 μg/mL	>14 μmol/L	>20 μg/mL

TABLE 4

VITAMINS AND SELECTED TRACE MINERALS

SPECIMEN	ANALYTE	REFERENCE RANGE	
		SI UNITS	CONVENTIONAL UNITS
Aluminum	S	<0.2 μmol/L	<5.41 μg/L
Arsenic	WB	0.03–0.31 μmol/L	2–23 μg/L
Cadmium	WB	<44.5 nmol/L	<5.0 μg/L
Coenzyme Q10 (ubiquinone)	P	433–1532 μg/L	433–1532 μg/L
β-Carotene	S	0.07–1.43 μmol/L	4–77 μg/dL
Copper	S	11–22 μmol/L	70–140 μg/dL
Folic acid	RC	340–1020 nmol/L cells	150–450 ng/mL cells
Folic acid	S	12.2–40.8 nmol/L	5.4–18.0 ng/mL
Lead (adult)	S	<0.5 μmol/L	<10 μg/dL
Mercury	WB	3.0–294 nmol/L	0.6–59 μg/L
Selenium	S	0.8–2.0 umol/L	63–160 μg/L
Vitamin A	S	0.7–3.5 μmol/L	20–100 μg/dL
Vitamin B_1 (thiamine)	S	0–75 nmol/L	0–2 μg/dL
Vitamin B_2 (riboflavin)	S	106–638 nmol/L	4–24 μg/dL
Vitamin B_6	P	20–121 nmol/L	5–30 ng/mL
Vitamin B_{12}	S	206–735 pmol/L	279–996 pg/mL
Vitamin C (ascorbic acid)	S	23–57 μmol/L	0.4–1.0 mg/dL
Vitamin D_3,1,25-dihydroxy, total	S, P	36–180 pmol/L	15–75 pg/mL
Vitamin D_3,25-hydroxy, total	P	75–250 nmol/L	30–100 ng/mL
Vitamin E	S	12–42 μmol/L	5–18 μg/mL
Vitamin K	S	0.29–2.64 nmol/L	0.13–1.19 ng/mL
Zinc	S	11.5–18.4 μmol/L	75–120 μg/dL

Abbreviations: P, plasma; RC, red cells; S, serum; WB, whole blood.

TABLE 5

CLASSIFICATION OF LDL, TOTAL, AND HDL CHOLESTEROL

LDL Cholesterol	
<70 mg/dL	Therapeutic option for very high risk patients
<100 mg/dL	Optimal
100–129 mg/dL	Near optimal/above optimal
130–159 mg/dL	Borderline high
160–189 mg/dL	High
≥190 mg/dL	Very high
Total Cholesterol	
<200 mg/dL	Desirable
200–239 mg/dL	Borderline high
≥240 mg/dL	High
HDL Cholesterol	
<40 mg/dL	Low
≥60 mg/dL	High

Abbreviations: LDL, low-density lipoprotein; HDL, high-density lipoprotein.
Source: Executive summary of the third report of the National Cholesterol Education Program (NCEP) expert panel on detection, evaluation, and treatment of high blood cholesterol in adults (adult treatment panel III). JAMA 2001; 285:2486–97. Implications of Recent Clinical Trials for the National Cholesterol Education Program Adult Treatment Panel III Guidelines. SM Grundy et al for the Coordinating Committee of the National Cholesterol Education Program: Circulation 110:227, 2004.

REFERENCE VALUES FOR SPECIFIC ANALYTES

TABLE 6

CEREBROSPINAL FLUID[a]

	REFERENCE RANGE	
CONSTITUENT	SI UNITS	CONVENTIONAL UNITS
Osmolarity	292–297 mmol/kg water	292–297 mOsm/L
Electrolytes		
Sodium	137–145 mmol/L	137–145 meq/L
Potassium	2.7–3.9 mmol/L	2.7–3.9 meq/L
Calcium	1.0–1.5 mmol/L	2.1–3.0 meq/L
Magnesium	1.0–1.2 mmol/L	2.0–2.5 meq/L
Chloride	116–122 mmol/L	116–122 meq/L
CO_2 content	20–24 mmol/L	20–24 meq/L
P_{CO_2}	6–7 kPa	45–49 mmHg
pH	7.31–7.34	
Glucose	2.22–3.89 mmol/L	40–70 mg/dL
Lactate	1–2 mmol/L	10–20 mg/dL
Total protein:		
Lumbar	0.15–0.5 g/L	15–50 mg/dL
Cisternal	0.15–0.25 g/L	15–25 mg/dL
Ventricular	0.06–0.15 g/L	6–15 mg/dL
Albumin	0.066–0.442 g/L	6.6–44.2 mg/dL
IgG	0.009–0.057 g/L	0.9–5.7 mg/dL
IgG index[b]	0.29–0.59	
Oligoclonal bands (OGB)	<2 bands not present in matched serum sample	
Ammonia	15–47 μmol/L	25–80 μg/dL
Creatinine	44–168 μmol/L	0.5–1.9 mg/dL
Myelin basic protein	<4 μg/L	
CSF pressure		50–180 mmH_2O
CSF volume (adult)	~150 mL	
Red blood cells	0	0
Leukocytes		
Total	0–5 mononuclear cells per μL	
Differential		
Lymphocytes	60–70%	
Monocytes	30–50%	
Neutrophils	None	

[a]Since cerebrospinal fluid concentrations are equilibrium values, measurements of the same parameters in blood plasma obtained at the same time are recommended. However, there is a time lag in attainment of equilibrium, and cerebrospinal levels of plasma constituents that can fluctuate rapidly (such as plasma glucose) may not achieve stable values until after a significant lag phase.
[b]IgG index = CSF IgG (mg/dL) × serum albumin (g/dL)/serum IgG (g/dL) × CSF albumin (mg/dL).

TABLE 7A

DIFFERENTIAL NUCLEATED CELL COUNTS OF BONE MARROW ASPIRATES[a]

	OBSERVED RANGE (%)	95% RANGE (%)	MEAN (%)
Blast cells	0–3.2	0–3.0	1.4
Promyelocytes	3.6–13.2	3.2–12.4	7.8
Neutrophil myelocytes	4–21.4	3.7–10.0	7.6
Eosinophil myelocytes	0–5.0	0–2.8	1.3
Metamyelocytes	1–7.0	2.3–5.9	4.1
Neutrophils			
Males	21.0–45.6	21.9–42.3	32.1
Females	29.6–46.6	28.8–45.9	37.4
Eosinophils	0.4–4.2	0.3–4.2	2.2
Eosinophils plus eosinophil myelocytes	0.9–7.4	0.7–6.3	3.5
Basophils	0–0.8	0–0.4	0.1
Erythroblasts			
Male	18.0–39.4	16.2–40.1	28.1
Females	14.0–31.8	13.0–32.0	22.5
Lymphocytes	4.6–22.6	6.0–20.0	13.1
Plasma cells	0–1.4	0–1.2	0.6
Monocytes	0–3.2	0–2.6	1.3
Macrophages	0–1.8	0–1.3	0.4
M:E ratio			
Males	1.1–4.0	1.1–4.1	2.1
Females	1.6–5.4	1.6–5.2	2.8

[a]Based on bone marrow aspirate from 50 healthy volunteers (30 men, 20 women).

Abbreviation: M:E, myeloid to erythroid ratio.

Source: BJ Bain: Br J Haematol 94:206, 1996.

TABLE 7B

BONE MARROW CELLULARITY

AGE	OBSERVED RANGE	95% RANGE	MEAN
Under 10 years	59.0–95.1%	72.9–84.7%	78.8%
10–19 years	41.5–86.6%	59.2–69.4%	64.3%
20–29 years	32.0–83.7%	54.1–61.9%	58.0%
30–39 years	30.3–81.3%	41.1–54.1%	47.6%
40–49 years	16.3–75.1%	43.5–52.9%	48.2%
50–59 years	19.7–73.6%	41.2–51.4%	46.3%
60–69 years	16.3–65.7%	40.8–50.6%	45.7%
70–79 years	11.3–47.1%	22.6–35.2%	28.9%

Source: From RJ Hartsock et al: Am J Clin Pathol 1965; 43:326, 1965.

TABLE 8

STOOL ANALYSIS

	REFERENCE RANGE	
	SI UNITS	CONVENTIONAL UNITS
Alpha-1-antitrypsin	≤540 mg/L	≤54 mg/dL
Amount	0.1–0.2 kg/d	100–200 g/24 h
Coproporphyrin	611–1832 nmol/d	400–1200 μg/24 h
Fat		
Adult		<7 g/d
Adult on fat-free diet		<4 g/d
Fatty acids	0–21 mmol/d	0–6 g/24 h
Leukocytes	None	None
Nitrogen	<178 mmol/d	<2.5 g/24 h
pH	7.0–7.5	
Potassium	14–102 mmol/L	14–102 mmol/L
Occult blood	Negative	Negative
Osmolality	280–325 mOsmol/kg	280–325 mOsmol/kg
Sodium	7–72 mmol/L	7–72 mmol/L
Trypsin		20–95 U/g
Urobilinogen	85–510 μmol/d	50–300 mg/24 h
Uroporphyrins	12–48 nmol/d	10–40 μg/24 h
Water	<0.75	<75%

Source: Modified from: FT Fishbach, MB Dunning III: *A Manual of Laboratory and Diagnostic Tests*, 7th ed. Philadelphia, Lippincott Williams & Wilkins, 2004.

TABLE 9

URINE ANALYSIS AND RENAL FUNCTION TESTS

	REFERENCE RANGE	
	SI UNITS	**CONVENTIONAL UNITS**
Acidity, titratable	20–40 mmol/d	20–40 meq/d
Aldosterone	Normal diet: 6–25 μg/d Low-salt diet: 17–44 μg/d High-salt diet: 0–6 μg/d	Normal diet: 6–25 μg/d Low-salt diet: 17–44 μg/d High-salt diet: 0–6 μg/d
Aluminum	0.19–1.11 μmol/L	5–30 μg/L
Ammonia	30–50 mmol/d	30–50 meq/d
Amylase		4–400 U/L
Amylase/creatinine clearance ratio [$(Cl_{am}/Cl_{cr}) \times 100$]	1–5	1–5
Arsenic	0.07–0.67 μmol/d	5–50 μg/d
Bence Jones protein, urine, qualitative	Not applicable	None detected
Bence Jones protein, urine, quantitative		
Free Kappa	1.4–24.2 mg/L	0.14–2.42 mg/dL
Free Lambda	0.2–6.7 mg/L	0.02–0.67 mg/dL
K/L ratio	2.04–10.37	2.04–10.37
Calcium (10 meq/d or 200 mg/d dietary calcium)	<7.5 mmol/d	<300 mg/d
Chloride	140–250 mmol/d	140–250 mmol/d
Citrate	320–1240 mg/d	320–1240 mg/d
Copper	<0.95 μmol/d	<60 μg/d
Coproporphyrins (types I and III)	0–20 μmol/mol creatinine	0–20 μmol/mol creatinine
Cortisol, free	55–193 nmol/d	20–70 μg/d
Creatine, as creatinine		
Female	<760 μmol/d	<100 mg/d
Male	<380 μmol/d	<50 mg/d
Creatinine	8.8–14 mmol/d	1.0–1.6 g/d
Dopamine	392–2876 nmol/d	60–440 μg/d
Eosinophils	<100 eosinophils/mL	<100 eosinophils/mL
Epinephrine	0–109 nmol/d	0–20 μg/d
Glomerular filtration rate	>60 mL/min/1.73 m^2 For African Americans multiply the result by 1.21	>60 mL/min/1.73 m^2 For African Americans multiply the result by 1.21
Glucose (glucose oxidase method)	0.3–1.7 mmol/d	50–300 mg/d
5-Hydroindoleacetic acid [5-HIAA]	0–78.8 μmol/d	0–15 mg/d
Hydroxyproline	53-328 μmol/d	53-328 μmol/d
Iodine, spot urine		
WHO classification of iodine deficiency:		
Not iodine deficient	>100 μg/L	>100 μg/L
Mild iodine deficiency	50–100 μg/L	50–100 μg/L
Moderate iodine deficiency	20–49 μg/L	20–49 μg/L
Severe iodine deficiency	<20 μg/L	<20 μg/L
Ketone (acetone)	Negative	Negative
17 Ketosteroids	3–12 mg/d	3–12 mg/d
Metanephrines		
Metanephrine	30–350 μg/d	30–350 μg/d
Normetanephrine	50–650 μg/d	50–650 μg/d

(continued)

TABLE 9

URINE ANALYSIS AND RENAL FUNCTION TESTS (*CONTINUED*)

	REFERENCE RANGE	
	SI UNITS	**CONVENTIONAL UNITS**
Microalbumin		
Normal	0.0–0.03 g/d	0–30 mg/d
Microalbuminuria	0.03–0.30 g/d	30–300 mg/d
Clinical albuminuria	>0.3 g/d	>300 mg/d
Microalbumin/creatinine ratio		
Normal	0–3.4 g/mol creatinine	0–30 μg/mg creatinine
Microalbuminuria	3.4–34 g/mol creatinine	30–300 μg/mg creatinine
Clinical albuminuria	>34 g/mol creatinine	>300 μg/mg creatinine
β_2-Microglobulin	0–160 μg/L	0–160 μg/L
Norepinephrine	89–473 nmol/d	15–80 μg/d
N-telopeptide (cross-linked), NTx		
Female, premenopausal	17–94 nmol BCE/mmol creatinine	17–94 nmol BCE/mmol creatinine
Female, postmenopausal	26–124 nmol BCE/mmol creatinine	26–124 nmol BCE/mmol creatinine
Male	21–83 nmol BCE/mmol creatinine	21–83 nmol BCE/mmol creatinine
BCE = bone collagen equivalent		
Osmolality	100–800 mOsm/kg	100–800 mOsm/kg
Oxalate		
Male	80–500 μmol/d	7–44 mg/d
Female	45–350 μmol/d	4–31 mg/d
pH	5.0–9.0	5.0–9.0
Phosphate (phosphorus) (varies with intake)	12.9–42.0 mmol/d	400–1300 mg/d
Porphobilinogen	None	None
Potassium (varies with intake)	25–100 mmol/d	25–100 meq/d
Protein	<0.15 g/d	<150 mg/d
Protein/creatinine ratio	Male: 15–68 mg/g Female: 10–107 mg/g	Male: 15–68 mg/g Female: 10–107 mg/g
Sediment		
Red blood cells	0–2/high-power field	
White blood cells	0–2/high-power field	
Bacteria	None	
Crystals	None	
Bladder cells	None	
Squamous cells	None	
Tubular cells	None	
Broad casts	None	
Epithelial cell casts	None	
Granular casts	None	
Hyaline casts	0–5/low-power field	
Red blood cell casts	None	
Waxy casts	None	
White cell casts	None	
Sodium (varies with intake)	100–260 mmol/d	100–260 meq/d
Specific gravity:		
After 12-h fluid restriction	>1.025	>1.025
After 12-h deliberate water intake	≤1.003	≤1.003
Tubular reabsorption, phosphorus	0.79–0.94 of filtered load	79–94% of filtered load
Urea nitrogen	214–607 mmol/d	6–17 g/d
Uric acid (normal diet)	1.49–4.76 mmol/d	250–800 mg/d
Vanillylmandelic acid (VMA)	<30 μmol/d	<6 mg/d

TABLE 10

NORMAL PRESSURES IN HEART AND GREAT VESSELS

PRESSURE (mmHg)	AVERAGE	RANGE
Right Atrium		
Mean	2.8	1–5
a wave	5.6	2.5–7
c wave	3.8	1.5–6
x wave	1.7	0–5
v wave	4.6	2–7.5
y wave	2.4	0–6
Right Ventricle		
Peak systolic	25	17–32
End-diastolic	4	1–7
Pulmonary Artery		
Mean	15	9–19
Peak systolic	25	17–32
End-diastolic	9	4–13
Pulmonary Artery Wedge		
Mean	9	4.5–13
Left Atrium		
Mean	7.9	2–12
a wave	10.4	4–16
v wave	12.8	6–21
Left Ventricle		
Peak systolic	130	90–140
End-diastolic	8.7	5–12
Brachial Artery		
Mean	85	70–105
Peak systolic	130	90–140
End-diastolic	70	60–90

Source: Reproduced from: MJ Kern *The Cardiac Catheterization Handbook*, 4th ed. Philadelphia, Mosby, 2003.

TABLE 11

CIRCULATORY FUNCTION TESTS

	RESULTS: REFERENCE RANGE	
TEST	**SI UNITS (RANGE)**	**CONVENTIONAL UNITS (RANGE)**
Arteriovenous oxygen difference	30–50 mL/L	30–50 mL/L
Cardiac output (Fick)	2.5–3.6 L/m^2 of body surface area per min	2.5–3.6 L/m^2 of body surface area per min
Contractility indexes		
Max. left ventricular *dp/dt* (*dp/dt*)	220 kPa/s (176–250 kPa/s)	1650 mmHg/s (1320–1880 mmHg/s)
DP when DP = 5.3 kPa	(37.6 ± 12.2)/s	(37.6 ± 12.2)/s
(40 mmHg) (DP, developed LV pressure)	3.32 ± 0.84 end-diastolic volumes per second	3.32 ± 0.84 end-diastolic volumes per second
Mean normalized systolic ejection rate (angiography)	1.83 ± 0.56 circumferences per second	1.83 ± 0.56 circumferences per second
Mean velocity of circumferential fiber shortening (angiography)		
Ejection fraction: stroke volume/end-diastolic volume (SV/EDV)	0.67 ± 0.08 (0.55–0.78)	0.67 ± 0.08 (0.55–0.78)
End-diastolic volume	70 ± 20.0 mL/m^2 (60–88 mL/m^2)	70 ± 20.0 mL/m^2 (60–88 mL/m^2)
End-systolic volume	25 ± 5.0 mL/m^2 (20–33 mL/m^2)	25 ± 5.0 mL/m^2 (20–33 mL/m^2)
Left ventricular work		
Stroke work index	50 ± 20.0 (g·m)/m^2 (30–110)	50 ± 20.0 (g·m)/m^2 (30–110)
Left ventricular minute work index	1.8–6.6 [(kg·m)/m^2]/min	1.8–6.6 [(kg·m)/m^2]/min
Oxygen consumption index	110–150 mL	110–150 mL
Maximum oxygen uptake	35 mL/min (20–60 mL/min)	35 mL/min (20–60 mL/min)
Pulmonary vascular resistance	2–12 (kPa·s)/L	20–130 (dyn·s)/cm^5
Systemic vascular resistance	77–150 (kPa·s)/L	770–1600 (dyn·s)/cm^5

Source: E Braunwald et al: *Heart Disease*, 6th ed. Philadelphia, W.B. Saunders Co., 2001.

TABLE 12

NORMAL ECHOCARDIOGRAPHIC REFERENCE LIMITS AND PARTITION VALUES IN ADULTS

	WOMEN REFERENCE RANGE	MILDLY ABNORMAL	MODERATELY ABNORMAL	SEVERELY ABNORMAL	MEN REFERENCE RANGE	MILDLY ABNORMAL	MODERATELY ABNORMAL	SEVERELY ABNORMAL
Left ventricular dimensions								
Septal thickness, cm	0.6–0.9	1.0–1.2	1.3–1.5	≥1.6	0.6–1.0	1.1–1.3	1.4–1.6	≥1.7
Posterior wall thickness, cm	0.6–0.9	1.0–1.2	1.3–1.5	≥1.6	0.6–1.0	1.1–1.3	1.4–1.6	≥1.7
Diastolic diameter, cm	3.9–5.3	5.4–5.7	5.8–6.1	≥6.2	4.2–5.9	6.0–6.3	6.4–6.8	≥6.9
Diastolic diameter/BSA, cm/m^2	2.4–3.2	3.3–3.4	3.5–3.7	≥3.8	2.2–3.1	3.2–3.4	3.5–3.6	≥3.7
Diastolic diameter/height, cm/m	2.5–3.2	3.3–3.4	3.5–3.6	≥3.7	2.4–3.3	3.4–3.5	3.6–3.7	≥3.8
Left ventricular volumes								
Diastolic, mL	56–104	105–117	118–130	≥131	67–155	156–178	179–201	≥202
Diastolic/BSA, mL/m^2	35–75	76–86	87–96	≥97	35–75	76–86	87–96	≥97
Systolic, mL	19–49	50–59	60–69	≥70	22–58	59–70	71–82	≥83
Systolic/BSA, mL/m^2	12–30	31–36	37–42	≥43	12–30	31–36	37–42	≥43
Left ventricular mass, 2D method								
Mass, g	66–150	151–171	172–182	≥183	96–200	201–227	228–254	≥255
Mass/BSA, g/m^2	44–88	89–100	101–112	≥113	50–102	103–116	117–130	≥131
Left ventricular function								
Endocardial fractional shortening (%)	27–45	22–26	17–21	≤16	25–43	20–24	15–19	≤14
Midwall fractional shortening (%)	15–23	13–14	11–12	≤10	14–22	12–13	10–11	≤9
Ejection fraction, 2D method (%)	≥55	45–54	30–44	≤29	≥55	45–54	30–44	≤29
Right heart dimensions (cm)								
Basal RV diameter	2.0–2.8	2.9–3.3	3.4–3.8	≥3.9	2.0–2.8	2.9–3.3	3.4–3.8	≥3.9
Mid-RV diameter	2.7–3.3	3.4–3.7	3.8–4.1	≥4.2	2.7–3.3	3.4–3.7	3.8–4.1	≥4.2
Base-to-apex length	7.1–7.9	8.0–8.5	8.6–9.1	≥9.2	7.1–7.9	8.0–8.5	8.6–9.1	≥9.2
RVOT diameter above aortic valve	2.5–2.9	3.0–3.2	3.3–3.5	≥3.6	2.5–2.9	3.0–3.2	3.3–3.5	≥3.6
RVOT diameter above pulmonic valve	1.7–2.3	2.4–2.7	2.8–3.1	≥3.2	1.7–2.3	2.4–2.7	2.8–3.1	≥3.2
Pulmonary artery diameter below pulmonic valve	1.5–2.1	2.2–2.5	2.6–2.9	≥3.0	1.5–2.1	2.2–2.5	2.6–2.9	≥3.0
Right ventricular size and function in 4-chamber view								
Diastolic area, cm^2	11–28	29–32	33–37	≥38	11–28	29–32	33–37	≥38
Systolic area, cm^2	7.5–16	17–19	20–22	≥23	7.5–16	17–19	20–22	≥23
Fractional area change, %	32–60	25–31	18–24	≤17	32–60	25–31	18–24	≤17
Atrial sizes								
LA diameter, cm	2.7–3.8	3.9–4.2	4.3–4.6	≥4.7	3.0–4.0	4.1–4.6	4.7–5.2	≥5.3
LA diameter/BSA, cm/m^2	1.5–2.3	2.4–2.6	2.7–2.9	≥3.0	1.5–2.3	2.4–2.6	2.7–2.9	≥3.0
RA minor axis, cm	2.9–4.5	4.6–4.9	5.0–5.4	≥5.5	2.9–4.5	4.6–4.9	5.0–5.4	≥5.5
RA minor axis/BSA, cm/m^2	1.7–2.5	2.6–2.8	2.9–3.1	≥3.2	1.7–2.5	2.6–2.8	2.9–3.1	≥3.2

(*continued*)

TABLE 12

NORMAL ECHOCARDIOGRAPHIC REFERENCE LIMITS AND PARTITION VALUES IN ADULTS (*CONTINUED*)

	WOMEN REFERENCE RANGE	MILDLY ABNORMAL	MODERATELY ABNORMAL	SEVERELY ABNORMAL	MEN REFERENCE RANGE	MILDLY ABNORMAL	MODERATELY ABNORMAL	SEVERELY ABNORMAL
LA area, cm²	<20	20–30	30–40	≥41	<20	20–30	30–40	≥41
LA volume, mL	22–52	53–62	63–72	≥73	18–58	59–68	69–78	≥79
LA volume/BSA, mL/m²	16–28	29–33	34–39	≥40	16–28	29–33	34–39	≥40
Aortic stenosis, classification of severity								
Aortic jet velocity, m/s		2.6–2.9	3.0–4.0	>4.0		2.6–2.9	3.0–4.0	>4.0
Mean gradient, mmHg		<20	20–40	>40		<20	20–40	>40
Valve area, cm²		>1.5	1.0–1.5	<1.0		>1.5	1.0–1.5	<1.0
Indexed valve area, cm²/m²		>0.85	0.60–0.85	<0.6		>0.85	0.60–0.85	<0.6
Velocity ratio		>0.50	0.25–0.50	<0.25		>0.50	0.25–0.50	<0.25
Mitral stenosis, classification of severity								
Valve area, cm²		>1.5	1.0–1.5	<1.0		>1.5	1.0–1.5	<1.0
Mean gradient, mmHg		<5	5–10	>10		<5	5–10	>10
Pulmonary artery pressure, mmHg		<30	30–50	>50		<30	30–50	>50
Aortic regurgitation, indices of severity								
Vena contracta width, cm		<0.30	0.30–0.60	≥0.60		<0.30	0.30–0.60	≥0.60
Jet width/LVOT width, %		<25	25–64	≥65		<25	25–64	≥65
Jet CSA/LVOT CSA, %		<5	5–59	≥60		<5	5–59	≥60
Regurgitant volume, mL/beat		<30	30–59	≥60		<30	30–59	≥60
Regurgitant fraction, %		<30	30–49	≥50		<30	30–49	≥50
Effective regurgitant orifice area, cm²		<0.10	0.10–0.29	≥0.30		<0.10	0.10–0.29	≥0.30
Mitral regurgitation, indices of severity								
Vena contracta width, cm		<0.30	0.30–0.69	≥0.70		<0.30	0.30–0.69	≥0.70
Regurgitant volume, mL/beat		<30	30–59	≥60		<30	30–59	≥60
Regurgitant fraction, %		<30	30–49	≥50		<30	30–49	≥50
Effective regurgitant orifice area, cm²		<0.20	0.20–0.39	≥0.40		<0.20	0.20–0.39	≥0.40

Abbreviations: BSA, body surface area; CSA, cross-sectional area; LA, left atrium; LVOT, left ventricular outflow tract; RA, right atrium; RV, right ventricle; RVOT, right ventricular outflow tract; 2D, 2-dimensional.

Source: Values adapted from: American Society of Echocardiography, Guidelines and Standards. *http://www.asecho.org/i4a/pages/index.cfm?pageid=3317*. Accessed Feb 23, 2010.

TABLE 13

SUMMARY OF VALUES USEFUL IN PULMONARY PHYSIOLOGY

	SYMBOL	TYPICAL VALUES: MAN AGED 40, 75 kg, 175 cm TALL	TYPICAL VALUES: WOMAN AGED 40, 60 kg, 160 cm TALL
Pulmonary Mechanics			
Spirometry—volume-time curves			
Forced vital capacity	FVC	5.0 L	3.4 L
Forced expiratory volume in 1 s	FEV_1	4.0 L	2.8 L
FEV_1/FVC	FEV_1%	80%	78%
Maximal midexpiratory flow rate	MMEF (FEF 25–75)	4.1 L/s	3.2 L/s
Maximal expiratory flow rate	MEFR (FEF 200–1200)	9.0 L/s	6.1 L/s
Spirometry—flow-volume curves			
Maximal expiratory flow at 50% of expired vital capacity	V_{max} 50 (FEF 50%)	5.0 L/s	4.0 L/s
Maximal expiratory flow at 75% of expired vital capacity	V_{max} 75 (FEF 75%)	2.1 L/s	2.0 L/s
Resistance to airflow:			
Pulmonary resistance	RL (R_L)	<3.0 (cmH_2O/s)/L	
Airway resistance	Raw	<2.5 (cmH_2O/s)/L	
Specific conductance	SGaw	>0.13 cmH_2O/s	
Pulmonary compliance			
Static recoil pressure at total lung capacity	Pst TLC	25 ± 5 cmH_2O	
Compliance of lungs (static)	CL	0.2 L cmH_2O	
Compliance of lungs and thorax	C(L + T)	0.1 L cmH_2O	
Dynamic compliance of 20 breaths per minute	C dyn 20	0.25 ± 0.05 L/cmH_2O	
Maximal static respiratory pressures:			
Maximal inspiratory pressure	MIP	>110 cmH_2O	>70 cmH_2O
Maximal expiratory pressure	MEP	>200 cmH_2O	>140 cmH_2O
Lung Volumes			
Total lung capacity	TLC	6.9 L	4.9 L
Functional residual capacity	FRC	3.3 L	2.6 L
Residual volume	RV	1.9 L	1.5 L
Inspiratory capacity	IC	3.7 L	2.3 L
Expiratory reserve volume	ERV	1.4 L	1.1 L
Vital capacity	VC	5.0 L	3.4 L
Gas Exchange (Sea Level)			
Arterial O_2 tension	Pa_{O_2}	12.7 ± 0.7 kPa (95 ± 5 mmHg)	
Arterial CO_2 tension	Pa_{CO_2}	5.3 ± 0.3 kPa (40 ± 2 mmHg)	
Arterial O_2 saturation	Sa_{O_2}	0.97 ± 0.02 (97 ± 2%)	
Arterial blood pH	pH	7.40 ± 0.02	
Arterial bicarbonate	HCO_3^-	24 + 2 meq/L	
Base excess	BE	0 ± 2 meq/L	
Diffusing capacity for carbon monoxide (single breath)	DL_{CO}	37 mL CO/min/mmHg	27 mL CO/min/mmHg
Dead space volume	V_D	2 mL/kg body wt	
Physiologic dead space; dead space-tidal volume ratio	V_D/V_T		
Rest		≤35% V_T	
Exercise		≤20% V_T	
Alveolar-arterial difference for O_2	$P(A - a)_{O2}$	≤2.7 kPa ≤20 kPa (≤24 mmHg)	

Source: Based on: AH Morris et al: *Clinical Pulmonary Function Testing. A Manual of Uniform Laboratory Procedures*, 2nd ed. Salt Lake City, Utah, Intermountain Thoracic Society, 1984.

TABLE 14

GASTROINTESTINAL TESTS

TEST	RESULTS	
	SI UNITS	CONVENTIONAL UNITS
Absorption tests		
D-Xylose: after overnight fast, 25 g xylose given in oral aqueous solution		
Urine, collected for following 5 h	25% of ingested dose	25% of ingested dose
Serum, 2 h after dose	2.0–3.5 mmol/L	30–52 mg/dL
Vitamin A: a fasting blood specimen is obtained and 200,000 units of vitamin A in oil is given orally	Serum level should rise to twice fasting level in 3–5 h	Serum level should rise to twice fasting level in 3–5 h
Bentiromide test (pancreatic function): 500 mg bentiromide (chymex) orally; *p*-aminobenzoic acid (PABA) measured		
Plasma		>3.6 (±1.1) μg/mL at 90 min
Urine	>50% recovered in 6 h	>50% recovered in 6 h
Gastric juice		
Volume		
24 h	2–3 L	2–3 L
Nocturnal	600–700 mL	600–700 mL
Basal, fasting	30–70 mL/h	30–70 mL/h
Reaction		
pH	1.6–1.8	1.6–1.8
Titratable acidity of fasting juice	4–9 μmol/s	15–35 meq/h
Acid output		
Basal		
Females (mean ± 1 SD)	0.6 ± 0.5 μmol/s	2.0 ± 1.8 meq/h
Males (mean ± 1 SD)	0.8 ± 0.6 μmol/s	3.0 ± 2.0 meq/h
Maximal (after SC histamine acid phosphate, 0.004 mg/kg body weight, and preceded by 50 mg promethazine, or after betazole, 1.7 mg/kg body weight, or pentagastrin, 6 μg/kg body weight)		
Females (mean ± 1 SD)	4.4 ± 1.4 μmol/s	16 ± 5 meq/h
Males (mean ± 1 SD)	6.4 ± 1.4 μmol/s	23 ± 5 meq/h
Basal acid output/maximal acid output ratio	≤0.6	≤0.6
Gastrin, serum	0–200 μg/L	0–200 pg/mL
Secretin test (pancreatic exocrine function): 1 unit/kg body weight, IV		
Volume (pancreatic juice) in 80 min	>2.0 mL/kg	>2.0 mL/kg
Bicarbonate concentration	>80 mmol/L	>80 meq/L
Bicarbonate output in 30 min	>10 mmol	>10 meq

TABLE 15

BODY FLUIDS AND OTHER MASS DATA

	REFERENCE RANGE	
	SI UNITS	CONVENTIONAL UNITS
Ascitic fluid		
Body fluid		
Total volume (lean) of body weight	50% (in obese) to 70%	
Intracellular	30–40% of body weight	
Extracellular	20–30% of body weight	
Blood		
Total volume		
Males	69 mL/kg body weight	
Females	65 mL/kg body weight	
Plasma volume		
Males	39 mL/kg body weight	
Females	40 mL/kg body weight	
Red blood cell volume		
Males	30 mL/kg body weight	1.15–1.21 L/m^2 of body surface area
Females	25 mL/kg body weight	0.95–1.00 L/m^2 of body surface area
Body mass index	18.5–24.9 kg/m^2	18.5–24.9 kg/m^2

TABLE 16

RADIATION-DERIVED UNITS

QUANTITY	MEASURES	OLD UNIT	SI UNIT	SPECIAL NAME FOR SI UNIT (ABBREVIATION)	CONVERSION
Activity	Rate of radioactive decay	curie (Ci)	Disintegrations per second (dps)	becquerel (Bq)	1 Ci = 3.7×10^{10} Bq 1 mCi = 37 MBq 1 Bq = 2.703×10^{-11} Ci
Exposure	Amount of ionizations produced in dry air by x-rays or gamma rays, per unit of mass	roentgen (R)	Coulomb per kilogram (C/kg)	none	1 C/kg = 3876 R 1 R = 2.58×10^{-4} C/kg 1 mR = 258 pC/kg
Air kerma	Sum of initial energies of charged particles liberated by ionizing radiation in air, per unit of mass	rad	Joule per kilogram (J/kg)	gray (Gy)	1 Gy = 100 rad 1 rad = 0.01 Gy 1 mrad = 10 μGy
Absorbed dose	Energy deposited per unit of mass in a medium, e.g., an organ/tissue	rad	Joule per kilogram (J/kg)	gray (Gy)	1 Gy = 100 rad 1 rad = 0.01 Gy 1 mrad = 10 μGy
Equivalent dose	Energy deposited per unit of mass in a medium, e.g., an organ/tissue, weighted to reflect type(s) of radiation	rem	Joule per kilogram (J/kg)	sievert (Sv)	1 Sv = 100 rem 1 rem = 0.01 Sv 1 mrem = 10 μSv
Effective dose	Energy deposited per unit of mass in a reference individual, doubly weighted to reflect type(s) of radiation and organ(s) irradiated	rem	Joule per kilogram (J/kg)	sievert (Sv)	1 Sv = 100 rem 1 rem = 0.01 Sv 1 mrem = 10 μSv

The contributions of Drs. Daniel J. Fink, Patrick M. Sluss, James L. Januzzi, and Kent B. Lewandrowski to this chapter in previous editions of Harrison's Principles of Internal Medicine are gratefully acknowledged. We also express our gratitude to Drs. Amudha Palanisamy and Scott Fink for careful review of tables and helpful suggestions.

REVIEW AND SELF-ASSESSMENT[a]

Charles Wiener ■ Cynthia D. Brown ■ Anna R. Hemnes

QUESTIONS

DIRECTIONS: Choose the **one best** response to each question.

1. During a neurologic examination, you ask a patient to stand with both arms fully extended and parallel to the ground with his eyes closed for 10 seconds. What is the name of this test?

   A. Babinski sign
   B. Dysdiadochokinesis
   C. Lhermitte symptom
   D. Pronator drift
   E. Romberg sign

2. This sign is considered positive if there is flexion at the elbows or forearms, or if there is pronation of the forearms. A positive test is a sign of:

   A. Abnormal sensation
   B. Early dementia
   C. Localized brainstem disease
   D. Potential weakness
   E. Underlying cerebellar dysfunction

3. A 55-year-old woman with known metastatic breast cancer presents to the emergency department complaining of new-onset weakness and numbness. The symptoms involve both arms and legs. She also has developed urinary incontinence over the past 24 hours. On physical examination, strength is 3/5 in the lower extremities and 4/5 in the upper extremities. Anal sphincter tone is decreased. Babinski sign is positive. Sensation is decreased in the extremities, but not in the face. Cranial nerves are symmetric and intact, and mental status is normal. Based on this information, what is the most likely site of the lesion causing the patient's symptoms?

   A. Brainstem
   B. Cerebrum
   C. Cervical spinal cord
   D. Lumbar spinal cord
   E. Neuromuscular junction

4. A 54-year-old woman presents to the emergency department complaining of the abrupt onset of what she describes as the worst headache of her life. You are concerned about the possibility of subarachnoid hemorrhage. What is the most appropriate initial test for diagnosis?

   A. Cerebral angiography
   B. CT of the head with IV contrast
   C. CT of the head without IV contrast
   D. Lumbar puncture
   E. Transcranial Doppler ultrasound

5. A 74-year-old woman has a recent diagnosis of small cell lung cancer. She is now complaining of headaches, and her family has noticed confusion as well. Metastatic disease to the brain is suspected. A mass lesion on magnetic resonance imaging (MRI) is demonstrated in the right parietal lobe. Which MRI technique would best identify the extent of the edema surrounding the lesion?

   A. MR angiography
   B. FLAIR
   C. T1-weighted
   D. T2-weighted
   E. B and D

6. Which of the following is a possible complication of administration of gadolinium to a patient with chronic kidney disease?

   A. Acute renal failure
   B. Hyperthyroidism
   C. Hypocalcemia
   D. Lactic acidosis
   E. Nephrogenic systemic sclerosis

7. In a patient with coma, an EEG showing triphasic waves is most suggestive of which of the following clinical disorders?

   A. Brain abscess
   B. Herpes simplex encephalitis
   C. Locked-in syndrome
   D. Metabolic encephalopathy
   E. Nonconvulsive status epilepticus

[a]Questions and answers were taken from Wiener C et al (eds): *Harrison's Principles of Internal Medicine Self-Assessment and Board Review*, 18th ed. New York: McGraw-Hill, 2012.

8. A 25-year-old woman becomes lightheaded and experiences a syncopal event while having her blood drawn during a cholesterol screening. She has no medical history and takes no medications. She experiences a brief loss of consciousness for about 20 seconds. She has no seizure-like activity and immediately returns to her usual level of functioning. She is diagnosed with vasovagal syncope, and no follow-up testing is recommended. Which of the following statements regarding neurally mediated syncope is TRUE?

A. Neurally mediated syncope occurs when there are abnormalities of the autonomic nervous system.
B. Proximal and distal myoclonus do not occur during neurally mediated syncope and should increase the likelihood of a seizure.
C. The final pathway of neurally mediated syncope results in a surge of the sympathetic nervous system with inhibition of the parasympathetic nervous system.
D. The primary therapy for neurally mediated syncope is reassurance, avoidance of triggers, and plasma volume expansion.
E. The usual finding with cardiovascular monitoring is hypotension and tachycardia.

9. A 76-year-old woman is brought to the emergency department after a syncopal event that occurred while she was singing in her church choir. She has a history of hypertension, diabetes mellitus, and chronic kidney disease (stage III). She does recall at least two prior episodes of syncope similar to this one. Her medications include insulin glargine 40 units daily, lispro insulin sliding scale, lisinopril 20 mg daily, and hydrochlorothiazide 25 mg daily. By the time she arrived in the emergency department, she reports feeling back to her usual self. She does recall feeling somewhat lightheaded before the syncopal events but does not recall the event itself. Witnesses report some jerking of her upper extremities. She regained full consciousness in less than 2 minutes. Her current vital signs include blood pressure of 110/62 mmHg, heart rate of 84 beats/min, respiratory rate of 16 breaths/min, and oxygen saturation of 95% on room air. She is afebrile. Her physical examination is unremarkable and includes a normal neurologic examination. Which of the following would be least helpful in determining the etiology of the patient's syncope?

A. CT scan of the head
B. Electrocardiogram
C. Fingerstick glucose measurement
D. Orthostatic blood pressure measurement
E. Tilt table testing

10. A 48-year-old man presents to the emergency department complaining of dizziness. He describes it as a sensation that the room is spinning. All of the following would be consistent with a central cause of vertigo EXCEPT:

A. Absence of tinnitus
B. Gaze-evoked nystagmus
C. Hiccups
D. Inhibition of nystagmus by visual fixation
E. Purely vertical nystagmus

11. A 62-year-old woman presents complaining of severe dizziness. She notes it especially when she turns over in bed and immediately upon standing. Her initial physical examination findings are normal. Upon further testing, you ask the patient to sit with her head turned 45 degrees to the right. You lower the patient to the supine position and extend the head backward 20 degrees. This maneuver immediately reproduces the patient's symptoms, and you note torsional nystagmus. What is the most appropriate next step in evaluation and treatment of this patient?

A. MRI of the brainstem
B. Methylprednisolone taper beginning at 100 mg daily
C. Repositioning (Epley) maneuvers
D. Rizatriptan 10 mg orally once
E. Valacyclovir 1000 mg three times daily for 7 days

12. A 42-year-old man presents complaining of progressive weakness over a period of several months. He reports tripping over his toes while walking and has dropped a cup of hot coffee on one occasion because he felt too weak to continue to hold it. A disorder affecting lower motor neurons is suspected. All of the following findings would be found in an individual with a disease primarily affecting lower motor neurons EXCEPT:

A. Decreased muscle tone
B. Distal greater than proximal weakness
C. Fasciculations
D. Hyperactive tendon reflexes
E. Severe muscle atrophy

13. A 78-year-old man is seen in clinic because of recent falls. He reports gait difficulties with a sensation of being off balance at times. One recent fall caused a shoulder injury requiring surgery to repair a torn rotation cuff. In epidemiologic case series, what is the most common cause of gait disorders?

A. Cerebellar degeneration
B. Cerebrovascular disease with multiple infarcts
C. Cervical myelopathy
D. Parkinson's disease
E. Sensory deficits

14. A 65-year-old man presents complaining of frequent falls and gait abnormalities. He first noticed the difficulty about 6 months ago. He has a history of hypertension and hypothyroidism and hyperlipidemia. His current medications include amlodipine 10 mg daily, simvastatin 20 mg daily, and levothyroxine 75 μg daily. On neurologic examination, you observe his gait to be wide based with short, shuffling steps. He has difficulty rising from his chair and initiating his gait. Upon turning, he takes multiple steps and appears unsteady. However, cerebellar testing results are normal, including heel-to-shin and Romberg testing. He has no evidence of sensory deficits in the lower extremities, and strength is 5/5 throughout all tested muscle groups. He shows no evidence of muscle spasticity on passive movement. His neurologic examination is consistent with which of the following causes?

A. Alcoholic cerebellar degeneration
B. Communicating hydrocephalus
C. Neurosyphilis
D. Multiple system atrophy
E. Lumbar myelopathy

15. A 74-year-old woman is admitted to the medical intensive care unit with confusion and sepsis from a urinary origin. Her initial blood pressure was 70/40 mmHg with a heart rate of 130 beats/min. She is volume resuscitated but requires dopamine to maintain an adequate blood pressure. Her mental status improved initially, but now she is agitated and pulling at her IV catheters. She is screaming that she is trapped, and she is not oriented to place or year. All of the following statements regarding the patient's condition are true EXCEPT:

A. An episode of delirium is associated with an in-hospital mortality rate of 25% to 33%.
B. A patient who has an episode of delirium in the hospital is more likely to be discharged to a nursing home.
C. Delirium is associated with an increased risk of all-cause mortality for at least 1 year after hospital discharge.
D. Delirium is typically short-lived and does not persist longer than several days.
E. Individuals who experience delirium have longer lengths of stay in the hospital.

16. You are covering the night shift at a local hospital and are called acutely to the bedside of a 62-year-old man to evaluate a change in his mental status. He was admitted 36 hours previously for treatment of community-acquired pneumonia. He received treatment with levofloxacin 500 mg daily and required oxygen 2 L/min. He has a medical history of tobacco abuse, diabetes mellitus, and hypertension. He reports alcohol intake of 2–4 beers daily. His vital signs at 10 pm were blood pressure of 138/85 mmHg, heart rate of 92 beats/min, respiratory rate of 20 breaths/min, temperature of 37.4°C (99.3°F), and SaO_2 of 92% on oxygen 2 L/min. Currently, the patient is agitated and pacing his room. He is reporting that he needs to leave the "meeting" immediately and go home. He states that if he does not do this, someone is going to take his house and car away. He has removed his IV and oxygen tubing from his nose. His last vital signs taken 30 minutes previously were blood pressure of 156/92 mmHg, heart rate of 118 beats/min, respiratory rate of 26 breaths/min, temperature of 38.3°C (100.9°F), and oxygen saturation of 87% on room air. He is noted to be somewhat tremulous and diaphoretic. All of the following should be considered as part of the patient's diagnostic work-up EXCEPT:

A. Arterial blood gas testing
B. Brain imaging with MRI or head CT
C. Fingerstick glucose testing
D. More thorough review of the patient's alcohol intake with his wife
E. Review of the recent medications received by the patient

17. Delirium, an acute confusional state, is a common disorder that remains a major cause of morbidity and mortality in the United States. Which of the following patients is at the highest risk for developing delirium?

A. A 36-year-old man admitted to the medical ward with a deep venous thrombosis
B. A 55-year-old man postoperative day 2 from a total colectomy
C. A 68-year-old woman admitted to the intensive care unit (ICU) with esophageal rupture
D. A 74-year-old woman in the preoperative clinic before hip surgery
E. An 84-year-old man living in an assisted living facility

18. A 28-year-old woman has severe head trauma after a motor vehicle accident. One year after the accident, she is noted to have spontaneous eye opening and is able to track an object visually at times. She does not speak or follow any commands. She breathes independently but is fed through a gastrostomy tube. She can move all extremities

18. (*Continued*)
spontaneously but without purposeful movement. What term best describes this patient's condition?

A. Coma
B. Locked-in
C. Minimally conscious state
D. Persistent vegetative state
E. Vegetative state

19. A 52-year-old man is evaluated after a large subarachnoid hemorrhage (SAH) from a ruptured cerebral aneurysm. There is concern that the patient has brain death. What test is most commonly used to diagnose brain death in this situation?

A. Apnea testing
B. Cerebral angiography
C. Demonstration of absent cranial nerve reflexes
D. Demonstration of fixed and dilated pupils
E. Performance of transcranial Doppler ultrasonography

20. Which of the following neurologic phenomena is classically associated with herniation of the brain through the foramen magnum?

A. Third-nerve compression and ipsilateral papillary dilation
B. Catatonia
C. "Locked-in" state
D. Miotic pupils
E. Respiratory arrest

21. Which of the following is the most common finding in aphasic patients?

A. Alexia
B. Anomia
C. Comprehension
D. Fluency
E. Repetition

22. A 65-year-old man experiences an ischemic cerebrovascular accident affecting the territory of the right anterior cerebral artery. After the stroke, an assessment reveals the findings shown in Figure 22. What diagnosis does this figure suggest?

A. Construction apraxia
B. Hemianopia
C. Hemineglect
D. Object agnosia
E. Simultanagnosia

23. A 42-year-old man is evaluated for excessive sleepiness that is interfering with his ability to work. He works at a glass factory that requires him to work rotating shifts. He typically cycles across day (7 am–3 pm), evening (3 pm–11 pm), and night (11 pm–7 am) shifts over the course of 4 weeks. He notes the problem to be most severe when he is on the night shift. Twice he has fallen asleep on the job. Although no accidents have occurred, he has been threatened with loss of his job if he

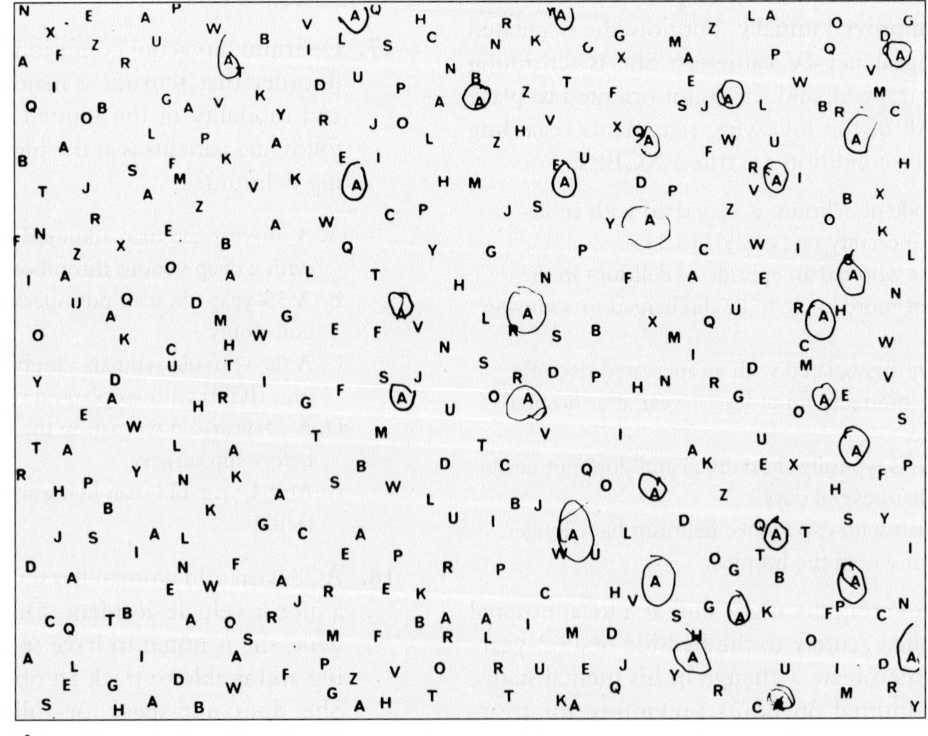

A

FIGURE 22

23. (*Continued*)
falls asleep again. His preferred sleep schedule is 10 pm until 6 am, but even when he is working day shifts, he typically only sleeps from about 10:30 pm until 5:30 am. However, he feels fully functional at work on day and evening shifts. After his night shifts, he states that he finds it difficult to sleep when he first gets home, frequently not falling asleep until 10 am or later. He is up by about 3 pm when his children arrive home from school. He drinks about 2 cups of coffee daily but tries to avoid drinking more than this. He does not snore and has a body mass index of 21.3 kg/m^2. All of the following are reasonable approaches to treatment in this man EXCEPT:

A. Avoidance of bright light in the morning after his shifts
B. Exercise in the early evening before going to work
C. Melatonin 3 mg taken at bedtime on the morning after a night shift
D. Modafinil 200 mg taken 30–60 minutes before starting a shift
E. Strategic napping of no more than 20 minutes during breaks at work

24. A 45-year-old woman presents for evaluation of abnormal sensations in her legs that keep her from sleeping at night. She first notices the symptoms around 8 pm when she is sitting quietly watching television. She describes the symptoms as "ants crawling in my veins." Although the symptoms are not painful, they are very uncomfortable and worsen when she lies down at night. They interfere with her ability to fall asleep about four times weekly. If she gets out of bed to walk or rubs her legs, the symptoms disappear almost immediately only to recur as soon as she is still. She also sometimes takes a very hot bath to alleviate the symptoms. During sleep, her husband complains that she kicks him throughout the night. She has no history of neurologic or renal disease. She currently is perimenopausal and has been experiencing very heavy and prolonged menstrual cycles over the past several months. The physical examination findings, including thorough neurologic examination, are normal. Her hemoglobin is 9.8 g/dL and hematocrit is 30.1%. The mean corpuscular volume is 68 fL. Serum ferritin is 12 ng/mL. Which is the most appropriate initial therapy for this patient?

A. Carbidopa/levodopa
B. Hormone replacement therapy
C. Iron supplementation
D. Oxycodone
E. Pramipexole

25. A 20-year-old man presents for evaluation of excessive daytime somnolence. He is finding it increasingly difficult to stay awake during his classes. Recently, his grades have fallen because whenever he tries to read, he finds himself drifting off. He finds that his alertness is best after exercising or brief naps of 10–30 minutes. Because of this, he states that he takes 5 or 10 "catnaps" daily. The sleepiness persists despite averaging 9 hours of sleep nightly. In addition to excessive somnolence, he reports occasional hallucinations that occur as he is falling asleep. He describes these occurrences as a voice calling his name as he drifts off. Perhaps once weekly, he awakens from sleep but is unable to move for a period of about 30 seconds. He has never had apparent loss of consciousness but states that whenever he is laughing, he feels heaviness in his neck and arms. Once he had to lean against a wall to keep from falling down. He undergoes an overnight sleep study and multiple sleep latency test. There is no sleep apnea. His mean sleep latency on five naps is 2.3 minutes. In three of the five naps, rapid eye movement sleep is present. Which of the following findings of this patient is most specific for the diagnosis of narcolepsy?

A. Cataplexy
B. Excessive daytime somnolence
C. Hypnagogic hallucinations
D. Rapid eye movement sleep in more than two naps on a multiple sleep latency test
E. Sleep paralysis

26. Which of the following is the most common sleep disorder in the U.S. population?

A. Delayed sleep phase syndrome
B. Insomnia
C. Obstructive sleep apnea
D. Narcolepsy
E. Restless legs syndrome

27. In which stage of sleep are the parasomnias somnambulism and night terrors most likely to occur?

A. Stage 1
B. Stage 2
C. Slow-wave sleep
D. Rapid eye movement sleep

28. A 44-year-old man is seen in the emergency department after a motor vehicle accident. The patient says, "I never saw that car coming from the right side." On physical examination, his pupils are equal and reactive to light. His visual acuity is normal; however, there are visual field defects in both eyes laterally (bitemporal hemianopia). Which of

28. (*Continued*)
the following is most likely to be found on further evaluation?

A. Retinal detachment
B. Occipital lobe glioma
C. Optic nerve injury
D. Parietal lobe infarction
E. Pituitary adenoma

29. A 42-year-old construction worker complains of waking up with a red, painful left eye. She often works without goggles at her construction site. Her history is notable for hypertension, inflammatory bowel disease, diabetes, and prior IV drug use. Her only current medication is lisinopril. On examination, the left eye is diffusely red and sensitive to light. The eyelids are normal. In dim light, visual acuity is normal in both eyes. All of the following diagnoses will explain her findings EXCEPT:

A. Acute angle-closure glaucoma
B. Anterior uveitis
C. Corneal abrasion
D. Posterior uveitis
E. Transient ischemic attack

30. A 75-year-old triathlete complains of gradually worsening vision over the past year. It seems to be involving near and far vision. The patient has never required corrective lenses and has no significant medical history other than diet-controlled hypertension. He takes no regular medications. Physical examination is normal except for bilateral visual acuity of 20/100. There are no focal visual field defects and no redness of the eyes or eyelids. Which of the following is the most likely diagnosis?

A. Age-related macular degeneration
B. Blepharitis
C. Diabetic retinopathy
D. Episcleritis
E. Retinal detachment

31. All of the following statements regarding olfaction are true EXCEPT:

A. Decrements in olfaction may lead to nutritional deficiency.
B. More than 40% of patients with traumatic anosmia will regain normal function over time.
C. Significant decrements in olfaction are present in more than 50% of the population 80 years and older.
D. The most common identifiable cause of long-lasting or permanent loss of olfaction in outpatients is severe respiratory infection.
E. Women identify odorants better than men at all ages.

32. A 64-year-old man is evaluated for hearing loss that he thinks is worse in his left ear. His wife and children have told him for years that he does not listen to them. Recently, he has failed to hear the chime of the alarm on his digital watch, and he admits to focusing on the lips of individuals speaking to him because he sometimes has difficulties in word recognition. In addition, he reports a continuous buzzing that is louder in his left ear. He denies any sensation of vertigo, headaches, or balance difficulties. He has worked in a factory for many years that makes parts for airplanes, and the machinery that he works with sits to his left primarily. He has no family history of deafness, although his father had hearing loss as he aged. He has a medical history of hypertension, hyperlipidemia, and coronary artery disease. You suspect sensorineural hearing loss related to exposure to the intense noise in the factory for many decades. Which of the following findings would you expect on physical examination?

A. A deep tympanic retraction pocket seen above the pars flaccida on the tympanic membrane.
B. Cerumen impaction in the external auditory canal.
C. Hearing loss that is greater at lower frequencies on pure tone audiometry.
D. Increased intensity of sound when a tuning fork is placed on the mastoid process when compared with placement near the auditory canal.
E. Increased intensity of sound in the right ear when a tuning fork is placed in the midline of the forehead.

33. All of the following neurologic conditions have a mechanistic association with abnormalities of ion channel function EXCEPT:

A. Epilepsy
B. Lambert-Eaton syndrome
C. Migraine
D. Parkinson's disease
E. Spinocerebellar ataxia

34. All of the following neurologic diseases are matched correctly with the neurotransmitter system that is dysfunctional EXCEPT:

A. Lambert-Eaton syndrome: acetylcholine
B. Myasthenia gravis: acetylcholine
C. Orthostatic tachycardia syndrome: serotonin
D. Parkinson's disease: dopamine
E. Stiff-person syndrome: GABA

35. An 18-year-old man seeks evaluation at his university health center for increasing episodes of sudden-onset smelling of burning kerosene. These episodes had occurred every few months during high school and he never told anyone. However, since starting college, he notes an increasing frequency, often

35. (*Continued*)
when sleep deprived. The episodes typically start without warning and he'll smell a distinct kerosene smell no matter the environment. The episodes last about 3–5 minutes and stop spontaneously. He has never lost consciousness. During the episodes, he can communicate with friends. An EEG during an episode shows abnormal discharges distinctly localized to an area of the frontal lobe. Which of the following is the most accurate classification of his seizure disorder?

A. Focal seizures with dyscognitive features
B. Focal seizures without dyscognitive features
C. Generalized seizure
D. Myoclonic seizures
E. Typical absence seizure

36. On the neurologic consultation service, you are asked to evaluate a patient with mesial temporal lobe epilepsy syndrome. The patient has a history of intractable focal seizures that rarely generalize. Her seizures often begin with an aura and commonly manifest as behavioral arrests, complex automatisms, and unilateral posturing. MRI findings include small temporal lobes and a small hippocampus with increased signal on T2-weighted sequences. Which of these additional historic factors is also likely to be present in this patient?

A. History of febrile seizures
B. Hypothyroidism
C. Neurofibromas
D. Recurring genital ulcers
E. Type 2 diabetes mellitus

37. You have just admitted a young man with a prior history of seizure disorder who was witnessed to have a seizure. His family's description suggests a focal seizure involving the left hand that spread to involve the entire arm. He did not lose consciousness. He was brought in 2 hours after symptom onset and is currently awake, alert, and oriented. He has not had any further seizures but has been unable to move his left hand since his seizure. His electrolytes and complete blood count are within normal limits. A noncontrast CT scan of his head is unremarkable. On examination, sensation is intact in the affected limb, but his strength is 0 out of 5 in the musculature of the left hand. What is the best course of action at this time?

A. Cerebral angiogram
B. Lumbar puncture
C. Magnetic resonance angiogram
D. Psychiatric evaluation
E. Reassess in a few hours

38. A 37-year-old man is witnessed by his family to have a generalized tonic-clonic seizure at a party. He does not have a known seizure disorder. There is no history of head trauma, stroke, or tumor. The patient is unemployed, married, and takes no medication. Physical examination shows no skin abnormalities and no stigmata of chronic liver or renal disease. The patient is postictal. His neck is difficult to maneuver due to stiffness. His white blood cell count is 19,000/μL, hematocrit 36%, and platelets 200,000/μL. Glucose is 102 mg/dL, sodium 136 meq/dL, calcium 9.5 mg/dL, magnesium 2.2 mg/dL, SGOT 18 U/L, blood urea nitrogen 7 mg/dL, and creatinine 0.8 mg/dL. Urine toxicology screen is positive for cocaine metabolites. Which next step is most appropriate in this patient's management?

A. Electroencephalogram (EEG)
B. IV loading with antiepileptic medication
C. Lumbar puncture
D. Magnetic resonance imaging
E. Substance abuse counseling

39. All of the following statements regarding epilepsy are true EXCEPT:

A. The incidence of suicide is higher in epileptic patients than it is in the general population.
B. Mortality is no different in patients with epilepsy than it is in age-matched controls.
C. A majority of patients with epilepsy that is completely controlled with medication eventually will be able to discontinue therapy and remain seizure-free.
D. Surgery for mesial temporal lobe epilepsy (MTLE) decreases the number of seizures in over 70% of patients.
E. Tricyclic antidepressants lower the seizure threshold and may precipitate seizures.

40. A 20-year-old woman is brought to the emergency department after a witnessed generalized tonic-clonic seizure. She has no identifying information, and her past medical history is unknown. What is the most likely cause of her seizure?

A. Amyloid angiopathy
B. Fever
C. Genetic disorder
D. Illicit drug use
E. Uremia

41. A 36-year-old man is brought to the emergency department because of a seizure. His family reports he has a history of seizure disorder but stopped his medications a month ago due to financial issues. He had a brief seizure at home that stopped within

41. (*Continued*)
a few minutes. However, 15 minutes later he began seizing again and the tonic-clonic activity has persisted for 30 minutes. On physical examination he is afebrile, hypertensive, and actively seizing. All of the following are potential therapies for his condition EXCEPT:

A. Carbamazepine
B. Fosphenytoin
C. Lorazepam
D. Phenobarbital
E. Valproate

42. The most common cause of a cerebral embolism is:

A. Atrial fibrillation
B. Cardiac prosthetic valves
C. Dilated cardiomyopathy
D. Endocarditis
E. Rheumatic heart disease

43. A 54-year-old male is referred to your clinic for evaluation of atrial fibrillation. He first noted the irregular heartbeat 2 weeks ago and presented to his primary care physician. He denies chest pain, shortness of breath, nausea, or gastrointestinal symptoms. Past medical history is unremarkable. There is no history of hypertension, diabetes, or tobacco use. His medications include metoprolol. The examination is notable for a blood pressure of 126/74 mmHg and a pulse of 64 beats/min. The jugular venous pressure is not elevated. His heart is irregularly irregular, with normal S_1 and S_2. The lungs are clear, and there is no peripheral edema. An echocardiogram shows a left atrial size of 3.6 cm. Left ventricular ejection fraction is 60%. There are no valvular or structural abnormalities. Which of the following statements regarding his atrial fibrillation and stroke risk is true?

A. He requires no antiplatelet therapy or anticoagulation because the risk of embolism is low.
B. Lifetime vitamin K antagonist therapy is indicated for atrial fibrillation in this situation to reduce the risk of stroke.
C. He should be admitted to the hospital for IV heparin and undergo electrical cardioversion; afterward there is no need for anticoagulation.
D. His risk of an embolic stroke is less than 1%, and he should take a daily aspirin.
E. He should be started on SC low-molecular-weight heparin and transitioned to warfarin.

44. All the following have been shown to reduce the risk of atherothrombotic stroke in primary or secondary prevention EXCEPT:

A. Aspirin
B. Blood pressure control
C. Clopidogrel
D. Statin therapy
E. Warfarin

45. A 57-year-old man is brought to the emergency department after falling while playing tennis and developing garbled speech. He has a past history of hypertension and hypercholesterolemia. His medications include atorvastatin and enalapril. On physical examination, his blood pressure is 210/115 mmHg with heart rate 105 beats/min, respirations 28 breaths/min, temperature 37°C (98.6°F), and oxygen saturation 94% on room air. He is alert but aphasic with upper and lower left extremity hemiparesis. He is able to move his right side normally. Based on the results of immediate imaging, all of the following are potential therapeutic considerations for his condition EXCEPT:

A. Anticoagulation
B. Blood pressure lowering
C. Hypothermia protocol
D. Intracerebral stent placement
E. IV thrombolysis

46. A 72-year-old right-handed male with a history of atrial fibrillation and chronic alcoholism is evaluated for dementia. His son gives a history of a stepwise decline in the patient's function over the last 5 years with the accumulation of mild focal neurologic deficits. On examination he is found to have a pseudobulbar affect, mildly increased muscle tone, and brisk deep-tendon reflexes in the right upper extremity and an extensor plantar response on the left. The history and examination are most consistent with which of the following?

A. Alzheimer's disease
B. Binswanger's disease
C. Creutzfeldt-Jakob disease
D. Multi-infarct dementia
E. Vitamin B_{12} deficiency

47. A 49-year-old woman presents for a second opinion regarding symptoms of tremors, difficulty with ambulation, and periodic flushing. Her symptoms originally began approximately 3 years ago. At that time, she was hospitalized for a syncopal episode, after which she was told to increase her salt intake. Since then, she has had progressive motor difficulties including bilateral tremors and a stiff, slow gait. She also has had several more episodes of syncope. She states that she knows when these syncopal events will occur because she feels faint and weak. She has never had an injury from syncope. A final recent symptom has been periodic flushing

47. (*Continued*)
and sweating. A neurologist previously diagnosed her with Parkinson's disease and prescribed therapy with ropinirole. Despite increasing doses, she does not feel improved, but rather has recently noticed uncontrollable movements that she describes as tics of her face. Her only other medical history is recent recurrent urinary tract infections. Her medications are ropinirole 24 mg daily and nitrofurantoin 100 mg daily. She reports no history of drug use. On physical examination, her blood pressure is 130/70 mmHg with a heart rate of 78 beats/min while sitting. Upon standing, her blood pressure drops to 90/50 mmHg with a heart rate of 110 beats/min. Her ocular movements are full and intact. She has recurrent motor movements of the right side of her face. Her neurologic examination shows increased muscle tone in the lower extremities with bilateral 4-Hz tremor. Deep tendon reflexes are brisk and 3+ in upper and lower extremities. Three beats of myoclonus are present at the ankles bilaterally. She walks with a spastic gait. Strength is normal. What is the most likely diagnosis?

A. Corticobasal degeneration
B. Diffuse Lewy body dementia
C. Drug-induced Parkinson's disease
D. Multiple system atrophy with parkinsonian features
E. Parkinson's disease with inadequate treatment

48. A 65-year-old man presents to your office complaining of a tremor and progressive gait abnormalities. He states that he first noticed a slowing of his gait approximately 6 months ago. He has difficulty rising to a standing position and states that he shuffles when he walks. In addition, he states that his right hand shakes more so than his left, and he is right handed. He believes it to be worse when not moving but states there are times when he spills his morning coffee because of the tremors. He has retired but states he is not able to play tennis and golf any longer because of his motor symptoms. He denies syncope or presyncope, difficulty swallowing, changes to his voice, or memory difficulties. His past medical history is significant for hypertension and hypercholesterolemia. His medications are hydrochlorothiazide 25 mg daily, ezetimibe 10 mg daily, and lovastatin 40 mg daily. He drinks a glass of wine with dinner daily and is a lifelong nonsmoker. On physical examination, he has masked facies. His gait shows decreased arm swing with slow shuffling steps. He turns en bloc. A pill-rolling tremor is present on the right side. There is cogwheel rigidity bilaterally. Eye movements are full and intact. There is no orthostatic hypotension. A

48. (*Continued*)
brain MRI with gadolinium shows no evidence of mass lesions, hydrocephalus, or vascular disease. You diagnose the patient with Parkinson's disease. The patient asks about his prognosis and likelihood of disability. Which of the following is correct about the clinical course and treatment of Parkinson's disease?

A. Early initiation of therapy with levodopa predisposes an individual to a higher likelihood of dyskinesias early in the disease.
B. Early therapy with bilateral deep-brain stimulation of the subthalamic nuclei slows the progression of Parkinson's disease.
C. Initial treatment with a dopamine agonist such as pramipexole is likely to be effective in controlling his motor symptoms for 1–3 years before the addition of levodopa or another agent is necessary.
D. Levodopa should be started immediately to prevent the development of disabling rigidity.
E. MAO inhibitors are contraindicated once the diagnosis of Parkinson's disease is established.

49. All of the following statements regarding restless legs syndrome (RLS) are true EXCEPT:

A. Dopamine antagonists are effective therapy.
B. Most patients develop symptoms before the age of 30 years old.
C. RLS may cause sleep disorder and daytime hypersomnolence.
D. RLS is more common in Asians than in the general U.S. population.
E. Symptoms may involve the upper extremity.

50. Which of the following statements regarding Alzheimer's disease is true?

A. Delusions are uncommon.
B. It accounts for over half of the cases of significant memory loss in patients over 70 years of age.
C. It typically presents with rapid (<6 months) significant memory loss.
D. Less than 5% of patients present with nonmemory complaints.
E. Pathologically, the most notable abnormalities are in the cerebellar regions.

51. A 63-year-old man seeks medical attention because of progressive weakness of the left foot and lower leg over the last 6 months. The progression has been gradual, and he only noticed it initially because of cramping and tripping while playing squash. He denies back pain. His only medication is atorvastatin. On physical examination, vital signs are normal and the only abnormalities are on neurologic examination. His left leg strength is notably

51. *(Continued)*
diminished in the hip flexors, hip adductors, quadriceps, and calf muscles. There is atrophy of the quadriceps and calf. His ankle and knee reflexes are increased on the left. He has subtle weakness on the right quadriceps. There are no sensory abnormalities in light touch, pinprick, temperature, or proprioception. There are occasional fasciculations of the abdominal muscles. Before diagnosing the patient with amyotrophic lateral sclerosis (ALS), all of the following alternative diagnoses should be ruled out EXCEPT:

A. Cervical spondylosis
B. Foramen magnum tumor
C. Lead poisoning
D. Multifocal motor neuropathy with conduction block
E. Vitamin C deficiency

52. A 42-year-old woman seeks medical attention for a 5- to 6-week history of marked fatigue that is affecting her work. She reports that she has felt some general fatigue but her symptoms are most notable when she starts moving around during the day. She has taken her pulse and it feels fast to her. She reports no loss of consciousness, but does say that she feels lightheaded and has blurred vision after arising. Sitting or lying down improves the symptoms. She has no notable past medical history and takes no medications other than a calcium/vitamin supplement. On physical examination, her supine heart rate is 90 beats/min with blood pressure of 110/70 mmHg. Upon standing her heart rate increases to 130 beats/min and is regular, and her blood pressure standing is 115/75 mmHg. She reports lightheadedness during the episode. An ECG while symptomatic shows sinus tachycardia without any conduction abnormalities. Which of the following is the most likely diagnosis?

A. Addison's disease
B. Autoimmune autonomic neuropathy
C. Diabetic neuropathy
D. Multisystem atrophy
E. Postural orthostatic tachycardia syndrome

53. A 45-year-old male complains of severe right arm pain. He gives a history of having slipped on the ice and severely contusing his right shoulder approximately 6 months ago. Soon thereafter, he developed sharp, knifelike pain in the right arm and forearm that lasted for a few months. There was some arm swelling and warmth. He was evaluated in an urgent care setting. There were no radiographic abnormalities and he was not treated. Since the injury, the pain and swelling have persisted.

53. *(Continued)*
Physical examination reveals a right arm that is more moist and hairy than the left arm. There is no specific weakness or sensory change. However, the right arm is clearly more edematous than the left, and the skin appears shiny and cool. The patient's pain most likely is due to:

A. Acromioclavicular separation
B. Brachial plexus injury
C. Cervical radiculopathy
D. Complex regional pain syndrome
E. Subclavian vein thrombosis

54. Which of the following criteria suggests the diagnosis of trigeminal neuralgia?

A. Deep-seated, steady facial pain
B. Elevated erythrocyte sedimentation rate (ESR)
C. Objective signs of sensory loss on physical examination
D. Response to gabapentin therapy
E. None of the above

55. A 72-year-old woman presents with recurrent episodes of incapacitating facial pain lasting from second to minutes and then dissipating. The episodes occur usually twice per day, usually without warning, but are also occasionally provoked by brushing of her teeth. On physical examination, she appears well with normal vital signs. Detailed cranial nerve examination reveals no sensory or motor abnormalities. The remainder of her neurologic examination is normal. What is the next step in her management?

A. Brain MRI
B. Brain MRI plus carbamazepine therapy
C. Carbamazepine therapy
D. Glucocorticoid therapy
E. Referral to Otolaryngology for surgical cure

56. A 72-year-old female presents with brief, intermittent excruciating episodes of lancinating pain in the lips, gums, and cheek. Touching the lips or moving the tongue can initiate these intense spasms of pain. The results of a physical examination are normal. MRI of the head is also normal. The most likely cause of this patient's pain is:

A. Acoustic neuroma
B. Amyotrophic lateral sclerosis
C. Meningioma
D. Trigeminal neuralgia
E. Facial nerve palsy

57. A 33-year-old woman presents with rapidly worsening pain at the top of the back over the last 3 days. The pain is not relieved by lying down or by wearing a soft neck collar. She notes that the pain is much worse with movement and has woken her

57. (*Continued*)
from sleep. The pain is severe and is impeding her daily activities. She denies any arm pain or weakness. There is no history of prior back or neck pain, trauma, or arthritis. She works as a postal delivery agent and her only physical activity is walking. She is monogamous with her husband and has no illicit activities. Her family history is notable for an aunt and mother with breast cancer. Her MRI is shown in Figure 57. Which is the most likely diagnosis?

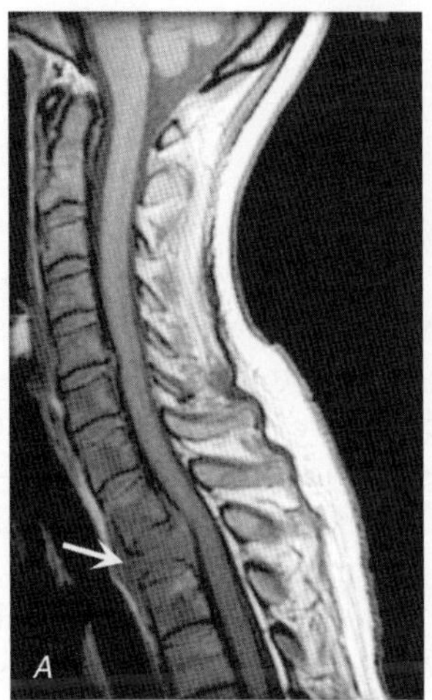

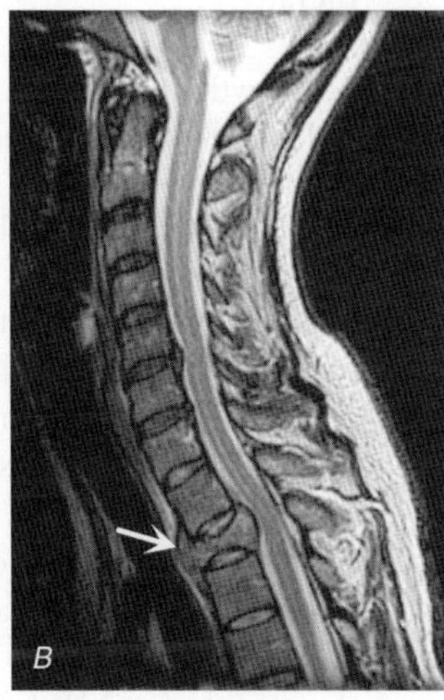

FIGURE 57

A. Cervical spondylosis
B. Hematomyelia
C. Metastatic breast cancer
D. Spinal epidural abscess
E. Spinal epidural hematoma

58. A 34-year-old female complains of lower extremity weakness for the last 3 days. She has noted progressive weakness in the lower extremities with loss of sensation "below the belly button" and incontinence. She had had some low-grade fevers for the last week. She denies recent travel. Past medical history is unremarkable. Physical examination is notable for a sensory level at the level of the umbilicus. The lower extremities show +3/5 strength bilaterally proximally and distally. Reflexes, cerebellar examination, and mental status are normal. All of the following are appropriate steps in evaluating this patient EXCEPT:

A. Antinuclear antibodies
B. Electromyography
C. Lumbar puncture
D. MRI of the spine
E. Viral serologies

59. Which of the following statements about syringomyelia is true?

A. More than half the cases are associated with Chiari malformations.

59. (*Continued*)

B. Symptoms typically begin in middle age.
C. Vibration and position sensation are usually diminished.
D. Syrinx cavities are always congenital.
E. Neurosurgical decompression is usually effective in relieving the symptoms.

60. A 17-year-old adolescent is seen in the clinic several weeks after he suffered a concussion during a high-school football game. At the time of the event, paramedics reported that he experienced no loss of consciousness but was confused for a period of about 10 minutes. Head imaging was normal. He describes a generalized headache that is present all the time since his trauma, and he occasionally feels dizzy. His mother is concerned that he is having a hard time concentrating in school and seems depressed to her lately; she describes him as being very energetic prior to his concussion. The patient's physical examination is entirely normal except for a somewhat flattened affect. Which of the following statements regarding his condition is true?

A. He has an excellent prognosis.
B. He meets the criteria for postconcussive syndrome and should improve over 1–2 months.
C. He should avoid contact sports for 2 weeks.
D. He is most likely malingering.
E. Low-dose narcotics should be started for headache.

61. A 68-year-old man is brought to the clinic by his wife for evaluation. She has noticed that over past 2–3 months her husband has had increasingly slowed thinking and a change in his personality in that he has become very withdrawn. His only complaint is a mild but persistent, diffuse headache. There is no history of head trauma, prior neurologic or psychiatric disease, or family history of dementia. Physical examination is only notable for a moderate cognitive deficit with a mini-mental examination of 19/30. His head CT is shown in Figure 61. What is the most likely diagnosis?

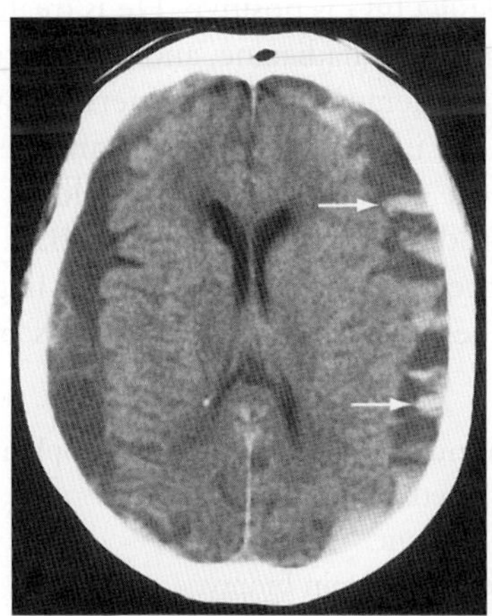

FIGURE 61

61. (*Continued*)

A. Acute epidural hematoma
B. Acute subarachnoid hemorrhage
C. Alzheimer's disease
D. Chronic subdural hematomas
E. Normal-pressure hydrocephalus

62. A 76-year-old nursing home resident is brought to the local emergency department after falling out of bed. The fall was not witnessed; however, she was suspected to have hit her head. She is not responsive to verbal or light tactile stimuli. At baseline she is able to converse but is frequently disoriented to place and time. She has a medical history that includes stable coronary disease, mild emphysema, and multi-infarct dementia. Immediately after triage she is taken for a CT scan of the head. Which of the following is true regarding head injury and hematomas?

A. More than 80% of patients with subdural hematomas will experience a lucid interval prior to loss of consciousness.
B. Epidural hematomas generally arise from venous sources.
C. Epidural hematomas are common among the elderly with minor head trauma.
D. Most patients presenting with epidural hematomas are unconscious.
E. Subdural hematomas lead to rapid increases in intracranial pressure and can require arterial ligation.

63. A 49-year-old man is admitted to the hospital with a seizure. He does not have a history of seizures and he currently takes no medications. He has AIDS and is not under any care at this time. His physical examination is most notable for small, shoddy lymphadenopathy in the cervical region. A head CT shows a ring-enhancing lesion in the right temporal lobe, with edema but no mass effect. A lumbar puncture shows no white or red blood cells, and the Gram stain is negative. His serum *Toxoplasma* IgG is positive. He is treated with pyrimethamine, sulfadiazine, and levetiracetam. After 2 weeks of therapy the central nervous system (CNS) lesion has not changed in size and he has not had any more seizures. All microbiologic cultures and viral studies, including Epstein-Barr virus DNA from the cerebrospinal fluid, are negative. What is the best course of action for this patient at this time?

A. Continue treatment for CNS toxoplasmosis.
B. Dexamethasone.
C. IV acyclovir.
D. Stereotactic brain biopsy.
E. Whole-brain radiation therapy.

64. A young man with a history of a low-grade astrocytoma comes into your office complaining of weight gain and low energy. He is status post resection of his low-grade astrocytoma and had a course of whole-brain radiation therapy (WBRT) 1 year ago. A laboratory workup reveals a decreased morning cortisol level of 1.9 μg/dL. In addition to depressed adrenocorticotropic hormone (ACTH) function, which of the following hormones is most sensitive to damage from whole-brain radiation therapy?

A. Growth hormone
B. Follicle-stimulating hormone
C. Prolactin
D. Thyroid-stimulating hormone

65. A 37-year-old woman with a history of 6 months of worsening headache is admitted to the hospital after a tonic-clonic seizure that occurred at work. The seizure lasted a short time and terminated spontaneously. On examination her vital signs are normal, she is somnolent but awake, and there are no focal abnormalities. Her initial CT scan showed no acute hemorrhage but was abnormal. An MRI is obtained and is shown in Figure 65. What is the most likely diagnosis in this patient?

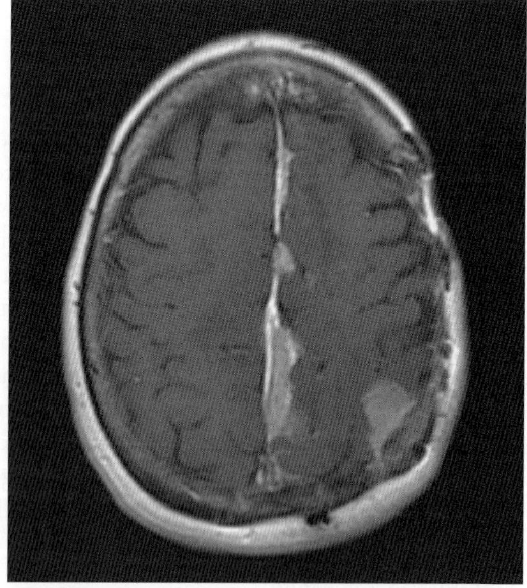

FIGURE 65

A. Brain abscess
B. Glioblastoma
C. Low-grade astrocytoma
D. Meningioma
E. Oligodendroglioma

66. All of the following hormones are produced by the anterior pituitary EXCEPT:

A. Adrenocorticotropic hormone
B. Growth hormone
C. Oxytocin
D. Prolactin
E. Thyroid-stimulating hormone

67. A 22-year-old woman who is otherwise healthy undergoes an uneventful vaginal delivery of a full-term infant. One day postpartum she complains of visual changes and severe headache. Two hours after these complaints, she is found unresponsive and profoundly hypotensive. She is intubated and placed on mechanical ventilation. Her blood pressure is 68/28 mmHg, heart rate is regular at 148 beats/min, and oxygen saturation is 95% on FiO_2 0.40. Physical exam is unremarkable. Her laboratories are notable for glucose of 49 mg/dL and normal hematocrit and white blood cell count. Which of the following is most likely to reverse her hypotension?

A. Activated drotrecogin alfa
B. Hydrocortisone
C. Piperacillin/tazobactam
D. T_4
E. Transfusion of packed red blood cells

68. A 45-year-old man reports to his primary care physician that his wife has noted coarsening of his facial features over several years. In addition, he reports low libido and decreased energy. Physical examination shows frontal bossing and enlarged hands. An MRI confirms that he has a pituitary mass. Which of the following screening tests should be ordered to diagnose the cause of the mass?

A. 24-hour urinary free cortisol
B. ACTH assay
C. Growth hormone level
D. Serum IGF-1 level
E. Serum prolactin level

69. All of the following are potential causes of hyperprolactinemia EXCEPT:

A. Cirrhosis
B. Hirsutism
C. Nipple stimulation
D. Opiate abuse
E. Rathke's cyst

70. A 28-year-old woman presents to her primary care physician's office with 1 year of amenorrhea. She reports mild galactorrhea and headaches. Although she is sexually active, a urine pregnancy test is negative. Serum prolactin level is elevated and she is subsequently diagnosed with a microscopic prolactinoma. Which of the following represents the primary goal of bromocriptine therapy for her condition?

A. Control of hyperprolactinemia
B. Reduction in tumor size
C. Resolution of galactorrhea
D. Restoration of menses and fertility
E. All of the above

71. A 58-year-old man undergoes severe head trauma and develops pituitary insufficiency. After recovery, he is placed on thyroid hormone, testosterone, glucocorticoids, and vasopressin. On a routine visit he questions his primary care physician regarding potential growth hormone deficiency. All of the following are potential signs or symptoms of growth hormone deficiency EXCEPT:

A. Abnormal lipid profile
B. Atherosclerosis
C. Increased bone mineral density
D. Increased waist:hip ratio
E. Left ventricular dysfunction

72. A 75-year-old man presents with development of abdominal obesity, proximal myopathy, and skin hyperpigmentation. His laboratory evaluation shows a hypokalemic metabolic alkalosis. Cushing's syndrome is suspected. Which of the following statements regarding this syndrome is true?

A. Basal ACTH level is likely to be low.
B. Circulating corticotropin-releasing hormone is likely to be elevated.
C. Pituitary MRI will visualize all ACTH-secreting tumors.
D. Referral for urgent performance of inferior petrosal venous sampling is indicated.
E. Serum potassium level below 3.3 mmol/L is suggestive of ectopic ACTH production.

73. A 23-year-old college student is followed in the student health center for medical management of panhypopituitarism after resection of craniopharyngioma as a child. She reports moderate compliance with her medications but feels generally well. A TSH is checked and is below the limits of detection of the assay. Which of the following is the next most appropriate action?

A. Decrease levothyroxine dose to half of current dose.
B. Do nothing.
C. Order free T_4 level.
D. Order MRI of her brain.
E. Order thyroid uptake scan.

74. A 23-year-old woman presents to the clinic complaining of months of weight gain, fatigue, amenorrhea, and worsening acne. She cannot precisely identify when her symptoms began, but she reports that without a change in her diet she has noted a 12.3-kg weight gain over the past 6 months. She has been amenorrheic for several months. On examination she is noted to have truncal obesity with bilateral purplish striae across both flanks. Cushing's syndrome is suspected. Which of the following tests should be used to make the diagnosis?

A. 24-hour urine free cortisol
B. Basal adrenocorticotropic hormone (ACTH)
C. Corticotropin-releasing hormone (CRH) level at 8 am
D. Inferior petrosal venous sampling
E. Overnight 1-mg dexamethasone suppression test

75. A patient visited a local emergency room 1 week ago with a headache. She received a head MRI, which did not reveal a cause for her symptoms, but the final report states, "An empty sella is noted. Advise clinical correlation." The patient was discharged from the emergency department with instructions to follow up with her primary care physician as soon as possible. Her headache has resolved, and the patient has no complaints; however, she comes to your office 1 day later very concerned about this unexpected MRI finding. What should be the next step in her management?

A. Diagnose her with subclinical panhypopituitarism, and initiate low-dose hormone replacement.
B. Reassure her and follow laboratory results closely.
C. Reassure her and repeat MRI in 6 months.
D. This may represent early endocrine malignancy—whole-body positron emission tomography/CT is indicated.
E. This MRI finding likely represents the presence of a benign adenoma—refer to neurosurgery for resection.

76. All of the following are frequent initial symptoms of multiple sclerosis EXCEPT:

A. Optic neuritis
B. Paresthesias
C. Sensory loss
D. Visual loss
E. Weakness

77. Which of the following is the most common clinical classification of multiple sclerosis?

A. Autoimmune autonomic neuropathy
B. Primary progressive
C. Progressive relapsing
D. Relapsing/remitting
E. Secondary progressive

78. Lumbar puncture should be preceded by CT or MRI in all of the following subsets of patients suspected of having meningitis EXCEPT those with:

A. Depressed consciousness
B. Focal neurologic abnormality
C. Known central nervous system (CNS) mass lesion
D. Positive Kernig's sign
E. Recent head trauma

79. A 78-year-old man with diabetes mellitus presents with fever, headache, and altered sensorium. On physical exam his temperature is 40.2°C (104.4°F), heart rate is 103 beats/min, and blood pressure is 84/52 mmHg. His neck is stiff and he has photophobia. His cerebrospinal fluid (CSF) examination shows 2100 cells/μL, with 100% neutrophils, glucose 10 mg/dL, and protein 78 mg/dL. CSF Gram stain is negative. In addition to empiric antibacterial antibiotics, initial therapy should include which of the following?

A. Acyclovir
B. Dexamethasone after antibiotics
C. Dexamethasone prior to antibiotics
D. IV γ globulin
E. Valacyclovir

80. Which of the following groups of patients should receive empirical antibiotic therapy that includes coverage of *Listeria monocytogenes* in cases of presumed meningitis?

A. Immunocompromised patients
B. Elderly patients
C. Infants
D. All of the above

81. Which of the following medicines has been most commonly implicated in the development of noninfectious chronic meningitis?

A. Acetaminophen
B. Acyclovir
C. β-lactam antibiotics
D. Ibuprofen
E. Phenobarbital

82. Variant Creutzfeldt-Jakob disease (vCJD) has been diagnosed in which of the following populations?

A. Family members with well-defined germ-line mutations leading to autosomal dominant inheritance of a fatal neurodegenerative disease
B. New Guinea natives practicing cannibalism
C. Patients accidentally inoculated with infected material during surgical procedures
D. Worldwide, in sporadic cases, mostly during the fifth and sixth decades of life
E. Young adults in Europe thought to have been exposed to tainted beef products

83. The presence of startle myoclonus in a 60-year-old man with rapidly progressive deficits in cortical dysfunction is which of the following?

A. Neither sensitive nor specific for Creutzfeldt-Jacob disease (CJD) but does represent grounds to explore further for this condition with an electroencephalogram (EEG)
B. Neither sensitive nor specific for CJD but does represent grounds to explore further for this condition with an EEG and brain MRI
C. Sensitive but not specific for CJD and is not enough to prompt a further workup for this condition unless other clinical criteria are met
D. Specific but not sensitive for CJD and should therefore prompt immediate referral for brain biopsy to confirm the diagnosis
E. Virtually diagnostic for CJD, and further workup including EEG, brain MRI, and perhaps brain biopsy serves only a prognostic purpose

84. A 55-year-old woman presents with progressive incoordination. Physical examination is remarkable for nystagmus, mild dysarthria, and past pointing on finger-to-nose testing. She also has an unsteady gait. MRI reveals atrophy of both lobes of the cerebellum. Serologic evaluation reveals the presence of anti-Yo antibody. Which of the following is the most likely cause of this clinical syndrome?

A. Non–small cell cancer of the lung
B. Small cell cancer of the lung
C. Breast cancer
D. Non-Hodgkin's lymphoma
E. Colon cancer

85. A 24-year-old man presents for evaluation of foot-drop. He has noted that for the last several months, he has had difficulty picking his feet up to walk up stairs and over thresholds. His right leg is more affected than his left leg. He has not noted any sensory changes. He has several family members with similar complaints. His exam is notable for distal leg weakness with reduced sensation to light touch in both lower extremities. Knee and ankle jerk reflexes are unobtainable. Calves are reduced in size bilaterally. Upper extremity examination is normal. Which of the following is the most likely diagnosis?

A. Charcot-Marie-Tooth syndrome
B. Fabry disease
C. Guillain-Barré syndrome
D. Hereditary neuralgic amyotrophy
E. Hereditary sensory and autonomic neuropathy

86. A 57-year-old immigrant from Vietnam is evaluated by his primary caregiver for dysesthesias that have been present in his hands and feet for the past several weeks. He also reports some difficulty walking. His past medical history is notable for hypertriglyceridemia, tobacco abuse, and a recently discovered positive PPD with sputum that is smear-negative for *Mycobacterium tuberculosis*. His medications include niacin, aspirin, and isoniazid. Which of the following is likely to reverse his symptoms?

A. Cobalamin
B. Levothyroxine
C. Neurontin
D. Pregabalin
E. Pyridoxine

87. A 52-year-old woman with long-standing, poorly controlled type 2 diabetes mellitus is evaluated for a sensation of numbness in her fingers and toes, as if she is wearing gloves and socks all the time. She also reports tingling and burning in the same location, but no weakness. Her symptoms have been intermittently present for the last several months. After a thorough evaluation, nerve biopsy is obtained and demonstrates axonal degeneration, endothelial hyperplasia, and perivascular inflammation. Which of the following statements regarding this condition is true?

A. Autonomic neuropathy is rarely seen in combination with sensory neuropathy.
B. The presence of retinopathy or nephropathy does not portend increased risk for diabetic neuropathy.
C. This is the most common cause of peripheral neuropathy in developed countries.
D. Tight glucose control from now on will reverse her neuropathy.
E. None of the above is true.

88. All the following cause primarily a sensory neuropathy EXCEPT:

A. Acromegaly
B. Critical illness
C. HIV infection
D. Hypothyroidism
E. Vitamin B_{12} deficiency

89. A 50-year-old male complains of weakness and numbness in the hands for the last month. He describes paresthesias in the thumb and the index and middle fingers. The symptoms are worse at night. He also describes decreased grip strength bilaterally. He works as a mechanical engineer. The patient denies fevers, chills, or weight loss. The examination is notable for atrophy of the thenar eminences bilaterally and decreased sensation in a median nerve distribution. You consider the diagnosis of carpal

89. (*Continued*)
tunnel syndrome. All the following are causes of carpal tunnel syndrome EXCEPT:

A. Amyloidosis
B. Chronic lymphocytic leukemia
C. Diabetes mellitus
D. Hypothyroidism
E. Rheumatoid arthritis

90. A 27-year-old woman is diagnosed with Guillain-Barré syndrome after presenting with flaccid paralysis and sensory disturbance several weeks after a diarrheal illness. Which of the following bacteria have been implicated in cases of Guillain-Barré syndrome?

A. *Bartonella* henselae
B. *Campylobacter jejuni*
C. *Escherichia coli*
D. *Proteus mirabilis*
E. *Tropheryma whippelii*

91. A 34-year-old female complains of weakness and double vision for the last 3 weeks. She has also noted a change in her speech, and her friends tell her that she is "more nasal." She has noticed decreased exercise tolerance and difficulty lifting objects and getting out of a chair. The patient denies pain. The symptoms are worse at the end of the day and with repeated muscle use. You suspect myasthenia gravis. All the following are useful in the diagnosis of myasthenia gravis EXCEPT:

A. Acetylcholine receptor (AChR) antibodies
B. Edrophonium
C. Electrodiagnostic testing
D. Muscle-specific kinase (MuSK) antibodies
E. Voltage-gated calcium channel antibodies

92. A 38-year-old female patient with facial and ocular weakness has just been diagnosed with myasthenia gravis. You intend to initiate therapy with anticholinesterase medications and glucocorticoids. All of the following tests are necessary before instituting this therapy EXCEPT:

A. MRI of mediastinum
B. Purified protein derivative skin test
C. Lumbar puncture
D. Pulmonary function tests
E. Thyroid-stimulating hormone

93. All of the following lipid-lowering agents are associated with muscle toxicity EXCEPT:

A. Atorvastatin.
B. Ezetimibe.
C. Gemfibrozil.
D. Niacin.
E. All of the above are associated with muscle toxicity.

94. All of the following endocrine conditions are associated with myopathy EXCEPT:

A. Hypothyroidism.
B. Hyperparathyroidism.
C. Hyperthyroidism.
D. Acromegaly.
E. All of the above are associated with myopathy.

95. A 34-year-old woman seeks evaluation for weakness. She has noted tripping when walking, particularly in her left foot, for the past 2 years. She recently also began to drop things, once allowing a full cup of coffee to spill onto her legs. In this setting, she also feels as if the appearance of her face has changed over the course of many years, stating that she feels as if her face is becoming more hollow and elongated, although she hasn't lost any weight recently. She has not seen a physician in many years and has no past medical history. Her only medications are a multivitamin and calcium with vitamin D. Her family history is significant for similar symptoms of weakness in her brother who is 2 years older. Her mother, who is 58 years old, was diagnosed with mild weakness after her brother was evaluated, but is not symptomatic. On physical examination, the patient's face appears long and narrow with wasting of the temporalis and masseter muscles. Her speech is mildly dysarthric, and the palate is high and arched. Strength is 4/5 in the intrinsic muscles of the hand, wrist extensors, and ankle dorsiflexors. After testing handgrip strength, you notice that there is a delayed relaxation of the muscles of the hand. What is the most likely diagnosis?

A. Acid maltase deficiency (Pompe's disease)
B. Becker muscular dystrophy
C. Duchenne muscular dystrophy
D. Myotonic dystrophy
E. Nemaline myopathy

96. An elevation in which of the following serum enzymes is the most *sensitive* indicator of myositis?

A. Aldolase
B. Creatinine kinase
C. Glutamic-oxaloacetic transaminase
D. Glutamate pyruvate transaminase
E. Lactate dehydrogenase

97. A 64-year-old woman is evaluated for weakness. For several weeks she has had difficulty brushing her teeth and combing her hair. She has also noted a rash on her face. Examination is notable for a heliotrope rash and proximal muscle weakness. Serum creatine kinase (CK) is elevated and she is

97. (*Continued*)
diagnosed with dermatomyositis. After evaluation by a rheumatologist, she is found to have anti-Jo-1 antibodies. She is also likely to have which of the following findings?

A. Ankylosing spondylitis
B. Inflammatory bowel disease
C. Interstitial lung disease
D. Primary biliary cirrhosis
E. Psoriasis

98. A 63-year-old woman is evaluated for a rash on her eyes and fatigue for 1 month. She reports difficulty with arm and leg strength and constant fatigue, but no fevers or sweats. She also notes that she has a red discoloration around her eyes. She has hypothyroidism but is otherwise well. On examination she has a heliotrope rash and proximal muscle weakness. A diagnosis of dermatomyositis is made after demonstration of elevated serum creatinine kinase and confirmatory EMGs. Which of the following studies should be performed as well to look for associated conditions?

A. Mammogram
B. Serum antinuclear antibody measurement
C. Stool examination for ova and parasites
D. Thyroid-stimulating immunoglobulins
E. Titers of antibodies to varicella zoster

99. You are seeing your patient with polymyositis for follow-up. He has been taking prednisone at high doses for 2 months, and you initiated mycophenolate mofetil at the last clinic visit for a steroid-sparing effect. He began a steroid taper 2 weeks ago. His symptoms were predominantly in the lower extremities and face, and he has improved considerably. He no longer needs a cane and his voice has returned to normal. Laboratory data show a creatine kinase (CK) of 1300 U/L, which is unchanged from 2 months ago. What is the most appropriate next step in this patient's management?

A. Continue current management.
B. Continue high-dose steroids with no taper.
C. Switch mycophenolate to methotrexate.
D. Repeat muscle biopsy.

100. A 45-year-old woman who is 6 months post–liver transplant is admitted to the hospital after two grand mal seizures in the last 45 minutes. For the last day she has complained about headache and confusion. Her medications include diltiazem, cyclosporine, prednisone, and mycophenolate mofetil. She is now awake but somnolent. Her vital signs are normal except a blood pressure of 150/90 mmHg.

100. (*Continued*)
There is bilateral afferent pupillary defect, and she reports she cannot see out of either eye. Hearing is intact. There is no nuchal rigidity. Her cyclosporine level is therapeutic. The FLAIR image of her MRI is shown in **Figure 100**. Which of the following is the most likely diagnosis?

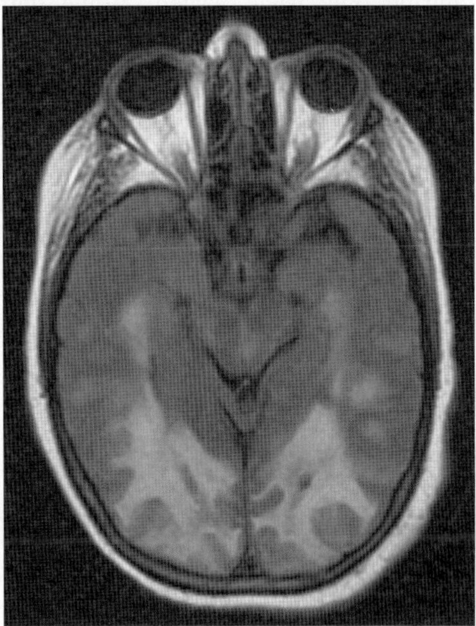

FIGURE 100

A. Acoustic neuroma
B. Calcineurin-inhibitor toxicity
C. Panhypopituitarism
D. Streptococcal meningitis
E. Tuberculous meningitis

101. A 77-year-old man undergoes coronary artery bypass grafting for refractory angina and three-vessel disease. Prior to surgery he still worked as a classics professor at a university teaching a renowned course on Dante's "Inferno." One month after surgery, his cardiac status is normal and his exercise tolerance is better than presurgery. However, his wife reports that he seems depressed and is often confused. His short-term memory is poor and he exhibits no enthusiasm for teaching. He has no fever or night sweats. Current medications include lovastatin and lisinopril. His physical examination is normal except for poor performance on serial 7 subtraction and only recalling 1 or 3 objects at 15 minutes. Which of the following is the most likely diagnosis?

A. Multiple sclerosis
B. Post–cardiac bypass brain injury
C. Streptococcal meningitis
D. Variant Creutzfeldt-Jacob disease
E. West Nile virus encephalitis

102. A 24-year-old man is recovering from ARDS due to severe influenza A infection. During his complicated 3-week course of respiratory failure, he was placed on high-frequency ventilation and prone positioning necessitating paralysis and heavy sedation. Passive splints were placed on his upper and lower extremities. He is now extubated and awake, requiring only nasal oxygen. While starting his physical therapy, it is noted that he has right foot-drop and numbness on the lateral leg. Additional examination reveals a unilateral right motor defect in foot dorsiflexion with intact inversion. There is sensory loss of the lateral aspect of the leg below the knee extending to the dorsum of the foot. The rest of the neurologic examination of the right leg and foot appears normal. Which of the following is the most likely etiology of his defects?

A. Cauda equina syndrome
B. Femoral nerve injury
C. L4 radiculopathy
D. L5 radiculopathy
E. Peroneal nerve injury

103. In the CDC diagnostic criteria for chronic fatigue syndrome, in addition to clearly delineated findings of fatigue, all of the following symptoms or findings must be concurrently present for at least 6 months EXCEPT:

A. Delusional disorder
B. Impaired memory or concentration
C. Muscle pain
D. Sore throat
E. Tender cervical or axillary lymph nodes

104. Which of the following is a beneficial therapy for chronic fatigue syndrome?

A. Bupropion
B. Cognitive behavioral therapy
C. Doxycycline
D. Fluoxetine
E. Olanzapine

105. A 26-year-old woman presents to the emergency department complaining of shortness of breath and chest pain. These symptoms began abruptly and became progressively worse over 10 minutes, prompting her to call 911. Over this same period, the patient describes feeling her heart pounding and states that she felt like she was dying. She feels lightheaded and dizzy. It is currently about 20 minutes since the onset of symptoms and the severity has abated, although she continues to feel not back to her baseline. She denies any immediate precipitating cause, although she has been under increased stress as her mother has been hospitalized recently with advanced breast cancer. She does not take any medications and has no medical history. She denies tobacco, alcohol, or drug use. On initial examination, she appears somewhat anxious and diaphoretic. Her initial vital signs show a heart rate of 108 beats/min, blood pressure 122/68 mmHg, and respiratory rate 20 breaths/min. She is afebrile. Her examination is normal. Her arterial blood gas shows a pH of 7.52, Pa_{CO_2} of 28 mmHg, and Pa_{O_2} of 116 mmHg. The ECG is normal as is a chest radiograph. What is the next best step in the management of this patient?

A. Initiate therapy with alprazolam 0.5 mg four times daily.
B. Initiate therapy with fluoxetine 20 mg daily.
C. Perform a CT pulmonary angiogram.
D. Reassure the patient and suggest medical and/or psychological therapy if symptoms recur on a frequent basis.
E. Refer for cognitive behavioral therapy.

106. All of the following antidepressant medications are correctly paired with their class of medication EXCEPT:

A. Duloxetine—Selective serotonin reuptake inhibitor
B. Fluoxetine—Selective serotonin reuptake inhibitor
C. Nortriptyline—Tricyclic antidepressant
D. Phenelzine—Monoamine oxidase inhibitor
E. Venlafaxine—Mixed norepinephrine/serotonin reuptake inhibitor and receptor blocker

107. A 42-year-old woman seeks your advice regarding symptoms concerning for post-traumatic stress disorder. She was the victim of a home invasion 6 months previously where she was robbed and beaten by a man at gunpoint. She thought she was going to die and was hospitalized with multiple blunt force injuries including a broken nose and zygomatic arch. She now states that she is unable to be alone in her home and frequently awakens with dreams of the event. She is irritable with her husband and children and cries frequently. She has worsening insomnia and often stays awake most of the night watching out her window because she is afraid her assailant will return. She has begun drinking a bottle of wine nightly to help her fall asleep, although she notes that this has worsened her nightmares in the early morning hours. You concur that post-traumatic stress disorder is likely. What treatment do you recommend for this patient?

A. Avoidance of alcohol
B. Cognitive behavioral therapy
C. Paroxetine 20 mg daily
D. Trazodone 50 mg nightly
E. All of the above

108. A 36-year-old man is being treated with venlafaxine 150 mg twice daily for major depression. He has currently been on the medication for 4 months. After 2 months, his symptoms were inadequately controlled, necessitating an increase in the dose of venlafaxine from 75 mg twice daily. He has had one prior episode of major depression when he was 25. At that time, he was treated with fluoxetine 80 mg daily for 12 months, but found the sexual side effects difficult to tolerate. He asks when he can safely discontinue his medication. What is your advice to the patient?

A. He should continue on the medication indefinitely as his depression is likely to recur.
B. The current medication should be continued for a minimum of 6–9 months following control of his symptoms.
C. The medication can be discontinued safely if he establishes a relationship with a psychotherapist who will monitor his progress and symptoms.
D. The medication can be discontinued safely now as his symptoms are well controlled.
E. The medication should be switched to fluoxetine to complete 12 months of therapy, as this was previously effective for him.

109. Which of the following will lead to a faster rate of absorption of alcohol from the gut into the blood?

A. Coadministration with a carbonated beverage
B. Concentration of alcohol of more than 20% by volume
C. Concurrent intake of a high-carbohydrate meal
D. Concurrent intake of a high-fat meal
E. Concurrent intake of a high-protein meal

110. Which of the following best reflects the effect of alcohol on neurotransmitters in the brain?

A. Decreases dopamine activity
B. Decreases serotonin activity
C. Increases γ-aminobutyric acid activity
D. Stimulates muscarinic acetylcholine receptors
E. Stimulates *N*-methyl-D-aspartate excitatory glutamate receptors

111. In an individual without any prior history of alcohol intake, what serum concentration of ethanol (in grams per deciliter) would likely result in death?

A. 0.02
B. 0.08
C. 0.28
D. 0.40
E. 0.60

112. All of the following statements regarding the epidemiology and genetics of alcoholism are true EXCEPT:

A. Among individuals who have demonstrated alcohol abuse, about 10% will develop true alcohol dependence.
B. Approximately 60% of the risk for alcohol abuse disorders is attributed to genetics.
C. Children of alcoholics have a 10-fold higher risk of alcohol abuse and dependence.
D. The presence of a mutation of aldehyde dehydrogenase that results in intense flushing with alcohol consumption confers a decreased risk of alcohol dependence.
E. The lifetime risk of alcohol dependence in most Western countries is about 10–15% for men and 5–8% for women.

113. A 42-year-old man with alcohol dependence is admitted to the hospital for acute pancreatitis. Upon admission, he has an abdominal CT scan that shows edema without necrosis or hemorrhage of the pancreas. He is treated with IV fluids with dextrose, multivitamins, thiamine 50 mg daily, pain control, and bowel rest. He typically drinks 24 12-ounce beers daily. Forty-eight hours after admission, you are called because the patient is febrile and combative with the nursing staff. His vital signs demonstrate a heart rate of 132 beats/min, blood pressure of 184/96 mmHg, respiratory rate of 32 breaths/min, temperature of 38.7°C (101.7°F), and oxygen saturation of 94% on room air. He is agitated, diaphoretic, and pacing his room. He is oriented to person only. His neurologic examination appears nonfocal, although he does not cooperate. He is tremulous. What is the next step in the management of this patient?

A. Administer a bolus of 1 L of normal saline and thiamine 100 mg IV.
B. Administer diazepam 10–20 mg IV followed by bolus doses of 5–10 mg as needed until the patient is calm but able to be aroused.
C. Perform an emergent head CT.
D. Perform two peripheral blood cultures and begin treatment with imipenem 1 g IV every 8 hours.
E. Place the patient in four-point restraints and treat with haloperidol 5 mg IV.

114. A 48-year-old woman is recovering from alcohol dependence and requests medication to help prevent relapse. She has a medical history of stroke occurring during a hypertensive crisis. Which of the following medications could be considered?

A. Acamprosate
B. Disulfiram

114. (*Continued*)

C. Naltrexone
D. A and C
E. All of the above

115. What is the most common initial illicit drug of abuse among U.S. adolescents?

A. Benzodiazepines
B. Heroin
C. Marijuana
D. Methamphetamines
E. Prescription narcotics

116. A 32-year-old woman is admitted to the hospital for drainage and treatment of a soft tissue abscess of her left forearm. She uses IV heroin on a daily basis, often spending $100 or more per day on drugs. Upon admission, she has a 4 × 2-cm fluctuant mass in the left forearm associated with fevers to 39.3°C (102.7°F) and tachycardia. The abscess is drained and packed, and the patient is initiated on therapy with IV clindamycin. About 10 hours after admission, you are called to the patient's bedside for a change in the patient's condition. You are suspecting narcotic withdrawal. All of the following symptoms are consistent with this diagnosis EXCEPT:

A. Hyperthermia
B. Hypotension
C. Piloerection
D. Sweating
E. Vomiting

117. A 24-year-old man is brought to the emergency department by emergency medical services (EMS) about 2 hours after an intentional overdose of sustained-release oxycodone that was taken in conjunction with alcohol. Upon arrival at the scene, emergency medical technicians found an empty bottle of sustained-release oxycodone tablets with a dose of 20 mg. It is unknown how many pills the patient ingested, but the prescription was written for 60 tablets. The patient was unresponsive with a respiratory rate of 4 breaths/min, blood pressure of 80/56 mmHg, heart rate of 65 beats/min, and oxygen saturation of 86% on room air. The patient was intubated in the field and naloxone 2 mg IM was administered. He is currently intubated and unresponsive without spontaneous respiration above the set ventilator rate. His blood pressure is 82/50 mmHg and heart rate is 70 beats/min. Which of the following is most appropriate at the present time in the evaluation and treatment of this patient?

A. Activated charcoal
B. IV saline bolus 1 L followed by repeated 500–1000 mL boluses to maintain adequate blood pressure
C. Naloxone continuous infusion at a rate of 0.4 mg/h
D. Urine drug screen, acetaminophen levels, and blood alcohol content
E. All of the above

118. Which of the following statements is TRUE with regard to the chronic effects of marijuana use?

A. Chronic use of marijuana is associated with low testosterone levels.
B. Chronic use of marijuana is the primary cause of amotivational syndrome.
C. Marijuana use is associated with an increased risk of psychotic symptoms in individuals with a past history of schizophrenia.
D. Physical and psychological tolerance does not develop in chronic users of marijuana.
E. There is no withdrawal syndrome associated with cessation of marijuana use.

ANSWERS

1 and 2. The answers are D and D, respectively. (*Chap. 1*) The ability to perform a thorough neurologic examination is an important skill for all internists to master. A careful neurologic examination can localize the site of the lesion and is important in directing further workup. The components of the neurologic examination include mental status, cranial nerves, motor, sensory, gait, and coordination. The motor examination is further characterized by appearance, tone, strength, and reflexes. Pronator drift is a useful tool for determining if upper extremity weakness is present. In this test, an individual is asked to stand with both arms fully extended and parallel to the floor while closing his or her eyes. If the arms flex at the elbows or fingers or there is pronation of the forearm, this is considered a positive test. Other tests of motor strength include tests of maximal effort in a specific muscle or muscle group. Most commonly this type of strength testing is graded from 0 (no movement) to 5 (full power) with varying degrees of weakness noted against resistance. However, many individuals find it more practical to use qualitative grading of strength, such as paralysis, severe weakness, moderate weakness, mild weakness, or full strength.

Babinski sign is a sign of upper motor neuron disease above the level of the S1 vertebra and is characterized by paradoxical extension of the great toe with fanning and extension of the other toes as well. Dysdiadochokinesis refers to the inability to perform rapid alternating movements and is a sign of cerebellar disease. Lhermitte symptom causes electric shock–like sensations in the extremities associated with neck flexion. It has many causes including cervical spondylosis and multiple sclerosis. Romberg sign is performed with an individual standing with feet together and arms at the side. The individual is then asked to close his or her eyes. If the individual begins to sway or fall, this is considered a positive test and is a sign of abnormal proprioception.

3. The answer is C.

(Chap. 1) This patient likely has metastatic disease to the cervical spinal cord. The patient's symptoms are bilateral with sparing of the cranial nerves and normal mental status, localizing the lesion below the level of the brainstem and cerebrum. The patient demonstrates mixed upper and lower motor neuron signs with decreased sphincter tone and a positive Babinski sign, placing the lesion at the level of the spinal cord. As the weakness is involving both the arms and legs, this would indicate a lesion in the lower cervical or upper thoracic spine. Symptoms of abnormalities at the level of the neuromuscular junction include bilateral weakness that can include the face having normal sensation.

4. The answer is C.

(Chap. 4) Appropriate and timely evaluation is needed to determine if a subarachnoid hemorrhage is present as it can be rapidly fatal if undetected. The procedure of choice for initial diagnosis is a CT of the head without IV contrast. On the CT, blood in the subarachnoid space would appear whiter compared to the surrounding brain tissue. The CT of the head is most sensitive when it is performed shortly after the onset of symptoms, but declines over several hours. It can also demonstrate the presence of mass effect and midline shift, factors that increase the severity of the underlying hemorrhage. In the situation where the CT head is negative but clinical suspicion is high, a lumbar puncture can be performed. This may demonstrate increased numbers of red blood cells that do not clear with successive aliquots of cerebrospinal fluid. If the lumbar puncture is performed more than 12 hours after a small subarachnoid hemorrhage, then the red blood cells may begin to decompose, leading to xanthochromia—a yellow to pink coloration of cerebrospinal fluid that can be measured spectrographically. A basic CT of the head with IV contrast is rarely useful in subarachnoid hemorrhage, as the brightness of the contrast material may make it difficult to identify blood in the subarachnoid space. However, a CT angiography that is performed with IV contrast can be useful in identifying the aneurismal vessel leading to the bleeding. Classic angiography is a more direct way to visualize the anatomy of the cranial vasculature and is now often combined with interventional procedures to coiling a bleeding vessel. Transcranial Doppler ultrasound is a test that measures the velocity of blood flow through the cranial vasculature. It is used in some centers following subarachnoid hemorrhage to assess for the development of vasospasm, which can worsen ischemia leading to increased damage to brain tissue following subarachnoid hemorrhage.

5. The answer is E.

(Chap. 4) Magnetic resonance imaging (MRI) is generated from the interaction between the hydrogen protons in biologic tissues, the magnetic field, and the radiofrequency (Rf) of waves generated by the coil placed next to the body part of interest. The Rf pulses transiently excite the protons of the body with a subsequent return to the equilibrium energy state, a process known as relaxation. During relaxation, the protons release Rf energy creating an echo that is then transformed via Fourier analysis to generate the MR image. The two relaxation rates that influence the signal intensity of the image are T1 and T2. T1 refers to the time in milliseconds that it takes for 63% of protons to return to their baseline state. T2 relaxation is the time for 63% of protons to become dephased owing to interactions among nearby protons. The intensity of the signal is also influenced by the interval between Rf pulses (TR) and the time between the Rf pulse and the signal reception (TE). T1-weighted images are produced by keeping both TR and TE relatively short, while T2-weighted images require long TR and TE times. Fat and subacute hemorrhages have relatively shorted TR and TE times and thus appear more brightly on T1-weighted images. Structures with more water such as cerebrospinal fluid or edema conversely have long T1 and T2 relaxation times, resulting in higher signal intensity on T2-weighted images. T2 images are also more sensitive for detecting demyelination, infarction, or chronic hemorrhage.

FLAIR stands for fluid-attenuated inversion recovery and is a type of T2-weighted image that suppresses the high-intensity signal of CSF. Because of this, images created by the FLAIR technique are more sensitive to detecting water-containing lesions or edema than the standard spin images.

MR angiography refers to several different techniques that are useful for assessing vascular structures, but does not provide details of the underlying brain parenchyma.

6. The answer is E.

(Chap. 4) For many years, MRI imaging was considered the modality of choice for patients with renal insufficiency because it does not lead to acute renal failure. However, gadolinium was recently linked to a rare disorder called nephrogenic systemic fibrosis. This newly described disorder results in widespread fibrosis in skin, skeletal muscle, bone, lungs, pleura, pericardium, myocardium, and many other tissues. Histologically, thickened collagen bundles

are seen in the deep dermis of the skin with increased numbers of fibrocytes and elastic fibers. There is no known medical treatment for nephrogenic systemic fibrosis (NSF), although improvement may be seen following kidney transplantation. It has only recently been linked to the receipt of gadolinium-containing contrast agents with a typical onset between 5 and 75 days following administration of the contrast. The incidence of NSF following administration of gadolinium in individuals with a glomerular filtration rate of less than 30 mL/min may be as high as 4% and is thus considered absolutely contraindicated in individuals with severe renal dysfunction.

Pseudohypocalcemia can occur following administration of gadolinium in individuals with renal dysfunction, but not true hypocalcemia. This occurs because of an interaction of the contrast dye with standard colorimetric assays for serum calcium that are commonly used. If ionized calcium is measured it would be normal, often in the face of very low levels of serum calcium.

The other reported complications can be seen following administration of iodinated contrast that is used for CT imaging. The most common complication of CT imaging outside of allergic reactions is the development of worsening renal function or acute renal failure. The risk of this can be minimized if the patient is adequately hydrated. Lactic acidosis is a rare but dreaded side effect of iodinated contrast that has been linked to the coadministration of metformin in diabetic patients. Typically a patient is asked to hold metformin for 48 hours before and after a CT scan. The reason for the development of lactic acidosis is actually related to the development of renal insufficiency and a subsequent buildup of lactic acid. In very rare instances, administration of iodinated contrast can unmask hyperthyroidism.

7. The answer is D.

(Chap. 5) While seldom diagnostic, the EEG can often provide clinically useful information in comatose patients. In patients with an altered mental state or some degree of obtundation, the EEG tends to become slower as consciousness is depressed, regardless of the underlying cause. The EEG generally slows in metabolic encephalopathies, and triphasic waves may be present. The findings do not permit differentiation of the underlying metabolic disturbance but help to exclude other encephalopathic processes by indicating the diffuse extent of cerebral dysfunction. As the depth of coma increases, the EEG becomes nonreactive and may show a burst-suppression pattern, with bursts of mixed-frequency activity separated by intervals of relative cerebral inactivity. The EEG is usually normal in patients with locked-in syndrome and helps in distinguishing this disorder from the comatose state with which it is sometimes confused clinically. Epileptiform activity characterized by bursts of abnormal discharges containing spikes or sharp waves may be useful to diagnose and treat nonconvulsive status in a presumed comatose patient. Patients with herpes simplex encephalitis may show a characteristic pattern of focal (often in the temporal regions) or lateralized periodic slow-wave complexes. Periodic lateralizing epileptiform discharges (PLEDs) are commonly found with acute hemispheric pathology such as a hematoma, abscess, or rapidly expanding tumor.

8. The answer is D.

(Chap. 10) Syncope is a common medical complaint that occurs when there is global cerebral hypoperfusion. Syncope accounts for 3% of all emergency department visits and 1% of all hospitalizations. Additionally, it is estimated that 35% of all individuals will experience at least one syncopal event in their lifetimes. The most common cause of syncope in young adults is neurally mediated syncope. The incidence of neurally mediated syncope is higher in females and has a familial predisposition. Neurally mediated syncope represents a complex reflex arc of the autonomic nervous system and inherently requires an intact autonomic nervous system to occur. The final pathway of neurally mediated syncope is a surge of parasympathetic activity with inhibition of the sympathetic nervous system. This results in hypotension with accompanying bradycardia. Syncope occurs when blood flow to the brain drops abruptly. Triggers of the reflex pathway are varied. Vasovagal syncope is one category without a clearly defined trigger but can occur with intense emotions, strong odors, or orthostatic stress. Individuals who faint at the sight of blood experience vasovagal syncope. Neurally mediated syncope can also be brought about by specific situations such as cough, micturition, swallowing, or carotid sensitivity. The primary symptoms of neurally mediated syncope include premonitory symptoms such as lightheadedness and dizziness as well as parasympathetic symptoms such as diaphoresis, pallor, hyperventilation, pallor, and palpitation. Myoclonic jerks of the extremities can occur and be difficult to distinguish from seizure activity. On rare occasions, an individual may experience urinary incontinence, but fecal incontinence does not occur. Individuals usually recover very quickly from neurally mediated syncope with a rapid return to consciousness and previous level of alertness. Reassurance and avoidance of triggers are the primary treatments. Liberal intake of fluids and salt expand plasma volume and are protective against syncopal events. In randomized controlled trials, isometric counterpressure maneuvers (leg crossing or handgrip) are also protective. In patients with refractory syncope, fludrocortisone, beta-blockers, or vasoconstricting agents have been used with clinical success, although there are no clinical trial data to support their use.

9. The answer is A.

(Chap. 10) The cornerstone of the evaluation of syncope is to perform an thorough history and examination. Clues to the cause of syncope include the presence of prodromal symptoms, presence of injury, and eyewit-

ness accounts of the event. Neurally mediated syncope is one of the most common causes of syncope and often has preceding lightheadedness or dizziness. Orthostatic hypotension is also frequently preceded by symptoms of lightheadedness and is more common in older individuals. Likewise, older individuals are at greater risk of cardiac syncope. Cardiac syncope needs to be considered as cardiac syncope caused by structural heart disease or primary arrhythmia is associated with an increased risk of sudden cardiac death. Cardiac syncope is more likely to occur without warning symptoms and is more likely to have associated serious injury. Hypoglycemia can present with syncope as well and needs to be considered in this case. Neurologic causes of syncope include seizures and vertebrobasilar insufficiency. A cerebrovascular accident does not commonly cause syncope because bihemispheric disruption of cerebral blood flow is necessary to cause loss of consciousness.

In this individual, evaluation should include fingerstick glucose measurement, orthostatic blood pressures, and an electrocardiogram. Tilt table testing can be considered, particularly because the patient has had recurrent episodes of syncope in the past. A head CT scan, however, should not be a routine part of the evaluation of syncope unless there is concern about a head injury that occurred as a result of the syncope.

10. The answer is D.

(Chap. 11) Dizziness is a common complaint affecting approximately 20% of the population over the course of the year. Most dizziness is benign, self-limited, and must be distinguished from vertigo. Although dizziness is often described as a sensation of lightheadedness, vertigo is more often described as a sensation that the room is spinning. Vertigo is most commonly from peripheral causes affecting labyrinths of the inner ear or the vestibular nerve. However, central lesions of the brainstem and cerebellum can also lead to vertigo. Features of the history and physical examination can be useful in determining central versus peripheral causes of vertigo. By history, deafness or tinnitus is typically absent with central lesions. On physical examination, spontaneous nystagmus is most often a sign of central vertigo, although it can be seen with acute vestibular neuritis. Specific patterns of vertigo that are characteristic of lesions in the cerebellar pathways are vertical nystagmus with a downward fast phase (downbeat nystagmus) and horizontal nystagmus that changes direction with gaze (gaze-evoked nystagmus). Alternatively, in peripheral vertigo, nystagmus typically is provoked by positional maneuvers and can be inhibited by visual fixation. Visual fixation does not, however, inhibit nystagmus in central lesions. Finally, central causes of nystagmus are more likely to be associated with other symptoms that would lead one to suspect a central cause. These include hiccups, diplopia, cranial neuropathies, and dysarthria.

11. The answer is C.

(Chap. 11) The symptoms and physical examination of this patient are typical of benign paroxysmal positional vertigo (BPPV). Episodes of BPPV are typically quite brief, lasting no more than 1 minute, and are brought about by changes in position relative to gravity. Typical movements that elicit the vertigo are lying down, rolling over in bed, rising from the supine position, and tilting the head to look upward. The labyrinth of the inner ear is responsible for process information with regards to position and movement. It consists of three semicircular canals: the superior canal, the posterior canal, and the horizontal canal. BPPV results when calcium carbonate crystals called otoconia migrate from the utricle of the inner ear into the semicircular canals. By far, the most commonly affected canal is the posterior one. When this occurs, vertigo is accompanied by nystagmus that beats upward and torsionally toward the affected ear. This can be brought about by the Dix-Hallpike maneuver, which is described in the clinical scenario. Less commonly, the horizontal canal is affected, leading to horizontal nystagmus. The primary treatment of BPPV is repositioning therapy that uses gravity to remove the otoconia from the affected canal. The Epley maneuver is the most common repositioning procedure.

The history and physical examination are not consistent with a central cause of vertigo; therefore, a brain MRI is not indicated. Methylprednisolone is the primary treatment of acute vestibular neuritis if used within the first 3 days of symptoms. Acute vestibular neuritis often presents with more prolonged symptoms that persist even when there is no movement of the head. Most patients recover spontaneously, but when used early, methylprednisolone will decrease the duration of symptoms. There is no indication for the use of antiviral therapy unless there is obvious herpes zoster infection. Likewise, the symptoms are not consistent with migrainous vertigo, which would be persistent for hours and not be affected by positional changes. Thus, the use of rizatriptan would not be helpful.

12. The answer is D.

(Chap. 12) Complaints of weakness in a patient have a multitude of causes, and it is important to perform a thorough history and physical examination to help localize the site of weakness. Lower motor neuron diseases occur when there is destruction of the cell bodies of the lower motor neurons in the brainstem or the anterior horn of the spinal cord. Lower motor neuron diseases can also occur because of direct axonal dysfunction and demyelination. The primary presenting symptoms are those of distal muscle weakness such as tripping or decreased hand grip strength. When a motor neuron becomes diseased, it may discharge spontaneously, leading to muscle fasciculations that are not seen in disease of the upper motor neurons or myopathies. Additionally, on physical examination, lower motor neuron disease leads to decreases in muscle tone and decreased or absent deep tendon reflexes. Over time,

severe muscle atrophy can occur. A Babinski sign should not be present. If there is evidence of a Babinski sign in the presence of lower motor neuron disease, this should raise the suspicion of a disorder affecting both upper and lower motor neurons such as amyotrophic lateral sclerosis.

13. The answer is E.
(Chap. 13) Approximately 15% of individuals older than 65 years have an identifiable gait disorder. By age 80 years, 25% of individuals require a mechanical aid to assist ambulation. Proper maintenance of gait requires a complex interaction between central nervous system centers to integrate postural control and locomotion. The cerebellum, brainstem, and motor cortex simultaneously process information regarding the environment and purpose of the motion to allow for proper gait and avoidance of falls. Any disorder affecting either sensory input regarding the environment or central nervous system output has the potential to affect gait. In most case series, the most common cause of gait disorders is a sensory deficit. The causes of sensory deficits can quite broad and include peripheral sensory neuropathy from a variety of causes, including diabetes mellitus, peripheral vascular disease, and vitamin B_{12} deficiency, among many others. Other common causes of gait disorders include myelopathy and multiple cerebrovascular infarcts. Although Parkinson's disease is almost inevitably marked by gait abnormalities, it occurs less commonly in the general population than the previously discussed disorders. Likewise, cerebellar degeneration is frequently associated with gait disturbance but is a less common disorder in the general population.

14. The answer is B.
(Chap. 13) Characteristics found during the neurologic examination can assist with the localization of disease in gait disorders. In this case, the patient presents with signs of a frontal gait disorder or parkinsonism. The specific characteristics that would be seen with a frontal gait disorder are a wide-based stance with slow and short shuffling steps. The patient may have difficulty rising from a chair and has a slow, hesitating start. Likewise, there is great difficult with turning with multiple steps required to complete a turn. The patient has very significant postural instability. However, cerebellar signs are typically absent. Romberg sign may or may not be positive, and seated cerebellar testing results are normal, including heel-to-shin testing and rapid alternating movements. Additionally, there should otherwise be normal muscle bulk and tone without sensory or strength deficits. The most common cause of frontal gait disorders (sometimes known as gait apraxia) is cerebrovascular disease, especially small vessel subcortical disease. Communicating hydrocephalus also presents with a gait disorder of this type. In some individuals, the gait disorder precedes other typical symptoms such as incontinence or mental status change.

Alcoholic cerebellar degeneration and multiple system atrophy present with signs of cerebellar ataxia. Characteristics of cerebellar ataxia include a wide-based gait with variable velocity. Gait initiation is normal, but the patient is hesitant during turns. The stride is lurching and irregular. Falls are a late event. The heel-to-shin test is abnormal, and the Romberg test is variably positive.

Neurosyphilis and lumbar myelopathy are examples of sensory ataxia. Sensory ataxia presents with frequent falls. The gait with sensory ataxia, however, is narrow based. Often the patient is noted to be looking down while walking. The patient tends to walk slowly but have path deviation. Gait is initiated normal, but the patient may have some difficulty with turning. The Romberg test is typically unsteady and may result in falls.

15. The answer is D.
(Chap. 16) Delirium is an acute confusional state that most frequently occurs in the context of an acute medical illness. Fluctuating levels of cognitive function with a particular deficit of attention are the primary clinical features of delirium. All levels of cognitive function, however, are invariably involved, including memory, language, and executive functioning. Other common associated symptoms are sleep–wake disturbances, hallucinations or delusions, affect changes, and changes in heart rate or blood pressure. Delirium remains a clinical diagnosis and is believed to affect as much as 50% of hospitalized patients. For elderly patients in intensive care, the incidence rises to between 70 and 87%. However, it has been estimated the diagnosis is missed in one-third of individuals with delirium. Once thought of as an acute but benign condition, increasing research is demonstrating delirium to have persisting effects on cognition and functioning. Delirium typically is short lived, but some episodes of delirium can last for weeks, months, or even years. When delirium persists for longer periods of time, it is thought to represent inadequate treatment of the cause of delirium or permanent neuronal damage from the episode. Delirium also has significant associated morbidity and mortality. A single episode of delirium in hospitalized patients has been associated with an in-hospital mortality rate as high as 25–33%. However, the increased mortality is not simply limited to the hospital stay. Individuals experiencing delirium in the hospital have increased mortality for the next several months to years. In addition, these individuals experience a longer hospital length of stay and are less likely to return to functional independence. Individuals who experience delirium are more likely to be discharged to nursing home care and are at increased risk of rehospitalization.

16. The answer is B.
(Chap. 16) This patient has features of acute delirium, which can be precipitated by many causes in hospitalized patients. Broad categories of causes of delirium include toxins, medication reactions, metabolic disorders, infec-

tions, endocrine disorders, cerebrovascular disorders (especially hypertensive encephalopathy), autoimmune disorders, seizures, neoplastic disorders, and hospitalization. Although the list of causes is broad, the initial history and physical examination are important to establish potential etiologies of delirium and guide further workup. In most patients with delirium, it is difficult to obtain an accurate history; therefore, it is important to seek out a spouse of family member to outline the history further. In this case, there are features that could suggest alcohol withdrawal (hypertension, tachycardia, fevers, tremors), and one should clarify his alcohol intake with his wife. Another primary consideration in determining the etiology of a delirium episode is the time course over which it evolves and the current medications. Particularly in older hospitalized individuals, common medications used as sleep aids, such as diphenhydramine, can have a paradoxical effect with delirium and agitation. It is estimated that as many as one-third of episodes of delirium in hospitalized patients are the result of medications. Worsening infection also needs to be considered because the change in the patient's vital signs could be indicative of an infectious source, although the elevated blood pressure is not consistent with this. Because the patient has required oxygen during his hospitalization, it is important to check an oxygen saturation or arterial blood gas because acute hypoxemia or hypercarbia can precipitate delirium. Likewise, given the patient's history of diabetes mellitus, a fingerstick glucose is necessary because hypoglycemia could also lead to alterations in mental status with evidence of tachycardia, tremor, and diaphoresis. Other initial tests to consider in an individual with delirium are electrolytes and basic liver and kidney function. Although commonly ordered, brain imaging is most often not helpful in the evaluation of delirium.

17. The answer is C.
(Chap. 16) Confusion is defined as a mental and behavioral state of reduced comprehension, coherence, and capacity to reason. *Delirium* is used to describe an acute confusional state. Delirium often goes unrecognized despite clear evidence that it is often a cognitive manifestation of many medical and neurologic illnesses. Delirium is a clinical diagnosis that may be hyperactive (e.g., alcohol withdrawal) or hypoactive (e.g., opiate intoxication). There is often dramatic fluctuation between states. Delirium is associated with a substantial mortality rate with in-hospital mortality estimates ranging from 25–33%. Overall estimates of delirium in hospitalized patients range from 15–55% with higher rates in elderly adults. Patients in the intensive care unit have especially high rates of delirium, ranging from 70–87%. The clinic setting represents the lowest risk. Postoperative patients, especially after hip surgery, have an incidence of delirium that is somewhat higher than patients admitted to the medical wards.

18. The answer is D.
(Chap. 17) Alterations in consciousness are among the most common reasons for admission to the hospital and occur frequently in seriously ill patients. When evaluating a patient with an alteration in consciousness, one must have a framework for understanding the spectrum of arousability one may encounter. *Coma* is a frequently misunderstood term that refers to a deep sleeplike state from which a patient cannot be aroused. A stuporous patient can be aroused briefly with noxious stimuli, and drowsiness refers to a patient who can be aroused easily with maintenance of attention for brief periods. Other conditions that alter the ability of a patient to respond appropriately to stimuli and are often confused with coma. A vegetative state is an awake but unresponsive condition that can occur in a patient who has emerged from a coma and is associated with extensive bilateral cerebral damage. A patient in a vegetative state can open the eyes spontaneously and often track objects. In addition, the patient has retention of respiratory and autonomic functions as well as spontaneous movement of extremities. However, meaningful responses to stimuli do not occur, and a vegetative state is sometimes referred to as an "awake coma." This patient would be characterized as being in a persistent vegetative state because the duration of the vegetative state has been 1 year. At this point, the likelihood of meaningful recovery of mental faculties is almost zero. A minimally conscious state is a less severe manifestation of bilateral cerebral injury. A patient in a minimally conscious state may have rudimentary vocal or motor behaviors and minimal responses to external stimuli. Other conditions that may be misinterpreted as a coma include akinetic mutism, catatonia, abulia, and locked-in syndrome.

19. The answer is A.
(Chap. 17) Brain death occurs when all cerebral function has ceased but the patient continues to have cardiac activity while supported by artificial means. If an individual is determined to have brain death, life-sustaining therapies are withdrawn. Although this can occur without the consent of the family, certainly it is important to have open communication with the family to allow the withdrawal of care without conflict. Most hospitals have developed specific protocols to diagnose a patient with brain death. Three essential elements should be demonstrated for the diagnosis of brain death. First, the patient should widespread cortical damage with complete absence of response to all external stimuli. Second, the patient should have no evidence of brainstem function with loss of oculovestibular and corneal reflexes and absent pupillary reaction to light. Finally, there should be no evidence of medullary activity manifested by apnea. When a brain death examination is performed, the patient should not be receiving any medications that could alter consciousness. The bedside examination will confirm absence of responsiveness to stimuli and lack of brainstem function. Apnea testing

is the final examination in the performance of the brain death examination. This test is important for documenting the absence of medullary function. For an apnea test result to be accurate, the carbon dioxide must be allowed to rise to a level that would stimulate respiration. When performing the test, the patient is preoxygenated with 100% oxygen, which is sustained throughout the test. At this point, ventilator support is stopped. In the absence of any respiration, carbon dioxide rises by 2–3 mmHg/min, and it is necessary for arterial partial pressure of carbon dioxide to rise to between 50–60 mmHg. If the patient has a normal $PaCO_2$ before beginning the apnea test, the test would typically need to continue for at least 5 minutes to be valid. The patient is observed for respiratory effort, and a $PaCO_2$ level is often measured at the end of the test to document that the rise in carbon dioxide is adequate to stimulate respiration. Some patients may have cardiovascular instability that makes the performance of apnea testing risky because one does not wish for the apnea test to lead to cardiovascular collapse. In this setting, an electroencephalogram demonstrating absence of electrical activity is used as an adjunctive diagnostic test. Newer methods of testing, including radionuclide brain scanning, cerebral angiography, and transcranial Doppler ultrasonography, may be used, but these tests are less well validated. In most cases, clinical evidence of brain death must be sustained for 6–24 hours before withdrawal of care.

20. The answer is E.

(Chap. 17) Foraminal herniation, which forces the cerebellar tonsils into the foramen magnum, leads to compression of the medulla and subsequent respiratory arrest. Central transtentorial herniation occurs when the medial thalamus compresses the midbrain as it moves through the tentorial opening; miotic pupils and drowsiness are the classic clinical signs. A locked-in state is usually caused by infarction or hemorrhage of the ventral pons; other causes include Guillain-Barré syndrome and use of certain neuromuscular blocking agents. Catatonia is a semi-awake state seen most frequently as a manifestation of psychotic disorders such as schizophrenia. Third-nerve palsies arise from an uncal transtentorial herniation in which the anterior medial temporal gyrus herniates into the anterior portion of the tentorial opening anterior to the adjacent midbrain. Coma may occur because of compression of the midbrain.

21. The answer is B.

(Chap. 18) When evaluating someone who reports difficulty with language, it is important to assess speech in several different domains, which are spontaneous speech, comprehension, repetition, naming, reading, and writing. *Anomia* refers to the inability to name common objects and is the most common finding in patients with aphasia. Indeed, anomia is present in all types of aphasia except pure word deafness or pure alexia. Anomia can present in many fashions, including complete an inability to name, provision of a related word ("pen" for "pencil"), a description of the word ("a thing for writing"), or the wrong word. Fluency is assessed by listening to spontaneous speech. Fluency is decreased in Broca's or global aphasia but is relatively preserved in other forms of aphasia. Comprehension is assessed by asking patients to follow conversation and provide simple answers (yes/no, pointing to appropriate objects). The most common aphasia presenting with deficits of comprehension is Wernicke's aphasia in which fluent but nonsensical spontaneous speech (word salad) is present. Repetition asks patients to repeat a string of words, sentences, or a single word and is impaired in many types of aphasia. In addition, repetition of tongue twisters can be useful in the evaluation of dysarthria or palilalia as well. Alexia refers to the inability to read aloud or comprehend written language.

22. The answer is C.

(Chap. 18) The parietofrontal area of the brain is responsible for spatial orientation. The major components of the network include the cingulate cortex, posterior parietal cortex, and the frontal eye fields. In addition, subcortical areas in the striatum and thalamus are also important. Together, these systems integrate information to maintain spatial cognition, and a lesion in any of these areas can lead to hemispatial neglect. In neglect syndromes, three behavioral manifestations are seen: Sensory events in the neglected hemisphere have less overall impact; there is a paucity of conscious acts directed toward the neglected hemisphere; and the patient behaves as if the neglected hemisphere is devalued. In Figure 22, almost all of the A's (the target) represented on the left half of the figure are missed. This is an example of a target detection task. Hemianopia alone is not sufficient to cause this finding because the individual can turn his or her head left and right to identify the targets.

Bilateral disorders of the parietofrontal area of the brain can lead to severe spatial disorientation known as Balint's syndrome. In Balint's syndrome, there is inability to orderly scan the environment (oculomotor apraxia) and inaccurate manual reaching for objects (optic apraxia). A third finding in Balint's syndrome is simultanagnosia. Simultanagnosia is the inability to integrate information in the center of the gaze with peripheral information. An example is a target detection test in which only the A's present in the outer portion of the figure would be indicated. Individuals with this finding also tend to miss the larger objects in a figure and would not be able to accurately identify the target when it was made much larger than the surrounding letters. Construction apraxia refers to the inability to copy a simple line drawing such as a house or star and occurs most commonly in association with parietal lesions. Object agnosia is the inability to name a generic object or describe its use in contrast to anomia when an individual should be able to describe the use of the object even if it cannot be named. The defect in the object agnosia is usually in the territory of the bilateral posterior cerebral arteries.

23. The answer is C.

(Chap. 20) Shift work sleep disorder is a disorder of the circadian rhythm that is common in any individual who has to commonly work at night. At present, an estimated 7 million individuals in the United States work permanently at night or on rotating shifts. Increasing research devoted to sleep disorders in night shift workers has demonstrated that the circadian rhythm never fully shifts to allow one to perform at full alertness at night. The reason for this is likely multifactorial and includes the fact that most individuals who work at night try to abruptly shift their sleep schedules to a more normal pattern on days when they are not working. Consequently, night shift workers often have chronic sleep deprivation, increased length of time awake before starting work, and misalignment of their circadian phase with the intrinsic circadian phase. The results of this lead to decreased alertness and increased errors during night shifts. In an estimated 5–10% of individuals working night shifts, the excessive sleepiness during the night and insomnia during the day are deemed to be clinically significant. Strategies for treating shift work sleep disorder use a combination of behavioral and pharmacologic strategies. Caffeine does promote wakefulness, but the effects are not long lasting, and tolerance develops over time. Brief periods of exercise frequently boost alertness and can be used before starting a night shift or during the shift at times of increased sleepiness. Many sleep experts support strategic napping during shifts for no more than 20 minutes at times of circadian nadirs. Naps longer than 20 minutes can lead to sleep inertia during which an individual may feel very disoriented and groggy and experience a decline in motor skills upon abrupt awakening from sleep. Bright lights before and during night shift work may improve alertness, but one must be careful to avoid bright lights in the morning after a night shift because light entrainment is a powerful stimulus of the internal circadian clock. If an individual is exposed to bright light in the morning, it will interfere with the ability to fall asleep during the day. Night shift workers should be encouraged to wear dark sunglasses in the morning on the way home. Sleep during the day is frequently disrupted in night shift workers. Creating a quiet, dark, and comfortable environment is important, and sleep should be a priority for the individual during the day. The only pharmacologic therapy approved by the Food and Drug Administration for treatment of shift work sleep disorder is modafinil 200 mg taken 20–30 minutes before the start of a night shift. Modafinil has been demonstrated to increase sleep latency and decrease attentional failures during night shifts but does not alleviate the feelings of excessive sleepiness. Melatonin is not one of the recommended therapies for shift work sleep disorder. If used, it should be taken 2–3 hours before bedtime rather than right before bedtime to simulate the normal peaks and troughs of melatonin secretion.

24. The answer is C.

(Chap. 20) This patient complains of symptoms that are consistent with restless legs syndrome (RLS). This disorder affects 1–5% of young to middle-aged individuals and as many as 20% of older individuals. The symptom of RLS is a nonspecific uncomfortable sensation in the legs that begins during periods of quiescence and is associated with the irresistible urge to move. Patients frequently find it difficult to describe their symptoms but usually describe the sensation as deep within the affected limb. Rarely is the sensation described as distinctly painful unless an underlying neuropathy is also present. The severity of the disorder tends to wax and wane over time and tends to worsen with sleep deprivation, caffeine intake, pregnancy, and alcohol. Renal disease, neuropathy, and iron deficiency are known secondary causes of RLS symptoms. In this patient, correcting the iron deficiency is the best choice for initial therapy because this may entirely relieve the symptoms of RLS. For individuals with primary RLS (not related to another medical condition), the dopaminergic agents are the treatment of choice. Pramipexole or ropinirole is recommended as first-line treatment. Although carbidopa/levodopa is highly effective, individuals have a high risk of developing augmented symptoms over time with increasingly higher doses needed to control the symptoms. Other options for treating RLS include narcotics, benzodiazepines, and gabapentin. Hormone replacement therapy has no role in the treatment of RLS.

25. The answer is A.

(Chap. 20) Narcolepsy is a sleep disorder characterized by excessive sleepiness with intrusion of rapid eye movement (REM) sleep into wakefulness. Narcolepsy affects about one in 4000 individuals in the United States with a genetic predisposition. Recent research has demonstrated that narcolepsy with cataplexy is associated with low or undetectable levels of the neurotransmitter hypocretin (orexin) in the CSF. This neurotransmitter is released from a small number of neurons in the hypothalamus. Given the association of narcolepsy with the major histocompatibility antigen human leukocyte antigen DQB1*0602, it is thought that narcolepsy is an autoimmune process that leads to destruction of the hypocretin-secreting neurons in the hypothalamus. The classic symptom tetrad of narcolepsy is (1) cataplexy, (2) hypnagogic or hypnopompic hallucinations, (3) sleep paralysis, and (4) excessive daytime somnolence. Of these symptoms, cataplexy is the most specific for the diagnosis of narcolepsy. Cataplexy refers to the sudden loss of muscle tone in response to strong emotions. It most commonly occurs with laughter or surprise but may be associated with anger as well. Cataplexy can have a wide range of symptoms from mild

sagging of the jaw lasting for a few seconds to a complete loss of muscle tone lasting several minutes. During this time, individuals are aware of their surroundings and are not unconscious. This symptom is present in 76% of individuals diagnosed with narcolepsy and is the most specific finding for the diagnosis. Hypnagogic and hypnopompic hallucinations and sleep paralysis can occur from any cause of chronic sleep deprivation, including sleep apnea and chronic insufficient sleep. Excessive daytime somnolence is present in 100% of individuals with narcolepsy but is not specific for the diagnosis because this symptom may be present with any sleep disorder as well as with chronic insufficient sleep. The presence of two or more REM periods occurring during a daytime multiple sleep latency test is suggestive but not diagnostic of narcolepsy. Other disorders that may lead to presence of REM during short daytime nap periods include sleep apnea, sleep phase delay syndrome, and insufficient sleep.

26. The answer is B.

(Chap. 20; http://www.sleepfoundation.org/site/c.huIXKj-M0IxF/b.2417355/k.143E/2002_Sleep_in_America_Poll.htm, accessed May 12, 2011) Insomnia is the most common sleep disorder in the population. In the 2002 Sleep in America Poll, 58% of respondents reported at least one symptom of insomnia on a weekly basis, and one-third of individuals experience these symptoms on a nightly basis. Insomnia is defined clinically as the inability to fall asleep or stay asleep, which leads to daytime sleepiness or poor daytime function. These symptoms occur despite adequate time and opportunity for sleep. Insomnia can be further characterized as primary or secondary. Primary insomnia occurs in individuals with an identifiable cause of insomnia and is often a long-standing diagnosis for many years. Within the category of primary insomnia is adjustment insomnia, which is typically of short duration with a well-defined stressor. Secondary causes of insomnia include comorbid medical or psychiatric conditions and can be related to caffeine or illegal and prescribed drugs. Obstructive sleep apnea is thought to affect as many as 10–15% of the population and is currently underdiagnosed in the United States. In addition, because of the rising incidence of obesity, obstructive sleep apnea is also expected to increase in incidence over the coming years. Obstructive sleep apnea occurs when there is ongoing effort to inspire against an occluded oropharynx during sleep. It is directly related to obesity and has an increased incidence in men and in older populations. Narcolepsy affects 1 in 4000 people and is caused by deficit of hypocretin (orexin) in the brain. Symptoms of narcolepsy include a sudden loss of tone in response to emotional stimuli (cataplexy), hypersomnia, sleep paralysis, and hallucinations with sleep onset and waking. Physiologically, there is intrusion or persistence of rapid eye movement sleep during wakefulness that accounts for the classic symptoms of narcolepsy. Restless legs syndrome is estimated to affect 1–5% of young to middle-aged adults and as many as 10–20% of elderly adults. Restless legs syndrome is marked by uncomfortable sensations in the legs that are difficult to describe. The symptoms have an onset with quiescence, especially at night, and are relieved with movement. Delayed sleep phase syndrome is a circadian rhythm disorder that commonly presents with a complaint of insomnia and accounts for as much as 10% of individuals referred to the sleep clinic for evaluation of insomnia. In delayed sleep phase syndrome, the intrinsic circadian rhythm is delayed such that sleep onset occurs much later than normal. When allowed to sleep according to the intrinsic circadian rhythm, individuals with delayed sleep phase syndrome sleep normally and do not experience excessive somnolence. This disorder is most common in adolescence and young adulthood.

27. The answer is C.

(Chap. 20) Parasomnias are abnormal behaviors or experiences that arise from slow-wave sleep. Also known as confusional arousals, the electroencephalogram during a parasomnia event frequently shows persistence of slow-wave (delta) sleep into arousal. Non–rapid eye movement (NREM) parasomnias may also include more complex behavior, including eating and sexual activity. Treatment of NREM parasomnias is usually not indicated, and a safe environment should be assured for the patient. When injury is likely to occur, treatment with a drug that decreases slow-wave sleep will treat the parasomnia. Typical treatment is a benzodiazepine. There are no typical parasomnias that arise from stage I or stage II sleep. REM parasomnias include nightmare disorder and REM-behavior disorder. REM-behavior disorder is increasingly recognized as associated with Parkinson's disease and other parkinsonian syndromes. This disorder is characterized by the absence of decreased muscle tone in REM sleep, which leads to the acting out of dreams, sometimes resulting in violence and injury.

28. The answer is E.

(Chap. 21) (See Figure 21-3.) Bitemporal hemianopia is caused by a lesion at the optic chiasm because fibers there decusate into the contralateral optic tract. Crossed fibers are more damaged by compression than uncrossed fibers. This finding is usually caused by symmetric compression in the sellar region by a pituitary adenoma, meningioma, craniopharyngioma, glioma, or aneurysm. These lesions are often insidious and may be unnoticed by the patient. They will escape detection by the physician unless each eye is tested separately. Lesions anterior to the chiasm (retinal injury, optic nerve injury) will cause unilateral impairment and an abnormal pupillary response. Postchiasmic lesions (temporal, parietal, occipital cortex) cause homonymous lesions (similar field abnormalities in both eyes) that vary with location. Occlusion of the posterior cerebral artery supplying the occipital lobe is a common cause of total homonymous hemianopia.

29. The answer is E.

(Chap. 21) The differential diagnosis of a red, painful eye is broad and includes corneal abrasion, subconjunctival hemorrhage, infective or allergic conjunctivitis (the most common cause of red, painful eye), keratoconjunctivitis sicca (medications, Sjögren's syndrome, sarcoidosis), keratitis (contact lens injury, trachoma, vitamin A deficiency), herpes infection, episcleritis (autoimmune, idiopathic), scleritis (autoimmune), uveitis, endophthalmitis, or acute angle-closure glaucoma. Uveitis requires slit-lamp examination for diagnosis. Anterior uveitis involving the iris is usually idiopathic but may be associated with sarcoidosis, ankylosing spondylitis, juvenile rheumatoid arthritis, inflammatory bowel disease, psoriasis, inflammatory arthritis, Behçet's disease, and a variety of infections. Posterior uveitis in the vitreous, retina, or choroid is more likely to be associated with a systemic disease or infection than anterior uveitis. Acute angle-closure glaucoma, although rare, is often misdiagnosed unless intraocular pressure is measured. Many physicians avoid dilating patients' pupils for fear of provoking acute angle-closure glaucoma. The risk is remote and rarely causes permanent vision loss. The value of a complete funduscopic examination outweighs the risk of this rare event. Transient ischemic attack (TIA) caused by temporary interruption of blood flow to the retina for more than a few seconds causes transient visual abnormality (amaurosis fugax). TIA is usually associated with atherosclerosis. If flow is restored quickly vision returns to normal.

30. The answer is A.

(Chap. 21) Age-related macular degeneration is a major cause of painless, gradual bilateral central visual loss. It occurs as nonexudative (dry) or exudative (wet) forms. Recent genetic data have shown an association with the alternative complement pathway gene for complement factor H. The mechanism link for that association is unknown. The nonexudative form is associated with retinal drusen that leads to retinal atrophy. Treatment with vitamin C, vitamin E, beta-carotene, and zinc may retard the visual loss. Exudative macular degeneration, which is less common, is caused by neovascular proliferation and leakage of choroidal blood vessels. Acute visual loss may occur because of bleeding. Exudative macular degeneration may be treated with intraocular injection of a vascular endothelial growth factor antagonist (bevacizumab or ranibizumab). Blepharitis is inflammation of the eyelids usually related to acne rosacea, seborrheic dermatitis, or staphylococcal infection. Diabetic retinopathy, now a leading cause of blindness in the United States, causes gradual bilateral visual loss in patients with long-standing diabetes. Retinal detachment is usually unilateral and causes visual loss and an afferent pupillary defect.

31. The answer is B.

(Chap. 23) A history of severe respiratory infection, including the common cold, influenza, pneumonia, or HIV, is the most common cause of long-lasting loss of smell. The mechanism, along with cases of chronic rhinosinusitis (another common cause) is likely related to permanent damage to the olfactory epithelium. Head trauma, causing shearing and scarring of olfactory fila at the cribriform plate, may cause anosmia. Fewer than 10% of patients with posttraumatic anosmia regain normal function. The severity of disease is associated with the likelihood of olfactory abnormality in trauma and chronic rhinosinusitis. Significant decrements in smell are present in more than 50% of people older than 65 years old. This finding may explain the common finding of loss of food flavor and nutritional deficiencies in elderly adults. Confirming popular wisdom studies have shown that at any age, women have a better ability to identify odorants than men (Figure 23-6).

32. The answer is E.

(Chap. 24) Hearing loss is a common complaint, particularly in older individuals. In this age group, 33% have hearing loss to a degree that requires hearing aids. When evaluating hearing loss, the physician should attempt to determine whether the cause is conductive, sensorineural, or mixed. Sensorineural hearing loss results from injury of the cochlear apparatus or disruption of the neural pathways from the inner ear to the brain. The primary site of damage is the hair cells of the inner ear. Common causes of hair cell injury include prolonged exposure to loud noises, viral infections, ototoxic drugs, cochlear otosclerosis, Ménière's disease, and aging. In contrast, conductive hearing loss results from impairment of the external ear and auditory canal to transmit and amplify sound through the middle ear to the cochlea. Causes of conductive hearing loss include cerumen impaction, perforations of the tympanic membrane, otosclerosis, cholesteatomas, large middle ear effusions, and tumors of the external auditory canal or middle ear among others. The initial physical examination can often differentiate between conductive or sensorineural hearing loss. Examination of the external auditory canal can identify cerumen or foreign body impaction. On otoscopic examination, it is more important to assess the topography of the tympanic membrane than to look for the presence of a light reflex. Of particular attention is the area in the upper third of the tympanic membrane known as the pars flaccida. This area can develop chronic retraction pockets that are indicative of Eustachian tube dysfunction or a cholesteatoma, a benign tumor composed of keratinized squamous epithelium. Bedside tests with a tuning fork also are useful for differentiating conductive from sensorineural hearing loss. In the Rinne's test, air conduction is compared with bony conduction of sound. A tuning fork is placed over the mastoid process and then in front of the external ear. In conductive hearing loss, the intensity of sound is louder when placed on the bone, but in sensorineural hearing loss, the intensity is greatest at the external ear. In the Weber test, the tuning fork is placed in the midline of the head. In unilateral conductive hearing

loss, the intensity of sound is loudest in the affected ear, but in unilateral sensorineural hearing loss, the intensity of sound is loudest in the unaffected ear. This patient reports left greater than right hearing loss that is suspected to be sensorineural in nature. Thus, the sound is expected to be greatest in the right ear on the Weber test. A more formal evaluation of hearing loss would include pure tone audiometry that plots hearing threshold versus frequency. Pure tone audiometry establishes the severity, type, and laterality of hearing loss. In this patient, high-frequency hearing loss would be expected based on his complaints of inability to hear the alarm tone of his digital watch.

33. The answer is D.

(Chap. 25) Channelopathies, disorders of ion channels that lead to disease, are a growing mechanism to explain a number of neurologic diseases. Most are caused by a mutation in the ion channel gene or by autoimmune alteration of ion channel proteins. Some forms of epilepsy, including benign neonatal familial convulsions and generalized epilepsy with febrile convulsions, are associated with genetic abnormalities of sodium or potassium channels. Familial hemiplegic migraines are associated with genetic abnormalities in sodium and calcium channels. Spinocerebellar ataxia and other ataxias are associated with genetic abnormalities in potassium or calcium channels. Lambert-Eaton syndrome is an example of autoimmune-related abnormalities in calcium channel function. Parkinson's disease is the classic example of neurotransmitter system–mediated disease.

34. The answer is C.

(Chap. 25) Synaptic neurotransmission is the predominant mechanism for neuronal communication. Therefore, it is not surprising that dysfunction with any step in the presynaptic synthesis, vesicular storage, and synaptic cleft release, and receptor binding in the postsynaptic cell may be associated with disease. Neurotransmitters bind to specific receptors that are either ionotropic or metabotropic. Functions related to ionotropic receptors are generally fast (<1 millisecond) and metabotropic receptors are more prolonged. Antibodies to the acetylcholine receptors or motor neuron calcium channels cause myasthenia gravis and Lambert-Eaton syndrome, respectively. Parkinson's syndrome is related to selective cell death in the nigrostriatal dopamine pathway. Stiff-person syndrome is related to antibodies to glutamic acid decarboxylase, the biosynthetic pathway for GABA. Orthostatic tachycardia syndrome is related to mutations in the norepinephrine transporter. Abnormalities with serotonin neurotransmitter function are implicated in mood disorders, migraine pain pathways, and somatic pain pathways.

35. The answer is B.

(Chap. 26) The International League against Epilepsy (ILAE) Commission on Classification and Terminology, 2005–2009, has provided an updated approach to the classification of seizures. This system is based on the clinical features of seizures and associated electroencephalographic findings. Seizures are classified as focal or generalized. Focal seizures arise from a neuronal network either discretely localized within one cerebral hemisphere or more broadly distributed but still within the hemisphere. They are frequently associated with a structural lesion. Generalized seizures are thought to arise at some point in the brain but immediately and rapidly engage neuronal networks in both cerebral hemispheres. Focal seizures are subdivided into those with or without dyscognitive features depending on the patient's ability to interact with the environment during an episode. The terms "simple partial seizure" and "complex partial seizure" have been eliminated. Typical absence seizures are characterized by sudden, brief lapses of consciousness without loss of postural control. The seizure typically lasts for only seconds, consciousness returns as suddenly as it was lost, and there is no postictal confusion. Myoclonus is a sudden and brief muscle contraction that may involve one part of the body or the entire body. Although the distinction from other forms of myoclonus (e.g., metabolic, degenerative neurologic disease, anoxic encephalopathy) is imprecise, myoclonic seizures are considered to be true epileptic events since they are caused by cortical dysfunction.

36. The answer is A.

(Chap. 26) Mesial temporal lobe epilepsy is the most common epilepsy syndrome associated with focal seizures with dyscognitive features. Patients are unable to respond to verbal or visual commands during the seizure and they often manifest complex automatisms or complex posturing. An aura is common before the seizures. There is postictal memory loss or disorientation. Patients often have a history of febrile seizures or a family history of seizures. MRI will show hippocampal sclerosis, a small temporal lobe, or enlarged temporal horn. Mesial temporal lobe epilepsy is important to recognize as a distinct syndrome because it tends to be refractory to treatment with anticonvulsants but responds extremely well to surgical intervention. Hypothyroidism, herpes virus infection, diabetes, and tuberous sclerosis are not associated with mesial temporal lobe epilepsy.

37. The answer is E.

(Chap. 26) Focal seizures without dyscognitive features cause motor, sensory, autonomic, or psychic symptoms without an obvious alteration in consciousness. The phenomenon of abnormal motor movements beginning in a restricted area then progressing to involve a larger area is termed *Jacksonian march*. The patient is describing Todd's paralysis, which may take minutes to many hours to return to normal. Although meningitis is a common cause of seizure in young patients, it is unlikely to be the cause in someone who has a known seizure disorder.

If his symptoms were to persist beyond many hours, it would be reasonable to investigate a different etiology of his hand weakness with imaging studies. Overt deficits in strength are not compatible with a primary psychiatric disorder. Magnetic resonance angiogram and cerebral angiogram are useful to evaluate for cerebrovascular disorders, but there is no evidence of subarachnoid bleeding or vasculitis.

38. The answer is C.

(Chap. 26) Nuchal rigidity and an elevated white blood cell count are very concerning for meningitis as the etiology for this patient, and lumbar puncture must be performed to rule this out. In addition, acute cocaine intoxication is a plausible reason for this new-onset seizure. Figure 26-2 illustrates the evaluation of the adult patient with a seizure. MRI would be indicated if the patient had a negative metabolic and toxicologic screening. Substance abuse counseling, while indicated, is not indicated at this point in his workup since he is postictal. The patient is not having seizures, does not have a known seizure disorder, and has not been treated for the underlying metabolic abnormality, making IV loading with an antiepileptic medication premature at this time.

39. The answer is B.

(Chap. 26) Optimal medical therapy for epilepsy depends on the underlying cause, type of seizure, and patient factors. The goal is to prevent seizures and minimize the side effects of therapy. The minimal effective dose is determined by trial and error. In choosing medical therapies, drug interactions are a key consideration. Certain medications, such as tricyclic antidepressants, may lower the seizure threshold and should be avoided. Patients who respond well to medical therapy and have completely controlled seizures are good candidates for the discontinuation of therapy, with about 70% of children and 60% of adults being able to discontinue therapy eventually. Patient factors that aid in this include complete medical control of seizures for 1–5 years, a normal neurologic examination, a normal EEG, and single seizure type. On the other end of the spectrum, about 20% of these patients are completely refractory to medical therapy and should be considered for surgical therapy. In the best examples, such as mesial temporal sclerosis, resection of the temporal lobe may result in about 70% of these patients becoming seizure-free and an additional 15–25% having a significant reduction in the incidence of seizures. In patients with epilepsy other considerations are critical. Psychosocial sequelae such as depression, anxiety, and behavior problems may occur. Approximately 20% of epileptic patients have depression, with their suicide rate being higher than that of age-matched controls. There is an impact on the ability to drive, perform certain jobs, and function in social situations. Furthermore, there is a two- to threefold increase in mortality for patients with epilepsy compared with age-matched controls. Although most of the increased mortality results from the underlying etiology of epilepsy, a significant number of these patients die from accidents, status epilepticus, and a syndrome known as sudden unexpected death in epileptic patients (SUDEP). A recent meta-analysis demonstrated that treatment of patients with refractory seizures with an antiepileptic drug could reduce the frequency of SUDEP (*Lancet Neurol 2011;10:961*).

40. The answer is D.

(Chap. 26) Adolescence and early adulthood mark the period where idiopathic or genetic epilepsy syndromes become less common and seizures due to acquired central nervous system (CNS) lesions become more common. The most common causes of seizures in the young adults are head trauma, CNS infections, brain tumors, congenital CNS lesions, illicit drug use, or alcohol withdrawal. Fever rarely causes seizure in patients older than 12 years. Amyloid angiopathy and uremia are more common in older adults.

41. The answer is A.

(Chap. 26) Status epilepticus refers to continuous seizures or repetitive, discrete seizures with impaired consciousness in the interictal period. The duration of seizure activity sufficient to meet the definition of status epilepticus has traditionally been specified as 15–30 minutes. Generalized convulsive status epilepticus (GCSE) is typically when seizures last beyond 5 minutes. GCSE is an emergency and must be treated immediately, since cardiorespiratory dysfunction, hyperthermia, and metabolic derangements can develop as a consequence of prolonged seizures, and these can lead to irreversible neuronal injury. Furthermore, CNS injury can occur even when the patient is paralyzed with neuromuscular blockade but continues to have electrographic seizures. The most common causes of GCSE are anticonvulsant withdrawal or noncompliance, metabolic disturbances, drug toxicity, CNS infection, CNS tumors, refractory epilepsy, and head trauma. GCSE is obvious when the patient is having overt convulsions. However, after 30–45 minutes of uninterrupted seizures, the signs may become increasingly subtle. Patients may have mild clonic movements of only the fingers or fine, rapid movements of the eyes. There may be paroxysmal episodes of tachycardia, hypertension, and pupillary dilation. In such cases, the EEG may be the only method of establishing the diagnosis. Thus, if the patient stops having overt seizures yet remains comatose, an EEG should be performed to rule out ongoing status epilepticus. The first steps in the management of a patient in GCSE are to attend to any acute cardiorespiratory problems or hyperthermia, perform a brief medical and neurologic examination, establish venous access, and send samples for laboratory studies to identify metabolic abnormalities. Anticonvulsant therapy should then begin without delay; a treatment approach is shown in Figure 26-3. Carbamazepine is a first-line therapy for focal seizures.

42. The answer is A.

(Chap. 27) Cardioembolism accounts for up to 20% of all ischemic strokes. Stroke caused by heart disease is due to thrombotic material forming on the atrial or ventricular wall or the left heart valves. If the thrombus lyses quickly, only a transient ischemic attack may develop. If the arterial occlusion lasts longer, brain tissue may die and a stroke will occur. Emboli from the heart most often lodge in the middle cerebral artery (MCA), the posterior cerebral artery (PCA), or one of their branches. Atrial fibrillation is the most common cause of cerebral embolism overall. Other significant causes of cardioembolic stroke include myocardial infarction, prosthetic valves, rheumatic heart disease, and dilated cardiomyopathy. Furthermore, paradoxical embolization may occur when an atrial septal defect or a patent foramen ovale exists. This may be detected by bubble-contrast echocardiography. Bacterial endocarditis may cause septic emboli if the vegetation is on the left side of the heart or if there is a paradoxical source.

43. The answer is D.

(Chap. 27) Nonrheumatic atrial fibrillation is the most common cause of cerebral embolism overall. The presumed stroke mechanism is thrombus formation in the fibrillating atrium or atrial appendage. The average annual risk of stroke is around 5%. However, the risk varies with the following factors: age, hypertension, left ventricular function, prior embolism, diabetes, and thyroid function. The risk of stroke can be estimated by calculating the CHADS2 score (see Table 27-3). Patients younger than 60 years of age without structural heart disease or without one of these risk factors have a very low annual risk of cardioembolism of less than 0.5%. Therefore, it is recommended that these patients only take aspirin daily for stroke prevention. Older patients with numerous risk factors may have annual stroke risks of 10–15% and must take a vitamin K antagonist indefinitely. Cardioversion is indicated for symptomatic patients who want an initial opportunity to remain in sinus rhythm. However, studies have shown that there is an increased stroke risk for weeks to months after a successful cardioversion, and these patients must remain on anticoagulation for a long period. Patients who do not respond to cardioversion and do not want catheter ablation have mortality and morbidity with rate control and anticoagulation similar to those of patients who opt for cardioversion. Low-molecular-weight heparin may be used as a bridge to vitamin K–antagonist therapy and may facilitate outpatient anticoagulation in selected patients.

44. The answer is E.

(Chap. 27) Numerous studies have identified key risk factors for ischemic stroke. Old age, family history, diabetes, hypertension, tobacco smoking, and cholesterol are all risk factors for atherosclerosis and therefore stroke. Hypertension is the most significant among these risk factors. All cases of hypertension must be controlled in the setting of stroke prevention. Antiplatelet therapy has been shown to reduce the risk of vascular atherothrombotic events. The overall relative risk reduction of nonfatal stroke is about 25–30% across most large clinical trials. The "true" absolute benefit is dependent on the individual patient's risk; therefore, patients with a low risk for stroke (e.g., younger patients with minimal cardiovascular risk factors) may have a relative risk reduction with antiplatelet therapy but a meaningless "benefit." Numerous studies have shown the benefit of statin therapy in the reduction of stroke risk even in the absence of hypercholesterolemia. Anticoagulation is the treatment of choice to prevent stroke in patients with atrial fibrillation and other potential causes of cardiocerebral emboli. However, data do not support the use of long-term vitamin K antagonists for preventing atherothrombotic stroke for either intracranial or extracranial cerebrovascular disease. The WARSS study found no benefit of warfarin (INR 1.4–2.8) over aspirin 325 mg for secondary prevention of stroke but did find a slightly higher bleeding rate in the warfarin group. A recent European study confirmed this finding. The Warfarin-Aspirin Symptomatic Intracranial Disease (WASID) study demonstrated no benefit of warfarin (INR 2–3) over aspirin in patients with symptomatic intracranial atherosclerosis, and also found higher rates of bleeding complications.

45. The answer is C.

(Chap. 27) Once the diagnosis of stroke is made, a brain imaging study is necessary to determine if the cause of stroke is ischemia or hemorrhage (Figure 27-1). There are no clinical findings that definitively distinguish ischemia from hemorrhage. If the stroke is ischemic, administration of recombinant tissue plasminogen activator (rtPA) or endovascular mechanical thrombectomy may be beneficial in restoring cerebral perfusion. Medical management to reduce the risk of complications becomes the next priority, followed by plans for secondary prevention. For ischemic stroke, several strategies can reduce the risk of subsequent stroke in all patients, while other strategies are effective for patients with specific causes of stroke such as cardiac embolus and carotid atherosclerosis. For hemorrhagic stroke, aneurysmal subarachnoid hemorrhage (SAH) and hypertensive intracranial hemorrhage are two important causes. The National Institute of Neurological Disorders and Stroke (NINDS) recombinant TPA (rtPA) Stroke Study showed a clear benefit for IV rtPA in selected patients with acute stroke. The NINDS study used IV rtPA (0.9 mg/kg to a 90-mg max; 10% as a bolus, then the remainder over 60 minutes) versus placebo in patients with ischemic stroke within 3 hours of onset. Subsequent studies using different dosing and timing ranges have not been as positive. rtPA is being reviewed for approval in the 3- to 4.5-hour window in Europe, but is only approved for 0–3 hours in the United States and Canada. Use of IV rtPA is considered a central component in primary stroke

centers as the first treatment proven to improve clinical outcomes in ischemic stroke and is cost-effective and cost saving. Because collateral blood flow within the ischemic brain is blood pressure dependent, there is controversy about whether blood pressure should be lowered acutely. Blood pressure should be lowered if there is malignant hypertension or concomitant myocardial ischemia or if blood pressure is above 185/110 mmHg and thrombolytic therapy is anticipated. When faced with the competing demands of myocardium and brain, lowering the heart rate with a β_1-adrenergic blocker (such as esmolol) can be a first step to decreasing cardiac work and maintaining blood pressure. Endovascular mechanical thrombectomy has recently shown promise as an alternative or adjunctive treatment of acute stroke in patients who are ineligible for, or have contraindications to, thrombolytics or in those who have failed to have vascular recanalization with IV thrombolytics. Studies have shown excellent acute and chronic recanalization rates and the FDA has approved some devices for intracerebral use. Hypothermia is a powerful neuroprotective treatment in patients with cardiac arrest and is neuroprotective in animal models of stroke, but it has not been adequately studied in patients with ischemic stroke.

46. The answer is D.

(Chap. 29) All the choices given in the question are causes of or may be associated with dementia. Binswanger's disease, the cause of which is unknown, often occurs in patients with long-standing hypertension and/or atherosclerosis; it is associated with diffuse subcortical white matter damage and has a subacute insidious course. Alzheimer's disease, the most common cause of dementia, is also slowly progressive and can be confirmed at autopsy by the presence of amyloid plaques and neurofibrillary tangles. Creutzfeldt-Jakob disease, a prion disease, is associated with a rapidly progressive dementia, myoclonus, rigidity, a characteristic EEG pattern, and death within 1–2 years of onset. Vitamin B_{12} deficiency, which often is seen in the setting of chronic alcoholism, most commonly produces a myelopathy that results in loss of vibration and joint position sense, and brisk deep tendon reflexes (dorsal column and lateral corticospinal tract dysfunction). This combination of pathologic abnormalities in the setting of vitamin B_{12} deficiency is also called subacute combined degeneration. Vitamin B_{12} deficiency may also lead to a subcortical type of dementia. Recent studies have demonstrated that elevated levels of MMA, which is a more sensitive measure of vitamin B_{12} deficiency, may increase the risk of cognitive decline in elderly patients. The therapeutic implications of this finding are not yet clear but emphasize the importance of adequate vitamin B_{12} intake. Multi-infarct dementia, as in this case, presents with a history of sudden stepwise declines in function associated with the accumulation of bilateral focal neurologic deficits. Brain imaging demonstrates multiple areas of stroke.

47. The answer is D.

(Chap. 30) The differential diagnosis of Parkinson's disease is broad, and the disease can be difficult to diagnose, with an estimated misdiagnosis of 10–25% even by experienced physicians. This patient exhibits several atypical features that should alert the physician to search for alternative diagnoses. These include early age of onset, prominent orthostasis, autonomic symptoms of flushing and diaphoresis, and failure to respond to dopaminergic agents. In addition, recurrent urinary tract infections should prompt an evaluation for urinary retention due to autonomic dysfunction in this patient. These symptoms are most consistent with multiple system atrophy with parkinsonian features (MSA-p). The average age of onset is 50 years, and these individuals more frequently present with bilateral, symmetric tremor and more prominent spasticity than those with Parkinson's disease. Orthostasis and autonomic symptoms are typically prominent. On MRI, one would expect to find volume loss and T2-hyperintensity in the area of the putamen, globus pallidus, and white matter. On pathologic examination, α-synuclein–positive inclusions would be seen in the affected areas. Median survival after diagnosis is 6–9 years. Dopaminergic agents are not helpful in the treatment of this disorder and are usually associated with drug-induced dyskinesias of the face and neck, rather than the limbs and trunk. Corticobasal degeneration is a sporadic tauopathy that presents in the sixth to seventh decades. In contrast to Parkinson's disease, this disorder is frequently associated with myoclonic jerks and involuntary purposeful movements of a limb. Its progressive nature leads to spastic paraplegia. Diffuse Lewy body disease has prominent dementia with parkinsonian features. Neuropsychiatric complaints including paranoia, delusions, and personality changes are more common than in Parkinson's disease. Drug-induced Parkinson's disease is not seen with nitrofurantoin, and the patient has no history of illicit drugs such as MTPT, which could cause Parkinson's disease. Finally, this is unlikely to be inadequately treated Parkinson's disease because one would expect at least an initial improvement on dopaminergic agents.

48. The answer is C.

(Chap. 30) Therapy for Parkinson's disease should be initiated when symptoms interfere with the patient's quality of life. Choice of initial drug therapy is usually with dopamine agonists, levodopa, or MAO inhibitors. The initial choice in most individuals is a dopamine agonist (pramipexole, ropinirole, rotigotine), and monotherapy with dopamine agonists usually controls motor symptoms for several years before levodopa therapy becomes necessary. Over this period, escalating doses are frequently required, and side effects may be limiting. It is thought that dopamine agonists delay the onset of dyskinesias and on-off motor symptoms such as freezing. By 5 years, over half of individuals will require levodopa to control motor symptoms. Levodopa remains the most effective

therapy for the motor symptoms of Parkinson's disease, but once levodopa is started, dyskinesias and on-off motor fluctuations become more common. MAO inhibitors (selegiline, rasagiline) work by decreasing the postsynaptic breakdown of dopamine. As monotherapy, these agents have only small effects and are most often used as adjuncts to levodopa. Surgical procedures such as pallidotomy and deep-brain stimulation are reserved for advanced Parkinson's disease with intractable tremor or drug-induced motor fluctuations or dyskinesias. In this setting, deep-brain stimulation can alleviate disabling symptoms.

49. The answer is D.

(Chap. 30) Restless legs syndrome (RLS) is a neurologic disorder that affects approximately 10% of the adult population, causing significant morbidity in some. It is rare in Asians. The four core symptoms required for diagnosis are as follows: an urge to move the legs, usually caused or accompanied by an unpleasant sensation in the legs; symptoms begin or worsen with rest; partial or complete relief by movement; worsening during the evening or night. Symptoms most commonly begin in the legs, but can spread to or even begin in the upper limbs. In about 80% of patients, RLS is associated with periodic leg movements (PLMs) during sleep and occasionally while awake. These involuntary movements are usually brief, lasting no more than a few seconds, and recur every 5–90 seconds. The restlessness and PLMs are a major cause of sleep disturbance in patients, leading to poor-quality sleep and daytime sleepiness. Primary RLS is genetic, and several loci have been found with an autosomal dominant pattern of inheritance, although penetrance may be variable. The mean age of onset in genetic forms is 27 years, although pediatric cases are recognized. The severity of symptoms is variable. Secondary RLS may be associated with pregnancy or a range of underlying disorders, including anemia, ferritin deficiency, renal failure, and peripheral neuropathy. The pathogenesis probably involves disordered dopamine function, which may be peripheral or central, in association with an abnormality of iron metabolism. Diagnosis is made on clinical grounds but can be supported by polysomnography and the demonstration of PLMs. The neurologic examination is normal. Secondary RLS should be excluded, and ferritin levels, glucose, and renal function should be measured. Most RLS sufferers have mild symptoms that do not require specific treatment. If symptoms are intrusive, low doses of dopamine (pramipexole, ropinirole) may be administered before bedtime. Levodopa can be effective but is frequently associated with augmentation (spread and worsening of restlessness and its appearance earlier in the day) or rebound (reappearance sometimes with worsening of symptoms at a time compatible with the drug's short half-life). Other drugs that can be effective include anticonvulsants, analgesics, and even opiates. Management of secondary RLS should be directed to correcting the underlying disorder.

50. The answer is B.

(Chap. 29) Approximately 10% of all persons over the age of 70 have significant memory loss, and in more than half the cause is Alzheimer's disease (AD). AD can occur in any decade of adulthood, but it is the most common cause of dementia in the elderly. AD most often presents with an insidious onset of memory loss followed by a slowly progressive dementia over several years. Pathologically, atrophy is distributed throughout the medial temporal lobes, as well as lateral and medial parietal lobes and lateral frontal cortex. Microscopically, there are neurofibrillary tangles composed of hyperphosphorylated tau filaments, and accumulation of amyloid in blood vessel walls in the cortex and leptomeninges. The cognitive changes of AD tend to follow a characteristic pattern beginning with memory impairment and spreading to language and visuospatial deficits. Yet approximately 20% of patients with AD present with nonmemory complaints such as word-finding, organizational, or navigational difficulty. In the early stages of the disease, the memory loss may go unrecognized or be ascribed to benign forgetfulness. Slowly the cognitive problems begin to interfere with daily activities, such as keeping track of finances, following instructions on the job, driving, shopping, and housekeeping. Some patients are unaware of these difficulties (*anosognosia*), while others remain acutely attuned to their deficits. Social graces, routine behavior, and superficial conversation may be surprisingly intact. Language becomes impaired—first naming, then comprehension, and finally fluency. In some patients, *aphasia* is an early and prominent feature. Word-finding difficulties and circumlocution may be a problem even when formal testing demonstrates intact naming and fluency. Visuospatial deficits begin to interfere with dressing, eating, or even walking, and patients fail to solve simple puzzles or copy geometric figures. Simple calculations and clock reading become difficult in parallel. Loss of judgment and reasoning is inevitable. Delusions are common and usually simple, with common themes of theft, infidelity, or misidentification. In end-stage AD, patients become rigid, mute, incontinent, and bedridden. Hyperactive tendon reflexes and myoclonic jerks may occur spontaneously or in response to physical or auditory stimulation. Generalized seizures may also occur. Often death results from malnutrition, secondary infections, pulmonary emboli, heart disease, or, most commonly, aspiration. The typical duration of AD is 8–10 years, but the course can range from 1 to 25 years. For unknown reasons, some AD patients show a steady decline in function, while others have prolonged plateaus without major deterioration.

51. The answer is E.

(Chap. 32) The combination of upper and lower motor neuron findings is highly suggestive of ALS. Indolent presentation is typical and many patients receive alternative diagnoses before defining ALS. There is currently

no curative therapy for ALS; therefore, treatable causes of motor nerve dysfunction should be ruled out. Compression of the cervical spinal cord or cervicomedullary junction from tumors in the cervical regions or at the foramen magnum or from cervical spondylosis with osteophytes projecting into the vertebral canal can produce weakness, wasting, and fasciculations in the upper limbs and spasticity in the legs, closely resembling ALS. Absence of pain or of sensory changes, normal bowel and bladder function, normal roentgenographic studies of the spine, and normal cerebrospinal fluid (CSF) all favor ALS. Another important entity in the differential diagnosis of ALS is multifocal motor neuropathy with conduction block (MMCB). In this disorder, remarkably focal blocks in conduction regionally and chronically disrupt lower motor neuron function. Many cases have elevated serum titers of mono- and polyclonal antibodies to ganglioside GM1; it is hypothesized that the antibodies produce selective, focal, paranodal demyelination of motor neurons. MMCB is not typically associated with corticospinal signs. In contrast with ALS, MMCB may respond dramatically to therapy such as IV immunoglobulin or chemotherapy; it is thus imperative that MMCB be excluded when considering a diagnosis of ALS. A diffuse, lower motor axonal neuropathy mimicking ALS sometimes evolves in association with hematopoietic disorders such as lymphoma or multiple myeloma. Lyme disease may also cause an axonal, lower motor neuropathy, although typically with intense proximal limb pain and a CSF pleocytosis.

Other treatable disorders that occasionally mimic ALS are chronic lead poisoning and thyrotoxicosis. Vitamin C deficiency may cause myalgias in addition to fatigue, lethargy, and skin findings, but motor neuron findings are not typical.

52. The answer is E.

(Chap. 33) Postural orthostatic tachycardia syndrome is characterized by symptomatic orthostatic intolerance and either an increase in heart rate to more than 120 beats/min or an increase of 30 beats/min with standing that subsides on sitting or lying down. There is no orthostatic hypotension. Women are affected approximately five times more often than men, and most develop the syndrome between the ages of 15 and 50. Approximately half of affected patients report an antecedent viral infection. Lightheadedness, weakness, and blurred vision combined with symptoms of autonomic over activity (palpitations, tremulousness, nausea) are common. Recurrent, unexplained episodes of dysautonomia and fatigue also occur. The pathogenesis is unclear in most cases; hypovolemia, deconditioning, venous pooling, impaired brainstem regulation, or adrenergic receptor supersensitivity may play a role. Although up to 80% of patients improve, only about 25% eventually resume their usual daily activities (including exercise and sports). Expansion of fluid volume and postural training are initial approaches to treatment. If these approaches are inadequate, then midodrine, fludrocortisone, phenobarbital, beta blockers, or clonidine may provide some benefit. Reconditioning and a sustained exercise program are very important. All of the other listed choices are associated with orthostatic hypotension.

53. The answer is D.

(Chap. 33) Complex regional pain syndrome (CRPS) types I and II are the terms that have replaced reflex sympathetic dystrophy (RSD) or causalgia because of the absence of a proven causative role for the autonomic nervous system. CRPS type I is a regional pain syndrome that usually develops after tissue trauma. Examples of associated trauma include myocardial infarction, minor shoulder or limb injury, and stroke. Allodynia, hyperpathia, and spontaneous pain occur. The symptoms are unrelated to the severity of the initial trauma and are not confined to the distribution of a single peripheral nerve. CRPS type II is a regional pain syndrome that develops after injury to a specific peripheral nerve, usually a major nerve trunk. Spontaneous pain initially develops within the territory of the affected nerve but eventually may spread outside the nerve distribution. Pain is the primary clinical feature of CRPS. Vasomotor dysfunction, sudomotor abnormalities, or focal edema may occur alone or in combination but must be present for diagnosis. Localized sweating and changes in blood flow may produce temperature differences between affected and unaffected limbs. CRPS type I has classically been divided into three clinical phases but is now considered to be more variable. Phase I consists of pain and swelling in the distal extremity occurring within weeks to 3 months after the precipitating event. The pain is diffuse, spontaneous, and either burning, throbbing, or aching in quality. The involved extremity is warm and edematous, and the joints are tender. Increased sweating and hair growth develop. In phase II (3–6 months after onset), thin, shiny, cool skin appears. After an additional 3–6 months (phase III), atrophy of the skin and subcutaneous tissue plus flexion contractures complete the clinical picture. A variety of surgical and medical treatments have been developed for CRPS, with conflicting reports of efficacy. Clinical trials suggest that early mobilization with physical therapy or a brief course of glucocorticoids may be helpful for CRPS type I. Other medical treatments include the use of adrenergic blockers, nonsteroidal anti-inflammatory drugs, calcium channel blockers, phenytoin, opioids, and calcitonin. Stellate ganglion blockade is a commonly used invasive technique that often provides temporary pain relief, but the efficacy of repetitive blocks is uncertain.

54. The answer is A.

(Chap. 34) Trigeminal neuralgia is a clinical diagnosis based entirely on patient history. The disorder is characterized by *paroxysms* of excruciating pain in the lips, gums, cheeks, and chin that resolves over seconds to minutes. It

is caused by ectopic action potentials in afferent pain fibers of the fifth cranial nerve, due either to nerve compression or other causes of demyelination. Symptoms are often, but not always, elicited by tactile stimuli on the face, tongue, or lips. An elevated ESR is not part of the clinical syndrome. Elevated ESR is associated with temporal arteritis, a vasculitis associated with jaw claudication, unilateral vision loss, and symptoms of polymyalgia rheumatica. Trigeminal neuralgia is specifically notable for a lack of sensory findings on examination, unless the diagnosis is made in conjunction with another disorder such as a midbrain mass lesion or aneurysm. Deep-seated facial and head pain is more commonly a feature of migraine headache, dental pathology, or sinus disease. First-line therapy is with carbamazepine, not gabapentin. It should be started and increased gradually until pain symptoms subside; 50–75% of patients will respond to this therapy. If treatment is effective, it is continued for 1 month then tapered.

55. The answer is C.

(Chap. 34) Trigeminal neuralgia is a clinical diagnosis based entirely on patient history, and as such should be treated once a patient presents with the virtually pathognomonic complaints of paroxysms of excruciating pain in the lips, gums, cheeks, and chin that resolve over seconds to minutes. Carbamazepine is first-line therapy. Oxcarbazepine likely has equivalent efficacy to carbamazepine with less toxicity. Lamotrigine, orphenytoin, and baclofen are other potential therapeutic options. Surgical approaches, such as radiofrequency thermal rhizotomy, gamma-knife radiosurgery, and microvascular decompression, should be considered only when medical options fail. Steroids have no therapeutic role, as trigeminal neuralgia is not an inflammatory condition. Neuroimaging is not indicated, unless other clinical features or a focal neurologic deficit elicited on history or physical examination suggest another possible diagnosis such as intracranial mass or multiple sclerosis.

56. The answer is D.

(Chap. 34) Brief paroxysms of severe, sharp pains in the face without demonstrable lesions in the jaw, teeth, or sinuses are called tic douloureux, or trigeminal neuralgia. The pain may be brought on by stimuli applied to the face, lips, or tongue or by certain movements of those structures. Aneurysms, neurofibromas, and meningiomas impinging on the fifth cranial nerve at any point during its course typically present with trigeminal neuropathy, which will cause sensory loss on the face, weakness of the jaw muscles, or both; neither symptom is demonstrable in this patient. Amyotrophic lateral sclerosis (ALS) is a motor neuron disease that may present with bulbar motor findings but sensory findings (in the absence of muscle spasms) are uncommon.

57. The answer is C.

(Chap. 35) The MRI shows an infiltrated and collapsed second thoracic vertebral body with posterior displacement and compression of the upper thoracic spinal cord due to metastatic breast cancer. The low-intensity bone marrow signal in panel A of Figure 57 signifies replacement by tumor. When a patient presents with possible myelopathy, the first priority is to distinguish between a compressive or noncompressive etiology. The common causes of compressive myelopathy are tumor, epidural abscess or hematoma, herniated disk, or vertebral pathology. Epidural compression due to malignancy or abscess often causes warning signs of neck or back pain, bladder disturbances, and sensory symptoms that precede the development of paralysis. MRI is the optimal diagnostic modality to image the spinal cord. In adults, most neoplasms are epidural in origin, resulting from metastases to the adjacent spinal bones. The propensity of solid tumors to metastasize to the vertebral column probably reflects the high proportion of bone marrow located in the axial skeleton. Almost any malignant tumor can metastasize to the spinal column, with breast, lung, prostate, kidney, lymphoma, and plasma cell dyscrasia occurring particularly frequently. The thoracic spinal column is most commonly involved; exceptions are metastases from prostate and ovarian cancer, which occur disproportionately in the sacral and lumbar vertebrae, probably resulting from spread through Batson's plexus, a network of veins along the anterior epidural space. Retroperitoneal neoplasms (especially lymphomas or sarcomas) enter the spinal canal through the intervertebral foramens and produce radicular pain with signs of root weakness prior to cord compression. Pain is usually the initial symptom of spinal metastasis and characteristically awakens patients at night. A recent onset of persistent back pain, particularly if in the thoracic spine (which is uncommonly involved by spondylosis), should prompt consideration of vertebral metastasis. Infections of the spinal column (osteomyelitis and related disorders) are distinctive in that, unlike tumor, they may cross the disk space to involve the adjacent vertebral body. Management of cord compression includes glucocorticoids to reduce cord edema, local radiotherapy (initiated as early as possible) to the symptomatic lesion, and specific therapy for the underlying tumor type. Spinal epidural abscess presents as a clinical triad of midline dorsal pain, fever, and progressive limb weakness. Risk factors include an impaired immune status (diabetes mellitus, renal failure, alcoholism, malignancy), IV drug abuse, and infections of the skin or other tissues. Two-thirds of epidural infections result from hematogenous spread of bacteria from the skin (furunculosis), soft tissue (pharyngeal or dental abscesses), or deep viscera (bacterial endocarditis). Hemorrhage into the epidural (or subdural) space causes acute focal or radicular pain followed by variable signs of a spinal cord or conus medullaris disorder. Therapeutic anticoagulation, trauma, tumor, or blood dyscrasias are predisposing conditions. Hemorrhage into the substance of the spinal cord is a rare result of trauma, intraparenchymal vascular malformation, vasculitis due to polyarteritis nodosa or systemic

lupus erythematosus (SLE), bleeding disorders, or a spinal cord neoplasm. Hematomyelia presents as an acute, painful transverse myelopathy.

58. The answer is B.
(Chap. 35) This patient has a history and examination consistent with a myelopathy. The rapidity of onset and the lack of other antecedent symptoms (e.g., pain) make a noncompressive etiology most likely. An MRI is the initial test of choice and will easily identify a structural lesion such as a neoplasm or subluxation. Noncompressive myelopathies result from five basic causes: spinal cord infarction; systemic disorders such as vasculitis, systemic lupus erythematosus (SLE), and sarcoidosis; infections (particularly viral); demyelinating disease such as multiple sclerosis; and idiopathic. Therefore, serologies for antinuclear antibodies, viral serologies such as HIV and HTLV-I, and lumbar puncture are all indicated. Because the clinical scenario is consistent with a myelopathy, an electromyogram is not indicated.

59. The answer is A.
(Chap. 35) Syringomyelia is a developmental, slowly enlarging cavitary expansion of the cervical cord that produces a progressive myelopathy. Symptoms typically begin in adolescence or early adulthood. They may undergo spontaneous arrest after several years. More than half are associated with Chiari malformations. Acquired cavitations of the spinal cord are referred to as syrinx cavities. They may result from trauma, myelitis, infection, or tumor. The classic presentation is that of a central cord syndrome with sensory loss of pain and temperature sensation, and weakness of the upper extremities. Vibration and position sensation are typically preserved. Muscle wasting in the lower neck, shoulders, arms, and hands with asymmetric or absent reflexes reflects extension of the cavity to the anterior horns. With progression, spasticity and weakness of the lower extremities, and bladder and bowel dysfunction may occur. MRI scans are the diagnostic modality of choice. Surgical therapy is generally unsatisfactory. Syringomyelia associated with Chiari malformations may require extensive decompressions of the posterior fossa. Direct decompression of the cavity is of debatable benefit. Syringomyelia secondary to trauma or infection is treated with decompression and a drainage procedure, with a shunt often inserted that drains into the subarachnoid space. Although relief may occur, recurrence is common.

60. The answer is A.
(Chap. 36) Concussions result from blunt head trauma that causes anterior-posterior movement of the brain within the skull. Transient loss of consciousness is common, as are confusion and amnesia. Many patients do not lose consciousness but feel dazed, stunned, or confused. A brief period of both retrograde and anterograde amnesia is characteristic of concussion and it recedes rapidly in alert patients. Head imaging is typically normal. Postconcussive syndrome is a constellation of symptoms including fatigue, headache, dizziness, and difficulty concentrating that follows a concussion. The patient described fits this diagnosis; strict diagnostic criteria do not exist. Typically patients will improve over a 6- to 12-month period. Patients who were energetic and highly functioning prior to their trauma have an excellent prognosis. Treatment is aimed at reassurance and relieving prominent symptoms. Dizziness can be treated with Phenergan, which acts as a vestibular suppressant. He should avoid contact sports at least until his symptoms resolve.

61. The answer is D.
(Chap. 36) The head CT (Figure 61) shows chronic bilateral subdural hematomas of varying age. The collections began as acute hematomas and have become hypodense in comparison to the adjacent brain. Some areas of resolving blood are contained in the more recently formed collection on the left. Acute hematomas (which would be as bright as the resolving blood shown in arrows) become hypodense in comparison with adjacent brain after approximately 2 months. During the isodense phase (2–6 weeks after injury), they may be difficult to discern. Chronic subdural hematoma may present without a history of trauma or injury in 20–30% of patients. Headache is common. Other symptoms may be vague, as in this case, or there may be focal signs including hemiparesis mimicking stroke. Underlying cortical damage may serve as a seizure focus. In relatively asymptomatic patients with small hematomas, observation and serial imaging may be reasonable; however, surgical evacuation is often necessary for large or symptomatic chronic hematomas.

62. The answer is D.
(Chap. 36) Hemorrhages beneath the dural layer (subdural) or between the skull and the dura (epidural) are common sequelae of head trauma. They can be life-threatening, and prompt evaluation and management are imperative. Several clinical features allow these conditions to be distinguished from one another. Acute subdural hematomas typically arise from venous sources, often the bridging veins located immediately under the dura mater. As the brain volume decreases with age, traction on these venous structures increases and even minor head trauma in the elderly can lead to a subdural hematoma. A "lucid interval" of several minutes to hours before coma supervenes is most characteristic of epidural hemorrhage, but it is still uncommon, and epidural hemorrhage is not the only cause of this temporal sequence. Subdural bleeding is typically slower than epidural bleeding due to their different sources. Small subdural bleeds are asymptomatic and often do not require evacuation. Epidural hematomas, on the other hand, can arise quickly and typically represent arterial bleeding. A lacerated middle meningeal artery from an overlying skull fracture often causes these. A rapid

increase in intracranial pressure from these bleeds can necessitate arterial ligation or emergent craniotomy. Most patients with epidural bleeding are unconscious when first evaluated; a "lucid interval" can occasionally be seen.

63. The answer is D.
(Chap. 37) Distinguishing CNS toxoplasmosis from primary CNS lymphoma in a patient with HIV infection is often difficult. The standard approach in a neurologically stable patient is to treat the patient for toxoplasmosis for 2–3 weeks then repeat neuroimaging. If the imaging shows clear improvement, continue antibiotics. If there is no response to therapy after 2 weeks, therapy does not need to be continued and a stereotactic brain biopsy is indicated. In this immunocompromised patient who has not responded to treatment for CNS toxoplasmosis, a positive CNS EBV DNA would be diagnostic of CNS lymphoma. Whole-brain radiation therapy is part of the treatment for CNS lymphoma, which is not yet diagnosed in this patient, and should not be instituted empirically. Treatments directed at viral infections of the CNS or CNS lymphomas are not indicated at this time since a diagnosis is still yet to be made. In the absence of a change in neurologic status or evidence of mass effect on CT, there is no indication for dexamethasone. Of note, the incidence of primary CNS lymphoma appears to be increasing in immunocompetent individuals for unclear reasons.

64. The answer is A.
(Chap. 37) Endocrine dysfunction resulting in hypopituitarism frequently follows exposure of the hypothalamus or pituitary gland to therapeutic radiation. Growth hormone is the most sensitive to the damaging effects of WBRT, and thyroid-stimulating hormone is the least sensitive. ACTH, prolactin, and gonadotropins have an intermediate sensitivity. Other complications of radiation therapy to the brain include acute radiation injury manifest by headache, sleepiness, and worsening of preexisting neurologic defects. Early delayed radiation injury occurs within the first 4 months after therapy. It is associated with increased white matter signal on MRI and is steroid responsive. Late delayed radiation injury occurs more than 4 months after therapy, typically 8–24 months. There may be dementia, gait apraxia, focal necrosis (after focal irradiation), or the development of secondary malignancies.

65. The answer is D.
(Chap. 37) The postgadolinium MRI shows multiple meningiomas along the falx and left parietal cortex. Meningiomas derive from the cells that give rise to the arachnoid granulations. They are now the most common primary brain tumor, accounting for approximately 32% of the total, and occur more commonly in women than men. They are usually benign (WHO classification grade 1) and attached to the dura. They rarely invade the brain. Meningiomas are diagnosed with increasing frequency as more people undergo neuroimaging studies for various indications. Their incidence increases with age, and they are more common in patients with a history of cranial irradiation. They are most commonly located over the cerebral convexities, especially adjacent to the sagittal sinus, but can also occur in the skull base and along the dorsum of the spinal cord. Many meningiomas are found incidentally following neuroimaging for unrelated reasons. They can also present with headaches, seizures, or focal neurologic deficits. On imaging studies they have a characteristic appearance usually consisting of a partially calcified, densely enhancing extra-axial tumor arising from the dura. The main differential diagnosis of meningioma is a dural metastasis. Total surgical resection of a meningioma is curative. Low-grade astrocytoma and high-grade astrocytoma (glioblastoma) often infiltrate into adjacent brain and rarely have the clear margins seen in Figure 65. Oligodendroma comprise approximately 15% of all gliomas and show calcification in roughly 30% of cases. They have a more benign course and are more responsive than other gliomas to cytotoxic therapy. For low-grade oligodendromas, the median survival is 7–8 years. Brain abscess will have distinctive ring-enhancing features with a capsule, will often have mass effect, and will have evidence of inflammation on MRI scanning.

66. The answer is C.
(Chap. 38) Hormones produced by the anterior pituitary include adrenocorticotropic hormone, thyroid-stimulating hormone, luteinizing hormone, follicle-stimulating hormone, prolactin, and growth hormone. The posterior pituitary produces vasopressin and oxytocin. The anterior and posterior pituitary has a separate vascular supply, and the posterior pituitary is directly innervated by the hypothalamic neurons via the pituitary stalk, thus making it susceptible to shear stress–associated dysfunction. Hypothalamic control of anterior pituitary function is through secreted hormones; thus it is less susceptible to traumatic injury.

67. The answer is B.
(Chap. 38) The patient has evidence of Sheehan's syndrome postpartum. In this syndrome, the hyperplastic pituitary postpartum is at increased risk for hemorrhage and/or infarction. This leads to bilateral visual changes, headache, and meningeal signs. Ophthalmoplegia may be observed. In severe cases, cardiovascular collapse and altered levels of consciousness may be observed. Laboratory evaluation commonly shows hypoglycemia. Pituitary CT or MRI may show signs of sellar hemorrhage if present. Involvement of all pituitary hormones may be seen, though the most acute finding is often hypoglycemia and hypotension from the failure of adrenocorticotropic hormone. The hypoglycemia and hypotension present in this case suggest failure of the glucocorticoid system; thus treatment with a corticosteroid is indicated. There is no

evidence of sepsis; thus antibiotics and drotrecogin alfa are not indicated. With a normal hematocrit and no reported evidence of massive hemorrhage, packed red cell transfusion is unlikely to be helpful. Although thyroid-stimulating hormone production is undoubtedly low in this patient, the most immediate concern is replacement of glucocorticoid.

68. The answer is D.

(Chap. 38) Functional pituitary adenoma presentations include acromegaly, as in this patient, prolactinomas, and Cushing's syndrome. Hypersecretion of growth hormone underlies this syndrome in patients with pituitary masses, though ectopic production of growth hormone, particularly by tumors, has been reported. Because growth hormone is secreted in a highly pulsatile fashion, obtaining random serum levels is not reliable. Thus, the downstream mediator of systemic effects of growth hormone, IGF-1, is measured to screen for growth hormone excess. IGF-1 is made by the liver in response to growth hormone stimulation. An oral glucose tolerance test with growth hormone obtained at 0, 30, and 60 minutes may also be used to screen for acromegaly, as normal persons should suppress growth hormone to this challenge. Serum prolactin level is useful to screen for prolactinomas; 24-hour urinary free cortisol and ACTH assay are useful screens for Cushing's disease.

69. The answer is B.

(Chap. 38) Hyperprolactinemia is the most common pituitary hormone hypersecretion syndrome in both men and women. Although pituitary adenoma is a frequent cause, there are several physiologic, medication-related, and potentially reversible etiologies. Prolactin is normally elevated during pregnancy and lactation, though levels should fall to normal within 6 months of cessation of breastfeeding. Nipple stimulation, sleep, and stress may all increase prolactin levels. Systemic disorders such as chronic renal failure and cirrhosis may also cause elevated prolactin levels. Prolactin levels are also typically elevated after generalized seizures, which may be useful in the evaluation of pseudoseizures. Drug-induced hypersecretion is associated with dopamine receptor blockers, dopamine synthesis inhibitors, opiates, H_2 antagonists, imipramines, selective serotonin reuptake inhibitors, and calcium channel blockers. Hypothalamic-pituitary stalk damage may also cause hyperprolactinemia. Rathke's cysts, which are benign intrasellar lesions, may produce endocrinologic abnormalities similar to pituitary adenomas.

70. The answer is E.

(Chap. 38) Tumors arising from the lactotrope cells of the pituitary account for half of all functioning pituitary tumors and most commonly affect women. The most common presentations are amenorrhea, infertility, and/or galactorrhea. Microadenomas rarely progress to become macroadenomas. For symptomatic disease, the primary goals of therapy are control of hyperprolactinemia, reduction of tumor size, restoration of menses and fertility, and resolution of galactorrhea. Usually oral dopamine agonists, such as cabergoline and bromocriptine, are used for this purpose.

71. The answer is C.

(Chap. 38) Adult growth hormone deficiency is usually caused by hypothalamic or pituitary damage. Because growth hormone is no longer important for achieving stature, the presentation is different from childhood growth hormone deficiency. Although growth hormone has direct tissue effects, it primarily acts through increasing secretion of IGF-1, which in turn stimulates lipolysis, increases circulating fatty acids, reduces omental fat mass, and enhances lean body mass. Thus, deficiency of growth hormone causes the opposite effects. In addition, hypertension, left ventricular dysfunction, and increased plasma fibrinogen levels may also be present with deficient growth hormone. Reduced, not increased, bone mineral density may also occur in adults with growth hormone deficiency.

72. The answer is E.

(Chap. 38) The patient has a clinical presentation consistent with Cushing's syndrome. Although many cases of inappropriate elevation of ACTH are due to pituitary tumors, a substantial proportion are due to ectopic ACTH secretion. Clues to this diagnosis include a rapid onset of hypercortisolism features associated with skin hyperpigmentation and severe myopathy. Additionally, hypertension, hypokalemic metabolic alkalosis, glucose intolerance, and edema are more prominent in ectopic ACTH secretion than in pituitary tumors. Serum potassium below 3.3 mmol/L is present in 70% of ectopic ACTH cases, but in less than 10% of pituitary-dependent Cushing's syndrome. ACTH levels will be high, as this is the underlying cause of both types of Cushing's syndrome. Corticotropin-releasing hormone is rarely the cause of Cushing's syndrome. Unfortunately, MRI of the pituitary gland will not visualize lesions less than 2 mm; thus occasional sampling of the inferior petrosal veins is required, but this is not indicated in the case presented at this time in the evaluation.

73. The answer is C.

(Chap. 38) The patient has panhypopituitarism and is unable to make TSH; thus her plasma TSH level will always be low, regardless of the adequacy of her T_4 replacement. A free T_4 level will allow the determination of whether her plasma level is in the normal range of thyroid hormone. This, coupled with her symptoms, will aid in the determination of proper levothyroxine dosing. There is no evidence of recurrent disease clinically; thus MRI is not useful. She is unlikely to have primary thyroid disease,

and T_4 level is unknown presently, so thyroid uptake scan is not indicated at this time.

74. The answer is A.

(*Chap. 38*) The diagnosis of Cushing's syndrome relies on documentation of endogenous hypercortisolism. Of the list of choices, the most cost-effective and precise test is the 24-hour urine free cortisol. Failure to suppress plasma morning cortisol after overnight suppression with 1 mg dexamethasone is an alternative. Most ACTH-secreting pituitary adenomas are less than 5 mm in diameter, and approximately half are not detected even with sensitive MRI. Further, because incidental microadenomas are common in the pituitary, the presence of a small pituitary abnormality on MRI may not establish the source of ACTH production. Basal plasma ACTH levels are used to distinguish between ACTH-independent (adrenal or exogenous glucocorticoid) and ACTH-dependent (pituitary, ectopic ACTH) sources of hypercortisolism. Mean basal ACTH levels are higher in patients with ectopic ACTH production than in patients with pituitary ACTH adenomas. There is significant overlap in ACTH levels, however, and this test should not be used as an initial diagnostic test. Rarely, patients have Cushing's syndrome and elevated ACTH due to a CRH-releasing tumor. In this case, CRH levels are elevated. Inferior petrosal venous sampling can be used to identify a pituitary source of ACTH secretion when imaging modalities do not reveal a source.

75. The answer is B.

(*Chap. 38*) The identification of an empty sella is often the result of an incidental MRI finding. Typically these patients will have normal pituitary function and should be reassured. It is likely that the surrounding rim of pituitary tissue is functioning normally. An empty sella may signal the insidious onset of hypopituitarism, and laboratory results should be followed closely. Unless her clinical situation changes, repeat MRI is not indicated. Endocrine malignancy is unlikely, and surgery is not part of the management of an empty sella.

76. The answer is D.

(Chap. 39) The onset of multiple sclerosis (MS) may be abrupt or insidious. Symptoms may be severe or seem so trivial that a patient may not seek medical attention for months or years. Indeed, at autopsy, approximately 0.1% of individuals who were asymptomatic during life will be found, unexpectedly, to have pathologic evidence of MS. Similarly, in the modern era, an MRI scan obtained for an unrelated reason may show evidence of asymptomatic MS. Symptoms of MS are extremely varied and depend on the location and severity of lesions within the CNS (see Table 39-2). Examination often reveals evidence of neurologic dysfunction, often in asymptomatic locations. For example, a patient may present with symptoms in one leg but signs in both.

77. The answer is D.

(Chap. 39) The four clinical types of multiple sclerosis (MS) include relapsing/remitting, secondary progressive, primary progressive, and progressive relapsing. Relapsing/remitting MS (RRMS) accounts for 85% of MS cases at onset and is characterized by discrete attacks that generally evolve over days to weeks (rarely over hours). There is often complete recovery over the ensuing weeks to months. However, when ambulation is severely impaired during an attack, approximately half will fail to improve. Between attacks, patients are neurologically stable. Secondary progressive MS (SPMS) always begins as RRMS. At some point, however, the clinical course changes so that the patient experiences a steady deterioration in function unassociated with acute attacks (which may continue or cease during the progressive phase). SPMS produces a greater amount of fixed neurologic disability than RRMS. For a patient with RRMS, the risk of developing SPMS is approximately 2% each year, meaning that the great majority of RRMS ultimately evolves into SPMS. SPMS appears to represent a late stage of the same underlying illness as RRMS. Primary progressive MS (PPMS) accounts for approximately 15% of cases. These patients do not experience attacks but only a steady functional decline from disease onset. Compared to RRMS, the sex distribution is more even, the disease begins later in life (mean age approximately 40 years), and disability develops faster (at least relative to the onset of the first clinical symptom). Despite these differences, PPMS appears to represent the same underlying illness as RRMS. Progressive/relapsing MS (PRMS) overlaps PPMS and SPMS and accounts for about 5% of MS patients. Like patients with PPMS, these patients experience a steady deterioration in their condition from disease onset. However, like SPMS patients, they experience occasional attacks superimposed upon their progressive course. Autoimmune autonomic neuropathy is a distinct clinical syndrome not related to MS. It presents with the subacute development of autonomic disturbances with orthostatic hypotension, enteric neuropathy (gastroparesis, ileus, constipation/diarrhea), and cholinergic failure; the latter consists of loss of sweating, sicca complex, and a tonic pupil. Autoantibodies against the ganglionic ACh receptor (A_3 AChR) are present in the serum of many patients and are now considered to be diagnostic of this syndrome.

78. The answer is D.

(Chap. 40) In a patient with suspected bacterial meningitis empirical therapy should be administered promptly to reduce mortality and morbidity. The decision to obtain an imaging study prior to lumbar puncture (LP) is based on the concern of precipitating herniation in a patient with elevated intracranial pressure or focal CNS lesions. Therefore, patients with the presence of papilledema on physical examination, history of recent head trauma, known or suspected intracranial lesions (immunosuppressed, known

malignancy), focal neurologic findings, or depressed level of consciousness should have a head CT or MRI prior to LP. In an immunocompetent patient with no known history of recent head trauma, a normal level of consciousness, and no evidence of papilledema or focal neurologic deficits, it is considered safe to perform LP without prior neuroimaging studies. Kernig's sign is elicited in a supine patient by flexing the thigh and knee. A positive sign occurs when the patient has head/neck pain when passively straightening the knee. The sensitivity and specificity of this sign (also Brudzinski's) for bacterial meningitis are unknown, but they imply meningeal irritation, not an intracranial lesion or elevated intracranial pressure. While cerebrospinal fluid cultures may be impacted by administration of antibiotics prior to LP, stains, antigen tests, and polymerase chain reaction tests will not be affected.

79. The answer is B.

(Chap. 40) The release of bacterial cell wall components after killing by antibiotics may evoke a marked inflammatory cytokine response in the subarachnoid space. This inflammation may lead to increased damage of the blood-brain barrier and central nervous system damage. Glucocorticoids can blunt this response by inhibiting tumor necrosis factor and interleukin-1. They work best if administered before antibiotics. Clinical trials have demonstrated that dexamethasone, 10 mg IV administered 20 minutes *before* antibiotics, reduced unfavorable outcomes, including death. The dexamethasone was continued for 4 days. The benefits were most striking in pneumococcal meningitis. Because this is the most common cause of meningitis in the elderly, empirical coverage should include this intervention as well. The efficacy of dexamethasone therapy in preventing neurologic sequelae is different between high- and low-income countries. Randomized trials in low-income countries (sub-Saharan Africa, Southeast Asia) failed to show benefit in subgroups of patients. The lack of efficacy of dexamethasone in these trials has been attributed to late presentation to the hospital with more advanced disease, antibiotic pretreatment, malnutrition, infection with HIV, and treatment of patients with probable, but not microbiologically proven, bacterial meningitis. The results of these clinical trials suggest that patients in sub-Saharan Africa and those in low-income countries with negative CSF Gram stain and culture should not be treated with dexamethasone. Empirical antibiotics in this case should include a third-generation cephalosporin, vancomycin, and ampicillin. However, dexamethasone may decrease vancomycin penetration into the CSF, so its use should be considered carefully in cases where the most likely organism requires vancomycin coverage. Acyclovir or valacyclovir may be used as initial empiric treatment in cases of suspected herpes CNS infection. However, in this case the LP is highly suggestive of acute bacterial infection. Intravenous gamma globulin is used as adjunctive therapy in children with known immunoglobulin deficiency who are at risk of viral meningitis/encephalitis.

80. The answer is D.

(Chap. 40) *Listeria* has become an increasingly important cause of bacterial meningitis in neonates (<1 month of age), pregnant women, individuals more than 60 years old, and immunocompromised individuals. Infection is acquired by eating contaminated foods such as unpasteurized dairy products, coleslaw, milk, soft cheeses, delicatessen meats, and uncooked hot dogs. Ampicillin is the agent most often added to the initial empirical regimen to cover *L. monocytogenes*.

81. The answer is D.

(Chap. 41) Ibuprofen, isoniazid, ciprofloxacin, tolmetin, sulfa-containing medicines, and phenazopyridine have been implicated in drug hypersensitivity leading to meningitis. The cerebrospinal fluid (CSF) will typically show neutrophils, but mononuclear cells or eosinophils are occasionally present. Most causes of chronic (not recurrent) meningitis cause a predominance of mononuclear cells. The differential for chronic meningitis is broad and a diagnosis is often difficult to make. The treating physician needs to consider a diverse array of viral, fungal, bacterial, mycobacterial, helminthic, and protozoal pathogens, both common and exotic, and therefore should obtain a detailed social history and consult an expert in the field. Recurrent meningitis is often due to herpes simplex virus type 2 infection and this should be ruled out, particularly if active genital ulcers develop concurrently. Malignancy, sarcoidosis, and vasculitis are all potential causes, and history, physical examination, and appropriate further testing should dictate the degree to which these possibilities are explored. Medications are often overlooked as a cause of chronic meningitis and should always be carefully considered. When CSF neutrophils predominate after 3 weeks of illness, *Nocardia*, *Actinomyces*, *Brucella*, tuberculosis (<10% of cases), and fungal and noninfectious causes of chronic meningitis should be considered.

82. The answer is E.

(Chap. 43) Prions are infectious particles that cause central nervous system degeneration. The human prion diseases described to date include Creutzfeldt-Jacob disease (CJD), kuru, Gerstmann-Straüssler-Scheinker disease, and fatal insomnia. The most common prion disease is sporadic CJD (sCJD), which occurs in a seemingly random pattern in adults in their fifth and sixth decades of life. sCJD accounts for about 85% of cases of CJD and occurs in approximately 1 per 1 million population. Variant CJD (vCJD) results from infection from bovine exposure to tainted beef from cattle with bovine spongiform encephalopathy (BSE). There has been a steady decline of cases of vCJD in Europe over the past decade. Infectious CJD (iCJD) has resulted from injection of tainted human growth hormone, as well

as transplant of infected dura mater grafts into humans. Familial CJD (fCJD) is due to germ-line mutations that follow an autosomal dominant inheritance. Kuru is due to infection through ritualistic cannibalism. Gerstmann-Straüssler-Scheinker disease and familial fatal insomnia (FFI) occur as dominantly inherited prion diseases. Sporadic cases of fatal insomnia (sFI) have been described.

83. The answer is B.

(Chap. 43) Startle myoclonus is a worrisome sign but is neither sensitive nor specific for CJD, though it is more worrisome if it occurs during sleep. The constellation of dementia, myoclonus, and periodic electrical bursts in an afebrile 60-year-old patient generally indicates CJD. Clinical abnormalities in CJD are confined to the CNS. Lewy body dementia, Alzheimer's disease, central nervous system infections, and myoclonic epilepsy can all cause myoclonus. Both EEG and MRI can help differentiate CJD from these disorders. The MRI finding of cortical ribboning and intensity in the basal ganglia on fluid-attenuated inversion recovery sequences is characteristic of CJD. EEG is useful if stereotypical periodic bursts every 1–2 seconds are present, but this is seen in only 60% of cases, and other findings may be less specific. Demonstration of specific immunoassays for proteolytic products of disease-causing prion proteins (PrP^{Sc}) at brain biopsy may be necessary to confirm diagnosis in some cases. However, these proteins are not uniformly distributed throughout the brain and false-negative biopsies occur. Both surgeons and pathologists must be warned to use standard precautions under these circumstances. These proteins cannot be measured from cerebrospinal fluid (CSF). CSF in CJD is usually normal except for a minimally elevated protein. Many patients with CJD have elevated CSF stress protein 14-3-3. This test alone is neither sensitive nor specific, as patients with herpes simplex virus encephalitis, multi-infarct dementia, and stroke may have similar elevations.

84. The answer is C.

(Chap. 44) One of the better characterized paraneoplastic neurologic syndromes is cerebellar ataxia caused by Purkinje cell drop-out in the cerebellum; it is manifested by dysarthria, limb and gait ataxia, and nystagmus. Radiologic imaging reveals cerebellar atrophy. Many antibodies have been associated with this syndrome, including anti-Yo, anti-Tr, and antibodies to the glutamate receptor. Although lung cancer, particularly small cell cancer, accounts for a large number of patients with neoplasm-associated cerebellar ataxia, those with the syndrome who display anti-Yo antibodies in the serum typically have breast or ovarian cancer. Cerebellar ataxia may also be seen in Hodgkin's lymphoma in association with anti-Tr antibodies.

85. The answer is A.

(Chap. 45) Charcot-Marie-Tooth (CMT) syndrome is the most common type of hereditary neuropathy. CMT is comprised of several similar but genetically distinct conditions with different associated mutations. CMT1 is the most common and is an inherited demyelinating sensorimotor neuropathy. CMT1 affects patients in the first to third decades of life with distal leg weakness, i.e., footdrop. Although patients generally do not complain of sensory symptoms, these can often be elicited on physical examination. Muscle stretch reflexes are unobtainable or reduced throughout and calves are often atrophied, which makes legs appear to have a so-called inverted champagne bottle appearance. Hereditary neuralgic amyotrophy (HNA) is an autosomal dominant disorder characterized by recurrent attacks of pain, weakness, and sensory loss in the distribution of the brachial plexus that often begins in childhood. Hereditary sensory and autonomic neuropathy (HSAN) is a very rare group of hereditary neuropathies in which sensory and autonomic dysfunction predominates over muscle weakness. This would not fit the clinical pattern described here. Guillain-Barré syndrome presents generally acutely with involvement of both proximal and distal weakness and sensory loss. The prolonged symptom period and distribution described here is not typical for Guillain-Barré syndrome. Fabry disease is an X-linked disorder in which men are more commonly affected than women. Patients have angiokeratomas, which are reddish-purple lesions usually found around the umbilicus, scrotum, and inguinal region. Burning pain in the hands and feet often is found in late childhood or early adult life. Patients also have premature atheroscloerosis from the underlying mutation in the alpha-galactosidase gene with accumulation of ceramide in nerves and blood vessels.

86. The answer is E.

(Chap. 45) One of the most common side effects of isoniazid treatment is peripheral neuropathy. The elderly, malnourished, and "slow acetylators" are at increased risk for developing the neuropathy. INH inhibits pyridoxal phosphokinase, resulting in pyridoxine (vitamin B_6) deficiency and the neuropathy. Prophylactic administration of pyridoxine can prevent the neuropathy from developing. Symptoms are generally dysesthesias and sensory ataxia. Impaired large-fiber sensory modalities are found on examination. Cobalamin (B_{12}) is not reduced in this condition and is unaffected by isoniazid. Neurontin and pregabalin may alleviate symptoms but will not reverse the neuropathy. There is no indication that hypothyroidism is present.

87. The answer is C.

(Chap. 45) Diabetes mellitus (DM) is the most common cause of peripheral neuropathy in developed countries and is associated with several different types of polyneuropathy including distal symmetric sensory or sensorimotor polyneuropathy, autonomic neuropathy, diabetic neuropathic cachexia, polyradiculoneuropathies, cranial neuropathies, and other mononeuropathies. Risk factors for the

development of neuropathy include long-standing and poorly controlled diabetes and the presence of retinopathy or nephropathy. The patient here appears to have diabetic distal symmetric sensory and sensorimotor polyneuropathy (DSPN), which is the most common form of diabetic neuropathy and presents with sensory loss beginning in the toes and gradually progresses over time up the legs and into the fingers and arms. Symptoms also may include tingling, burning, and deep, aching pains. Nerve biopsy, though rarely indicated, often shows axonal degeneration, endothelial hyperplasia, and occasionally perivascular inflammation. Tight glucose control prevents the development of disease but does not reverse established disease. Diabetic autonomic neuropathy is often seen in combination with DSPN and manifests by abnormal sweating, dysfunctional thermoregulation, dry eyes and mouth, postural hypotension, gastrointestinal abnormalities including gastroparesis, and genitourinary dysfunction.

88. The answer is B.

(Chap. 45) Peripheral neuropathy is a general term indicating peripheral nerve disorders of any cause. The causes are legion, but peripheral neuropathy can be classified by a number of means: axonal versus demyelinating, mononeuropathy versus polyneuropathy versus mononeuritis multiplex, sensory versus motor, and by the tempo of the onset of symptoms. Mononeuropathy typically results from local compression, trauma, or entrapment of a nerve. Polyneuropathy often results from a more systemic process. The distinction between axonal and demyelinating can often be made only with nerve conduction studies. HIV infection causes a common, distal, symmetric, mainly sensory polyneuropathy. Vitamin B_{12} deficiency typically causes a sensory neuropathy that predominantly involves the dorsal columns. Hypothyroidism and acromegaly may both cause compression and swelling of nerve fibers, resulting first in sensory symptoms and later in disease with motor symptoms. Critical illness polyneuropathy is predominantly motor in presentation. Patients typically present with weakness that can be profound. These patients may recover over the course of weeks to months. The etiology is unknown, but an association may exist with prolonged immobilization, severity of illness, neuromuscular blockade, and corticosteroids.

89. The answer is B.

(Chap. 45) Carpal tunnel syndrome is caused by the entrapment of the median nerve at the wrist. Symptoms begin with paresthesias in the median nerve distribution. With worsening, atrophy and weakness may develop. This condition is most commonly caused by excessive use of the wrist and situations involving repetitive motion. Most cases are idiopathic other than those related to occupational or environmental associations. Less commonly, systemic disease may result in carpal tunnel syndrome related to nerve compression or infiltrative disease. This may be suspected when bilateral disease is apparent. Tenosynovitis with arthritis, as in the case of rheumatoid arthritis, and thickening of the connective tissue, as in the case of amyloid or acromegaly, may cause carpal tunnel syndrome. Other systemic diseases, such as hypothyroidism and diabetes mellitus, are also possible etiologies. Acute or chronic leukemia is not typically associated with carpal tunnel syndrome.

90. The answer is B.

(Chap. 46) Guillain-Barré syndrome (GBS) is an acute, severe polyradiculoneuropathy that is autoimmune in nature. GBS manifests as rapidly evolving, areflexic motor paralysis with or without sensory disturbance, usually with ascending paralysis developing over several days. Approximately 70% of GBS cases occur 1–3 weeks after an acute infectious process, usually respiratory or gastrointestinal. Twenty to thirty percent of cases in North America, Europe, and Australia are preceded by infection or reinfection with *Campylobacter jejuni.* Other implicated infections include Epstein-Barr virus, CMV, and *Mycoplasma pneumoniae. T. whippelii* is the etiologic agent of Whipple's disease and *B. henselae* is implicated in cat-scratch fever.

91. The answer is E.

(Chap. 47) Myasthenia gravis (MG) is a neuromuscular disorder characterized by weakness and fatigability of skeletal muscles. The primary defect is a decrease in the number of acetylcholine receptors at the neuromuscular junction secondary to autoimmune antibodies. MG is not rare, affecting at least 1 in 7500 individuals. Women are affected more frequently than men. Women typically present in the second and third decades of life, and men present in the fifth and sixth decades. The key features of MG are weakness and fatigability. Clinical features include weakness of the cranial muscles, particularly the eyelids and extraocular muscles. Diplopia and ptosis are common initial complaints. Weakness in chewing is noticeable after prolonged effort. Speech may be affected secondary to weakness of the palate or tongue. Swallowing may result from weakness of the palate, tongue, or pharynx. In the majority of patients the weakness becomes generalized. The diagnosis is suspected after the appearance of the characteristic symptoms and signs. Edrophonium is an acetylcholinesterase inhibitor that allows ACh to interact repeatedly with the limited number of AChRs, producing improvement in the strength of myasthenic muscles. False-positive tests may occur in patients with other neurologic diseases. Electrodiagnostic testing may show evidence of reduction in the amplitude of the evoked muscle action potentials with repeated stimulation. Testing for the specific antibodies to AChR are diagnostic. In addition to anti-AChR antibodies, antibodies to MuSK have been found in some patients with clinical MG. Antibodies to voltage-gated calcium channels are found in patients with the Lambert-Eaton syndrome.

92. The answer is C.
(Chap. 47) Except for lumbar puncture, all of the options listed are indicated at this time. Thymic abnormalities are present in 75% of patients with myasthenia gravis. A CT or MRI of the mediastinum may show enlargement or neoplastic changes in the thymus and is recommended upon diagnosis. Hyperthyroidism occurs in 3–8% of patients with myasthenia gravis and may aggravate weakness. Testing for rheumatoid factor and antinuclear antibodies should also be obtained because of the association of myasthenia gravis to other autoimmune diseases. Due to side effects of immunosuppressive therapy, a thorough evaluation should be undertaken to rule out latent or chronic infections such as tuberculosis. Measurements of ventilatory function are valuable as a baseline because of the frequency and seriousness of respiratory impairment in myasthenic patients, and they can be used as an objective measure of response to therapy.

93. The answer is E.
(Chap. 48) All classes of lipid-lowering agents have been implicated in muscle toxicity including fibrates, HMG-CoA reductase inhibitors, niacin, and ezetimibe. Myalgia, malaise, and muscle tenderness are the most common manifestations, and muscle pain may be exacerbated by exercise. Proximal weakness may be found on examination. In severe cases, rhabdomyolysis and myoglobinuria may occur, though most cases are mild. Concomitant use of statins with fibrates and cyclosporine are more likely to cause adverse muscle reactions. Elevated serum CK is often identified, and muscle weakness is evidenced by myopathic EMG studies and myonecrosis on muscle biopsy. Severe myalgias, muscle weakness, and significant elevations in CK ($>3 \times$ upper limit of normal) and myoglobinuria are indications for stopping. After cessation, improvement generally occurs after several weeks.

94. The answer is E.
(Chap. 48) A number of endocrinologic conditions are associated with myopathy. Both hypo- and hyperthyroidism are associated with proximal muscle weakness. Hypothyroidism is frequently associated with an elevated CK, even with minimal clinical evidence of muscle disease. Thyrotoxic patients may have fasciculations in addition to proximal myopathy, but in contrast to hypothyroid patients, CK is not generally elevated. Hyperparathyroidism is associated with muscle weakness that is generally proximal. Muscle wasting and brisk reflexes are also generally present. Serum CK levels may be normal or slightly elevated. Serum calcium and phosphate levels show no correlation with clinical weakness. Hypoparathyroid patients also often have myopathy due to hypocalcemia. Patients with acromegaly usually have mild proximal weakness without atrophy. The duration of acromegaly, not the serum growth hormone levels, correlate with the degree of myopathy. Diabetes mellitus is a very rare cause of myopathy, generally due to ischemic infarction of muscle and not a primary myopathy. Finally, vitamin D deficiency is associated with muscle weakness, as are glucocorticoid excess states, e.g., Cushing's disease.

95. The answer is D.
(Chap. 48) There are two recognized clinical forms of myotonic dystrophy, both of which are characterized by autosomal dominant inheritance. Myotonic dystrophy 1 (DM1) is the most common form and the most likely disorder in this patient. Characteristic clinical features of this disorder include a "hatchet-faced" appearance, due to wasting of the facial muscles, and weakness of the neck muscles. In contrast to the muscular dystrophies (Becker and Duchenne), distal limb muscle weakness is more common in DM1. Palatal, pharyngeal, and tongue involvement are also common and produce the dysarthric voice that is frequently heard. The failure of relaxation after a forced hand-grip is characteristic of myotonia. Percussion of the thenar eminence can also elicit myotonia. In most individuals, myotonia is present by age 5, but clinical symptoms of weakness that lead to diagnosis may not be present until adulthood. Cardiac conduction abnormalities and heart failure are also common in myotonic dystrophy. Diagnosis can often be made from clinical features alone in an individual with classic symptoms and a positive family history. An electromyogram would confirm myotonia. Genetic testing for DM1 would show a characteristic trinucleotide repeat on chromosome 19. Genetic anticipation occurs with an increasing number of repeats and worsening clinical disease over successive generations. Myotonic dystrophy 2 (DM2) causes primarily proximal muscle weakness and is also known by the name proximal myotonic myopathy (PROMM). Other features of the disease overlap with DM1. Acid maltase deficiency (glucosidase deficiency, or Pompe's disease) has three recognized forms, only one of which has onset in adulthood. In the adult-onset form, respiratory muscle weakness is prominent and often is the presenting symptom. As stated previously, Becker and Duchenne muscular dystrophies present with primarily proximal muscle weakness and are X-linked recessive disorders. Becker muscular dystrophy presents at a later age than Duchenne muscular dystrophy and has a more prolonged course. Otherwise, their features are similar. Nemaline myopathy is a heterogeneous disorder marked by the threadlike appearance of muscle fibers on biopsy. Nemaline myopathy usually presents in childhood and includes a striking facial appearance similar to that in myotonic dystrophy with a long, narrow face. This disease is inherited in an autosomal dominant fashion.

96. The answer is B.
(Chap. 49) When patients present with proximal muscle weakness and myositis, whether polymyositis, dermatomyositis, or inclusion body myositis, the diagnosis is

confirmed by analysis of serum muscle enzymes, EMG findings, and muscle biopsy. The most sensitive serum enzyme is creatinine kinase (CK), which can be elevated as much as 50-fold in active disease. CK levels usually parallel disease activity, but can be normal in some patients with inclusion body myositis or dermatomyositis. CK is always elevated in active polymyositis and thus is considered most sensitive. Other enzymes may be elevated as well including glutamic-oxaloacetic transaminase, glutamate pyruvate transaminase, lactate dehydrogenase, and aldolase.

97. The answer is B.

(Chap. 49) Various autoantibodies against nuclear antigens, e.g., ANAs, and cytoplasmic antigens are found in up to 20% of patients with inflammatory myopathies. The antibodies to cytoplasmic antigens are directed against ribonucleoproteins involved in protein synthesis (antisynthetases) or translational transport (anti–signal-recognition particles). The antibody directed against the histidyl-transfer RNA synthetase, called anti-Jo-1, accounts for 75% of all the antisynthetases and is clinically useful because up to 80% of patients with this autoantibody will have interstitial lung disease. Patients with anti-Jo-1 may also have Raynaud's phenomenon, nonerosive arthritis, and the MHC molecules DR3 and DRw52. Interstitial lung disease associated with anti-Jo-1 is often rapidly progressive and fatal, even if treated aggressively with cyclophosphamide or other immunosuppressants.

98. The answer is A.

(Chap. 49) Dermatomyositis is associated with malignancy in up to 15% of cases, thus age-appropriate cancer screening is indicated when this diagnosis is made. Exhaustive cancer searches are not recommended, however. Dermatomyositis may be associated occasionally with scleroderma and mixed connective tissue disease, but less frequently with systemic lupus erythematosus, rheumatoid arthritis, or Sjögren's syndrome, which are more closely associated with polymyositis or inclusion body myositis (IBM). Viruses may be associated with IBM and polymyositis, but are not proven to be associated with dermatomyositis. Parasites and bacteria such as cestodes and nematodes are associated with polymyositis, but not other forms of inflammatory myopathy. Finally, thyroid-stimulating immunoglobulins are not known to be associated with dermatomyositis.

99. The answer is A.

(Chap. 49) A common mistake in the management of patients with inflammatory myopathy is to "chase the CK" instead of adjusting therapy based on the clinical response. The goal of therapy is to improve strength. If that goal is being achieved, no augmentation of therapy is necessary. In this case, the plan to switch to long-term maintenance with steroid-sparing immunosuppressants should still be pursued. There have been no controlled studies comparing mycophenolate to methotrexate for long-term use in polymyositis, and in the absence of an adverse reaction to mycophenolate, therapy should not be changed. Despite an elevated CK, patients with polymyositis who are responding to therapy do not need a repeat muscle biopsy.

100. The answer is B.

(Chap. 50) The FLAIR MRI shows increased signal bilaterally in the occipital lobes predominantly involving the white matter. This pattern is typical of a hyperperfusion state, in this case secondary to calcineurin-inhibitor toxicity. This clinical-radiographic abnormality was previously described as reversible posterior leukoencephalopathy. However, this characterization is no longer utilized because the syndrome may not be reversible, the territory may not be confined posteriorly, and gray matter may be involved. Hyperperfusion syndrome may be due to a hydrostatic elevation in cerebral capillary pressure or disorders with endothelial dysfunction and capillary leakage. Hydrostatic causes include hypertensive encephalopathy, post–carotid endarterectomy syndrome, (pre)eclampsia, and high-altitude cerebral edema. Endothelial dysfunction causes include calcineurin-inhibitor toxicity, other chemotherapeutic agent toxicity, HELLP syndrome, TTP, SLE, or granulomatosis with polyangiitis (Wegener's). The diagnosis is clinical and radiographic. CSF findings are nonspecific. In the case of cyclosporine the syndrome may occur with therapeutic serum levels and sporadically after years of treatment. Acoustic neuroma would present on MRI with a discrete mass. The radiologic and clinical appearance is not consistent with pituitary apoplexy. Post–liver transplant patients are at risk of acute (streptococcal) and chronic (tuberculous) meningitis, but the clinical and radiologic findings in this case would not be typical.

101. The answer is B.

(Chap. 50) Acute neurologic events, such as encephalopathy or stroke (often related to intraoperative hypotension or embolism), are common after open heart surgery or coronary artery bypass graft (CABG). Additionally, a chronic syndrome of cognitive impairment is now increasingly recognized after surgery. Small or microemboli during surgery are thought to be the etiology of a hyper- or hypoactive confusional state in the postoperative period. A smaller burden of microemboli may be responsible for the more subtle post–cardiac surgery syndrome characterized by confusion and depressive symptoms as described in this case. Cardiac surgery may also unmask the early manifestations of vascular dementia or Alzheimer's disease. Off-pump CABG patients have a shorter length of hospital stay and fewer perioperative complications. Recent studies do not confirm the hypothesis that off-pump surgery results in less cognitive impairment than on-pump surgery. Ongoing studies are testing the efficacy of microfilters to capture emboli and

reduce CNS complications. Given the temporal relation to CABG surgery and the lack of temporal variability, multiple sclerosis is not likely in this case. Similarly, in the absence of meningitis or encephalitis signs or symptoms, streptococcal or West Nile virus disease is unlikely. vCJD is associated with ingestion of prion-contaminated product. It is characterized by rapidly developing delirium and dementia, often associated with myoclonic jerks.

102. The answer is E.

(Chap. 50) The peroneal nerve winds around the head of the fibula below the lateral aspect of the knee. This superficial location makes it vulnerable to trauma. Poorly applied leg braces, fibular fracture, tight-fitting stockings, or casts may cause peroneal nerve injury and neuropathy. Patients may present with footdrop (dorsiflexion defect) with weakness of foot eversion. Intact foot inversion at the ankle distinguishes peroneal nerve injury from L5 radiculopathy, which involves the muscles innervated by the tibial nerve. Sensory loss due to peroneal nerve injury involves the lateral aspect of the leg below the knee and the dorsum of the foot. Cauda equina syndrome is caused by compression of the spinal nerve roots of the lumbar plexus usually due to tumor, trauma, or spinal stenosis. It typically presents with weakness of the muscles innervated by the involved nerves, incontinence, and decreased anal sphincter tone. Cauda equina syndrome is usually a medical emergency to avoid permanent functional loss. The femoral nerve branches into anterior and posterior portions in the leg. Injury of the anterior branches may lead to sensory findings in the thigh and muscular findings in the sartorius and the quadriceps. L4 radiculopathy causes symptoms in the anterior thigh and knee extensors (including the patellar reflex).

103. The answer is A.

(Chap. 52) Chronic fatigue syndrome (CFS) is a disorder characterized by persistent and unexplained fatigue resulting in severe impairment in daily functioning. Besides intense fatigue, most patients with CFS report concomitant symptoms such as pain, cognitive dysfunction, and unrefreshing sleep. Additional symptoms can include headache, sore throat, tender lymph nodes, muscle aches, joint aches, feverishness, difficulty sleeping, psychiatric problems, allergies, and abdominal cramps. Criteria for the diagnosis of CFS have been developed by the U.S. Centers for Disease Control and Prevention (see Table 52-1). CFS is seen worldwide, with adult prevalence rates varying between 0.2% and 0.4%. In the United States, the prevalence is higher in women, members of minority groups (African and Native Americans), and individuals with lower levels of education and occupational status. Approximately 75% of all CFS patients are women. The mean age of onset is between 29 and 35 years. It is probable that many patients go undiagnosed and/or do not seek help.

104. The answer is B.

(Chap. 52) Cognitive behavioral therapy (CBT) and graded exercise therapy (GET) have been found to be the only beneficial interventions in chronic fatigue syndrome (CFS). CBT is a psychotherapeutic approach directed at changing condition-related cognitions and behaviors. CBT for CFS aims at changing a patient's perpetuating factors by exploiting various techniques and components. The intervention, which typically consists of 12–14 sessions spread over 6 months, helps CFS patients gain control over their symptoms. GET is based on the model of deconditioning and exercise intolerance and usually involves a home exercise program that continues for 3–5 months. Walking or cycling is systematically increased, with set target heart rates. Evidence that deconditioning is the basis for symptoms in CFS is lacking, however. The primary component of CBT and GET that results in a reduction in fatigue is a change in the patient's perception of fatigue and focus on symptoms. CBT is generally the more complex treatment, which might explain why CBT studies tend to yield better improvement rates than GET trials. Not all patients benefit from CBT or GET. Predictors of poor outcome are somatic comorbidity, current disability claims, and severe pain. CBT offered in an early stage of the illness reduces the burden of CFS for the patient as well as society in terms of decreased medical and disability-related costs. Full recovery from untreated CFS is rare: the median annual recovery rate is 5% (range 0–31%) and the improvement rate 39% (range 8–63%). Major depressive disorder, bipolar disorder, eating disorder, and schizophrenia are exclusion criteria for the diagnosis of chronic fatigue syndrome.

105. The answer is D.

(Chap. 54) This patient is experiencing her first episode of a panic attack and does not meet the criteria for panic disorder. In this situation, no specific treatment is required. The patient should be reassured in a manner that is empathetic and supportive that she does not have any evidence of a serious medical disorder. Panic attacks are common, with about 1–3% of the population experiencing at least one panic attack. Panic attacks begin abruptly, most commonly without an immediate precipitating cause, and peak in severity over 10 minutes. The symptoms usually subside spontaneously over the course of an hour. Diagnostic criteria for a panic attack include a minimum of four of the following criteria: palpitations or racing heart, sweating, trembling, shortness of breath, feeling of choking, chest pain, nausea or GI distress, dizziness, derealization, fear of losing control, fear of dying, paresthesias, or chills/hot flushes. If a patient subsequently develops panic disorder, a variety of treatment options can be pursued. Panic disorder is marked by at least 1 month of recurrent panic attacks associated with excessive worry about or change in behavior as a result of the attacks. The goals of therapy for panic attacks are to decrease the frequency of attacks and

the severity of symptoms during the attack. Antidepressant medications are the cornerstone of therapy with selective serotonin reuptake inhibitors being the most frequently used class of medication. The dose of medication for panic disorder is typically lower than the antidepressant dose. For fluoxetine, this would be 5–10 mg daily. As these medications take 2–6 weeks to become effective, they are often combined with benzodiazepines to be used on an as-needed basis for immediate relief of attacks. Alprazolam and clonazepam are common agents used for panic disorder, although alprazolam may have more associated dependence with the need for escalating doses of medications. In combination with pharmacologic therapy, psychotherapy and education are also useful for the treatment of panic disorder. The therapy often includes breathing techniques, cognitive behavioral therapy, and even homework assignments.

106. The answer is A.

(Chap. 54) There are increasing numbers of antidepressant medications available in a variety of classes. Selective serotonin reuptake inhibitors (SSRIs) are the most commonly used antidepressant drugs. This class of medications includes fluoxetine, sertraline, paroxetine, fluvoxamine, citalopram, and escitalopram. These medications are taken once daily and have side effects including sexual dysfunction, headache, and insomnia. Tricyclic antidepressants were commonly used in past decades for the treatment of depression. However, overdoses can be lethal, and anticholinergic side effects including dry mouth, constipation, and urinary retention can limit the dose. Medications in the tricyclic class of antidepressants include amitriptyline, nortriptyline, imipramine, desipramine, doxepin, and clomipramine. Mixed norepinephrine/serotonin reuptake inhibitors and receptor blockers are a newer class of medications. These medications are increasing in use as they are quite effective and do not have the same frequency of sexual dysfunction. Medications in this class include venlafaxine, desvenlafaxine, duloxetine, and mirtazapine. Monoamine oxidase inhibitors were once a common antidepressant class of medication, but these medications are now only rare used. There is a wide range of drug and food interactions that can lead to hypertensive crises. Examples of medication in this class include phenelzine, tranylcypromine, and isocarboxazid. A final class of antidepressants is called simply mixed action drugs and includes trazodone, bupropion, and nefazodone.

107. The answer is E.

(Chap. 54) Post-traumatic stress disorder (PTSD) was only added as a discrete disorder in 1980. The diagnostic criteria for PTSD are long and require that an individual experiences an event where there was an actual or perceived threat of death or serious injury and that the individual's reaction included intense fear or helplessness. Following the event, the individual continues to re-experience the event and avoids stimuli associated with the trauma. In association with this, there is also often a generalized withdrawal and decrease in responsiveness. At the same time, the patient exhibits an increase in arousal that is often exhibited by insomnia, irritability, hypervigilance, and difficulty concentrating. Treatment of PTSD is almost always multifactorial, including both pharmacotherapy and psychotherapy. It is not uncommon for an individual with PTSD to develop a dependence on drugs or alcohol as an attempt to control the symptoms, and any substance abuse issues need to be treated simultaneously as well. This patient's treatment would include avoidance of alcohol and intensive substance abuse treatment as needed. Treatment with antidepressant medications can decrease anxiety and avoidance behaviors. Trazodone is often given at night for its sedating properties. Psychotherapeutic strategies include cognitive behavioral therapy to overcome avoidance behaviors as well.

108. The answer is B.

(Chap. 54) Fifteen percent of the population will experience at least one episode of major depression over the course of a lifetime, and most episodes of major depression are treated by primary care practitioners. Treatment can be any of a number of medications across a variety of classes. Despite the popularity of newer antidepressants, there is no evidence that these medications are more efficacious than older drugs like tricyclic antidepressants. Indeed, 60–70% of patients will respond to any drug chosen if given in a sufficient dose for 6–8 weeks. Once a patient has been on treatment for about 2 months, the response should be evaluated, and if there has been an insufficient response, a dosage increase should be considered. In this patient, a dosage increase yielded control of depressive symptoms at 4 months. Once control of symptoms has been achieved, the drug should be continued for an additional 6–9 months to prevent relapse. If a patient experiences any additional episodes of major depression, he or she will likely require indefinite maintenance treatment.

109. The answer is A.

(Chap. 56) Alcohol is primarily absorbed through the proximal small intestine, but small to moderate amounts can also be absorbed in the mouth, esophagus, stomach, and large intestines. Several factors can increase the rate of absorption. One factor that increases absorption is rapid gastric emptying, which can be induced by concurrent consumption of carbonated beverages. Another factor that increases absorption from the gut to the blood is the ingestion of alcohol in the absence of other calorie sources such as proteins, fat, or carbohydrates. A final factor that can increase absorption is to drink alcohol that is diluted to a modest concentration (~20% or less). At high

alcohol concentrations absorption is decreased, although high blood levels may be achieved because the amount of alcohol ingested is high.

110. The answer is C.

(Chap. 56) Alcohol has effects on many neurotransmitters in the brain. The predominant effect of alcohol lies in its ability to cause the release of γ-aminobutyric acid (GABA) and acts primarily at the $GABA_A$ receptors. GABA is the primary inhibitory neurotransmitter in the brain and is associated with the sedative effects of alcohol. Many other drugs affect the GABA system including benzodiazepines, nonbenzodiazepine sleep aids such as zolpidem, anticonvulsants, and muscle relaxants. The euphoric effects of alcohol consumption are related to increases in dopamine, which is common to all pleasurable activities. The effects on dopamine are thought to be important in alcohol craving and relapse. In addition, alcohol alters opioid receptors and can lead to a release of beta endorphins during acute ingestion. In addition to these effects, alcohol also inhibits postsynaptic *N*-methyl-D-aspartate excitatory glutamate receptors. Glutamate is the primary excitatory neurotransmitter of the brain, and its inhibition further contributes to the sedative effects of alcohol. Additional important effects on neurotransmitters include increased serotonin activity and decreased nicotinic acetylcholine receptors.

111. The answer is D.

(Chap. 56) The acute effects of any drug depend on many factors including amount consumed and absorbed, presence of other drugs, and past experience with the drug. In an individual who is naïve to alcohol, drug levels as low as 0.02 g/dL can lead to a decrease in inhibitions and a slight feeling of intoxication. In the United States, "legal" intoxication occurs at a blood alcohol level of 0.08 g/dL in most states. At this level, decreases in cognitive and motor abilities are seen. Once an alcohol level of 0.20 g/dL is achieved, an individual is obviously impaired with slurred speech, poor judgment, and impaired coordination. Light coma and depression of respiratory rate, blood pressure, and pulse occur at levels of around 0.30 g/dL, and death is likely to occur at levels of 0.40 g/dL. However, in individuals who drink heavily, tolerance begins to develop to alcohol. After a period of 1–2 weeks of daily alcohol consumption, liver metabolism of alcohol increases by as much as 30%, but disappears quite quickly with abstinence. Cellular or pharmacodynamic tolerance also occurs and refers to the neurochemical changes that allow an individual to maintain more normal physiologic functioning despite the presence of alcohol.

112. The answer is C.

(Chap. 56) Alcohol abuse is defined as repetitive problems in any one of four life areas that can be attributed to alcohol. The four life areas that can be affected by alcohol include social, interpersonal, legal, or occupational. In addition, an individual who repetitively engages in hazardous behaviors while under the influence of alcohol would be considered to suffer from alcohol abuse. However, this is to be differentiated from alcohol dependence. Alcohol dependence is defined in the DSM-IV as repeated alcohol-related difficulties in three of seven life areas and includes the development of tolerance and dependence. If tolerance or dependence is present, this predicts a more severe clinical course, and the presence of alcohol dependence decreases overall life span by about a decade. Only about 50% of individuals with alcohol abuse will continue to experience similar alcohol-related problems 3–5 years later, and only 10% will go on to develop alcohol dependence. The lifetime risk of alcohol dependence in most Western countries is about 10–15% in men and 5–8% in women. However, there may be higher rates in Ireland, France, and Scandinavian countries. In addition, native cultures appear to be especially susceptible to problems with alcohol dependence. This has been seen in Native Americans, Maoris, and the aboriginal tribes of Australia.

About 60% of the risk for alcohol use disorders is attributed to genetic influences. Children of alcoholics do have a higher risk of alcohol abuse and dependence; however, this risk is about 4 times higher, not 10. Identical twins also exhibit a higher risk of concurrent alcohol abuse and dependence when compared to fraternal twins. The genetic factors that appear to be most strongly linked to alcohol use disorders include genes that are linked to impulsivity, schizophrenia, and bipolar disorder. In addition, genes that affect alcohol metabolism or sensitivity to alcohol also contribute to the genetics of alcoholism. A mutation in aldehyde dehydrogenase that is more common in individuals of Asian descent results in intense flushing when alcohol is consumed and confers a decreased risk of alcohol dependence. Conversely, genetic variants that lead to a low sensitivity to alcohol increase the risk of subsequent alcohol abuse and dependence, as higher and higher doses of alcohol are required to achieve the same effects.

113. The answer is B.

(Chap. 56) Individuals with alcohol dependence are susceptible to alcohol withdrawal when alcohol intake is stopped abruptly. The individual in this case scenario is likely alcohol dependent given his large amount of alcohol intake on a daily basis. Symptoms of alcohol withdrawal can range from mild tremulousness to hallucinations, seizures, or the development of delirium tremens. Other clinical features of alcohol withdrawal include anxiety, insomnia, and autonomic nervous system overactivity manifested as tachycardia, tachypnea, elevated blood pressure, and fever. This patient exhibits symptoms of the more severe delirium tremens, with mental confusion, agitation, and fluctuating levels of consciousness. While minor symptoms of alcohol withdrawal may begin

as soon as 5–10 hours after cessation of alcohol intake, the symptoms do not peak for 48–72 hours, putting this patient in the appropriate time frame for alcohol withdrawal.

The best approach for the alcohol-dependent patient who abruptly stops all alcohol intake is to take a prophylactic approach and screen early for symptoms of alcohol withdrawal. Tools such as the Revised Clinical Institute for Withdrawal Assessment for Alcohol (CIWA-Ar) may help clinicians and nurses screen for the early development of symptoms and allow intervention before symptoms escalate. In this setting, most experts recommend the use of oral long-acting benzodiazepines such as chlordiazepoxide or diazepam beginning on the first day. However, in this case, the patient received no such treatment and is now experiencing severe alcohol withdrawal and delirium tremens. Intravenous medications that have a rapid onset of action and can be titrated for more aggressive symptom management are often employed in this setting. Thus, the use of IV lorazepam or diazepam is preferred in this patient. Following an initial bolus, repeated doses can be used in short intervals until the patient is calm but arousable. In some instances a continuous infusion may be required, although bolus dosing is preferred. In the most severe cases, propofol or barbiturates may be required, although the patient would most likely need to be intubated for airway protection with use of these medications.

The other options listed are not appropriate for initial management of this patient. Intravenous fluids and thiamine had been administered since hospital admission. Administration of glucose-containing fluids without thiamine in the alcohol-dependent patient can precipitate Wernicke's encephalopathy, which would present with ophthalmoparesis, ataxia, and encephalopathy. Given the patient's fever, an infectious etiology can be considered, and it would be appropriate to perform blood cultures in this patient. However, given the clear symptoms of alcohol withdrawal and lack of necrotizing pancreatitis on CT abdomen, empiric treatment with antibiotics is not required. Likewise, without focal neurologic findings, a head CT would be a low-yield diagnostic procedure that would be difficult to perform in the patient's current agitated condition and would only delay appropriate therapy. Finally, restraints are best avoided if the patient's safety can be ensured through the appropriate use of benzodiazepines, as restraints are only likely to make the patient's agitation worse and may lead to iatrogenic harm. Haloperidol may have some sedative effect on the patient, but could lead to torsades de pointe arrhythmia as this patient is at risk for electrolyte deficiencies from his alcoholism and pancreatitis.

114. The answer is D.

(Chap. 56) In individuals recovering from alcoholism several medications may have a modest benefit in increasing abstinence rates. The two medications with the best risk-benefit ratio are acamprosate and naltrexone. Acamprosate inhibits NMDA receptors, decreasing symptoms of prolonged alcohol withdrawal. Naltrexone is an opioid antagonist than can be administered orally or as a monthly injection. It is thought to act by decreasing activity in the dopamine-rich ventral tegmental area of the brainstem and subsequently decreasing the pleasurable feelings associated with alcohol consumption. There is some research to suggest that the use of these medications in combination may be more effective than either one alone. Disulfiram is an aldehyde dehydrogenase inhibitor that has been used for many years in the treatment of alcoholism. However, it is no longer a commonly used drug due to its many side effects and risks associated with treatment. The primary mechanism by which it acts is to create negative effects of vomiting and autonomic nervous system hyperactivity when alcohol is consumed concurrently with use of the medication. As it inhibits an enzyme that is part of the normal metabolism of alcohol, it allows the buildup of acetaldehyde, which creates these symptoms. Because of the autonomic side effects, it is contraindicated in individuals with hypertension, a history of stroke, heart disease, or diabetes mellitus.

115. The answer is E.

(Chap. 57) Prescription drug abuse has increased dramatically among all age groups and is strikingly common in teenagers. Since 2007, prescription opiates have passed marijuana as the most common illicit drugs that adolescents initially abuse. This has occurred at the same time as rates of prescription narcotic abuse have increased across all age groups. The annual prevalence of heroin abuse is approximately 0.14% of the population. In contrast, this prevalence is only one-third the rate of prescription opiate abuse. Among prescription narcotics, oxycodone is the single most commonly abused drug. Other common prescription narcotics that are abused include morphine and hydrocodone. Among health care professionals, meperidine and fentanyl are more frequently abused.

116. The answer is B.

(Chap. 57) Tolerance and withdrawal begin within 6–8 weeks of chronic daily opioid use. Tolerance develops not because of increased metabolism, but through a change in the pharmacodynamics of the drugs, requiring increasing doses to achieve the euphoric effects and prevent withdrawal. With the abrupt cessation of narcotics, acute withdrawal symptoms begin within 8–10 hours after the last dose. While the symptoms of narcotic withdrawal are noxious, they are not life threatening, as is the case with benzodiazepine or barbiturate withdrawal. The primary symptoms of opiate withdrawal are related to over activity of the autonomic nervous system. This manifests as increased lacrimation, rhinorrhea, and sweating. In addition, patients frequently will have diffuse piloerection (chill bumps), giving rise to the term "cold turkey." As

withdrawal symptoms progress, patients appear restless with myalgias, nausea, vomiting, and diarrhea. Hypertension, hyperthermia, and tachypnea can occur as well. Hypotension is not a symptom of opioid withdrawal. A patient with known infection and new-onset hypotension should be evaluated for systemic infection, not withdrawal.

117. The answer is E.

(Chap. 57) The patient is presenting with an acute overdose of an unknown quantity of extended-release opioid medications taken with alcohol. When evaluating and treating a patient with an intention overdose, the first priority is to stabilize the patient's condition. The patient was appropriately given the opiate antagonist naloxone by emergency responders as the patient was near-apneic. In addition, the patient was also appropriately intubated and stabilized for transport to the hospital. In the emergency room, however, the patient remained hypotensive and unresponsive. At this point, the next step in stabilizing the patient is to support the blood pressure with bolus fluid resuscitation, and if the patient fails to respond, IV vasopressors would be required. Given his ongoing unresponsive state and the expected long duration of effect with a sustained-release preparation, it is appropriate to initiate a continuous infusion of naloxone. After a bolus dose, the expected onset of action is 1–2 minutes, but the duration of effect is only a few hours. Some care must be taken when giving naloxone as one only wants to reverse the respiratory and cardiovascular depression associated with the overdose. Particularly in chronic drug abusers, high doses of naloxone can precipitate the distressing symptoms of narcotic withdrawal. When long-acting preparations of opioids are taken, activated charcoal and gastric lavage are appropriate considerations to decrease the absorption of any undigested pills. While the patient is being stabilized from a cardiovascular and respiratory standpoint, it is important that the clinician consider if any other concurrent ingestion may have occurred that would affect the patient's outcome. As the patient is unable to provide any history and the overdose was not witnessed, one must not focus solely on the opioids. The appropriate approach is to perform a comprehensive toxicology evaluation that should include a urine drug screen, blood alcohol level, and acetaminophen levels, at a minimum. One could also consider sending for levels of aspirin or tricyclic antidepressants.

118. The answer is C.

(Chap. 58) Marijuana is the most commonly used illegal drug in the United States with over 6% of all individuals reporting current usage in 2009 (http://www.whitehousedrugpolicy.gov/publications/pdf/nsduh.pdf, accessed July 25, 2011). In part, the prevalence of marijuana use is related to the widespread belief that marijuana is thought to have few negative health effects. Acutely, marijuana causes a sense of relaxation and mild euphoria, not unlike that of alcohol intoxication. In addition, impaired judgment, cognition, and psychomotor performance are seen. Occasionally, acute intoxication can lead to negative emotional responses as well. A consensus about the chronic effects of marijuana usage is not clearly defined. Traditionally, marijuana usage has been linked with an "amotivational syndrome." While it is true that chronic users of marijuana may lose interest in day-to-day activities and spend more time using the drug, this is certainly not specific for marijuana uses, and a specific "amotivational syndrome" is not defined with chronic marijuana use. Other symptoms that have been attributed to chronic marijuana use that lack good evidence for causation include depression and maturational dysfunction. In individuals with a history of schizophrenia, however, chronic marijuana use has been associated with an increased risk of psychotic symptoms.

The physical effects of chronic marijuana use are also not clearly known. Acutely, marijuana causes increased heart rate, but tolerance for this effect occurs rapidly. Acute ingestion can also precipitate angina. The chronic effects on lung function are not known, as tobacco products are frequent confounders. Acute decreases in vital capacity and diffusion capacity are seen, but whether this translates into an increased risk of emphysema has not yet been determined. Most studies have not found an association with emphysema. A variety of other adverse physical effects have been described but not confirmed in a systematic fashion. This includes reports of low testosterone levels, decreased sperm count, impaired fetal growth, and chromosomal abnormalities.

Contrary to popular belief, chronic use of marijuana is associated with the development of tolerance as well as a withdrawal syndrome. Signs of physical tolerance include tolerance to the development of tachycardia and conjunctival injection. The psychological tolerance that develops is more prominent and predictable. This occurs rapidly, with individuals often seeking more potent compounds or smoking the drug more frequently. With cessation of marijuana use, a withdrawal syndrome can be demonstrated with irritability, anorexia, and sleep disturbance.

INDEX

Bold page number indicates the start of the main discussion of the topic; page numbers with "f" and "t" refer to figures and tables, respectively.

AAN (autoimmune autonomic neuropathy), 387
Abdominal aortic aneurysm, 81
Abducens nerve, examination of, 6
Abducens nerve palsy, 194
Abducens nerve paresis, 194
A-beta (Aβ) fibers, 40
Abetalipoproteinemia, 368
Aβ protein, 312t, 319, 319f
Abscess
 brain. *See* Brain abscess
 epidural. *See* Epidural abscess
Absence seizures, 233
Abstract thought, assessment of, 6
Abulia, 132, 276f
Acalculia, 147
Acamprosate, in alcoholism management, 760, 849
Acanthamoeba infections, chronic meningitis in, 530t
Acephalic migraine, 56, 257
Acetaminophen
 adverse effects of, 45
 for back pain, 82
 for migraine, 57, 58t
 for pain, 45, 46t
 for spinal stenosis, 78
 for tension-type headache, 122
Acetaminophen-aspirin-caffeine, for migraine, 57, 58t
Acetazolamide
 for acute angle-closure glaucoma, 182
 for altitude illness, 164
 for hypokalemic periodic paralysis, 642
 for pseudotumor cerebri, 186
 for raised CSF pressure headache, 68
Acetylcholine
 anatomic and clinical aspects of, 222t, 380
 deficiency of, in delirium, 126–127
 structure of, 222t
Acetylcholine receptor, in myasthenia gravis, 609–610
Acetylcholinesterase test, in myasthenia gravis, 611
Achromatopsia, 152, 177
Acoustic neuroma. *See* Vestibular schwannoma (acoustic neuroma)
Acoustic reflex, 214
Acoustic reflex decay, 214
Acromegaly, **462**
 clinical features of, 463, 463f
 diagnosis of, 463–464
 etiology of, 462–463, 462t
 familial, 447
 laboratory evaluation of, 463–464
 screening tests for, 451t
 treatment of, 464–465, 465f
Acrylamide, 587t
ACTH. *See* Adrenocorticotropic hormone (ACTH)
Actinomycosis, chronic meningitis in, 529t
Acupuncture, for back pain, 82
Acute disseminated encephalomyelitis (ADEM), **491**
 clinical features of, 492
 diagnosis of, 492
 etiology of, 491
 neuroimaging in, 693f
 pathophysiology of, 491
 treatment of, 492
Acute inflammatory demyelinating polyneuropathy (AIDP), 600–601, 600t, 602t, 604t
Acute necrotizing myopathy, paraneoplastic, 565
Acyclovir
 for Bell's palsy, 396
 for ocular HSV infections, 181
Acyclovir (*Cont.*):
 for viral encephalitis, 512–513
 for viral meningitis, 507
AD. *See* Alzheimer's disease (AD)
ADAMTS13, 775t
A-delta (Aδ) fibers, 40, 41
ADEM. *See* Acute disseminated encephalomyelitis (ADEM)
Adenovirus infections, conjunctivitis, 180
Adhesive arachnoiditis, lumbar, 80
Adie's syndrome, 176
Adolescents, seizures in, 238t
Adrenalectomy, for Cushing's syndrome, 469
Adrenal insufficiency
 delirium in, 129
 muscle weakness in, 644
Adrenocorticotropic hormone (ACTH), **465**
 action of, 466
 deficiency of, 446t, 466
 ectopic production of, 468t
 laboratory evaluation of, 445t
 secretion of, 466
 synthesis of, 465–466
Adrenoleukodystrophy, 575–576, 575t
Adrenomyeloneuropathy, 412, 575–576
Adult growth hormone deficiency
 clinical features of, 460–461, 461t, 813, 839
 laboratory evaluation of, 461, 461t
 treatment of, 461–462, 462f
Adult Tay-Sachs disease, 374t, 377
Advanced sleep phase disorder, **172**
AEDs. *See* Antiepileptic drugs (AEDs)
Aerophobia, 512
Aging
 olfactory function and, 202, 202f, 206
 sleep patterns and, 158, 159, 159f
Agnosia, object, 152, 278, 826
Agoraphobia, 102, 721, 721t
Agrammatism, 145, 148
Agraphesthesia, 122
Agraphia, 144
AIDP (acute inflammatory demyelinating polyneuropathy), 600–601, 600t, 602t, 604t
AIDS, 536, 537t. *See also* HIV infection
AIDS dementia complex (HIV-associated dementia), 541–543, 542f, 542t
Air-conduction threshold, 213
Akathisia, 354, 740
Akinetic mutism, 132
Albendazole, for cysticercosis, 522
Alcohol, **752**. *See also* Alcohol use
 absorption of, 752–753, 819, 847–848
 abuse of. *See* Alcohol abuse or dependence (alcoholism)
 actions of, 221, 718t, 848
 blood levels of, in absence of tolerance, 753, 753t
 metabolism of, 752–753, 753f, 819, 847–848
 pharmacology of, 752–753, 753f
 tolerance of, 753–754, 848
Alcohol abuse or dependence (alcoholism), **756**
 acute intoxication, 113
 adverse effects of, 166
 chronic, dementia due to, 328
 definition of, 756, 848
 genetic factors in, 757, 848
 insomnia in, 165
 lifetime risk for, 756–757
 myopathy in, 646, 756
 natural history of, 757
 neuropathy in, 387
 ocular involvement in, 196
Alcohol abuse or dependence (alcoholism) (*Cont.*):
 olfactory/taste dysfunction in, 205
 psychiatric comorbidity with, 754–755
 treatment of, 758–760
  acute intoxication, 758
  alcohol withdrawal in. *See* Alcohol withdrawal syndrome
  AUDIT in, 758, 758t
  identification of alcoholic in, 757–758, 758t
  interventions, 758
  rehabilitation, 759–760
  relapse prevention, 759–760, 819–820, 849
Alcoholic myopathy, 756
Alcoholic neuropathy, 387
Alcohol-induced psychotic disorders, 755
Alcohol use
 behavioral effects of, 753–754, 753t, 848
 nutritional impact of, 752–753
 in pregnancy, 756
 sleep disturbances and, 166
 systemic effects of, 752–753
Alcohol Use Disorder Screening Test (AUDIT), 758, 758t
Alcohol Use Disorders Identification Test-Consumption (AUDIT-C) module, 746, 747t
Alcohol withdrawal syndrome, 125, 128–129, 759, 819, 848–849
Alexia, 144, 144t, 146–147
Alien hand (limb) syndrome, 147, 325
Allodynia, 44, 117, 389
Almotriptan, for migraine, 58t, 59, 59t
α_2-adrenergic agonists
 for acute angle-closure glaucoma, 182
 for opiate detoxification, 764–765
α-adrenergic antagonists, adverse effects of, 95
α-lipoic acid, for olfactory dysfunction, 206
α motor neurons, 106f
Alport syndrome, hearing loss in, 212, 212t
Alprazolam
 for generalized anxiety disorder, 725t
 for panic disorder, 722
 pharmacology of, 725t
ALS. *See* Amyotrophic lateral sclerosis (ALS)
ALS/parkinsonian/dementia complex of Guam, 330
Alternative splicing, 219
Aluminum toxicity, 329
Alvimopan, 48
Alzheimer's disease (AD), **316**
 aphasia in, 146, 149
 Bálint's syndrome in, 151–152
 clinical features of, 317, 834
 cost of care for, 316
 diagnosis of, 318f, 833
 differential diagnosis of, 311t, 317–318, 318f
 early onset, 320
 epidemiology of, 318
 frontal lobe syndromes in, 155, 156
 genetic factors in, 228, 319–320, 319f
 Lewy body variant of, 326
 memory loss in, 153–154, 156
 molecular basis of, 312t
 neurotransmitter systems in, 221
 olfactory dysfunction in, 199, 202–203, 206
 pathology of, 316, 318–319, 319f, 834
 presenilins in, 319–320
 risk factors for, 318
 treatment of, 320–322
 trisomy 21 and, 319

Amacrine cells, of retina, 174
Amantadine
for fatigue in MS, 490
for PD, 342, 346
for SSRI-related sexual dysfunction, 733
Amaurosis fugax, 182–183, 269
Amblyopia, 193
American trypanosomiasis. *See* Chagas' disease
Aminoglutethimide, for Cushing's syndrome, 469
Aminoglycosides, 209
4-Amino pyridine, for weakness in MS, 489
Amiodarone, adverse effects of
myopathy, 645t, 647
neuropathy, 586t, 589
optic neuropathy, 185
Amitriptyline
adverse effects of, 61t, 206, 723t
for chronic daily headache, 65
for depression, 723t
dosage of, 723t
for insomnia, 164
for migraine prevention, 60, 61t
for olfactory dysfunction, 206
for pain, 46t, 490
for posttraumatic headache, 68
for tension-type headache, 122
Amnesia, **152**
anterograde, 153
caring for patient with, 155–156
clinical examination in, 153
etiology of, 153–154
after head injury, 415
psychogenic, dementia due to, 330
retrograde, 153
transient global, 154, 329–330
video library, 157
Amnestic state, 152
Amoxapine, for depression, 723t, 732
Amphetamine(s)
action of, 221, 718t
adverse effects of, 166
Amphotericin B
for *Cryptococcus* infections, 516
for *Histoplasma* infections, 516
Ampicillin, for meningitis, 499t, 501
Amygdalohippocampectomy, for epilepsy, 251
Amyloid angiopathy, 319
Amyloidosis
autonomic dysfunction in, 387
neuropathy in, 387, 577
ocular involvement in, 176
pathophysiology of, 387
Amyloid polyneuropathy, familial, 575t, 577
Amyloid precursor protein (APP), 318–319, 319f
Amyotrophic lateral sclerosis (ALS), **370,** 834–835
clinical features of, 371–372
"definite," criteria for, 372
diagnosis of, 86, 371–372, 372f
differential diagnosis of, 371t, 373, 376
epidemiology of, 371–372
familial, 228, 373, 374t
pathogenesis of, 376
pathology of, 370–371
treatment of, 377t
Amyotrophic lateral sclerosis (ALS)/parkinsonian/dementia complex of Guam, 330
Amyotrophy, 370
definition of, 370
diabetic, 579, 644
Analgesia (sensory abnormality), 117
Analgesics
for lumbar puncture, 35
medication-overuse headache and, 60, 66
Anaplasma spp. infections, 500
Andersen syndrome (type IV glycogenosis), 637
Andersen-Tawil syndrome, 641t, 643
Anemia
delirium in, 129
sideroblastic, 364t
Anesthesia (sensory abnormality), 117
Aneurysm
abdominal aortic, 81
cerebral, 15f, 69
mycotic, circle of Willis, 305
repair of, 307, 307f
saccular, 304–305
Angelman syndrome, imprinting in, 219
Angiitis, chronic meningitis in, 532t
Angina pectoris, in orthostatic hypotension, 94
Angiography
cerebral, in stroke, 285
complications, 25
CT, 14, 15f
in neurologic disease, **25**
spinal, 25
Angioma, cavernous, 292–293
Angiopathy
amyloid, 319
cerebral amyloid, 322
Angiostrongylus spp. infections, chronic meningitis in, 530t
Anisocoria, 176
Ankylosing spondylitis
back pain in, 79
diagnosis of, 79
neck pain in, 86
ocular involvement in, 181
pathogenesis of, 79
treatment of, 79
Anomia, 143, 152, 826
color, 147, 177
finger, 147
Anosognosia, 150, 256, 317
Anterior cerebral artery
lesion in territory of, 107, 146, 153
occlusion of, 275–276, 276f
Anterior choroidal artery, occlusion of, 276, 277f
Anterior dens dislocation, 698f
Anterior horn cell disorders, weakness in, 106, 107, 109
Anterior ischemic optic neuropathy, 184, 184f
Anterior pituitary, disorders of, **441**
Anterior spinal artery syndrome, 403
Anterocollis, 349
Anterolateral system, 118
Anti-AChR antibody, 559t
Anti-AMPA receptor antibodies, 559t, 562
Anti-amphiphysin, 559t
Antiarrhythmics, for pain, 46t, 50
Antibacterial drugs, for bacterial meningitis, 499t, 500–502, 501t
Antibody(ies), in neurologic paraneoplastic syndromes, 559t
Anticardiolipin antibodies, 183, 183f
Anticholinergics, 126–127
Anticoagulant(s)
intracerebral hemorrhage due to, 289
for ischemic stroke, 261
in stroke prevention, 271–272
for suppurative thrombophlebitis, 526
Anti-CV$_2$/CRMP5 antibody, 559t, 561
Antidepressants. *See also specific drugs*
actions of, 716
adverse effects management, 724t
adverse effects of, 723t
classification of, 818, 847
for depression, 723t, 731–733, 732f
dosage of, 723t
for pain, 46t, 49–50, 49t, 490
Antiepileptic drugs (AEDs). *See also specific drugs*
adverse effects of, 247–249t, 254–255
for brain abscess, 521
breast-feeding and, 255
discontinuation of, 250–251
drug interactions of, 247–249t, 255
for focal seizures, 246, 250
for generalized anxiety disorders, 726
for generalized seizures, 350
initiation of, 245
mechanisms of action of, 240–241
monitoring of, 250
oral contraceptives and, 255
Antiepileptic drugs (AEDs) (*Cont.*):
for pain, 46t, 50
pharmacology of, 247–249t
for refractory epilepsy, 251
selection of, 245–246
Anti-GABA antibodies, 559t, 562
Anti-GAD antibody, 559t, 562
Anti–glycolipid antibodies, in immune neuropathies, 600–601, 602f
Antihistamines
for insomnia, 163
for vertigo, 102t
Anti-Hu antibody, 559t, 561
Anti-Hu paraneoplastic neuropathy, **607**
Anti-Jo-1, 651
Anti-Ma proteins, 559t, 561, 561f
Antineuronal antibodies, 559t
Anti-NMDA receptor antibodies, 559t, 560f, 562
Antinucleosides, adverse effects of, 587t
Antiphospholipid antibody(ies), testing for, 775t
Antiplatelet agents
for ischemic stroke, 260–261
in stroke/TIA prevention, 270–271
Antipsychotics
action of, 738–739
for acute alcohol intoxication, 758
in AD, 321–322
adverse effects of, 354, 739t, 740
for schizophrenia, 738–740, 739t
Anti-Ri antibody, 559t, 563
Antithrombin deficiency, 183
Antithrombotic drugs
chronic use in cardiac conditions, 264t
for ischemic stroke, 260–261
Anti-Tr antibody, 559t, 562
Anti-VGCC antibodies, 559t
Anti-VGKC-related proteins, 559t, 562
Anti-Yo antibody, 559t, 562
Anton's syndrome, 278
Anxiety, vs. syncope, 96
Anxiety disorders, **720**
generalized anxiety disorder, 722–725, 725t
insomnia in, 165
panic disorder, 721–722, 721t
phobic disorders, 726–727
stress disorders, 727–728, 727t
vertigo in, 101–102
AOA1 (ataxia with oculomotor apraxia), 363t
AOA2 (ataxia with oculomotor apraxia), 363t
Aortic aneurysm, abdominal, 81
Aortic regurgitation, 796t
Aortic stenosis
antithrombotic prophylaxis for, 264t
echocardiography in, 796t
severity classification, 796t
APC gene, 425t
Aphasia, **142,** 804, 826
anomic, 144t, 146
Broca's, 144t, 145
caring for patient with, 155–156
conduction, 144t, 145–146
crossed, 143
fluent transcortical, 144t, 146
global, 144t, 145
isolation, 144t, 146
jargon, 144
nonfluent transcortical, 144t, 146
primary progressive, 148–149, 156, 323
progressive nonfluent, 148
subcortical, 148
video library, 157
Wernicke's, 144–145, 144t
Aphemia, 147
Apnea testing, 140, 826
ApoE gene, 320
Apomorphine
adverse effects of, 341
for PD, 341, 343t
Aponeurotic ptosis, 192
Apoplexy, pituitary, 443–444
Apoptosis
mitochondria in, 226–227
in neurologic disease, 226–227, 295

APP (amyloid precursor protein), 319, 319f
Apraxia, 103, 147
buccofacial, 147
construction, 150
dressing, 150
gait, 112
ideational, 147
ideomotor, 147
limb, 147
limb-kinetic, 147
ocular, 195
oculomotor, 150
Aprosodia, 148
Aquaporins, 491
Arachnoid cysts, 448
Arachnoiditis, lumbar, 80
Argyll Robertson pupil, 176
Aripiprazole, for schizophrenia, 739t, 740
Arousal
confusional, 170
level of, in coma, 136
ARSACS (autosomal recessive spastic ataxia of Charlevoix-Saguenay), 362t
Arsenic exposure/poisoning
clinical features of, 329
laboratory evaluation of, 788t
neuropathies in, 588t, 590–591
optic neuropathy in, 185
Arterial blood gases, reference values, 779t
Arteriovenous fistula
dural, 293
weakness in, 107
Arteriovenous malformation (AVM)
cerebral, 292
dural, 191
spinal cord, 49–410, 410f
Arteritis, stroke due to, 267
Artery of Percheron, occlusion of, 278
Artery-to-artery embolic stroke, 263–265
Arthritis, back pain in, 79
Arthrogryposis, 630
Artificial saliva, 205
Artificial tears, 180
Ashkenazi Jewish population
dystonia in, 348
hearing loss in, 212
Asimultanagnosia, 278
Asparaginase, 438t
Aspergillus infections
cerebral, 676–677f
chronic meningitis in, 530t
sinonasal, 677–678f
Aspirin
adverse effects of, 45
as antithrombotic in cardiac conditions, 264t
for ischemic stroke, 260–261
for migraine, 57, 59
for pain, 45, 46t
for stroke/TIA prevention, 270–271
for tension-type headache, 122
Association cortex, 142, 143f
Associative prosopagnosia, 152
Astasia-abasia, 113
Astereognosis, 122
Asterixis, 115, 136
Asthenia, 620
Asthma, sleep disruption in, 165
Astigmatism, 175
Astrocytoma
high-grade, 427–428, 427f, 428f
intramedullary, 405, 405f
low-grade, 426–427, 426f
Ataxia, **357**
approach to the patient, 357
autosomal dominant, 358, 359–361t, 364
autosomal recessive, 361–364t. *See also* Ataxia telangiectasia (AT); Friedreich's ataxia
cerebellar, 112, 113t, 842
early-onset, 363t
etiology of, 357, 358t
with muscle coenzyme Q deficiency, 363t
Ataxia (*Cont.*):
chemotherapy-induced, 438t
clinical features of, 357–358
episodic, 220t, 362–363t, 367
focal, 358
Friedreich's. *See* Friedreich's ataxia
inherited, **358**
ion channel defects causing, 220t
mitochondrial, 368
in MS, 478, 489
neoplastic, 561
ocular/optic, 150, 195
sensory, 112, 113t, 118
spinocerebellar. *See* Spinocerebellar ataxia
symmetric, 357–358
treatment of, 368–369
with vitamin E deficiency, 368
Ataxia telangiectasia (AT)
clinical features of, 363t, 368
genetic factors in, 363t, 368
treatment of, 368–369
Ataxia with oculomotor apraxia (AOA1), 363t
Ataxia with oculomotor apraxia (AOA2), 363t
Ataxin-1, 365
Ataxin-3, 366
Atherosclerosis
carotid. *See* Carotid atherosclerosis
intracranial, 265, 273
risk factors for, 269–270
Athetosis, 347t
Athlete(s), concussion in, 420, 420t
Atlastin gene, 374t, 378–379
ATM gene, 368
Atonic seizures, 234
Atrial fibrillation
chronic use of antithrombotics in, 264t
stroke and, 262–263, 265t, 808, 832
Atrophy
dentatorubropallidoluysian, 361t, 366–367
muscle, 622
spinal muscle, 370, 374t, 377–378
Atropine, ocular effects of, 176
Attention, assessment of, 127
Attentional deficit, 155
Audiogram, 213
Audiometry, 213–214
AUDIT (Alcohol Use Disorder Screening Test), 758, 758t
AUDIT-C (Alcohol Use Disorders Identification Test-Consumption) module, 746, 747t
Auditory brainstem responses, 214
Auditory cortex, 143f
Auditory nerve, 207
Aura, 232
Autism spectrum disorders, **710**
epidemiology of, 710
genetic factors in, 711–712, 711t
neuropathology of, 710–711
pathogenesis of, 712
Autoantibody(ies), in inflammatory myopathies, 651
Autoimmune autonomic neuropathy (AAN), 387
Automatisms, 232
Autonomic dysfunction, **380**
acute syndromes of, 389
in alcoholic neuropathy, 387
in amyloidosis, 387
approach to the patient, 383–385, 385t
in autoimmune autonomic neuropathy, 387
autonomic testing in, 384–385, 385t
in botulism, 387–388
classification of, 380, 382t
clinical evaluation of, 381–383, 382t
clinical features of, 381–383
in CRPS, 389–390
in diabetes mellitus, 386
drug-related, 383, 384t
in Guillain-Barré syndrome, 386
heart rate variation with deep breathing in, 384, 385t
in inherited disorders, 388
in multiple system atrophy, 385–386, 386f
in neuromuscular junction disorders, 386–388
orthostatic blood pressure recordings in, 385
orthostatic hypotension and, 383, 383t
Autonomic dysfunction (*Cont.*):
in PD, 345
in porphyrias, 386
in postural orthostatic tachycardia syndrome, 388
in primary hyperhidrosis, 388
in pure autonomic failure, 388
in reflex sympathetic dystrophy, 389–390
spinal cord lesions and, 386
sudomotor function in, 384–385, 385t
syndromes of, **385**
tilt table testing for syncope in, 385, 385t
treatment of, 390–391, 390t
Valsalva response in, 384, 385t
Autonomic dysreflexia, 386, 414
Autonomic failure, pure, 388
Autonomic nervous system, 380, 381f, 381t
disorders of. *See* Autonomic dysfunction
Autonomic neuropathy
autoimmune, 387
diabetic, 578–579
paraneoplastic, 564–565
Autonomic storm, 389
Autophagy, 228
Autoregulation, 295
Autosomal dominant nocturnal frontal lobe, 235t
Autosomal dominant partial epilepsy with auditory features, 235t
Autosomal recessive spastic ataxia of Charlevoix-Saguenay (ARSACS), 362t
AVM. *See* Arteriovenous malformation (AVM)
Azathioprine
for inflammatory myopathies, 658
for MS, 489
for myasthenia gravis, 615
for neuromyelitis optica, 491
AZT (zidovudine), 645t, 646

Babinski sign, 8, 104, 104t, 133, 820–821
Back pain, **71**
in ankylosing spondylitis, 79
approach to the patient, 72–75
in arthritis, 79
breakaway weakness in, 74
in cancer patient, 79
in cauda equina syndrome, 77–78
causes of, 75t
chronic, 82–84
in congenital anomalies of lumbar spine, 75–76, 75t
costs of, 71
in degenerative conditions, 75t, 78–79, 78f, 79f
diagnosis of, 74–75
electromyography in, 75
idiopathic, 81
imaging in, 75
in infections/inflammation, 75t, 80
local, 72
in lumbar disk disease. *See* Intervertebral disk, herniation of
metabolic causes of, 75t, 80
with muscle spasm, 73
nerve conduction studies in, 75
patient education in, 82
physical examination in, 73–74, 74t
postural, 81
in psychiatric disease, 81
radicular, 72
referred, 72, 80–81
risk factors for structural cause, 73t
of spine origin, 72
in sprains and strains, 76
trauma-related, 75t, 76
treatment of, 82–84
acute pain without radiculopathy, 82
chronic pain without radiculopathy, 82–84
pain with radiculopathy, 84–85
types of, 72–73
in vertebral fracture, 76, 80
Baclofen
for dystonia, 349
for spasticity in neurologic disease, 414, 489
for stiff-person syndrome, 563
for tardive dyskinesia, 354
for trigeminal neuralgia, 393

Bacterial endocarditis. *See* Infective endocarditis
Bacterial meningitis. *See* Meningitis, bacterial
BAEPs (brainstem auditory evoked potentials), 29–30, 214–215
Balamuthia
in chronic meningitis, 530t
in encephalitis, 511
Balance
anatomy and physiology of, 111
disorders of, 111–112, **114**. *See also* Fall(s)
standing, 110
Bálint's syndrome, 150–151, 195, 278, 826
Baló's concentric sclerosis, 694–695f
Baltic myoclonus, 362t
Bamboo spine, 79
Bannwarth's syndrome, 529t
Barbiturates, for epilepsy, 250
Bardet-Biedl syndrome, 442
Baroreceptors, 90, 91f
Basal cell nevus syndrome, 425t
Basal ganglia, 335f, 339f
Basal meningitis, 528
Basic fibroblast growth factor (bFGF), 447
Basilar artery
ischemia in territory of, 195
occlusion of, 210, 279–282, 281–284f
Basilar skull fracture, 417
Bassen-Kornzweig disease, 190
Baylisascaris procyonis infections
chronic meningitis in, 531t
encephalitis in, 511
BCNU (carmustine), adverse effects of, 438t
Beck Depression Inventory, 48
Becker's disease, 643
Becker's muscular dystrophy, **628**
clinical features of, 625t, 628, 844
genetic factors in, 625t
laboratory evaluation of, 628
treatment of, 628
Becquerel (Bq), 799t
Bed rest, for back pain, 82
Bedwetting, 170
Beevor's sign, 401
Behavioral modification/behavioral therapy
for insomnia, 164
for sleep enuresis, 170
Behçet's syndrome
chronic meningitis in, 532t
neurologic involvement in, 678f
ocular involvement in, 181, 182
Bell's palsy, **395**
clinical features of, 395
differential diagnosis of, 395–396
incidence of, 395
laboratory evaluation of, 396, 396f
neuroimaging in, 691f
pathophysiology of, 395
taste disorders in, 204
treatment of, 396
Bell's phenomenon, 394
Benedikt's syndrome, 193
Benign familial neonatal convulsions, 235t
Benign forgetfulness of the elderly, 311
Benign hereditary chorea of childhood, 352
Benign paroxysmal positional vertigo, 99t, 100, 802, 823
Benserazide/levodopa, for PD, 339, 343t
Benznidazole, for Chagas' disease, 548
Benzodiazepine(s)
for acute alcohol intoxication, 758
adverse effects of, 128, 166
for delirium, 131
dosage of, 725t
for generalized anxiety disorder, 725t, 726
in opiate overdose management, 764
pharmacology of, 725t
for restless legs syndrome, 166
withdrawal from, 128–129, 726
Benzodiazepine receptor agonists, for insomnia, 164–165
Benztropine
for extrapyramidal symptoms, 740
for PD, 342
Beriberi, 591. *See also* Thiamine (vitamin B_1), deficiency of
β-adrenergic antagonists (beta blockers)
for acute angle-closure glaucoma, 182
for glaucoma, 188
for migraine prevention, 60
for phobic disorders, 726
for syncope, 92
β-carotene, for macular degeneration, 189
Bethanechol
for bladder dysfunction in MS, 490
for SSRI-related sexual dysfunction, 733
Bevacizumab
adverse neurologic effects of, 438, 438t
for macular degeneration, 189
bFGF (basic fibroblast growth factor), 447
Bilateral simultaneous stimulation test, 122
Biliary disease, back pain in, 81
Binswanger's disease, 112, 322, 833
Biofeedback training, for migraine, 57
Bipolar cell antibodies, 559t
Bipolar disorder, **733**
clinical features of, 733–734
diagnosis of, 734, 734t
differential diagnosis of, 734
etiology of, 734
pathophysiology of, 734
treatment of, 734–735, 735t, 736t
Bipolar II disorder, 734
Bitter taste sensation, 201
Blackout, 754
Bladder dysfunction, in neurologic disease, 413, 478
Bladder training, for sleep enuresis, 170
Blastomyces spp. infections, chronic meningitis in, 530t
Blepharitis, 180
Blepharoptosis, 191–192
Blepharospasm, 348–349
Blessed Dementia Rating Scale, 127
Blindness
color, 177
cortical, 179
in diabetic retinopathy, 189
legal, 175
transient monocular, 182–184
Blind spot, 179
Blink reflexes, 34
Blood, reference values, 775–778t
Blood pressure
changes during Valsalva maneuver, 384, 385t
during sleep, 161
Body fluids, reference values, 799t
Bone-anchored hearing aid, 215
Bone-conduction threshold, 213
Bone disease, neck pain in, 87
Bone marrow/bone marrow examination, normal, 790t
Bone spicules, 189–190, 190f
BOR (branchio-oto-renal) syndrome, 212t
Bortezomib, adverse effects of, 438, 438t, 585t
Botulinum toxin
for dystonia, 349–350
for hemifacial spasm, 397
for hyperhidrosis, 388
for Tourette's syndrome, 353
Botulism
autonomic dysfunction in, 387–388
clinical features of, 387–388, 613
diplopia in, 193
pathogenesis of, 613
treatment of, 613
Bound morphemes, 145
Bourneville's disease. *See* Tuberous sclerosis
Bovine spongiform encephalopathy, 550, 550t, 554
Bq (becquerel), 799t
Brachial neuritis, 87
Brachial plexopathy
immune-mediated, 87, 595
neoplastic, 595–596
neuroimaging in, 697–698f
Brachial plexus
anatomy of, 595, 596f
injury to, neck pain in, 87
Bradyarrhythmia, syncope in, 95
Bradykinesia, 103
Bradykinin, 42f
Brain
alcohol effects on, 752–753
inferior aspect of, 277f
Brain abscess, **518**
approach to the patient, 493–494, 494–495f
clinical features of, 519–520
definition of, 518
diagnosis of, 18f, 520, 520f
differential diagnosis of, 520
epidemiology of, 518
etiology of, 518–519
pathogenesis of, 519
prognosis of, 521
treatment of, 521
Brain biopsy
in dementia, 316
in viral encephalitis, 510
Brain death, criteria for, 140, 804, 825–826
Brain edema, 294
Brain germ cell tumors, 448–449
Brain hemorrhage, 416, 416f
Brain injury. *See also* Head injury
caring for patient with, 155–156
post-cardiac bypass, 662–663, 662f, 817, 845–846
post-solid organ transplantation, 663
Brainstem accessory optic system, 174
Brainstem auditory evoked potentials (BAEPs), 29–30, 214–215
Brainstem disorders/lesions
clinical features of, 10t
sensory abnormalities in, 123
weakness in, 106
Brainstem ischemia, bilateral, 281
Brainstem reflexes, examination in coma, 136–138, 137f
Brain tumors, **423**
amnesia in, 153
approach to the patient, 423–424
clinical features of, 423–424, 423t
extrinsic "benign," **430**
craniopharyngioma. *See* Craniopharyngioma
meningioma. *See* Meningioma
pituitary tumors. *See* Pituitary tumors (adenomas)
schwannoma, 431–432, 431f
headache in, 51t, 53
hemorrhage into, 289
intrinsic malignant, **426**
astrocytoma. *See* Astrocytoma
ependymoma, 429
medulloblastoma, 430
oligodendroglioma, 428–429
pineal region tumors, 176, 195, 430
primary lymphoma, 429–430, 429f
metastatic, **433,** 433t
diagnosis of, 433–434, 434f
epidural. *See* Spinal cord compression, neoplastic
leptomeningeal, 435–436, 435f
treatment of, 434
neuroimaging of, 424
primary, **424**
genetic syndromes associated with, 425t
pathogenesis of, 424–426, 425t, 426f
treatment of, 424
Branching enzyme deficiency (type IV glycogenosis), 637
Branchio-oto-renal (BOR) syndrome, 212t
Branch retinal vein occlusion, 183
Breast cancer
alcohol effects on, 755
metastatic
to CNS, 403, 404f, 433t, 801, 810–811, 811f, 821, 836
to eye, 190
paraneoplastic syndromes in, 559t
Breast-feeding, AEDs and, 255
Broca's aphasia, 144t, 145
Broca's area, 142, 149f

Bromocriptine
for acromegaly, 465
adverse effects of, 457
for prolactinoma, 457
Brown-Séquard syndrome, 106, 123, 402
Brucella spp. infections
chronic meningitis in, 529t
ocular involvement in, 182
Brudzinski's sign, 493
Brugada syndrome, 95
Bruns-Garland syndrome, 579
Bruxism, 170
Bulbospinal pathway, 105f
Bulimia nervosa, 204
Buprenorphine
as maintenance drug, 765
for opiate detoxification, 764
in opiate overdose management, 764
Bupropion
adverse effects of, 723t
for depression, 723t, 732
for SSRI-related sexual dysfunction, 733
Burning mouth syndrome (glossodynia), 206
Buspirone
for generalized anxiety disorder, 725t, 726
for SSRI-related sexual dysfunction, 733
Busulfan, adverse effects of, 438t
Butorphanol
for migraine, 58t, 60
other opioids and, 50
for pain, 46t, 47

Cabergoline
for acromegaly, 465
adverse effects of, 457
for prolactinoma, 457
Cachectic myopathy, 304
CADASIL (cerebral autosomal dominant arteriopathy with subcortical infarcts and leukoencephalopathy), 268, 323, 685f
Cadmium exposure/poisoning, 788t
Caffeine
action of, 160
adverse effects of, 165–166
for hypnic headache, 70
for migraine, 58t
for shift-work disorder, 172
Calcinosis, dermatomyositis and, 659
Calcitonin gene-related peptide, 42
Calcium channel(s), disorders of, 640–642, 641t
Calculation ability, assessment of, 6
Caloric irrigation, 138, 195
Campylobacter spp. infections, Guillain-Barré syndrome and, 600, 601f
Cancer
alcohol effects on, 755
chronic meningitis in, 532t
depression in, 729
inflammatory myopathies and, 650
neuropathies associated with, 583–584
recurrent, 597–598
Cancer chemotherapy
neurologic complications of, 438, 438t, 584–585t
timing of, 173
Candida spp. infections
chronic meningitis in, 530t
in newborn, 675f
Cannabinoid(s), 769
Capgras syndrome, 312
Capillary telangiectasias, 292
Capsaicin, for neuropathy, 578t
Carbamazepine
adverse effects of
common, 393, 735t
hematologic, 246
liver dysfunction, 246, 578t
neurologic, 247t, 578t
rare, 735t
systemic, 247t
for bipolar disorder, 735, 735t
dosage of, 247t, 578t
drug interactions of, 247t
for epilepsy, 246, 247t
Carbamazepine (*Cont.*):
for focal seizures, 246
for neuromyotonia, 565
for neuropathy, 578t
for pain, 46t, 50, 489
pharmacology of, 246, 247t, 735t
for trigeminal neuralgia, 393
Carbidopa/levodopa, for PD, 339, 343t
Carbon disulfide, 588t
Carbonic anhydrase inhibitors, for glaucoma, 188
Carbon monoxide poisoning
aphasia in, 146
complications of, 300
hypoxia in, 299
optic neuropathy in, 185
treatment of, 300
Carcinoid tumors, 565
Cardiac arrhythmias, syncope in, 95–96
Cardiac catheterization , normal values, 793t
Cardiac output, calculation and normal values, 794t
Cardiac syncope, 93t, 95–96
Cardioembolic stroke, 261–263, 263t
Cardiomyopathy, syncope in, 96
Cardiopulmonary bypass, brain injury after, 662–663, 662f, 817, 845–846
Cardiopulmonary resuscitation, 299, 299f
Cardiovascular disease
depression in, 729
embolic stroke in, 261–263, 263t
syncope in, 95–96
Cardiovascular system
alcohol effects on, 755
in sleep, 161
Carmustine (BCNU), adverse effects of, 438t
Carney syndrome
clinical features of, 447t
pituitary tumors in, 447, 447t
Carnitine palmitoyltransferase deficiency, 638
Carotid artery
occlusion of, 276–277, 277f
stenosis, 69, 183, 265t
Carotid atherosclerosis
asymptomatic, surgical treatment of, 272
stroke due to, 263–265, 265t
treatment of, 272
endovascular therapy in, 273
extracranial-to-intracranial bypass surgery in, 273
surgical, 272–273
Carotid cavernous fistula, 191
Carotid sinus massage, 97
Carpal tunnel syndrome, 87, 815–816, 843
Caspase, 226
Catamenial epilepsy, 254
Cataplexy, 96, 163t, 168t, 169
Cataract, 187–188
Catatonia, 132
Catecholaminergic polymorphic ventricular tachycardia, 95
Catechol-O-methyltransferase (COMT) inhibitors, for PD, 342, 343t
Cat-scratch disease, 182
Cauda equina syndrome
clinical features of, 77–78, 402, 846
diagnosis of, 77
treatment of, 78
weakness in, 107
Causalgia, 45
Cavernous angiomas, 292–293
Cavernous malformations, 20f
Cavernous sinus syndrome, 399, 399f
CBT. *See* Cognitive behavioral therapy (CBT)
Cefepime, 501
Cefepime, for meningitis, 499t, 500
Cefotaxime, for meningitis, 499t, 501
Ceftazidime, for meningitis, 499t
Ceftriaxone, for meningitis, 499t, 501
Celecoxib, 45, 46t
Celiac disease (gluten-induced enteropathy), 580
Cellulitis, orbital, 191
Central cord syndrome, 402
Central core disease, **635**
Central fever, 135
Central nervous system (CNS)
alcohol effects on, 754
electrodiagnostic studies of, **26**. *See also specific technique and* Electrodiagnostic studies
paraneoplastic syndromes of, 558t
vasculitis of, 329, 686f
Central nervous system (CNS) cancer
dementia in, 329
lymphoma, 429–430, 429f, 545, 545f
primary and metastatic tumors, **423**. *See also specific types and sites*
approach to the patient, 423–424
clinical features of, 423–424, 423t
Central nervous system (CNS) infections
brain abscess. *See* Brain abscess
cranial epidural abscess, **524,** 524f
dementia due to, 328–329
empyema. *See* Subdural empyema
encephalitis. *See* Encephalitis
meningitis. *See* Meningitis
nonbacterial causes of, **521**
sarcoidosis, 532t
treatment of, 494–495f
Central pontine myelinolysis, 301, 302f
Central retinal artery occlusion, 183–184, 183f
Central retinal vein occlusion, 183–184, 184f
Central sensitization, 41
Central sleep apnea, 169
Central transtentorial herniation, 133f, 134
Centronuclear (myotubular) myopathy, **636**
Cerebellar arteries, occlusion of, 279
Cerebellar degeneration/atrophy
alcohol and, 754
gait disorders in, 111t, 112
paraneoplastic, 559t, 562
Cerebellar gait ataxia, 112, 113t
Cerebral amyloid angiopathy, 289, 322
Cerebral aneurysm, 69
Cerebral angiography, in stroke, 268f, 285
Cerebral artery(ies)
aneurysm of, 15f
anterior. *See* Anterior cerebral artery
middle. *See* Middle cerebral artery
posterior. *See* Posterior cerebral artery
stenosis, neuroimaging in, 683f
Cerebral autosomal dominant arteriopathy with subcortical infarcts and leukoencephalopathy (CADASIL), 268, 323, 685f
Cerebral blood flow, autoregulation of, 295, 296f
Cerebral glioma, 21f
Cerebral hemispheres, anatomy of, 143f, 274f, 275f, 276f
Cerebral ischemia, 256, 258f
Cerebral palsy, 111
Cerebral perfusion pressure, 295, 296f
Cerebral venous sinuses, 525–526, 525f
Cerebritis, 518
Cerebrospinal fluid (CSF)
leakage of, 67–68, 67f
low volume, headache with, 67–68
raised pressure. *See* Intracranial pressure, increased
Cerebrospinal fluid (CSF) analysis
in bacterial meningitis, 498–499, 499t
in chronic meningitis, 533–534
in coma, 138–139
in delirium, 130
in MS, 480t, 482
normal values, 38, 38t
reference values, 789t
in viral encephalitis, 508–509
in viral meningitis, 504
Cerebrovascular disease, **256**. *See also* Stroke
approach to the patient, 256–257, 257f
definition of, 256
dementia associated with, **322**
imaging studies of, **282**
incidence of, 256
seizures due to, 238
types of, 256
Cerumen impaction, 213
Cervical angina syndrome, 87
Cervical collar, 88
Cervical dystonia, 349

Cervical radiculopathy, 86t
Cervical spine
disk disease, 85–86, 86t
lesions of, 401
trauma to, 85
C fibers, 40, 41
CHADS2 score, 262, 264t
Chagas' disease, in HIV infection, 547–548
Chalazion, 180
Channelopathy(ies), 806, 830
muscular, 640–642, 641t, 642f
neurologic, 220, 220t
Charcot-Marie-Tooth (CMT) disease, **571,** 815, 842
CMT1, 572–574, 572t
CMT1A, 219, 572t, 574
CMT1X, 572t, 574
CMT2, 572t, 574
CMT3, 573t, 574
CMT4, 574, 574t
connexin in, 221
genetic factors in, 572–573t
Chemical restraints, 131
Cheyne-Stokes respiration, in coma, 138
Chiari malformation, 196
headache in, 67
syringomyelia associated with, 410, 411f
Chiasmal tumor, 190
Children
GH deficiency in, 459–460
seizures in, 238t
Chiropractic, 82
Chlamydia trachomatis infections, 180
Chloramphenicol
adverse effects of, 185
therapeutic monitoring of, 786t
Chlordiazepoxide, 725t, 758
Chlorhexidine mouthwash, 205
Chloride channel disorders, **643**
Chloroquine, adverse effects of
myopathy, 645t, 647
neuropathy, 585, 586t
ocular, 190
Chlorpromazine
for medication-overuse headache, 66
for migraine, 58t, 60
Cholesteatoma, 209
Cholinergics, for glaucoma, 188
Cholinesterase inhibitors
for dementia, 331
for dementia with Lewy bodies, 326
for myasthenia gravis, 614
Chorda tympani nerve, 201f, 202
Chordoma, 448
Chorea(s), 347t, **350**
disorders associated with, 352
paraneoplastic, 352, 559t
Sydenham's, 352
Chorea-acanthocytosis, 352
Choriocarcinoma, parasellar, 448–449
Choriomeningitis, lymphocytic, 531t
Chorioretinopathy, central serous, 189
Choroidal artery, occlusion of, 276, 277f
CHRNA4 gene, 235t
Chronic cerebrospinal insufficiency, in MS, 489
Chronic fatigue syndrome, **704,** 818, 846
definition of, 704
diagnosis of, 704t, 705–706
epidemiology of, 704
etiology of, 704–705, 705t
pathophysiology of, 705
prognosis of, 707
treatment of, 706–707, 706f
Chronic inflammatory demyelinating polyneuropathy (CIDP), **605**
clinical features of, 605
diagnosis of, 605
vs. Guillain-Barré syndrome, 605
pathogenesis of, 602t, 605
treatment of, 606
Chronic kidney disease (CKD)
laboratory evaluation of, 791–792t
Chronic kidney disease (CKD) (*Cont.*):
neuromuscular disorders in
back pain, 81
coma, 134–135
delirium, 129, 129t
gait disorders, 113
neuropathy, 580
Chronic obstructive pulmonary disease (COPD), sleep disorders in, 165
Chronic progressive external ophthalmoplegia, 192
Chronic wasting disease, 550, 550t
Cidofovir, for viral encephalitis, 513, 514
CIDP. *See* Chronic inflammatory demyelinating polyneuropathy (CIDP)
Cingulate cortex, 149
Ciprofloxacin, 185
Circadian pacemaker, 172–173
Circadian rhythmicity
medical implications of, 173
physiology of, 160–161, 160f
Circadian rhythm sleep disorders, **170**
Cisplatin, adverse effects of
hearing loss, 209
neurologic, 438, 438t, 584t
Cisternography, CT, 14
Citalopram, 723t
CKD. *See* Chronic kidney disease (CKD)
Cladribine, for MS, 486t, 487–488
Clasp-knife phenomenon, 103
Claude's syndrome, 193, 278
Claudication, neurogenic, 78
Clinical Dementia Rating, 127
Clinical laboratory tests, reference values
body fluids, 799t
bone marrow aspirates, 790t
cerebrospinal fluid, 789t
cholesterol, 789t
circulatory function, 794t
clinical chemistry and immunology, 778–785t
echocardiographic reference limits and partition values, 795–796t
gastrointestinal tests, 798t
hematology and coagulation, 775–778t
normal pressures in heart and great vessels, 793t
pulmonary physiology, 797t
radiation derived units, 799t
stool analysis, 790t
toxicology and therapeutic drug monitoring, 786–788t
urine analysis and renal function, 791–792t
vitamins and trace minerals, 788t
Clomipramine
adverse effects of, 723t
for depression, 723t
for narcolepsy, 169
for obsessive-compulsive disorder, 728
Clonazepam
adverse effects of, 248t
for ataxia/tremor, 489
for epilepsy, 248t
for generalized anxiety disorder, 725t
for myoclonus, 353
for pain, 46t
for panic disorder, 722
pharmacology of, 248t
for posthypoxic myoclonus, 300
for REM sleep behavior disorder, 170
for tardive dyskinesia, 354
for vertigo, 102t
Clonidine, for opioid withdrawal syndrome, 66, 764
Clopidogrel, for stroke/TIA prevention, 270
Clozapine
adverse effects of, 739t
for Huntington's disease, 351
for schizophrenia, 739, 739t
Club drugs, 128
Cluster headache, 51t, **63**
clinical features of, 63t
insomnia in, 165
neuroimaging in, 56f
prevention of, 64, 64t
treatment of, 64
Cluster-tic, 393
CMDs (congenital muscular dystrophies), 625t, **630,** 631t
CMS (congenital myasthenic syndromes), 610–611, 612t
CMT disease. *See* Charcot-Marie-Tooth (CMT) disease
CMV. *See* Cytomegalovirus (CMV) infections
CNS. *See* Central nervous system (CNS)
Coagulation disorders, laboratory evaluation of, 775–778t
Coats' disease, 632
Cobalamin (vitamin B_{12})
deficiency of, 411–412
delirium in, 129
dementia in, 328, 833
frontal lobe syndrome in, 155
gait disorders in, 112
neuropathies in, 411–412, 591, 843
olfactory dysfunction in, 206
optic neuropathy in, 185
orthostatic hypotension, 95
sensory disturbances in, 122
malabsorption of, 206
reference range for, 788t
Cobblestone papillae, 180
Cocaine, **767**
action of, 221, 718t
acute and chronic intoxication, 767–768, 807, 831
adverse effects of, 767
autonomic, 389
insomnia, 166
myopathy, 645t, 646
intracerebral hemorrhage due to, 289
reinforcing effects of, 767
systemic effects of, 767–768
Coccidioides spp. infections. *See also* Meningitis
chronic meningitis in, 530t, 674f
neuroimaging in, 674f
ocular involvement in, 182
subacute meningitis in, 514–515
Cochlea, 207, 207f
Cochlear implant, 210, 215–216
Codeine, for pain, 46t
Cognitive behavioral therapy (CBT)
for back pain, 83
for chronic fatigue syndrome, 706–707, 846
for PTSD, 748
Cognitive dysfunction
alcohol and, 754
caring for patient with, 155–156
delirium and, 126
in MS, 478
Cognitive evoked potentials, 30
Cognitive function assessment, 127
Cognitive rehabilitation procedures, 156
Colchicine, adverse effects of
myopathy, 645t, 647
neuropathy, 585, 586t
Collier's sign, 195
Colloid cysts, 115, 432
Color anomia, 177
Color blindness, 177
Colorectal cancer, back pain in, 81
Color vision, assessment of, 177
Coma, **132**
anatomy of, 133–135
approach to the patient
brainstem reflexes, 136–138, 137f
history, 135
level of arousal, 136
neurologic examination, 136
physical examination, 135–136
brain death determination in, 140
definition of, 132
differential diagnosis of, 139, 139t
due to cerebral mass lesions and herniations, 133–134, 133f
due to metabolic disorders, 134–135
due to widespread cerebral damage, 135
EEG in, 28
epileptic, 135
imaging in, 138–139
laboratory studies in, 138–139
prognosis of, 141
toxic/drug-induced, 135
treatment of, 141

Combination antiretroviral therapy (cART), 589
Common carotid artery, occlusion of, 277
Common cold, 203
Complement factor H, in macular degeneration, 189
Complex febrile seizures, 238
Complex partial status epilepticus, 329
Complex regional pain syndrome (CRPS), 45, 389–390, 810, 835
Comprehension, assessment of, 143
Comprehensive stroke centers, 285
Compression fracture, 698f
Computed tomography (CT)
in cerebral artery occlusion, 16f, 285f
in cerebral contusion, 416f
in CNS vasculitis, 686f
in coma, 137
in diffuse axonal injury, 416f
in epidural hematoma, 418f, 699f
in hearing loss, 215
in Huntington's disease, 690f
in lacunar infarction, 684f
in neurologic critical illness, 296–297
in neurologic disease, **13**
complications of, 14–17, 17t
guidelines for, 14t
indications for, 14, 14t
premedication guidelines for patients with prior contrast allergy, 17t
technique, 13–14, 15f
in stroke, 282–284, 285f
in subarachnoid hemorrhage, 306–307, 307f, 821
in subdural hematoma, 418f, 419f
in superior sagittal sinus thrombosis, 687f
in viral encephalitis, 510
Computed tomography (CT) angiography, 14, 15f
Computed tomography (CT) cisternography, 14
Computed tomography (CT) myelography, 14, 24
COMT (catechol-O-methyltransferase) inhibitors, for PD, 342, 343t
Concussion, **418**
definition of, 415, 837
mechanics of, 415
vs. moderate/severe head injury, 745t. *See also* Head injury
sports-related, 420, 420t
treatment of, 837
in war veterans, 744–745, 745t, 749
Cone(s), 174, 177
Confabulation, 153
Confusion, **125,** 825
Confusion Assessment Method, 127
Congenital amaurosis. *See* Leber hereditary optic neuropathy (congenital amaurosis)
Congenital heart disease, brain abscess and, 519
Congenital motor nystagmus, 196
Congenital muscular dystrophy(ies) (CMDs), 625t, **630,** 631t
Congenital myasthenic syndromes (CMS), 611–612, 612t
Congenital myopathies, **635**
Congenital myotonic dystrophy, 631
Congenital sensory nystagmus, 196
Congenital vascular malformations, 292
Conjugate eye movement, 137
Conjunctivitis, 180
Connexin(s), 221
Connexin 26, 212
Consciousness, assessment of, 5
Constipation
in MS, 478
opioid-induced, 48
treatment of, 48
Contact lenses, 180
Contraception, AEDs and, 255
Contracture, 622
Contrast agents
adverse effects of
nephrogenic systemic fibrosis, 19–21, 821–822
nephropathy, 15, 822
precautionary measures for, 17t
Contusion, cerebral, 416, 416f
Conus medullaris syndrome, 401–402
Convergence-projection hypothesis, of referred pain, 42f
Conversion disorder, 736
Convulsion, 417
Coordination, assessment of, 9
COPD (chronic obstructive pulmonary disease), sleep disorders in, 165
Copper
deficiency of, 592
reference values, 788t
Corneal blink reflex, 137f
Corneal light reflex, 177
Cortical venous thrombosis, 107
Corticobasal degeneration, 112, 147, 325, 336
Corticospinal pathway, 105f
Corticosteroids. *See* Glucocorticoid(s)
Corticotrope, 439t, 446t
Cotton-wool spots, 186f
Cough Assist Device, for ALS, 377
Cough headache, primary, **69**
Cover test, 177, 192
Cowden syndrome, 425t
COX inhibitors. *See* Cyclooxygenase (COX) inhibitors
Coxsackievirus, in meningitis, 505
Cramps, muscle, 622
Cranial epidural abscess
clinical features of, 524–525
definition of, 524, 524f
diagnosis of, 525
etiology of, 524
pathophysiology of, 524
prognosis of, 525
treatment of, 525
Cranial nerve examination, 6–7
Cranial nerve injuries, 417
Cranial nerve palsies, 398–399, 399f
Cranial nerve syndromes, 397–398, 398t
Craniopharyngioma
clinical features of, 432, 447–448
ocular signs in, 179
treatment of, 432
C-reactive protein (CRP), 780t
Creatine kinase, CK-MB, 780t
CREB protein, 718
Creutzfeldt-Jakob disease
clinical course of, 555
clinical features of, 314t, 549, 554–555, 833, 842
dementia due to, 326
diagnosis of, 555, 556f
differential diagnosis of, 555
after dura matter grafts, 553
after human growth hormone therapy, 553
iatrogenic, 553
laboratory evaluation of, 555–556, 556f
molecular basis of, 312t
myoclonus in, 554–555, 842
neuropathology of, 554
after pituitary gonadotropin therapy, 553
prevention of, 557
as prion disease, 549, 841–842
prions associated with, 555–556
treatment of, 556, 557
variant, 554
Critical illness myopathy, 304
Critical illness polyneuropathy, 304, 581
Critically ill patient
neurologic disorders in, 295t
approach to the patient, 296
diagnostic studies, 296–297
elevated ICP treatment, 297–298, 298t
ICP monitoring, 297, 297f
secondary brain insults, 299–300
central pontine myelinolysis, 301, 302f
delirium, 125, 131, 300–301
hypoxic-ischemic encephalopathy, 299–300, 300f
metabolic encephalopathies, 300–301
myopathy, 304
neuromuscular transmission disorders, 303–304
neuropathy, 303, 581
pathophysiology of
brain edema, 294
cerebral perfusion and autoregulation, 295, 296f
Critically ill patient, neurologic disorders in, pathophysiology of (*Cont.*):
CSF and intracranial pressure, 295–296, 296f
ischemic cascade and cellular injury, 294–295
peripheral nervous system, 295t, 303–304
respiratory evaluation in, 303
sepsis-associated encephalopathy, 301
status epilepticus, 297, 300
Wernicke's disease, 302–303, 302f
Crohn's disease, ocular involvement in, 182f
Crossed aphasia, 143
Crossed straight-leg raising sign, 74
Crow-Fukase syndrome (POEMS syndrome), 564
CRPS (complex regional pain syndrome), 45, 389–390, 810, 835
Cryptococcus spp. infections
chronic meningitis in, 530t
in HIV infection, 545–546
subacute meningitis in, 514–515
Cryptogenic sensory and sensorimotor polyneuropathy (CSPN), 593
CSF. *See* Cerebrospinal fluid (CSF)
CSTB gene, 235t
CT. *See* Computed tomography (CT)
Cushing response, 136
Cushing's disease, 451t
Cushing's syndrome, **467**
caused by ectopic ACTH production
diagnosis of, 468, 468t, 840
clinical features of, 467, 467t
differential diagnosis of, 468t, 813, 839–840
etiology of, 467
inferior petrosal venous sampling in, 468
laboratory evaluation of, 467–468
prevalence of, 467
treatment of, 469, 469f
Cutaneous reflexes, 9, 104
Cyanide poisoning, 300
Cyclobenzaprine
for back pain, 82
for spasticity in MS, 489
Cyclooxygenase (COX) inhibitors
adverse effects of, 45
opioid combinations, 48
for pain, 45
Cyclopentolate hydrochloride, for red or painful eye, 179
Cyclophosphamide
for cerebellar degeneration, 564
for inflammatory myopathies, 658
for MS, 489
for myasthenia gravis, 616
Cyclosporine
for inflammatory myopathies, 658
for myasthenia gravis, 616
therapeutic monitoring of, 786t
Cyclothymic disorder, 734
Cyproheptadine
for Cushing's syndrome, 469
for migraine prevention, 60
Cystatin B, 235t
Cysticercosis
chronic meningitis in, 530t
clinical features of, 521
diagnosis of, 521–522
etiology of, 521
ocular involvement in, 182, 195
treatment of, 522
Cytarabine, 438t, 585t
Cytomegalovirus (CMV) infections
myelopathy and polyradiculopathy in, 543
neuropathy in, 583
Cytotoxic edema, 294

Dabigatran, for stroke prevention, 271
Dacarbazine (DTIC), adverse effects of, 438t
Dacryocystitis, 180
Dalfampridine, for weakness in MS, 489
Dantrolene, for spasticity in neurologic disease, 414, 489
Dapsone, 587t
Daytime sleepiness, 163t, 166–168, 173
DDAVP. *See* Desmopressin (DDAVP)

ddC (zalcitabine), adverse effects of, 589
Debranching enzyme deficiency (type III glycogenosis), 637
Decerebrate rigidity, 136
Decorticate rigidity, in coma, 136
Decubitus ulcers, prevention of, 413
Deep brain stimulation (DBS)
  for dystonia, 350
  for headache, 64
  for PD, 343, 346
Dehydration, delirium in, 128
Déjérine-Roussy syndrome, 123, 288
Delayed puberty, anosmia in, 205
Delayed sleep phase disorder, **172**
Delirium, **125**
  approach to the patient, 127–130, 130t, 803, 824–825
  clinical features of, 125
  in critically ill patient, 125, 131, 300–301
  dementia and, 126
  diagnosis of, 130, 130t, 824–825
  drug-induced, 126–127, 129t
  in elderly, 126
  epidemiology of, 126
  etiology of, 128–130, 129t, 825–826
  history in, 127–128
  hyperactive, 125
  hypoactive, 125
  pathogenesis of, 126–127
  physical examination in, 128
  postoperative/ICU, 125, 131, 824
  prevention of, 131
  reversibility of, 125
  risk factors for, 125–126
  screening tools for, 127–128
  treatment of, 131
Delirium Detection Score, 127
Delirium Rating Scale, 127
Delirium tremens, 125, 759
Demecarium bromide, 177
Dementia, **310**. *See also specific types*
  in alcoholism, 328
  ALS/parkinsonian/dementia complex of Guam and, 330
  aphasia in, 149
  approach to the patient, 312, 314t, 808, 833
  caring for patient with, 155–156
  clinical features of, 314t
  in CNS infections, 328–329
  in CNS neoplasms, 329
  cognitive examination in, 314–315, 315t
  in corticobasal degeneration, 325
  in Creutzfeldt-Jakob disease, 326
  definition of, 310
  delirium and, 126–127
  differential diagnosis of, 311t
  etiology of, 310–312, 311t
  frontotemporal. *See* Frontotemporal dementia
  functional anatomy of, 310
  head trauma–related, 329
  HIV-associated, 541–543, 542f, 542t
  in Huntington's disease, 326–327
  insomnia in, 165
  in isolated vasculitis of CNS, 329
  in Korsakoff's syndrome, 328
  laboratory tests in, 314t, 315–316
  memory loss in, 156
  metal exposure and, 329
  molecular basis of, 312t
  multi-infarct, 322
  neurologic examination in, 313–314, 314t
  in nicotinic acid deficiency, 328
  in normal-pressure hydrocephalus, 327–328, 327f
  patient history in, 312–313, 314t
  in PD, 326, 344–345
  physical examination in, 313–314, 314t
  in Pick's disease, 324, 325f
  prevalence of, 310
  in prion diseases, 326
  in progressive supranuclear palsy, 325
  in psychiatric diseases, 330–331
  in seizure disorders, 329
  semantic, 152
Dementia (*Cont.*):
  transient global amnesia and, 329–330
  treatment of, 331–332
  types of, 312, 312t
  vascular, 310, **322,** 322f
  in vitamin B_1 deficiency, 328
  in vitamin B_{12} deficiency, 328
Dementia pugilistica, 329, 744
Dementia with Lewy bodies, **326**
  clinical features of, 126, 312, 314t, 326
  molecular basis of, 312t
  neuropathology of, 326
  olfactory dysfunction in, 203
  orthostatic hypotension in, 95
  vs. Parkinson's disease dementia, 344
  treatment of, 326
Dentatorubropallidoluysian atrophy, 361t, 366–367
Dependence
  alcohol. *See* Alcohol abuse or dependence (alcoholism)
  physical, 716
  psychological (motivational), 716
  substance, vs. substance abuse, 716. *See also* Substance use disorders
Depression/depressive disorders, **730**
  agitated, 734
  chemosensory alterations in, 205
  clinical features of, 730–731
  diagnosis of, 730t
  dizziness in, 101
  drug-related, 729
  in epilepsy, 253
  etiology of, 731
  headache and, 52
  insomnia in, 164–165
  major depression, 730, 730t, 732f, 819, 847
  medical illness–related, 729
  minor depression, 730–731
  in MS, 478, 490
  neural circuitry of, 715f
  pain and, 48
  pathophysiology of, 731
  in PD, 344
  treatment of
    algorithm for, 732f
    antidepressants, 723t, 724t, 731–733
    in cerebral function disorders, 156
    consensus guidelines on, 736t
    supportive, 731
  unipolar, 731
  in war veterans, 748
Dermatomes, 120f, 121f
Dermatomyositis, **648,** 817, 845
  calcinosis in, 659
  clinical features of, 109, 648, 649, 649t
  diagnosis of, 655–657, 656t, 657f
  differential diagnosis of, 653–655
  drug-induced, 655
  immunopathogenesis of, 650–652, 651f
  malignancies associated with, 650
  prognosis of, 659
  treatment of, 657–659
Dermatomyositis sine myositis, 649
Dermoid cysts, 432
Desipramine
  adverse effects of, 723t
  for depression, 723t
  dosage of, 723t
  for pain, 46t, 49, 50, 490
Desmopressin (DDAVP)
  for orthostatic hypotension, 95
  for sleep enuresis, 170
Desvenlafaxine, for depression, 723t
Detrusor hyperreflexia, 490
Devic's syndrome, 490
Dexamethasone
  for bacterial meningitis, 502–503
  for brain abscess, 521
  for cerebral edema, 424
  for increased intracranial pressure, 298t
Dextroamphetamine, for narcolepsy, 169
Diabetes mellitus (DM)
  autonomic dysfunction in, 386
  depression in, 730
Diabetes mellitus (DM) (*Cont.*):
  myopathy in, 644
  neuropathy in. *See* Diabetic neuropathy
  ocular involvement in
    abducens nerve palsy, 194
    cataracts, 187–188
    epiretinal membrane, 190
    mydriasis, 176
    myopia, 175
    oculomotor nerve palsy, 193
    optic neuropathy, 184
    retinal hemorrhage, 182
    retinal vein occlusion, 184
    tonic pupil, 176
    vitreous degeneration, 187
  stroke risk in, 265t
  taste disorders in, 204
  type 2, in schizophrenia, 740
Diabetic amyotrophy, 579, 644
Diabetic autonomic neuropathy, 578–579
Diabetic neuropathy, 842–843
  autonomic, 578–579
  distal symmetric sensory and sensorimotor polyneuropathy, 578, 843
  mononeuropathy, 579
  pathophysiology of, 44
  polyneuropathy, 578
  radiculoplexus neuropathy, 579
  treatment of, 49, 578t
Diabetic radiculoplexus neuropathy, 579
Diazepam
  for alcohol withdrawal, 758
  in cocaine abuse management, 768
  dosage of, 725t
  for generalized anxiety disorder, 725t
  pharmacology of, 725t
  for spasticity in MS, 489
  for stiff-person syndrome, 563
  for vertigo, 102t
Dichloralphenazone, for migraine, 58t, 60
Dichromat, 177
Diffuse axonal injury, 416
Diffuse Lewy body disease, 326
Diffuse white matter disease, 322, 322f
Diffusion-perfusion mismatch, 286f
Diffusion tensor imaging (DTI), 23
Diffusion tractography, in cerebral glioma, 21f
DiGeorge region deletions, 713
Digitalis, 185
Digit span tests, 128, 154
Dihydroergotamine
  for exertional headache, 69
  for medication-overuse headache, 66
  for migraine, 58t, 59–60, 59t
  nasal spray, 58t, 59
Diltiazem, for sex headache prevention, 70
Dimenhydrinate. for vertigo, 102t
Dimethyl fumarate, for MS, 490
Diphtheria, neuropathy in, 581
Diplopia, **192,** 478
Dipyridamole, for stroke/TIA prevention, 270–271
DISC1, 713
Discectomy with fusion, cervical, 88
Discography, 24, 83
Disequilibrium, **114**. *See also* Balance
Distal myopathies, **633,** 634t
Disulfiram
  adverse effects of, 185, 587t, 849
  in alcoholism management, 760
Diuretics
  adverse effects of
    hearing loss, 209
  for Ménière's disease, 210
  for vertigo, 102t
Dix-Hallpike maneuver, 99–100, 802, 823
Dizziness, **98**
  approach to the patient, 98–100, 802, 823
  history in, 98–99
  physical examination in, 99–100
  psychosomatic, 101–102
  in vascular disorders, 98
  vestibular causes, 99
DJ-1, 228

DM. *See* Diabetes mellitus (DM)
Docetaxel, 584t
"Doll's eyes," 137
Domestic abuse/violence, 741
Domoic acid intoxication, 239
Domperidone, for nausea, 66
Donepezil
- for AD, 206, 321
- for Parkinson's disease dementia, 345

Dopamine
- anatomic and clinical aspects of, 222t
- in migraine, 54
- in schizophrenia, 713
- structure of, 222t

Dopamine agonists
- for acromegaly, 464
- adverse effects of, 341, 457
- for PD, 341, 343t, 346f
- for prolactinoma, 456–457

Dopamine antagonists, for migraine, 54, 58t, 60
Dopa-responsive dystonia, 348
Doppler echocardiography, 795–796t
Dorsal midbrain syndrome (Parinaud's syndrome), 195
Dorsal root ganglia, 40, 41f3f, 42–43
Dorsal root ganglionopathy, 563–564
Dothiepin, for migraine prevention, 61t
Doublecortin gene, 235t
Downbeat nystagmus, 196
Down syndrome (trisomy 21), AD and, 319
Doxepin
- adverse effects of, 723t
- for depression, 723t
- dosage of, 723t
- for insomnia, 164
- for pain, 46t

Driving ability/privileges
- epilepsy and, 254
- sleep disorders and, 167

Drop attacks, 115
Drowsiness, 132
Drp1, 228
Drug(s)
- autonomic function effects of, 383, 384t
- therapeutic monitoring, reference values, 786–788t
- time-of-day effects on, 173

Drusen, 186
- in macular degeneration, 189, 189f
- optic disc, 186, 186f

Dry beriberi, 591
Dry eye (keratoconjunctivitis sicca), 180
DSPN (diabetic distal symmetric sensory and sensorimotor polyneuropathy), 578
DTI (diffusion tensor imaging), 23
DTIC (dacarbazine), adverse effects of, 438t
Dual task walking, 111
Duchenne's muscular dystrophy, **624**
- clinical features of, 624, 625t, 844
- genetic factors in, 625t
- incidence of, 624
- laboratory evaluation of, 624–626
- pathogenesis of, 626, 628f
- treatment of, 28

Duloxetine
- adverse effects of, 578t
- for neuropathy, 578t
- for pain, 46t, 49, 50

Dura, vascular malformations of, 49–410, 293, 410f
Dural arteriovenous fistulas, 293
Dural sinus thrombosis, 273
Dura matter grafts, Creutzfeldt-Jakob disease after, 553
Dynamic visual acuity, 100
Dysarthria, 143
Dysembryoplastic neuroepithelial tumors, 432
Dysesthesia, 117
Dysgerminoma, brain, 448
Dysgraphia, 147
Dyskinesia(s)
- diphasic, levodopa-related, 340
- paroxysmal, 352
- tardive, 112, 354, 740

Dyslexia, 149
Dysphagia, 397–398, 398t
Dysphonia, 397–398, 398t
Dysplasia(s)
- fibromuscular, 267
- pituitary, 442

Dyspnea
- in orthostatic hypotension, 94
- paroxysmal nocturnal, 165

Dysproteinemia, 183
Dysreflexia, autonomic, 386
Dysthymic disorder, 730
Dystonia, 111, 347t, **348**
- cervical, 349
- clinical features of, 348
- dopa responsive, 348
- drug-induced, 354
- focal, 348–349
- idiopathic torsion, 348
- limb, 349
- Oppenheim's, 348
- oromandibular, 349
- pathophysiology of, 349
- primary, 348
- secondary, 349
- Segawa variant, 348
- spasmodic, 348
- treatment of, 349–350

Dystonia plus syndromes, 349
Dystonic storm, 350
Dystrophin, 626, 628f, 629f
DYT1 gene, 348

Ear, 207, 207f
Ear canal, atresia of, 215
Eating disorders, sleep-related, 170
EBV infections. *See* Epstein-Barr virus (EBV) infections
Echocardiography, 795–796t
Echolalia, 144t, 146
Echo-planar magnetic resonance imaging, 23
Echovirus infections, chronic meningitis in, 531t
Ecstasy (MDMA), 128, 129t, 770
Ectropion, 180
ED. *See* Erectile dysfunction (ED)
Edema
- brain, 294
- cytotoxic, 294
- vasogenic, 294

Edinger-Westphal nuclei, 174
EDSS (Expanded Disability Status Score), 484t
EEG. *See* Electroencephalography (EEG)
Ehrlichia chaffeensis, 500
Elderly. *See also* Aging
- benign forgetfulness of, 311
- cerumen impaction in, 213
- delirium in, 126
- falls in, 110, 114. *See also* Fall(s)
- hearing loss in, 209–210
- olfactory dysfunction in, 202, 202f, 206
- seizures in, 238t

Electrocochleography, 214
Electroconvulsive therapy, for depression, 733
Electrodiagnostic studies, **26**
- electroencephalography. *See* Electroencephalography (EEG)
- electrophysiologic studies. *See* Electrophysiologic studies
- evoked potentials. *See* Evoked potentials
- magnetoencephalography, 29, 243
- in myasthenia gravis, 611
- in myopathies, 623
- in myopathy, 623
- nerve conduction studies. *See* Nerve conduction studies
- in peripheral neuropathy, 568–570, 570t

Electroencephalography (EEG), **26,** 27f, 801, 822
- in brain death, 140
- in coma, 28, 138
- continuous monitoring, 29
- in delirium, 126
- in epilepsy, 8f, 26–28
- in neurologic critical illness, 297
- in seizures, 233, 234, 241–243

Electrolyte disturbances
- delirium in, 129, 129t
- neurologic complications of, 663–665
- weakness in, 108t

Electromyography (EMG)
- in back pain, 75
- in peripheral neuropathy, 570, 570t
- principles of, 31–32, 31f
- single-fiber, 34

Electrophysiologic studies, **31**
- blink reflexes, 34
- F-wave studies, 33
- H-reflex studies, 33
- muscle response to repetitive nerve stimulation, 33–34
- in seizures, 241–243

Eletriptan, for migraine, 58t, 59, 59t
Embolic stroke
- artery-to-artery, 263–265
- prevention of, 271–272

Embryonal carcinoma, parasellar, 448
Emery-Dreifuss muscular dystrophy, **629**
- clinical features of, 625t, 629
- genetic factors in, 625t, 629
- laboratory evaluation of, 629, 629f
- treatment of, 629

Emetine, 185
EMG. *See* Electromyography (EMG)
Emmetropia, 175
Empty sella, 444, 840
Encephalitis
- amnesia in, 153
- approach to the patient, 493–494, 494–495f
- brainstem, 558t, 561
- chronic, **516**
  - progressive multifocal leukoencephalopathy. *See* Progressive multifocal leukoencephalopathy (PML)
  - progressive rubella panencephalitis, 518
  - subacute sclerosing panencephalitis, 517–518
- cortical, 561
- delirium in, 129, 129t
- focal, 561–562
- limbic, 329, 668–669f
- paraneoplastic, 329, 558t, 561–562
- viral, **508**
  - approach to the patient, 493–494, 494–495f
  - clinical features of, 508
  - definition of, 508
  - diagnosis of, 510f, 511t
    - brain biopsy in, 510
    - CSF analysis in, 508–509
    - CT in, 510
    - MRI in, 510, 510f, 511t
    - serologic studies and antigen detection in, 509–510
  - differential diagnosis of, 510–512
  - enteroviral, 505
  - etiology of, 503t, 508
  - HSV
    - differential diagnosis of, 500, 511, 511t
    - memory loss in, 153
    - MRI in, 19f
  - sequelae of, 514
  - treatment of, 512–514
  - West Nile virus, 511–512, 511t

Encephalomyelitis
- acute disseminated. *See* Acute disseminated encephalomyelitis (ADEM)
- definition of, 561
- experimental allergic, 224, 224f
- paraneoplastic, 559t, 561–562
- postinfectious, 491

Encephalopathy, 125. *See also* Delirium
- chemotherapy-induced, 438t
- Hashimoto's, 555, 696f
- HIV, 541–543, 542f, 542t
- hypertensive, 129t, 289
- hypoxic-ischemic, 256, 299–300, 300f
- metabolic, 146, 155, 300–301
- sepsis-associated, 301

Endarterectomy, carotid, 273
Endocrine myopathies, **643**

Endolymphatic hydrops. *See* Ménière's disease
Endometrial cancer, back pain in, 81
Endometriosis, back pain in, 81
Endophthalmitis, 182
Endovascular procedures
  for carotid atherosclerosis, 273
  for ischemic stroke, 259–260
Enophthalmos, 190
Entacapone, for PD, 342, 343t
Enteroviruses, in meningitis, 505
Entrapment neuropathy, 665
Entropion, 180
Enuresis, sleep, 170
Environmental factors, in neuropathy, 588t, 589–591
Enzyme(s), in myopathy, 622–623
Ependymoma, 429
Epidermoid cyst, 432
Epidural abscess
  cranial, 524–525, 524f
  spinal, 78, 405–406, 406f
  weakness in, 107
Epidural hematoma
  clinical features of, 418–419, 837
  neuroimaging in, 418f, 699f
  spinal, 406
  treatment of, 419
  weakness in, 107
Epidural metastases, 436, 436f
Epidural spinal hemorrhage, 290
Epidural tumor, 107
Epigenetics, 219
Epilepsia partialis continua, 232, 561
Epilepsy, **231**. *See also* Seizure(s)
  adverse effects of, 253
  autonomic, 96
  catamenial, 254
  coma in, 135
  definition of, 231
  EEG in, 8f, 26–28
  employment and, 254
  etiology of, 236–237
    age-related, 237–238, 238t
    drug-related, 239, 239t
    genetic, 235t, 240
  incidence of, 231
  insomnia in, 165
  ion channel defects causing, 220t
  loss of driving privileges in, 254
  mortality of, 253–254
  pregnancy and, 254–255
  prevalence of, 231
  psychiatric disorders associated with, 253
  psychosocial issues in, 254
  refractory, 251–252
  taste disorders in, 204
  treatment of, **245,** 807, 831
    antiepileptic drugs, 245–251, 247–249t
    avoidance of precipitating factors in, 245
    surgical, 251–252
    underlying conditions–related, 245
  in women, 254–255
Epilepsy syndromes, 231, **234**
  genetic, 235t
  juvenile myoclonic epilepsy, 234, 236
  Lennox-Gastaut syndrome, 236
  mesial temporal lobe epilepsy, 236, 236f, 236t, 807, 830
Epileptic spasms, 234
Epileptiform activity, 26, 243
Epileptogenesis, 240
Epiretinal membrane, 190
Episcleritis, 181
Episodic ataxia, 220t, 362–363t, 367
Epley maneuver, 100, 823
EPM2A gene, 235t
Epstein-Barr virus (EBV) infections
  meningitis, 506
  neuropathy in, 583
Erectile dysfunction (ED)
  autonomic dysfunction and, 381
  cocaine and, 768
Ergotamine
  for cluster headache prevention, 64–123
  for exertional headache, 69
  for migraine, 58t, 59, 59t
  for sex headache prevention, 70
Ergotism, 64
Erythrocyte sedimentation rate, in temporal arteritis, 53
Erythromycin, for blepharitis, 180
Erythropoietin therapy, for orthostatic hypotension, 95, 390
Escitalopram, for depression, 321, 331, 723t
Esophageal cancer, alcohol effects on, 755
Esophagus, alcohol effects on, 755
Essential tremor, 347
Estrogen therapy
  for AD prevention, 321
  for migraine prevention, 59t
Eszopiclone, 164, 204
Ethacrynic acid, 209
Ethambutol
  adverse effects of, 185, 587t
  for tuberculous meningitis, 515
Ethanol. *See* Alcohol
Ethchlorvynol, 185
Ethosuximide, 247t, 250
Ethylene glycol poisoning
  delirium in, 129t
  optic neuropathy in, 185
Ethylene oxide, 588t
Etomidate, for Cushing's syndrome, 469
Etoposide, 585t
Euphoria, 716
Eustachian tube dysfunction, 209
Eustachian tube obstruction, 214
Evoked potentials, 29–31
  cognitive, 30
  motor, 30
  in MS, 480t, 482
  somatosensory, 30
Excitotoxicity, 226
Executive functions, 154
Exercise
  for back pain, 82, 83
  in PD, 345
  for prevention of falls, 115
  for spinal stenosis, 78
Exertional headache, primary, 51t, **69**
Exophthalmos, 190
Expanded Disability Status Score (EDSS), 484t
Experimental allergic neuritis, 600
Extensor plantar response, 8
Extinction (sensory phenomenon), 122, 150
Extracranial-to-intracranial bypass surgery, 273
Extramedullary syndromes, 403
Eye(s). *See also* Ocular disorders
  alignment of, 177
  dry (keratoconjunctivitis sicca), 180
  melanoma of, 190, 190f
  movements of, 174
    in coma, 137–138, 137f
    in dizziness evaluation, 99
    video library, 198
  painful or red, 179–182, 806, 829
  physiology of, 174
  tumors of, 190
Eye fields, frontal, 149, 149f
Eyelids, disorders of, 180, 191–192
Ezetimibe, 645t, 646

Fabry disease, 575, 575t
Face recognition, 152
Facet fracture, 698f
Facet joint, 71, 79
Facial hemiatrophy, 397
Facial myokymia, 397, 479
Facial nerve
  anatomy of, 201f, 395f
  examination of, 6
  injury to, 210
  in taste sensation, 201
Facial numbness, **392**
Facial pain, **392**
Facial weakness, **394**
  anatomic considerations in, 394–395, 395f
  facial hemiatrophy, 397
  facial myokymia, 397
  hemifacial spasm, 397
  in MS, 478
Facioscapulohumeral muscular dystrophy, 620f, 625t, **632**
Factitious illness
  characteristics of, 736
  visual loss, 187
Factor V, screening assays, 776t
Factor VII, screening assays, 776t
Factor VIII, screening assays, 776t
Fall(s), **114**
  collapsing, 115
  drop attacks, 115
  in elderly, 110, 114
  epidemiology of, 110, 114
  gait freezing and, 115
  mechanical, 115
  prevention of, 115
  recurrent, 114
  reducing injury risk in, 115
  risk factors for, 114, 114t
  sensory deficits and, 115
  slipping and tripping, 115
  toppling, 115
  weakness and frailty and, 115
Famciclovir, for viral meningitis, 507
Familial amyloid polyneuropathy, 575t, 577
Familial amyotrophic lateral sclerosis, 372, 374t
Familial spastic paraplegia, 374–376t, 378–379, 412
Fasciculations, 104, 104t
Fatal familial insomnia, 165
Fatigue
  definition of, 620
  increased fatigability, 103
  in MS, 477, 490
  myasthenic, 610
  vs. sleepiness, 166–167
Fazio-Londe syndrome, 378
Felbamate, 249t
Femoral neuropathy, 594
Fenoprofen, for pain, 46t
Fentanyl
  for pain, 46t, 47
  transdermal, 47, 50
Fetal alcohol spectrum disorder, 756
Fetal alcohol syndrome, 756
Fetal nigral dopamine cells, for PD, 344
Fetal posterior cerebral artery, 277
Fever
  central, 135
  in coma, 135
  quadriplegic, 413
Fibric acid derivatives, adverse effects of, 645t, 844
Fibrillation potential, 104
Fibromuscular dysplasia, 267
Fibromyalgia, 621
Fila, 199
Finger anomia, 147
Fingolimod
  action of, 487
  for MS, 486t, 487
Fisher's syndrome, 194–195
Fistula(s), dural arteriovenous, 293
Flaccidity, 103
Flavor enhancers, 205
Floaters, 186
Fludarabine, 438, 438t
Fludrocortisone
  for orthostatic hypotension, 95, 345, 390
  for syncope, 92
Fluid-attenuated inversion recovery (FLAIR), 18, 821
  in brain tumors, 424, 427f
  in Creutzfeldt-Jakob disease, 556f
  in diffuse white matter disease, 322f
  in Huntington's disease, 351f
  in hyperperfusion syndrome, 817, 817f, 845
  in limbic encephalitis, 560f, 668–669f
  in MS, 481f

Fluid-attenuated inversion recovery (FLAIR) (*Cont.*):
  in seizures, 243
  in viral encephalitis, 500, 510, 510f, 511t
Flumazenil, in opiate overdose management, 764
Flunarizine
  adverse effects of, 61t
  for chronic daily headache, 66
  for hypnic headache, 70
  for migraine prevention, 60, 61t
Flunitrazepam, abuse of, 772
Fluoride, for otosclerosis, 209
5-Fluorouracil (5-FU), 438t
Fluoxetine
  adverse effects of, 723t
  for depression, 723t, 732
  dosage of, 723t
  for narcolepsy, 169
  for obsessive-compulsive disorder, 728
  for pain, 49
  for panic disorder, 722, 847
  pharmacology of, 732
Fluphenazine, 739t
Flurazepam
  for generalized anxiety disorder, 725t
  pharmacology of, 725t
Fluvoxamine
  for depression, 723t
  for obsessive-compulsive disorder, 728
Focal seizures. *See* Seizure(s), focal
Folate
  deficiency of, 185
  reference values, 788t
Folinic acid, for megaloblastic anemia prophylaxis, 522
Follicle-stimulating hormone (FSH), **469**
  action of, 470
  deficiency of, 446t
  reference values, 781t
  secretion of, 469–470
  synthesis of, 469–470
Foramen magnum syndrome, 403
Forearm exercise test, 623–624
Foreign body, in eye, 179
Fortification spectra, 4, 187
Foscarnet, for viral encephalitis, 513
Foster Kennedy syndrome, 205
Fovea, 174
Foveation, 174
Foville's syndrome, 194
Fragile X pre-mutation, 112
Fragile X tremor/ataxia syndrome, 363t
Frataxin gene, 368
Freezing episodes, in PD, 345
Frenzel eyeglasses, 100
Friedreich's ataxia, 367
  clinical features of, 361t, 367
  genetic factors in, 228, 361t, 368
  imaging of, 367f
  locus and phenotype of, 361t
  treatment of, 368–369
Frontal abulic syndrome, 154, 155
Frontal bone fractures, 417
Frontal disinhibition syndrome, 154, 155
Frontal eye field, 195
Frontal gait disorder, 112, 113t
Frontal network syndrome, 155
Frontotemporal degenerations, 149
Frontotemporal dementia (FTD), **323**
  behavioral variant, 155
  clinical features of, 155, 312, 314t, 323
  functional anatomy of, 310, 323
  genetic factors in, 219, 228, 323
  imaging in, 323–324, 324f
  molecular basis of, 312t
  olfactory dysfunction in, 202–203
Frontotemporal lobar degeneration (FTLD), 229, 324
Frovatriptan, for migraine, 58t, 59, 59t
FSH. *See* Follicle-stimulating hormone (FSH)
FTD. *See* Frontotemporal dementia (FTD)
Fukitin-related protein deficiency, 630, 631t
Fukuyama congenital muscular dystrophy, 630, 631t
Functional Status (FS) Score, 484t
Fundus examination, 182
Fungal infections, chronic meningitis in, 530t
Furosemide, 209
FUS gene, 228, 312t, 323
FUS/TLS gene, 373, 374t
F-wave studies, 33

GABA. *See* γ-aminobutyric acid (GABA)
Gabapentin
  adverse effects of, 61t, 248t, 578t
  for chronic daily headache, 66
  for cluster headache prevention, 64t
  for epilepsy, 248t
  for migraine prevention, 60, 61t
  for neuropathy, 578t
  for pain, 46t, 50, 489–490
  pharmacology of, 248t
  for posttraumatic headache, 68
  for restless legs syndrome, 166
  for SUNCT/SUNA prevention, 65
GAD1 gene, 712
Gadolinium contrast, 18–21, 801, 821–822. *See also* Contrast agents
Gag reflex, 7
Gait
  anatomy and physiology of, 110–111
  disorders, **111,** 111t
    approach to the patient, 113, 802, 824
    cautious gait, 111
    cerebellar gait ataxia, 112, 113t
    freezing gait, 112, 115. *See also* Parkinson's disease (PD)
    frontal, 112, 113t, 802, 824
    in neuromuscular disease, 113
    psychogenic, 113
    sensory ataxia, 112, 113t
    slowly progressive, 113
    spastic, 111
    spastic-ataxic, 111
    stiff-legged, 111
    in toxic and metabolic disorders, 113
    video library, 116
  examination of, 9
Gait apraxia, 112
Gait cycle, 110
Galactorrhea, 455
Galactosemia, ocular involvement in, 188
Galantamine, for AD, 321
Gallium nitrate, 438t
γ-aminobutyric acid (GABA)
  alcohol effects on, 753
  anatomic and clinical aspects of, 222t
  structure of, 222t
γ-hydroxybutyric acid (GHB)
  abuse of, 128, 129t, 772
  for narcolepsy, 169
Gamma knife surgery, for trigeminal neuralgia, 393
γ motor neurons, 106f
Ganciclovir, for viral encephalitis, 513
Gangliocytomas, 448
Gangliogliomas, 429
Ganglion cells, of retina, 174
Ganglionopathy, dorsal root, **564**
Gap junctions, 221
Gardner's syndrome, brain tumors and, 425t
Gas exchange, reference values, 797t
Gastric juice, 798t
Gaze disorders
  horizontal, 195, 196f
  in MS, 478
  supranuclear, 195
  vertical gaze, 195
Gaze stabilization reflex, 174
GBA gene, 338
GBS. *See* Guillain-Barré syndrome (GBS)
Gegenhalten, 103
Generalized anxiety disorder, **722**
  clinical features of, 722
  diagnosis of, 725t
  etiology of, 724
  pathophysiology of, 724
  treatment of, 724–726
Generalized convulsive status epilepticus, **252**
Generalized epilepsy with febrile seizures, 235t
Generalized tonic-clonic status epilepticus, 252, 253f
Gene therapy, for PD, 344
Genome-wide association studies, 218
Gentamicin
  intratympanic, for Ménière's disease, 210
  for meningitis, 499t, 502
German measles (rubella), congenital, 518
Germinoma, parasellar, 448
Gerstmann's syndrome, 147
Gerstmann-Straüssler-Scheinker (GSS) disease, 550, 550t, 554, 842
GHB. *See* γ-hydroxybutyric acid (GHB)
Giant cell arteritis (temporal arteritis)
  clinical features of, 53
  erythrocyte sedimentation rate in, 53
  headache in, 53
  ocular involvement in, 183, 184, 184f, 194
  stroke due to, 267
Gingivitis, taste disorders in, 204
Gingko biloba, 321
Glasgow Coma Scale, 421, 421t
Glatiramer acetate
  adverse effects of, 486
  for MS, 486, 486t
Glaucoma, **188,** 188f
  acute angle-closure, 182, 188
  headache in, 53
  low-tension, 188
  treatment of, 188
  visual field assessment in, 178–179
Glioblastoma(s), 425–426, 426f, 427–428, 427f, 428f
Glioma
  cerebral, 21f
  hypothalamic, 448
  ocular signs in, 179
  optic, 448
Gliomatosis cerebri, 129t, 428
Gliosarcoma(s), 429
Glossodynia (burning mouth syndrome), 206
Glossopharyngeal nerve
  anatomy of, 201f
  examination of, 7
  in taste sensation, 201
Glossopharyngeal neuralgia, 397, 398t, 479
Glucocorticoid(s)
  for ACTH deficiency, 466
  adverse effects of
    cataracts, 188
    myopathy, 645t, 646, 658
  for allergic conjunctivitis, 180
  for anterior ischemic optic neuropathy, 184
  for brain abscess, 521
  for CIDP, 606
  for cluster headache prevention, 64–123
  for Cushing's syndrome, 469
  epidural
    for back pain, 82, 83, 84
    for neck pain, 88
  for episcleritis and scleritis, 181
  for inflammatory myopathies, 658
  intranasal, for sinusitis, 206
  for MS, 485
  for muscular dystrophy, 628
  for myasthenia gravis, 615
  for neck pain, 88
  for neuromyelitis optica, 491
  for optic neuritis, 185
  for orbital pseudotumor, 191
  systemic
    for Ménière's disease, 210
    for sinusitis, 202
  topical
    for herpes simplex keratitis, 181
    for uveitis, 181
Glucose-6-phosphate dehydrogenase (G6PD) deficiency, 776t
Glue sniffer's neuropathy, 589–590
Glutamate
  anatomic and clinical aspects of, 222t
  as neurotransmitter, 42
  structure of, 222t
Gluten-free diet, for ataxic disorders, 369
Glycine, 222t

Glycine receptor, 559t
Glycogen storage diseases, **636**
with exercise intolerance, 637
with skeletal myopathy/progressive weakness, 636–637
type II (acid maltase deficiency), 636–637
type III (debranching enzyme deficiency), 637
type IV (branching enzyme deficiency), 637
type V (myophosphorylase deficiency), 637
type VII (phosphofructokinase deficiency), 637
Glycolysis, abnormalities of, 637
Glycopyrrolate, for primary hyperhidrosis, 388
Gnathostoma spinigerum/gnathostomiasis, chronic meningitis in, 530t
Gold therapy, adverse effects of, 588t
Gonadotrope, 439t, 446t
Gonadotropin(s), **469**
action of, 470
deficiency of, 470–471
synthesis of, 469–470
Gonadotropin-releasing hormone (GnRH), 441f
Go-no-go test, 155
Gorlin's syndrome (nevoid basal cell carcinoma syndrome), 425t
Gottron's sign, 649
Gowers' sign, 618, 621f
G protein–coupled receptors (GPCRs), in taste sensation, 201
Graded exercise therapy, for chronic fatigue syndrome, 706–707, 846
Gradenigo's syndrome, 194, 526
Granisetron, for nausea and vomiting, 66
Granulomatosis with polyangiitis (Wegener's)
chronic meningitis in, 533t
ocular disease in, 181
Graphesthesia, 122
Graves' ophthalmopathy, 191, 644
Gray (radiation unit), 799t
Greater petrosal nerve, 202
GRN gene, 323
Growth
disorders of, 459–460
somatic, skeletal maturation and, 459
Growth hormone (GH), **458**
Creutzfeldt-Jakob disease after treatment with, 553
insensitivity, 460
laboratory evaluation of, 445t
recombinant
for adult growth hormone deficiency, 461–462, 462f
adverse effects of, 462
for growth hormone deficiency in children, 460
secretion of, 458
synthesis of, 458
Growth hormone (GH) deficiency
in adults. *See* Adult growth hormone deficiency
in children, 446t, 459–460
idiopathic, 460
Growth hormone (GH) receptor antagonists, for acromegaly, 465
Growth hormone-releasing hormone (GHRH) receptor mutations, 460
Guanfacine, for Tourette's syndrome, 353
Guillain-Barré syndrome (GBS), **599**
antecedent events, 600, 816, 843
autonomic dysfunction in, 387
vs. CIDP, 605
clinical features of, 599–600, 600t
cranial nerve palsies in, 399
diagnosis of, 603, 604t
facial nerve disorders in, 397
immunopathogenesis of, 62t, 600–603, 601f
laboratory evaluation of, 603
paraneoplastic, 565
pathophysiology of, 603
prevalence of, 599
prognosis of, 604–605
recovery from, 605
subtypes of, 599–600, 600t
treatment of, 603–604
weakness in, 108, 109
Gynecomastia, cocaine and, 768
Haemophilus influenzae infections, 495, 496. *See also* Meningitis
Hallucinations
alcohol and, 755
chemosensory, 205
hypnagogic, 163t, 168, 168t
hypnopompic, 168
in PD, 344–345
Hallucinosis, peduncular, 278
Haloperidol
for acute alcohol intoxication, 758
adverse effects of, 739t
for delirium, 301
Hamartin, 433
Hamartoma, hypothalamic, 448
Hand, mechanic's, 649
Hand-Schüller-Christian disease, 448
Hashimoto's encephalopathy, 555, 696f
Hashish, 769
Haw River syndrome, 367
Headache, **51**
acute, new-onset, 52, 52t, 305
anatomy and physiology of, 51–52
with autonomic symptoms, 52
in brain abscess, 519
in brain tumor, 51t, 53
chronic daily, **65**
classification of, 65, 66t
diagnosis of, 65–66
from medication overuse, 60, 66
cluster. *See* Cluster headache
depression and, 52
in glaucoma, 53
in head injury, 51t, 68
hemicrania continua, 66t, 68–69
hypnic, **70**
in intracranial hemorrhage, 52–53
medication-overuse, 60, **66**
in meningitis, 52
migraine. *See* Migraine
new daily persistent, **66**
clinical features of, 66–67
diagnosis of, 67t
low CSF volume headache, 67–68, 67f
posttraumatic, 51t, 68
raised CSF pressure headache, 68
in papilledema, 185
paroxysmal hemicrania, 64–65, 66t
post–lumbar puncture, 37–38, 37t
primary, 51, 51t, **53**
primary cough, **69**
primary exertional, 51t, **69**
primary sex, **70**
primary stabbing, 51t, **69**
primary thunderclap, **70**
secondary, 51, 51t, **52**
in subarachnoid hemorrhage, 51t, 52, 305
SUNCT/SUNA, 65, 66t
symptoms of serious underlying disorder, 52t
tension-type. *See* Tension-type headache
Head drop, 648
Head impulse test, 99
Head injury, **415**. *See also specific types*
amnesia in, 153
aphasia in, 145
autonomic storm following, 389
brain hemorrhage in, 416, 416f, 812, 837
clinical syndromes of, **419**
concussion in. *See* Concussion
contusion in, 416, 416f
convulsions after, 417
cranial nerve injuries, 417
diffuse axonal injury in, 416, 416f
emergency care of, 415
grading of, 421, 421t
headache in, 51t, 68
of intermediate severity, 420–421
intracerebral hemorrhage due to, 289
minor injury, 419–420
olfactory dysfunction in, 202
postconcussion syndrome, 421–422, 837
prevalence of, 415
prognosis of, 421
Head injury (*Cont.*):
recurrent, dementia due to, 329
seizures and, 237, 417–418
severe injury, 421
skull fractures in, 417
types of, **415**
in war veterans, 744–745, 745t, 749
Head tilt test, 194
Head-up tilt test, 385, 385t
Health care workers, shift-work disorder in, 171
Hearing, 207
Hearing aid, 210, 215
Hearing loss, **208,** 806, 829–830
approach to the patient, 207f, 212–213
audiologic assessment of, 213–214
conductive, 208–209
drug-induced, 209
evoked responses in, 214–215
genetic causes of, 211–212, 211t, 212t
imaging studies in, 215
ion channel defects causing, 220t
mixed, 210
noise-induced, 213, 216
prevention of, 216
sensorineural, 209–210
treatment of, 215–216
Heart, normal pressures in, 793t
Heart failure (HF), cerebral symptoms of, 129, 129t
Heart rate
response to deep breathing, 384, 385t
during sleep, 161
Heat sensitivity, in MS, 478–479
Hematocrit, normal, 777t
Hematologic disease, reference values, 775–778t
Hematoma
epidural. *See* Epidural hematoma
spinal, 406
subdural. *See* Subdural hematoma
Hematomyelia, 406
Hematopoietic stem cell transplantation, complications of, 583
Hemianopia, 178f
bitemporal, 179
homonymous, 178f, 179
Hemiatrophy, facial, 397
Hemiballismus, 165, 352
Hemicrania continua, 66t, **68**
Hemifacial spasm, 394, 397, 479
Hemilaminectomy, in lumbar disk disease, 85
Hemineglect, 804, 826
Hemiparesis, **106**
acute or episodic, 106
cerebral artery occlusion and, 16f
chronic, 107
subacute, 106–107
Hemispherectomy, for refractory epilepsy, 151
Hemoglobin, normal, 777t
Hemorrhage
brain, traumatic, 416, 416f
epidural spinal, 290
intracranial. *See* Intracranial hemorrhage
subconjunctival, 179
Heparin, monitoring treatment with, 776t
Hepatic encephalopathy
coma in, 134–135
delirium in, 129t
Hepatitis, neuropathy in, 583
Hereditary endotheliopathy, retinopathy, nephropathy, and stroke (HERNs), 268
Hereditary myopathies, **624,** 625t. *See also* Muscular dystrophy
Hereditary neuropathy(ies)
approach to, 568, 568t
Charcot-Marie-Tooth disease. *See* Charcot-Marie-Tooth (CMT) disease
Fabry disease, 575, 575t
familial amyloid polyneuropathy, 575t, 577
hereditary neuralgic amyotrophy, 573t, 574–575, 842
hereditary neuropathy with liability to pressure palsies, 572t, 574
porphyria, 575t, 576–577
Tangier disease, 575t, 576

Hereditary sensory and autonomic neuropathy (HSAN)
  autonomic dysfunction in, 388
  clinical features of, 575, 842
  genetic factors in, 388, 573t
  orthostatic hypotension in, 95
Herniation, cerebral, 133–134, 133f, 804, 826
HERNS (hereditary endotheliopathy, retinopathy, nephropathy, and stroke), 268
Heroin
  adverse effects of, 177, 645t, 646
  systems effects of, 763
Herpes simplex virus (HSV) infections
  encephalitis
    memory loss in, 153
    vs. meningitis, 500
    MRI in, 19f
  keratitis, 181
  meningitis, 506, 531t
  uveitis, 181
Herpes zoster (shingles)
  clinical features of
    glossopharyngeal neuropathy, 397
    neck pain, 86
    neuropathy, 582–583
    ocular, 181
    postherpetic neuralgia, 583
  pathogenesis of, 44
Herpes zoster ophthalmicus, 181
Hertel exophthalmometer, 191
HESX1 gene, 442
Heterotropia, 177
Hexacarbons, neuropathies due to, 588t, 589–590
High-altitude illness, sleep impairment in, 164
Hip pain, 74
Hippocampus, in mood disorders, 715
Histamine, pain and, 42f
Histiocytosis, neuroimaging in, 683f
Histiocytosis X, 443, 448
Histoplasma spp. infections
  chronic meningitis in, 530t
  ocular involvement in, 182
  of pons, MRI in, 673f
  subacute meningitis in, 514–515
HIV
  replication cycle of, 538–540
  structure of, 538, 538f
HIV-1, 536–538
HIV-2, 538
HIV infection
  classification of, 536, 537t
  depression in, 729
  hearing loss in, 210
  lymphoma in, 544–545
  neurologic manifestations of, 536t, **541**
    Chagas' disease, 547–548
    chronic meningitis, 531t, 534–535
    CNS lymphoma, 545, 545f
    cognitive impairment, 541
    cryptococcosis, 545–546
    HIV-associated dementia, 541–543, 542f, 542t
    meningitis, 506, 543
    myelopathy, 543
    myopathy, 544
    neuropathy, 582
    pathogenesis of, 540–541
    peripheral neuropathy, 543–544
    progressive multifocal leukoencephalopathy, 517, 547
    seizures, 548
    stroke, 548
    toxoplasmosis, 546–547, 547f
  olfactory dysfunction in, 202
  opportunistic/disseminated infections in, 545, 546f
  orthostatic hypotension in, 95
  pathophysiology of, 540
  weakness in, 107
HNPP (hereditary neuropathy with liability to pressure palsies), 572t, 574
Hodgkin's disease, paraneoplastic syndromes in, 563
Hollenhorst plaque, 183, 183f
Homeless, mental health problems in, 741
Homer-Wright rosettes, 430
Hordeolum, 180
Horizontal cells, of retina, 174
Hormone(s), alcohol effects on, 756
Hormone replacement therapy, for hypopituitarism, 444, 446t
Horner's syndrome
  in cervical cord lesions, 401
  ocular manifestations of, 176, 192
"Hot cross buns sign," 386, 386f
H-reflex studies, 33
HSAN. *See* Hereditary sensory and autonomic neuropathy (HSAN)
HSV infections. *See* Herpes simplex virus (HSV) infections
Human chorionic gonadotropin (hCG), reference values, 782t
Human T-cell lymphotropic virus-I (HTLV-I) infections, myelopathy and, 410
Humoral autoimmunity, in MS, 476–477
Hunt-Hess scale, for subarachnoid hemorrhage, 305, 306t
huntingtin gene, 350–351
Huntington's disease, **350**
  clinical features of, 350
  dementia in, 310, 326–327
  etiology of, 350–351
  frontal lobe syndrome in, 155
  functional anatomy of, 310
  gait disorders in, 112
  insomnia in, 165
  neuroimaging in, 351f, 690f
  neuropathology of, 228, 350
  ocular involvement in, 195
  olfactory dysfunction in, 202
  prevalence of, 350
  treatment of, 351
Huntington's disease–like 1, 351
Huntington's disease–like 2, 351
Hutchinson's sign, 181
Hydrocephalus
  balance disorders in, 114
  coma in, 139
  gait disorders in, 111t, 112
  normal-pressure, dementia due to, 327–328, 327f
  obstructive, ocular involvement in, 176, 195
  after subarachnoid hemorrhage, 306
  weakness in, 107
Hydrocortisone, for ACTH deficiency, 466
Hydromorphone, for pain, 46t
Hydrophobia, in rabies, 512
Hydroxychloroquine, adverse effects of
  myopathy, 645t, 647
  neuropathy, 585, 586t
  ocular, 190
Hypalgesia, 117
Hyperaldosteronism, weakness in, 644
Hyperalgesia, 41, 117
Hyperarousal, 163
Hypercalcemia, neurologic consultation for, 665
Hypercarbia, delirium in, 129, 129t
Hypercoagulable state, stroke due to, 267
Hypereosinophilic syndrome, 580
Hyperesthesia, 117
Hyperglycemia, myopia in, 175
Hyperhidrosis, primary, **388**
Hyperkalemia, neurologic consultation for, 664–665
Hyperkalemic periodic paralysis (HyperKPP), 220t, 641t, 642
Hyperkinetic movement disorders, **346,** 347t, 355
Hyperkyphosis, 73
Hyperlordosis, 73
Hypermagnesemia, neurologic consultation for, 665
Hypernatremia, neurologic consultation for, 663–664
Hyperopia, 175
Hyperosmolality, neurologic consultation for, 663–664
Hyperparathyroidism
  delirium in, 129t
  muscle weakness in, 644
Hyperpathia, 44, 118, 389
Hyperperfusion states
  diagnosis of, 661, 661f, 817, 817f, 845
  etiology of, 660, 661t
  neurologic consultation for, 660–662
  treatment of, 661–662
Hyperprolactinemia, **453,** 813, 839
  clinical features of, 454–455
  diagnosis of, 454–455
  etiology of, 453–454, 454t
  galactorrhea and, 455
  laboratory studies of, 455
  treatment of, 455
Hyperprolactinemia, cocaine and, 768
Hypersensitivity reactions, chronic meningitis due to, 532t
Hypertension
  optic neuropathy in, 184
  retinopathy in, 183, 183f
  stroke risk in, 265t
  supine, 94
Hypertensive encephalopathy, 129t, 289
Hyperthermia, delirium in, 129t
Hyperthyroidism
  delirium in, 129, 129t
  muscle involvement in, 644
Hypertonic saline, for increased intracranial pressure, 298t
Hypertrophic cardiomyopathy, syncope in, 96
Hypesthesia, 117
Hypnic headache, **70**
Hypnosis, 57
Hypocalcemia, neurologic consultation for, 665
Hypoceruloplasminemia, 364t
Hypochondriasis, 736
Hypocupric myelopathy, 412
Hypoesthesia, 117
Hypoglossal nerve, 7
Hypoglycemia
  Bálint's syndrome in, 151
  syncope and, 96
Hypogonadotropic hypogonadism
  clinical features of, 470
  diagnosis of, 470
  isolated, 470
  treatment of, 470–471
Hypokalemia, neurologic consultation for, 664
Hypokalemic periodic paralysis (HypoKPP), 220t, 640–642, 642f
Hypomagnesemia, neurologic consultation for, 665
Hypomania, 165
Hyponatremia
  neurologic consultation for, 664
  after subarachnoid hemorrhage, 306
Hypoparathyroidism, muscle weakness in, 644
Hypophysitis, 443
Hypopituitarism, **441**
  anterior pituitary insufficiency and, 441
  clinical features of, 444
  diagnosis of, 444, 445t
  etiology of, 441t
    acquired, 443–444, 838, 839
    developmental and genetic, 442–443
  treatment of, 444, 446t
Hypotension, in coma, 136
Hypothalamic disease
  hypopituitarism due to, 443
  metabolic effects of, 449
Hypothalamic gliomas, 448
Hypothalamic hamartomas, 448
Hypothalamic-pituitary vasculature, 440f
Hypothalamus
  developmental dysfunction of, 442–443
  in sleep onset, 159
Hypothermia
  coma and, 136
  delirium in, 129t
  for hypoxic-ischemic encephalopathy, 300
Hypothyroidism
  depression in, 729
  muscle disorders in, 644
  neuropathy in, 579
Hypoxia, delirium in, 129, 129t
Hypoxic-ischemic encephalopathy, 256, 299–300, 300f

IBD. *See* Inflammatory bowel disease (IBD)
IBPN (immune-mediated brachial plexus neuropathy), 595
Ibuprofen
  for migraine, 58t
  for pain, 46t
ICAM-1 (intercellular adhesion molecule-1), 540
ICP. *See* Intracranial pressure (ICP)
Ideational apraxia, 147
Ideomotor apraxia, 147
Idiopathic growth hormone deficiency (IGHD), 460
Idiopathic torsion dystonia, 348
Ifosfamide, 438, 438t
IKBKAP gene, 388
Ileus, postoperative, 48
Iloperidone, 739t
Imipramine
  adverse effects of, 723t
  for depression, 723t, 732
  dosage of, 723t, 732
  for pain, 46t
  for sleep enuresis, 170
Immune-mediated brachial plexus neuropathy (IBPN), 595
Immune myelopathies, 407–409
Immune neuropathies, 601–602, 602f
Immune response/immune system, reference values, 778–785t
Immunocompromised patient, primary CNS lymphoma in, 429–430
Immunodeficiency viruses, 536
Immunoglobulin(s), reference values, 782t
Immunomodulators, for inflammatory myopathies, 658
Immunosuppressive therapy
  chronic meningitis associated with, 534–535
  for myasthenia gravis, 615
Implicit memory, 153
Imprinting, 219
Inclusion body myositis, **648**
  clinical features of, 648, 649–650, 649t
  diagnosis of, 655–657, 656t, 657f
  differential diagnosis of, 653–655
  drug-induced, 655
  genetic factors in, 650
  muscle damage in, 652, 652f
  nonimmune factors in, 653
  prognosis of, 659
  treatment of, 657–659
  viral infections and, 653
Indomethacin
  for cough headache, 69
  for exertional headache, 69
  for hemicrania continua, 69
  for pain, 46t
  for paroxysmal hemicrania, 65
  for sex headache, 70
  for stabbing headache, 69
Infants, seizures in, 238t
Infective endocarditis
  retinal hemorrhage in, 182
  stroke and, 263
Inferior petrosal venous sampling, in Cushing's syndrome, 468
Inferior pontine syndrome, lateral/medial, 281f
Inflammation, nociceptor-induced, 41
Inflammatory bowel disease (IBD)
  neuropathy in, 580
  ocular involvement in, 181, 182, 182f
Inflammatory mediators, in sensitization, 40–41
Inflammatory myelopathies, 407–409
Inflammatory myopathies
  autoantibodies in, 651, 816–817, 845
  clinical features of, 648–650, 649t
  diagnosis of, 655–657, 656f, 656t, 657f
  differential diagnosis of, 653–655
  drug-induced, 655
  immunogenetics in, 651
  immunopathologic mechanisms in, 651–652, 652f
  malignancies associated with, 650
  overlap syndrome, 650
  pathogenesis of, 650–653
  prevalence of, 648
  prognosis of, 659
Inflammatory myopathies (*Cont.*):
  treatment of, 657–659
  viral infections associated with, 653
Influenza, 202
Influenza vaccine, Guillain-Barré syndrome and, 600
Insomnia
  adjustment (acute), 164
  altitude, 164
  drug-induced, 165–166
  evaluation of, 162–163, 163t
  fatal familial, 165
  long-term (chronic), 162
  in medical disorders, 165
  in mental disorders, 164–165
  in neurologic disease, 165
  paradoxical, 163
  primary, 163–164
  psychophysiologic, 164
  rebound, 164, 166
  short-term, 162
  sleep maintenance, 162
  sleep offset, 162
  sleep onset, 162
  transient, 162
  treatment of, 163–164, 163t
Insomnia phobia, 164
Insulin-like growth factor I (IGF-I), 459
Intercellular adhesion molecule 1 (ICAM-1), 540
Interferon-β (IFN-β), for MS, 485–486, 486t
Interferon-β1a (IFN-β1a)
  for MS, 485–486, 486t
  for optic neuritis, 185
Interferon-β1b (IFN-β1b), for MS, 485–486, 486t
Internal carotid artery, occlusion of, 276–277, 276f, 277f
Internuclear ophthalmoplegia, 195, 196f
Interventional neuroradiology, 25
Intervertebral disk
  anatomy of, 71, 72f
  herniation of
    diagnosis of, 76–77
    imaging in, 77, 77f
    nerve compression in, 73f
    pain mechanism in, 75t, 76–77
    physical examination in, 74t, 76–77
    weakness in, 107
  replacement, 84
Intracranial atherosclerosis, 273
Intracranial hemorrhage, **286**
  anticoagulant therapy and, 289
  aphasia in, 145
  brain tumor and, 289
  in cerebral amyloid angiopathy, 289
  clinical outcomes of, 291t
  in cocaine users, 289
  etiology of, 256, 287t, 289–290
  headache in, 52–53
  head injury and, 289
  hypertensive encephalopathy and, 289–290
  intraparenchymal, 288–289, 288f
  laboratory/imaging evaluation of, 290
  lobar, 289
  prevention of, 291
  primary intraventricular, 290
  prognosis of, 291t
  treatment of, 287, 290–291
Intracranial meningitis, 527–528
Intracranial pressure (ICP)
  increased
    in bacterial meningitis, 498, 503
    headache with, 68
    in intracranial hemorrhage, 291
    monitoring of, 297, 297f
    ocular manifestations of, 185–186, 186f, 194
    pathophysiology of, 295, 296f
    signs of, 298
    treatment of, 297–298, 298t
  low, ocular manifestations of, 194
Intramedullary syndromes, 403
Intraocular pressure, increased, 182, 188
Intraparenchymal hemorrhage, hypertensive, 288–289, 288f
Intravenous immunoglobulin (IVIg)
  for CIDP, 606
  for dermatomyositis, 658
Intravenous immunoglobulin (IVIg) (*Cont.*):
  for GBS, 604
  for MS, 489
  for myasthenia gravis, 616
  for stiff-person syndrome, 563
Ion channels, disorders of, 220, 220t
Ionotropic receptors, 221
Iridectomy, laser, 182
Iritis. *See* Uveitis
Iron, brain accumulation of, 352
Isaacs' syndrome, 564, 622
Ischemia
  bilateral brainstem, 281
  cerebral, 256, 258f
Ischemic cascade, 294–295
Ischemic heart disease
  insomnia in, 165
  neck pain in, 87
Ischemic penumbra, 257
Ischemic stroke, **257**
  etiology of, 261, 263t, 808, 832
    artery-to-artery embolic, 263–265
    cardioembolic, 261–263, 262f
  pathophysiology of, 257–258, 258f, 262f
  risk factors for, 808, 832
  treatment of, **258**
    anticoagulants in, 261
    antiplatelet agents in, 260–261
    approach to, 257, 257f, 258
    endovascular techniques in, 259–260
    intravenous thrombolysis in, 259, 260t
    medical support in, 258–259
    neuroprotective agents in, 261
    rehabilitation in, 261
    rtPA in, 259, 260t
    stroke centers in, 261
Ishihara color plates, 177
Isocarboxazid, for depression, 723t
Isometheptene, for migraine, 58t, 60
Isoniazid
  adverse effects of
    neuropathy, 587t, 589, 842
    optic neuropathy, 185
  for tuberculous meningitis, 515
Isoprinosine, for subacute sclerosing panencephalitis, 518
IVIg. *See* Intravenous immunoglobulin (IVIg)

"Jacksonian march," 232, 830
Jactatio capitis nocturna, 170
JC virus infection, in HIV infection, 517, 547
Jefferson fracture, 699f
Jerk nystagmus, 196
Jervell and Lange-Nielsen syndrome, 212, 212t, 220t
Jet lag disorder, **170**
Joint(s), position testing of, 118, 120t
Joubert syndrome, 363t
Juvenile myotonic epilepsy, 234, 236

KAL gene, 442
Kallmann syndrome, 205, 442
Kayser-Fleischer ring, in Wilson disease, 356
KCNQ2 gene, 235t
Kearns-Sayre syndrome
  clinical features of, 362t, 639
  diagnosis of, 639
  genetic factors in, 362t, 639
  mitochondrial DNA mutation in, 639
  ocular manifestations of, 190, 192
  treatment of, 639
Kennedy's disease, 374t, 377
Keratic precipitates, 181
Keratitis, 180–181
Keratoconjunctivitis, 180
Keratoconjunctivitis sicca, 180
Keratoconus, 192
Kernig's sign, 493, 841
Kernohan-Woltman sign, 134
Ketamine, abuse of, 128, 129t, 772
Ketoconazole
  adverse effects of, 469
  for Cushing's syndrome, 469
Ketorolac
  for conjunctivitis, 180
  for pain, 45, 46t

Korsakoff 's psychosis, 302
Korsakoff's syndrome, 328, 754
Kugelberg-Welander disease, 377
Kuru, 550, 550t
Kussmaul respiration, 138

Labyrinthectomy, for Ménière's disease, 210
Labyrinthine infarction, 210
Lacosamide, 249t
Lacrimal system, obstruction of, 180
Lacrimation, with headache, 51–52
Lactotrope, 439t, 446t
Lacunar infarction, 265, 684f
Lacunar syndromes, 266
LaFora's disease, 235t
Laforin, 235t
Laing's distal myopathy, 633, 634t
Lambert-Eaton myasthenic syndrome (LEMS)
  cranial nerve palsy in, 194, 612
  diagnosis of, 612–613
  in lung cancer, 561
  muscle response to repetitive nerve stimulation in, 34
  paraneoplastic, 561
  reflex responses in, 104
  treatment of, 613
  weakness in, 108t
Laminectomy, for neck pain, 88
Lamotrigine
  adverse effects of, 246, 247t, 735t
  dosage of, 247t, 735t
  for epilepsy, 247t
  for focal seizures, 246
  for generalized seizures, 250
  pharmacology of, 247t, 735t
  for SUNCT/SUNA prevention, 65
  for trigeminal neuralgia, 393
Lancinations, 117
Language
  assessment of, 5, 143–144
  perisylvian network for, **142**
Lanreotide, for acromegaly, 464
Laser iridectomy, 182
Laser therapy, for neck pain, 88
LASIK, 175
Lateral femoral cutaneous neuropathy, 67, 594, 666f
Lateral geniculate body, 174, 179
Lateral medullary syndrome, 279, 280f
Lateral sclerosis, 370, 412
Latex agglutination assay, 499
LCM (lymphocytic choriomeningitis), 507, 531t
Lead poisoning
  clinical features of, 329
  diagnosis of, 788t
  neuropathy in, 588t, 590
  optic neuropathy in, 185
  treatment of, 329
Leber hereditary optic neuropathy (congenital amaurosis)
  clinical features of, 185
  genetic factors in, 185
  visual fields in, 179
Leflunomide, 587t
Leg cramps, nocturnal, 170
LEMS. *See* Lambert-Eaton myasthenic syndrome (LEMS)
Lennox-Gastaut syndrome, 236
Lenticulostriate arteries, 274
Lentiviruses, 536
Leprosy
  complications of, 181
  neuropathy in, 581
  ocular involvement in, 181
Leptin
  deficiency of, 442
  mutations, hypopituitarism due to, 442
Leptomeningeal metastases, 435–436, 435f
Leptospira/leptospirosis, 529t
Leukemia, ocular invasion by, 190
Leukoaraiosis, 268
Leukodystrophy(ies), 330
Leukoencephalopathy, reversible posterior, 268, 290
Leukotrienes, pain and, 41
Levetiracetam, 249t
Levodopa
  action of, 338–339
  adverse effects of, 339–341, 340f, 345
  for dystonia, 349
  for PD, 338–341, 340f, 343t, 346, 346f
Levorphanol, for pain, 46t, 50
Lewis-Sumner syndrome, 605
Lewy body disease, diffuse, 326
Lewy body variant of AD, 326
LGI1 gene, 235t
LGMD. *See* Limb-girdle muscular dystrophy (LGMD)
LH. *See* Luteinizing hormone (LH)
Lhermitte's sign/symptom, 4, 85, 123, 479, 821
Lidocaine
  for neuropathy, 50, 578t
  for SUNCT/SUNA, 65
Lidoderm patch, 578t
Li-Fraumeni syndrome, brain tumors and, 425t
Ligament(s), injury to, 700f
Light-headedness, 98
Limb(s)
  alien, 147, 325
  apraxia, 147
  dystonias of, 349
Limb-girdle muscular dystrophy (LGMD)
  autosomal dominant, 625t
  autosomal recessive, 626t
  classification of, 628–629
Limbic encephalitis
  clinical features of, 329, 561
  neuroimaging of, 560f, 668–669f
  pathogenesis of, 559t
Limbic network, for memory, 152–153
Limulus amebocyte lysate assay, 499
LINGO1 gene, 347
Lingual nerve, 202
Lipid(s)
  defects in metabolism of, 637–638
  as energy source, 637–638
Lipoprotein disorders, laboratory evaluation of, 789t
Lip reading, 216
Lissencephaly, classic, 235t
Listeria monocytogenes infections, 495, 496, 501t, 502, 841. *See also* Meningitis
Lithium
  action of, 716
  adverse effects of
    common, 735, 735t
    nystagmus, 196
    rare, 735t
  for bipolar disorder, 734–735, 735t, 736t
  clinical pharmacology of, 735t
  for cluster headache prevention, 64, 64t
  dosage of, 735, 735t
  for hypnic headache, 70
Liver, alcohol effects on, 755
Liver disease/failure
  delirium in, 129, 129t
  neuropathy in, 581
Lobar hemorrhage, 289
Lobectomy, temporal, 151
Locked-in state, 133, 279
Locus coeruleus, opiate action in, 718, 719f
Long QT syndrome, 95
Loop diuretics, 209
Lorazepam
  for acute alcohol intoxication, 758
  for generalized anxiety disorder, 725t
  for insomnia, 164
  pharmacology of, 725t
Lordotic posture, 620, 621f
Lower motor neuron diseases, 374t, 377–378. *See also* Amyotrophic lateral sclerosis (ALS)
Lower motor neuron pathways, 106f
Lower motor neuron (neuropathic) weakness, 104, 104t
Loxapine, 739t
LRRK2 gene, 334, 338
LSD (lysergic acid diethylamide), **771**
Lumbar fusion, 84
Lumbar puncture, **35**
  analgesia for, 35
  in coma, 138–139
  headache following, 37–38, 37t, 67
  imaging and laboratory studies prior to, 35
  in meningitis, 498
  needles for, 37–38, 38f
  in neurologic critical illness, 297
  normal values, 38, 38t
  patient positioning for, 35–36, 36f
  technique, 36–37
Lumbar spinal stenosis, 78, 78f
Lumbosacral plexopathy, 597, 597t
Lumbosacral plexus, 596f, 597f
Lumbosacral radiculopathy, 74t
Lung cancer
  metastatic, 190, 433t, 434f
  small cell, 561, 608
Lung volume(s), reference values, 797t
Lupus erythematosus
  delirium in, 129t
  ocular involvement in, 181, 183
Luteinizing hormone (LH), **469**
  action of, 470
  deficiency of, 446t
  laboratory evaluation of, 445t
  reference values, 783t
  secretion of, 469–470
  synthesis of, 469–470
Lyme borreliosis (Lyme disease)
  chronic meningitis in, 529t
  neuropathy in, 581
  ocular involvement in, 181
Lymphocytic choriomeningitis (LCM), 507, 531t
Lymphocytic hypophysitis, 443
Lymphocytic meningitis, 532t
Lymphoid malignancies
  CNS, primary, 429–430, 429f, 545, 545f, 838
  in HIV infection, 544–545, 838
  metastatic, 190
  neuropathy in, 583–584
  paraneoplastic syndromes in, 564
  weakness in, 107
Lysergic acid diethylamide (LSD), **771**

Machado-Joseph disease, 359t, 365–366
Macula, 174, 177
Macular degeneration, **188,** 189f, 806, 829
  dry (nonexudative), 189
  treatment of, 189
  wet (exudative), 189
Macular hole, 190
Magnesium supplements, for migraine, 206
Magnetic resonance angiography (MRA)
  in neurologic disease, **22,** 683f
  phase-contrast, 22
  TOF imaging, 22
Magnetic resonance imaging (MRI), **17,** 821
  in acute transverse myelitis, 692f
  in AD, 318f
  in ADEM, 693f
  in amyotrophic lateral sclerosis, 372f
  in arteriovenous malformation in spine, 410f
  in astrocytoma, 427f
  in Behçet's syndrome, 678f
  in Bell's palsy, 396f, 691f
  in brachial plexopathy, 697–698f
  in brain abscess, 520, 520f
  in brain metastases, 434f
  in brain tumors, 424, 427f, 428f
  in CADASIL, 685f
  in candidiasis, 675f
  in central pontine myelinolysis, 301, 302f
  in cerebral abscess, 18f
  in cerebral artery stenosis, 683f
  in CNS aspergillosis, 676–678f
  in CNS tuberculosis, 669–670f
  in CNS vasculitis, 686f
  complications of, 21–22
  contraindications to, 22, 22t
  contrast agents, 18–21
  in Creutzfeldt-Jakob disease, 556f
  in diffuse white matter disease, 322f
  diffusion tensor, 23

Magnetic resonance imaging (MRI) (*Cont.*):
in epidural metastases, 436f
in epidural spinal compression, 404f
in FTD, 324f
functional, 23, 96, 149f, 229–230, 229f
in glioblastoma, 427f, 428f
guidelines for, 14t
in Hashimoto's encephalopathy, 696f
in hearing loss, 215
in histiocytosis, 683f
in histoplasmosis of the pons, 673f
in Huntington's disease, 351f, 690f
in hypoxic-ischemic encephalopathy, 300f
in intramedullary astrocytoma, 405f
in lacunar infarction, 684f
in leptomeningeal metastases, 435f
in limbic encephalitis, 668–669f
in low CSF volume headache, 67f
in meningioma, 431f
in meningitis, 499–500, 674f
in mesial temporal lobe epilepsy, 236f
in MS, 480t, 481–482, 481f, 694–695f
in multiple system atrophy, 386f, 689f
in neurosarcoid, 678–682f
in neurosyphilis, 670–672f
in paraneoplastic encephalitis, 561f
perfusion, 23
in pituitary tumors, 450, 450f
in primary central nervous system lymphoma, 429, 429f, 533f, 545, 545f
in progressive multifocal leukoencephalopathy, 517
relaxation times, 17t
in SCA1, 365f
in seizures, 243
in spinal cord infarction, 692f
in spinal epidural abscess, 406f
in stroke, 286, 286f
in subdural empyema, 523, 523f
in subdural hematoma, 701f
in superior sagittal sinus thrombosis, 687 688f
in syringomyelia associated with Chiari malformation, 411f
T1 and T2 relaxation times, 17–18, 17t, 821
technique, 17–21, 17t, 18–21f
in thoracic meningioma, 405f
in vestibular schwannoma, 431f
in viral encephalitis, 18f, 510, 510f, 511t
in Wernicke's disease, 302f
Magnetic resonance neurography, 23
Magnetoencephalography (MEG), 29, 243
Major depression, 730, 730t, 732f, 819, 847
Malabsorption syndromes, ataxia due to, 369
Malingering, 187, 737
Mania
acute, treatment of, 736t
insomnia in, 165
mixed, 734
Mannitol, for increased intracranial pressure, 298t
MAO-B inhibitors. *See* Monoamine oxidase type B (MAO-B) inhibitors
MAOIs. *See* Monoamine oxidase inhibitors (MAOIs)
MAPT gene, 323
Marburg's variant, MS, 491
Marchiafava-Bignami disease, 328
Marcus Gunn pupil, 176, 176f
Marijuana, 769, 850
dependence on, 770
initial actions of, 718t
physical effects of, 769–770
THC in, 221, 769
therapeutic applications, 770
tolerance to, 770
Marijuana use/abuse, **769**
acute and chronic intoxication, 769
adverse effects of, 770, 850
prevalence of, 769
withdrawal signs, 770
Marinesco-Sjögren syndrome, 362t
Markesbery-Griggs distal myopathy, 633, 634t
"Master gland," 439
Mastoiditis, 194, 518–519
MBP (myelin basic protein), 223f
McArdle disease (myophosphorylase deficiency), 637
McCune-Albright syndrome, 447
MCI (mild cognitive impairment), 311
MCTD (mixed connective tissue disease), 580
MDCT (multidetector computed tomography), 13–14, 15f
MDMA (ecstasy), 128, 129t, 770
Measles (rubeola), complications of, 491, 518
Mechanical ventilation, in coma, 140
Mechanic's hands, 649
Mechlorethamine (nitrogen mustard), 438t
Medial medullary syndrome, 279, 280f
Median neuropathy, 593
Median preoptic nucleus, of hypothalamus, 159
Medication-overuse headache, 60, **66**
Medulloblastoma, 430
MEG (magnetoencephalography), 29, 243
Meibomian gland carcinoma, 180
Meibomitis, 180
Melanoma
of eye, 190, 190f
metastatic to CNS, 433t
retinopathy in, 559t, 565
Melanopsin, 174
MELAS (mitochondrial myopathy, encephalopathy, lactic acidosis, and stroke) syndrome
clinical features of, 362t, 640
genetic factors in, 362t
hearing loss in, 212
mitochondrial DNA mutation in, 640
Melatonin
for circadian sleep disorders, 173
for cluster headache prevention, 64t
secretion of, 161
Melkersson-Rosenthal syndrome, 396
Melodic intonation therapy, 145
Memantine, for AD, 321, 331
Memory
assessment of, 5, 154–155, 229–230
implicit, 153
limbic network for, 152–153
retentive, 155
working, 155
MEN 1. *See* Multiple endocrine neoplasia type 1 (MEN 1)
Ménière's disease
clinical features of, 101, 210
diagnosis of, 101, 214–215
dizziness in, 98
epidemiology of, 210
hearing loss in, 210, 213, 214
nystagmus in, 196
pathophysiology of, 101, 210
treatment of, 101, 210
Meningeal biopsy, in chronic meningitis, 534
Meningioma, 812, 838
clinical features of, 430–431
imaging in, 215, 431, 431f, 812, 812f, 838
ocular signs in, 179
parasagittal, 108
pathophysiology of, 430–431
sellar, 448
thoracic, 405, 405f
treatment of, 431
Meningitis
approach to the patient, 493–494, 494–495f, 807, 831
bacterial, **494,** 814, 840–841
chronic, 529t
clinical features of, 498
definition of, 494–495
diagnosis of, 498–500, 499t
differential diagnosis of, 500
epidemiology of, 495
etiology of, 495–496
gram-negative, 501t, 502
H. influenzae, 495, 496
incidence of, 495–496
increased ICP in, 503
L. monocytogenes, 495, 496, 501t, 502, 841
M. tuberculosis, 514–515
meningococcal, 495–496, 501, 501t
mortality data, 503
pathophysiology of, 496–498, 497f
pneumococcal, 495, 501–502, 501t
Meningitis (*Cont.*):
prognosis of, 503
staphylococcal, 496, 501t, 502
treatment of, 841
adjunctive therapy in, 502–503
algorithm for, 494–495f
antimicrobial therapy based on pathogen, 501–502, 501t
dexamethasone, 502–503
empirical antimicrobial therapy, 499t, 500–501
ICP-related, 503
basal, 528
chronic, **527,** 814, 841
approach to the patient, 528, 531
clinical features of, 527–528, 527t
CSF analysis in, 533–534
epidemiology of, 528
in HIV infection, 534–535
imaging in, 533, 533f
in immunosuppressed patients, 534–535
infectious causes of, 528, 529–531t
laboratory studies in, 534
meningeal biopsy in, 534
noninfectious causes of, 532–533t
pathophysiology of, 527–528
systemic manifestations of, 528
treatment of, 534
Coccidioides, 530t, 674f
Cryptococcus, 514–515, 530t, 545–546
delirium in, 129, 129t
fungal, 515
headache in, 52
hearing loss in, 209
intracranial, 527–528
Mollaret's, 532t
in neurosyphilis, 516
spinal, 528
subacute, **514**
viral, **503**
arborvirus, 505–506
clinical features of, 503
differential diagnosis of, 505
EBV, 506
enteroviral, 505
epidemiology of, 504
etiology of, 503, 504t, 505–507
in HIV infection, 506, 543
HSV, 506, 531t, 841
laboratory evaluation of, 504–505
lymphocytic choriomeningitis, 507
in mumps infection, 506–507
prevention of, 507
prognosis of, 507
treatment of, 507
VZV, 506
weakness in, 107
Menstrual disorders, 81
Mental status assessment, 5–6
Meperidine
adverse effects of, 646
for migraine, 60
for pain, 46t
Meralgia paresthetica, 594
Mercury exposure/poisoning
clinical features of, 329
neuropathy due to, 588t, 590
reference range for, 788t
Meropenem, for meningitis, 499t, 501
Merosin deficiency, 630, 631t
MERRF (myoclonic epilepsy and ragged red fiber) syndrome
clinical features of, 362t, 639–640
diagnosis of, 640
genetic factors in, 362t
hearing loss in, 212
mitochondrial DNA mutation in, 640
Mesial temporal lobe epilepsy, 236, 236f, 236t, 807, 830
Metabolic disease, coma due to, 134–135
Metabolic encephalopathy, 146, 155, 300–301
Metabolic myopathies, **643**
Metabotropic receptors, 221
Metachromatic leukodystrophy (MLD), 330
Metamorphopsia, 189, 190

Metastatic disease
  to brain. *See* Brain tumors, metastatic
  to eye, 190, 191
  to spine, 79, 810–811, 811f, 836
    epidural, 436, 436f
    leptomeningeal, 435–436, 435f
Methadone
  as maintenance drug, 765
  for opiate detoxification, 764
  for pain, 46t, 50
Methamphetamine
  abuse of, 770
  actions of, 718t
  intracerebral hemorrhage due to, 289
Methanol poisoning, 185
Methocarbamol, for back pain, 82
Methotrexate
  adverse effects of, 438t
  for inflammatory myopathies, 658
  for MS, 489
  for primary central nervous system lymphoma, 430
  therapeutic monitoring of, 787t
Methylnaltrexone, 48, 50
Methylphenidate
  for fatigue in MS, 490
  for narcolepsy, 163t, 169
Methylprednisolone
  for MS, 485, 489
  for optic neuritis, 184
  for vertigo, 102t
Methysergide
  adverse effects of, 61t, 62
  for chronic daily headache, 66
  for cluster headache, 64
  for cluster headache prevention, 64t
  for exertional headache, 69
  for hypnic headache, 70
  for migraine prevention, 61t, 62
Metoclopramide, for migraine, 58t, 60
Metronidazole
  adverse effects of, 586t
  for meningitis, 499t, 501
Metyrapone
  adverse effects of, 469
  for Cushing's syndrome, 469
Mexiletine
  adverse effects of, 578t
  for neuropathy, 578t
  for pain, 50, 490
Meyer's loop, 179
Midbrain syndrome, lateral/medial, 284f
Middle cerebral artery
  lesion in territory of, 145, 146
  occlusion of, 16f, 262, 274–275, 275f, 285f
  stenosis of, 683f
Midodrine, for orthostatic hypotension, 95, 390
Midpontine syndrome, lateral/medial, 282f
Migraine, 51t, **53**
  acephalic, 56, 257
  autonomic symptoms in, 51–52
  chronic, 56
  clinical features of, 54–56, 54t
  diagnosis of, 54–56, 56t
  familial hemiplegic, 54
  insomnia in, 165
  ion channel defects causing, 220t
  memory loss in, 154
  neuroimaging in, 54, 55f
  ocular manifestations of, 187
  pathogenesis and pathophysiology of, 44, 54, 54f
  prevention of, 59t, 60, 61t, 62
  retinal, 183
  taste disorders in, 204
  treatment of, 56–62
    5-HT_1 agonists, 58t, 59–60
    acute attack therapies, 57, 58t, 59t
    dopamine antagonists, 58t, 60
    nonpharmacologic, 56–57
    nonsteroidal anti-inflammatory drugs, 57, 58t, 59
  triggers, 53
  vertigo in, 98, 100–101
Migraine aura, 54
Migraine Disability Assessment Score, 56, 57f
Mild cognitive impairment (MCI), 311, 316f
Millard-Gubler syndrome, 194
Miller Fisher syndrome, 599–600, 602t
Mineral(s), reference ranges, 788t
Minimally conscious state, 132
Mini-Mental Status Examination (MMSE)
  in delirium evaluation, 128
  in dementia, 314, 315t
  in neurologic examination, 5–6
Minor depression, 730–731
Mirror neuron systems, 229–230, 229f
Mirtazapine, 517, 723t, 733
Misonidazole, 586t
Mitochondria
  in apoptosis, 226–227, 227f
  dysfunction, in neurodegenerative disease, 228
Mitochondrial ataxias, 368
Mitochondrial DNA diseases, 640
Mitochondrial DNA skeletal muscle–central nervous system syndromes, **639**
Mitochondrial myopathy(ies), **638**
  drug-induced, 646
  genetic factors in, 638
  pathogenesis of, 638
  progressive external ophthalmoplegia syndromes, 185, 639. *See also* Kearns-Sayre syndrome
  pure myopathy syndromes, 640
  skeletal muscle-CNS syndromes
    MELAS syndrome. *See* MELAS (mitochondrial myopathy, encephalopathy, lactic acidosis, and stroke) syndrome
    MERRF syndrome. *See* MERRF (myoclonic epilepsy and ragged red fiber) syndrome
Mitochondrial myopathy, encephalopathy, lactic acidosis, and stroke (MELAS) syndrome. *See* MELAS (mitochondrial myopathy, encephalopathy, lactic acidosis, and stroke) syndrome
Mitotane
  adverse effects of, 469
  for Cushing's syndrome, 469
Mitoxantrone
  action of, 487
  adverse effects of, 487
  for MS, 486t, 487
Mitral cells, 199
Mitral regurgitation, 264t, 796t
Mitral stenosis, 264t, 796t
Mitral valve prolapse, 264t
Mixed connective tissue disease (MCTD), 580
Mixed mania, 734
Miyoshi's myopathy, 633, 634t
MLD (metachromatic leukodystrophy), 330
MMSE. *See* Mini-Mental Status Examination (MMSE)
Modafinil
  for fatigue in MS, 490
  for narcolepsy, 163t, 169
  for shift-work disorder, 172
Moffett's position, 206
MOG (myelin oligodendrocyte glycoprotein), 223f
Molindone, 739t
Mollaret's meningitis, 532t
Monoamine oxidase inhibitors (MAOIs)
  adverse effects of, 723t, 733
  for depression, 733
  drug interactions of, 733
  for panic disorder, 722
Monoamine oxidase type B (MAO-B) inhibitors
  action of, 341
  adverse effects of, 341–342
  for PD, 341–342, 343t, 346, 346f
Monoclonal antibodies, anti-CD3, 185
Monoclonal antibodies, anti-CD20
  for MS, 490
  for neuromyelitis optica, 491
Monoclonal antibodies, anti-CD52, 490
Monoclonal gammopathy of undetermined significance (MGUS), 584, **607**
Mononeuropathy
  diabetic, 579
  multiple, HIV-related, 544, 582
Monoparesis, 108–109
Monosodium glutamate, 205
Mood disorders, **714, 729**. *See also specific disorders*
  bipolar disorder. *See* Bipolar disorder
  epidemiology of, 714
  genetic factors in, 714
  in the homeless, 741
  neuroimaging of, 714
  neuropathology of, 714, 715f
  pathogenesis of, 714–716, 715f
  personality disorders, **737**
  schizophrenia. *See* Schizophrenia
  somatoform disorders, **736**
Mood stabilizers, 735t
Morphine
  adverse effects of, 177
  for pain, 46t, 47
  sustained-release, 46t, 50
Morvan's syndrome, 562
Motivational dependence, 716
Motor cortex, 142, 143f
Motor evoked potentials, 30
Motor examination, 7–9
Motor neuron disorders
  differential diagnosis of, 371t
  etiology of, 371t
  genetic, 374–376t
  lower, 374t, 377–378
  sporadic, 372t
  upper, 374–376t, 378–379
Motor neuropathy
  multifocal, **606**
  subacute, paraneoplastic, 563
Motor tic, 353
Motor vehicle accidents, 167
Movement disorders
  drug-induced, **354**
    acute, 354
    subacute, 354
    tardive syndromes, 354–355
  Huntington's disease. *See* Huntington's disease
  hyperkinetic, **346,** 347t. *See also specific disorders*
  PD. *See* Parkinson's disease (PD)
  psychogenic, 356
  tics, 347t, 352–353
  Tourette's syndrome. *See* Tourette's syndrome
Moyamoya disease, 268, 290
MPTP, 336–337
MRA. *See* Magnetic resonance angiography (MRA)
MRF (myelin gene regulatory factor), 224
MRI. *See* Magnetic resonance imaging (MRI)
MS. *See* Multiple sclerosis (MS)
MSA. *See* Multiple system atrophy (MSA)
Multidetector computed tomography (MDCT), 13–14, 15f
Multifocal motor neuropathy, 602t, **606**
Multifocal motor neuropathy with conduction block, 373, 378, 835
Multi-infarct dementia, 322
Multiple endocrine neoplasia type 1 (MEN 1), 425t
  clinical features of, 447t
  pituitary tumors in, 447
Multiple hamartoma syndrome (Cowden syndrome), 425t
Multiple myeloma
  neuropathy in, 584, **606**
  paraneoplastic syndromes in, 564
Multiple sclerosis (MS), **474,** 814, 840
  acute, 491
  acute myelitis in, 408
  anatomy of, 474
  chronic cerebrospinal insufficiency in, 489
  chronic myelopathy in, 411
  clinical features of, 477–479, 477t
  clinical variants of, 490–491
  course of, 479, 479f
  diagnosis of, 86, 480, 480t
    CSF analysis in, 482
    evoked potentials in, 482
    neuroimaging in, 481–482, 481f, 694–695f
  differential diagnosis of, 482–483, 482t
  epidemiology of, 475–476
  frontal lobe syndrome in, 155
  gait disorders in, 111
  genetic factors in, 219, 476–477, 476t

Multiple sclerosis (MS) (*Cont.*):
hearing loss in, 210
immunology of, 476–477
Marburg's variant, 491
myelitis in, 408
neurodegeneration in, 477
ocular involvement in, 182, 184–185, 195, 196
olfactory dysfunction in, 203
pathogenesis of, 223f, 474–477, 475f
physiology of, 474–475, 475f
pregnancy and, 483
primary progressive, 479, 479f, 488f, 489
prognosis of, 483
progressive/relapsing, 479, 479f
relapsing/remitting, 479, 479f, 488f
risk factors for, 475, 476t
scoring systems for, 483, 484t
secondary progressive, 479, 479f, 488–489, 488f
taste disorders in, 204
treatment of
acute attacks, 483, 485
changing of, 488, 488f
cladribine in, 487–488
dietary therapies in, 489
disease-modifying therapies in, 484–488, 485, 486t, 488f
experimental therapies in, 489
fingolimod in, 487
glatiramer acetate in, 486
glucocorticoids in, 485
INF-β in, 485–486
initial demyelinating episodes, 483, 485
initiation of, 488, 488f
mitoxantrone hydrochloride in, 487
natalizumab in, 486–487
off-label options in, 489
symptomatic therapy in, 489–490
triggers of, 477
types of, 479, 479f, 840
weakness in, 107, 108t
Multiple sleep latency test, 168
Multiple system atrophy (MSA)
autonomic dysfunction in, 385–386, 386f
clinical features of, 386
gait disorders in, 112
neuroimaging in, 386f, 689f
olfactory dysfunction in, 203
orthostatic hypotension in, 94
parkinsonism in, 335–336, 337t
treatment of, 386
Mumps, meningitis in, 506–507, 531t
Munchausen syndrome, 737
Mu receptors, 761–762, 761t
Muscle(s)
atrophy of, 622
calcium channel disorders of, **640**
contracture of, 622
electrophysiologic studies of. *See* Electromyography (EMG)
enlargement of, 622
response to repetitive nerve stimulation, 33–34
sodium channel disorders of, **642**
Muscle biopsy
in dermatomyositis, 656t, 657f
in inclusion body myositis, 656t, 657f
in myopathy, 623
in polymyositis, 656t, 657f
Muscle bulk, 103
Muscle contracture, 622
Muscle cramps, 622
Muscle disorders
energy metabolism disorders, **636**. *See also* Glycogen storage diseases
membrane excitability disorders, **640,** 641t
muscle fiber disorders. *See* Myopathy(ies)
muscular dystrophy. *See* Muscular dystrophy
Muscle-eye-brain disease, 630, 631t
Muscle pain
drugs causing, 621, 621t
in myopathy, 620–622
weakness due to, 655
Muscle relaxants, for back pain, 82
Muscle-specific tyrosine kinase (MuSK), in myasthenia gravis, 610–611
Muscle spindle, 106f
Muscle stiffness, 622
Muscle stretch (tendon) reflexes, 8, 104, 104t, 106f
Muscle tone, 103, 104t
Muscle weakness
acute, differential diagnosis of, 654
diagnostic evaluation of, 618–620, 619f, 620f, 620t
in parathyroid disorders, 644
subacute or chronic progressive, differential diagnosis of, 653–654
Muscular dystrophy, **618**
Becker's. *See* Becker's muscular dystrophy
congenital, 625t, **630,** 631t
congenital myopathies, **635**
cramps in, 622
distal myopathies, **633,** 634t
Duchenne's. *See* Duchenne's muscular dystrophy
Emery-Dreifuss. *See* Emery-Dreifuss muscular dystrophy
facioscapulohumeral, 625t, **632**
gait disorders in, 113
hereditary myopathies, 625t
laboratory evaluation of, 619f, 622
DNA analysis, 623
electrodiagnostic studies, 623
forearm exercise test, 623–624
muscle biopsy, 624
serum enzymes, 622–623
limb-girdle, 628–629
autosomal dominant, 626t
autosomal recessive, 627t
muscle pain in, 620–622, 621t
muscle weakness in, 618–620, 619f, 620f, 620t, 621f
myotonic. *See* Myotonic dystrophy
oculopharyngeal, 192, 625t, 633
progressive, 625t
proteins associated with, 626, 628f, 629f
stiffness in, 622
MuSK (muscle-specific tyrosine kinase), in myasthenia gravis, 610–611
Mutism, 143, 147
Myalgia. *See* Muscle pain
Myasthenia gravis, **609,** 816, 843
ACh test in, 611
antibodies to AChR or MuSK, 610–611
clinical features of, 610
diagnosis of, 610–612, 611t, 612t, 613t, 843
differential diagnosis of, 612–613
diplopia in, 193
disorders associated with, 63–614, 613t
drugs affecting, 616
drugs to avoid in, 616, 617t
electrodiagnostic studies in, 611
muscle response to repetitive nerve stimulation in, 33–34
nystagmus in, 196
ocular, 610
pathophysiology of, 609–6110, 609f
ptosis in, 192
reflex responses in, 104
treatment of, **614**
algorithm for, 614f
azathioprine, 615–616
cyclosporine, 616
glucocorticoids, 615
immunosuppression, 615–616
IVIg, 616
mycophenolate mofetil, 615–616
patient assessment in, 616–617, 617f
plasmapheresis, 616
pyridostigmine, 614
tacrolimus, 616
thymectomy, 614–615
weakness in, 107, 108t, 109
Myasthenic crisis, 616
Myasthenic fatigue, 610
Mycobacterium spp. infections, 514–515, 529t. *See also* Meningitis
Mycophenolate mofetil
for inflammatory myopathies, 658
for myasthenia gravis, 615–616
for neuromyelitis optica, 491
Mycotic aneurysm, circle of Willis, 305
Mydriasis, 176
Myelin basic protein (MBP), 223f
Myelin defects, in neurologic disease, 223–224, 223f, 224f
Myelin gene regulatory factor (MRF), 224
Myelin oligodendrocyte glycoprotein (MOG), 223f
Myelin sheath, 223f
Myelitis, 407–409
acute infectious, 409
acute transverse
MRI in, 692f
weakness in, 107
neuromyelitis optica, 408, 490–491
paraneoplastic syndromes, 561, 563
postinfectious, 408–409
Myelography, 23–24
Myeloma
multiple. *See* Multiple myeloma
sclerotic, 565
Myelopathy
acute transverse, 407t
chemotherapy-induced, 438t
chronic, **409**
adrenomyeloneuropathy, 412
familial spastic paraplegia, 378–379, 412
hypocupric, 412
in multiple sclerosis, 411
primary lateral sclerosis, 378, 412
spondylitic, 409
syringomyelia, 86, 410–411, 411f
in tabes dorsalis, 412
tethered cord syndrome, 76, 412
toxic causes of, 413
in vascular malformations of cord and dura, 409–410, 410f
in vitamin B_{12} deficiency, 411–412, 591
compressive. *See* Spinal cord compression
evaluation of, 811, 837
gait disorders in, 111t
HIV-associated, 543
immune, 407–408
inflammatory, 408–409
noncompressive, **406**
vs. compressive, 403
evaluation of, 407t
spinal cord infarction, 407, 692f
paraneoplastic, 563
Myoadenylate deaminase deficiency, 638
Myocardial infarction (MI), circadian variations in, 173
Myoclonic dystonia, 348
Myoclonic epilepsy, juvenile, 234, 236
Myoclonic epilepsy and ragged red fiber syndrome. *See* MERRF
Myoclonic seizures, 234
Myoclonus, 347t, **353**
Baltic, 362t
clinical features of, 353
in Creutzfeldt-Jakob disease, 554–555
nocturnal (periodic limb movement disorder), 166
posthypoxic, 300
startle, 815, 842
treatment of, 353
Myofascial pain syndrome, 48
Myofasciitis, 654
Myofibrillar myopathies, 633, 634t
Myogenic ptosis, 192
Myokymia, 397, 622
Myopathy(ies)
acute quadriplegic, 304
alcoholic, 646, 756
autoimmune, 647
centronuclear (myotubular), **636**
congenital, **635**
in critical/systemic illness, 304, 645
distal, **633,** 634t
drug-induced, **645,** 645t, 655
drugs of abuse and, 645t, 646
endocrine, **643,** 816, 844
gait disorders in, 113
glucocorticoid-related, 645t, 646, 658
hereditary, **624,** 625t. *See also* Muscular dystrophy
HIV-related, 544

Myopathy(ies) (*Cont.*):
inflammatory. *See* Inflammatory myopathies
laboratory evaluation of, 619f, 622
DNA analysis, 623
electrodiagnostic studies, 623
forearm exercise test, 623–624
muscle biopsy, 624
serum enzymes, 622–623
metabolic, **643**
mitochondrial. *See* Mitochondrial myopathy(ies)
muscle enlargement and atrophy in, 622
muscle pain in, 620–622, 621t
muscle weakness in, 105–106, 109, 618–620, 619f, 620f, 620t
nemaline, **635**
paraneoplastic, 563
proximal myotonic, 622
Myophosphorylase deficiency (type V glycogenosis), 637
Myopia, 175
Myositis, necrotizing, 654
Myotonia
conditions associated with, 622
definition of, 622
ion channel defects causing, 220t
nondystrophic, 641t
potassium-aggravated, 642
Myotonia congenita, 220t, 622
Myotonic disorders, 623t
Myotonic dystrophy, **630,** 816, 844
clinical features of, 625t, 630–631
congenital, 631
laboratory features of, 631–632
ocular involvement in, 188, 192
treatment of, 632
Myotubular myopathy, **636**
Myxoma, syncope in, 96

Naegleria infection, in encephalitis, 511
Nafcillin, for meningitis, 499t, 502
Naloxone
as opiate antagonist, 47
for opioid overdose, 764
Naltrexone, in alcoholism management, 760, 849
Naming deficit, 143
Naproxen
for migraine, 58t, 59
for pain, 46t
Naratriptan, for migraine, 58t, 59, 59t
Narcolepsy, **168**
clinical features of, 159, 168t, 827–828
diagnosis of, 168–169, 828
genetic factors in, 168
olfactory dysfunction in, 204
treatment of, 169
Narcolepsy-cataplexy syndrome, 163t
NARP (neuropathy, ataxia, retinitis pigmentosa) syndrome, 362t
Nasal congestion, with headache, 51–52
Natalizumab
adverse effects of, 487
for MS, 486t, 487–488
Neck pain, **85**
in ankylosing spondylitis, 86
in brachial plexus injury, 87
in cancer, 86–87
in carpal tunnel syndrome, 87
in cervical disk disease, 85–86, 86t
in cervical spine trauma, 85
in cervical spondylosis, 86
in herpes zoster, 86
in orthostatic hypotension, 94
in peripheral nerve disorders, 87
physical examination in, 86t
in rheumatoid arthritis, 86
in thoracic outlet syndrome, 87
treatment of, 87–88
Neck weakness, 398, 398t
Necrotizing arteritis, 267
Necrotizing fasciitis, 654
Necrotizing myositis, 654
Nefazodone, for depression, 723t
Neglect (sensory phenomenon), 122, 150
caring for patient with, 155–156
hemispatial, 149–150, 149f, 151f, 804, 826

Neisseria meningitidis infections
meningitis. *See* Meningitis
Nelson syndrome, 469
Nemaline myopathy, **635,** 844
Neonate(s)
Candida infections in, 675f
seizures in, 238t
Nephrogenic systemic fibrosis, 19–21, 821–822
Nephrolithiasis, back pain in, 81
Nephropathy, contrast-induced, 15
Nerve biopsy, in peripheral neuropathy, 571
Nerve conduction studies
in back pain, 75
in peripheral neuropathy, 570, 570t
principles of, 32–33, 32f
Nerve growth factor, 41
Neural foraminal narrowing with radiculopathy, 78–79, 79f
Neuralgia(s)
glossopharyngeal, 397, 398t
trigeminal. *See* Trigeminal neuralgia
Neural network, large-scale, 142
Neurasthenia, 613
Neuritic plaque, in AD, 318–319, 319f
Neuroacanthocytosis, 352
Neuroblastoma, paraneoplastic syndromes in, 563
Neurocutaneous syndromes, **432**
Neurocysticercosis. *See* Cysticercosis
Neurodegeneration
in MS, 477
protein aggregation and, 227–229
Neurofibromatosis type 1 (NF1)
brain tumors and, 425t
clinical features of, 433
genetic factors in, 433
skin manifestations of, 433
Neurofibromatosis type 2 (NF2)
brain tumors and, 425t
clinical features of, 433
genetic factors in, 433
hearing loss in, 212
ocular involvement in, 188
Neurofibromin, 432
Neurogenetics, **218**
Neurogenic ptosis, 192
Neuroimaging, **13**. *See also specific disorders*
atlas of, 668–701f
CT. *See* Computed tomography (CT)
echo-planar MR imaging, 23
interventional neuroradiology, 25
magnetic resonance neurography, 23
MRA. *See* Magnetic resonance angiography (MRA)
MRI. *See* Magnetic resonance imaging (MRI)
myelography, 23–24
PET. *See* Positron emission tomography (PET)
spine interventions, 24–25
Neuroleptic malignant syndrome (NMS)
clinical features of, 355, 389
treatment of, 355
Neuroleptics. *See also* Antipsychotics
adverse effects of, 355
for dystonia, 349
for Tourette's syndrome, 353
Neurologic disease, **218**. *See also specific diseases*
angiography in, **25**
apoptosis in, 226–227
approach to the patient. *See* Neurologic examination/consultation
cell death in, 226–227
channelopathies, 220, 220t
in critically ill patient. *See* Critically ill patient, neurologic disorders in
depression in, 729
gene transcription disorders, 223
genome-wide association studies of, 218–219
imaging studies. *See* Neuroimaging
insomnia in, 165
ion channel disorders, 220, 220t
localization of, 9–10, 10t
mechanisms of, **218**
myelin disorders, 223–224, 223f, 224f
neurotransmitter/neurotransmitter receptor disorders, 221, 222t

Neurologic disease (*Cont.*):
neurotrophic factors in, 224–225, 224t
prevalence of, 2, 2t
protein aggregation in, 227–229
signaling pathway defects, 223
stem cell therapy for, 225–226
Neurologic examination/consultation, **4, 11, 12**
in back pain, 74
after cardiac bypass, 662–663, 662f
in CNS dysfunction, 660–663, 661t, 662f
in coma, 136–139
coordination examination, 9
cranial nerve examination, 6–7
in delirium, 127–128
in dizziness and vertigo, 99–100
in electrolyte disturbances, 663–665
gait examination, 9
in headache, 52
imaging studies. *See* Neuroimaging
localization of findings in nervous system, 9–10, 10t
mental status examination, 5–6
motor examination, 7–9, 801, 820
neurologic history in, **3**
neurologic method in, **2**
in olfactory/taste dysfunction, 204–205
in peripheral nervous system dysfunction, 665–667
sensory examination, 8–9
after solid organ transplantation, 663
video library, 11, 12
Neuromuscular blocking agents, 303–304, 645t
Neuromuscular jitter, 34
Neuromuscular junction disorders, **609**
autonomic dysfunction in, 386–388
clinical features of, 10t
reflex responses in, 104
weakness in, 108t, 109
Neuromyelitis optica, 408, 490–491
Neuromyotonia, 564, 622
Neuropathic pain, **44,** 50
Neuropathic (lower motor neuron) weakness, 104, 104t
Neuropathy(ies). *See also specific types and disorders*
alcoholic, 387
anti-Hu paraneoplastic, **607**
approach to, 568t
autoimmune autonomic, 387
autonomic, 578–59
chemotherapy-related, 438, 438t
diabetic. *See* Diabetic neuropathy
diphtheritic, 581–582
entrapment, 665
femoral, 594
gastric surgery–related, 592–593
hereditary. *See* Hereditary neuropathy(ies)
in hypothyroidism, 579
immune, 601–602, 602f
lateral femoral cutaneous, 594, 666f, 667
median, 593
with monoclonal gammopathy, **606**
multifocal motor, **606**
obstetric, 667
optic. *See* Optic neuropathy
paraneoplastic syndromes, 564–565
peripheral. *See* Peripheral neuropathy
peroneal, 594–595, 666, 666f
proximal femoral, 666, 666f
radial, 594, 665, 666f
in rheumatoid arthritis, 579
sciatic, 594
sensory, 579
sensory deficits in, 122–123
in systemic sclerosis, 580
trigeminal, **394,** 394t
ulnar, 594–595, 665–666, 666f
uremic, 580
vasculitic, **607**
Neuropathy, ataxia, retinitis pigmentosa (NARP) syndrome, 362t
Neuroprotective agents
for ischemic stroke, 261
for PD, 342
Neurosarcoid, 678–682f
Neurostimulation therapy
for cluster headache, 64
for SUNCT/SUNA, 65

Neurosyphilis
  clinical features of, 112
  neuroimaging in, 670–672f
  vs. viral meningitis, 505
Neurotransmitter(s)
  clinical aspects, 221, 222t, 806, 830
  functions, 221
  inotropic, 221
  metabotropic, 221
Neurotransmitter receptors, 221, 222t
Neurotrophic factors, in neurologic disease, 224–225, 224t
NF1. *See* Neurofibromatosis type 1 (NF1)
NF1 gene, 425t, 432
NF2. *See* Neurofibromatosis type 2 (NF2)
NF2 gene, 433
Nicotinamide adenine dinucleotide dehydrogenase (NADH) deficiency, 185
Nicotine, 221, 718t
Nicotinic acid, 645t, 646
  deficiency of. *See* Pellagra
Nifurtimox, for Chagas' disease, 548
Nightmares, 169
Night work, 171–172
Nimodipine
  for primary thunderclap headache, 70
  after subarachnoid hemorrhage, 308
Nitrates, 95
Nitrofurantoin, 587t
Nitroprusside, therapeutic monitoring of, 787t
NMDA receptors, 226, 560f
  antibodies to. *See* Anti-NMDA receptor antibodies
Nocardia spp. infections, chronic meningitis in, 529t
Nocebo effect, 43
Nociceptor(s), primary afferent, 40, 41f3f, 42f
Nociceptor-induced inflammation, 41
Non-24 hour sleep-wake disorder, **172**
Nonaka's distal myopathy, 633, 634t
Noncompressive myelopathies, 403, **406**
Nonsteroidal anti-inflammatory drugs (NSAIDs)
  for AD, 321
  adverse effects of, 45
  for back pain, 82
  for episcleritis and scleritis, 181
  for migraine, 58t
  for neck pain, 88
  for pain, 45, 46t
  for spinal stenosis, 78
  for tension-type headache, 122
  topical, for conjunctivitis, 180
Norepinephrine, 222t, 380
Normal-pressure hydrocephalus, 327–328, 327f
Normeperidine, 47
Norrie disease, 212t
Nortriptyline
  adverse effects of, 723t
  for depression, 723t
  dosage of, 723t
  for migraine prevention, 60, 61t
  for pain, 46t, 49, 50, 490
Notch-3, 268
Nothnagel's syndrome, 193
NREM sleep, 158, 159f
NRG1, 713
NSAIDs. *See* Nonsteroidal anti-inflammatory drugs (NSAIDs)
Nucleus accumbens, 715–716
Nucleus of the solitary tract (NTS), 201f, 202
Numbness, **117**. *See also* Sensation
Nutritional diseases, neuropathies in, 591–592
Nutritional short stature, 460
Nutritional support/therapy, for MS, 489
Nystagmus, 99, 99t, **195,** 823

Object recognition, 152
Obsessive-compulsive disorder (OCD), **728**
Obstetric neuropathies, 667
Obstructive sleep apnea, 169, 828
  daytime sleepiness in, 166
  diagnosis of, 163t
  polysomnography in, 167f
  treatment of, 163t
Occipital lobe stroke, 187
Occipital nerve stimulation
  for cluster headache, 64
  for hemicrania continua, 69
  for SUNCT/SUNA prevention, 65
Occipitotemporal network, 152
Occupational illness
  hearing loss, 216
  shift-work disorder, 171–172, 804–805, 827
Octreotide
  for acromegaly, 464
  adverse effects of, 464
  for postprandial orthostatic hypotension, 391
Ocular alignment, 177
"Ocular bobbing," 137
"Ocular dipping," 137
Ocular disorders, **179**. *See also* Visual loss
  in myasthenia gravis, 610
  painful or red eye, 179–182, 806, 829
  video library, 198
Ocular flutter, 197
Ocular lubricants, 180
Oculocephalic reflexes, 137
Oculomotor nerve, 6
Oculomotor nerve palsy, 176, 193
Oculomotor nerve paresis, 176
Oculopharyngeal dystrophy, 192, 625t, 633
Odontoid fracture, 700f
Olanzapine
  for acute alcohol intoxication, 758
  adverse effects of, 739t
  for schizophrenia, 739t, 740
Olfactory bulb, 199, 200f
Olfactory disorders, **202**
  diseases and conditions associated with, 202–204, 203t, 806, 829
  epidemiology of, 202, 202f
  etiology of, 202, 203t
  evaluation of, 204–205
  taste disorders and, 204
  treatment of, 205–206
Olfactory nerve, 6
Olfactory system, 199–200, 200f
Olig 2 gene, 224
Oligodendroglioma, 428–429
Oligomer(s), 228
Olivopontocerebellar degeneration, 190, 195
Onchocerca volvulus/onchocerciasis, 181, 182
Ondansetron
  for ataxia/tremor in MS, 489
  for nausea, 66
One-and-a-half syndrome, 195
Opa1, 228
Ophthalmopathy, Graves', 191, 644
Ophthalmoplegia
  internuclear, 195, 196f
  neuromuscular causes of, 618, 620t
Opioid(s)
  action of, 47, 221, 718t, 719f
  administration of
    intrathecal, 48
    intravenous, 47
    patient-controlled, 47
  adverse effects of, 761
    delirium, 128, 129t
    management of, 48
    respiratory depression, 47
  for back pain, 82
  COX inhibitor combinations, 48
  endogenous, 44
  for migraine, 58t, 60
  most commonly abused, 761
  neurobiology of, 761–762, 761t
  overdosage/poisoning with, 763–765, 764, 820, 850
  for pain, 46t, 47–48, 50
  pharmacology of, 762–763
  for restless legs syndrome, 166
  systems effects of, 763
  toxicity of, 763
  withdrawal from, 764, 849–850
Opioid abuse/dependence, **761,** 849–850
  diagnosis of, 761
  prevention of, 766
  treatment of, **764**
    agonist medications in, 764–765
    antagonist medications in, 764–765
    medication-free, 766
    residential program in, 766
    withdrawal management in, 764
Opioid receptors, 47, 761–762, 761t
Oppenheim's dystonia, 348
Opsoclonus, 197, 563
Opsoclonus-myoclonus syndrome, paraneoplastic, 563
Optic atrophy, 185, 185f, 205
Optic chiasm, 174, 828
Optic cup, 188, 188f
Optic disc
  drusen, 179, 186, 186f
  edema, 185–186, 186f
Optic gliomas, 448
Optic nerve, 174
  disorders of, visual field defects in, 178–179
  examination of, 6
Optic neuritis, 176, **184**
  color desaturation in, 177
  in MS, 184–185, 478
  paraneoplastic, 565
  retrobulbar, 176, 184, 185f
  visual field defects in, 179
Optic neuropathy
  anterior ischemic, 184, 184f
  compressive, 179
  drug-induced, 185
  Leber, 179, 185
  nutritional, 179
  posterior ischemic, 184
  toxic, 179, 185
Optokinetic reflex, 174
Oral cancer, alcohol effects on, 755
Oral contraceptives, drug interactions of, 255
Orbit, 191
Orexin, 160, 168, 204
Organic Brain Syndrome Scale, 127
Organ of Corti, 207, 207f
Organophosphates, 588t
Orgasm, headaches associated with, 70
Oromandibular dystonia, 349
Orthostatic hypotension
  approach to the patient, 383–385
  in autonomic dysfunction, 383, 383t
  causes of, 93t, 383t
  clinical features of, 94, 383t
  dizziness in, 98
  falls and, 115
  neurogenic, 94–95
  nonneurogenic, 383t
  pathophysiology of, 90, 93–94, 94f
  in PD, 345
  prevalence of, 383t
  treatment of, 95, 390–391, 390t
Oscillopsia, 98, 196
Osler-Weber-Rendu syndrome (hereditary hemorrhagic telangiectasia), 292
Osteoarthritis
  back pain in, 79
  neck pain in, 86
Osteogenesis imperfecta, otosclerosis in, 209
Osteomyelitis, vertebral, 80
Osteoporosis
  back pain in, 80
  treatment of, 80
  vertebral fracture in, 80
Osteosclerosis, 80
Otitis media
  brain abscess associated with, 518–519
  hearing loss in, 209
Otoacoustic emissions, 214
Otoconia, 100
Otosclerosis, 209, 213
Otoscopy, 209
Ovarian cancer, paraneoplastic syndromes in, 564
Ovary, teratoma of, 560f, 563
Overlap syndrome, in inflammatory myopathy, 650

- Oxazepam, 725t
- Oxcarbazepine
  - adverse effects of, 249t, 735t
  - for bipolar disorder, 735, 735t
  - for epilepsy, 249t
  - for focal seizures, 246
  - for pain, 46t
  - pharmacology of, 249t, 735t
  - for trigeminal neuralgia, 393
- Oxidative phosphorylation, 638
- Oxybutynin
  - for detrusor spasticity, 413, 490
  - for sleep enuresis, 170
- Oxycodone, for pain, 46t

- P1 syndromes, 276f, 277f, 278
- P2 syndromes, 276f, 277f, 278
- *p53* gene, 425t
- Paclitaxel, 584t
- Paget's disease of bone, back pain in, 80
- Pain
  - acute, treatment of, **45**
  - chronic, **48**
    - treatment of, **49**
      - anticonvulsants and antiarrhythmics for, 50
      - antidepressants for, 49–50, 49t
      - opioids for, 50
  - depression and, 48
  - modulation in different situations/individuals, 43–44
  - in MS, 489–490
  - neuropathic, **44,** 50
  - pathophysiology of, **40**
    - ascending pathways, 43, 43f
    - central mechanisms, 42–43, 42f
    - pain sensory system, 40–42
    - peripheral mechanisms, 41f, 42f
  - perception of, 51
  - psychological variables, 43–44
  - sympathetically maintained, 45
  - testing sense of, 119, 120t
- Palinopsia, 278
- Paliperidone, 739, 739t
- Pallister-Hall syndrome, 448
- Pancoast tumor, 87
- Pancreas, alcohol effects on, 755
- Pancreatic disease, back pain in, 81
- Pancuronium, 303
- Panencephalitis
  - progressive rubella, 518
  - subacute sclerosing, 517–518
- Panic attack, 818, 846
- Panic disorder, **721,** 846–847
  - clinical features of, 721
  - diagnosis of, 721–722, 721t
  - etiology of, 722
  - pathology of, 722
  - treatment of, 722
- Panuveitis, 182
- Papilledema, 185–186, 186f, 205
- Paralysis, **103**
  - periodic. *See* Periodic paralysis
  - sleep, 163t, 168
  - Todd's, 232
  - tongue, 398
- Paramyotonia congenita, 220t, 622, 641t, 642–643
- Paraneoplastic syndromes
  - ataxia in, 368–369
  - ion channel defects causing, 220t
  - limbic encephalitis, 329
  - neurologic, **558,** 558t, 842
    - acute necrotizing myopathy, 565
    - approach to the patient, 559–561
    - cerebellar degeneration, 562
    - CNS and dorsal root ganglia, 559–560
    - incidence of, 558
    - nerve and muscle, 560–561
    - opsoclonus-myoclonus syndrome, 563
    - pathogenesis of, 558–559, 559t, 560f
    - peripheral neuropathies, 564–565
    - sensory neuronopathy, 563–564
    - in spinal cord disease/injury, 563
    - stiff-person syndrome, 563
    - visual, 559t, 565
- Paraparesis, 107–108
- Paraphasia, 143
- Paraplegia(s), spastic familial, 378–379, 412
- *Paraplegin* gene, 379
- Parasomnias, **169,** 805, 828
- Parathyroid disease, muscle weakness in, 644
- Paratonia, 103
- Parcopa, for PD, 343t
- Paresis, 103
- Paresthesia, 117
- Parietal cortex, posterior, 149, 149f
- Parietal lesions, 195
- Parietofrontal network, **149,** 149f
- Parinaud's syndrome, 195, 430
- *parkin* gene, 334–335, 338
- Parkinsonian dementia syndromes, **326**
- Parkinsonism
  - atypical, 335–336, 335t, 337t
  - disorders associated with, 355
  - drug-induced, 355
  - gait disorders in, 111t, 112
  - lower body, 112
  - secondary, 335–336, 335t, 337t
- Parkinson's disease (PD), **333**
  - autonomic disturbances in, 345
  - clinical features of, 333, 334t
  - delirium in, 127
  - dementia in, 325, 344–345
  - depression in, 344
  - differential diagnosis of, 333–336, 335f, 335t, 336f, 337t, 808–809, 833
  - etiology of, 336–338, 337f
  - falls in, 115
  - familial, 228
  - frontal lobe syndrome in, 155
  - gait disorders in, 112
  - genetic factors in, 228, 337t, 338
  - hallmark features of, 333, 334f
  - nondopaminergic features of, 344–345
  - nonmotor features of, 344–345
  - ocular involvement in, 195
  - olfactory dysfunction in, 199, 203–204
  - orthostatic hypotension in, 95
  - pathogenesis of, 336–338, 337f
  - pathophysiology of, 338, 339f
  - prevalence of, 333
  - vs. progressive supranuclear palsy, 325
  - psychoses in, 344
  - REM sleep behavior disorder in, 170, 345
  - sleep disorders in, 165, 345
  - treatment of, **338,** 833–834
    - amantadine, 342
    - benztropine, 342
    - COMT inhibitors, 342, 343t
    - current methods, 345–346, 346f
    - deep brain stimulation, 343, 346
    - dopamine agonists, 341, 343t, 346
    - levodopa, 338–341, 340f, 343t, 346
    - MAO-B inhibitors, 341–342, 343t, 346
    - neuroprotective agents, 342
    - nonmotor and nondopaminergic features, 344–345
    - nonpharmacologic, 345
    - surgical, 342–344
    - trihexyphenidyl, 342
  - tremor in, 347
- Parkinson's disease dementia (PDD), **326,** 344–345
- Paroxetine, 722, 723t
- Paroxysmal dyskinesias, 352
- Paroxysmal hemicrania, 51, 63t, 64–65, 66t
- Paroxysmal nocturnal dyspnea, 165
- Paroxysmal nonkinesigenic dyskinesia (PNKD), 352
- Parsonage-Turner syndrome, 595
- Pars planitis, 182
- Patent foramen ovale, 264t
- Patient-controlled analgesia, 47
- Patient Health Questionnaire-2, in war veterans, 746, 747t
- Patrick sign, 74
- Pavor nocturnus, 169
- PD. *See* Parkinson's disease (PD)
- PDD (Parkinson's disease dementia), **326,** 344–345
- Peduncular hallucinosis, 278
- Pegvisomant, for acromegaly, 464
- Pellagra
  - clinical features of, 328
  - global considerations, 592
  - treatment of, 592
- Pendred syndrome, 212, 212t
- D-Penicillamine, adverse effects of
  - myopathy, 645t, 647
  - optic neuropathy, 185
- Penicillin G, for meningitis, 499t, 501
- Pentazocine, 50
- Penumbra, 294
- Perfusion magnetic resonance imaging, 23
- Perilymphatic fistula, 210
- Perimeter, computer-driven, 177, 178f
- Periodic hypothermia syndrome, 449
- Periodic limb movement disorder, **166**
- Periodic limb movements of sleep, 166, 167f, 834
- Periodic paralysis
  - clinical features of, 641t
  - hyperkalemic, 642
  - hypokalemic, 640–642, 642f
  - ion channel defects causing, 220t
- Peripheral nerve(s)
  - components, 41f
  - cutaneous fields of, 120f
  - pain mechanisms, 40–42
- Peripheral neuropathy, **566,** 843. *See also specific disorders*
  - alcohol and, 754
  - approach to, **566,** 567f, 568t
    - distribution of weakness, 566–567
    - hereditary neuropathy, 568
    - medical conditions, 568
    - pattern recognition, 568, 569t
    - sensory involvement, 567–568
    - systems involved, 566
    - temporal evolution, 568
    - upper motor neuron involvement, 568
  - CSPN, 594
  - drug-induced, 438t, 584–585t, 585–590, 586–587t
  - electrodiagnostic studies in, 568–570, 570t
  - EMG in, 570, 570t
  - gait disorders in, 113
  - hereditary. *See* Hereditary neuropathy(ies)
  - HIV-related, 543–544
  - laboratory evaluation of, 570–571, 570t
  - malignancy-related, 583–584
  - nerve biopsies in, 571
  - nerve conduction studies in, 570, 570t
  - nutritional, 591–592
  - painful sensory, 578t
  - paraneoplastic, 564–565
  - skin biopsies in, 571
  - toxic causes of, 585–591, 586–588t
  - weakness in, 106, 108, 566–567
- Peripheral sensitization, 41
- Perisylvian network, **142**
- Periventricular white matter disease, 268
- Permeability transition pore, 227, 227f
- Peroneal neuropathy, 594–595, 666, 666f, 818, 846
- PERRLA, 176
- Persistent vegetative state, 132, 803–804, 825
- Personality disorders, **737**
- PET. *See* Positron emission tomography (PET)
- Petrous bone fractures, 417
- PGC-1α, 228
- Phakomatosis(es), **432**
- Phencyclidine (PCP)
  - abuse/overdose of, 771
  - actions of, 718t, 771
  - adverse effects of, 129t
- Phenelzine
  - adverse effects of, 62, 723t
  - for depression, 723t
  - for migraine prevention, 62
  - for posttraumatic headache, 68
- Phenobarbital, 248t
- Phenothiazines, adverse effects of
  - ocular, 190
  - orthostatic hypotension, 95

Phenytoin
adverse effects of, 246
hepatotoxicity, 578t
long-term, 246
neurologic, 247t, 578t, 587t
systemic, 247t
dosage of, 247t
drug interactions of, 247t
for epilepsy, 247t
for neuromyotonia, 565
for neuropathy, 578t
for pain, 46t, 50, 489
pharmacology of, 247t
therapeutic monitoring of, 787t
for trigeminal neuralgia, 393
Pheochromocytoma, headache in, 69
Phobic disorders, **726**
Phosphofructokinase deficiency (type VII glycogenosis), 637
Photopigments, 177
Photoreceptors, 174
Phototherapy
for circadian rhythm sleep disorders, 172–173
for shift-work disorder, 172
Physical dependence, 716
Physical restraints, in delirium, 126, 131
Physical therapy
for back pain, 82
for vertigo, 102t
Physostigmine, for anticholinergic overdose, 140
Pick bodies, 149
Pick's disease, 324, 325f
Pilizaeus-Merzbacher disease, 379
Pilocarpine
for acute angle-closure glaucoma, 182
adverse effects of, 177
in diagnosis of tonic pupil, 176
Pineal region tumors, 176, 195, 430
Pinguecula, 179–180
PINK1, 228, 338
Piracetam, for myoclonus, 353
Piroxicam, for paroxysmal hemicrania, 65
PIT-1, 441, 442
Pituitary apoplexy, 190, 443–444
Pituitary axes, 440f
Pituitary disorders, muscle weakness in, 644
Pituitary gland
anatomy of, 440–441, 440f
basic fibroblast growth factor in, 447
development of, 439t, 441
dysplasia, 442
hormones produced by, 439–440
tests of function of, 445t
Pituitary hormones
expression and regulation of, 439t, 813, 838
secretion of, 439–440, 440f
Pituitary tumors (adenomas), **444,** 813, 839
in Carney syndrome, 447, 447t
classification of, 432, 444, 446t
diagnosis of, **449**
histologic evaluation in, 451
laboratory studies in, 450, 451t
local mass effects, 449–450, 449t
MRI in, 450, 450f
ophthalmologic evaluation in, 450
etiology of, 446–447
in familial acromegaly, 447, 447t
gonadotropin-producing, 471–472
hormone-excess syndromes due to, 440
local mass effects of, 449–450, 449t
in McCune-Albright syndrome, 447
in MEN 1, 447, 447t
metabolic effects of, 449
metastatic, 448
nonfunctioning, 432, 471–472, 472f
ocular signs in, 179, 190
pathogenesis of, 446–447
sellar mass lesions, 448, 449t
treatment of, 432, 448, 451–453, 452f
TSH-secreting, 473
Pizotifen, for migraine prevention, 61t
Placebo effect, 43, 44f
Plaque, neuritic, 319, 319f
Plaques jaunes, 416
Plasmapheresis
for Guillain-Barré syndrome, 604
for myasthenia gravis, 616
Platelet(s), reference values for, 777t
Pleconaril, for viral meningitis, 507
Pleomorphic xanthoastrocytomas, 429
Plexopathy
brachial, 595–596, 697–698f
evaluation and treatment of, 598
lumbosacral, 597, 597t
perioperative, 596
radiation-induced, 597
PML (progressive multifocal leukoencephalopathy), 516–517
Pneumococcal infections
meningitis. *See* Meningitis
Pneumonia
delirium in, 129, 129t
olfactory dysfunction and, 202
PNKD (paroxysmal nonkinesigenic dyskinesia), 352
Podophyllin, adverse effects of, 586t
POEMS syndrome (Crow-Fukase syndrome), 564
Poisoning/drug overdose, laboratory evaluation in, 786–788t
Poliovirus infection, weakness in, 108
Polyarteritis nodosa
neuropathy in, 607
ocular involvement in, 181
Polydrug abuse, 772
Polymyalgia rheumatica, 184, 621
Polymyositis, **648**
clinical features of, 109, 648–649, 649t
diagnosis of, 655–657, 656f, 656t, 844–845
differential diagnosis of, 653–655
drug-induced, 655
muscle damage in, 652, 652f
prognosis of, 659
treatment of, 657–659, 817, 845
viral infections and, 653
Polymyxin-bacitracin, for conjunctivitis, 180
Polyneuropathy
acute inflammatory demyelinating, 600t, 601–602
acute toxic, 109
critical illness, 581
cryptogenic sensory and sensorimotor, 594
distal symmetric, HIV-related, 582
familial amyloid, 575t, 577
large-fiber, 122–123
sensory deficits in, 122–123
small-fiber, 123
weakness in, 109
Polyradiculopathy, in HIV infection, 582
Polysomnography
definition, 158
in obstructive sleep apnea, 167f
in periodic limb movements of sleep, 166, 167f
in sleep disorder evaluation, 162–163, 163t
POMC gene, 466
Pompe disease (acid maltase deficiency; type II glycogenosis), 636–637
Pons
histoplasmosis of, 673f
inferior of, 281f
mid, 282f
superior, 283f
Porphyria(s)
autonomic dysfunction in, 387
clinical features of, 576
neuropathy in, 575t, 576–577
Positron emission tomography (PET)
in cluster headache, 56f
in migraine, 54, 55f
in mild cognitive impairment, 316f
in neurologic disease, 23
in PD, 334, 336f
in stroke, 286
Postconcussion syndrome, 421–422, 837
Posterior cerebral artery
fetal, 277
lesion in territory of, 147, 152, 154
occlusion of, 179, 277–2778, 277f
Posterior column-medial lemniscal pathway, 118, 119f
Posterior cortical atrophy syndrome, 151
Posterior fossa brain tumor, 53
Postictal state, 135
Postinfectious myelitis, 408–409
Posttraumatic stress disorder (PTSD)
biological correlates of, 743–744
clinical features of, 743–744
definition of, 743
diagnosis of, 727t, 818, 847
etiology of, 727–728
pathophysiology of, 727–728
treatment of, 728
in war veterans, 743–744, 748–749
Postural control, 110, 114
Postural orthostatic tachycardia syndrome, 67, **388,** 810, 835
Potassium channels, disorders of, **643**
Pott's disease, 80
Prader-Willi syndrome, 219
genetic factors in, 443
hypopituitarism due to, 443
Pramipexole
adverse effects of, 341
for PD, 341, 343t
for restless legs syndrome, 163t, 166, 355
Praziquantel, for cysticercosis, 522
Prednisone
for ACTH deficiency, 466
adverse effects of, 646, 658
for Bell's palsy, 396
for cluster headache prevention, 64, 64t
for Duchenne's muscular dystrophy, 628
for Graves' ophthalmopathy, 191
for sinusitis with hyposmia, 206
for vasculitic neuropathy, 607
Prefrontal network, 154
Pregabalin
adverse effects of, 578t
for neuropathy, 578t
for pain, 46t, 50, 490
Pregnancy
alcohol use in, 756
epilepsy in, 254–255
in MS, 483
prolactinoma in, 457–458
retinal artery occlusion in, 183
Presbycusis, 209
Presbyopia, 175
Presbyosmia, 202
Presenilin, in AD, 319–320
Pressure ulcers, prevention of, 413
Presynaptic rundown, 610
Presyncope, 89
Primary afferent(s), 40, 41f
Primary afferent nociceptors, 40, 41f, 42f
Primary Care PTSD Screen, 746, 747t
Primary cough headache, **69**
Primary exertional headache, **69**
Primary intraventricular hemorrhage, 290
Primary lateral sclerosis, 378, 412
Primary olfactory cortex, 199–200, 200f
Primary progressive aphasia, 148–149, 156, 323
Primary sex headache, **70**
Primary stabbing headache, **69**
Primary taste cortex (PTC), 202
Primary thunderclap headache, **70**
Primate immunodeficiency viruses, 53
Primidone
adverse effects of, 248t
for essential tremor, 348
for myoclonus, 353
pharmacology of, 248t
Primitive reflexes, 8
Prion(s)
decontamination of, 556
definition of, 549
terminology related to, 549t
transmissibility of, 550–551
Prion disease(s), **549,** 841–842. *See also* Creutzfeldt-Jakob disease
clinical features of, 554–555
dementia due to, 326
diagnosis of, 555

Prion disease(s) (*Cont.*):
differential diagnosis of, 555
epidemiology of, 550–551, 550t
human *PRNP* gene polymorphisms in, 553
infectious, **553,** 556f
inherited, 552–553
laboratory evaluation of, 555–556, 556f
neuropathology of, 554
pathogenesis of, 551–552, 551f, 552t
prevention of, 557
prion strains in, 551–552, 552t
species barrier in, 552
spectrum of, 550
sporadic, 552–553
treatment of, 557
types of, 550, 550t
Prion-like proteins, 557
Prion proteins, 549, 549f
Prion strains, 551–552, 552t
PRNP gene, 549t, 553
Procarbazine, 438t
Prochlorperazine, for migraine, 58t, 120
Progranulin, in FTD, 323
Progressive external ophthalmoplegia, **639**
clinical features of, 639
differential diagnosis of, 613
genetic factors in, 639
hearing loss in, 212
with ragged red fibers, 639
Progressive multifocal leukoencephalopathy (PML), 516–517, 547
Progressive muscular atrophy, 370
Progressive muscular dystrophies, 625t
Progressive myoclonus epilepsy, 235t
Progressive polyradiculopathy, HIV-related, 582
Progressive rubella panencephalitis, 518
Progressive supranuclear palsy
balance disorders in, 114
clinical features of, 325
falls in, 114
gait disorders in, 112
parkinsonism in, 336
pathology of, 325, 337t
vs. PD, 325
Prolactin, **453**
action of, 453
laboratory evaluation of, 445t
secretion of, 453
synthesis of, 453
Prolactinoma, **455**
clinical features of, 455–456
diagnosis of, 455–456
etiology of, 455
during pregnancy, 457–458
prevalence of, 455
screening tests for, 451t
treatment of, 456–458, 456f
Promitochondrial agents, for Huntington's disease, 351
PROMM (proximal myotonic myopathy), 622
Pronator drift, 7, 820, 821
PROP-1, 441, 442
Propranolol
adverse effects of, 61t
for ataxia/tremor in MS, 489
for essential tremor, 347–348
for migraine prevention, 60, 61t
for phobic disorders, 726
for sex headache prevention, 70
Proprioception, 118
Proptosis, 190–191
Prosody, 148
Prosopagnosia, 152, 177
Prostaglandin(s), pain and, 41, 42f
Prostaglandin analogues
for acute angle-closure glaucoma, 182
for glaucoma, 188
Prostate cancer
back pain in, 81
CNS metastases in, 433t
paraneoplastic syndromes in, 565
Prostate-specific antigen (PSA), reference values, 784t
Prostatitis, back pain in, 81
Prosthetic heart valve, antithrombotic prophylaxis for, 264t
Protein(s)
aggregation of, in neurologic disease, 227–229
muscular dystrophy-associated, 627, 628f, 629f
prion, 549, 549f
prion-like, 557
Protein C, reference values, 777t
Protein C deficiency, 183
Protein S
deficiency, 183
reference values, 777t
Protriptyline, for narcolepsy, 163t, 169
Proximal femoral neuropathy, 666, 666f
Proximal myotonic myopathy (PROMM), 622
PrP amyloid, 549t
PS-1, 319
PS-2, 319–320
Pseudoathetosis, 118
Pseudobulbar palsy, 104
Pseudodementia(s), 330
Pseudoephedrine, for orthostatic hypotension, 95
Pseudopapilledema, 186
Pseudotumor, orbital, 191
Pseudotumor cerebri, 67, 68, 186, 186f
Psoriasis, ocular involvement in, 181
Psychiatric/psychological disorders, **720**. *See also specific disorders*
back pain in, 81
biology of, **710**
classification of, 720
dementia due to, 330–331
gait disorders in, 113
in the homeless, 741
insomnia in, 164–165
prevalence of, 720
primary care physician's responsibility in, 720
syncope in, 96, 97
in war veterans. *See* War veterans, neuropsychiatric illnesses in
Psychogenic amnesia, 330
Psychogenic movement disorders, 356
Psychogenic seizures, 244
Psychological (motivational) dependence, 716
Psychosis(es)
in epilepsy, 253
in PD, 344
Psychosocial short stature, 460
Psychostimulants, 718t
Psychotherapy
for depression, 731
for generalized anxiety disorder, 724
for panic disorder, 722
for phobic disorders, 727
referral for, 720
for stress disorders, 728
PTEN gene mutations, 425t
Pterygium, 180, 192
Ptosis, 191–192, 618, 620t
PTSD. *See* Posttraumatic stress disorder (PTSD)
"Puff of smoke" lesion, 268
Pulmonary embolism (PE), after subarachnoid hemorrhage, 308–309
Pulmonary function tests, reference values, 797t
"Punch drunk" syndrome, 329
Pupil(s), 175–177
Argyll Robertson, 176
in coma, 136–137
inequality in size of, 176
Marcus Gunn, 176, 176f
tonic, 176
Pupillary defect, afferent, 176
Pure alexia without agraphia, 144t, 146–147
Pure autonomic failure
autonomic dysfunction in, 388
orthostatic hypotension in, 95
Pure motor hemiparesis, 266
Pure myopathy syndromes, **640**
Pure sensory stroke, 266
Pure tone audiometry, 213
Pure word deafness, 144t
Pyramidal (corticospinal) system, 105f
Pyrazinamide, for tuberculous meningitis, 515
Pyridostigmine
for myasthenia gravis, 614
for orthostatic hypotension, 95, 390
Pyridoxine (vitamin B_6)
deficiency of, 592
reference range for, 788t
toxicity of, 587t, 589
for tuberculous meningitis, 515
Pyrimethamine, for toxoplasmosis, 522

Quadrantanopia, 178f
Quadriparesis, 108
Quadriplegic fever, 413
Quantitative sudomotor axon reflex test, 384–385, 385t
Quetiapine
adverse effects of, 739t
for dementia, 331
for psychosis in Huntington's disease, 351
for schizophrenia, 739t, 740
Quinine, 209

Rabies, 512
Rad, 799t
Radial neuropathy, 594, 665, 666f
Radiation-derived units, 799t
Radiation dose, 799t
Radiation therapy
for acromegaly, 464
adverse effects of
cataract, 188
neurologic, 437
pituitary, 443, 452, 812, 838
plexopathy, 597
for metastatic brain tumors, 434
for pituitary tumors, 452
Radiculopathy, 71, 595, 595t
Radiofrequency denervation, 83–84
Radiofrequency thermal rhizotomy, for trigeminal neuralgia, 393
Ragged-red fibers, 192
Ramsay Hunt syndrome, 100, 396
Ranibizumab, for macular degeneration, 189
RAS (reticular activating system), 133
Rasagiline, for PD, 341–342, 343t
Rathke's cyst, 448
Reactive arthritis (Reiter's syndrome), 181
Reading, assessment of, 144
Recoverin, 559t
Reelin, 713–714
Referred pain, 43
to back, 72, 80–81
convergence-projection hypothesis of, 42f
Reflex(es), testing of, 8. *See also specific reflexes*
Reflex sympathetic dystrophy, 45, 389–390
Reflex syncope, 89
Refractive state, 175
Refsum disease, 190, 575t, 576
Rehabilitation
of alcoholics, 759–760
in ischemic stroke management, 261
in opiate abusers, 766
of spinal cord disorders, **413,** 413t
Relapsing polychondritis, 181
Relative afferent pupil defect, 176, 176f
Relaxation rate, 17
Rem, 799t
REM sleep, 158, 159f
REM sleep behavior disorder, 160, 170, 204, 312, 345, 828
Repetition, assessment of, 144
Resistance strength training, 115
Respiratory function, during sleep, 161
Respiratory tract infections
mastoiditis, 194, 518–519
olfactory disorders in, 202
Restless legs syndrome, 163t, **166, 355,** 805, 809, 827, 834
Reticular activating system (RAS), 133
Reticulospinal pathway, 105f
Retina, 174
detached, 178, 187, 187f
infarction of, 183
lesions of, 178

Retinal artery occlusion, 183, 183f
Retinal vein occlusion, 183–184, 184f
Retinitis pigmentosa, 19–190, 190f
Retinoids, for olfactory dysfunction, 206
Retinopathy
cancer-associated (paraneoplastic), 565
hypertensive, 183, 183f
Retrobulbar tumor, 190
Retrocollis, 349
Retroperitoneal hemorrhage, 81
Retropharyngeal soft tissue mass, 699f
Retrovirus(es), myopathies associated with, 409, 653
Rett syndrome, 223
Reverse straight-leg raising sign, 74
Reverse transcriptase enzyme, HIV, 538
Reversible posterior leukoencephalopathy, 268, 290
Rheumatic fever, prophylaxis for cardiac complications of, 264t
Rheumatoid arthritis
juvenile, 181
neck pain in, 86
neuropathy in, 579
ocular involvement in, 181
Ribavirin, for viral encephalitis, 514
Riboflavin (vitamin B_2)
reference range for, 788t
supplements, for migraine, 206
Rifampin
prophylactic, 501
for tuberculous meningitis, 515
Right-left confusion, 147
Rigidity, 103
Riley-Day syndrome, 388
Riluzole, for ALS, 377
Rinne test, 213
Risperidone
adverse effects of, 739t
for psychosis in Huntington's disease, 351
for schizophrenia, 739t, 740
Rituximab
for cerebellar degeneration, 563
for inflammatory myopathies, 658
Rivastigmine
for AD, 321
for Parkinson's disease dementia, 345
Rizatriptan, for migraine, 58t, 59, 59t
Rocky Mountain spotted fever (RMSF), 500
Rod(s), 174
Romberg maneuver, 9
Romberg's sign, 114, 118, 821
Ropinirole
adverse effects of, 341
for PD, 341, 343t
for restless legs syndrome, 163t, 166, 355
Rosenbaum card, 175, 175f
Roth's spots, 182
Rotigotine
adverse effects of, 341
for PD, 341, 343t
Rubella (German measles), congenital, 518
Rubeola (measles), complications of, 518
Rubrospinal pathway, 105f
Rufinamide, 249t

Saccades, 177
Saccadomania, 197
Saccular aneurysm, 304–305
Sacral insufficiency fracture, 700f
Sacral pain, 81
Sagittal sinus thrombosis, Bálint's syndrome in, 151
St. Vitus' dance, 352
Salicylates, 209
Saliva, artificial, 205
Salt therapy, for syncope, 92
Salty taste sensation, 201
SANDO (sensory ataxic neuropathy and ophthalmoparesis), 361t
Sandostatin-LAR, for acromegaly, 464
Sarcoidosis
clinical features of, 443
MRI in, 678–682f

Sarcoidosis (*Cont.*):
neurologic features of
chronic meningitis, 532t
myelopathy, 408
peripheral neuropathy, 580
ocular involvement in, 180, 181, 182
weakness in, 107
SCA. *See* Spinocerebellar ataxia (SCA)
SCAN1 (spinocerebellar ataxia with neuropathy), 364t
Schirmer strip, 180
Schistosomiasis, myelitis in, 409
Schizoaffective disorder, 738
Schizophrenia, **712, 738**
catatonic-type, 738
CATIE study of, 740
chemosensory alterations in, 204
clinical features of, 712, 738
diabetes mellitus type 2 in, 740
differential diagnosis of, 738
disorganized-type, 738
epidemiology of, 712, 738
genetic factors in, 713
insomnia in, 165
neuroimaging of, 712
neuropathology of, 712
paranoid-type, 738
pathogenesis of, 713–714
pathophysiology of, 738
residual-type, 738
treatment of, 738–740, 739t
types of, 738
Schizophreniform disorder, 738
Schwannoma, 431–432, 431f
Schwannomatosis, familial, 425t
Sciatica, 84–85
Sciatic neuropathy, 594
Scleritis, 181
Scleroderma. *See* Systemic sclerosis (scleroderma)
SCN1B gene, 235t
Scopolamine
ocular effects, 177
for vertigo, 102t
Scotoma, 178f, 179, 187
Seasonal affective disorder, 731
Secondary taste cortex, 202
Second impact syndrome, 420
Segawa variant dystonia, 348
Seizure(s), **231**. *See also* Epilepsy
absence, 233
approach to the patient, 241, 242f, 831–832
atonic, 234
in brain abscess, 519
in brain tumor, 424
chemotherapy-induced, 438t
classification of, 231t, 232–233, 807–808, 830
coma in, 135
complex febrile, 238
definition of, 231
delirium and, 129, 129t, 329
differential diagnosis of, 243–244, 244t
EEG studies in, 241–243
electrographic, 8f, 26–27
electrophysiologic studies in, 241–243
etiology of, 236–239, 238t, 239t
focal, **232,** 807, 830
AEDs for, 246, 250
with dyscognitive features, 232–233
evolution to generalized seizures, 233
without dyscognitive features, 232
focal sensory, 124
generalized, **233**
absence, 233
AEDs for, 250
atonic, 234
evolution from focal seizures, 233
myoclonic, 234
tonic-clonic, 233–234
after head injury, 417–418
history and examination in, 241
in HIV infection, 548
interictal behavior related to, 53
laboratory evaluation of, 241
magnetoencephalography in, 29, 243

Seizure(s) (*Cont.*):
mechanisms of, **239**
epileptogenesis in, 240
initiation phase, 239–240
propagation phase, 239–240
in meningitis, 498
neuroimaging in, 243
nocturnal, 170
psychogenic, 245
vs. syncope, 96, 243–244, 244t
temporal lobe, 154
treatment of, **245,** 807, 831
avoidance of precipitating factors in, 245
underlying conditions–related, 245
unclassifiable, 234
Selective serotonin reuptake inhibitors (SSRIs)
adverse effects of, 723t, 732–733
serotonin syndrome, 732
sexual dysfunction, 732–733
for depression, 321, 331, 723t, 732–733, 732f
drug interactions of, 724t
for narcolepsy, 169
for neuropathic pain, 50
for panic disorder, 722
pharmacology of, 732–733
for PTSD, 748
for vertigo, 101, 102t
Selegiline
adverse effects of, 341–342
for depression, 723t
for PD, 341, 343t
Selenium, reference range for, 788t
Sella chordomas, 448
Sellar mass lesions, 448, 449t, 828
Semantic dementia, 152
Semantic paraphasia, 143
Sensation
abnormalities of, **116**
in brainstem lesions, 123
in cortical lesions, 123
falls and, 115
focal seizures, 124
localization of, 121f, **122**
in nerve and root lesions, 121f, 122
in spinal cord lesions, 123
in thalamic lesions, 123
anatomy of, 118, 119f
examination of, **118,** 120t
cortical, 122
primary, 119–121
quantitative sensory, 122
positive and negative phenomena, 117
terminology in, 117–118
Sensorimotor neuropathy, paraneoplastic, 563–564
Sensory area, primary, 142
Sensory ataxia, 112, 113t, 118
Sensory ataxic neuropathy and ophthalmoparesis (SANDO), 361t
Sensory balance training, 115
Sensory dissociation, 123
Sensory examination, **8**
Sensory neuropathy
autoimmune subacute, 114
HIV-related, 582
painful, 579
paraneoplastic, 563–564
Sentinel bleeds, in subarachnoid hemorrhage, 305
Sepsis/septic shock
delirium in, 129, 129t
encephalopathy in, 301
Septic cavernous sinus thrombosis, 526
Septic myopathy, 304
Septic thrombosis, of superior sagittal sinus, 526
Septo-optic dysplasia, 442
Serotonin (5-HT)
anatomic and clinical aspects of, 222t
in migraine, 54
pain and, 42f
structure of, 222t
Serotonin (5-HT_1) agonists, for migraine, 57, 58t, 59–60
Serotonin (5-HT_3) antagonists, for nausea and vomiting, 66
Serotonin norepinephrine reuptake inhibitors, for PTSD, 748

Serotonin syndrome, 355, 732
Sertraline
  adverse effects of, 723t
  for depression, 723t
  dosage of, 723t
  for obsessive-compulsive disorder, 728
  for panic disorder, 722
Setting sun sign, 195
Sex headache, primary, **70**
Sexual dysfunction
  alcohol and, 756
  cocaine and, 768
  in MS, 478, 490
Shawl sign, 649
Sheehan's syndrome, 443–444, 813, 838–839
Shift-work disorder, **171,** 804–805, 827
Shortened Fatigue Questionnaire, 706, 706f
Short stature
  clinical features of, 460
  etiology of, 459–460
  laboratory evaluation of, 460
  nutritional, 460
  psychosocial, 460
  treatment of, 460
Shoulder pain, 87
Sialadenitis, 204
Sickle cell anemia
  ocular involvement in, 187
  stroke due to, 267
Sideroblastic anemia, 364t
Sievert (Sv), 799t
Signal transduction pathway defects, 223
Silent nociceptors, 41
Simultanagnosia, 150, 151f, 195, 826
Simultaneous bilateral stimulation test, 150
Single-fiber electromyography, 34
Sinusitis
  brain abscess and, 519
  olfactory dysfunction in, 202, 206
  subdural empyema and, 522–523
Sinus thrombosis
  cavernous, 526
  superior sagittal, 526, 687–689f
  transverse, 526
Sirolimus, therapeutic monitoring of, 787t
Sjögren syndrome
  neuropathy in, 579
  ocular involvement in, 180
Skeletal maturation, somatic growth and, 459
Skew deviation, 195
Skin biopsy, 571
Skull fractures, 417
Sleep, **158**
  age-related changes in, 158, 159, 159f
  behavioral changes in, 161
  circadian rhythmicity in, 160–161, 160f
  neuroanatomy of, 159–160
  neurochemistry of, 160
  nonrestorative, 162
  NREM, 158
  organization of, 158–159
  physiology of, 158–162
  REM, 158, 159f
  states and stages of, 158, 161–162
Sleep apnea, **169**
  central, 169
  daytime sleepiness and, 166
  diagnosis of, 163t
  mixed, 169
Sleep bruxism, 170
Sleep disorder(s), **162,** 805, 828
  approach to the patient, 162, 163t
  circadian rhythm, **170**
  daytime sleepiness in, 166–168
  driving rights and, 167
  insomnia. *See* Insomnia
  narcolepsy. *See* Narcolepsy
  parasomnias, 169–170
  in PD, 345
  periodic limb movement disorder, **166**
  restless legs syndrome, **166**
  in war veterans, 749
Sleep enuresis, 170
Sleep hygiene, 163–164
Sleep paralysis, 163t, 169
Sleep-promoting substances, 160
Sleep terrors, 169–170
Sleep-wake cycle, 160–161, 160f
Sleepwalking, 169
Slipping clutch syndrome, 112
Slit-lamp examination, 177, 181
SMA (spinal muscle atrophy), 370, 374t, 377–378
Small-vessel stroke, 263t, **265**
  clinical features of, 266
  definition of, 265
  pathophysiology of, 265–266, 266f
Smoking
  insomnia and, 166
  stroke risk and, 265t
Snellen chart, 175, 175f
Snoring, 163t
Social jet lag, 71
SOD1, 373
Sodium channel disorders, of muscle, **642**
Solid organ transplantation, brain injury after, 663
Solitary tract nucleus, 201f, 202
Somatization disorder, 736, 736t
Somatoform disorders, **736**
Somatosensory cortex, 43, 43f, 143f
Somatosensory evoked potentials (SSEPs), 30
Somatosensory pathways, 119f
Somatostatin, 458
Somatostatin analogues
  for acromegaly, 464, 465f
  adverse effects of, 464
  for TSH-secreting adenomas, 473
Somatotrope, 439t, 446t
Somnambulation, 169
Sour taste sensation, 201
Spasmodic dystonia, 349
Spasms
  hemifacial, 394, 397
  in MS, 478, 489–490
  muscle, 622
Spasticity, 103, 111, 115, 414
Spastic paraplegia, familial, 111, 378–379, 412
Spastin gene, 374t, 378
Spatial orientation, 149–152, 149f
Speech
  assessment of, 5
  spontaneous, 143
Speech audiometry, 214
Speech reception threshold, 214
Sphingosine-1-phosphate receptor antagonists, 490
Spina bifida occulta, 76
Spinal accessory nerve, 7
Spinal angiography, 25
Spinal cord
  disorders of. *See* Spinal cord disease/injury
  pain mechanisms of, 42–43, 43f
  transverse section through, 402f
  vascular malformations of, 409–410, 410f
Spinal cord compression
  in hematomyelia, 406
  neoplastic, 810–811, 811f, 836
    clinical features of, 403–404
    diagnosis of, 404, 404f
    intradural mass lesions, 404–405, 404f
    pathogenesis of, 403–404
    in primary intramedullary tumors, 405, 405f
    treatment of, 404–405
  in spinal epidural abscess, 80, 405–406, 406f, 836
  in spinal epidural hematoma, 406
Spinal cord disease/injury, **400**
  acute, **403**
  anatomy related to, 400–401, 401t, 402f
  approach to the patient, 400–403, 400t
  autonomic dysfunction in, 386
  bladder dysfunction in, 413
  cervical cord, 85, 401
  chronic myelopathies, **409**
    adrenomyeloneuropathy, 412
    familial spastic paraplegia, 378–379, 412
    hypocupric, 412
    in multiple sclerosis, 411
    primary lateral sclerosis, 378, 412
Spinal cord disease/injury, chronic myelopathies (*Cont.*):
    retrovirus-associated, 410
    spondylitic myelopathy, 409
    syringomyelia, 86, 410–411, 411f
    in tabes dorsalis, 412
    tethered cord syndrome, 76, 412
    toxic causes of, 413
    in vascular malformations of cord and dura, 409–410, 410f
    in vitamin B_{12} deficiency, 411–412, 591
  compressive vs. noncompressive myelopathy, 403
  extramedullary syndromes, 403
  infarction, 107, 692f
  intramedullary syndromes, 403
  level of lesion in, 10t, 401–402
  lumbar cord, 401
  meningitis, 528. *See also* Meningitis
  noncompressive myelopathies, **406**
    evaluation of, 407t
    spinal cord infarction, 407, 692f
  paraneoplastic syndromes and, 563
  patterns of, 402–403
  rehabilitation of, **413,** 413t
  sacral cord/conus medullaris, 401–402
  sensory abnormalities in, 123
  subacute, 403
  thoracic cord, 401
Spinal epidural abscess, 80, 405–406, 406f, 836
Spinal epidural hematoma, 406
Spinal fusion, 84
Spinal muscle atrophy (SMA), 370, 374t, 377–378
Spinal stenosis
  acquired, 78
  back pain in, 78
  congenital, 78
  lumbar, 78, 78f
  treatment of, 78
Spine
  anatomy of, 71, 72f
  bamboo, 79
  lumbar
    congenital anomalies of, 75–76
  pain sensitive structures in, 71
Spinobulbar muscular atrophy, 374t, 377
Spinocerebellar ataxia (SCA)
  classification of, 358, 359–364t, 364
  clinical features of, 359–364t, 364–366
  genetic factors in, 220t, 359–364t, 364–366
  infantile-onset, 364t
  with neuropathy (SCAN1), 364t
  SCA1, 359t, 364–365, 365f
  SCA2, 359t, 365–366
  SCA3, 359t, 365–366
  SCA5, 359t
  SCA6, 220t, 359t, 366
  SCA7, 359t, 366
  SCA8, 359t, 366
  SCA10 through SCA12, 359t
  SCA13 through SCA23, 360t
  SCA25 through SCA31, 361t
  treatment of, 369
Spinothalamic tract, 43, 43f, 118, 119f
Spirometry, reference values for, 797t
Spondylitic myelopathy, 409
Spondylolisthesis, back pain in, 6
Spondylolysis, vertebral, 75–76
Spondylosis
  back pain in, 79
  cervical, 86, 111
Spontaneous speech, 143
Sporothrix infections, chronic meningitis in, 530t
Sprain, low back, 76
Spurling's sign, 85
SSEPs (somatosensory evoked potentials), 30
SSPE (subacute sclerosing panencephalitis), 517–518
SSRIs. *See* Selective serotonin reuptake inhibitors (SSRIs)
Stabbing headache, primary, **69**
Stapedectomy, 209, 215
Stapes, 207, 207f
Staphylococcus aureus infections
  meningitis. *See* Meningitis, bacterial

Statins
for AD, 321
adverse effects of, 645–646, 645t, 816, 844
for stroke prevention, 269–270
Status epilepticus, **252,** 807–808, 831
complex partial, 329
in critically ill patient, 297, 300
definition of, 252
delirium in, 129, 129t
generalized convulsive, 252
generalized tonic-clonic, 252, 253f
nonconvulsive, 252
Stem cell(s), in neurologic disease, 225–226
Stem cell therapy
for Huntington's disease, 225
for PD, 225, 344
sources of cells for, 228
Stereognosis, 122
Stereopsis, 177
Stiff-person syndrome
clinical features of, 622
gait disorders in, 111
paraneoplastic, 559t, 563
pathogenesis of, 622
Stokes-Adams attack, 95
Stomach, alcohol effects on, 755
Stool analysis, reference ranges, 790t
Strabismus, 192–193
Straight-leg raising sign, 74, 74t
Strain, low back, 76
Strength testing, 7–8
Streptococcal infections
meningitis. *See* Meningitis
Streptomycin, 185
Stress disorders, **727,** 727t
Stroke, **257**. *See also* Cerebrovascular disease; Stroke syndromes
aphasia in, 145, 148
in CADASIL, 268
cardioembolic, 261–263, 263t
circadian variations in, 173
clinical features of, 256
definition of, 256
delirium in, 129, 129t
drugs and, 268
embolic, artery-to-artery, 263–265
etiology of, 257f, 262f, 263t
fibromuscular dysplasia and, 267
gait disorders in, 111
hearing loss in, 213
hypercoagulable disorders and, 267
imaging studies in, **282,** 808, 832
cerebral angiography, 268f, 285
CT, 282–284, 285f
MRI, 286, 286f
PET, 286
ultrasound, 286
intracranial hemorrhage in. *See* Intracranial hemorrhage
ischemic. *See* Ischemic stroke
leukoaraiosis and, 268
in Moyamoya disease, 268
necrotizing arteritis and, 267
noncardiogenic, prevention of, 272
ocular manifestations of, 177, 187, 196
prevention of, 269–272
primary CNS vasculitis and, 267–268, 268f
reversible posterior leukoencephalopathy and, 268
with right hemiplegia but preserved language, 285f
risk factors for, 265t, 808, 832
small-vessel, 263t, 265–266, 266f
taste disorders in, 204
temporal (giant cell) arteritis and, 267
after TIA, 269, 269t
treatment of, 257, 257f, 832–833
venous sinus thrombosis and, 267
weakness in, 106
Stroke centers
comprehensive, 285
in ischemic stroke management, 261
Stroke syndromes, **273**
within anterior circulation, 274
anterior cerebral artery, 275–276, 276f
anterior choroidal artery, 276, 277f
common carotid artery, 277
internal carotid artery, 276–277, 276f, 277f
middle cerebral artery, 274–275, 275f
within posterior circulation, 277
basilar artery, 279–282, 281–284f
P1 syndrome, 278
P2 syndrome, 278
posterior cerebral artery, 276f, 277–278, 277f
vertebral artery, 278–279, 280f
Stupor, 132
Sty (hordeolum), 180
Subacute combined degeneration, 411–412
Subacute sclerosing panencephalitis (SSPE), 517–518
Subarachnoid hemorrhage
clinical features of, 305, 821
in critically ill patient, 304
delayed neurologic deficits after, 305–306
DVT prophylaxis after, 308–309
ECG in, 307
etiology of, 304–305
fundus examination in, 136
grading of, 305, 306t
headache in, 51t, 52, 305, 801
hyponatremia in, 306
imaging in, 306–307, 307f
laboratory evaluation of, 306–307
pathophysiology of, 305
saccular aneurysms in, 304–305
treatment of, 307–309
Subclavian artery, occlusion of, 279
Subconjunctival hemorrhage, 179
Subdural empyema, **522**. *See also* Epidural abscess
approach to the patient, 493–494, 494–495f
clinical features of, 523
definition of, 522, 522f
diagnosis of, 523–524, 523f
differential diagnosis of, 524
epidemiology of, 522
etiology of, 523
pathophysiology of, 523
prognosis of, 524
treatment of, 524
Subdural hematoma
acute, 418, 418f, 837
chronic, 419, 419f, 811, 837
coma in, 134
neuroimaging in, 134f, 419f, 701f, 811f
weakness in, 107
Substance P, pain and, 41, 42f
Substance use disorders, **716**. *See also specific substances*
delirium in, 128–129, 129t
epidemiology of, 717
genetic factors in, 717
neural circuitry of, 715f
neuroimaging of, 717
neuropathology of, 221
pathogenesis of, 717–718, 718t, 719f
vs. substance dependence, 716
Sudden cardiac death, circadian variations in, 173
Sudomotor function, in autonomic dysfunction, 384–385, 385t
Sulfacetamide, for conjunctivitis, 180
Sulfadiazine, for CNS toxoplasmosis, 522
Sulfonamides, 185
Sumatriptan
for cluster headache, 64
for migraine, 58t, 59–60, 59t
nasal spray, 58t, 59–60
SUNCT/SUNA, 63t, 65
Sundowning, 127, 131, 165
Superior oblique muscle paresis, 109
Superior pontine syndrome, lateral/medial, 283f
Superior sagittal sinus thrombosis
clinical features of, 526
neuroimaging in, 687–689f
Supine hypertension, 94
Suppurative thrombophlebitis, intracranial. *See* Venous thromboembolism (VTE), suppurative intracranial
Suprachiasmatic nucleus, 174
Suprascapular neuropathy, 87
Suramin, 438t, 585t
Swinging flashlight test, 176, 176f
Sydenham's chorea, 352
Sympathetic postganglionic neuron, 41f
Syncope, **89**
approach to the patient, 96–97, 802, 822–823
in arrhythmias, 93t, 95–96
in cardiovascular disease, 93t, 95–96
in carotid sinus hypersensitivity, 97
definition of, 89
diagnosis of, 802, 822–823
ECG in, 97
epidemiology of, 89
vs. falls in neurologic disease, 96
high-risk features of, 90t
hypoglycemia and, 96
natural history of, 89
neurally mediated
causes of, 93t
classification of, 90–91
clinical features of, 91–92, 822
pathophysiology of, 90, 92f
treatment of, 92
in orthostatic hypotension. *See* Orthostatic hypotension
pathophysiology of, 90
in psychiatric disorders, 96, 97
vs. seizure, 96, 243–244, 244t
tilt table testing for, 385
treatment of, 92
vasovagal
causes of, 90, 93t
Synkinesis, 394
Syntax, 142
Syphilis, secondary
neurologic manifestations of
chronic meningitis, 529t
subacute meningitis, 515, 516
ocular involvement in, 181
Syringomyelia
Chiari malformation and, 410, 411f
clinical features of, 410–411, 811, 837
diagnosis of, 86, 837
treatment of, 410–411
Systemic lupus erythematosus (SLE), neurologic manifestations of, 352, 408/, 532t, 579–580
Systemic sclerosis (scleroderma)
facial hemiatrophy in, 397
neuropathy in, 580
Systems neuroscience, 229–230, 229f

Tabes dorsalis, 412
Tachyarrhythmias, syncope in, 95
Tachycardia-bradycardia syndrome, 95
Tacrine, for AD, 321
Tacrolimus
for myasthenia gravis, 616
therapeutic monitoring of, 787t
Tamoxifen, 438t
Tangier disease (ABCA1 deficiency), 575t, 576
Tardive dyskinesia, 112, 354, 740
Tardive syndromes, 354–355
Tarui disease (phosphofructokinase deficiency), 637
Taste buds, 200, 201f, 204
Taste disorders
diseases and conditions associated with, 204
drug-related, 204
etiology of, 204
evaluation of, 204–205
olfactory dysfunction and, 204
treatment of, 205–206
Taste pore, 201, 201f
Taste system, 200–202
Tau protein, 312t, 316
Taxanes, 584t
Tay-Sachs disease, adult, 374t, 377
TCAs. *See* Tricyclic antidepressants (TCAs)
T cell(s), autoreactive, in MS, 476
TDP-43 gene, 228, 312t

Teardrop fracture, 701f
Telangiectasia(s), capillary, 292
Telmisartan, for stroke/TIC prevention, 271
Temazepam
  for generalized anxiety disorder, 725t
  for insomnia, 164
  pharmacology of, 725t
Temperature sense, testing of, 119, 120t
Temporal arteritis. *See* Giant cell arteritis (temporal arteritis)
Temporal bone
  CT scan of, 215
  fracture of, 210
Temporal lobectomy, for refractory epilepsy, 251
Tension-type headache, 51t, **62**
  clinical features of, 62
  diagnosis of, 62
  pathophysiology of, 62
  treatment of, 62
Teratoma
  ovarian, 560f, 563
  parasellar, 448–449
Terazosin, for urinary dyssynergia, 413, 490
Terbinafine, 204
Teriflunomide, for MS, 487
Terminally ill patient, delirium in, 129t, 130
Terminal restlessness, 130
Testosterone therapy, for hypogonadism, 470–471
Tethered cord syndrome, 76, 412
Tetrabenazine
  adverse effects of, 354
  for dystonia, 349
  for tardive dyskinesia, 354
Tetracycline(s), for meibomitis, 180
Tetrahydrocannabinol (THC), 769
Thalamic Déjérine-Roussy syndrome, 278, 288
Thalamus
  lesions of, sensory disturbances in, 123
  in olfaction, 199
Thalidomide, adverse effects of, 438, 586t, 589
Thallium poisoning, 185, 588t, 590
THAP1 gene, 348
Theophylline, 163t
  adverse effects of, 165
  therapeutic monitoring of, 788t
Thermoregulation, 162
Thiamine (vitamin B_1)
  deficiency of
    delirium in, 129
    dementia in, 328
    neuropathies in, 591
    optic neuropathy in, 185
    Wernicke's disease, 302–303, 302f
  reference range for, 788t
Thioridazine, 739t
Thiotepa, 438t
Thiothixene, 739t
Third window, inner ear, 209
Thomsen disease, 643
Thoracic outlet, 87
Thoracic outlet syndrome, 87
Thrombolytic therapy, for ischemic stroke, 261–262
Thrombophlebitis. *See* Venous thromboembolism (VTE)
Thrombosis
  dural sinus, 273
  venous sinus, 267
Thunderclap headache, primary, **70**
Thymectomy, for myasthenia gravis, 614–615
Thymoma, paraneoplastic syndromes in, 565
Thyroid disorders, muscle disorders and, 643–644
Thyroid-stimulating hormone (TSH), **472**
  action of, 472
  deficiency of, 446t, 472–473
  laboratory evaluation of, 445t
  secretion of, 472
  synthesis of, 472
Thyroid-stimulating hormone (TSH)–secreting adenomas, 473
Thyrotrope, expression and regulation of, 439t
Thyrotropin-releasing hormone (TRH), 453, 472–473
TIA. *See* Transient ischemic attack (TIA)
Tiagabine
  for epilepsy, 248t
  for stiff-person syndrome, 563
Tibial muscular dystrophy (Udd's distal myopathy), 633, 634t
Tic(s), **352**
  definition of, 347t
  motor, 353
  in Tourette's syndrome, 352–353
  vocal, 353
Ticlopidine, in stroke/TIA prevention, 270
Tilt table test, 97, 385, 385t
Time-of-flight (TOF) imaging, 22
Timolol, for migraine prevention, 60
Tingling, **117**. *See also* Sensation
Tinnitus, 210, 216
Tinnitus masker, 216
Tizanidine, for spasticity in neurologic disease, 414, 489
Todd's paralysis, 232, 807, 830
TOF (time-of-flight) imaging, 22
Tolcapone, for PD, 342, 343t
Tolerance, definition of, 716
Tolfenamic acid, for migraine, 58t
Tolosa-Hunt syndrome, 191, 193, 194, 399
Tone, 103, 104t
Tongue paralysis, 398
Tonic-clonic seizures. *See also* Seizure(s)
  characteristics of, 233–234
  vs. syncope, 243–244, 244t
Tonic pupil, 176
Topiramate
  adverse effects of, 61t, 246, 248t
  for chronic daily headache, 66
  for cluster headache prevention, 64t
  for epilepsy, 248t
  for hemicrania continua, 69
  for migraine prevention, 60, 61t
  pharmacology of, 248t
  for posttraumatic headache, 68
  for raised CSF pressure headache, 68
  for SUNCT/SUNA prevention, 65
"Top of the basilar" syndromes, 279
Torsades de pointes, 95
Torsin A, 348
Torticollis, 349
Touch localization test, 122
Touch sensation, testing of, 120t, 121
Tourette's syndrome, 352–353
  etiology of, 353
  pathophysiology of, 353
  prevalence of, 352–353
  sleep disturbances in, 165
  treatment of, 353
Toxins, neuropathies due to, 588t, 589–591
Toxoplasma gondii infection
  cerebral/CNS, 521, 546–547, 547f, 812, 838
  chronic meningitis in, 530t
  ocular, 182
  treatment of, 522
  weakness in, 107
Trachoma, 180
Tractography, diffusion, 21f
Tramadol
  adverse effects of, 578t
  for back pain, 82
  for neuropathy, 578t
  for pain, 46t
Transcendental meditation, for migraine, 57
Transcranial magnetic stimulation, for depression, 733
Transfalcial herniation, 133f, 134
Transient global amnesia, 329–330
Transient ischemic attack (TIA), **268**
  definition of, 256
  pathophysiology of, 268–269
  prevention of, 269
    anticoagulants in, 271–272
    antiplatelet agents in, 270–271
  risk factors for, 269–270
  stroke following, 269, 269t
Transient ischemic attack (TIA) (*Cont.*):
  treatment of, 257f
  visual symptoms of, 187
  weakness in, 108t
Transsphenoidal surgery
  for acromegaly, 464
  for Cushing's syndrome, 469
  for pituitary tumors, 451–452, 452f, 473
Transtentorial herniation, 133
Transverse sinus thrombosis, 526
Tranylcypromine, for depression, 723t
Trauma
  back pain following, 75t, 76
  cervical spine, 85
Traumatic brain injury (TBI). *See* Head injury
Trazodone
  adverse effects of, 723t
  for depression, 723t
  for insomnia, 164
  for stress disorders, 728
Treacher Collins syndrome, 212t
Tremor(s), **347**
  clinical features of, 347
  essential, 347
  etiology of, 347
  pathophysiology of, 347
  in PD, 347
  prevalence of, 347
  treatment of, 347–348
  in Wilson's disease, 356
TRH (thyrotropin-releasing hormone), 453, 472–473
Triazolam
  for generalized anxiety disorder, 725t
  for insomnia, 164
  pharmacology of, 725t
Trichinella/trichinellosis, chronic meningitis in, 531t
Trichromat, 177
Tricyclic antidepressants (TCAs)
  adverse effects of, 49, 578t, 723t
    orthostatic hypotension, 95
  for chronic daily headache, 65–66
  contraindications to, 732
  for depression, 723t, 731–732, 732f
  for migraine prevention, 61t
  for narcolepsy, 169
  for neuropathy, 578t
  for pain, 46t, 49, 49t
  pharmacology of, 732
  for posttraumatic headache, 68
Trigeminal autonomic cephalalgia, 51, **62,** 63t
Trigeminal nerve
  disorders of, 394t
  examination of, 6
  sensory divisions of, 392f
Trigeminal neuralgia, **392,** 835–836
  clinical features of, 392
  diagnosis of, 65
  differential diagnosis of, 393
  incidence of, 392
  laboratory evaluation of, 393
  in MS, 479
  with paroxysmal hemicrania, 65
  pathophysiology of, 393
  treatment of, 50, 393, 810, 836
Trigeminal neuropathy, **394,** 394t, 836
Trigeminovascular system, 51
Trigger(s), migraine, 53
Trigger point injections, 83
Trihexyphenidyl
  for dystonia, 349
  for extrapyramidal symptoms, 740
  for PD, 342
Trilostane, for Cushing's syndrome, 469
Trimethoprim-polymyxin, for conjunctivitis, 180
Trimethoprim-sulfamethoxazole (TMP-SMZ), for meningitis, 502
Triptans, for migraine, 58t, 59
Trismus, 394
Trochlear nerve, 6
Trochlear nerve palsy, 194
Trypanosoma spp. infections
  chronic meningitis in, 530t. *See also* Meningitis
  in HIV infection, 547–548

TSC1 gene, 425t, 433
TSC2 gene, 425t, 433
TSH. *See* Thyroid-stimulating hormone (TSH)
Tuberculosis (TB), extrapulmonary
  meningitis, 529t
  ocular manifestations, 181
  spinal/skeletal, 406, 406f, 669–670f
Tuberous sclerosis
  brain tumors and, 425t, 433
  clinical features of, 433
  pathogenesis of, 433
  seizures in, 433
Tufted cells, 199
Tullio phenomenon, 209
Turcot's syndrome, 425t
Two-point discrimination test, 122
Tympanic membrane, 207, 207f
  assessment of, 213
  perforation of, 209, 215
Tympanogram, 214
Tympanometry, 214
Tympanoplasty, 209, 215
Tympanostomy tubes, 215
Tyramine, MAOIs and, 341

Udd's distal myopathy (tibial muscular dystrophy), 633, 634t
Ulnar nerve, motor conduction studies of, 32f
Ulnar neuropathy, 593–594, 665–666, 666f
Ultrasonography
  in neurologic disease, 14t
  in stroke, 286
Umami, 201
Uncal transtentorial herniation, 133, 133f
Unipolar depressive disorders, 731
University of Pennsylvania Smell Identification Test, 202f, 205
Unthoff's symptom, 478
Unverricht-Lundborg disease, 235t, 362t
Upper motor neuron diseases, 374–376t, 378–379
Upper motor neuron pathways, 105f
Upper motor neuron weakness, 104, 104t
Uremia, delirium in, 129t
Urinalysis, reference ranges for, 791–792t
Urinary tract infections (UTIs)
  delirium in, 129, 129t
  in MS, 490
Usher syndrome, 212, 212t
Uterosacral ligament, disorders involving, 81
Uveitis, 181, 182f, 188, 829
  anterior, 181
  intermediate, 182
  paraneoplastic, 565
  posterior, 182

Vagus nerve
  anatomy of, 201f
  diseases of, 397
  examination of, 7
  stimulation
    for depression, 733
    for epilepsy, 252
  in taste sensation, 201
Valacyclovir
  for Bell's palsy, 396
  for viral encephalitis, 513
  for viral meningitis, 507
Valdecoxib, 46t
Valproate/valproic acid
  action of, 716
  adverse effects of, 61t, 735t
    bone marrow suppression, 250
    common, 735t
    hepatotoxicity, 250
    neurologic, 247t
    rare, 735t
    systemic, 247t
    teratogenic, 254
  for bipolar disorder, 735, 735t
  for chronic daily headache, 66
  dosage of, 247t, 735t
  drug interactions of, 247t
  for epilepsy, 247t, 250
Valproate/valproic acid (*Cont.*):
  for focal seizures, 250
  for generalized seizures, 250
  for migraine prevention, 60, 61t
  for myoclonus, 353
  pharmacology of, 247t, 735t
  for posthypoxic myoclonus, 300
  for posttraumatic headache, 68
  for stiff-person syndrome, 563
  for tardive dyskinesia, 354
  therapeutic monitoring of, 788t
Valsalva response, in autonomic dysfunction, 384, 385t
Vancomycin
  for meningitis, 499t, 501, 502
  therapeutic monitoring of, 788t
Varicella (chickenpox), complications of, 491, 492
Varicella-zoster virus (VZV) infections
  meningitis, 506
  neuropathy in, 582–583
Vascular anomalies, 291–293
Vascular dementia, 310, 314t, **322,** 322f
Vascular endothelial growth factor (VEGF) inhibitors, 189
Vasculitic neuropathy, **607**
Vasculitis
  CNS
    angiography in, 686f
    CT in, 686f
    stroke due to, 267–268, 268f
  isolated, dementia due to, 329
  of nerve and muscle, 564
  paraneoplastic, 564
Vasoactive intestinal peptide (VIP), 453
Vasogenic edema, 294
Vasospasm, after subarachnoid hemorrhage, 306, 307–308
Vegetative state, 132
Venlafaxine
  adverse effects of, 578t, 723t
  for depression, 723t, 733
  dosage of, 723t
  for neuropathy, 578t
  for pain, 46t, 49, 50, 490
  for panic disorder, 722
  pharmacology of, 733
Venous anomalies, 292
Venous sinus thrombosis, stroke due to, 267
Venous thromboembolism (VTE)
  with brain tumor, 424
  suppurative intracranial
    anatomy of, 525–526, 525f
    clinical features of, 526
    definition of, 525
    diagnosis of, 526
    pathophysiology of, 525–526
    treatment of, 526
Ventricular tachycardia, syncope in, 95
Ventriculostomy, for ICP and brain tissue monitoring, 297, 297f
Ventrolateral preoptic hypothalamus, 159
VEPs (visual evoked potentials), 29
Verapamil
  adverse effects of, 64
  for cluster headache prevention, 64, 64t
  for hypnic headache, 70
Vertebrae, anatomy of, 71, 72f
Vertebral artery, occlusion of, 278–279
Vertebral fractures
  neuroimaging in, 700f, 701f
  in osteoporosis, 80
  pain in, 76, 80
Vertebrobasilar insufficiency, 69
Vertigo, **98**
  acute prolonged, 100
  approach to the patient, 98–100, 823
  benign paroxysmal positional, 99t, 100
  central, 99t
  evoked by loud sounds, 209
  in migraine, 98, 100–101
  in MS, 478
  peripheral, 99t
  prevention of, 102
Vertigo (*Cont.*):
  psychosomatic, 101–102
  treatment of, 102, 102t
  in vestibular dysfunction, 99t, 100
Vestibular dysfunction
  balance disorders in, 101, 114
  clinical features of, 101
  evaluation of, 100
  vertigo in, 99t, 100
Vestibular-evoked myogenic potential test, 215
Vestibular nerve section, for Ménière's disease, 210
Vestibular neuritis, 99t, 100
Vestibular nystagmus, 196
Vestibular rehabilitation therapy, 101–102
Vestibular schwannoma (acoustic neuroma)
  diagnosis of, 101, 214–215, 431–432, 431f
  facial nerve involvement in, 396
  hearing loss in, 101, 210, 213, 214
  imaging in, 215, 431, 431f
Vestibulocochlear nerve, 7
Vestibuloocular reflex, 99
Vestibulospinal pathway, 105f
Vibration sense, 120t, 121
Vigabatrin, for stiff-person syndrome, 563
Vincristine, adverse effects of, 438, 438t
Violence, assessment of, 741
Visual acuity, 100, 175, 175f
Visual aura, 187
Visual blurring, in MS, 478
Visual cortex, 143f
Visual evoked potentials (VEPs), 29
Visual fields, assessment of, 177–179, 178f
Visual function, assessment of
  color vision, 177
  eye movements and alignment, 177
  pupils, 175–177, 176f
  refractive state, 175
  stereopsis, 177
  visual acuity, 175, 175f
  visual fields, 177–179, 178f
Visual loss
  chemotherapy-induced, 438t
  chronic, 187–190
  factitious, 187
  in pituitary tumors, 449
  transient or sudden, 182–187
Visual object agnosia, 152
Visual target cancellation test, 150
Visual vertigo, 101
Vitamin(s), reference ranges for, 788t
Vitamin A
  deficiency of, 181
  reference range for, 788t
  for retinitis pigmentosa, 190
  supplements, for olfactory dysfunction, 206
Vitamin B_1. *See* Thiamine
Vitamin B_2. *See* Riboflavin
Vitamin B_6. *See* Pyridoxine
Vitamin B_{12}. *See* Cobalamin
Vitamin C
  for macular degeneration, 189
  reference range for, 788t
Vitamin D
  deficiency of, 645
  reference range for, 788t
Vitamin E
  deficiency of
    ataxic disorders in, 368, 369
    neuropathies in, 591–592
  for macular degeneration, 189
  reference range for, 788t
Vitamin K
  reference range for, 788t
Vitreous degeneration, 186–187
Vitreous detachment, 186
Vitreous hemorrhage, 187
Vocal tic, 353
Vogt-Koyanagi-Harada syndrome, 182, 532t
von Hippel-Lindau disease
  brain tumors in, 425t
  clinical features of, 362t
  genetic factors in, 362t
V sign, 649